FOURTH EDITION

Clinical Manual for the
ONCOLOGY ADVANCED PRACTICE NURSE

EDITED BY
Dawn Camp-Sorrell, MSN, CRNP, AOCN®
Rebecca A. Hawkins, MSN, ARNP
Diane G. Cope, PhD, APRN, BC, AOCNP®

Oncology Nursing Society
Pittsburgh, Pennsylvania

ONS Publications Department
Publisher and Director of Publications: William A. Tony, BA, CQIA
Senior Editorial Managers: Lisa M. George, MPH, BA, CHES, and Sean Pieszak, BA
Acquisitions Editor: John Zaphyr, BA, MEd
Staff Editor: Andrew Petyak, BA
Associate Staff Editor: Casey S. Kennedy, BA
Design and Production Administrator: Dany Sjoen
Editorial Assistant: Rachel Geffrey, BFA

First printing, February 2022; second printing, May 2023

Library of Congress Cataloging-in-Publication Data
Names: Camp-Sorrell, Dawn, editor. | Cope, Diane G., editor. | Hawkins,
  Rebecca A. (Rebecca Ann), 1957- editor. | Oncology Nursing Society,
  issuing body.
Title: Clinical manual for the oncology advanced practice nurse / edited by
  Dawn Camp-Sorrell, Diane G. Cope, Rebecca A. Hawkins.
Description: Fourth edition. | Pittsburgh, Pennsylvania : Oncology Nursing
  Society, [2022] | Includes bibliographical references and index
Identifiers: LCCN 2021031325 (print) | LCCN 2021031326 (ebook) | ISBN
  9781635930450 (paperback) | ISBN 9781635930467 (ebook)
Subjects: MESH: Neoplasms--nursing | Advanced Practice Nursing--methods |
  Oncology Nursing--methods | Handbook
Classification: LCC RC266 (print) | LCC RC266 (ebook) | NLM WY 49 | DDC
  616.99/40231--dc23
LC record available at https://lccn.loc.gov/2021031325
LC ebook record available at https://lccn.loc.gov/2021031326

Publisher's Note
    This book is published by the Oncology Nursing Society (ONS). ONS neither represents nor guarantees that the practices described herein will, if followed, ensure safe and effective patient care. The recommendations contained in this book reflect ONS's judgment regarding the state of general knowledge and practice in the field as of the date of publication. The recommendations may not be appropriate for use in all circumstances. Those who use this book should make their own determinations regarding specific safe and appropriate patient care practices, taking into account the personnel, equipment, and practices available at the hospital or other facility at which they are located. The editors and publisher cannot be held responsible for any liability incurred as a consequence from the use or application of any of the contents of this book. Figures and tables are used as examples only. They are not meant to be all-inclusive, nor do they represent endorsement of any particular institution by ONS. Mention of specific products and opinions related to those products do not indicate or imply endorsement by ONS. Websites mentioned are provided for information only; the hosts are responsible for their own content and availability. Unless otherwise indicated, dollar amounts reflect U.S. dollars.
    ONS publications are originally published in English. Publishers wishing to translate ONS publications must contact ONS about licensing arrangements. ONS publications cannot be translated without obtaining written permission from ONS. (Individual tables and figures that are reprinted or adapted require additional permission from the original source.) Because translations from English may not always be accurate or precise, ONS disclaims any responsibility for inaccuracies in words or meaning that may occur as a result of the translation. Readers relying on precise information should check the original English version.

Printed in the United States of America

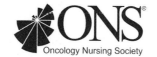

Innovation • Excellence • Advocacy

Contributors

Editors

Dawn Camp-Sorrell, MSN, CRNP, AOCN°
Oncology Nurse Practitioner
Children's Hospital of Alabama
Birmingham, Alabama
Chapter 1. Hiccups (Singultus); Chapter 135. Dystonia

Rebecca A. Hawkins, MSN, ARNP
Director, Compassionate Care
Providence St. Joseph Health
Pendleton, Oregon
Chapter 55. Constipation; Chapter 158. Hypothyroidism

Diane G. Cope, PhD, APRN, BC, AOCNP°
Oncology Nurse Practitioner
Director of Nursing
Florida Cancer Specialists and Research Institute
Fort Myers, Florida
Chapter 71. Gastroesophageal Reflux Disease; Chapter 112. Lymphedema

Authors

Kristine Deano Abueg, RN, MSN, OCN°, CBCN°
Nurse Navigator, Leukemia and Lymphoma Center
Kaiser Permanente
Roseville, California
Chapter 123. Essential Thrombocythemia; Chapter 129. Thrombocytopenia

Jeannine M. Brant, PhD, APRN, AOCN°
Oncology Clinical Nurse Specialist
Director and Lead Scientist
Collaborative Science and Innovation
Billings Clinic
Billings, Montana
Chapter 53. Abdominal Pain; Chapter 97. Bone Pain

Bradley Burton, PharmD, BCOP
Clinical Pharmacy Specialist, Medical Oncology
The Johns Hopkins Hospital
Baltimore, Maryland
Treatment Section Reviewer

Myriam J. Cadet, PhD, APRN, MSN, FNP-C
Adjunct Assistant Professor
SUNY Downstate Health Sciences University
Brooklyn, New York
Chapter 87. Benign Prostatic Hyperplasia

Constance Dahlin, MSN, ANP-BC, ACHPN, FPCN, FAAN
Palliative Nurse Practitioner
Mass General Brigham, Salem Hospital
Salem, Massachusetts
Consultant
Center to Advance Palliative Care
New York, New York
Chapter 133. Confusion/Delirium; Chapter 161. Anxiety; Chapter 162. Depression

Mary Elizabeth Davis, DNP, RN, CHPN, AOCNS°
Clinical Nurse Specialist
Memorial Sloan Kettering Cancer Center
New York, New York
Chapter 142. Neurotoxicity

R. Tim Davis, MSN, APRN
Gastroenterology and Interventional Radiology
Moffitt Cancer Center
Tampa, Florida
Chapter 70. Diverticulitis; Chapter 77. Pancreatitis

Deena Damsky Dell, MSN, APRN, AOCN°, LNC
Nursing Professional Development Specialist
Brian D. Jellison Cancer Center, Sarasota Memorial Hospital
Sarasota, Florida
Chapter 69. Cirrhosis

Corazon Lauren Delumpa, MSN, RN, FNP-C
Assistant Professor of Nursing
University of St. Thomas Peavy School of Nursing
Clinical Instructor
University of Texas at Houston Cizik School of Nursing-
Houston, Texas
Chapter 136. Foot Drop; Chapter 139. Syncope; Chapter 143. Peripheral Neuropathy

Kristine Dukart-Harrington, DNP, RN, AGNP-C, ACHPN
Assistant Professor
University of Portland School of Nursing
Oncology Palliative Care Nurse Practitioner
Providence Franz Cancer Center
Portland, Oregon
Chapter 16. Pruritus; Chapter 99. Muscle Cramps; Chapter 149. Thirst

Mary W. Dunn, MSN, RN, OCN®, NP-C
Adult Nurse Practitioner, Department of Urology and Division of Oncology
UNC Lineberger Comprehensive Cancer Center
University of North Carolina at Chapel Hill
Chapel Hill, North Carolina
Chapter 86. Acute Kidney Injury; Chapter 89. Lower Urinary Tract Infection (Cystitis); Chapter 94. Pyelonephritis

Beth Faiman, PhD, MSN, APRN-BC, AOCN®, FAAN
Nurse Practitioner, Department of Hematologic Oncology and Blood Disorders
Cleveland Clinic, Taussig Cancer Institute
Cleveland, Ohio
Chapter 43. Deep Venous Thrombosis; Chapter 113. Anemia of Chronic Disease; Chapter 115. Cobalamin (Vitamin B$_{12}$) Deficiency; Chapter 122. Hypercoagulable State; Chapter 124. Immune Thrombocytopenia; Chapter 126. Monoclonal Gammopathy of Undetermined Significance; Chapter 130. Thrombotic Thrombocytopenia Purpura

Christina Ferraro, MSN, APRN-CNP, BMTCN®
BMT/Apheresis Nurse Practitioner
Cleveland Clinic, Taussig Cancer Institute
Cleveland, Ohio
Chapter 7. Cataracts; Chapter 111. Lymphadenopathy; Chapter 127. Neutropenia; Chapter 147 Fever; Chapter 150. Anaphylaxis

Rachael Fornwalt, MSN, AG-ACNP
Oncology Critical Care Nurse Practitioner
Johns Hopkins Hospital, Sidney Kimmel Comprehensive Cancer Center
Baltimore, Maryland
Chapter 48. Hypotension; Chapter 159. Rhabdomyolysis; Chapter 160. Shock

Renee Genther, MSN, ANP-C, AOCNP®
Oncology Nurse Practitioner/Hospitalist
Florida Cancer Specialists
Ocala, Florida
Chapter 40. Stable Angina; Chapter 42. Congestive Heart Failure

Jeanne Held-Warmkessel, MSN, RN, AOCN®, ACNS-BC
Clinical Nurse Specialist
Fox Chase Cancer Center
Philadelphia, Pennsylvania
Chapter 13. Hyperpigmentation; Chapter 56. Diarrhea; Chapter 59. Hematemesis; Chapter 62. Melena; Chapter 64. Rectal Bleeding (Hematochezia); Chapter 67. Bowel Obstruction/Ileus; Chapter 78. Peptic Ulcer Disease

Keri McLendon Hyde, DNP, MBA, FNP-C, AOCNP®
Nurse Practitioner
Grandview Medical Center
Adjunct Clinical Instructor
University of Alabama at Birmingham School of Nursing
Birmingham, Alabama
Chapter 47. Hypertension

Stephanie Jackson, DNP, MSN, RN, AOCNS®, BMTCN®
Oncology Clinical Nurse Specialist
Hematology/Stem Cell Transplant Unit
Ronald Reagan UCLA Medical Center
Los Angeles, California
Chapter 80. Amenorrhea; Chapter 90. Menopausal Symptoms and Menopause

Santosh Kesari, MD, PhD, FANA, FAAN
Chair of Translational Neurosciences and Neurotherapeutics
Director of Neuro-Oncology
Pacific Neuroscience Institute and Saint John's Cancer Institute at Providence Saint John's Health Center
Santa Monica, California
Chapter 101. Fibromyalgia Syndrome; Chapter 104. Lyme Disease; Chapter 105. Osteoarthritis; Chapter 107. Restless Legs Syndrome; Chapter 108. Rheumatoid Arthritis; Chapter 109. Sciatica; Chapter 110. Systemic Lupus Erythematosus

Deborah Kirk, DNP, FNP-BC, NP-C, AOCN®, FAANP
Associate Dean/Associate Professor/Nurse Practitioner
Edith Cowan University, School of Nursing and Midwifery
Joondalup, Western Australia
Chapter 40. Stable Angina; Chapter 41. Cardiomyopathy; Chapter 42. Congestive Heart Failure; Chapter 44. Dyslipidemia; Chapter 47. Hypertension; Chapter 51. Peripheral Vascular Disease; Chapter 52. Pulmonary Hypertension; Chapter 120. Disseminated Intravascular Coagulation; Chapter 121. Hemochromatosis

Sandra Kurtin, PhD, ANP-C, AOCN®
Director, Advanced Practice and Clinical Integration
Nurse Practitioner, Clinical Assistant Professor of Medicine
University of Arizona and Arizona Cancer Center
Tucson, Arizona
Chapter 151. Diabetes Mellitus, Types 1 and 2; Chapter 152. Hypocalcemia/Hypercalcemia; Chapter 153. Hypokalemia/Hyperkalemia; Chapter 154. Hypomagnesemia/Hypermagnesemia; Chapter 155. Hyponatremia/Hypernatremia; Chapter 156. Hypophosphatemia/Hyperphosphatemia; Chapter 157. Hyperthyroidism

Heather T. Mackey, MSN, RN, ANP-BC, AOCN®
Scientific Director
Haymarket Medical Education
Paramus, New Jersey
Chapter 114. Aplastic Anemia; Chapter 116. Folate (Vitamin B₉) Deficiency Anemia; Chapter 117. Hemolytic Anemia; Chapter 118. Iron-Deficiency Anemia; Chapter 119. Sickle Cell Disease; Chapter 125. Leukocytosis; Chapter 128. Polycythemia Vera

Laurl A. Matey, MSN, RN-BC, CHPN
Medical Director
National Association of Continuing Education
Plantation, Florida
Chapter 164. Phlebitis

Kristina Mathey, MS, APRN-CNP, AOCNP®
Advanced Practice Clinical Educator
Oncology Advanced Practice Provider Fellowship
    Program Manager
Gastrointestinal Medical Oncology Nurse Practitioner
Arthur G. James Cancer Hospital and Richard J. Solove
    Research Institute
The Ohio State University
Columbus, Ohio
Chapter 54. Ascites; Chapter 57. Dysphagia; Chapter 58. Heartburn/Ingestion/Dyspepsia; Chapter 63. Nausea and Vomiting; Chapter 65. Splenomegaly; Chapter 66. Anorexia/Cachexia; Chapter 72. Gastritis; Chapter 76. Irritable Bowel Syndrome

Leslie Matthews, MS, ANP-BC, AOCNP®
Professor, Clinical
Molloy College
Barbara H. Hagan School of Nursing and Health Sciences
Rockville Centre, New York
Chapter 24. Dyspnea; Chapter 27. Wheezing; Chapter 28. Chronic Obstructive Pulmonary Disease; Chapter 37. Upper Respiratory Infection

Cecile B. Miller, MSN, CRNP
Adult Oncology Nurse Practitioner
Home-Based Palliative Care Practice
Main Line Health
Wayne, Pennsylvania
Chapter 81. Dysuria; Chapter 82. Hematuria; Chapter 92. Prostatitis/Lower Urinary Tract Symptoms

Faith A. Mutale, MSN, CRNP
Advanced Practice Oncology Nurse Practitioner, Head
    and Neck and Thoracic Oncology
Abramson Cancer Center
University of Pennsylvania
Philadelphia, Pennsylvania
Chapter 81. Dysuria; Chapter 82. Hematuria; Chapter 88. Hemorrhagic Cystitis; Chapter 92. Prostatitis/Lower Urinary Tract Symptoms

Enza Esposito Nguyen, DNP, RN, ANP-BC, AOCNP®
Project Consultant
Austin, Texas
Chapter 29. Pleural Effusion; Chapter 34. Sleep Apnea (Sleep Disorder Breathing); Chapter 35. Systemic Capillary Leak Syndrome

Kimberly A. Noonan, DNP, ANP-BC, AOCN®
Nurse Practitioner
Dana-Farber Cancer Institute
Boston, Massachusetts
Chapter 96. Arthralgia; Chapter 100. Myalgia; Chapter 102. Fractures; Chapter 103. Gout; Chapter 140. Tremor

Patricia A. Obulaney, DNP, APRN, ANP-C
Clinical Associate Professor
University of Houston College of Nursing
Houston, Texas
Chapter 146. Stroke

Richard Ornato, PA-C
Physician Assistant
Gastro Health
Fort Myers, Florida
Chapter 60. Hepatomegaly; Chapter 61. Jaundice; Chapter 68. Cholecystitis

Kristin Ownby, PhD, RN, AOCN®, ANP-BC, ACHPN
Associate Professor of Clinical Nursing
University of Texas Health Science Center at Houston
Cizik School of Nursing
Houston, Texas
Chapter 146. Stroke

Karen L. Pitman, RN, MSN, ARNP, NP-C
Director of Occupational Health and Wellness, Leave
    Administration and Worker's Compensation
Florida Cancer Specialists
Tampa, Florida
Chapter 36. Tuberculosis; Chapter 74. Hepatitis

Elena C. Prendergast, DNP, APRN, FNP-C, ACHPN
Assistant Professor
Clinical Nurse Leader, Program Director
Augusta University College of Nursing
Augusta, Georgia
Tree of Life Health Consultant, Owner
Augusta, Georgia
Chapter 133. Confusion/Delirium; Chapter 161. Anxiety; Chapter 162. Depression

Catherine Reavis, EdD, FNP-BC, FAANP
Professor, Clinical
Retired
University of Texas Health Sciences Center
Cizik School of Nursing
Houston, Texas
Chapter 134. Dizziness/Vertigo

Karen A. Roesser, MSN, RN, AOCNS®
Director of Oncology Practice
Sarah Cannon Cancer Institute at Johnston-Willis
    Hospital
Richmond, Virginia
Chapter 12. Stomatitis/Xerostomia; Chapter 73. Hemorrhoids; Chapter 75. Hepatotoxicity; Chapter 85. Vaginitis

Beth Sandy, MSN, CRNP
Nurse Practitioner
Abramson Cancer Center, University of Pennsylvania
Philadelphia, Pennsylvania
Chapter 33. Pulmonary Embolism

Marlene SanFilippo, MSN, ARNP, FNP-C, AOCNP®
Hematology-Oncology Nurse Practitioner
Kadlec Clinic Hematology and Oncology
Kennewick, Washington
Chapter 17. Rash; Chapter 21. Furuncle; Chapter 22.
Herpes Zoster; Chapter 106. Osteoporosis

Marlon Garzo Saria, PhD, RN, FAAN
Oncology Clinical Nurse Specialist
Director of Clinical Education and Professional Practice
Pacific Neuroscience Institute and Saint John's Cancer
Institute at Providence Saint John's Health Center
Santa Monica, California
Chapter 101. Fibromyalgia Syndrome; Chapter 104. Lyme
Disease; Chapter 105. Osteoarthritis; Chapter 107.
Restless Legs Syndrome; Chapter 108. Rheumatoid
Arthritis; Chapter 109. Sciatica; Chapter 110. Systemic
Lupus Erythematosus

Raymond Scarpa, DNP, APNC, AOCN®
Head and Neck Oncology Program Manager
Department of Otolaryngology Head and Neck Surgery
University Hospital
Newark, New Jersey
Chapter 2. Hoarseness/Dysphonia; Chapter 4. Sore
Throat (Pharyngitis/Tonsillitis); Chapter 5. Tinnitus;
Chapter 6. Allergic Rhinitis; Chapter 8. Conjunctivitis;
Chapter 11. Rhinosinusitis

Christa Seligman, MSN, APRN, AGNP-C
Neurology Nurse Practitioner
Ascension Seton Medical Center
Austin, Texas
Chapter 131. Ataxia/Incoordination; Chapter 137. Headache

Brenda K. Shelton, DNP, APRN-CNS, RN, CCRN, AOCN®
Clinical Nurse Specialist
Sidney Kimmel Comprehensive Cancer Center
Johns Hopkins University School of Nursing
Baltimore, Maryland
Chapter 38. Palpitations; Chapter 45. Dysrhythmias;
Chapter 46. Endocarditis; Chapter 49. Myocardial
Infarction/Acute Coronary Syndromes; Chapter 50.
Pericarditis/Pericardial Effusion/Pericardial Tamponade

Gary Shelton, DNP, MSN, NP, ANP-BC, AOCNP®, ACHPN
Oncology Clinical Nurse Specialist and Adult Health Nurse
Practitioner
Mount Sinai Hospital System
New York, New York
Chapter 83. Oliguria/Anuria/Azotemia; Chapter 91. Ne-
phrotic Syndrome; Chapter 93. Proteinuria; Chapter 95.
Syndrome of Inappropriate Antidiuretic Hormone

Victoria Sherry, DNP, CRNP, AOCNP®
Oncology Nurse Practitioner
Abramson Cancer Center, University of Pennsylvania
Medical Center
Faculty, University of Pennsylvania School of Nursing
Philadelphia, Pennsylvania
Chapter 23. Cough; Chapter 25. Hemoptysis; Chapter
26. Orthopnea; Chapter 30. Pneumonia; Chapter 31.
Pneumothorax; Chapter 32. Pulmonary Edema

Marcel Smith, RN, MS, FNP-BC
Nurse Practitioner—Department of Neurology
Memorial Sloan Kettering Cancer Center
New York, New York
Chapter 141. Meningitis

Allison Strider, MSN, AGNP-BC, AOCNP®
Oncology Nurse Practitioner
O'Neal Comprehensive Cancer Center at the University of
Alabama at Birmingham
Birmingham, Alabama
Chapter 44. Dyslipidemia

Lindsay Tedder, MSN, APRN, WHNP-BC
Nurse Practitioner
Moffit Cancer Center
Tampa, Florida
Chapter 79. Abnormal Vaginal Bleeding (Menorrhagia)

Jennifer A. Tschanz, MSN, FNP, AOCNP®, ACHPN
Nurse Practitioner
Department of Hematology and Oncology
Naval Medical Center San Diego
San Diego, California
Chapter 163. Fatigue

Wendy H. Vogel, MSN, FNP, AOCNP®
Executive Director
Advanced Practitioner Society for Hematology and
Oncology
Lawrenceville, New Jersey
Chapter 3. Ear Pain (Otalgia); Chapter 9. Otitis Externa;
Chapter 10. Otitis Media; Chapter 39. Peripheral Edema;
Chapter 84. Urinary Incontinence; Chapter 148. Flu-Like
Syndrome

Kathryn R. Waitman, DNP, MSN, FNP-C, AOCNP
Advanced Practice Nurse
CompHealth Locum Company
Billings Clinic
Billings, Montana
Chapter 98. Low Back Pain; Chapter 145. Spinal Cord
Compression

Julie G. Walker, PhD, APRN, FNP-C
Advanced Practice Registered Nurse
University of Texas MD Anderson Cancer Center
Houston, Texas
Chapter 138. Paresthesia; Chapter 144. Seizures

Mailey Wilks, DNP, MSN, APRN, NP-C
Nurse Practitioner, Department of Hematologic Oncology
and Blood Disorders
Outpatient APRN/PA Coordinator
Cleveland Clinic, Taussig Cancer Institute
Cleveland, Ohio
Chapter 43. Deep Venous Thrombosis; Chapter 113.
Anemia of Chronic Disease; Chapter 115. Cobalamin
(Vitamin B_{12}) Deficiency; Chapter 122. Hypercoagulable
State; Chapter 124. Immune Thrombocytopenia; Chap-
ter 130. Thrombotic Thrombocytopenia Purpura

Tracy C. Wyant, DNP, AOCN®, CHPN, GERO-BC, CPPS, EBP-C
Senior Director, Medical Content
Office of Cancer Research and Implementation
American Cancer Society
Atlanta, Georgia
Chapter 14. Nail Changes; Chapter 15. Pressure Injuries
(Pressure Ulcers/Sores); Chapter 18. Atopic Dermatitis;
Chapter 19. Cellulitis; Chapter 20. Contact Dermatitis;
Chapter 132. Blurred Vision

Disclosure

Editors and authors of books and guidelines provided by the Oncology Nursing Society are expected to disclose to the readers any significant financial interest or other relationships with the manufacturer(s) of any commercial products.

A vested interest may be considered to exist if a contributor is affiliated with or has a financial interest in commercial organizations that may have a direct or indirect interest in the subject matter. A "financial interest" may include, but is not limited to, being a shareholder in the organization; being an employee of the commercial organization; serving on an organization's speakers bureau; or receiving research funding from the organization. An "affiliation" may be holding a position on an advisory board or some other role of benefit to the commercial organization. Vested interest statements appear in the front matter for each publication.

Contributors are expected to disclose any unlabeled or investigational use of products discussed in their content. This information is acknowledged solely for the information of the readers.

The contributors provided the following disclosure and vested interest information:

Jeannine M. Brant, PhD, APRN, AOCN®: Advanced Practitioner Society for Hematology and Oncology, NRG Oncology, SWOG Cancer Research Network, *Journal of the Advanced Practitioner in Oncology*, *JCO Global Oncology*, employment or leadership positions; Hospice and Palliative Nurses Association, consultant or advisory role; Carevive Systems, stock ownership; Daiichi Sankyo, AstraZeneca, Northwestern University, Harborside, Oncology Nursing Society, Elsevier, honoraria; Fabry Registry, AstraZeneca, NIH Cancer Moonshot, research funding

Mary Elizabeth Davis, DNP, RN, CHPN, AOCNS®: Oncology Nursing Society New York City Chapter, employment or leadership position

Deena Damsky Dell, MSN, APRN, AOCN®, LNC: Elsevier, Relias, honoraria

Mary W. Dunn, MSN, RN, OCN®, NP-C: American Urological Association, honoraria

Jeanne Held-Warmkessel, MSN, RN, AOCN®, ACNS-BC: Oncology Nursing Society, other remuneration

Stephanie Jackson, DNP, MSN, RN, AOCNS®, BMTCN®: Oncology Nurse News, employment or leadership position; Jazz Pharmaceuticals, consultant or advisory role

Sandra Kurtin, PhD, ANP-C, AOCN®: Advanced Practitioner Society for Hematology and Oncology, MDS Foundation, employment or leadership position; Abbvie, Amgen, AstraZeneca, Bristol Myers Squibb, Celgene, GlaxoSmithKline, Incyte, Pharmacyclics, Takeda Pharmaceutical Company, consultant or advisory role

Heather T. Mackey, MSN, RN, ANP-BC, AOCN®: Elsevier, employment or leadership position

Laurl A. Matey, MSN, RN-BC, CHPN: Haymarket Medical Education, employment or leadership position; Elsevier, honoraria

Enza Esposito Nguyen, DNP, RN, ANP-BC, AOCNP®: AstraZeneca, employment; AstraZeneca, stock ownership

Beth Sandy, MSN, CRNP: AstraZeneca, Jazz Pharmaceuticals, Merck, Takeda Pharmaceutical Company, honoraria

Marlon Garzo Saria, PhD, RN, FAAN: CureScience, employment or leadership position; CancerLife, NeuraMetrix, consultant or advisory role; CancerLife, Headspace, NeuraMetrix, Tower Cancer Research Foundation, research funding

Victoria Sherry, DNP, CRNP, AOCNP®: AstraZeneca, consultant or advisory role; O'Bryan, Brown & Toner PLLC, expert testimony

Lindsay Tedder, MSN, APRN, WHNP-BC: Society of Gynecologic Oncology, employment or leadership position; University of Tampa, honoraria

Wendy H. Vogel, MSN, FNP, AOCNP®: Advanced Practitioner Society for Hematology and Oncology, employment or leadership position

Mailey Wilks, DNP, MSN, APRN, NP-C: Kent State University, employment or leadership position; Oncology Nursing Society, honoraria

Licensing Opportunities

The Oncology Nursing Society (ONS) produces some of the most highly respected educational resources in the field of oncology nursing, including ONS's award-winning journals, books, online courses, evidence-based resources, core competencies, videos, and information available on the ONS website at www.ons.org. ONS welcomes opportunities to license reuse of these intellectual properties to other organizations.

Licensing opportunities include the following:
- **Reprints**—Purchase high-quality reprints of ONS journal articles, book chapters, and other content directly from ONS, or obtain permission to produce your own reprints.
- **Translations**—Translate and then resell or share ONS resources internationally.
- **Integration**—Purchase a license to incorporate ONS's oncology-specific telephone triage protocols or other resources into your institution's EMR or EHR system.
- **Cobranding**—Display your company's logo on ONS resources for distribution to your organization's employees or customers.
- **Educational reuse**—Supplement your staff or student educational programs using ONS resources.
- **Customization**—Customize ONS intellectual property for inclusion in your own products or services.
- **Bulk purchases**—Buy ONS books and online courses in high quantities to receive great savings compared to regular pricing.

As you read through the pages of this book, think about whether any of these opportunities are the right fit for you as you consider reusing ONS content—and the contents of this book—for your organization.
Contact licensing@ons.org with your licensing questions or requests.

Contents

Preface

As we reflect on the completion of the fourth edition of the *Clinical Manual for the Oncology Advanced Practice Nurse*, we are nothing short of amazed. When we published the first edition in 2000, we never dreamt that we would see multiple editions. We simply wanted to publish the manual we so desperately needed—a quick reference that bridged the gap of how to treat patients with cancer who present with a variety of medical issues. We found as new oncology nurse practitioners that the medical textbooks and references were helpful but did not account for the nuances of the patient with cancer who was currently in treatment or had completed treatment. So, we had a dream to make the manual a reality, and with help from the Oncology Nursing Society (ONS) and numerous writers, we did—four times!

As with previous editions, the manual has undergone extensive revisions to reflect current patient care practice, including six new chapters. Tables, figures, and appendices have been updated to provide easy access to important concepts discussed throughout the manual. As with previous editions, leading experts in oncology nursing have authored each chapter.

The fourth edition continues with the tradition of being a quick reference guide for the diagnosis and treatment of acute and chronic problems occurring in the patient with cancer. The format is extensively cross-referenced to allow easy identification of symptoms to determine the medical diagnosis. Although the information is not all-inclusive, the manual provides a comprehensive resource to guide the busy practitioner within their practice.

This is a time of reflection for us as we publish this edition. When creating the first edition, we were young, ambitious, and novice oncology nurse practitioners. There were only a handful of nurse practitioners in the United States. Basically, we were "flying by the seat of our pants." Today, we are nearing the end of our careers. We have seen so much through the years—changes in therapies and diagnostic techniques, an increase in overall survival in cancer, changes in our career paths, and numerous personal changes, as have many of you have.

It is a bit overwhelming to look back and realize we have spent our entire careers being passionate about caring for those with cancer and for our advanced practice colleagues who have revolutionized cancer care. It is with grateful hearts that we will pass the baton to our good friend and colleague, Diane G. Cope, to keep the manual alive for its subsequent editions.

We close in gratitude to the ONS Publications Department for taking a chance on our idea and keeping that dream alive. We are grateful to all of the numerous writers and contributors of the manual who have made this publication the most sought-after reference. Lastly, we are grateful for our friendships that started within ONS and have lasted all these years. What an unintended blessing we never could have imagined.

Dawn, Becca, and Diane

List of Abbreviations

ABG—arterial blood gas
ACD—anemia of chronic disease
ACE—angiotensin converting enzyme
ADH—antidiuretic hormone
ADLs—activities of daily living
AIDS—acquired immunodeficiency syndrome
AKI—acute kidney injury
ALT—alanine aminotransferase
ANC—absolute neutrophil count
aPTT—activated partial thromboplastin time
ARB—angiotensin II receptor blocker
ASA—aspirin
AST—aspartate transaminase
ATP—adenosine triphosphate
AV—atrioventricular
BMI—body mass index
BNP—B-type natriuretic peptide
BPH—benign prostatic hyperplasia
bpm—beats per minute
BUN—blood urea nitrogen
CAD—coronary artery disease
CAR—chimeric antigen receptor
CBC—complete blood count
CBD—common bile duct
CDC—Centers for Disease Control and Prevention
CHF—congestive heart failure
CIPN—chemotherapy-induced peripheral neuropathy
cGy—cenitgray
CKD—chronic kidney disease
CMV—cytomegalovirus
CNS—central nervous system
COPD—chronic obstructive pulmonary disease
CRP—C-reactive protein
CSF—cerebrospinal fluid
CT—computed tomography
CTLA-4—cytotoxic T-lymphocyte antigen 4
DEXA—dual energy x-ray absorptiometry
DIC—disseminated intravascular coagulation
DVT—deep venous thrombosis
ECG—electrocardiogram
EGD—esophagogastroduodenoscopy
EGFR—epidermal growth factor receptor
EPO—erythropoietin
ESR—erythrocyte sedimentation rate
ET—essential thrombocythemia
FDA—U.S. Food and Drug Administration

FEV$_1$—forced expiratory volume in one second
FMS—fibromyalgia syndrome
FSH—follicle-stimulating hormone
FVC—forced vital capacity
G-CSF—granulocyte–colony-stimulating factor
GERD—gastroesophageal reflux disease
GFR—glomerular filtration rate
GI—gastrointestinal
GU—genitourinary
GVHD—graft-versus-host disease
Gy—gray
HDL—high-density lipoprotein
HEENT—head, ears, eyes, nose, and throat
Hgb—hemoglobin
HIV—human immunodeficiency virus
HLA—human leukocyte antigen
HSCT—hematopoietic stem cell transplantation
HSV—herpes simplex virus
HZV—herpes zoster virus
IBS—irritable bowel syndrome
ICP—intracranial pressure
ICU—intensive care unit
IFN—interferon
Ig—immunoglobulin
IL—interleukin
IM—intramuscular
INR—international normalized ratio
IT—primary immune thrombocytopenia
ITP—immune thrombocytopenia
IV—intravenous
IVC—inferior vena cava
IVIg—intravenous immunoglobulin
JVD—jugular venous distention
LDH—lactate dehydrogenase
LDL—low-density lipoprotein
LES—lower esophageal sphincter
LFT—liver function test
LLN—lower limit of normal
LMWH—low-molecular-weight heparin
mcg—microgram
MGUS—monoclonal gammopathy of undetermined significance
MI—myocardial injury
MMA—methylmalonic acid
MRI—magnetic resonance imaging
MRSA—methicillin-resistant *Staphylococcus aureus*

NCCN—National Comprehensive Cancer Network
NCI CTEP—National Cancer Institute Cancer
  Therapy Evaluation Program
NG—nasogastric
NPO—nothing by mouth
NSAID—nonsteroidal anti-inflammatory drug
OA—osteoarthritis
OE—otitis externa
OM—otitis media
PD-1—programmed cell death protein 1
PD-L1—programmed cell death-ligand 1
PE—pulmonary embolism
PET—positron-emission tomography
PH—pulmonary hypertension
PNS—peripheral nervous system
PPI—proton pump inhibitor
PRN—as needed
PT—prothrombin time
PTH—parathyroid hormone
PTT—partial thromboplastin time
QOL—quality of life
RA—rheumatoid arthritis

RBC—red blood cell
SCC—spinal cord compression
SIADH—syndrome of inappropriate antidiuretic
  hormone
SLE—systemic lupus erythematosus
SPEP—serum protein electrophoresis
SSRI—selective serotonin reuptake inhibitor
STI—sexually transmitted infection
SVC—superior vena cava
T_3—triiodothyronine
T_4—thyroxine
TB—tuberculosis
TIPS—transjugular intrahepatic portosystemic shunt
TKI—tyrosine kinase inhibitor
TMJ—temporomandibular joint
TNF—tumor necrosis factor
TSH—thyroid-stimulating hormone
ULN—upper limit of normal
URI—upper respiratory infection
UTI—urinary tract infection
VZV—varicella zoster virus
WBC—white blood cell

Head and Neck

SYMPTOMS

MEDICAL DIAGNOSES

CHAPTER 1

Hiccups (Singultus)

Dawn Camp-Sorrell, MSN, CRNP, AOCN®

I. Definition: An involuntary, intermittent, spasmodic contraction of the diaphragm and intercostal muscles (Gonella & Gonella, 2015; Hernandez et al., 2015; Jeon et al., 2018; Karakonstantis et al., 2018; Kohse et al., 2017)
  A. Bout: Episode persisting as long as 48 hours
  B. Persistent: Episode persisting longer than 48 hours but less than one month
  C. Intractable: Episode occurring continuously for months or years

II. Physiology/Pathophysiology (Gonella & Gonella, 2015; Karakonstantis et al., 2018; Kim et al., 2018; Rouse & Wodziak, 2018; Steger et al., 2015; Zhang et al., 2018)
  A. Normal: Glottis pertains to the area of the vocal cords. The diaphragm separates the abdomen from the thoracic cavity. Intercostal muscles (external and internal) are located on the outer layer and between the ribs.
  B. Pathophysiology
    1. Synchronous clonic spasm of the intercostal muscles and diaphragm causes sudden inspiration followed by prompt closure of the glottis, causing the hiccup sound and inhibiting respirations.
    2. Hiccups are a reflex arc traveling an afferent pathway over vagal sympathetic and sensory fibers of the phrenic nerve. It is thought that the central connection for hiccups involves an interaction among the medulla oblongata and reticular formation of the brain stem, phrenic nerve nuclei, and the hypothalamus.
      a) The afferent pathway of hiccup reflex encompasses the phrenic and vagus nerves and the sympathetic chain arising from the thoracic (T) segments T6–T12.
      b) The primary efferent reflex branch is the phrenic nerve; however, the glottis and accessory muscles of the respiratory nerves have been suggested as the efferent pathway.
      c) The hiccup center is thought to be between cervical (C) segment C3–C5 and the brain stem.
    3. Hiccups most often occur during inspiration and are inhibited by elevations in carbon dioxide.

III. Clinical features: Hiccups are a transient, innocuous symptom, but they can become exhausting and disabling (e.g., respiratory insufficiency, fatigue) if they persist. They are classified as psychogenic (associated with stress, anxiety, or excitement), organic (cause from irritation of phrenic and/or vagus nerve), and idiopathic (cause unidentified). Serious consequences can result with refractory hiccups, including malnutrition, dehydration, insomnia, and decreased QOL. Hiccups occur more frequently in men, and they serve no known physiologic function. Hiccups tend to occur with a frequency of 4–60 per minute (Gardecki et al., 2017; Gonella & Gonella, 2015; Jeon et al., 2018; Kohse et al., 2017; Rouse & Wodziak, 2018; Steger et al., 2015).

A. Etiology
   1. Vagus and phrenic nerve irritation
     a) Esophagitis
     b) Intraoperative manipulation
     c) Intubation
     d) Pharyngitis
     e) Laryngitis
     f) Mediastinal mass
     g) Goiter
     h) Tumors of the neck that stimulate the laryngeal nerve
   2. CNS disorder
     a) Head trauma
     b) Multiple sclerosis
     c) Encephalitis
     d) Meningitis
     e) Hydrocephalus
   3. Metabolic
     a) Uremia
     b) Alcohol intoxication
     c) Anesthesia
     d) Drug induced: Corticosteroids, benzodiazepines, hydrocodone
     e) Chemotherapy induced: Cisplatin, carboplatin, etoposide, irinotecan, docetaxel, paclitaxel, gemcitabine, vinorelbine
     f) Hypokalemia
     g) Hypocalcemia
     h) Hyperventilation
   4. GI
     a) Distension from overeating or fluid buildup such as ascites
     b) GERD
     c) *Helicobacter pylori* infection
     d) Gastric cancer
     e) Abdominal abscesses
     f) Gallbladder disease
     g) Pancreatitis
     h) Pancreatic cancer
     i) Inflammatory bowel disease
     j) Hepatitis
   5. Cardiac disorders: MI, pericarditis
   6. Thoracic disorders
     a) Lymphadenopathy secondary to infection or neoplasm
     b) Pneumonia
     c) Empyema
     d) Asthma
     e) Mediastinal tumors
   7. Other: Excessive drinking, excessive smoking, sudden excitement or stress
B. History
   1. History of cancer and cancer treatment

    2. Current medications: Prescribed, over the counter

    3. History of presenting symptoms: Precipitating factors, onset, location, duration

    4. Changes in ADLs

    5. Past medical history: Recent abdominal, thoracic, or neurologic surgery; emotional problems

    6. Social history: Alcohol use, tobacco use

C. Signs and symptoms of intractable hiccups

    1. Dyspnea

    2. Anorexia

    3. Weight loss

    4. Fatigue and exhaustion

    5. Insomnia

    6. Heartburn (from severe gastric reflux)

    7. Depression

    8. Dehydration

    9. Chest pain

D. Physical examination

    1. HEENT: Evidence of trauma or infection

        a) Mucous membranes: Dehydration

        b) Nuchal rigidity, thyromegaly, cervical adenopathy

        c) Trauma or foreign body in external ear canals

        d) Thyromegaly and lymphadenopathy on neck palpation

    2. Integument: Wound dehiscence as a secondary problem from hiccups

    3. Pulmonary

        a) Evidence of reduced diaphragmatic excursion on chest percussion

        b) Abnormal sounds indicating infiltrate, effusion, or pleuritis on auscultation

    4. Abdominal: Distention, organomegaly

    5. Neurologic examination

        a) Mental changes indicating stroke, brain metastasis, dehydration, or trauma

        b) Assessment of cranial nerves for changes indicating structural lesions (see Appendix A)

IV. Diagnostic tests (Gardecki et al., 2017; Karakonstantis et al., 2018; Kohse et al., 2017)

A. Laboratory

    1. Serum *H. pylori* if suspected GERD

    2. CBC to evaluate for infection with increased WBC count

    3. Thyroid studies to evaluate for thyroid disorder

    4. Complete metabolic panel to evaluate for electrolyte imbalances and hyperglycemia; liver function tests, amylase, and lipase to evaluate for GI causes

    5. Uric acid to evaluate for uremia

B. Radiology

    1. Chest x-ray to evaluate for pulmonary, mediastinal, or cardiac abnormalities capable of irritating the phrenic nerve, vagal nerve, or diaphragm

    2. CT scan

        a) Abdominal CT scan to evaluate for abnormalities of the subdiaphragmatic region

        b) Head CT scan to evaluate for lesions or bleeds

    3. MRI of the head to evaluate for lesions or bleeds

C. Other

    1. ECG to evaluate for heart block or bradyarrhythmia

    2. Lumbar puncture to evaluate for CNS infection or malignancy

V. Differential diagnosis (Kohse et al., 2017; Rouse & Wodziak, 2018; Steger et al., 2015)
   A. Structural defect
      1. Pericarditis (see Chapter 50)
      2. Malignancy
      3. Subdiaphragmatic abscess
      4. Hiatal hernia
      5. MI (see Chapter 49)
      6. Peritonitis
      7. Pancreatitis (see Chapter 77)
      8. Biliary tract disease
   B. Metabolic disturbances
      1. Uremia
      2. Diabetes mellitus (see Chapter 151)
      3. Alcoholism
      4. Goiter (see Chapters 157 and 158)
      5. Electrolyte imbalances (see Chapters 152–156)
   C. CNS disorders: Infection or multiple sclerosis
   D. Thorax related
      1. Ulcer
      2. Abscess
      3. Aneurysm
      4. Pleuritis
      5. Pneumonia (see Chapter 30)
   E. Drug induced
      1. Corticosteroids: Dexamethasone, methylprednisolone
      2. Benzodiazepines: Midazolam, chlordiazepoxide
      3. Anesthesia
      4. Chemotherapy induced
   F. Psychogenic disease
      1. Hysteria
      2. Anorexia nervosa (see Chapter 66)
      3. Anxiety (see Chapter 161)

VI. Treatment: The overall goal is to relieve the patient of discomfort and to correct the underlying discomfort (Gardecki et al., 2017; Hernandez et al., 2015; Jeon et al., 2018; Kim et al., 2018; Kohse et al., 2017; Rouse & Wodziak, 2018; Zhang et al., 2018).
   A. Nonpharmacologic measures: Many without scientifically proven efficacy
      1. Nasopharyngeal stimulation
         a) Perform intranasal application of vinegar or similar smell.
         b) Inhale smelling salt or similar irritant.
         c) Stimulate oropharynx (e.g., ice water, vinegar, granulated sugar).
         d) Lift uvula with a spoon.
      2. Vagal stimulation
         a) Apply cold compress to face.
         b) Give carotid massage.
         c) Induce fright.
         d) Induce vomiting.
      3. Respiratory maneuvers
         a) Hold breath.
         b) Perform rebreathing.

   c) Perform Valsalva maneuver.
  4. Phrenic nerve transmission disruption
   a) Rhythmically tap over fifth cervical vertebra.
   b) Apply ice to skin over phrenic nerve.
   c) Apply electric stimulation over phrenic nerve.
   d) Stimulate phrenic nerve.
  5. Counterirritation of the diaphragm
   a) Pull knees to chest.
   b) Lean forward to compress chest.
   c) Apply pressure at points of diaphragmatic insertion.
  6. Hypnosis
  7. Peppermint facilitates belching by relaxing the lower esophageal sphincter.
  8. Acupuncture has been found to improve intractable hiccups.
   a) Most acupoints for hiccups are located near dermatomes (see Appendix B) related to afferent and efferent pathways. Secondary synapses or nuclei are involved in the hiccup reflex arc.
   b) Acupuncture may modulate any portion of the hiccup reflex arc locally by changing blood perfusion, activating the autonomic nervous system, regulating inflammatory mediators, or altering axonal excitability.

B. Pharmacologic measures: To interrupt afferent and efferent pathways
  1. Miscellaneous agents
   a) Metoclopramide: 10 mg PO three times a day
   b) Baclofen: 10 mg PO three times a day; thought to block the hiccup stimulus arc
   c) PPI for GERD: Omeprazole 20–40 mg PO daily
   d) Sertraline: 50 mg PO daily; may inhibit the hiccup reflex arc by affecting $5\text{-}HT_3$ (serotonin) receptors in GI tract; ironically, hiccups can be an adverse reaction to sertraline.
   e) Simethicone: To relieve gastric distention
   f) Benzonatate: 100 mg PO every 4 hours, not to exceed 600 mg in 24 hours
   g) Gabapentin: 300 mg PO one to three times a day
  2. For intractable hiccups, hospital admission may be warranted to use IV or oral agents because of the side effects and drug interactions associated with these agents.
   a) Antipsychotics act centrally by dopamine antagonism in the hypothalamus.
    (1) Chlorpromazine: 25–50 mg PO initially with maintenance therapy of 25 mg four times a day
    (2) Haloperidol: 2–5 mg IM initially with maintenance of 1–4 mg PO three times a day
   b) Anticonvulsants have been effective in treating intractable hiccups.
    (1) Valproic acid: 250 mg PO daily in divided doses for two weeks; no long-term use because of potential hepatotoxicity; thought to block hiccup stimulus
    (2) Phenytoin: 200 mg IV initially, followed by maintenance dose of 300 mg PO daily
   c) If a patient is hospitalized and if necessary, give a large dose of metoclopramide IV (2 mg/kg). This may reduce esophageal contraction. Large doses are associated with tardive dyskinesia. After loading dose, begin oral dosing as listed.

C. Surgical infiltration of the phrenic nerve: When other measures have not been successful; some benefit with ultrasound guidance

      1. Injection of long-acting anesthetic or alcohol has been effective in treatment of intractable hiccups.
      2. Surgical procedure of crushing or cutting the phrenic nerve has been effective in controlling intractable hiccups.
      3. Continuous cervical epidural block at the level of C3–C5 for refractory hiccups has been reported beneficial. When hiccups subside for 48 hours, cervical epidural catheter is removed, and oral medication is given.
   D. General anesthesia for intractable hiccups as a last resort

VII. Follow-up: Dependent on etiology and occurrence of hiccups
   A. For persistent and intractable hiccups, see patient daily until interventions have been successful and maintenance dose is managed.
   B. Follow up for recurrence of hiccups PRN.
   C. Hospitalization may be warranted to aggressively manage symptom if patient has persistent or intractable hiccups.

VIII. Referrals
   A. Surgeon: If invasive procedure is necessary
   B. Anesthesiologist: For phrenic nerve block or general anesthesia
   C. Behavioral therapy: For identified triggers (e.g., stress, anxiety)

References

Gardecki, J., Espinosa, J., Lucerna, A., & Bernhardt, J. (2017). Singultus: Avoiding a hiccup in care. *American Journal of Emergency Medicine, 35*(6), 938.E1–938.E3. https://doi.org/10.1016/j.ajem.2016.12.056

Gonella, S., & Gonella, F. (2015). Use of vinegar to relieve persistent hiccups in an advanced cancer patient. *Journal of Palliative Medicine, 18*(5), 467–470. https://doi.org/10.1089/jpm.2014.0391

Hernandez, S.L., Fasnacht, K.S., Sheyner, I., King, J.M., & Stewart, J.T. (2015). Treatment of refractory hiccups with amantadine. *Journal of Pain and Palliative Care Pharmacotherapy, 29*(4), 374–377. https://doi.org/10.3109/15360288.2015.1101640

Jeon, Y.S., Kearney, A.M., & Baker, P.G. (2018). Management of hiccups in palliative care patients. *BMJ Supportive and Palliative Care, 8*(1), 1–6. https://doi.org/10.1136/bmjspcare-2016-001264

Karakonstantis, S., Pitsigavdaki, S., Korela, D., & Galani, D. (2018). Lower lobe pneumonia presenting as singultus (hiccups). *Caspian Journal of Internal Medicine, 9*(4), 403–405. https://doi.org/10.22088/cjim.9.4.403

Kim, J.E., Lee, M.K., Lee, D.K., Choi, S.S., & Park, J.S. (2018). Continuous cervical epidural block: Treatment for intractable hiccups. *Medicine, 97*(6), e9444. https://doi.org/10.1097/MD.0000000000009444

Kohse, E.K., Hollmann, M.W., Bardenheuer, H.J., & Kessler, J. (2017). Chronic hiccups: An underestimated problem. *Anesthesia and Analgesia, 125*(4), 1169–1183. https://doi.org/10.1213/ANE.0000000000002289

Rouse, S., & Wodziak, M. (2018). Intractable hiccups. *Current Neurology and Neuroscience Reports, 18,* 51. https://doi.org/10.1007/s11910-018-0856-0

Steger, M., Schneemann, M., & Fox, M. (2015). Systemic review: The pathogenesis and pharmacological treatment of hiccups. *Alimentary Pharmacology and Therapeutics, 42*(9), 1037–1050. https://doi.org/10.1111/apt.13374

Zhang, Y., Duan, F., & Ma, W. (2018). Ultrasound-guided phrenic nerve block for intraoperative persistent hiccups: A case report. *BMC Anesthesiology, 18,* 123. https://doi.org/10.1186/s12871-018-0589-2

CHAPTER 2

Hoarseness/Dysphonia

Raymond Scarpa, DNP, APNC, AOCN®

I. Definition: Hoarseness is a symptom of altered voice quality (Cooper & Quested, 2016; Stachler et al., 2018; Stinnett et al., 2018).
   A. Dysphonia: Impaired voice production characterized by altered pitch quality, loudness, or vocal effort that impairs communication
   B. Dysarthria: Speech disorder related to impaired movement of the structures used for speech
   C. Muscle tension dysphonia: Altered laryngeal muscle tension despite normal laryngeal anatomy; also known as functional dysphonia

II. Physiology/Pathophysiology (Cooper & Quested, 2016; Hoover, 2018; House & Fisher, 2017; Reiter et al., 2015; Stinnett et al., 2018)
   A. Normal: Voice production
      1. Synchronization of optimal vocal cord positioning with optimal control of airflow from lung to oropharynx
      2. Proper vocal fold performance to ensure optimal dynamic vibratory characteristics of the vocal cords
      3. Anatomy
         a) The larynx is composed of the three distinct regions: the supraglottis, glottis, and subglottis.
         b) The primary function of the larynx is to protect the airway during swallowing and breathing and to produce sound for speech.
         c) The vocal cords, located in the glottis, are composed of five layers (deep to superficial): thyroarytenoid muscle, deep lamina propria, intermediate lamina propria, superficial lamina propria, and the squamous epithelium. These layers extend from the arytenoids posteriorly to the midline thyroid cartilage anteriorly.
         d) The false vocal cords located in the supraglottis are situated superior to the true vocal cords and are termed *ventricular folds*. They also protect the airway with a minimal role in phonation.
         e) True vocal cords are the narrowest part of the upper aerodigestive system.
   B. Pathophysiology: Hoarseness is a principal symptom of dysphonia. It is manifested by irregular oscillation of the vocal cords. This results in excessive tension on the vocal cords, incomplete closure of the glottis when speaking, or an increase in bulk of the vocal cords.

III. Clinical features: Hoarseness may be from a functional or organic cause (Cooper & Quested, 2016; Hoover, 2018; Stinnett et al., 2018; Zhang, 2016).
   A. Etiology by voice sound: Voice is produced at the glottis level.
      1. Breathy voice sounds are caused by incomplete glottis closure.

2. A constrained or pressed voice is caused by tight vocal cord closure, resulting in a rough, raspy voice (e.g., spasmodic dysphonia).

3. Weakened muscle (as in aging), neurologic impairment, or muscle atrophy can result in insufficient glottal closure during phonation. This can cause a shaky or muffled voice (e.g., phonasthenia).

4. Hoarseness that is worse earlier in the day may be reflux; hoarseness late in day may indicate neurologic etiology.

5. A honking quality may signify sarcoidosis.

6. Low-pitched vocalization may be secondary to hypothyroidism, reflux, leukoplakia, muscle tension, dysphonia, edema, or vocal cord paralysis.

B. History

1. History of cancer and cancer treatment

2. Current medications: Prescribed, over the counter, herbal

3. History of presenting symptoms: Precipitating factors, onset, location, duration, timing of initial and progressive changes in voice, associated symptoms (e.g., sore throat, fever, chills, dysphagia, otalgia, odynophagia)

4. Changes in ADLs

5. Past medical history: Recent URI, thyroid disorders, myalgia (self or family member), sarcoidosis, trauma, injury to upper chest
   a) Neurologic disorders: Stroke, amyotrophic lateral sclerosis, Parkinson disease, multiple sclerosis, myasthenia gravis
   b) GI conditions: Reflux, hernias, GERD

6. Past surgical history: Neck, oral cavity or thoracic surgery, difficult intubation, prolonged intubations, thyroid or parathyroid surgery

7. Social history: Alcohol use, tobacco use, recreational drug use (e.g., vaping)

8. Occupational history: Exposure to dust, fire, smoke, or irritant fumes

C. Signs and symptoms

1. Quality of voice: Completely lost, raspy, breathy, coarse, stridor
   a) Changes in volume, quality, flexibility, or pitch
   b) Continuous or intermittent; sudden onset, progressive, or chronic
   c) Vocal tremor

2. Nasal or pharyngeal drainage or congestion

3. Shortness of breath

4. Neck swelling

5. Hemoptysis

6. Difficulty swallowing

7. Indigestion

8. Sore throat

9. Trismus

10. Referred ear pain (otalgia)

D. Physical examination

1. HEENT
   a) Inspection of nose, paranasal sinuses, nasopharynx, and ears: Abnormal anatomy, excess tissue, abnormal growths, mechanical obstruction/foreign objects, inflammation, infection, injury
   b) Palpation of thyroid, head and neck lymph nodes, and oral cavity: Abnormal anatomy, excess tissue, abnormal growths, lymphadenopathy, asymmetry, inflammation, infection, injury
   c) Oral: Dentition, tongue mobility, symmetry of palatal tonsils, oral cavity architecture, buccal mucosa

    2. Pulmonary: Absence of lung sounds or adventitious sounds indicating possible source

    3. Abdominal: Tenderness in the mid-upper region indicating possible gastric reflux

    4. Neurologic: Head, face, and neck examination for abnormal response to expected normal neurologic examination, focusing on cranial nerves I–XII (see Appendix A) suggestive of Parkinson disease, multiple sclerosis, or other

IV. Diagnostic tests (Cooper & Quested, 2016; Frances & Smith, 2019)

    A. Laboratory: Thyroid function studies (e.g., TSH, serum T_4), calcitonin, thyroglobulin, and PTH (if enlarged thyroid) to evaluate for thyroid disease

    B. Radiology

        1. Chest x-ray (posterior anterior and lateral) for suspected malignancy or nerve or chest involvement

        2. CT scan of head and neck or chest only for suspected malignancy

        3. MRI or PET scan of head and neck only if CT scan results are inconclusive

        4. Ultrasound thyroid or ultrasound-guided fine needle aspiration of suspicious clinical findings

    C. Other

        1. Flexible fiberoptic laryngoscopy: Essential with a history of hoarseness for greater than two weeks; visualizes the nasal cavity, nasopharynx, pharynx, lingual tonsil, supraglottis, and glottis to detect obstruction, inflammation or infection, incomplete closure of vocal cords, abnormal anatomy, excess tissue, or abnormal growths; performed in office suite

        2. Direct laryngoscopy to visualize larynx and vocal cords, especially for patients experiencing hoarseness for more than two weeks with unknown etiology

        3. Measurement of acoustic parameters (audiogram)

        4. EGD for GERD

        5. Biopsy: Required for all suspicious lesions

V. Differential diagnosis (House & Fisher, 2017; Stinnett et al., 2018)

    A. Neoplastic and dysplastic

        1. Vocal cord malignancy

        2. Supraglottic cancer with muscle invasion

        3. Leukoplakia/dysplasia

        4. CNS tumor affecting cranial nerve X

        5. Multiple myeloma

    B. Nonmalignant etiology

        1. Infectious, inflammatory, or irritant

        2. Viral laryngitis

        3. Bacterial or fungal tracheitis or laryngitis

        4. Croup/pertussis

        5. Papillomatosis

        6. Upper respiratory allergies (see Chapter 37)

        7. Environmental irritants: Smoke

        8. Medications: Inhaled corticosteroids

        9. Laryngopharyngeal or gastric reflux (see Chapter 71)

      10. Vocal cord nodules or polyp

      11. External laryngeal trauma

      12. Senile atrophy

      13. Thoracic aortic dissection

14. Vocal abuse
15. Direct trauma
C. Neurologic
    1. Tumor compression: Glomus, thyroid, pulmonary, esophageal
    2. Trauma to nerves: Vagus or laryngeal
    3. Neural tumors
    4. Neuromuscular disease: Parkinsonism, tremor of cords, spasmodic dysphonia, muscular sclerosis, myasthenia gravis
    5. Spasmodic dystonia
    6. Cerebrovascular accident (see Chapter 146)
    7. Muscle tension dysphonia
D. Functional
    1. Hysterical aphonia: Absence of voice from psychiatric hysteria
    2. Ventricular dysphonia
    3. Hyperkinetic dysphonia
    4. Vocal abuse: Overuse or exaggerated use, such as screaming
E. Endocrine-associated systemic diseases
    1. Hypothyroidism (see Chapter 158)
    2. Adrenal insufficiency
    3. Acromegaly
    4. Hormones: Oral contraceptives, menopause
    5. Menopause (see Chapter 90)
    6. Amyloidosis
    7. Inflammatory arthritis with cricoarytenoid joint involvement
    8. Sarcoidosis
    9. SLE (see Chapter 110)

VI. Treatment (Cooper & Quested, 2016; Frances & Smith, 2019; Hoover, 2018; House & Fisher, 2017; Stachler et al., 2018)
    A. Treatment for simple hoarseness is dependent on the resolution of etiologic factors, as well as localized, symptomatic relief.
        1. Treat the underlying infectious process with antibiotics (see Appendix C).
        2. Eliminate causative factors (e.g., smoking, exposure to chemical toxins, overuse or abuse of vocal cords).
        3. Patients must drink plenty of fluids, rest the voice for 24–72 hours, and use a humidifier, especially at night.
        4. In severe laryngitis, inhaled or systemic corticosteroids may effectively assist rapid resolution.
        5. Vocal hygiene, voice therapy involving teaching techniques to minimize harmful behaviors, and altering voice production may be effective for select conditions, such as vocal cord nodules and functional voice disorders.
    B. When reflux is identified as the causative factor, use aggressive therapy to reduce the acid production and acid splash (see Chapter 71).
    C. Avoid exposure to tobacco and secondhand smoke.

VII. Follow-up
    A. Short term: Follow-up should occur within 48 hours of initial contact to verify partial or complete resolution of symptoms.
    B. Long term: Follow-up is dependent on etiology and causative factors, as well as the persistence of symptoms.

VIII. Referrals (Cooper & Quested, 2016)
  A. No referral: For patients who improve significantly or spontaneously resolve within 48 hours (without evidence of underlying disease)
  B. Family/General practice physician: For patients who do not improve or resolve after 48 hours
  C. Otolaryngologist: For hoarseness lasting longer than two weeks; complete examination recommended, including a flexible fiberoptic laryngoscopy for removal of mass, nodules, or polyps
  D. Pulmonologist: May be required in cases with concurrent dyspnea
  E. Speech pathologist: May be helpful to retrain the voice through vocal therapy, as well as for measurement of acoustic parameters
  F. Gastroenterologist: If GERD is uncontrolled, may require a GI examination

The author would like to acknowledge Joanne Lester, PhD, CNP, AOCN®, for her contribution to this chapter that remains unchanged from the previous edition of this book.

References

Cooper, L.N., & Quested, R.A. (2016). Hoarseness: An approach for the general practitioner. *Australian Family Physician, 45*(6), 378–381.

Frances, D.O., & Smith, L.J. (2019). Hoarseness guidelines redux: Toward improved treatment of patients with dysphonia. *Otolaryngologic Clinics of North America, 52*(4), 597–605. https://doi.org/10.1016/j.otc.2019.03.003

Hoover, L. (2018). Dysphonia (hoarseness): AAO-HNSF releases updated clinical guideline for treatment. *American Family Physician, 98*(10), 606–607. https://www.aafp.org/afp/2018/1115/afp20181115p606.pdf

House, S.A., & Fisher, E.L. (2017). Hoarseness in adults. *American Family Physician, 96*(11), 720–728. https://www.aafp.org/afp/2017/1201/p720.html

Reiter, R., Hoffmann, T.K., Pickhard, A., & Brosch, S. (2015). Hoarseness: Causes and treatments. *Deutsches Ärzteblatt International, 112*(19), 329–237. https://doi.org/10.3238/arztebl.2015.0329

Stachler, R.J., Francis, D.O., Schwartz, S.R., Damask, C.C., Digoy, G.P., Krouse, H.J., … Nnacheta, L.C. (2018). Voice problems: Updates to treatment and care of patients with hoarseness. *American Academy of Otolaryngology—Head and Neck Surgery*. https://www.eurekalert.org/pub_releases/2018-03/aaoo-vpu022718.php

Stinnett, S., Chmielewska, M., & Akst, L.M. (2018). Update on management of hoarseness. *Medical Clinics of North America, 102*(6), 1027–1040. https://doi.org/10.1016/j.mcna.2018.06.005

Zhang, Z. (2016). Mechanics of human voice production and control. *Journal of the Acoustical Society of America, 140*(4), 2614–2635. https://doi.org/10.1121/1.4964509

CHAPTER 3

Ear Pain (Otalgia)

Wendy H. Vogel, MSN, FNP, AOCNP®

I. Definition: The sensation of pain localizing to the ear (Earwood et al., 2018; Harrison & Cronin, 2016)
   A. Primary otalgia: Pain that originates within the ear
   B. Referred otalgia: Pain that originates outside the ear

II. Physiology/Pathophysiology (Anwar et al., 2019; Earwood et al., 2018; Harrison & Cronin, 2016)
   A. Normal
      1. The external ear includes the auricle, external ear canal, and the lateral surface of the tympanic membrane. The outer cartilaginous canal structures include cerumen glands, sebaceous glands, and hair follicles.
         a) The external canal is a cylinder measuring approximately 2.5 cm in length, extending from the conchal cartilage of the auricle to the tympanic membrane.
         b) The inferior tympanic recess is a small depression in the inferior medial aspect of the ear canal, adjacent to the tympanic membranes. Debris can collect in the area, leading to ear infection.
      2. Nerves innervating the auricle or external auditory canal include cranial nerves V, VII, IX, and X and cervical nerves C1, C2, and C3.
      3. Otalgia sensation is believed to originate in the spinal tract nucleus of cranial nerve V.
      4. These nerves also innervate the pharynx, potentially causing referred pain.
   B. Pathophysiology: Nerves innervating the auricle or external canal (or distant branches of these nerves) may be stimulated or compressed by inflammation, tumor, or infection.

III. Clinical features: Earache is a common presentation in the HEENT outpatient clinic. The severity of otalgia does not reflect the seriousness of the etiology, as serious pathology can develop without otalgia (Anwar et al., 2019; Bradley, 2019; Earwood et al., 2018; Fenton et al., 2018; Gauer & Semidey, 2015; Harrison & Cronin, 2016; Vlastarakos et al., 2019).
   A. Risk factors
      1. Recent swimming or deep-sea diving
      2. Injuries to the ear
      3. Recent travel in an airplane
      4. Frequent tonsillitis
      5. Inflammation/irritation of the tongue, palate, pharynx, nasopharynx, or larynx
      6. Head and neck cancers
      7. Poor dentition
      8. Alcohol or tobacco abuse

      9. Age older than 50 years

     10. Recent URI, OE, acute OM, or HZV

  B. Etiology

      1. Primary otalgia originates in ear, usually via infection, trauma, or foreign body. It is usually detected by otoscopy (OM and OE).

      2. Referred otalgia may not have distinct otologic etiology but originates outside the ear. Fifty percent of adult patients have referred otalgia.

         a) Most referred cases are of benign etiology (e.g., TMJ syndrome, dental infections).

         b) Maintain high suspicion for necrotizing (malignant) OE with persistent, severe pain that worsens at night.

  C. History

      1. History of cancer and cancer treatment

      2. Current medications: Prescribed, over the counter

      3. History of presenting symptoms: Precipitating factors, onset, location, radiation, duration, intensity, associated symptoms

         a) Characteristics of pain often correlate with etiology. For example, pain associated with infection is usually continuous and progressive.

         b) Intermittent pain is likely to be related to musculoskeletal disorders. Duration of pain points differentiates an acute or chronic condition.

         c) Associated symptoms include dysphonia, dysphagia, hearing loss (especially unilateral), ringing in the ears, disequilibrium, ear drainage, itching, painful teeth, pain with chewing or swallowing, ears popping, and tinnitus.

         d) Associated symptoms that might cause suspicion for malignancy include weight loss, odynophagia, dysphagia, or hoarseness.

      4. Changes in ADLs or mental status

      5. Past medical history: Previous episodes, injuries to the ear, infections, surgeries, diabetes, thyroid diseases, cardiac disease, dermatologic disorders, immunocompromised states, tobacco or alcohol use, gastroesophageal reflux, sinusitis, dental procedures, unexplained weight loss

      6. History of recent air travel or swimming

  D. Signs and symptoms: Ear pain

  E. Physical examination

      1. HEENT

         a) External ear and external auditory canal

            (1) Inspection of auricle, tragus, and periauricular region examination for edema, erythema (indicating cellulitis), lacerations, purulent green or yellow discharge (indicating OE), furuncle (tender meatal swelling), cholesteatoma (abnormal skin growth in middle ear), or foreign body

            (2) Inspection of auricle, periauricular region, and tragus palpation for pain, tenderness, warmth, and postaural edema

         b) Otoscopic examination: Tympanic membrane

            (1) Hemorrhagic vessels or blebs indicating bullous myringitis or HZV oticus

            (2) Erythema or bulging tympanic membrane with or without yellow pus indicating OM or possible neoplasm (e.g., glomus tumor)

            (3) Blue tympanic membrane (from hemorrhage) indicating old blood, often from barotrauma (i.e., from air travel or diving)

            (4) Perforation

            (5) Poor mobility when pneumatic pressure applied per pneumatic otoscope

    c) Hearing

        (1) Whisper test: To ascertain hearing alteration; if positive, perform Rinne and Weber tests with a 512 hertz tuning fork.

        (2) Rinne and Weber tests: To compare hearing by bone and air conduction (see Appendices A and D)

    d) Oral cavity

        (1) Erythematous posterior pharynx or exudate indicating pharyngitis or tonsillitis

        (2) Base-of-tongue abnormalities: Neoplasm, ulceration

        (3) Gingival and dental inspection and palpation observation for pain on palpation or percussion of teeth and signs of abscess or infection

        (4) Swelling, tenderness, or mass in parotid gland with lack of expressible saliva or purulent exudate from the Stensen duct (located high in cheek behind second molar and carries saliva from the parotid gland to the mouth) indicating neoplasm, calculus, or infection

        (5) Vocal hoarseness or breathiness indicating laryngeal pathology

  2. Neurologic: Cranial nerves (see Appendix A)

  3. Lymph node: Lymphadenopathy indicating infection or neoplasm (see Appendix D)

  4. Musculoskeletal

    a) Cervical spine pain or crepitus indicating cervical spine lesion

    b) Palpation of TMJ for tenderness and crepitus while having the patient open and close the mouth; malocclusion or trismus possibly indicative of TMJ dysfunction causing pain

  5. Vital signs: Fever indicating infectious source

IV. Diagnostic tests: When diagnosis is not apparent from otoscopy, further workup may be required (Earwood et al., 2018; Harrison & Cronin, 2016).

  A. Laboratory

    1. Myringotomy with culture of middle-ear fluid

    2. In recurrent otalgia, such as in chronic otitis, glucose level to evaluate for possible diabetes

  B. Radiology

    1. X-ray of the mastoid to evaluate for mastoid or middle ear disease

    2. CT scan of the temporal bone to evaluate for changes, inflammation, or infection

    3. CT scan of the head and neck to evaluate for pathologic bone changes (e.g., mastoiditis, OE, subperiosteal abscess), periodontal disease, and infectious or inflammatory processes

    4. MRI to evaluate for intracranial complications such as brain abscess, head and neck masses or inflammations, disorders of the cervical spine, and mastoiditis

    5. Panorex imaging to evaluate dentition and malocclusion

    6. Chest x-ray to evaluate for lung carcinomas presenting as otalgia

  C. Other diagnostic tests

    1. Audiometry: Conductive versus sensorineural hearing loss

    2. Fine needle aspiration of neck or parotid mass

    3. Nasolaryngoscopy to evaluate structural defect, tumor, and infection

V. Differential diagnosis (Bradley, 2019; Canzano et al., 2019; Earwood et al., 2018; Gauer & Semidey, 2015; Harrison & Cronin, 2016; Vlastarakos et al., 2019)

  A. Primary otalgia

    1. OE (see Chapter 9)

    2. Furunculosis (see Chapter 21)

    3. Malignant OE

    4. Acute or chronic OM (see Chapter 10)

    5. Eustachian tube dysfunction

    6. Mastoiditis

    7. Bullous myringitis

    8. Impacted cerumen

    9. Foreign bodies

    10. Malignancy: Head and neck

  B. Referred otalgia: Not all-inclusive listing

    1. Sinusitis, pharyngitis, tonsillitis (see Chapters 4 and 11)

    2. Dental disease (e.g., caries, periodontal abscesses, impacted third molars) or teeth grinding

    3. Malignancy: Head and neck, upper respiratory, brain

    4. TMJ disorder

    5. Acoustic neuroma

    6. Neuralgias: Glossopharyngeal, trigeminal neuralgia

    7. Parapharyngeal, retropharyngeal, or peritonsillar abscess

    8. HZV oticus: Ramsay Hunt syndrome

    9. Mastoiditis

    10. Trauma

    11. Cholesteatomas

    12. Bell's palsy

    13. Temporal arteritis

    14. Thyroiditis (see Chapters 157 and 158)

    15. MI (see Chapter 49)

    16. Disorders of the pharynx or larynx: Ulcers, inflammation, neoplasms

    17. Osteonecrosis of the auditory canal

VI. Treatment (Earwood et al., 2018; Harrison & Cronin, 2016)

  A. Treat the cause of the otalgia, if found.

  B. Prescribe topical and/or systemic analgesics.

VII. Follow-up: Close follow-up after treatment is necessary to evaluate response to therapy (Earwood et al., 2018; Harrison & Cronin, 2016).

VIII. Referrals

  A. Otolaryngologist: For most primary otalgia

  B. Dentist: For treatment of dental causes

  C. Neurosurgeon: If intracranial abnormality is found on radiologic examination

  D. Oral surgeon/neurologist: To evaluate a suspicious mass or lesion or for TMJ disorder

References

Anwar, K., Khan, S., Shahabi, I., & Niazi, Z.B. (2019). The frequency of involvement of head and neck sites in referred otalgia: An experience at a tertiary care hospital. *Pakistan Journal of Medical Sciences, 35*(4), 1138–1142. https://doi.org/10.12669/pjms.35.4.236

Bradley, P.J. (2019). Symptoms and signs, staging and co-morbidity of hypopharyngeal cancer. *Advanced Otorhinolaryngology, 83,* 15–26. https://doi.org/10.1159/000492304

Canzano, F., Di Lella, F., Manuguerra, R., & Vincenti, V. (2019). Osteonecrosis of the external auditory canal associated with oral sorafenib therapy: Sorafenib and temporal bone osteonecrosis. *Otology and Neurotology, 40*(8), e812–e815. https://doi.org/10.1097/MAO.0000000000002344

Earwood, J.S., Rogers, T.S., & Rathjen, N.A. (2018). Ear pain: Diagnosing common and uncommon causes. *American Family Physician, 97*(1), 20–27. https://www.aafp.org/afp/2018/0101/afp20180101p20.pdf

Fenton, J.E., Uzomefuna, V., O'Rourke, C., & Kaare, M. (2018). Applying the Ts of referred otalgia to a cohort of 226 patients. *Clinical Otolaryngology, 43*(3), 937–940. https://doi.org/10.1111/coa.13069

Gauer, R.L., & Semidey, M.J. (2015). Diagnosis and treatment of temporomandibular disorders. *American Family Physician, 91*(6), 378–386. https://www.aafp.org/afp/2015/0315/afp20150315p378.pdf

Harrison, E., & Cronin, M. (2016). Otalgia. *Australian Family Physician, 45*(7), 493–497.

Vlastarakos, P., Gkouvali, A., & Katsochi, D. (2019). Attitudes and parameters affecting the behavior toward precursor symptoms of head and neck cancer. *Ear, Nose and Throat Journal, 98*(6), E58–E63. https://doi.org/10.1177/0145561319840881

CHAPTER 4

Sore Throat (Pharyngitis/Tonsillitis)

Raymond Scarpa, DNP, APNC, AOCN®

I. Definition: A sore throat is a feeling of pain in the upper aerodigestive tract ranging from mild to severe (Farooqui et al., 2017; Ruppert & Vaunette, 2015).
   A. Pharyngitis: Inflammation of the tissues of the upper aerodigestive tract, including the pharynx, larynx, and posterior nasal cavity
   B. Tonsillitis: Inflammation of the palatal tonsils, which may extend to the adenoid and lingual tonsils; termed *pharyngitis* if extensive

II. Physiology/Pathophysiology (Fossum et al., 2017; Klein, 2019)
   A. Normal: The oropharynx is lined by nonkeratinized, stratified squamous epithelium cells. In the regions of the palatine and lingual tonsils, discrete nodules of lymphoid tissue are situated under the epithelium.
      1. The oropharynx is located posterior to the oral cavity and is continuous with, but inferior to, the nasopharynx.
      2. It is divided into four distinct areas: the base of the tongue, the soft palate, the palatine tonsillar fossa, and the pharyngeal wall known as Waldeyer's ring.
      3. The palatal tonsils lie in the cavity between the pillars. Crypts are located on the tonsils which increase the surface area and interact with antigens.
      4. Waldeyer's ring safeguards the oropharynx. This is where the immune system facilitates the interaction between its cells and pathogens.
   B. Pathophysiology
      1. Organisms that enter the oropharynx stimulate an immune response. The tonsils are the immune system's first line of defense from external factors (e.g., physical, chemical, microbial) entering the oropharynx.
      2. Both viral and bacterial infections can cause acute sore throat, resulting in cellular inflammation and discomfort.

III. Clinical features: Acute sore throat with or without dysphagia is classified as acute tonsillitis, acute pharyngitis, or acute tonsillopharyngitis and is usually caused by a viral infection. Chronic pharyngitis is rarely infectious in nature. In adult patients with exudative pharyngitis with fever, adenopathy, and absence of URI symptoms such as cough, 5%–15% will have a positive streptococcal culture. A positive culture does not mean a streptococcal infection; the patient can be a carrier (Klein, 2019; Luo et al., 2019; Reinholdt et al., 2019; Stelter, 2014; Windfuhr et al., 2016).
   A. Risk factors
      1. Chronic exposure to irritants

2. Tobacco use
3. Dehydration
4. Allergies
5. Immunocompromise from chemotherapy, HIV, or other immunosuppressive medications
6. Frequent exposure to pathogens, such as with daycare workers, teachers, or parents

B. Etiology: The most common infectious causes are respiratory virus and group A *Streptococcus*.
   1. Common viral causes are adenovirus, Epstein-Barr virus, human herpesvirus, influenza A and B virus, Coxsackievirus, CMV, and HIV.
   2. *Streptococcus pyogenes* (group C or G) is the most common bacterial source in adults.
   3. Other infective organisms
      a) *Fusobacterium necrophorum*: Can cause abscess formation along with thrombosis
      b) Rare pathogens causing tonsillitis: *Corynebacterium ulcerans, Arcanobacterium haemolyticum, Francisella tularensis, Yersinia pestis, Yersinia enterocolitica, Treponema pallidum, Mycoplasma pneumoniae, Chlamydia pneumoniae, Chlamydia psittaci*
      c) STIs: *Neisseria gonorrhoeae, Treponema pallidum*
   4. Patients receiving 5-fluorouracil, methotrexate, cyclophosphamide, anthracyclines, cisplatin, or radiation therapy to the head and neck area may experience pharyngitis caused by inflammation and cellular death, creating open lesions.

C. History
   1. History of cancer and cancer treatment
   2. Current medications: Prescribed, over the counter, current measures to relieve throat pain
   3. History of presenting symptoms: Precipitating factors, onset, location, duration, exposure to infections
   4. Changes in ADLs
   5. Past medical history: Immune disorders, STIs, human papillomavirus vaccine
   6. Social history: Alcohol use, tobacco use, sexual history (e.g., oral sex)

D. Signs and symptoms: Symptoms of bacterial and viral pharyngitis are similar, making it difficult to differentiate by examination alone.
   1. Fever, headache, malaise, chills
   2. Sore throat
   3. Nonproductive cough: More common in viruses
   4. Anorexia
   5. Rhinorrhea indicating a viral infection
   6. Otalgia: Referred ear pain

E. Physical examination
   1. Vital signs: Elevated temperature
   2. HEENT
      a) Ears: Inspection for erythema, drainage, and alteration of landmarks
      b) Oropharynx
         (1) Enlarged tonsils
         (2) Pharyngeal redness
         (3) Tonsillar exudates
         (4) Soft palate petechiae
         (5) Oral lesions: Aphthous ulcers, candidiasis, herpetic lesions

(6) Trismus

(7) Small vesicles on pharynx, buccal mucosa, or tonsils

3. Integument: Color, exanthema, rash, hydration status

4. Lymph node: Enlarged cervical, submandibular, and periauricular lymph nodes on palpation (see Appendix D)

5. Neck: Nuchal rigidity

6. Cardiac and pulmonary: Abnormal sounds indicating pulmonary infection, rheumatic fever, or concurrent URI

IV. Diagnostic tests (Klein, 2019; Stelter, 2014; Windfuhr et al., 2016)

A. Laboratory: No laboratory parameter allows for a reliable differentiation between bacterial and viral etiology of tonsillopharyngitis. Routine laboratory work regarding CRP and eosinophil sedimentation rate is not recommended in suspected or present tonsillitis.

1. Throat culture: Perform if fever and cervical adenopathy are present in the absence of cough, rhinorrhea, or conjunctivitis.

a) Rapid streptococcal testing has a positive predictive value of 90%–96%.

b) Throat culture specificity is 76%–99%.

c) Neither the rapid streptococcal test nor throat culture will detect *Chlamydia*, *Mycoplasma*, or viral infections.

d) A streptococcal antigen test is specific for streptococci, although not sensitive.

2. CBC with differential: WBC count is increased in bacterial infection.

a) CBC has low predictive value.

b) It may help in differentiating between viral and bacterial etiologies but is not definitive.

c) Pharyngitis is common in neutropenic patients, even in the absence of an apparent causative factor, and resolves when counts normalize.

3. Culture for gonorrhea or syphilis: Consider if patient practices oral genital sex.

4. Mononucleosis spot: Perform if Epstein-Barr virus infection is suspected.

5. Recurrent infections may be a sign of immunodeficiency; tests for Epstein-Barr virus or HIV may be indicated.

B. Radiology: It is usually not indicated unless peritonsillar abscess is suspected.

C. Other: For patients with persistent sore throat or hoarseness lasting more than two to three weeks or accompanied by signs and symptoms suggestive of a more serious process (e.g., weight loss, dysphagia, mass), perform flexible laryngoscopy to evaluate for presence or absence of masses and vocal cord mobility.

V. Differential diagnosis (Klein, 2019; Luo et al., 2019; Stelter, 2014; Windfuhr et al., 2016)

A. Stomatitis (see Chapter 12)

B. Epiglottitis: Urgent patient care issue

C. Allergic rhinitis with postnasal drip (see Chapter 6)

D. Rhinosinusitis (see Chapter 11)

E. Viral infection: Herpangina, mononucleosis, Coxsackievirus, influenza

F. Bacterial infection: Group A beta-hemolytic *Streptococcus, N. gonorrhoeae, Corynebacterium diphtheriae*

1. Peritonsillar abscess

2. Retropharyngeal abscess

G. Fungal infections: *Candida albicans*

H. Mouth breathing causing dryness and irritation of mucous membranes

I. Trauma from thermal chemical irritants

J. Infectious mononucleosis: Epstein-Barr virus

K. HIV

L. Aphthous ulcers (i.e., canker sores): Usually numerous, small, ulcerated lesions on tongue, palate, and buccal mucosa associated with viral infections (e.g., Coxsackievirus A, HSV) or antineoplastic therapy

M. Pemphigus: Bullae or vesicle formation on skin or mucous membranes

N. Erythema multiforme

O. Blood dyscrasia including leukemia and lymphoma

P. Carcinoma of the tonsil, tongue, soft palate, or supraglottic larynx

Q. Salivary gland tumors

R. Acute rheumatic fever

S. Palatal cellulitis

T. Plaut-Vincent angina: Mucosal aphthous caused by *Treponema vincentii* and fusiform *Fusobacterium*

U. Gingivitis: "Trench mouth" and tooth decay

V. GERD (see Chapter 71)

W. Diphtheria: Gray membranes across the tonsils and back of the throat

X. Scarlet fever: Exotoxin-mediated systemic disease caused by streptococci; different from streptococcal tonsillitis, as it is associated with a skin rash

VI. Treatment: Acute tonsillitis should be treated with steroids, NSAIDs, and antibiotics. No difference exists between short-term and 10-day therapy (Harris et al., 2016; Luo et al., 2019; Reinholdt et al., 2019; Stelter, 2014).

A. For viral pharyngitis, treatment is aimed at symptomatic pain relief.

1. Teach patients to maintain adequate fluid intake and to avoid alcohol use and irritating liquids.

2. Patients should use acetaminophen or NSAIDs for fever or pain (see Appendix E). Severe mucositis from chemotherapy or radiation may require opioids for pain relief (see Appendix F).

3. Patients may use over-the-counter lozenges, normal saline gargles, or commercially available oral analgesic rinses to relieve pain.

4. Viscous lidocaine to swish in oral cavity may be prescribed to relieve severe pain, but the effect will not last long.

5. Encourage smoking cessation.

6. Humidified air with cool mist may offer symptomatic relief.

7. Instruct patients to seek immediate medical attention if swallowing is impaired.

8. Patients should avoid alcohol-based mouth care products.

B. For streptococcal infections and other bacterial infections, antibiotics are needed to reduce the unlikely possibility of suppurative complications, decrease the risk of rheumatic fever, and avoid disease transmission or the development of rare but life-threatening complications. Avoid antibiotic overtreatment. Unless the patient has no concurrent cold symptoms (e.g., cough, rhinorrhea, conjunctivitis), antibiotics should not be given empirically except if patients are immunocompromised (see Table 4-1).

C. If patients have *C. albicans* related to neutropenia, it may resolve with return to normal WBC. Antifungals may be used (see Table 4-1).

D. If patients are immunocompromised or at high risk for recurrent infections, they should avoid contact with infected individuals. They should also discard toothbrushes of family members with infections.

E. Patients with epiglottitis need urgent and constant monitoring for airway compromise. Hospitalization is needed for administration of IV antibiotics and steroids.

TABLE 4-1   Pharmacologic Therapy in Pharyngitis

Type	Drug Therapy	Dose and Frequency	Side Effects	Considerations
Group A beta-hemolytic *Streptococcus*	Azithromycin	500 mg PO day 1, then 250 mg days 2–5	Gastrointestinal (GI) upset, allergies	–
	Cefaclor	250–500 mg PO every 8 hours for 10 days	GI upset	–
	Cefuroxime	125–250 mg PO every 12 hours for 10 days	–	–
	Erythromycin	250 mg PO 4 times a day for 10 days	Superinfection, GI upset, anaphylaxis, urticaria	Consider as an alternative in patients with penicillin allergy.
	Penicillin G	1.2 million units intramuscular (IM) for 1 dose only	Superinfection, anaphylaxis, urticaria	–
	Penicillin VK	250 mg PO 4 times a day for 10 days	Superinfection, anaphylaxis, urticaria	–
Gonococcal infection of pharynx	Ceftriaxone	250 mg IM for 1 dose	Local reaction, anaphylaxis	–
Pharyngitis	Cefadroxil	1 g PO daily or 500 mg PO 2 times a day for 10 days	–	–
	Cefixime	400 mg PO for 1 dose	Diarrhea, GI upset, rash	Use caution in patients with penicillin allergy.
	Ceftriaxone	250 mg IM for 1 dose	Local reaction, anaphylaxis	–
Candidiasis	Clotrimazole troche	10 mg PO 5 times a day for 14 days	Nausea, vomiting	Drug should be dissolved slowly.
	Fluconazole	200 mg initially, 100 mg PO each day for 14 days	Nausea, rash, headache, diarrhea, hepatotoxicity	May need loading dose of 400 mg PO. Monitor liver function in prolonged use. Potentiates warfarin, oral hypoglycemic agents, and theophylline.
	Nystatin suspension: 100,000 units/ml	5–15 ml PO 4 times a day for 10 days, swish and swallow	Diarrhea, nausea, vomiting	Instruct patient to retain in mouth as long as possible.
Chlamydia trachomatis	Azithromycin	1 g PO for 1 dose	Diarrhea, GI distress	Consider counseling for sexually transmitted infections.

(Continued on next page)

TABLE 4-1	Pharmacologic Therapy in Pharyngitis *(Continued)*			
Type	Drug Therapy	Dose and Frequency	Side Effects	Considerations
Chlamydia trachomatis (cont.)	Doxycycline	100 mg PO 2 times a day for 7 days	Diarrhea, GI distress	–
	Erythromycin	500 mg PO 4 times a day for 7 days	Superinfection, diarrhea, GI distress	–
	Levofloxacin	500 mg PO daily for 7 days	GI distress, headache, dizziness	–
	Ofloxacin	300 mg PO 2 times a day for 7 days	GI distress, headache, dizziness	–
Mycoplasma pneumoniae	Azithromycin	500 mg PO day 1, 250 mg on days 2–5	GI upset	Patient should take on an empty stomach.
	Erythromycin	250 mg PO 3 times a day or 4 times a day for 10 days	Superinfection, anaphylaxis, GI upset, urticaria	–
Viral	None, pain relief measures	–	–	–

Note. Based on information from Klein, 2019; Luo et al., 2019; Reinholdt et al., 2019; Woodhead et al., 2011.

    F. Indications for surgery (tonsillectomy) include seven infections diagnosed in one year, five infections diagnosed in two consecutive years, or three infections diagnosed in three consecutive years.

VII. Follow-up
    A. Short term: Not necessary in uncomplicated cases
        1. Instruct patients to call for reevaluation if symptoms do not resolve in three to four days.
        2. Assume patients are noninfectious after 24 hours of antibiotic therapy if the infection was caused by a bacterial source.
        3. Patients with infections from gonorrhea and chlamydia should be counseled about STI transmission and should be referred to the health department or local STI clinic.
    B. Long term
        1. Repeat throat cultures are indicated only in patients who are at high risk for rheumatic fever or are symptomatic after treatment.
        2. Monitor nutritional status and weight of patients with chronic pharyngitis or acute or severe pharyngitis related to cancer therapy.

VIII. Referrals
    A. Otolaryngologist: For patients with peritonsillar abscess or epiglottitis for evaluation, possible IV antibiotics, or surgical intervention
    B. Surgeon
        1. To evaluate lesions that may indicate malignancy for biopsy
        2. For patients meeting criteria for tonsillectomy

C. Specialist: For suspected immunodeficiency and to identify appropriate physician (e.g., infectious disease, HIV/AIDS specialist)
D. Dietitian: For chronic or severe pharyngitis that affects patient ability to maintain adequate nutritional intake or hydration

The author would like to acknowledge Miriam Rogers, EdD, APRN, AOCN®, CNS, for her contribution to this chapter that remains unchanged from the previous edition of this book.

References

Farooqui, I.A., Akram, T., & Zaka, M. (2017). Incidence and empiric use of antibiotics therapy for tonsillitis in children. *International Journal of Applied Science, 3*(12), 323–327. http://www.allresearchjournal.com/archives/2017/vol3issue12/PartE/3-12-10–802.pdf

Fossum, C.C., Chintakuntlawar, A.V., Price, D.L., & Garcia, J.J. (2017). Characterization of the oropharynx: Anatomy, histology, immunology, squamous cell carcinoma and surgical resection. *Histopathology, 70*(7), 1021–1029. https://doi.org/10.1111/his.13140

Harris, A.M., Hicks, L.A., & Qaseem, A. (2016). Appropriate antibiotic use for acute respiratory tract infection in adults: Advice for high-value care from the American College of Physicians and the Centers for Disease Control and Prevention. *Annals of Internal Medicine, 164*(6), 425–434. https://doi.org/10.7326/M15-1840

Klein, M.R. (2019). Infections of the oropharynx. *Emergency Medicine Clinics of North America, 37*(1), 69–80. https://doi.org/10.1016/j.emc.2018.09.002

Luo, R., Sickler, J., Vahidnia, F., Lee, Y.-C., Frogner, B., & Thompson, M. (2019). Diagnosis and management of group a streptococcal pharyngitis in the United States, 2011–2015. *BMC Infectious Diseases, 19*(1), 193. https://doi.org/10.1186/s12879-019-3835-4

Reinholdt, K.B., Rusan, M., Hansen, P.R., & Klug, T.E. (2019). Management of sore throat in Danish general practices. *BMC Family Practice, 20*(1), 75. https://doi.org/10.1186/s12875-019-0970-3

Ruppert, S., & Vaunette, F. (2015). Pharyngitis: Soothing the sore throat. *Nurse Practitioner, 40*(7), 18–25. https://doi.org/10.1097/01.NPR.0000466498.57296.60

Stelter, K. (2014). Tonsillitis and sore throat in children. *GMS Current Topics in Otorhinolaryngology: Head and Neck Surgery, 13,* Doc07. https://doi.org/10.3205/cto000110

Windfuhr, J.P., Toepfner, N., Steffen, G., Waldfahrer, F., & Berner, R. (2016). Clinical practice guideline: Tonsillitis I. Diagnostic and nonsurgical management. *European Archives of Oto-Rhino-Laryngology, 273,* 973–987. https://doi.org/10.1007/s00405-015-3872-6

Woodhead, M., Blasi, F., Ewig, S., Garau, J., Huchon, G., Ieven, M., ... Verheij, T.J.M. (2011). Guidelines for the management of adult lower respiratory tract infections. *Clinical Microbiology and Infection, 17*(Suppl. 6), E1–E59. https://doi.org/10.1111/j.1469–0691.2011.03672.x

CHAPTER 5

Tinnitus

Raymond Scarpa, DNP, APNC, AOCN®

I. Definition: Tinnitus is the perception of sound without external stimulation. It can be classified as nonpulsatile, which is subjective, or pulsatile, which is usually objective (Wu et al., 2018).
   A. Subjective nonpulsatile tinnitus is the most common and heard only by the patient.
   B. Objective pulsatile tinnitus is caused by an internal vibration or noise and, at times, can be heard by an examiner.

II. Physiology/Pathophysiology (López de Nava & Lasrado, 2020; Salehi et al., 2019; Tang et al., 2019)
   A. Normal
      1. The outer ear is known as the auricle. The helix, antihelix, tragus, and antitragus are the anatomical structures that compose the outer ear.
      2. The middle ear is an air-filled space that contains the malleus, incus, and stapes. These ossicles transmit vibrations to the inner ear.
      3. The inner ear is a membranous, curved cavity inside a bony labyrinth consisting of the vestibule, semicircular canals responsible for vestibular function, and the cochlea.
      4. The cochlea is referred to as the organ of hearing. It contains the organ of Corti, which transmits sound impulses to cranial nerve VIII.
   B. Pathophysiology
      1. Tinnitus may be caused by a lack of neural input from the auditory receptors to the cochlear nerve. When a region of the cochlea is damaged, neurons in the area increase the rate and frequency of firing, or neuronal hyperactivity.
      2. Damage can occur from loud noise causing damage or death to stereocilia (i.e., microscopic appendages of hair cells in the cochlea).
      3. Other theories include overactivation of the CNS resulting in tinnitus.

III. Clinical features: It is estimated that 6.4% of the adult population has experienced tinnitus at some point. Tinnitus is poorly understood and is best described as a nonspecific manifestation of pathology of the inner ear, cranial nerve VIII, or central auditory mechanism (Aazh et al., 2020; Bhatt et al., 2017; Tang et al., 2019; Vecchiarelli et al., 2017; Wu et al., 2018).
   A. Etiology: Pathologic conditions of the external ear canal, middle ear, auditory nerve, brain stem, and cerebral cortex
      1. Exact cause is unknown in a large percentage of patients.
      2. Possible causes
         a) Spontaneous otoacoustic emissions from the cochlea
         b) Spontaneous electrical activity in cranial nerve VIII
         c) Electrophysiologic events in the brain stem and cerebral cortex

        d) Anxiety

        e) Depression

        f) Insomnia

        g) Eustachian tube dysfunction

    3. Persistent tinnitus is usually associated with sensory hearing loss.

    4. Most tinnitus is bilateral.

    5. If unilateral or asymmetric, consider a lesion proximal to the cochlea.

B. History

    1. History of cancer and cancer treatment

    2. Current medications: Prescribed, over the counter

    3. History of presenting symptoms: Precipitating factors, onset, location, duration, associated symptoms (e.g., vertigo, other focal neurologic deficits)

    4. Changes in ADLs

    5. Past medical history: Exposure to ototoxic agents or events (see Figure 5-1), repetitive loud noises, head trauma, psychiatric disorders (e.g., anxiety, depression)

C. Signs and symptoms

    1. High-pitched ringing, buzzing, humming, or whining sound in the ears or head are described by patients (e.g., crickets, cicadas, blowing, whistling).

        a) Unilateral or bilateral

        b) Continuous or intermittent

        c) Description of the tinnitus: Pulsatile versus nonpulsatile, rhythmicity, pitch, and quality

    2. Intermittent periods of mild, high-pitched tinnitus for several minutes are normal and not diagnostic of tinnitus.

    3. Mood disorders can result from severe and persistent tinnitus.

D. Physical examination: In rare cases of objective tinnitus, the sound perceived is audible to the examiner regarding vascular or mechanical disorders. Pulsatile tinnitus is associated with vascular abnormalities, including arterial bruits, arteriovenous shunts, paraganglioma, and venous hum. Muscular tinnitus can include spasms of the muscles of the inner ear or myoclonus of the palatal muscles.

    1. HEENT

        a) External ear should reveal normal anatomy.

FIGURE 5-1   **Factors Contributing to the Development of Tinnitus**

Medications
- Aminoglycosides
- Angiotensin inhibitors
- Calcium channel blockers
- Cisplatin
- Clarithromycin
- Fluoroquinolones
- Ifosfamide
- Loop diuretics
- Nonsteroidal anti-inflammatory drugs
- Oral contraceptives
- Quinine/antimalarials
- Salicylates
- Sertraline

Noise Trauma
- Industrial noise
- Loud music
- Weapons

Physical Trauma
- Cerumen impaction/extraction
- Head injury
- Radiation therapy
- Recurrent infections, especially otitis media, meningitis, syphilis, measles, rubella, cytomegalovirus, Lyme disease
- Temporomandibular joint syndrome
- Whiplash

Note. Based on information from Salehi et al., 2019; Tunkel et al., 2014; Wu et al., 2018.

        b) Canal and tympanic membrane should be intact and reveal normal anatomy.

        c) Palpate TMJ for smooth range of motion, snapping, or clicking.

        d) Jaw clenching and eye movements should not increase tinnitus.

    2. Neurologic examination (see Appendices A and D)

        a) Cranial nerve assessment should be normal.

        b) Hearing may be normal or decreased based on the whisper test.

        c) Weber test should be negative.

        d) Air conduction is greater than bone conduction on the Rinne test.

    3. Auscultation can be performed to assess carotid bruits, which can be inferred as tinnitus or ear noise.

IV. Diagnostic tests (Aazh et al., 2020; Tang et al., 2019; Wu et al., 2018)

    A. Laboratory: Typically not indicated for tinnitus

    B. Radiology

        1. MRI or CT scan of head to rule out intracranial lesions

        2. CT angiography/venography to rule out vascular lesions

    C. Other

        1. Audiometry

            a) Perform baseline audiometry if using ototoxic agents; serial measurements may be necessary.

            b) Perform baseline for new onset of tinnitus to evaluate for hearing loss (sensorineural loss with aging or acquired high frequency loss).

        2. Test auditory brain stem evoked response to rule out lesion.

        3. Consider Doppler studies if tinnitus is pulsatile or objective to evaluate vascular causes.

V. Differential diagnosis (Iliescu et al., 2015; Ralli et al., 2018; Vecchiarelli et al., 2017; Wu et al., 2018)

    A. Structural lesions

        1. Malignant or benign cochlear tumor

        2. Malignant or benign glomus tumor

        3. Acoustic neuroma

        4. Meningioma

        5. TMJ syndrome

        6. Metastatic tumors

        7. Middle ear muscle myoclonus

        8. Eustachian tube dysfunction

        9. Sarcoidosis

    B. Metabolic derangements

        1. Diabetes mellitus (see Chapter 151)

        2. Hypothyroidism (see Chapter 158)

        3. Dyslipidemia (see Chapter 44)

        4. Renal failure (see Chapter 86)

        5. Anemia (see Chapters 113–118)

        6. Hyperparathyroidism

    C. Infections

        1. Otitis media (see Chapter 10)

        2. Mumps

        3. Measles

        4. Syphilis

        5. Meningitis (see Chapter 141)

  6. Lyme disease (see Chapter 104)

  7. CMV

 D. Autoimmune disorders

  1. Polyarteritis nodosa

  2. SLE (see Chapter 110)

  3. Giant cell arteritis

  4. RA (see Chapter 108)

  5. Cogan syndrome

  6. Sarcoidosis

  7. Behçet disease

  8. Sjögren syndrome

  9. Myasthenia gravis

  10. Multiple sclerosis

  11. Relapsing polychondritis

  12. Vogt-Koyanagi-Harada disease

 E. Vascular anomalies

  1. Arteriovenous malformation

  2. Aneurysm

  3. Paraganglioma

  4. Cerebral vascular accident (see Chapter 146)

  5. Glomus jugulare

  6. Carotid body tumor

  7. Vascular anomalies of the middle ear

 F. Cardiovascular

  1. Hypertension (see Chapter 47)

  2. Arteriosclerosis/carotid artery occlusion

 G. Migraine headache (see Chapter 137)

 H. Cerumen impaction

 I. Ménière disease

 J. Otosclerosis

 K. Multiple sclerosis

VI. Treatment (Aazh et al., 2020; Dang & Liu, 2019; Folmer et al., 2014; Mielczarek & Olszewski, 2014; Salehi et al., 2019; Servais et al., 2017; Tang et al., 2019; Tunkel et al., 2014)

 A. Prevention

  1. Avoid exposure to ototoxic agents (see Figure 5-1).

  2. Reduce dose of causative agents if possible.

  3. Monitor serum peaks/troughs of ototoxic medications and adjust as necessary.

  4. Avoid concomitant use of ototoxic agents.

  5. Reduce dose of ototoxic agents in patients with renal impairment.

  6. Use caution and appropriate technique for cerumen removal.

 B. Nonpharmacologic measures: Tinnitus is usually an irreversible condition. Treatment is focused on decreasing awareness of the symptom and increasing QOL.

  1. Obtain a comprehensive audiologic examination in patients with tinnitus that is unilateral, associated with hearing difficulties, or persistent (six months or longer).

  2. Hearing aids can be used to amplify normal sounds and block high-frequency noises.

  3. Music or other ambient sounds (e.g., waves, rain, white noise) can mask tinnitus.

  4. Counseling, reassurance, or cognitive behavioral therapy can be considered.

  5. Tinnitus retraining therapy is used to train the individual to become unaware of the presence of tinnitus by changing the emotional response to the sound.

      6. Biofeedback can prove useful in distraction.

      7. Hypnosis can alleviate awareness.

      8. Patients should be encouraged to limit caffeine and sodium intake.

      9. Patients should be advised to stop tobacco use.

    10. Clinicians should not recommend *Ginkgo biloba*, melatonin, zinc, or other dietary supplements for treating patients with persistent, bothersome tinnitus.

    11. Clinicians should not recommend transcranial magnetic stimulation for the treatment of patients with persistent, bothersome tinnitus.

    12. Treat TMJ syndrome PRN with NSAIDs, mouth guards, and physical therapy.

C. Pharmacologic measures

    1. Clinicians should not routinely recommend antidepressants, anticonvulsants, anxiolytics, or intratympanic medications for treating persistent, bothersome tinnitus.

    2. Acamprosate, a medication used to treat alcohol dependence, regulates gamma-aminobutyric acid– and glutamate-mediated neurotransmission.

    3. Two randomized controlled trials for treatment of tinnitus showed favorable results, but evidence is still insufficient to recommend treatment.

D. Experimental therapies: Most invasive treatments for tinnitus should be avoided because of limited evidence supporting efficacy. Risk with invasive procedures is much greater than that posed with tinnitus.

    1. Cochlear implants for severe hearing loss can reduce tinnitus in some patients but may cause it in others.

    2. Botulinum toxin injection may be helpful for tinnitus caused by myoclonus of palatal or inner ear muscles.

    3. Intratympanic injection of dexamethasone was shown to be effective with coexisting sensorineural hearing loss or autoimmune inner ear disease.

    4. Electrical stimulation of the cochlea by direct electrode placement on the bony cochlea improved tinnitus in patients with hearing loss.

    5. Repetitive transcranial magnetic stimulation uses magnetic stimulation to the left temporal or temporoparietal cortex and should not be used for treatment.

VII. Follow-up

A. Short term: Evaluate for progression of symptoms during therapy for possible dose reduction.

B. Long term: Evaluate for progression at long-term follow-up visits.

VIII. Referrals (Tunkel et al., 2014)

A. Audiologist: For audiometry

B. Otolaryngologist: For conductive hearing loss

C. Psychiatrist/psychologist: For habituation therapy

D. Neurotologist, neurologist, or neurosurgeon: If tumor is suspected or to assess abnormal cranial nerve

The author would like to acknowledge Kristine Turner Story, RN, MSN, APRN, BC, for her contribution to this chapter that remains unchanged from the previous edition of this book.

References

Aazh, H., Heinonen-Guzejev, M., & Moore, B.C.J. (2020). The relationship between hearing loss and insomnia for patients with tinnitus. *International Journal of Audiology, 59*(1), 68–72. https://doi.org/10.1080/14992027.2019.1654621

Bhatt, J.M., Bhattacharyya, N., & Lin, H.W. (2017). Relationships between tinnitus and the prevalence of anxiety and depression. *Laryngoscope, 127*(2), 466–469. https://doi.org/10.1002/lary.26107

Dang, J., & Liu, Y.-C.C. (2019). Treatment of objective tinnitus with transpalatal Botox® injection in a pediatric patient with middle ear myoclonus: A case report. *International Journal of Pediatric Otorinholaryngology, 116,* 22–24. https://doi.org/10.1016/j.ijporl.2018.09.024

Folmer, R.L., Theodoroff, S.M., Martin, W.H., & Shi, Y. (2014). Experimental, controversial, and futuristic treatments for chronic tinnitus. *Journal of the American Academy of Audiology, 25*(01), 106–125. https://doi.org/10.3766/jaaa.25.1.7

Iliescu, D.A., Timaru, C.M., Batras, M., De Simone, A., & Stefan, C. (2015). Cogan's syndrome. *Romanian Journal of Ophthalmology, 59*(1), 6–13.

López de Nava, A.S., & Lasrado, S. (2020, September 2). Physiology, ear. In *StatPearls.* https://www.ncbi.nlm.nih.gov/books/NBK540992

Mielczarek, M., & Olszewski, J. (2014). Direct current stimulation of the ear in tinnitus treatment: A double-blind placebo-controlled study. *European Archives of Oto-Rhin-Laryngology, 271*(6), 1815–1822. https://doi.org/10.1007/s00405-013-2849-6

Ralli, M., D'Aguanno, V., Di Stadio, A., De Virgilio, A., Croce, A., Longo, L., ... de Vincentiis, M. (2018). Audiovestibular symptoms in systemic autoimmune diseases. *Journal of Immunology Research, 2018,* 5798103. https://doi.org/10.1155/2018/5798103

Salehi, P.P., Kasle, D., Torabi, S.J., Michaelides, E., & Hildrew, D.M. (2019). The etiology, pathogeneses, and treatment of objective tinnitus: Unique case series and literature review. *American Journal of Otolaryngology, 40*(4), 594–597. https://doi.org/10.1016/j.amjoto.2019.03.017

Servais, J.J., Hörmann, K., & Wallhäusser-Franke, E. (2017). Unilateral cochlear implantation reduces tinnitus loudness in bimodal hearing: A prospective study. *Frontiers in Neurology, 8*(60), 1–10. https://doi.org/10.3389/fneur.2017.00060

Tang, D., Li, H., & Chen, L. (2019). Advances in understanding, diagnosis, and treatment of tinnitus. *Advances in Experimental Medicine and Biology, 1130,* 109–128. https://doi.org/10.1007/978-981-13-6123-4_7

Tunkel, D.E., Bauer, C.A., Sun, G.H., Rosenfeld, R.M., Chandrasekhar, S.S., Cunningham, E.R., Jr., ... Whamond, E.J. (2014). Clinical practice guideline: Tinnitus. *Otolaryngology–Head and Neck Surgery, 151*(Suppl. 2), S1–S40. https://doi.org/10.1177/0194599814545325

Vecchiarelli, K., Amar, A.P., & Emanuele, D. (2017). Increasing awareness with recognition of pulsatile tinnitus for nurse practitioners in the primary care setting: A case study. *Journal of the American Association of Nurse Practitioners, 29*(9), 506–510. https://doi.org/10.1002/2327-6924.12476

Wu, V., Cooke, B., Eitutis, S., Simpson, M.T.W, & Beyea, J.A. (2018). Approach to tinnitus management. *Canadian Family Physician, 64*(7), 491–495.

CHAPTER 6

Allergic Rhinitis

Raymond Scarpa, DNP, APNC, AOCN®

I. Definition (Eifan & Durham, 2016; Wheatley & Togias, 2015)
   A. Rhinitis is a common chronic disorder defined as an inflammation of the nasal mucosa and characterized by the presence of one or more assorted nasal symptoms inclusive of sneezing, itching, nasal discharge, and nasal blockage.
   B. Allergic rhinitis is the most common form of noninfectious rhinitis. It is caused by an IgE-mediated reaction to inhaled allergens and involves nasal mucosal inflammation driven by helper T2 cells. Symptoms include sneezing, nasal pruritus, airflow obstruction, and watery nasal discharge.
      1. Seasonal (intermittent): Symptoms occur at a particular time of year related to airborne allergens.
      2. Perennial (persistent): Persistent nasal symptoms lasting more than two hours a day for nine months a year.
   C. Vasomotor rhinitis is caused by increased sensitivity of the Vidian nerve and is a common cause of clear rhinorrhea in older adults.
   D. Atrophic rhinitis is a chronic nasal condition with an unknown cause. It is characterized by progressive atrophy of the nasal mucosa and underlying bone.

II. Physiology/Pathophysiology (Bjermer et al., 2019; Eguiluz-Gracia et al., 2019; Eifan & Durham, 2016)
   A. Normal
      1. The nasal cavity is divided by the nasal septum composed of bone and cartilage. The superior, middle, and inferior turbinates are located laterally and lined with pseudostratified columnar respiratory epithelium. The mucosa regulates inhaled air temperature and humidification and filters the inspired air.
      2. Healthy nasal airway epithelium is comprised of ciliated cells, mucous-secreting goblet cells, and basal cells, which represent 50%–90% of airway epithelial cell population and form the connection between environmental exposure and the immune system.
      3. Parasympathetic cholinergic nerve stimulation leads to dilation of blood vessels and results in mucosal thickening, mucus production, and congestion.
      4. Stimulation of the sympathetic nerves results in vasoconstriction, which increases nasal patency by opening the nasal airway.
   B. Pathophysiology
      1. Primary exposure to allergens
         a) Soluble allergens are inhaled and invade nasal mucosa and diffuse across the nasal membranes.

   b) Antigen-presenting cells (macrophages and dendritic cells) process the allergen and present to helper T cells, then B cells, triggering both cytotoxic and humoral immune responses.

   c) If an individual is genetically predisposed, cytokines are generated and released, which induce B-cell production of antigen-specific IgE.

   d) IgE antibodies attach to receptors on mast cells in respiratory mucosa and basophils in the peripheral blood, sensitizing the individual.

  2. Subsequent exposure

   a) Allergen diffuses over nasal membrane and bridges IgE molecules, causing degranulation of mast cells.

   b) Inflammatory mediators are released, including histamine, tryptase, helper T cells, and others.

  3. Immediate response

   a) Histamine causes increased epithelial permeability, vasodilation, and stimulation of the parasympathetic reflex, resulting in rhinorrhea, swelling with congestion, and itching of the nose, eyes, and palate.

   b) This leads to acetylcholine release, hypersecretion of mucus, and increased blood flow.

   c) CNS is activated, resulting in sneezing.

  4. Recruitment phase

   a) Adhesion markers on the endothelium are upregulated.

   b) Chemoattraction of eosinophils, basophils, and helper T cells to the nasal epithelium are increased.

   c) Mediators are released, leading to a late-phase response.

  5. Late-phase response: Symptoms recur 6–12 hours later, with basophil cell activation and cytokine release.

  6. Chronic phase: Mucosal mast cells, eosinophils, and helper T cells infiltrate the mucosa, resulting in chronic inflammation.

III. Clinical features: Between 10%–40% of adults in industrialized nations experience allergic rhinitis. Symptoms vary based on seasonal changes and exposure to allergens. For adults, observed patterns of presentation reveal that the adjusted prevalence rate was 9.6% for nonallergic rhinitis and 29.8% for allergic rhinitis (Baptist & Nyenhuis, 2018; Carroll et al., 2019; Eguiluz-Gracia et al., 2019; Eifan & Durham, 2016; May & Dolen, 2019; Small et al., 2018).

 A. Risk factors

  1. Family or personal history of atopic disease, including dermatitis, asthma, and food allergies

  2. Occupational exposures

   a) Dust mites in flour (baker's rhinitis)

   b) Latex allergy

   c) Paint

  3. Exposure to smoke and secondhand smoke

  4. Presence of allergen-specific IgE

 B. Etiology

  1. Seasonal allergens are predictable regionally, occurring during the same time each year (e.g., tree and grass pollen [spring]; plants and grass [summer]; ragweed and mold [fall]).

  2. Perennial allergens (e.g., environmental—dust mites, animal dander, mold spores, cockroach antigen) occur year-round.

3. Continuous positive airway pressure–associated rhinitis can occur.
4. Medicamentosa can occur because of nasal decongestant or cocaine abuse.

C. History
    1. History of cancer and cancer treatment
    2. Current medications: Prescribed, over the counter
    3. History of presenting symptoms: Precipitating factors, onset, location, duration
    4. Changes in ADLs: Impact on sleep, performance at school or work
    5. Past medical history: Eczema, dermatitis, urticaria, hives, asthma, food and other allergies
    6. Social history: Occupational exposure to irritants, exposure to smoke, home environment (e.g., animals)

D. Signs and symptoms
    1. Nasal congestion
    2. Rhinorrhea
    3. Postnasal drainage
    4. Paroxysmal sneezing
    5. Itchy nose, ears, or throat
    6. Watery, itchy eyes
    7. Headache or facial pressure
    8. Altered sense of smell and taste
    9. Cough
    10. Periorbital and eyelid edema
    11. Halitosis cause by mouth breathing
    12. Sneezing
    13. Frequent sniffing or throat clearing

E. Physical examination
    1. HEENT
        a) Nose
            (1) Assessment for excoriation of external nares
            (2) Transverse nasal crease across lower half of nose caused by "allergic salute," frequent upward wiping of the nose
            (3) Reduced nasal airflow as indicator of congestion
        b) Nasal passages
            (1) Turbinate hypertrophy: Classic examination finding (one-third of cases)
            (2) Nasal polyps: Clear to grey boggy masses of hypertrophic mucosa related to long-term allergic rhinitis
            (3) Watery discharge
            (4) Red mucosa with thickened strands of mucus across turbinates (one-third of cases); more common in infectious etiology
            (5) Bluish-gray mucosa when edema is severe
        c) Oral cavity
            (1) Nasal mucous drainage in posterior pharynx
            (2) Lymphoid hyperplasia in posterior pharynx
            (3) Persistent mouth breathing resulting in hypognathous, mandibular deformity, or bite abnormalities
            (4) Posterior pharyngeal wall cobble stoning
            (5) Palatal tonsil hypertrophy
            (6) Palatal tonsil exudate
        d) Eyes
            (1) Conjunctiva and scleral injection of the eyes

(2) Infraorbital edema with darkening circles under the eyes ("allergic shiners" caused by subcutaneous dilation) and prominent skin creases below the lower lids (Dennie-Morgan folds)

e) Sinus: Tenderness or bogginess with palpation

f) Ears: Pneumatic otoscopy to assess eustachian tube patency and tympanic membrane; possible OM

2. Integument: Excoriation and/or crusting of external nares and evidence of atopic changes

IV. Diagnostic tests: Seasonal allergic rhinitis can be diagnosed based on symptoms and history alone (Eguiluz-Gracia et al., 2019; Heffler et al., 2018; Small et al., 2018).

A. Laboratory

1. Nasal cytology of nasal secretions

a) Collect by having patients blow nose directly onto wax paper or cellophane.

b) Presence of eosinophils in clumps or more than 10% of total WBCs indicates a probable allergic process.

2. Immunologic testing: Reserve for those not responding to symptomatic therapy. This testing has demonstrated improved outcomes in patients with poor symptom control, coexistent asthma, or recurrent infections.

a) Skin testing: Discontinue antihistamines three to five days prior to testing, depending on agent. Low cost and high sensitivity make it preferable over other methods. Avoid during peak of allergy season.

(1) Allergens are applied by intracutaneous or scratch techniques.

(2) Allergen is identified, and degree of sensitivity is evaluated.

b) Immunoassay for antigen-specific IgE (radioallergosorbent test): Draw blood sample.

(1) Measures the level of IgE for a specific allergen

(2) Less sensitive and more expensive than skin test

(3) Limited selection of antigens available

c) Nasal allergen provocation test: Identify allergens.

3. Thyroid panel to evaluate for thyroid disorders

B. Radiology

1. Waters view x-ray to evaluate for sinusitis

2. CT scan of sinuses, if indicated, to evaluate for sinusitis or other causes

3. MRI of head and sinuses for soft tissue evaluation

C. Other: With flexible fiber-optic or ridged endoscopic nasal examination, clear rhinorrhea may be visible anteriorly. If nasal obstruction is present, posterior drainage may be visualized across pharynx, which has cobblestone appearance because of lymphoid hyperplasia. Masses, lesions, or polyps may be identified.

V. Differential diagnosis (Carroll et al., 2019; Heffler et al., 2018; Wheatley & Togias, 2015)

A. Infectious

1. Acute rhinitis: Common cold

a) Viral sinusitis: Erythematous turbinates

b) Bacterial sinusitis: Related to allergic rhinitis obstruction of ostiomeatal complex

c) Fungal

d) Granulomatous infections: TB, leprosy, syphilis

2. Rhinosinusitis: Chronic rhinosinusitis can coexist with allergic rhinitis and should be evaluated when symptoms do not improve (see Chapter 11).

B. Structural

1. Deviated septum

2. Hypertrophy of tissues: Turbinates, adenoids, fleshy components, nasal valve
3. Tumor: Benign or malignant
4. Foreign body

C. Hormonal: Metabolic
1. Pregnancy: Prominent nasal mucosal edema
2. Hypothyroidism (see Chapter 158)
3. Acromegaly

D. Neurologic involvement
1. Vasomotor rhinitis (e.g., perennial nonallergic rhinitis): Increased nociceptive nerve sensitivity to strong odors, wine, weather changes, smoke, and other inhalants; present in more than 50% of people with allergic rhinitis and 10%–15% of the rest of the population
2. Horner syndrome
3. Cholinergic rhinitis
   a) Gustatory: "Salsa sniffles"
   b) Cold air: "Ski-bunny rhinitis"
4. Medications: Drug induced
   a) Antihypertensive agents
      (1) Beta-blockers
      (2) Alpha-blockers
      (3) Reserpine
      (4) ACE inhibitors
   b) ASA/NSAIDs (see Appendix E)
   c) Estrogen and progesterone
   d) Phosphodiesterase: Erectile dysfunction
   e) Glaucoma medications
5. Rhinitis medicamentosa
   a) Chronic use of topical alpha-adrenergic agonists: Decongestant sprays cause rebound hyperemia.
   b) Cocaine use

E. Occupational rhinitis caused by workplace stimuli

F. Other
1. Wegener granulomatosis
2. Nonallergic rhinitis with eosinophilia syndrome
3. Bright light induced
4. Emotional
5. Asthma

VI. Treatment (Brożek et al., 2017; Eguiluz-Gracia et al., 2019; May & Dolen, 2019; Small et al., 2018)
A. Environmental modification: Patient education is key.
1. Seasonal
   a) Stay indoors.
   b) Filter room air using high-efficiency particulate absorbing filters or electrostatic furnace filters.
   c) Keep windows closed and air conditioner on.
2. Perennial
   a) Eliminate dust traps in the home (e.g., rugs, curtains, feather pillows).
   b) Remove sources of mold spores (e.g., house plants).
   c) Control dust mites.

    (1) Regularly wash curtains.

    (2) Use water-sealed vacuum cleaner.

    (3) Encase mattress, box spring, and pillows in plastic.

    (4) Wash sheets in hot water (at least 130°F [54.4°C]) weekly.

    (5) Keep humidity less than 50%.

   d) Eliminate pets from the home or minimize pet dander.

    (1) Wash pets weekly.

    (2) Keep pets out of bedrooms.

   e) Eliminate other irritants, such as cigarette smoke.

 B. Pharmacologic

  1. Intranasal glucocorticoids (see Appendix G): Evidence demonstrates that intranasal glucocorticoids are effective and less sedating and may be less expensive than antihistamines. Symptom relief may be delayed by up to two weeks. All agents are equally effective when used as prescribed. Later generations have less systemic uptake and decreased side effects. Taper dose when symptoms decrease.

   a) Beclomethasone (first generation): 42 mcg spray two times a day per nostril

   b) Budesonide (second generation; 10%–34% bioavailability): 100 mcg spray two times a day per nostril

   c) Flunisolide (generic; first generation; 40%–50% bioavailability): 25 mcg spray two times a day per nostril

   d) Fluticasone propionate (generic; third generation; less than 2% bioavailability): 50 mcg spray (two sprays) once daily; decreased to one spray per nostril once daily for maintenance

   e) Mometasone furoate (third generation; undetectable): 50 mcg spray (two sprays per nostril) once daily

  2. Antihistamines (see Appendix H): These drugs provide rapid, though temporary, relief of symptoms but are less effective than intranasal glucocorticoids in treating allergic rhinitis. Primary side effect is sedation, although second-generation agents cause fewer side effects than first-generation agents. Second-generation antihistamines are an option for patients with mild or intermittent symptoms and are more efficacious than cromolyn sodium.

   a) Oral

    (1) Loratadine: 10 mg PO once daily

    (2) Cetirizine: 10 mg PO once daily

    (3) Fexofenadine: 60 mg PO two times a day or up to 180 mg once daily

    (4) Desloratadine: 5 mg PO once daily

    (5) Brompheniramine or chlorpheniramine: 4 mg PO every six to eight hours or sustained-release 8 or 12 mg PO every 8–12 hours

   b) Intranasal antihistamine spray: It can improve nasal congestion. A combination of topical antihistamine and a topical glucocorticoid may be helpful in patients who do not obtain sufficient relief with one agent.

    (1) Azelastine hydrochloride: One or two sprays in each nostril two times a day

    (2) Olopatadine: Two sprays in each nostril two times a day

  3. Decongestants (see Appendix I): Decongestants are less effective than antihistamines in relieving the symptom cluster of itching, sneezing, and rhinorrhea. Use of phenylephrine is less effective for allergic rhinitis symptoms. Decongestants must be used with caution in a number of conditions (e.g., hypertension).

  4. Mast cell stabilizer: Cromolyn sodium inhibits intermediate pathways and ultimately inhibits release of histamine and inflammatory mediators. It blocks immediate and late symptoms and should be used 30 minutes prior to exposure. This

makes it useful for patients who experience known episodes of exposure, such as cat dander. Evidence shows it is less effective than intranasal glucocorticoids and second-generation antihistamines. Its required use is four times a day.

    a) The antileukotriene medication montelukast used in asthma has demonstrated to be more effective than placebo but less effective than intranasal glucocorticoids and second-generation antihistamines.

    b) When montelukast is combined with antihistamines, the result is synergistic. For patients who cannot tolerate intranasal glucocorticoids or have asthma, montelukast is an option.

    c) Side effect profile includes alteration in mood, and patients should be counseled appropriately.

5. Intranasal anticholinergic agents: Ipratropium bromide 0.03% spray and other agents may be helpful to decrease persistent rhinorrhea.

6. Ocular medications
    a) If symptoms do not improve with antihistamines
    b) Cromolyn ophthalmic: One or two drops in each eye four to six times a day

7. Nasal saline irrigation: It is used to mechanically flush allergens from nasal cavity. Nasal saline irrigation may help symptoms and has been studied with positive results. Patients can use commercially available kits or prepare it themselves. They should be cautioned not to use tap water (unless boiled) to decrease any risk of primary amoebic meningoencephalitis. It is effective for patients with severe, uncontrolled symptoms and helpful for those with a comorbid condition (e.g., asthma). It has also proven to reduce circulating IgE levels and requirements for medication.

8. Specific therapies based on results of radioallergosorbent testing or skin testing by allergist: Weekly injection of allergen decreases sensitivity over an extended period (years).

9. Management of asthma (see Chapter 28)

VII. Follow-up
  A. Short term: Assess response to therapy. If no change within two to three weeks, try alternative treatments or refer.
  B. Long term
    1. Prevent seasonal allergies with premedication.
    2. Prevent and monitor for development of asthma.

VIII. Referrals
  A. Otolaryngologist
    1. If anatomic (polyposis) or secondary disorder is suspected
    2. To provide additional treatment options if initial therapy has failed
    3. If patients have unilateral symptoms, which rarely indicates allergy as the source
  B. Allergist: For testing to isolate a definitive cause if initial therapy is not effective
  C. Pulmonologist: For asthma management

The author would like to acknowledge Patricia A. Spencer-Cisek, MS, APN-BC, AOCN®, for her contribution to this chapter that remains unchanged from the previous edition of this book.

References

Baptist, A.P., & Nyenhuis, S.M. (2018). Rhinitis of the elderly. In J.A. Bernstein (Ed.), *Rhinitis and related upper respiratory conditions: A clinical guide* (pp. 123–136). Springer.

Bjermer, L., Westman, M., Holmström, M., & Wickman, M.C. (2019). The complex pathophysiology of allergic rhinitis: Scientific rationale for the development of an alternative treatment plan. *Allergy, Asthma and Clinical Immunology, 15,* 24. https://doi.org/10.1186/s13223-018-0314-1

Brożek, J.L., Bousquet, J., Agache, I., Agarwal, A., Bachert, C., Bosnic-Anticevich, S., ... Schünemann, H.J. (2017). Allergic rhinitis and its impact on asthma (ARIA) guidelines—2016 revision. *Journal of Allergy and Clinical Immunology, 140*(4), 950–958. https://doi.org/10.1016/j.jaci.2017.03.050

Carroll, M.P., Jr., Bulkhi, A.A., & Lockey, R.F. (2019). Rhinitis and sinusitis. In J.A. Namazy & M. Schatz (Eds.), *Asthma, allergic and immunologic diseases during pregnancy: A guide to management* (pp. 61–86). Springer.

Eguiluz-Gracia, I., Pérez-Sánchez, N., Bogas, G., Campo, P., & Rondón, C. (2019). How to diagnose and treat local allergic rhinitis: A challenge for clinicians. *Journal of Clinical Medicine, 8*(7), E1062. https://doi.org/10.3390/jcm8071062

Eifan, A.O., & Durham, S.R. (2016). Pathogenesis of rhinitis. *Clinical and Experimental Allergy, 46*(9), 1139–1151. https://doi.org/10.1111/cea.12780

Heffler, E., Landi, M., Caruso, C., Fichera, S., Gani, F., Guida, G., ... Gelardi, M. (2018). Nasal cytology: Methodology with application to clinical practice and research. *Clinical and Experimental Allergy, 48*(9), 1092–1106. https://doi.org/10.1111/cea.13207

May, J.R., & Dolen, W.K. (2019). Evaluation of intranasal corticosteroid sensory attributes and patient preference for fluticasone furoate for the treatment of allergic rhinitis. *Clinical Therapeutics, 41*(8), 1589–1596. https://doi.org/10.1016/j.clinthera.2019.05.017

Small, P., Keith, P.K., & Kim, H. (2018). Allergic rhinitis. *Allergy, Asthma and Clinical Immunology, 14,* 51. https://doi.org/10.1186/s13223-018-0280-7

Wheatley, L.M., & Togias, A. (2015). Allergic rhinitis. *New England Journal of Medicine, 372*(5), 456–463. https://doi.org/10.1056/NEJMcp1412282

CHAPTER 7

Cataracts

Christina Ferraro, MSN, APRN-CNP, BMTCN®

I. Definition: Opacity of the lens of the eye causing blurred or distorted vision, glare, or blindness if left untreated (Crispim & Chamon, 2017; Y.-C. Liu et al., 2017)

II. Physiology/Pathophysiology (Thompson & Lakhani, 2015)
   A. Normal: Lenses of the eye appear transparent because they are composed of cells that contain a high content of cytoplasmic protein.
   B. Pathophysiology
      1. Lenses are unable to shed nonviable cells, which compresses them over time and causes a loss of transparency.
      2. Degenerative effects of aging on the cell structure contribute to protein accumulation, which produces a fibrous, thickened lens that obscures vision.
      3. Single fraction dosing versus hyperfractionated total body irradiation has a higher risk of cataract formation.

III. Clinical features: Cataracts typically occur in individuals who are older than age 60 years. They are the major cause of reversible visual changes in the world. Cataracts present in 33% of patients with altered vision. Over the next 20 years, this number is anticipated to climb as the life expectancy of the population increases. Cataracts are the leading cause of blindness (50%) in low- to middle-income countries, although this rate has decreased. In developed countries, the rate of blindness associated with cataracts is 5%. Cataracts are frequently associated with intraocular inflammation and glaucoma (Alloin et al., 2014; Crispim & Chamon, 2017; Dest, 2016; Haupt et al., 2018; Huillard et al., 2014; Inamoto et al., 2019; E. Liu & Kopani, 2016; Y.-C. Liu et al., 2017; Majhail et al., 2012; Starr et al., 2019; Thompson & Lakhani, 2015; Vrooman et al., 2017).
   A. Etiology: Environmental stressors causing formation of toxins or impairment of antioxidants
      1. Trauma
      2. Uveitis
      3. Scleritis
      4. Medication induced: Topical, inhaled, and systemic corticosteroids; phenothiazine; topical anticholinesterases; rociletinib, an EGFR inhibitor; imatinib, a TKI
      5. Total body irradiation and CNS radiation
   B. Risk factors
      1. Age
      2. Tobacco use
      3. Alcohol use
      4. Sunlight or radiation exposure

5. Low education level
6. Poor lifestyle: Malnutrition, sedentary behaviors
7. Metabolic syndrome
8. Diabetes
9. HIV/AIDS
10. Systemic corticosteroids
11. Statin use

C. History
1. History of cancer and cancer treatment
2. Current medications: Prescribed, over the counter
3. History of presenting symptoms: Precipitating factors, onset, location, duration, associated symptoms (e.g., night vision, altered vision)
4. Changes in ADLs: Difficulty driving
5. Past medical history: Trauma, diabetes, glaucoma
6. Social history: Environmental exposures; alcohol, tobacco, and illicit drug use; sun exposure; diet recall

D. Signs and symptoms
1. Painless, bilateral progression of impaired vision, especially night vision
2. Myopic shift (improved nearsightedness) prior to progressive deterioration
3. Decreased QOL caused by altered vision
4. Severe difficulty with glare
5. Altered color perception

E. Physical examination
1. Fundoscopic examination with direct ophthalmoscope: Reveals darkening or opacity in the red reflex or obscuration of ocular fundus examination
   a) Nuclear sclerosis: Slowly progressing, dulling white color
   b) Cortical spoking: Slowly progressing component without symptoms
   c) Posterior subcapsular haze: Progresses quickly and can cause disabling glares with sunlight and headlights
   d) A mature cataract has absence of red reflex, and an immature cataract has present red reflex.
2. Cranial nerve examination with visual fields (see Appendix A)
3. Evaluation for possible associated diagnoses, including glaucoma

IV. Diagnostic tests (Y.-C. Liu et al., 2017; Starr et al., 2019; Thompson & Lakhani, 2015)
A. Laboratory: Not indicated
B. Radiology: Not indicated

V. Differential diagnosis (Thompson & Lakhani, 2015)
A. Diabetic retinopathy (see Chapter 151)
B. Refractory errors
C. Macular or corneal degeneration
D. Glaucoma
E. Retinal detachment
F. Retinitis

VI. Treatment: The goal of treatment is to restore vision (Brandsdorfer & Kang, 2018; Chen et al., 2017; Crispim & Chamon, 2017; Grimfors et al., 2018; Y.-C. Liu et al., 2017; Starr et al., 2019).
A. Microsurgical techniques combined with intraocular lens implantation can restore normal vision.

        1. Initial complications
           a) Macular edema: Treated with NSAIDs, topical steroids
           b) Infection: Preventable with topical antibiotics
           c) Lens dislocation: May need to sleep with eye protection
           d) Toxic anterior segment syndrome: Inflammation of the anterior segment of the eye caused by equipment, solutions, or supplies during the procedure
        2. Delayed complications
           a) Retinal detachment
           b) Posterior capsule opacification
           c) Macular degeneration
  B. Techniques
        1. Phacoemulsification: Small incision surgery where the lens is removed using a 1–3 mm tipped tool and vibration to break up and evacuate the remnants of the lens nucleus
        2. Standard extracapsular cataract extraction: Removal of lens nucleus in one piece
        3. Synthetic lens: Placed during phacoemulsification and extracapsular cataract extraction procedures
        4. No impact on outcomes with delayed treatment
  C. Surgery
        1. Typically, surgery lasts 10–20 minutes.
        2. Local anesthesia is used in most situations but general anesthesia is used in patients with cognitive impairment or communication barriers.
        3. The procedure is generally safe and effective, with 84%–94% of patients achieving best-corrected visual acuity of 20/30 around six months after surgery.
  D. Complications can occur intraoperatively or in the early or late postoperative phases.
        1. Most common intraoperative complication is posterior capsule rupture, which occurs in 0.5%–5.2% of cases. Rupture can increase risk of endophthalmitis and retinal detachment.
        2. Early postoperative complications
           a) Postoperative corneal edema can occur immediately after surgery and can be resolved within two to four weeks.
           b) Endophthalmitis is the most serious postoperative complication. Inflammation of the interior of the eye can lead to blindness.
           c) Transient elevated intraocular pressure occurs in about 0.3%–18.1% of patients requiring no intervention.
        3. Late postoperative complications
           a) Posterior capsule opacification can occur.
           b) Clinical cystoid macular edema can occur in around four to six weeks after surgery, which typically spontaneously resolves within six months.
        4. Pain management: Mild pain is possible within the first 24 hours and usually is relieved by acetaminophen.

VII. Follow-up (Chen et al., 2017; Y.-C. Liu et al., 2017)
  A. Postoperative follow-up occurs 24 hours, 7 days, and 30 days after surgery.
  B. Resume all medication, including antithrombotics and anticoagulants.
  C. Activities such as watching television and reading can be resumed the evening after surgery.
  D. Strenuous activity, including sex and exercise, may be resumed two to six weeks after surgery, as recommended by an ophthalmologist.

VIII. Referrals: An ophthalmologist should be seen at least yearly for vision screening and dilated fundoscopic eye examination (Haupt et al., 2018; Majhail et al., 2012; Vrooman et al., 2017).

References

Alloin, A.-L., Barlogis, V., Auquier, P., Contet, A., Poiree, M., Demeocq, F., ... Michel, G. (2014). Prevalence and risk factors of cataract after chemotherapy with or without central nervous system irradiation for childhood acute lymphoblastic leukaemia: An LEA study. *British Journal of Haematology, 164*(1), 94–100. https://doi.org/10.1111/bjh.12598

Brandsdorfer, A., & Kang, J.J. (2018). Improving accuracy for intraocular lens selection in cataract surgery. *Current Opinion in Ophthalmology, 29*(4), 323–327. https://doi.org/10.1097/ICU.0000000000000493

Chen, H., Lin, H., Chen, W., Zhang, B., Xiang, W., Gao, Q., ... Liu, Y. (2017). Preoperative and postoperative measurements of retinal vessel oxygen saturation in patients with different grades of cataracts. *Acta Ophthalmologica, 95*(6), e436–e442. https://doi.org/10.1111/aos.13332

Crispim, J., & Chamon, W. (2017). Lens: Management of cataract surgery, cataract prevention, and floppy iris syndrome. In S. Whitcup & D. Azar (Eds.), *Handbook of experimental pharmacology: Vol. 242. Pharmacologic therapy of ocular disease* (pp. 163–177). Springer. https://doi.org/10.1007/164_2016_90

Dest, V.M. (2016). Neurologic, ocular, and dermatologic toxicities. In B.H. Gobel, S. Triest-Robertson, & W.H. Vogel (Eds.), *Advanced oncology nursing certification review and resource manual* (2nd ed., pp. 577–641). Oncology Nursing Society.

Grimfors, M., Lundström, M., Höijer, J., & Kugelberg, M. (2018). Intraoperative difficulties, complications and self-assessed visual function in cataract surgery. *Acta Ophtalmologica, 96*(6), 592–599. https://doi.org/10.1111/aos.13757

Haupt, R., Essiaf, S., Dellacasa, C., Ronckers, C.M., Caruso, S., Sugden, E., ... Ladenstein, R. (2018). The 'Survivorship Passport' for childhood cancer survivors. *European Journal of Cancer, 102,* 69–81. https://doi.org/10.1016/j.ejca.2018.07.006

Huillard, O., Bakalian, S., Levy, C., Desjardins, L., Lumbroso-Le Rouic, L., Pop, S., ... Le Tourneau, C. (2014). Ocular adverse events of molecularly targeted agents approved in solid tumours: A systematic review. *European Journal of Cancer, 50*(3), 638–648. https://doi.org/10.1016/j.ejca.2013.10.016

Inamoto, Y., Petriček, I., Burns, L., Chhabra, S., DeFilipp, Z., Hematti, P., ... Valdés-Sanz, N. (2019). Non-graft-versus-host disease ocular complications after hematopoietic cell transplantation: Expert review from the Late Effects and Quality of Life Working Committee of the Center for International Blood and Marrow Transplant Research and the Transplant Complications Working Party of the European Society for Blood and Marrow Transplantation. *Biology of Blood and Marrow Transplantation, 25*(5), e145–e154. https://doi.org/10.1016/j.bbmt.2018.11.033

Liu, E., & Kopani, K. (2016). Rapidly progressive cataract formation associated with non-small-cell lung cancer therapy. *Journal of Cataract Refractive Surgery, 42*(12), 1838–1840. https://doi.org/10.1016/j.jcrs.2016.11.006

Liu, Y.-C., Wilkins, M., Kim, T., Malyugin, B., & Mehta, J.S. (2017). Cataracts. *Lancet, 390*(10094), 600–612. https://doi.org/10.1016/S0140-6736(17)30544-5

Majhail, N.S., Rizzo, J.D., Lee, S.J., Aljurf, M., Atsuta, Y., Bonfim, C., ... Tichelli, A. (2012). Recommended screening and preventive practices for long-term survivors after hematopoietic cell transplantation. *Biology of Blood and Marrow Transplantation, 18*(3), 348–371. https://doi.org/10.1016/j.bbmt.2011.12.519

Starr, C.E., Gupta, P.K., Farid, M., Beckman, K.A., Chan, C.C., Yeu, E., ... Mah, F.S. (2019). An algorithm for the preoperative diagnosis and treatment of ocular surface disorders. *Journal of Cataract and Refractive Surgery, 45*(5), 669–684. https://doi.org/10.1016/j.jcrs.2019.03.023

Thompson, J., & Lakhani, N. (2015). Cataracts. *Primary Care: Clinics in Office Practice, 42*(3), 409–423. https://doi.org/10.1016/j.pop.2015.05.012

Vrooman, L.M., Millard, H.R., Brazauskas, R., Majhail, N.S., Battiwalla, M., Flowers, M.E., ... Duncan, C. (2017). Survival and late effects after allogeneic hematopoietic cell transplantation for hematologic malignancy at less than three years of age. *Biology of Blood and Marrow Transplantation, 23*(8), 1327–1334. https://doi.org/10.1016/j.bbmt.2017.04.017

CHAPTER 8

Conjunctivitis

Raymond Scarpa, DNP, APNC, AOCN®

I. Definition: Conjunctivitis is an inflammatory process involving the bulbar and/or palpebral conjunctiva of the eye. This transparent, lubricating mucous membrane covers the surface of the eye and the lining of the undersurface of the eyelids (Alfonso et al., 2015; Ridolo et al., 2019; Streitz, 2018; Watson et al., 2018).
   A. Keratoconjunctivitis: An inflammatory process that involves the conjunctiva and the superficial cornea
   B. Blepharitis: An inflammatory process that affects the area around the base of the eyelashes

II. Physiology/Pathophysiology (Bielory et al., 2020; Chigbu & Labib, 2018; Ridolo et al., 2019; Streitz, 2018)
   A. Normal
      1. The conjunctiva is a thin, transparent membrane composed of a nonkeratinized squamous epithelium and the substantia propria, which is highly vascularized. It is the site of immunologic activity and covers the anterior surface of the eye and the inner surface of the eyelid. Tears lubricate the eye and are composed of three layers called the tear film.
         a) The lacrimal gland produces the watery part of the tears.
         b) The meibomian gland produces the oily part of the tear film.
         c) The lacrimal duct drains tears away from the eye.
      2. The portion covering the globe is the bulbar conjunctiva, and the portion lining the lids is the tarsal conjunctiva.
      3. Hematologic immune mechanisms found in the conjunctival vasculature, tear film Igs, and lysozyme help to protect the eye. The action of lacrimation and blinking provide additional protection.
   B. Pathophysiology
      1. Disruption of normal flora in the epithelial layer covering the conjunctiva can lead to inflammation from irritants, allergens, or bacterial, viral, chlamydial, or fungal infections.
      2. Hemorrhage can result from trauma to the conjunctiva by laceration, contusion, coagulopathies, or concomitant infection.
      3. Systemic disorders causing degenerative, inflammatory, or infiltrative changes can result in opacification of the conjunctiva, causing a white, yellow, or fleshy appearance.

III. Clinical features: Conjunctivitis may be acute or chronic. It is highly transmissible via direct contact with contaminated items. Conjunctivitis is the most likely diagnosis in a patient with red eye and discharge. Most cases are viral etiology. Infectious keratitis can cause blindness and is an emergency requiring specialist treatment (Alfonso et al., 2015; Arshad et al., 2020; Bielory et al., 2020; Castillo et al., 2015; NCCN, 2021; Ridolo et al., 2019; Sacchetti et al., 2018; Streitz, 2018; Watson et al., 2018; Zahler et al., 2019).

A. Etiology: The three main etiologies, viral, bacterial, and allergic, can be divided into infectious and noninfectious causes.

1. Common infectious bacterial pathogens: *Staphylococcus aureus*, *Streptococcus pneumoniae*, *Haemophilus influenzae*, *Moraxella catarrhalis*, *Pseudomonas* species, *Neisseria gonorrhoeae*, *Chlamydia trachomatis*

2. Common infectious viral pathogens: Adenovirus (commonly type 3, 4, or 7), picornavirus, enterovirus, HSV type 1

3. Radiation induced from treatment of head and neck cancers

4. Chemotherapy induced
   a) Docetaxel and paclitaxel
   b) Cytarabine
   c) 5-Fluorouracil
   d) Methotrexate
   e) Ifosfamide and cyclophosphamide
   f) Nitrosourea
   g) Tamoxifen
   h) Rituximab
   i) Cisplatin
   j) Vinblastine and vincristine
   k) Immune checkpoint inhibitors: Ipilimumab, nivolumab, pembrolizumab, cemiplimab, avelumab, durvalumab, atezolizumab

5. IFN-induced immunotherapy

6. Chronic contact lenses wear

B. History

1. History of cancer and cancer treatment

2. Current medications: Prescribed, over the counter

3. History of presenting symptoms: Precipitating factors, onset, location, duration, associated symptoms (e.g., visual changes, foreign body sensation, photophobia)

4. Changes in ADLs

5. Past medical history: Eye trauma, eye infections, STIs

6. History of wearing eyeglasses or contact lenses

7. Recent close contact with person with conjunctivitis

C. Signs and symptoms: Most conjunctivitis is self-limiting and presenting signs and symptoms may not always point to the causative factor.

1. Bacterial conjunctivitis
   a) Acute-onset mucopurulent drainage (green or yellow): It is usually unilateral at onset, with transmission to the unaffected eye in two to five days. Discharge continues throughout the day and reappears within minutes of wiping eyes.
   b) Foreign body sensation: Common
   c) Lid edema with matting of lashes, especially upon awakening
   d) Itching, redness, burning
   e) Corneal ulcerations or infiltration
   f) *Neisseria* species: A sight-threatening hyperacute bacterial conjunctivitis can occur that is characterized by a striking amount of purulent discharge within 12 hours of inoculation. This requires immediate ophthalmologic referral.

2. Viral conjunctivitis
   a) Marked conjunctival injection
   b) Watery or mucoid discharge
   c) Coexisting symptoms of fever and pharyngitis: Common
   d) Second eye involved in 24–48 hours but may be unilateral
   e) Tarsal conjunctiva with possible pebbly appearance
3. Allergic conjunctivitis
   a) Itchy eyes: Cardinal symptom
   b) Edematous lids
   c) Watery discharge
   d) Potentially severe chemosis: Conjunctival edema
   e) Coexisting systemic allergic symptoms: Sneezing, rhinorrhea; common
   f) Allergic shiners
   g) Usually bilateral at onset
4. Chlamydial conjunctivitis
   a) Thin, mucoid discharge
   b) Photophobia
   c) Moderate eyelid edema
5. Conjunctivitis caused by HSV
   a) Vesicle on skin of lids
   b) Coexisting fever blisters on the lips or face: Common
6. Chemical conjunctivitis
   a) Burning, itching sensation
   b) Redness extending to lids
   c) Watery discharge or excessive dryness

D. Physical examination
   1. Vital signs: May have elevated temperature
   2. HEENT
      a) Pupils: Equal, round, reactive to light and accommodation
      b) EOMs: Intact
      c) Funduscopic examination usually normal; potential ulceration
      d) Normal visual acuity or slightly blurred vision
      e) Clear corneas: Dendrite corneal lesions possible with herpes
      f) Conjunctiva
         (1) More injected around periphery with extension toward the iris
         (2) Follicles (small sacs or gland that secrete) or papillae (small, rounded pro-tuberance) can be a sign of viral infections and can occur with chronic allergic or hypersensitivity conjunctivitis.
      g) Eyelid drainage and edema
         (1) Discharge: Bacterial conjunctivitis can be more purulent than viral conjunctivitis and is generally seen as white, green, or yellow mucous discharge of the eyelid margins.
         (2) Difficulty getting the eyelids open following sleep: Patients may report waking up with their eyes "glued" or "crusted" shut.
         (3) Eyelid edema: It is often present in bacterial conjunctivitis but mild in most cases. Severe eyelid edema in the presence of copious purulent discharge raises the suspicion of N. gonorrhoeae infection.
      h) Oral examination
         (1) Posterior pharynx inflammation with viral infection
         (2) Black eschar in the oral cavity hard palate or in the nose

       i) Nasal mucosa: Pale and edematous
   3. Lymph node: Enlarged preauricular and neck nodes (see Appendix D)
      a) Large preauricular lymph nodes: Associated with viral infection
      b) Enlarged preauricular lymph nodes: Common in viral conjunctivitis and unusual in bacterial conjunctivitis, although found in severe bacterial conjunctivitis caused by *N. gonorrhoeae*

IV. Diagnostic tests (Arshad et al., 2020; Kam et al., 2015; Sacchetti et al., 2018; Streitz, 2018; Watson et al., 2018)
   A. Laboratory: Culture and sensitivity; gram stain of discharge only if gonorrhea, syphilis, or chlamydia is suspected or treatment resistant
     1. A rapid test for adenoviral infections (AdenoPlus®) is available to help distinguish viral from bacterial infections.
     2. Eversion of the eyelid when performing a slit lamp examination is indicated when a foreign body is suspected.
     3. Dendrites on slit lamp examination can be seen in CMV and adenovirus, not just with HSV or HZV infections.
   B. Radiology: Noncontributory
   C. Other: Fluorescein dye stain if history of trauma is present, if corneal abrasion is suspected, or to diagnose HSV (will see dendritic pattern on stain)

V. Differential diagnosis: It is imperative that urgent cases of red eye be ruled out before treatment (Alfonso et al., 2015; Bielory et al., 2020; Ridolo et al., 2019; Sacchetti et al., 2018; Streitz, 2018; Watson et al., 2018).
   A. Subconjunctival hemorrhage
   B. Systemic illnesses
     1. Stevens-Johnson syndrome
     2. SLE (see Chapter 110)
     3. Sarcoidosis
     4. Ankylosing spondylitis
     5. Behçet syndrome
     6. Thyroid disease (see Chapters 157 and 158)
   C. Infectious diseases
     1. Reiter syndrome
     2. Mumps
     3. Rubella
     4. HZV
     5. Viral illnesses: CMV
     6. STIs: Syphilis, gonorrhea, chlamydia
   D. Vitamin A deficiency
   E. Chemotherapy-induced ocular toxicities
   F. Radiation-induced ocular toxicities secondary to head and neck cancers

VI. Treatment (Arshad et al., 2020; Bielory et al., 2020; Castillo et al., 2015; Chigbu & Labib, 2018; Ridolo et al., 2019; Sacchetti et al., 2018; Streitz, 2018; Watson et al., 2018)
   A. Never patch an infected eye.
   B. Avoid prescribing topical anesthetics.
   C. Do not use topical steroids; reserve for use only by ophthalmologist.
   D. Symptomatic measures
     1. Apply cool compresses two to four times a day.

2. Clean lids and eyelashes with diluted baby shampoo two times a day.

3. Wash hands well and dispose of used tissues; do not share washcloths, linens, or similar materials.

4. Dispose of used eye makeup.

5. Do not wear contact lenses until 24 hours after infection clears and use a new pair after infection clears.

6. Advise patients to return to school or work after drainage has cleared or after at least 24 hours of treatment.

E. Medication is based on causative agent (see Figure 8-1).

   1. Bacterial conjunctivitis

      a) Bacterial conjunctivitis is self-limiting; patients improved after one to two weeks. Delaying antibiotics may be an option, but patient immune status should be considered in the decision.

      b) First-line treatment should be with inexpensive, nontoxic topical antibiotics such as erythromycin ophthalmic ointment or sulfa drops or polymyxin/trimethoprim drops.

      c) Alternatives include bacitracin ointment, sulfacetamide ointment, polymyxin/bacitracin ointment, fluoroquinolone drops, or azithromycin drops.

FIGURE 8-1   **Ophthalmic Therapies for Conjunctivitis**

Allergic Conjunctivitis
- Antihistamine/mast cell stabilizers
  - Alcaftadine 0.25% solution 1 drop daily
  - Azelastine 0.05% solution 1 drop two times a day
  - Bepotastine besilate 1.5% solution 1 drop two times a day
  - Epinastine 0.05% solution 1 drop two times a day
  - Ketotifen 0.025% solution 1–2 drops every 8 hours as needed
  - Naphazoline/pheniramine solution 1–2 drops every 4–6 hours as needed
  - Olopatadine 0.1% solution 1 drop two times a day
- Mast cell stabilizers
  - Lodoxamide 0.1% solution 1–2 drops four times a day
  - Nedocromil sodium 2% solution 1–2 drops two times a day
- Nonsteroidal anti-inflammatories
  - Diclofenac 0.1% solution 1 drop four times a day
  - Ketorolac 0.5% solution 1 drop four times a day

Bacterial Conjunctivitis
- Azithromycin 1% solution 1 drop two times a day for 2 days then 1 drop daily for 5 days
- Besifloxacin 0.6% solution 1 drop three times a day for 7 days
- Ciprofloxacin 0.3% solution 1–2 drops every 2 hours for 2 days then four times a day for 5 days
- Erythromycin 0.5% ointment 0.5 inch three times a day for 7 days
- Gatifloxacin 0.3% solution 1 drop three times a day for 7 days
- Gentamicin 0.3% ointment 0.5 inch four times a day for 7 days
- Gentamicin 0.3% solution 1–2 drops four times a day for 7 days
- Levofloxacin 0.5% solution 1–2 drops four times a day for 7 days
- Moxifloxacin 0.5% solution 1 drop three times a day for 7 days
- Ofloxacin 0.3% solution 1–2 drops four times a day for 7 days
- Sulfacetamide 10% ointment 0.5 inch four times a day for 7 days
- Sulfacetamide 10% solution 1–2 drops every 2–3 hours for 7 days
- Tobramycin 0.3% ointment 0.5 inch three times a day for 7 days
- Tobramycin 0.3% solution 1–2 drops four times a day for 7 days
- Trimethoprim/polymyxin B solution 1–2 drops four times a day for 7 days

---

Note. Based on information from Castillo et al., 2015; Streitz, 2018.

        d) Avoid aminoglycoside drops because of corneal toxicity.

        e) Fluoroquinolones or aminoglycoside can also be considered for therapy.

        f) Concurrent chlamydial infection for patients and their sexual partners should be managed with one of the following.

            (1) Azithromycin: 1,000 mg PO single dose

            (2) Doxycycline: 100 mg PO two times a day for seven days

            (3) Tetracycline: 250 mg PO four times a day for seven days

            (4) Erythromycin: 500 mg PO four times a day for seven days

        g) Avoid preparations containing neomycin because they can cause hypersensitivity.

2. Viral conjunctivitis: Treatment is symptomatic. Complications should be investigated if symptoms do not resolve after 7–10 days.

        a) Antihistamine/decongestant drops for symptom relief

        b) Nonantibiotic lubricating drops/saline eye drops

        c) Cool compresses

3. Allergic conjunctivitis: Treatment is symptomatic or removal of offending agent.

        a) Oral antihistamines (see Appendix H)

        b) Saline eye drops: 1–2 drops every two to four hours PRN; may avoid need for costly eye drops

        c) Mast cell stabilizer eye drops

        d) Antihistamine/mast cell stabilizer eye drops

        e) Nonsteroidal anti-inflammatory eye drops

        f) Cyclosporine 0.05% ophthalmologic suspension (Restasis®): One drop every 12 hours; may be helpful in nonresponsive cases

        g) Surface-acting steroids: Fluorometholone, rimexolone

4. Herpes simplex conjunctivitis

        a) Refer to ophthalmologist for treatment.

        b) Avoid steroids.

        c) Topical and oral antivirals are recommended to shorten the course of the disease.

            (1) Acyclovir

                (a) 3% ophthalmic ointment: 200, 400, or 800 mg five times a day for 10 days

                (b) 200 mg/5 ml suspension

                (c) 400 mg five times a day for 10 days

                (d) 5% dermatologic ointment six times a day for seven days

            (2) Ganciclovir: 0.15% topical ophthalmic gel five times a day until epithelium heals, then three times a day for seven days

5. Chemical-induced conjunctivitis

        a) Topical lubricants

        b) Refer to ophthalmologist for possible steroid drops.

F. Foul-smelling discharge with pre-septal cellulitis is more likely to have an anaerobic infection.

G. Patients who report a history of diabetes, abuse alcohol, or are immunocompromised should consider mucormycosis. This will require surgical intervention with debridement.

VII. Follow-up

  A. Short term

    1. See patient in office if no improvement in 48 hours.

    2. Follow-up on mild cases is not needed if resolved.

    3. Follow-up should occur in 7–10 days for severe cases.

  B. Long term: Follow-up is unnecessary unless repeat occurrences.

VIII. Referral: Refer to ophthalmologist for diagnosis and management for suspected keratitis or iritis, acute angle glaucoma, STIs, cancer treatment–induced conjunctivitis, ulceration, HSV conjunctivitis, and treatment failures (Alfonso et al., 2015; Bielory et al., 2020).

The author would like to acknowledge Kristine Turner Story, RN, MSN, APRN, BC, for her contribution to this chapter that remains unchanged from the previous edition of this book.

References

Alfonso, S.A., Fawley, J.D., & Lu, X.A. (2015). Conjunctivitis. *Primary Care: Clinics in Office Practice, 42*(3), 325–345. https://doi.org/10.1016/j.pop.2015.05.001

Arshad, J.I., Saud, A., White, D.E., Afshari, N.A., & Sayegh, R.R. (2020). Chronic conjunctivitis from a retained contact lens. *Eye and Contact Lens, 46*(1), e1–e4. https://doi.org/10.1097/ICL.0000000000000587

Bielory, L., Delgado, L., Katelaris, C.H., Leonardi, A., Rosario, N., & Vichyanoud, P. (2020). ICON: Diagnosis and management of allergic conjunctivitis. *Annals of Allergy, Asthma and Immunology, 124*(2), 118–134. https://doi.org/10.1016/j.anai.2019.11.014

Castillo, M., Scott, N.W., Mustafa, M.Z., Mustafa, M.S., & Azuara-Blanco, A. (2015). Topical antihistamines and mast cell stabilisers for treating seasonal and perennial allergic conjunctivitis. *Cochrane Database of Systematic Reviews, 2015*(6). https://doi.org/10.1002/14651858.CD009566.pub2

Chigbu, D.I., & Labib, B.A. (2018). Pathogenesis and management of adenoviral keratoconjunctivitis. *Infection and Drug Resistance, 11,* 981–993. https://doi.org/10.2147/IDR.S162669

Kam, K.Y.R., Ong, H.S., Bunce, C., Ogunbowale, L., & Verma, S. (2015). Sensitivity and specificity of the AdenoPlus point-of-care system in detecting adenovirus in conjunctivitis patients at an ophthalmic emergency department: A diagnostic accuracy study. *British Journal of Ophthalmology, 99*(9), 1186–1189. https://doi.org/10.1136/bjophthalmol-2014-306508

National Comprehensive Cancer Network. (2021). *NCCN Clinical Practice Guidelines in Oncology (NCCN Guidelines®): Management of immunotherapy-related toxicities* [v.3.2021]. https://www.nccn.org/professionals/physician_gls/pdf/immunotherapy.pdf

Ridolo, E., Kihlgren, P., Pellicelli, I., Nizi, M.C., Pucciarini, F., & Incorvaia, C. (2019). Atopic keratoconjunctivitis: Pharmacotherapy for the elderly. *Drugs and Aging, 36*(7), 581–588. https://doi.org/10.1007/s40266-019-00676-7

Sacchetti, M., Abicca, I., Bruscolini, A., Cavaliere, C., Nebbioso, M., & Lambiase, A. (2018). Allergic conjunctivitis: Current concepts on pathogenesis and management. *Journal of Biological Regulators and Homeostatic Agents, 32*(Suppl. 1), 49–60.

Streitz, M. (2018). Eye infections. In B. Long & A. Koyfman (Eds.), *Handbook of emergency ophthalmology* (pp. 161–190). Springer.

Watson, S., Cabrera-Aguas, M., & Khoo, P. (2018). Common eye infections. *Australian Prescriber, 41*(3), 67–72. https://doi.org/10.18773/austprescr.2018.016

Zahler, S., Ghazi, N.G., & Singh, A.D. (2019). Principles and complications of chemotherapy. In A.D. Singh & B.E. Damato (Eds.), *Clinical ophthalmic oncology: Basic principles* (pp. 129–142). Springer.

CHAPTER 9

Otitis Externa

Wendy H. Vogel, MSN, FNP, AOCNP®

I. Definition: Inflammation and/or infection of the auricle or external auditory canal (Magliocca et al., 2018; Rosenfeld et al., 2014; Szmuilowicz & Young, 2019; Wiegand et al., 2019)
   A. Acute diffuse: Most common, often seen in swimmers
   B. Acute localized: Furunculosis
   C. Chronic: Lasting more than six weeks
   D. Herpetic: Ramsay Hunt syndrome
   E. Otomycosis: Fungal
   F. Necrotizing: Malignant; extends into deeper tissues, primarily in immunocompromised individuals
   G. Radiation associated
   H. Eczematous: Psoriasis, atopic dermatitis, and eczema

II. Physiology/Pathophysiology
   A. Normal (Eguchi et al., 2018; Koltsidopoulos & Skoulakis, 2020; Szmuilowicz & Young, 2019; Szymanski & Geiger, 2019)
      1. The external ear includes the auricle, external ear canal, and the lateral surface of the tympanic membrane. The outer cartilaginous canal structures include cerumen glands, sebaceous glands, and hair follicles.
         a) The external canal is a cylinder measuring approximately 2.5 cm in length, extending from the conchal cartilage of the auricle to the tympanic membrane.
         b) The inferior tympanic recess is a small depression in the inferior medial aspect of the ear canal, adjacent to the tympanic membranes. Debris can collect in the area, leading to ear infection.
      2. The skin of the cartilaginous canal has unique qualities.
         a) Self-debridement, shedding, and migration of cells occurs into the canal; cells are trapped by cerumen, which has antibacterial properties, and are expelled.
         b) Both aerobic and anaerobic bacteria normally colonize the ear canal, but organisms primarily are gram positive (e.g., staphylococci).
      3. Boundaries of the ear canal are important in understanding potential complications of OE.
         a) Superiorly by the middle cranial fossa
         b) Anteriorly by the temporomandibular and parotid region
         c) Medially by the tympanic membrane
         d) Posteriorly by the mastoid cavity
         e) Inferiorly by skull base and soft tissues of the neck
      4. Aging effects of ear and ear canal
         a) Subcutaneous tissue, overlying skin: Atrophy, thinning

       b) Skin: Dry, prone to breakdown or trauma

       c) Cerumen: Concentrated; possibly hard and impacted

       d) Increase in ear size, cartilage growth, and pendulous lobule elongation

  B. Pathophysiology

    1. Breakdown of the skin and cerumen barrier may occur from excess moisture, trauma, or contact dermatitis.

    2. Inflammation and edema of the skin lead to pruritus and obstruction. Scratching may lead to further injury. Exudate and pus may be present.

    3. Alteration of cerumen production occurs; impaired epithelial migration and increased pH of the ear canal result in an ideal environment for numerous organisms to breed.

    4. Compression of the cranial nerve can occur.

    5. Radiation can cause ischemic changes of the ear canal, altering cerumen production and epithelium migration.

III. Clinical features: OE can occur in all age groups, with 5% of cases occurring in those aged 20 years or older. OE is more likely to occur in the summer, which could be related to the increase in humidity and participation in water activities (Eguchi et al., 2018; Koltsidopoulos & Skoulakis, 2020; Magliocca et al., 2018; Mustafa et al., 2015; Rosenfeld et al., 2014; Shukla et al., 2017; Szmuilowicz & Young, 2019; Wiegand et al., 2019).

  A. Risk factors

    1. Swimming

    2. Tendency to retain water in the ear canal caused by small or tortuous canal anatomy

    3. Hot, humid climates

    4. Trauma to the ear: Commonly self-induced with cotton-tipped applicators, bobby pins, or paper clips

    5. Radiation to the head

    6. Age older than 65 years

    7. Diabetes

    8. Immunocompromised state

    9. Prolonged use of topical antibiotics and steroid preparations

    10. Occlusion of the ear canal from devices such as hearing aids and earphones, or from bone growth (i.e., swimmer's ear)

    11. Dermis abnormalities: SLE, psoriasis, eczema

  B. Etiology

    1. Acute diffuse (swimmer's ear): *Pseudomonas aeruginosa, Staphylococcus aureus*

    2. Acute localized (furunculosis): *S. aureus,* typically from infected hair follicle, precipitated by excessive moisture in or trauma to the external auditory canal

    3. Chronic: Persistent low-grade infection and inflammation

    4. Herpetic OE: HZV

    5. Otomycosis: Primary fungal infection, secondary to a bacterial infection, or from prolonged use of topical antibiotics and steroid preparations; usually from *Aspergillus* and *Candida* infection in patients with hearing aids

    6. Necrotizing: Persistent OE; usual from *P. aeruginosa;* associated with high mortality unless treated early; occurs more often in older adults, diabetics, and immunocompromised individuals

    7. Radiation induced

       a) Inflammatory changes in the tympanic membrane may cause erythema or congestion and may result in visual changes within the middle ear.

        b) External auditory canal develops inflammation and erythema caused by radiation exposure.

        c) Canal may develop stenosis or necrosis from radiation effect.

        d) Ototoxicity may occur in contralateral or ipsilateral ear following head and neck irradiation.

        e) *P. aeruginosa* is the most commonly isolated pathogen.

    8. Eczematous: Results from several dermatologic disorders (e.g., SLE, seborrheic dermatitis, atopic dermatitis, psoriasis, neurodermatitis)

C. History

    1. History of cancer and cancer treatment

    2. Current medications: Prescribed, over the counter, local remedies for ear disturbances

    3. History of presenting symptoms: Precipitating factors, onset, location, duration, associated symptoms (e.g., fever, chills, pruritus, erythema, scaling, crusting)

    4. Changes in ADLs

    5. Past medical history: Ear infections; ear surgery; self-induced trauma (use of cotton swabs); recent change of soap, lotion, hairspray, shampoo, or earrings; comorbidities (e.g., diabetes, HIV/AIDS, other immunosuppressed states); dermatologic history (e.g., SLE, eczema, psoriasis)

    6. Exposure to water: Swimming, surfing, diving

D. Signs and symptoms

    1. Pruritus: External auditory canal and auricle

    2. Pain: Increased with movement of ear or swallowing

    3. Muffled hearing: From edema within canal

    4. Discharge

    5. Ear fullness, pressure, or tinnitus

    6. Radiation induced: Initial dry desquamation; pruritus may develop into moist desquamation or false membrane formation.

E. Physical examination

    1. HEENT: External ear examination

        a) Skin of the auditory canal: May be edematous, erythematous, fissured; may be indicative of deeper infection or topical allergic reaction

        b) Debris in canal: Scales or crusts

        c) Discharge: May range from green, indicating bacterial infection, to dark, indicating fungal infection

        d) Pain with manipulation of auricle: Differentiates OE from OM; response is best elicited by pushing on the tragus; pulling back on the helix is less sensitive.

        e) Assessment for cellulitis of the face/neck

    2. Otoscopic examination: Remove cerumen, desquamated skin, and purulent material from ear canal to increase visualization and penetration of ear drops. Then, distinguish among OE, OM, or other ototoxicity.

        a) Furunculosis: Pustules or furuncles in outer third of ear canal

        b) Eczematous: Erythema, scaling, crusting, and fissuring in ear canal

        c) Acute diffuse

            (1) Erythema and edema of external canal

            (2) Dull or infected tympanic membrane

            (3) Narrowing or occlusion of the canal

            (4) Serous or purulent drainage

        d) Otomycosis: Fungal growth appears in a variety of colors, most often white or gray.

            (1) *Pseudomonas* infection appears green or yellow.

            (2) *Aspergillus* appears as a white mat topped with black spheres.

        e) Chronic
- (1) Dry, atrophic canal
- (2) Lack of cerumen
- (3) Thickened, narrowing lumen of ear canal

        f) Necrotizing
- (1) Erythema, edema of the ear canal
- (2) Classic finding: Granulation tissue on floor of canal and bone-cartilage junction
- (3) Ulceration of the necrotic soft tissue at the bone-cartilage junction
- (4) Purulent drainage, less as infection advances
- (5) Frank necrosis of ear canal

        g) Radiation induced: Erythema, dry or moist desquamation, ulceration of the skin, late changes (e.g., atrophy, ulceration, canal stenosis, decreased cerumen)

        h) Tympanic membrane: Could be perforated; presence of air-fluid level along tympanic membrane indicative of underlying OM

   3. Lymph nodes examination: Lymphadenopathy of preauricular, cervical, and submental nodes (see Appendix D)

   4. Neurologic examination: Cranial nerve impairment (VII, IX, X, XI and XII; see Appendix A)

 IV. Diagnostic tests: The diagnosis of OE is clinically based (Morales et al., 2019; Mustafa et al., 2015; Szmuilowicz & Young, 2019).

   A. Laboratory

     1. CBC, ESR, glucose and creatinine levels to evaluate for infection if necrotizing OE is suspected; ESR is often elevated in malignant OE.

     2. Culture and sensitivity of ear discharge for severe cases if patient is immunosuppressed or does not respond to treatment

     3. Potassium hydroxide, microscopic evaluation, or microscopic culture if fungal cause is suspected

     4. Viral cultures of ear drainage if HZV is suspected

   B. Radiology

     1. CT scan to evaluate for cartilage and bone invasion if necrotizing OE is suspected

     2. MRI to evaluate soft tissue changes

   C. Biopsy if melanoma or metastatic disease is suspected

 V. Differential diagnosis (Wiegand et al., 2019)

   A. Contact dermatitis (see Chapter 20): Often caused by ototopical agents such as neomycin, benzocaine, or propylene glycol

   B. Acute or chronic suppurative OM (see Chapter 10)

   C. Foreign bodies

   D. Mastoiditis

   E. Impetigo: Superficial, spreading infection; may involve concha and auricle

   F. Bullous myringitis

   G. HZV (see Chapter 22)

   H. Carcinoma or melanoma

   I. Seborrheic dermatitis, psoriasis

   J. Perichondritis or chondritis

   K. Erysipelas: Infection caused by group A *Streptococcus*; may involve concha, canal, dermis, and deeper tissues

VI. Treatment (Demirci & O'Brien, 2019; Hajioff & MacKeith, 2015; Koltsidopoulos & Skou-lakis, 2020; Suyama et al., 2019; Szmuilowicz & Young, 2019; Wiegand et al., 2019)

  A. Cleansing of ear canal

    1. Proper cleansing is necessary, especially if accumulated debris prevents solution from contacting affected area. Use gentle suction or cotton-tipped applicator.

    2. Irrigate with warm saline or diluted hydrogen peroxide solution (1:1 dilution of 3%) if necessary.

    3. Dry with gentle suction if necessary.

  B. Medications

    1. Topical antimicrobial is often combined with steroids or 2% acetic acid solution (combinations and dosing varies) usually for 10–14 days. Acetic acid solution inhibits growth of bacteria and fungi. Do not use if perforation of tympanic membrane is suspected. Apply with a cotton wick if canal is narrowed or occluded.

      a) Neomycin otic solutions/suspensions: Several drops in affected ear three to four times a day

      b) Quinolone solution: Ofloxacin 0.3% or ciprofloxacin 0.3% with or without corticosteroid

      c) Antifungals: Amphotericin B 3% lotion, clotrimazole 1% solution (has the broadest spectrum of activity for common fungi), or tolnaftate 1% (dosing varies)

      d) No significant difference exists in antibiotic choices. Treatment is personalized based on toxicity profile of the agent.

      e) Patients should be taught how to properly instill ear drops: Tilt the head toward opposite shoulder, pull superior aspect of auricle upward, then fill the ear canal with drops. Patient should lie on side for 20 minutes or place a cotton ball in ear canal for 20 minutes to maximize medication exposure.

    2. Use oral antibiotics if cellulitis or systemic symptoms are present or if patient is in immunocompromised state (see Chapter 19 and Appendix C).

      a) Reserve for severe cases, such as *P. aeruginosa* or *S. aureus.*

      b) Ciprofloxacin or levofloxacin may be used orally.

      c) Dicloxacillin or cephalexin are used for *S. aureus.*

    3. Necrotizing

      a) Ciprofloxacin is the antibiotic of choice and is usually initiated at 400 mg IV every 8 hours, then stepped down to 500 mg PO every 12 hours; treat for six to eight weeks.

      b) Necrotizing OE requires IV antibiotics (antipseudomonal beta-lactam with or without aminoglycoside) that cover *Pseudomonas* and must be given for 6–12 weeks.

      c) In some cases, oral quinolones may be used.

      d) IV antipseudomonal with or without aminoglycosides is appropriate.

      e) Local debridement may be necessary.

    4. Furunculosis does not require antibiotics unless the surrounding tissue is inflamed. Applying heat can cause spontaneous eruption. Incision and drainage may be required.

    5. Pain management may include NSAIDs to opioids (see Appendices E and F), as well as topical corticosteroids to reduce swelling and inflammation.

  C. Prevention

    1. Tight-fitting bathing caps and tight-fitting earplugs should be encouraged in swimmers who are prone to recurrent infections. Patients should avoid water sports for 7–10 days.

    2. Instruct patients to dry the ear canal after water exposure.

a) With acetic acid solution or Burow's solution

b) Hair dryer set on low and held about 12 inches from ear

c) Shaking ear dry after swimming

3. Patients should avoid scratching or traumatizing the ear (i.e., using cotton-tipped applicators).

4. Teach proper ear hygiene.

a) Ear is self-cleaning.

b) Fingers, cotton swabs, or foreign objects should not be used to clean ears.

VII. Follow-up

A. In three to five days, follow up with patients if they do not respond to therapy or if oral antibiotics are required. Maintain high index of suspicion for necrotizing OE in patients with persistent otalgia, history of diabetes, or compromised immunologic status.

B. In 7–14 days, assess response to treatment.

C. Necrotizing OE requires frequent and prolonged follow-up.

VIII. Referrals (Szmuilowicz & Young, 2019)

A. Otolaryngologist: If necrotizing OE is suspected and patient is immunocompromised or diabetic; if no response to treatment; the patient has severe pain; or the tympanic membrane is ruptured

B. Audiologist: If sensorineural hearing loss is suspected

References

Demirci, T., & O'Brien, S. (2019). Complicated necrotizing otitis externa progressing to coalescent mastoiditis and temporal lobe abscess. *American Journal of Medicine, 132*(2), E39–E40. https://doi.org/10.1016/j.amjmed.2018.10.005

Eguchi, T., Basugi, A., Kanai, I., Miyata, Y., Nasuno, T., & Hamada, Y. (2018). Malignant external otitis following radiotherapy for oral cancer: A case report. *Medicine, 97*(21), e10898. https://doi.org/10.1097/MD.0000000000010898

Hajioff, D., & MacKeith, S. (2015). Otitis externa. *British Medical Journal of Clinical Evidence, 6,* 510. https://www.ncbi.nlm.nih.gov/pmc/articles/PMC4466798/pdf/2015–0510.pdf

Koltsidopoulos, P., & Skoulakis, C. (2020). Otomycosis with tympanic membrane perforation: A review of the literature. *Ear, Nose, and Throat Journal, 99*(8), 518–521. https://doi.org/10.1177/0145561319851499

Magliocca, K.R., Vivas, E.X., & Griffith, C.C. (2018). Idiopathic, infectious and reactive lesions of the ear and temporal bone. *Head and Neck Pathology, 12,* 328–349. https://doi.org/10.1007/s12105-018-0952-0

Morales, R.E., Eisenman, D.J., & Raghavan, P. (2019). Imaging necrotizing otitis externa. *Seminars in Roentgenology, 54*(3), 215–226. https://doi.org/10.1053/j.ro.2019.04.002

Mustafa, M., Patawari, P., Sien, M.M., Muniandy, R.K., & Zinatara, P. (2015). Acute otitis externa: Pathophysiology, clinical presentation, and treatment. *Journal of Dental and Medical Sciences, 14*(7), 73–78. https://www.iosrjournals.org/iosr-jdms/papers/Vol14-issue7/Version-1/O014717378.pdf

Rosenfeld, R.M., Schwartz, S.R., Cannon, C.R., Roland, P.S., Simon, G.R., Kumar, K.A., ... Robertson, P.J. (2014). Clinical practice guideline: Acute otitis externa executive summary. *Otolaryngology–Head and Neck Surgery, 150*(2), 161–168. https://doi.org/10.1177/0194599813517659

Shukla, R., Easto, R., & Williams, R. (2017). Conditions of the external and middle ear: An overview of presentation, management and associated complications. *Journal of the Royal Naval Medical Service, 103*(1), 49–55.

Suyama, Y., Okada, M., Nozaki, T., & Furukawa, K. (2019). Necrotizing otitis externa. *Internal Medicine, 58*(6), 895–896. https://doi.org/10.2169/internalmedicine.1684-18

Szmuilowicz, J., & Young, R. (2019). Infections of the ear. *Emergency Medicine Clinics of North America, 37*(1), 1–9. https://doi.org/10.1016/j.emc.2018.09.001

Szymanski, A., & Geiger, Z. (2019). Anatomy, head and neck, ear. In *StatPearls.* https://www.ncbi.nlm.nih.gov/books/NBK470359

Wiegand, S., Berner, R., Schneider, A., Lundershausen, E., & Dietz, A. (2019). Otitis externa: Investigation and evidence-based treatment. *Deutsches Ärzteblatt International, 116*(13), 224–234. https://doi.org/10.3238/arztebl.2019.0224

CHAPTER 10

Otitis Media

Wendy H. Vogel, MSN, FNP, AOCNP®

I. Definition: Presence of fluid in the middle ear associated with signs and symptoms of inflammation (Dickson, 2014; Gaddey et al., 2019; Roditi et al., 2017)
   A. Acute otitis media (AOM): Acute onset, presence of middle ear effusion, and signs of middle ear inflammation
   B. Otitis media with effusion (OME): Presence of fluid in the middle ear without signs or symptoms of acute ear infection
   C. Chronic otitis media (COM): Chronic ear infections with perforated tympanic membrane and chronic purulent drainage
   D. OE: Infection or irritation of the outer third of the ear canal

II. Physiology/Pathophysiology (Akazawa et al., 2018; Christensen et al., 2018; Dickson, 2014; Earwood et al., 2018; Harrison & Cronin, 2016; Islam et al., 2018; Roditi et al., 2017; Young, 2019)
   A. Normal: The middle ear consists of the tympanic membrane, auditory ossicles (malleus, incus, and stapes), and the eustachian tube. The middle ear is lined with mucous-secreting epithelium. The eustachian tube connects the middle ear to the nasopharynx.
      1. Eustachian tube function includes equalizing pressure on both sides of the tympanic membrane.
      2. The eustachian tube normally is in a collapsed, closed position, which protects the middle ear from reflux of nasopharyngeal debris.
      3. Secretions move through the tube into the nasopharynx by way of ciliary action.
      4. Normal transmission of sound to the tympanic membrane requires a patent eustachian tube.
   B. Pathophysiology
      1. AOM occurs when the normal eustachian tube is obstructed, resulting in fluid retention and entrance of pathogens and inflammatory mediators into the middle ear and causing inflammation, erythema, and edema.
      2. Abnormal eustachian tube reflux and obstruction caused by viral nasopharyngitis are the major pathogenetic factors. Bacteria or viruses can ascend from the nasopharynx, leading to infection.
      3. Radiation therapy negatively affects eustachian tube function and may result in OME.
      4. OME may be sterile fluid secondary to URI and eustachian tube dysfunction. OME may be residual fluid after an episode of AOM.

III. Clinical features: It is important to distinguish AOM from OME. OME can result in deafness, tinnitus, and pain. OME may follow AOM but may result from barotraumas (as with scuba diving or air travel) or allergies. Many patients with nasopharyngeal carcinoma have

OME before treatment and could develop it after treatment. More than one-half of patients will report radiation-induced ear dysfunction after nasopharyngeal cancer treatment ("Acute otitis media in adults," 2019; Akazawa et al., 2018; Burrows et al., 2013; Gaddey et al., 2019; Islam et al., 2018; Young, 2019).

A. Risk factors
   1. Eustachian tube dysfunction: More common in children and declines with age
   2. Higher occurrence in males than females
   3. Recent URI
   4. Smoking/secondhand smoke exposure
   5. Previous episodes of AOM or OME
   6. Allergies
   7. Enlarged adenoid
   8. Alaska Native/Native American heritage
   9. Nasopharyngeal tumor and/or history of nasopharyngeal irradiation
   10. Immunocompromised status
   11. Strong family history
   12. Fall, winter, or early spring seasons
   13. Radiation to head and neck

B. Etiology
   1. AOM may be preceded by URI that often is viral.
   2. Almost one-half of patients have acute middle ear effects during radiation therapy; severity is affected by radiation dose and tumor site close to the ear.
   3. OME may occur spontaneously because of poor eustachian tube function or as an inflammatory response after AOM, allergic rhinitis, or URI.
   4. OME may be a presenting symptom in nasopharyngeal carcinoma.
   5. Most common bacterial pathogens
      a) *Streptococcus pneumoniae* (up to 50%): Least likely to resolve without treatment; now increasingly penicillin resistant (8%–34%)
      b) *Haemophilus influenzae* (20%–30%)
      c) *Moraxella catarrhalis* (10%–15%)
      d) Group A *Streptococcus* (rare): May cause sensorineural hearing impairment and more-severe clinical case
   6. Other infrequently cultured pathogens include *Mycoplasma pneumoniae,* group A beta-hemolytic *Streptococcus, Staphylococcus aureus, Chlamydia trachomatis,* and anaerobic bacteria (chronic infections).
   7. Potential viral etiologies include respiratory syncytial virus, rhinovirus, adenovirus, and influenza viruses.
   8. Fungal etiologies such as *Candida* and *Aspergillus* may also be considered.

C. History
   1. History of cancer and cancer treatment
   2. Current medications: Prescribed, over the counter
   3. History of presenting symptoms: Precipitating factors, onset, location, radiation, duration, intensity
      a) Associated symptoms include dysphonia, dysphagia, hearing loss, ringing in the ears, disequilibrium, ear drainage, itching, painful teeth, pain with chewing or swallowing, ears popping, and tinnitus.
      b) Associated symptoms that might cause suspicion for malignancy include weight loss, odynophagia, dysphagia, or hoarseness.
      c) Characteristics of pain often correlate with etiology. For example, pain associated with infection is usually continuous and progressive.

    d) Intermittent pain is more likely to be related to musculoskeletal disorders.

    e) Duration of pain points differentiates an acute or chronic condition.

  4. Changes in ADLs

  5. Past medical history: Injuries to the ear, infections, surgeries, comorbidities (e.g., diabetes, thyroid diseases, dermatologic disorders, immunocompromised states), recent URI

  6. History of recent air travel or swimming

D. Signs and symptoms

  1. Otalgia: Ear pain; may be aggravated by swallowing or belching and spread to temporal region

  2. Otorrhea: Inflammation of ear with drainage

  3. Hearing loss, ear fullness, or "popping"

  4. Vertigo

  5. Tinnitus

  6. Systemic symptoms: Fever, rhinitis, sore throat, dizziness

  7. Disturbed sleep, lethargy

  8. Irritability

  9. Loss of appetite

  10. Nausea/vomiting

  11. Usual signs and symptoms absent in neutropenic patients

  12. Increased pressure sensation in the ears

E. Physical examination

  1. Vital signs: Elevated temperature

  2. HEENT

    a) External ear: Inspect auricle, tragus, and periauricular region for edema, erythema (indicating cellulitis), lacerations, purulent green or yellow discharge (indicating OE), furuncle (tender meatal swelling), cholesteatoma (abnormal skin growth in middle ear), or foreign body. Assess for pain with tugging.

    b) Pneumatic otoscopic examination: Remove cerumen that is partially or completely obstructing the ear canal and preventing adequate visualization.

      (1) Mobility of the tympanic membrane

        (a) Bulging with no mobility indicating pus or fluid in the middle ear

        (b) Retracted with no mobility indicating obstruction of the eustachian tube with or without fluid

        (c) Mobility with negative pressure only indicating obstruction of the eustachian tube

        (d) Excess mobility (flaccid tympanic membrane) indicating healed perforation or patulous eustachian tube

      (2) Color

        (a) Amber indicating serous fluid in middle ear

        (b) Blue or deep red indicating blood or erythema

        (c) Chalky white indicating infection

        (d) Redness indicating infection or scarring of the middle ear

        (e) Dullness indicating fibrosis or effusion

        (f) White flakes or dense white plaques indicating healed inflammation or cholesteatoma

      (3) Other findings

        (a) Fluid line indicating fluid behind middle ear

        (b) Dark area on tympanic membrane indicating perforation

        (c) Bullae or blisters indicating infection

(*d*) Discharge indicating infection or perforation

(*e*) Air bubbles indicating serous fluid

(*f*) Diminished light reflex

(*g*) Purulent drainage indicating ruptured tympanic membrane

IV. Diagnostic tests (Burrows et al., 2013)

    A. Laboratory

       1. CBC to evaluate for leukocytosis with polymorphonuclear elevation

       2. Culture of ear drainage or nasopharynx to document infection: Approximately 45% predictive value from culture

    B. Radiology: CT or MRI if a complication such as CNS infection, mastoiditis, cholesteatoma, facial nerve paralysis, or labyrinthitis is suspected

    C. Other

       1. Impedance tympanometry

          a) Measurement of resonance of ear canal to changes in air pressure

          b) Sensitive and reliable method of detecting an effusion

          c) Useful for COM

       2. Acoustic reflectometry: Sonar measurement of sound reflected back from the tympanic membrane

       3. Tympanocentesis: A surgical puncture of the tympanic membrane with or without placement of pressure-equalizing tube

          a) Procedure is usually not necessary unless patient is immunosuppressed, develops antibiotic resistance (no response in 48–72 hours), or is septic.

          b) One-third of cultures show no growth.

V. Differential diagnosis: The etiology of otorrhea can be OE or OM with perforation (Burrows et al., 2013; Gaddey et al., 2019; see Table 10-1).

    A. Myringitis: Red tympanic membrane without exudate

    B. Pharyngitis (see Chapter 4)

    C. Tonsillitis (see Chapter 4)

    D. TMJ syndrome

    E. Mastoiditis

    F. Foreign body

    G. Dental abscess

    H. Furuncle (see Chapter 21)

    I. Tumor (external compression)

    J. Trauma

    K. Ototoxicity from medications or cancer treatments

       1. Radiation therapy to the ear region

       2. Chemotherapy: Cisplatin

       3. Other: Aminoglycosides, salicylates, quinidine, furosemide

    L. Referred pain: May be from but not limited to the mouth, nasopharynx, tonsils, or other parts of the upper respiratory tract; dental disease; malignancy; TMJ syndrome; or HZV oticus (i.e., Ramsay Hunt syndrome)

VI. Treatment (Burrows et al., 2013; Gaddey et al., 2019; Islam et al., 2018; Roditi et al., 2017; Spurling et al., 2017)

    A. AOM

       1. Observation for 48–72 hours may be employed instead of immediate prescription of antibiotic. Unlike children, no data exist for observation over antibiotic treatment

TABLE 10-1	Otitis Media Versus Otitis Externa	
Symptom/Sign	Otitis Media	Otitis Externa
Auricle motion tenderness	None	Extreme
Canal edema	None	Present
Decreased hearing	May be present	May be present
Ear pain	With swallowing or belching	With moving jaw or auricle
Exudate	Only with perforation	May be minimal
Lymphadenopathy	None	Regional
Systemic signs	Fever, upper respiratory infection	None
Tympanic membrane	Fluid line, may be perforated	Normal or inflamed, no fluid line

Note. Based on information from Burrows et al., 2013; Mustafa et al., 2017.

for adults; therefore, as it is unusual for an adult to have AOM, it is appropriate to treat with an antibiotic. This is an option only for certain patients.
   a) Those who can be monitored and have ready access to health care
   b) Patients in whom AOM is not severe
   c) Patients who are not immunocompromised or do not have underlying conditions that could alter the natural course of AOM, such as immune system disorders or cochlear implants
2. Ibuprofen or acetaminophen should provide pain relief in the first 24 hours, as antibiotics have a minimal effect on pain (see Appendix E).
3. First-line antibiotic of choice is amoxicillin for uncomplicated infection (see Appendix C). Antibiotics are appropriate if the patient is toxic or has a high fever.
   a) Amoxicillin: 500–875 mg PO every 12 hours or 250–500 mg PO every eight hours; some recommendations for doses of 1–2 g every eight hours
   b) Treatment duration: 5–7 days for mild to moderate disease; 10 days for more severe disease
   c) Patients allergic to penicillin: May treat with erythromycin combined with sulfisoxazole, azithromycin, or clarithromycin
4. Treatment failure is defined as no improvement in 48–72 hours, and treatment should be redirected to cover drug-resistant *S. pneumoniae,* beta-lactamase–producing strains of *H. influenzae,* or *M. catarrhalis.* Acceptable antibiotics might include amoxicillin/clavulanate, cefuroxime, cefaclor, cefixime, and ceftriaxone.
5. If penicillin resistant, *S. pneumoniae* is suspected.
   a) Azithromycin: 500 mg PO on day 1, then 250 mg PO every day for four days
   b) Clarithromycin: 250–500 mg PO every 12 hours for 7–14 days
   c) Levofloxacin and moxifloxacin: May be considered
B. OME
1. Long-term benefits of antimicrobial therapy are unproven, and it is appropriate only if OME is persistent beyond three months. Most effusions will spontaneously resolve.
2. Antihistamines (see Appendix H) and decongestants (see Appendix I) may cause some symptom relief by decreasing nasal congestion.

3. Autoinsufflation (pinch the nose while exhaling gently) may push air back through the eustachian tube and repressurize the ear.

VII. Follow-up ("Acute otitis media in adults," 2019; Burrows et al., 2013; Spurling et al., 2017)
  A. Continue to monitor for potential severe complications, such as CNS infection, mastoiditis, or cholesteatoma.
  B. Physical examination
    1. Conduct three to four weeks after start of therapy to assess for persistent effusion.
    2. Evaluate symptomatic patients sooner, within 48–72 hours if symptoms have not improved.
    3. Assess for hearing loss (see Appendix D). Consider audiology evaluation.
  C. Education
    1. Discuss strategies for optimizing the listening and learning environment until the effusion resolves.
    2. Instruct family members, coworkers, and others to face the patient, speak clearly, and speak in close proximity to the patient.
    3. Preferential classroom or work seating may be necessary.
    4. Influenza and pneumococcal vaccines have shown some benefits in preventing AOM and should be considered.

VIII. Referrals
  A. Otolaryngologist
    1. For OME lasting more than 12 weeks or severe cases that need prompt pain relief to accelerate the resolution of infection in AOM or for adults with more than one episode
    2. If surgery is indicated to remove infected tissue in the middle ear or mastoid, and to repair ear damage that results in hearing loss
    3. For chronic tympanic membrane perforation persisting six weeks or longer
  B. Audiologist: When OME lasts more than three months or if language delays, learning problems, or suspected hearing loss is present

References

Acute otitis media in adults. (2019). In *Evidence-based medicine guidelines*. Duodecim Medical Publications. https://evidence.unboundmedicine.com/evidence/view/EBMG/455364/all/Acute_otitis_media_in_adults

Akazawa, K., Doi, H., Ohta, S., Terada, T., Fujiwara, M., Uwa, N., ... Sakagami, M. (2018). Relationship between eustachian tube dysfunction and otitis media with effusion in radiotherapy patients. *Journal of Laryngology and Otology, 132*(2), 111–116. https://doi.org/10.1017/S0022215118000014

Burrows, H.L., Blackwood, R.A., Cooke, J.M., Harrison, R.V., Harmes, K.M., & Passaman, P.P. (2013). *Guidelines for clinical care ambulatory: Otitis media*. University of Michigan. http://www.med.umich.edu/1info/FHP/practiceguides/om/OM.pdf

Christensen, J.G., Wessel, I., Gothelf, A.B., & Homøe, P. (2018). Otitis media with effusion after radiotherapy of the head and neck: A systematic review. *Acta Oncologica, 57*(8), 1011–1016, https://doi.org/10.1080/0284186X.2018.1468085

Dickson, G. (2014). Acute otitis media. *Primary Care: Clinics in Office Practice, 41*(1), 11–18. https://doi.org/10.1016/j.pop.2013.10.002

Earwood, J.S., Rogers, T.S., & Rathjen, N.A. (2018). Ear pain: Diagnosing common and uncommon causes. *American Family Physician, 97*(1), 20–27. https://www.aafp.org/afp/2018/0101/p20.html

Gaddey, H.L., Wright, M.T., & Nelson, T.N. (2019). Otitis media: Rapid evidence review. *American Family Physician, 100*(6), 350–356. https://www.aafp.org/afp/2019/0915/p350.html

Harrison, E., & Cronin, M. (2016). Otalgia. *Australian Family Physician, 45*(7), 493–497. https://www.racgp.org.au/afp/2016/july/otalgia

Islam, M.A., Hague, S., Ahmed, K., Bari, M.S., Hogue, M.M., Khan, M.K., … Kobir, M.S. (2018). Outcome of surgery in chronic inactive mucosal otitis media. *Mymensingh Medical Journal, 27*(3), 617–625.

Mustafa, M., Patawari, P., Sien, M.M., Muniandy, R.M., & Zinatara, P. (2017). Acute otitis externa: Pathophysiology, clinical presentation, and treatment. *IOSR Journal of Dental and Medical Sciences, 14*(7), 73–78. http://www.iosrjournals .org/iosr-jdms/papers/Vol14-issue7/Version-1/O014717378.pdf

Roditi, R.E., Rosenfeld, R.M., & Shin, J.J. (2017). Otitis media with effusion: Our national practice. *Otolaryngology—Head and Neck Surgery, 157*(2), 171–172. https://doi.org/10.1177/0194599817703056

Spurling, G.K.P., Del Mar, C.B., Dooley, L., Foxlee, R., & Farley, R. (2017). Delayed antibiotic prescriptions for respiratory infections. *Cochrane Database of Systematic Reviews, 2017*(9). https://doi.org/10.1002/14651858.CD004417.pub5

Young, Y.-H. (2019). Irradiated ears in nasopharyngeal carcinoma survivors: A review. *Laryngoscope, 129*(3), 637–642. https://doi.org/10.1002/lary.27303

CHAPTER 11

Rhinosinusitis

Raymond Scarpa, DNP, APNC, AOCN®

I. Definition: Inflammation of the mucous membranes of the paranasal sinuses and the nasal cavity (Al-Sayed et al., 2017; Rosenfield et al., 2015; Syke et al., 2018)

II. Physiology/Pathophysiology (Al-Sayed et al., 2017; Craig, 2019; London & Ramanathan, 2018; Rosenfield et al., 2015; Sedaghat, 2017)
   A. Normal
      1. Sinuses are air-filled spaces in the bones of the skull that are lined with respiratory epithelia.
      2. Mucous membranes warm and moisten the air passing through the sinuses.
      3. Mucous membranes create slightly sticky mucus that gathers dust, smoke, bacteria, or virus particles to cleanse the air.
      4. Tiny hairs, or cilia, move the mucus through the sinuses and out the nares.
   B. Pathophysiology
      1. Bacteria or allergens invade the sinus cavities, causing acute or chronic manifestations.
      2. Inflammation occurs with resultant edema, causing obstruction to the flow of secretions and a decrease in mucociliary action.
      3. Inflammation of the mucous membranes causes an increase in mucus production, creating an environment that facilitates bacterial growth within the sinus cavities.
      4. Acute sinusitis is distinguished from chronic sinusitis by the type of cytokine involved, despite bacterial or viral etiology.
         a) Acute is characterized by an increase in neutrophils, IL-1α, IL-6, and IL-8.
         b) Chronic is characterized by lymphocytic infiltrates. If an allergic component is noted, then high levels of helper T1 cells and helper T2 cells are present.

III. Clinical features: Chronic sinusitis often is not associated with an infection and generally does not include fever. The maxillary and frontal sinuses are most frequently involved. Acute bacterial rhinosinusitis should be suspected if an acute URI has not improved or is worse after 10–14 days. It can range from acute viral rhinitis to acute bacterial rhinosinusitis. The most recent guidelines published by the American Academy of Otolaryngology–Head and Neck Surgery do not recognize subacute sinusitis as a distinct clinical entity. It was defined by symptoms lasting for 4–12 weeks. Most common fungal infections are caused by *Aspergillus*, *Fusarium*, and *Mucorales*. Bacterial sources are most commonly *Streptococcus pneumoniae*, *Haemophilus influenzae*, and *Moraxella catarrhalis* (Al-Sayed et al., 2017; Craig, 2019; Lam et al., 2015; London & Ramanathan, 2018; Rosenfield et al., 2015; Sedaghat, 2017).
   A. Risk factors
      1. Congenital bone, cartilage, or ciliary anomalies

    2. Nasal polyps

    3. Cystic fibrosis

    4. Recent URI

    5. Allergic rhinitis

    6. Orofacial trauma

    7. Recent dental procedure

    8. Cigarette smoking

    9. Diabetes mellitus

    10. Swimming, diving, or high-altitude climbing

    11. Sarcoidosis

    12. Immunodeficiency

    13. Mold exposure

    14. Dental infection

B. Classifications

    1. Acute rhinosinusitis

      a) Onset: Rapid

      b) Duration: Four weeks or less

      c) Symptoms: Presence of purulent nasal discharge or nasal obstruction and congestion

    2. Acute bacterial rhinosinusitis

      a) Onset: Gradual

      b) Duration: Purulent drainage after five days lasting longer than 10 days

      c) Symptoms: Complete resolution usually with medical interventions

    3. Subacute rhinosinusitis

      a) Onset: Rapid

      b) Duration: 4–12 weeks

      c) Symptoms: Complete resolution with medical interventions

    4. Recurrent acute rhinosinusitis: Four or more acute episodes annually

      a) Onset: Rapid

      b) Duration: Seven days

      c) Symptoms: Complete resolution usually without medical interventions

    5. Chronic rhinosinusitis

      a) Onset: Rapid or gradual

      b) Duration: 12 weeks or longer

      c) Symptoms: Persists with medical interventions

C. Etiology: Chronic rhinosinusitis can be categorized based on the presence or absence of polyps. The most prominent environmental factors are considered to be microbial, including both fungi and bacteria. Genetic disorders, autoimmune disorders, and immunodeficiency conditions can exhibit symptoms of chronic rhinosinusitis.

D. History

    1. History of cancer and cancer treatment

    2. Current medications: Prescribed, over the counter

    3. History of presenting symptoms: Precipitating factors, onset, location, duration, associated symptoms (e.g., fever, headache, drainage)

    4. Changes in ADLs

    5. Social history: Tobacco use

    6. History of recent URI or dental procedure

E. Signs and symptoms

    1. Pain

      a) In maxillary teeth

  b) Over sinuses

  c) Increased when bending over

2. Nasal obstruction

3. Nasal or postnasal discharge

4. Hyposmia/anosmia: Defect in sense of smell

5. Thick, purulent nasal drainage

6. Headache

7. Low-grade or absent fever: Fever in acute bacterial rhinosinusitis only

8. Halitosis

9. Fatigue

10. Cough with or without sputum production

11. Sore throat

12. Inability to expel nasal secretions

13. Ear pain, pressure, or fullness

F. Physical examination

  1. Vital signs: Low-grade or absent fever

  2. HEENT

    a) Maxillary or frontal sinus

      (1) Tenderness to percussion

      (2) Sinus opacity on transillumination

    b) Ethmoid or sphenoid sinus

      (1) Retro-orbital pain

      (2) Mild palpebral edema

    c) Nares

      (1) Edematous, erythematous inferior turbinate

      (2) Thick or crusty purulent nasal drainage

      (3) Anosmia: Decreased or loss of smell

    d) Oral cavity/oropharynx

      (1) Purulent nasal drainage

      (2) Pharyngeal erythema

      (3) Examination of maxillary teeth with tongue blade to assess for dental source

      (4) Speech indicating fullness of the sinuses

    e) Ears: Presence of middle ear effusions

  3. Pulmonary: Adventitious sounds on auscultation

  4. Neurologic: Cranial nerves (e.g., I [olfactory nerve]), anosmia (see Appendix A)

IV. Diagnostic tests: Not indicated in patients with uncomplicated rhinosinusitis (London & Ramanathan, 2018; Rosenfield et al., 2015; Syke et al., 2018)

A. Laboratory: Anterior nasal cultures are not accurate because of nasal contaminants.

B. Radiology: It is not indicated in patients who meet the diagnostic criteria for acute rhinosinusitis unless a complication or alternative diagnosis is suspected.

  1. Sinus plain films: Typically, films are specific for maxillary sinusitis. Sphenoid sinus is visualized by including a submentovertex view. It has a poor view of ethmoid and frontal sinuses.

  2. CT scan: A scan should be performed if symptoms persist after medical management or recurrence of more than three times a year. Careful observation for unilateral disease, sinus expansion, and bony erosion should occur.

    a) Images the frontal, maxillary, sphenoid, and ethmoid sinuses

    b) 90%–100% sensitivity

      3. MRI: Imaging is not recommended if patients are overly sensitive to mucosal changes and fail to demonstrate bony anatomy of the osteomeatal complex

  C. Other

      1. Flexible rhinopharyngoscopy by otolaryngologist or allergist

      2. Sinus tap to obtain material for culture, especially in neutropenic patients

      3. Testing for allergy and immune function to evaluate patients with chronic rhinosinusitis or recurrent acute rhinosinusitis

      4. Transillumination performed in a dark room with bright light: Findings are recorded as normal (typical light transmission), dull (reduced light transmission), or opaque (no light transmission). This method is only useful for examining maxillary and frontal sinuses.

V. Differential diagnosis: Assess patients with chronic rhinosinusitis or recurrent acute rhinosinusitis for other multiple chronic conditions that would modify management, such as asthma, cystic fibrosis, immunocompromised state, and ciliary dysfunction (Lam et al., 2015; Rosenfield et al., 2015; Syke et al., 2018).

  A. Inflammatory

      1. Allergic/atopic rhinitis (see Chapter 6)

      2. Wegener granulomatosis

      3. Sarcoidosis

      4. OM (see Chapter 10)

      5. Gastroesophageal reflux (see Chapter 71)

  B. Noninflammatory

      1. Idiopathic vasomotor rhinitis

      2. Drug-induced vasomotor rhinitis

      3. Hormone-induced rhinitis: From pregnancy

      4. Nasal drying: Sjögren syndrome, keratoconjunctivitis

  C. Mechanical

      1. Deviated septum

      2. Nasal polyps

      3. Tumor

      4. Foreign body

  D. Barotrauma: Bleeding into sinuses caused by negative pressure

  E. Other causes of headache/facial pain

      1. Temporomandibular disorder

      2. Migraine (see Chapter 137)

      3. Dental pathology

      4. Neuralgia

      5. CNS tumor

      6. Temporal arteritis

  F. Genetic

      1. Cystic fibrosis

      2. Ciliary dyskinesia/immobile cilia

      3. Ataxia-telangiectasia

      4. Kartagener syndrome

      5. Wiskott-Aldrich syndrome

VI. Treatment: Recommended treatment may include analgesics, topical intranasal steroids, and/or nasal saline irrigation for symptomatic relief of viral rhinosinusitis and bacterial rhinosinusitis (Craig, 2019; Lemiengre et al., 2018; Lin & Kacker, 2019; London &

Ramanathan, 2018; Rosenfield et al., 2015; Sedaghat, 2017; Smith et al., 2017; Syke et al., 2018).

A. Decongestants: Expert opinion suggests that decongestants may improve drainage and decrease nasal congestion. Topical decongestant use should be limited to three days because of possible rebound vasodilation (e.g., rhinitis medicamentosa) or atrophic rhinitis (see Appendix I).

B. Antihistamines (see Appendix H): These medications may have anticholinergic properties and provide symptom relief. Their effectiveness in treating acute rhinosinusitis in nonatopic individuals is not established. Second-generation antihistamines are less likely to be effective for diminishing rhinorrhea, and first-generation versions may cause sedation and impair psychomotor ability.

    1. Diphenhydramine: 25–50 mg PO every four to six hours PRN

    2. Chlorpheniramine maleate: 4 mg PO every four to six hours PRN

    3. Loratadine: 10 mg PO daily

C. Antibiotics (see Appendix C): Approximately 70% of patients with acute bacterial rhinosinusitis improve within two weeks without antibiotics; approximately 85% improve with appropriate antibiotics.

    1. Acute sinusitis: Amoxicillin, with or without clavulanate, for 5–10 days is first-line therapy for most adult patients.

        a) Amoxicillin/clavulanate: 500 mg/125 mg or 875 mg/125 mg PO two times a day for five to seven days (first-line antibiotic therapy)

            (1) High-dose amoxicillin/clavulanate: 2 g PO two times a day; recommended as empiric therapy in geographic regions where rates of penicillin-resistant *S. pneumoniae* exceed approximately 10%

            (2) For patients who meet any of the following: Age older than 65 years, recently hospitalized, treated with an antibiotic in previous month, immunocompromised

        b) Levofloxacin/moxifloxacin are reasonable alternatives for penicillin-allergic patients.

    2. Recurrent or chronic sinusitis: Cover for beta-lactamase, *H. influenzae,* or *M. catarrhalis.*

        a) Amoxicillin/clavulanate: 500 mg PO every eight hours or 875 mg every 12 hours for two weeks, or 1,000 mg extended release two times a day

        b) For penicillin-allergic patients or if suspicion for MRSA: Clindamycin 450 mg PO three times a day

        c) Bacterial resistance has increased in recent years to both penicillin and cephalosporin.

        d) Moxifloxacin: 400 mg PO every day for two weeks

        e) Levofloxacin: 500 mg PO every day for two weeks

D. Sinus surgery/balloon sinuplasty: In cases of recurrent acute rhinosinusitis with associated septal deviations, consider septoplasty.

E. Antifungals

    1. Initial therapy includes amphotericin B or voriconazole (mucormycosis).

    2. Clinicians should not prescribe topical or systemic antifungal therapy for patients with chronic rhinosinusitis.

F. Pain

    1. Acetaminophen: 325 mg (two tablets) PO every four to six hours PRN

    2. Ibuprofen: 200–400 mg PO every four to six hours PRN

G. Nasal saline: Irrigation and nasal sprays are helpful in all types of sinusitis.

H. Intranasal glucocorticoid nasal sprays: Budesonide, fluticasone propionate, or mometasone furoate are given as one or two sprays per nostril daily (see Appendix G).

I. Functional endoscopic sinus surgery: Procedure should be used for chronic sinus disease or removal of polyps.

J. Special considerations

    1. Neutropenic or immunocompromised patients

        a) Antibiotic therapy is used for recurrent or chronic sinusitis.

        b) Consider G-CSF support.

        c) Irrigation of sinus may be needed for symptomatic relief.

        d) Consider gamma globulin infusion for patients with hypogammaglobulinemia or with frequent recurrent infections.

    2. Neutropenic population is at a greater risk for complications (e.g., orbital cellulitis, frontal sinus abscess, cavernous sinus thrombosis).

K. Vitamin C, zinc gluconate lozenges, and Echinacea extract provided symptom relief in some studies.

L. Expectorants may thin secretions and improve mucus clearance, though evidence is lacking.

M. Oral corticosteroids have no proven benefit; however, they may decrease mucosal inflammation.

N. Relief of facial pain and overall symptoms in patients with chronic rhinosinusitis was reported in patients treated with multimodal vibration ultrasound at a 1 MHz frequency.

VII. Follow-up

A. Short term: Improvement in symptoms should be noted within two to three days of initiating treatment.

B. Long term: Chronic infections require appropriate referrals.

VIII. Referrals

A. Otolaryngologist or allergist: For complicated sinusitis, recurrent infections, or chronic sinus disease

B. Neurologist: If any indication of CNS involvement

C. Allergist: For atopic allergy testing

The author would like to acknowledge Diane G. Cope, PhD, ARNP-BC, AOCNP®, for her contribution to this chapter that remains unchanged from the previous edition of this book.

References

Al-Sayed, A.A., Aug, R.U., & Massoud, E. (2017). Models for the study of nasal and sinus physiology in health and disease: A review of the literature. *Laryngoscope Investigative Otolaryngology, 2*(6), 398–409. https://doi.org/10.1002/lio2.117

Craig, J.R. (2019). Updates in management of acute invasive fungal rhinosinusitis. *Current Opinion in Otolaryngology and head and neck surgery, 27*(1), 29–36. https://doi.org/10.1097/MOO.0000000000000507

Lam, K., Schleimer, R., & Kern, R.C. (2015). The etiology and pathogenesis of chronic rhinosinusitis: A review of current hypotheses. *Current Allergy and Asthma Reports, 15*(7), 41. https://doi.org/10.1007/s11882-015-0540-2

Lemiengre, M.B., van Driel, M.L., Merenstein, D., Liira, H., Mäkelä, M., & De Sutter, A.I.M. (2018). Antibiotics for acute rhinosinusitis in adults. *Cochrane Database of Systematic Reviews, 2018*(9). https://doi.org/10.1002/14651858. CD006089.pub5

Lin, J., & Kacker, A. (2019). Management strategies for recurrent acute rhinosinusitis. *Laryngoscope Investigative Otolaryngology, 4*(4), 379–382. https://doi.org/10.1002/lio2.294

London, N.R., Jr., & Ramanathan, M., Jr. (2018). Sinuses and common rhinologic conditions. *Medical Clinics of North America, 102*(6), 993–1000. https://doi.org/10.1016/j.mcna.2018.06.003

Rosenfield, R.M., Piccirillo, J.F., Chandrasekhar, S.S., Brook, I., Kumar, K.A., Kramper, M., ... Corrigan, M.D. (2015). Clinical practice guideline (update): Adult sinusitis. *Otolaryngology—Head and Neck Surgery, 152*(2 Suppl.), s1–s39. https://doi.org/10.1177/0194599815572097

Sedaghat, A.R. (2017). Chronic rhinosinusitis. *American Family Physician, 98*(8), 500–506. https://www.aafp.org/afp/2017/1015/p500.html

Smith, M., Berenger, P.G., Bonutti, P., Ramakrishnan, A.P., Beyers, J., & Ramakrishnan, V. (2017). Multimodal frequency treatment for facial pain caused by chronic rhinosinusitis: A pilot study. *Sinusitis, 2*(3), 5. https://doi.org/10.3390/sinusitis2030005

Syke, E.P., Harrison, R.V., Terrell, J.E., & Zao, D.H. (2018). *Guidelines for clinical care ambulatory: Acute rhinosinusitis in adults.* University of Michigan. https://www.med.umich.edu/1info/FHP/practiceguides/Rhino/rhino.pdf

CHAPTER 12

Stomatitis/Xerostomia

Karen A. Roesser, MSN, RN, AOCNS®

I. Definition: Diffuse ulcerative condition of oral mucosa most commonly occurring in non-keratinized cells (National Cancer Institute, 2016; Peterson et al., 2015; Villa et al., 2015)
  A. Mucositis: Inflammatory process involving the mucous membranes of the oral cavity and GI tract from the mouth to the anus; refers to process resulting from chemotherapy agents or ionizing radiation
  B. Xerostomia: Refers to dry mouth; may be related to qualitative and/or quantitative changes in the composition of saliva; may or may not accompany mucositis
  C. Stomatitis: Inflammatory condition of oral tissue including mucosa, dentition/periapices, and periodontium; includes infections of oral tissues as well as mucositis; should be used for oral complaints not related to chemotherapy agents or ionizing radiation (e.g., targeted agents)

II. Physiology/Pathophysiology (Al-Ansari et al., 2015; Maria et al., 2017; Sonis, 2009; Stringer & Logan, 2015; Villa & Sonis, 2016)
  A. Normal: The oral cavity is composed of rapidly dividing epithelial cells. Major salivary glands produce 90% of secretions.
  B. Pathophysiology
    1. A complex interaction between epithelia and connective tissue results in destruction of epithelial stem cells and interruption of epithelial renewal.
    2. Ulceration of the oral cavity occurs within five to seven days of chemotherapy drug administration and heals in approximately 7–10 days.
    3. With radiation therapy, the first clinical sign of mucositis can be observed after the patient has received 15 Gy (the second week of treatment) and reaches full severity at 30 Gy. After completion of treatment, mucositis will generally subside in two to four weeks but may last longer with extended radiation treatment protocols.
    4. Xerostomia (dryness of oral cavity) contributes to the development of stomatitis; radiation alters the amount of saliva and its buffering capacity.
    5. Five phases have been identified as leading to oral mucositis.
      a) Initiation: Generation of oxygen free radicals that damage DNA
      b) Upregulation (signaling): Activation of transcription factors
      c) Message generation: Message amplification and generation
      d) Ulceration: Bacterial colonization, inflammation, and pain
      e) Healing: Spontaneous recovery of mucosal tissue

III. Clinical features: The mouth is the most frequently documented source of infection in immunosuppressed patients. Stomatitis typically involves the labial and buccal mucosa and tongue with adjacent tissue appearing healthy. The cause of cancer treatment–induced stomatitis is poorly understood (Chaveli-López & Bagán-Sebastián, 2016; De Sanctis et al., 2016; NCI CTEP, 2017; Sibaud et al., 2017; Stringer & Logan, 2015).

A. Risk factors
   1. Chemotherapy
      a) Plant alkaloids
         (1) Docetaxel
         (2) Paclitaxel
      b) Antitumor antibiotics
         (1) Dactinomycin
         (2) Doxorubicin
         (3) Epirubicin
         (4) Idarubicin
      c) Antimetabolites
         (1) Capecitabine
         (2) Cytarabine
         (3) 5-Fluorouracil
         (4) Methotrexate
      d) Alkylating agents: In high doses
         (1) Cyclophosphamide
         (2) Melphalan
   2. Targeted therapy
      a) Mechanistic target of rapamycin (mTOR) inhibitors: Everolimus
      b) TKIs: EGFR inhibitors (e.g., erlotinib)
   3. Immunotherapy agents: PD-1/PD-L1 inhibitor therapy (e.g., nivolumab)
   4. Intensive systemic chemotherapy: Type, dose, and duration of therapy (e.g., bolus 5-fluorouracil more stomatotoxic than continuous infusion)
   5. Previous cancer treatment: Previous history of problems with mucositis
   6. Radiation therapy to oral cavity
   7. HSCT (allogeneic carries greater risk than autologous), GVHD
   8. Multimodal therapy: Combined chemotherapy and radiation therapy to the head and neck region
   9. Recent oral surgery
   10. Alteration in saliva production and composition
   11. Poor oral hygiene: Gingivitis, caries, periodontitis
   12. Genetic risk for mucositis: Genetic variants of difluoropyrimidine dehydrogenase, which influence development of stomatitis with 5-fluorouracil; increased sensitivity to oromucosal toxicity of methotrexate in patients with Down syndrome
   13. Health conditions that may increase risk: Psoriasis (presumably due to preexisting epithelial dysfunction), Addison disease (presumably due to preexisting inflammatory condition), diabetes mellitus (increased risk of denture stomatitis)
   14. Renal impairment and hepatic impairment: May delay elimination of anticancer treatments
   15. Smoking: Affects microcirculation and potentially delays healing
   16. Mucosal trauma: Ill-fitting dentures
   17. Chronic alcohol use: Affects mucosal atrophy and hyper-regeneration of the basal layer cells, thereby increasing susceptibility of the mucosa
   18. Dehydration
   19. Other factors: Age (increased risk in very young and old age), body size (increased risk in patients with low BMI), gender (females have worse stomatitis with 5-fluorouracil and methotrexate than males)

B. Etiology
   1. Poor nutritional status
   2. Poor oral hygiene
   3. Vitamin deficiency
   4. Infection: *Candida albicans*, *Streptococcus*, HSV, mononucleosis, Coxsackievirus
   5. Cancer therapy: Radiation, chemotherapy, targeted therapy, immunotherapy
C. History
   1. History of cancer and cancer treatment
   2. Current medications: Prescribed, over the counter
   3. History of presenting symptoms: Precipitating factors, onset, location, duration
   4. Changes in ADLs
   5. Past medical history: HIV, poor dentition
   6. Social history: Tobacco use, alcohol use
   7. History of nutritional intake: Current diet, weight loss, current oral hygiene practices
D. Signs and symptoms
   1. Erythema
   2. Ulceration
   3. Swelling
   4. Pale mucosa
   5. Xerostomia
   6. Fever
   7. Pain
   8. Dysphagia
   9. Hoarseness
   10. Difficulty speaking
   11. Abnormal taste sensation
   12. Difficulty in wearing dentures
   13. Change in consistency of saliva: Watery versus thick and ropy
   14. Burning sensation of oral cavity
E. Physical examination
   1. HEENT
      a) Removal of dentures and oral prostheses to visualize oral cavity
      b) Oral cavity condition and presence of lesions
         (1) Gray-white lesions with necrotic clusters are typical appearance of stomatitis.
         (2) Raised, white curd-like areas indicative of *C. albicans* are the most frequently observed fungal infection of the oral cavity.
         (3) Croppy, painful vesicular lesions with ulceration seen unilaterally and on the palate indicate herpes infection.
         (4) White, lacy keratotic lesions with erosive or painful bullous lesions are typical of the oral manifestations of GVHD.
         (5) Stomatitis associated with mTOR inhibitors is characterized by discrete, ovoid ulcers with characteristic erythematous halos and appears identical to idiopathic aphthous stomatitis in otherwise healthy individuals.
         (6) EGFR inhibitor–associated stomatitis is characterized by erythema, inflammation, or demarcated ulceration, such as aphthous-like lesions.
         (7) Immune checkpoint inhibitor therapy–associated toxicity has been associated with numerous discrete whitish raised papules, reticular streaks on lips, tongue, and buccal mucosa, and xerostomia.

       c) Presence, absence, and character of saliva

       d) Ease of swallowing

       e) Assessment tools: Assist in evaluating the grade of stomatitis (e.g., Common Terminology Criteria for Adverse Events)

    2. Lymph node: Cervical and submandibular lymph nodes palpation to evaluate for enlargement (see Appendix D)

IV. Diagnostic tests (Mortazavi et al., 2016)

    A. Laboratory

       1. CBC to assess for neutropenia

       2. Culture of oral lesions to identify organism

       3. Blood cultures if systemic sepsis is suspected or fever is present

       4. HSV antibody status

       5. HIV status, if indicated

    B. Radiology: Not indicated

V. Differential diagnosis (Mortazavi et al., 2016)

    A. Poor oral hygiene

    B. Kaposi sarcoma

    C. Infections: Candida, herpes, Coxsackievirus, syphilis, HIV

    D. Aphthous ulcers: Canker sores

    E. Trauma to oral mucosa

    F. Oral cancers: Squamous cell carcinoma

    G. Leukoplakia

    H. Reiter syndrome: Triad of symptoms—conjunctivitis, urethritis, and arthritis with oral, genital, or mucocutaneous lesions

    I. Behçet syndrome: Triad of symptoms—iritis, oral lesions, and genital lesions

    J. SLE (see Chapter 110)

    K. Acute GVHD

VI. Treatment: The goal of treatment is to prevent and/or minimize the oral consequences of cancer therapy (Al-Ansari et al., 2015; Chaveli-López & Bagán-Sebastián, 2016; Crimi et al., 2019; De Sanctis et al., 2016; Maria et al., 2017; NCCN, 2021; Pappas et al., 2016; Stringer & Logan, 2015).

    A. Thorough dental examination: Conduct prior to initiation of therapy.

       1. Caries or gum disease should be corrected.

       2. Necessary teeth extractions should occur with 10–14-day delay to start of treatment.

    B. Prophylactic basic oral hygiene

       1. Patients should brush teeth at least two times a day using a soft toothbrush. Toothbrush should be air dried before storing and replaced regularly.

       2. Toothbrush and foam oral swabs should be used during aplasia rather than replacing toothbrushes with oral swabs. Toothbrushes are necessary for adequate cleaning of the enamel surfaces of teeth, and oral swabs are beneficial for cleaning the mucous membranes during mucotoxic therapy.

       3. Bland mouth rinses include a diluted bicarbonate solution, which increases the local pH, making the mouth unfavorable to microbial growth; sodium chloride 0.9% for irrigation, which is used at least four to six times a day or more frequently; and a saline and sodium bicarbonate mixture, usually ¼ teaspoon each of salt and/or bicarbonate per cup of tap water.

       4. Patients should avoid harsh chemicals or irritants (e.g., alcohol-containing mouthwashes, irritating foods, alcohol, tobacco), as well as acidic, hot, rough, or spicy foods.

5. Water-based moisturizers can provide lip protection.
6. Soft, nutritious foods are preferred, and patients should limit sucrose intake.
7. Prostheses should be removed until healing occurs.
8. Prophylactic antivirals are included in some protocols (e.g., HSCT, multimodal), as HSV infection is implicated in stomatitis (see Appendix J).
   a) Prophylactic treatment should be targeted to specific high-risk patients. Dosage is acyclovir 400–800 mg PO two times a day.
   b) In non-HSCT, high-risk patients, prophylaxis should be administered to patients who are seropositive for HSV.
   c) In HSCT recipients, prophylaxis is only indicated if either the donor or recipient is seropositive for HSV.
9. Palifermin, a recombinant human keratinocyte growth factor, decreases the incidence and duration of severe oral mucositis in patients with hematologic malignancies receiving high-dose chemotherapy or total body irradiation followed by autologous HSCT. The dose is 60 mcg/kg IV daily three days prior to HSCT conditioning and is continued three days after transplantation.
10. Cryotherapy may be used to reduce stomatitis following IV bolus administration of 5-fluorouracil. This requires patients to hold ice chips in their mouth starting five minutes prior to beginning chemotherapy administration and continuing for up to 30 minutes after drug administration.
11. Dexamethasone mouthwash (0.1 mg/ml) is recommended for patients receiving mTOR inhibitors.
12. Low-level laser therapy (wavelength at 650 nm, power of 40 mW, and each square centimeter treated with the required time to a tissue energy dose of 2 J/cm^2) may reduce oral mucositis in patients receiving high-dose chemotherapy with or without total body irradiation before autologous HSCT and may also be used in patients with head and neck cancer who are receiving radiation therapy without concomitant chemotherapy.
13. Benzydamine mouthwash is recommended in patients with head and neck cancer receiving moderate-dose radiation therapy (up to 50 Gy).

C. Pain management: All treatments listed can be used before meals and at bedtime.
   1. Lidocaine rinses are given at 5–15 ml and swished and expectorated.
   2. Systemic analgesics may be indicated, including the use of patient-controlled analgesia with morphine or hydromorphone or the use of fentanyl (see Appendix F).
   3. The use of a special "magic mouthwash" consisting of diphenhydramine, aluminum hydroxide, magnesium hydroxide, and viscous lidocaine (15–30 ml; swished and swallowed) is not recommended in the prevention or treatment of mucositis.

D. Xerostomia management
   1. Artificial saliva
   2. Sucrose-free lemon drops
   3. Frequent intake of fluids: 2 liters a day (eight 8 oz glasses)
   4. Water-based moisturizers to protect lips
   5. Pilocarpine: 5–10 mg PO three times a day for at least three months to stimulate salivary flow during radiation treatment; should be used with caution in patients with cardiovascular disease
   6. Cevimeline: 30 mg PO three times a day for at least three months
   7. Sugarless gum

E. Infection
   1. Candidiasis: Treatment is for seven days or until tests indicate that active fungal infection has subsided.

       a) Nystatin oral suspension: 400,000–600,000 units (4–6 ml) swished and swallowed four times a day and continued for at least 48 hours after symptoms resolve

       b) Fluconazole

          (1) Oropharyngeal candidiasis: Fluconazole 100–200 mg PO daily for 7–14 days for moderate to severe cases

          (2) Esophageal candidiasis: 200–400 mg PO daily for 14–21 days

          (3) Monitoring for drug–drug interactions

       c) Clotrimazole: One lozenge (i.e., troche) four to five times a day, dissolved slowly in mouth, and continued for at least 48 hours after symptoms resolve

    2. HSV infections in immunocompetent patients: Famciclovir 250 mg PO three times a day for 7–10 days, or valacyclovir 1 g PO three times a day, or acyclovir 5 mg/kg IV every eight hours for 7–10 days or until lesions crust over

       a) Recurrent episodes: Beginning when prodrome occurs or within two days of onset of lesion; acyclovir 200 mg PO five times a day or 800 mg PO two times a day for five days

       b) Suppressive therapy, as warranted: Acyclovir 200 mg PO two to five times a day for one year or 400 mg two times a day for one year; therapy individualized to patient circumstances or per institution

    3. If bacterial infection is suspected, consider coverage with amoxicillin/clavulanate (if not penicillin allergic) 875 mg PO two times a day for 10 days.

    4. Keep oral cavity clean by rinsing with saline solution four to six times a day or more often (1 L saline with 1 teaspoon bicarbonate of soda; swished and expectorated).

  F. Complementary therapies

    1. Meditation

    2. Relaxation

    3. Acupuncture

VII. Follow-up

  A. During the acute phase of stomatitis, inspect the oral cavity at least once a day.

  B. Carefully follow patients who have had stomatitis, particularly with HSV infection, when subsequent treatment begins, as viral reactivation is possible.

  C. Patients should report a history of stomatitis and oral cavity irradiation to their dentist, as subsequent dental work may require antibiotic prophylaxis if permanent dryness or changes in the oral cavity exist.

VIII. Referrals

  A. Dentist: To evaluate for dental caries or other dental concerns

  B. Dietitian: To maintain adequate food and fluid intake

References

Al-Ansari, S., Zecha, J.A.E.M., Barasch, A., de Lange, J., Rozema, F.R., & Raber-Durlacher, J.E. (2015). Oral mucositis induced by anticancer therapies. *Current Oral Health Reports, 2*(4), 202–211. https://doi.org/10.1007/s40496-015-0069-4

Chaveli-López, B., & Bagán-Sebastián, J.V. (2016). Treatment of oral mucositis due to chemotherapy. *Journal of Clinical and Experimental Dentistry, 8*(2), e201–e209. https://doi.org/10.4317/jced.52917

Crimi, S., Fiorillo, L., Bianchi, A., D'Amico, C., Amoroso, G., Gorassini, F., ... Cicciu, M. (2019). Herpes virus, oral clinical signs and QOL: Systematic review of recent data. *Viruses, 11*(5), E463. https://doi.org/10.3390/v11050463

De Sanctis, V., Bossi, P., Sanguineti, G., Trippa, F., Ferrari, D., Bacigalupo, A., ... Lalla, R.V. (2016). Mucositis in head and neck cancer patients treated with radiotherapy and systemic therapies: Literature review and consensus statements. *Critical Reviews in Oncology/Hematology, 100,* 147–166. https://doi.org/10.1016/j.critrevonc.2016.01.010

Maria, O.M., Eliopoulos, N., & Muanza, T. (2017). Radiation-induced oral mucositis. *Frontiers in Oncology, 7,* 89. https://doi.org/10.3389/fonc.2017.00089

Mortazavi, H., Safi, Y., Baharvand, M., & Rahmani, S. (2016). Diagnostic features of common oral ulcerative lesions: An updated decision tree. *International Journal of Dentistry, 2016,* 7278925. https://doi.org/10.1155/2016/7278925

National Cancer Institute. (2016). Oral complications of chemotherapy and head/neck radiation (PDQ®) [Health professional version]. https://www.cancer.gov/about-cancer/treatment/side-effects/mouth-throat/oral-complications-hp-pdq

National Cancer Institute Cancer Therapy Evaluation Program. (2017). *Common terminology criteria for adverse events* [v. 5.0]. https://ctep.cancer.gov/protocoldevelopment/electronic_applications/docs/CTCAE_v5_Quick_Reference_8.5x11.pdf

National Comprehensive Cancer Network. (2021). *NCCN Clinical Practice Guidelines in Oncology (NCCN Guidelines®): Prevention and treatment of cancer-related infections* [v.1.2021]. https://www.nccn.org/professionals/physician_gls/pdf/infections.pdf

Pappas, P.G., Kauffman, C.A., Andes, D.R., Clancy, C.J., Marr, K.A., Ostrosky-Zeichner, L., … Sobel, J.D. (2016). Executive summary: Clinical practice guideline for the management of candidiasis: 2016 update by the Infectious Diseases Society of America. *Clinical Infectious Diseases, 62*(4), 409–417. https://doi.org/10.1093/cid/civ1194

Peterson, D.E., Boers-Doets, C.B., Bensadoun, R.J., & Herrstedt, J. (2015). Management of oral and gastrointestinal mucosal injury: ESMO clinical practice guidelines for diagnosis, treatment, and follow-up. *Annals of Oncology, 26*(Suppl. 5), v139–v151. https://doi.org/10.1093/annonc/mdv202

Sibaud, V., Eid, C., Belum, V.R., Combemale, P., Barres, B., Lamant, L., … Lacouture, M.E. (2017). Oral lichenoid reactions associated with anti-PD1/PD-L1 therapies: Clinicopathological findings. *Journal of the European Academy of Dermatology and Venereology, 31*(10), e464–e469. https://doi.org/10.1111/jdv.14284

Sonis, S.T. (2009). Mucositis: The impact, biology and therapeutic opportunities. *Oral Oncology, 45*(12), 1015–1020. https://doi.org/10.1016/j.oraloncology.2009.08.006

Stringer, A.M., & Logan, R.M. (2015). The role of oral flora in the development of chemotherapy-induced oral mucositis. *Journal of Oral Pathology and Medicine, 44*(2), 81–87. https://doi.org/10.1111/jop.12152

Villa, A., Connell, C., & Abati, S. (2015). Diagnosis and management of xerostomia and hyposalivation. *Therapeutics and Clinical Risk Management, 11,* 45–51. https://doi.org/10.2147/TCRM.S76282

Villa, A., & Sonis, S.T. (2016). Pharmacotherapy for the management of cancer regimen-related oral mucositis. *Expert Opinion on Pharmacotherapy, 17*(13), 1801–1807. https://doi.org/10.1080/14656566.2016.1217993

Integument

CHAPTER 13

Hyperpigmentation

Jeanne Held-Warmkessel, MSN, RN, AOCN®, ACNS-BC

I. Definition: Darkening of the skin, mucous membranes, or nails; may be localized or diffuse (Meys, 2017)

II. Physiology/Pathophysiology (Cestari et al., 2014; Di Tullio et al., 2018; Kanlayavattanakul & Lourith, 2018; Nicolaidou & Katsambas, 2014; Noori et al., 2017; Pillaiyar et al., 2017; Schalka, 2017; Speeckaert et al., 2014; Wu et al., 2016)
   A. Normal
      1. Normal pigmentation is derived from endogenous sources, including amino acids, melanin, and blood proteins.
      2. Multiple transcription factors are involved in pigment signaling pathways.
      3. Melanin accumulates in keratinocytes of the skin and retina in response to exposure to sunlight.
      4. Melanin protects the skin from the damage of sun exposure by trapping the injurious free radicals produced by the action of ultraviolet light on the skin.
   B. Pathophysiology
      1. Hyperpigmentation develops because of the following.
         a) Increased rate of melanin production and deposition
         b) Increased amount of melanosome transferred to keratinocytes
         c) Increased size and melanization of the melanosome, or when the pigment is deposited in anomalous sites
         d) Increased melanocyte size or activity
         e) Increased number of melanocytes
      2. Mechanisms that produce hyperpigmentation include the following.
         a) Elevated adrenocorticotropic hormone: Stimulates melanocytes
         b) Direct stimulation of melanocytes
         c) Inflammatory changes: Stimulates melanin formation, possibly from cytokines
         d) Drug induced (e.g., chemotherapy, antimalarials, tetracyclines, heavy metal therapy): Induces pigmentation through an increased deposit of melanin in the skin and mucous membranes; reduces melanin clearance
         e) Cytotoxic agents: Increases pigmentation by a direct stimulatory or toxic effect on melanocytes, by slowing the turnover rate of epithelial cells thereby allowing more time for the transfer of melanin to occur, or by affecting the blood vessel endothelium
         f) Targeted therapies (e.g., imatinib): Increases melanin production from melanocyte stimulation and causes melanotic macules
         g) Melanocyte-stimulating hormone receptors: Increases in oral cavity and skin hyperpigmentation

      h) Tumor mediated: Releases hormones or cytokines

      i) Ultraviolet (UV) exposure: Increases melanocortin in melanocytes and keratinocytes

III. Clinical features: Hyperpigmentation is a common, usually harmless condition in which patches of skin or nails become discolored or darker in color than the surrounding skin. Hyperpigmentation can occur from many different conditions (Di Tullio et al., 2018; Kutlubay et al., 2015; Meys, 2017; Nicolaidou & Katsambas, 2014; Noori et al., 2017).

  A. Etiology

    1. Drug induced

    2. Autoimmune disease

    3. Nutritional deficits

    4. Systemic disease

  B. History

    1. History of cancer and cancer treatment

    2. Current medications: Prescribed, over the counter, oral contraceptives

    3. History of presenting symptoms: Precipitating factors, onset, location, duration, sudden onset of seborrheic keratoses (may be malignancy associated)

    4. Changes in ADLs

    5. Past medical history: Skin problems, adrenal insufficiency, thyroid or liver disease, inflammation

    6. Sun exposure history

    7. Family history: Familial cancer syndromes

  C. Signs and symptoms

    1. Diffuse melanosis: Generalized darkening of the skin that is evenly distributed

    2. Local area of pigmentation

    3. Circumscribed

      a) Actinic keratosis: Flattened papule, dry, tan, or gray

      b) Actinic or solar lentigines: Macule on the dorsum of the hand and/or wrist; often termed *liver spots*

      c) Chloasma or melasma: Nonuniform, hyperpigmented flat spots seen on the face, often on the forehead, cheeks, chin, and upper lip

      d) Nevus: Slightly elevated, round, evenly pigmented

      e) Nodules: Deep, firm, raised lesion greater than 0.5 cm

      f) Ochronosis: Bluish-black or brown pigmented area of the sclerae, ears, skin, or nails

      g) Tinea pityriasis versicolor: Patchy, yellow-brown pigmented area over the trunk

    4. Reticulate: Net-like pattern of hyperpigmentation

    5. Serpentine: Hyperpigmentation of skin overlying the peripheral veins used for chemotherapy administration

  D. Physical examination

    1. Integument

      a) Skin and scalp: Assessment for color, moisture, temperature, texture, mobility, and turgor

      b) Lesions: Location, onset, size, color, border, distribution

      c) Specifics of skin

        (1) Increased carotene ingestion: Orange tone

        (2) GVHD: Acral erythema

        (3) Hepatic insufficiency: Jaundice

        (4) Porphyria cutanea: Diffuse hyperpigmentation

(5) Scleroderma: Thick, tight skin
(6) Acanthosis nigricans: Velvety pigmented patches in flexures on the neck, axillae, and groin
   (a) Multiple types
   (b) May be malignancy associated and may precede, follow, or most often, occur with the diagnosis
   (c) Other types: Benign in origin, as well as from obesity and insulin resistance
(7) Neurofibromatosis: Freckling, brown spots on skin
(8) Chemotherapy-induced pigmentation
   (a) Generalized hyperpigmentation
   (b) Localized patterns of hyperpigmentation
   (c) Mucosal pigmentation
(9) Targeted therapy–induced hyperpigmentation: Imatinib resulting in hyperpigmentation of the hard palate, oral mucosa, skin, and nails
2. Nails: Assessment for color, shape, and lesions
3. Oral mucosa: Mucous membrane for color, moisture, and lesions
4. Eyes: Conjunctivae for increase of pigmentation

IV. Diagnostic tests
   A. Laboratory
      1. Usually not indicated
      2. Biopsy of areas suspicious for malignancy, infection, and skin disorders or when an accurate diagnosis is needed to determine therapy
   B. Radiology: Usually not indicated

V. Differential diagnosis (Cestari et al., 2014; Lee, 2015; Meys, 2017; Nicolaidou & Katsambas, 2014; Noori et al., 2017; Sardon & Dempsey, 2017; Speeckaert et al., 2014; Wu et al., 2016)
   A. Genetic factors
      1. Melasma (chloasma): This condition is especially associated with chronic UV exposure, female sex hormones, and inflammation.
      2. Wilson disease: Skin manifestations include acanthosis nigricans.
      3. Peutz-Jeghers syndrome: This genetic disorder is characterized by mucocutaneous pigmented macules/spots causing patches of hyperpigmentation in the mouth and on the hands and feet. This syndrome carries a high risk of developing GI and pancreatic cancer.
      4. McCune-Albright syndrome: This genetic disorder is characterized by bone, skin, and hormonal problems, along with premature puberty. Café-au-lait skin pigmentation develops unilaterally on the body.
   B. Endocrine
      1. Addison disease: Hyperpigmentation of creases, pressure areas, and nipples
      2. Hypothyroidism (see Chapter 158)
      3. Pregnancy
      4. Use of oral contraceptives
      5. Primary adrenal insufficiency
      6. Nelson syndrome
      7. Cushing syndrome
      8. Polycystic ovary syndrome
      9. Acromegaly
   C. Metabolic

    1. Biliary cirrhosis (see Chapter 69)

    2. Gaucher disease

    3. Hemosiderosis

    4. Ochronosis

    5. Obesity related

    6. Diabetes related (see Chapter 151)

D. Nutritional

    1. Excessive carotene ingestion

    2. Folate deficiency (see Chapter 116)

    3. Malabsorption

    4. Pellagra: Niacin (vitamin B_3) deficiency

    5. Vitamin B_{12} deficiency (see Chapter 115)

E. Systemic

    1. GVHD

    2. Hemochromatosis (see Chapter 121)

    3. Hepatic insufficiency

    4. Porphyria cutanea tarda

    5. RA (see Chapter 108)

    6. Scleroderma

    7. Acanthosis nigricans: May be associated with diabetes, endocrine disorders, and malignancies

    8. Progressive systemic sclerosis

F. Malignancy associated/paraneoplastic

    1. Adrenocorticotropic hormone–producing tumors, melanocyte-stimulating hormone–producing tumors, pheochromocytoma

    2. Carcinoid syndrome

    3. Cutaneous malignancies, melanoma

    4. Neurofibromatosis

    5. Multicentric Castleman disease

    6. GI tract cancer

    7. Hodgkin lymphoma

    8. Sign of Leser-Trélat: Sudden increase in number and size of seborrheic keratosis indicating an internal malignancy

G. Medications

    1. Chemotherapy (single agent and combination therapy) and targeted therapy: Bleomycin, busulfan, cisplatin, cyclophosphamide, dacarbazine, dactinomycin, daunorubicin, doxorubicin, 5-fluorouracil, hydroxyurea, 6-mercaptopurine, mitomycin, methotrexate, pemetrexed, thiotepa, vinblastine, vinorelbine

    2. Topical benzoyl peroxide

    3. Tretinoin

    4. Multiple nonantineoplastic agents: NSAIDs, amiodarone, antibiotics, antimalarials, anticonvulsants

H. Radiation: Acute and late effects; UV radiation (UV exposure)

I. Aging

J. Vascular: Chronic venous insufficiency

K. Postinflammation hyperpigmentation: Common; area of prior inflammation becomes hyperpigmented.

L. Infection: Whipple disease (*Tropheryma whipplei*), leishmaniasis

M. Metal exposure: Arsenic

N. New malignancy: Melanoma

VI. Treatment (Cestari et al., 2014; Chaowattanapanit et al., 2017; Hexsel et al., 2015; Kanlaya-vattanakul & Lourith, 2018; Kwon et al., 2016; Meys, 2017; Nicolaidou & Katsambas, 2014; Plensdorf et al., 2017)

 A. Treatment usually is not necessary.

 B. Hyperpigmentation may or may not be reversible and often is permanent after the patient undergoes radiation therapy. Chemotherapy-induced hyperpigmentation usually resolves several months after treatment or when nail grows.

 C. Patients should be reassured that these changes are an adverse effect of the treatment and not progression of disease.

 D. Makeup for pigmented facial spots may minimize the appearance of lesions.

 E. Melasma management

 1. Bleaching preparations consisting of hydroquinone cream may lighten the lesion if the pigment is in the epidermis but can be irritating to the skin.

 2. Triple combination products of tretinoin (0.05%; an antiwrinkle and hypopigmentation agent) or retinoic acid (0.05%), with hydroquinone cream (4%), and fluocinolone acetonide (0.01%) in a hydrophilic cream/ointment can be used to lighten the lesion but can be irritating to the skin.

 3. Excessive pigmented lesions can be minimized with mid-depth trichloroacetic acid, glycolic acid chemical peels, or laser or light therapies.

 4. Causative medication should be discontinued, if applicable.

 F. Postinflammatory hyperpigmentation: Topical hydroquinone and tretinoin, either alone or together; glycolic acid or salicylic acid peels; topical hydroquinone, retinoic acid, and corticosteroid cream

 G. Solar lentigines: Mequinol (2%) and tretinoin (0.01%) cream

 H. Patient education

 1. Avoid sun exposure, UV light, photosensitizers, trauma to the skin, and radiation.

 2. Protect skin with hats, clothing, and sunscreen with SPF 30 and higher with UVA/UVB protection. Physical and visible light-blocking agents should be used for both prevention and management of hyperpigmentation.

 3. Soy-based topical products (e.g., creams, lotions) may be useful.

 4. Multiple cosmetic companies have products available for the face/neck to manage hyperpigmentation appearance.

VII. Follow-up: Periodic evaluation of the skin should be performed at consecutive visits. Monitor for change in appearance of skin lesions.

VIII. Referrals: Patients with any skin lesion suspicious of malignancy should undergo biopsy and be referred to a dermatologist. Patients interested in laser or light therapy should also see a dermatologist.

References

Cestari, T.F., Dantas, L.P., & Boza, J.C. (2014). Acquired hyperpigmentation. *Anais Brasileiros de Dermatologia, 89*(1), 11–25. https://doi.org/10.1590/abd1806-4841.20142353

Chaowattanapanit, S., Silpa-archa, N., Kohli, I., Lim, H.W., & Hamzavi, I. (2017). Postinflammatory hyperpigmentation: A comprehensive overview: Treatment options and prevention. *Journal of the American Academy of Dermatology, 77*(4), 607–621. https://doi.org/10.1016/j.jaad.2017.01.036

Di Tullio, F., Mandel, V.D., Scotti, R., Padalino, C., & Pellacani, G. (2018). Imatinib-induced diffuse hyperpigmentation of the oral mucosa, the skin, and the nails in the patient affected by chronic myeloid leukemia: Report of a case and review of the literature. *International Journal of Dermatology, 57*(7), 784–790. https://doi.org/10.1111/ijd.13931

Hexsel, D., Hexsel, C., Porto, M.D., & Siega, C. (2015). Triple combination as adjuvant to cryotherapy in the treatment of solar lentigines: Investigator-blinded, randomized clinical trial. *European Academy of Dermatology and Venerology, 29*(1), 129–133. https://doi.org/10.1111/jdv.12484

Kanlayavattanakul, M., & Lourith, N. (2018). Plants and natural products for the treatment of skin hyperpigmentation—A review. *Planta Medica, 84*(14), 988–1006. https://doi.org/10.1055/a-0583-0410

Kutlubay, Z., Engin, B., Bairamov, O., & Tüzün, Y. (2015). Acanthosis nigricans: A fold (intertriginous dermatosis). *Clinics in Dermatology, 33*(4), 466–470. https://doi.org/10.1016/j.clindermatol.2015.04.010

Kwon, S.-H., Hwang, Y.-J., Lee, S.-K., & Park, K.C. (2016). Heterogeneous pathology of melasma and its clinical implications. *International Journal of Molecular Sciences, 17*(6), 824. https://doi.org/10.3390/ijms17060824

Lee, A.-Y. (2015). Recent progress in melasma pathogenesis. *Pigment Cell and Melanoma Research, 28*(6), 648–660. https://doi.org/10.1111/pcmr.12404

Meys, R. (2017). Skin pigmentation. *Medicine, 45*(7), 438–442. https://doi.org/10.1016/j.mpmed.2017.04.011

Nicolaidou, E., & Katsambas, A.D. (2014). Pigmentation disorders: Hyperpigmentation and hypopigmentation. *Clinics in Dermatology, 32*(1), 66–72. https://doi.org/10.1016/j.clindermatol.2013.05.026

Noori, M., Hunter-Ellul, L., & Kelly, B. (2017). Serpentine supravenous hyperpigmentation following cisplatin and pemetrexed chemotherapy. *Cutis, 99*(4), E20–E22. https://www.mdedge.com/dermatology/article/137206/pigmentation-disorders/serpentine-supravenous-hyperpigmentation-following

Pillaiyar, T., Manickam, M., & Jung, S.-H. (2017). Downregulation and melanogenesis: Drug discovery and therapeutic options. *Drug Discovery Today, 22*(2), 282–298. https://doi.org/10.1016/j.drudis.2016.09.016

Plensdorf, S., Livieratos, M., & Dada, N. (2017). Pigmentation disorders: Diagnosis and management. *American Family Physician, 96*(12), 797–804. https://www.aafp.org/afp/2017/1215/p797.html

Sardon, C., & Dempsey, T. (2017). The Leser-Trélat sign. *Cleveland Clinic Journal of Medicine, 84*(12), 918. https://doi.org/10.3949/ccjm.84a.17021

Schalka, S. (2017). New data on hyperpigmentation disorders. *Journal of the European Academy of Dermatology and Venerology, 31*(Suppl. 5), 18–21. https://doi.org/10.1111/jdv.14411

Speeckaert, R., Van Gale, M., Speeckaert, M.M., Lambert, J., & van Geel, N. (2014). The biology of hyperpigmentation syndromes. *Pigment Cell and Melanoma Research, 27*(4), 512–524. https://doi.org/10.1111/pcmr.12235

Wu, F., Su, C., Liu, L., & Xu, J. (2016). Hyperpigmentation in palms associated with lung adenocarcinoma resolving after chemotherapy. *Clinical Respiratory Journal, 10*(3), 368–370. https://doi.org/10.1111/crj.12226

CHAPTER 14

Nail Changes

Tracy C. Wyant, DNP, AOCN®, CHPN, GERO-BC, CPPS, EBP-C

I. Definition: Alterations in the nail unit or nail beds (Baran et al., 2014)

II. Physiology/Pathophysiology (Baran et al., 2014; Dunne et al., 2015; Lacouture & Sibaud, 2018; Maddy & Tosti, 2018; Matthews et al., 2020; Murdan, 2016; Robert et al., 2015; Zawar et al., 2019)

   A. Normal
      1. The nail protects the terminal phalanx and aids in perception of fine touch and the ability to perform motor skills such as to pick, lift, and scratch.
      2. The nail unit consists of the nail plate and epithelial tissues and is supported by the distal phalanx of each finger and toe.
      3. The nail plate is composed of keratin and is attached to and receives nutrients from the vascular nail bed. The blood supply originates from two main arterial arches, which are branches of the digital arteries.
      4. The nail root is the living nail layer. The root lies under the proximal nail fold and extends out to form the lunula (white moon).
      5. Cuticles form a seal between the nail fold and the plate, protecting this space from external moisture. The plate side is covered by the lateral nail fold.
      6. The nail apparatus consists of a horny dead product, the nail plate, and four specialized epithelial structures: the proximal nail fold, the nail matrix, the nail bed, and the hyponychium.
      7. Chemical composition shows that a normal nail contains approximately 18% water.
      8. Nail plate grows continuously from the nail root or matrix at a rate of 3 mm for fingernails and 1 mm for toenails per month. Growth decreases with age; after approximately 25 years, the rate tends to decrease by approximately 0.5% per year.

   B. Pathophysiology
      1. Pigmentary changes (e.g., hyperpigmentation) are caused by the absence of melanin or an increased, decreased, or altered distribution of melanin.
      2. Cytotoxic agents are toxic to the mitotically active cells of the nail matrix, which cease growing or have incomplete formation of the nail plate, leading to Beau lines or other alterations.
      3. EGFR agents penetrate the nail plate, leading to periungual inflammation in the fingers and toes.
      4. Disruption of the differentiation of nail keratinocytes can produce an abnormal nail plate.
      5. Nail changes are common with aging, as calcium content increases and iron content decreases in the nail.
         a) Keratinocytes of the nail plate increase in size with aging.

    b) Nail bed dermis shows thickening of the blood vessels and elastic tissue with aging.

   6. Infection of nails can alter the nail fold, nail matrix, nail bed, or hyponychium.

    a) Bacterial growth from *Staphylococcus aureus* is the most common.

    b) Fungal (dermatophytes) and yeast growth also can occur.

III. Clinical features: Nail changes can occur in many local or systemic disorders. Assessment should begin early and continue regularly. Changes should be correlated with other clinical findings. Clinical presentation varies depending on which nail structure is affected and the severity of insult. Nail changes may involve some or all nails. Changes may be asymptomatic and limited to cosmetic concerns; however, severe effects can cause pain and discomfort. Onychomycosis is the most frequently diagnosed nail condition (Baran et al., 2014; Charles et al., 2016; Dunne et al., 2015; Gupta & Stec, 2019; Lacouture & Sibaud, 2018; Lipner et al., 2021; Matthews et al., 2020; McFarlane et al., 2020; Robert et al., 2015; Sibaud, 2018; Zawar et al., 2019).

  A. Etiology: Similar nail changes may occur in different conditions because the nails have a limited response capability.

    1. Trauma to nail

    2. Infection

    3. Dermatologic disease or disorder

    4. Systemic disease

    5. Paraneoplastic syndrome

    6. Medications

    7. Nutritional deficiencies: Kwashiorkor; marasmus; iron, calcium, or vitamin deficiencies

    8. Impaired circulation of the distal extremities

  B. History

    1. History of cancer and cancer treatment

    2. Current medications: Prescribed, over the counter, supplements

    3. History of presenting symptoms: Precipitating factors, onset, location, duration, frequency

    4. Changes in ADLs: Family/social roles, effects on QOL

    5. Past medical history of recent trauma or chemical contact to the nails or frequent wetting of the nails

  C. Signs and symptoms

    1. Painful or cold fingers/toes

    2. Discoloration of fingers/toes

    3. Inflammation, markings, and other changes in nail bed

    4. Hyperpigmentation

    5. Slowed nail growth rate

  D. Physical examination: Inspect and palpate nails, noting color, shape, and lesions. Inspect tissue surrounding the nail for erythema or swelling.

    1. Beau lines: Transverse linear depression of the nails emerging from under the proximal nail folds growing out with the nails; usually follows one month after an acute illness or associated with chronic alcoholism, protein deficiency, or MI

    2. Brittle dry nails: Split or break easily indicating nutritional deficiencies, anorexia, advanced age, drug-induced changes, or thyroid disorders

    3. Clubbing: Rounded and bulbous distal phalanx; convex nail plate; angle between distal phalanx and nail bed greater than 180° possibly associated with tobacco use or iodine deficiency

4. Ridging: Normal finding with advanced age, with color varying from yellow to gray
5. Discoloration: Typically drug induced
6. Hyperpigmentation bands: Dark brown or blue transverse lines across nail plate associated with vitamin deficiency or drug-induced changes
7. Koilonychia (spoon nail): Concave malformation of outer surface of the nail indicating chronic anemia or iron-deficiency anemia
8. Leukonychia: White spots that grow out with the nail associated with hypoalbuminemia, calcium deficiency, or vitamin deficiency
9. Subungual hematoma: Painful red subungual discoloration typically from trauma; discoloration suggestive of melanocytic lesion
10. Mees lines: Transverse white lines emerging from the proximal nail folds that grow out with the nail without palpable ridges; may indicate heart failure, Hodgkin lymphoma, or renal failure
11. Nail atrophy or dystrophy: Observed in malabsorption syndromes
12. Onychauxis: Thickened nail plates seen in older adults normally; could indicate infection or drug-induced changes
13. Onycholysis: Distal separation of the nail plate from the nail bed suggestive of iron deficiency, drug-induced changes, infection, or thyroid disorders
14. Paronychia: Inflammation and erythema of the proximal and lateral nail folds suggestive of bacterial or fungal infection; can mimic ingrown nails
15. Pitting: Small pits in the nail indicative of drug-induced changes, psoriasis, or sarcoidosis
16. Splinter hemorrhages: Thin, longitudinal red or brown bands seen in endocarditis, SLE, renal failure, or cirrhosis
17. Subungual or periungual lesions: Growth of tissue under or within the nail indicative of melanoma
18. Terry nails: White with a distal band of reddish brown; nonvisible lunula indicative of malnutrition
19. Yellow nail syndrome: Nail yellowing and ceasing growth indicative of liver disease, diabetes, or respiratory disease
20. Fissured nails and impaired nail growth: Noted in marasmus
21. Onychorrhexis: Longitudinal splitting that begins at the free edge and extends proximally; indicative of malnutrition, iron deficiency, or calcium deficiency
22. Onychoschizia: Lamellar peeling of the free edge of the nail plate seen in malnutrition
23. Onychocryptosis: Ingrown toenail; penetrates the adjacent lateral nail fold secondary to nail plate over curvature, inflamed lateral nail fold

IV. Diagnostic tests: Not necessary for treatment-related nail changes (Alessandrini et al., 2017; Baran et al., 2014; Dunne et al., 2015; Matthews et al., 2020; Robert et al., 2015)
   A. Laboratory
      1. CBC to evaluate for anemia
      2. ESR to evaluate for inflammatory process
      3. Serum iron and iron-binding capacity to detect iron-deficiency anemia
      4. Culture of nail or surrounding tissue for fungus or bacteria
      5. Biopsy of nail or surrounding tissue if malignancy is suspected
      6. Potassium hydroxide examination of scrapings to evaluate for onychomycosis
      7. Vitamin levels to detect deficiencies, such as D or B
   B. Radiology: Chest x-ray to evaluate clubbing from cardiopulmonary disorders or lung cancer
   C. Other: Dermoscopy to evaluate nail plate surface

V. Differential diagnosis: Comorbid conditions should be considered. Nail changes must be correlated with other findings to accurately diagnose (Alessandrini et al., 2017; Baran et al., 2014; Dunne et al., 2015; Gupta & Stec, 2019; Lacouture & Sibaud, 2018; Matthews et al., 2020; McFarlane et al., 2020; Robert et al., 2015; Sibaud, 2018).

A. Medication-induced nail changes can vary.
   1. Antimalarials: Blue-gray to yellow discoloration
   2. Antibiotics
      a) Demethylchlortetracycline and doxycycline may cause painful photo-onycholysis and yellow pigmentation.
      b) Cloxacillin and cephaloridine may cause temporary nail loss.
   3. Arsenic, thallium, or fluoride: Transverse white lines
   4. Beta-blockers
      a) Practolol: Psoriasiform nail dystrophy, onycholysis, subungual hyperkeratosis
      b) Propranolol: Psoriasiform eruptions with thickening, pitting, and discoloration of nails
      c) Metoprolol: Beau lines
      d) Timolol maleate eye drops: Pigmentation
   5. Chemotherapy, targeted therapy, and immunotherapy
      a) Antiangiogenic multikinase inhibitors (e.g., sorafenib, sunitinib): Subungual hemorrhage
      b) Bleomycin: Nail loss and dark pigmentation
      c) Capecitabine: Hyperpigmentation
      d) Cyclophosphamide: Hyperpigmentation, transverse ridging
      e) Dacarbazine and daunorubicin: Hyperpigmentation, onycholysis
      f) Doxorubicin: Hyperpigmentation of nail beds, paronychia, dermal creases
      g) 5-Fluorouracil: Nail loss, brittleness, cracking, separation, pigmentation
      h) EGFR inhibitors, such as TKIs (e.g., erlotinib, gefitinib, dacomitinib) and monoclonal antibodies (e.g., cetuximab, necitumumab, panitumumab): Hyperpigmentation, paronychia, onychodystrophy
      i) Hydroxyurea: Longitudinal pigmented nail bands, pigmentation
      j) Idarubicin: Transverse pigmented bands, hyperpigmentation
      k) Ifosfamide: Nail ridging
      l) Melphalan, mechlorethamine, methotrexate, and mitomycin: Hyperpigmentation and dark half-circles
      m) Mitoxantrone: Onycholysis
      n) Taxanes: Darkening of nail, brittleness
B. Infection
   1. Candidiasis: Onycholysis invading the superficial aspect of the undersurface of the nail along the distal and lateral borders
   2. Onychomycosis: Distal subungual, proximal subungual, or white superficial
   3. HIV: Hyperpigmentation, transverse and longitudinal ridging
   4. Paronychia: Redness, swelling, and tenderness at the lateral fold
   5. Tinea unguium: Hyperkeratosis at the lateral or distal margin of the plate progressing to fragmentation of the nail plate
C. Benign growths
   1. Warts, periungual fibroma: Fibrous tissue growing from the lateral nail fold
   2. Subungual exostosis: Firm swelling of the great toe below the nail tip, displacing the nail
   3. Pigmented nevus: Longitudinal band of pigment in nail plate caused by junctional nevus in matrix

D. Malignancy associated
1. Epithelioma: Chronic paronychia
2. Melanoma
3. Kaposi sarcoma
4. Squamous cell carcinoma
5. Bronchopulmonary cancer clubbing
E. Nail changes associated with systemic disease and comorbidities
1. Vitamin B_{12} deficiency: Digital and nail pigmentation (see Chapter 115)
2. Digital artery insufficiency: Permanent loss of nail in a single digit
3. Diabetes mellitus (see Chapter 151)
4. Cardiovascular or pulmonary disease: Clubbing, cyanosis
5. Chronic anemia: Brittle, spooning (see Chapter 113)
6. Endocarditis: Splinter hemorrhages (see Chapter 46)
7. Hyperparathyroidism: Nail dystrophy, onycholysis
8. Hyper/hypothyroidism: Brittleness, onycholysis (see Chapters 157 and 158)
9. Hypopituitarism: Dystrophy, loss of lunula, spooning
10. Peripheral neuropathy: Nail dystrophy (see Chapter 143)
11. Raynaud phenomenon: Longitudinal ridging, nail splitting, koilonychia, onycholysis, sclerodactyly
12. Arthritis: Rheumatoid—ridging and beading (see Chapter 108)
13. Scleroderma: Partial or total loss of nail, sclerodactyly
14. SLE: Clubbing, splinter hemorrhage, nail fold infarcts, onycholysis, pitting, ridging, sclerodactyly (see Chapter 110)
15. Febrile illness: Beau lines
16. MI: Beau lines (see Chapter 49)
17. Psoriasis: Irregular large and deep nail pits
18. Renal failure: Splinter hemorrhages, hyperkeratosis, onychomycosis (see Chapter 86)
19. Lichen planus: Nail thinning, ridging, and fissuring
F. Trauma-associated nail changes
1. Ingrown nail: Nail plate grows into the lateral nail folds; progresses to form granulation tissue and possibly infection
2. Loss, chipping, and splitting of nail: Occurs from direct blow to nail or excessive exposure to water or irritants

VI. Treatment (Baran et al., 2014; Dunne et al., 2015; Gupta & Stec, 2019; Lacouture & Sibaud, 2018; Leggit, 2017; Matthews et al., 2020; Mayeaux et al., 2019; McFarlane et al., 2020; Robert et al., 2015; Sibaud, 2018)
A. Treatment is directed at the underlying medical conditions, which may or may not result in improvement of nail condition.
B. Nonpharmacologic
1. Educate the patient regarding potential nail toxicities and strategies for prevention, if appropriate.
2. Encourage appropriate nail cutting and moisturizing.
C. Drug-induced changes do not require treatment and usually improve when the drug is discontinued and the nail regrows. Severe cases may warrant dose or drug change.
1. Reassure the patient that nail changes are an expected adverse effect and are not cancer related.
2. Educate the patient that it takes approximately 5.5 months for fingernails to completely regrow and 12–18 months for toenails to regrow.

D. Primary nail conditions
  1. Onychomycosis (fungal infection): Successful treatment is difficult.
    a) Terbinafine (first-line therapy): 250 mg PO every day for six weeks for finger-nails and three months for toenails
    b) Itraconazole: For fingernail treatment, give 200 mg two times a day for one week per month for two months. For toenail treatment, give 200 mg two times a day for one week per month for three months.
    c) Ciclopirox: An 8% solution (nail lacquer) is applied once daily on the top and underside of affected nails. The nail is wiped clean with alcohol once weekly, and the unattached infected part of the nail is removed periodically. Treatment is continued until the nail clears or for up to 48 weeks.
  2. Warts
    a) Fulguration or cryosurgery
    b) Keratolytic agents and occlusions
    c) Operative removal
  3. Paronychia: Lance the fold. Keep hands dry. Apply topical boric acid ointment directly once or twice daily.
    a) Soak nail in warm saline water for 15 minutes four times a day and cover with a nonocclusive dressing.
    b) Chronic paronychia: Avoid excessive exposure to water and irritants.
    c) Topical corticosteroids may be helpful if inflammation is present (see Appendix K).
    d) If abscessed, consider opening area to facilitate drainage and antibiotics given depending on the severity of inflammation and presence of cellulitis.
      (1) Trimethoprim/sulfamethoxazole: 1 double-strength tablet PO two times a day for 10 days
      (2) Cephalexin: 500 mg PO every six hours for 7–10 days
      (3) Clindamycin: 150–450 mg PO four times a day for 7–10 days
  4. Onycholysis: To prevent secondary bacterial infection, perform careful debridement, manicuring, and reduction of irritant exposure.
  5. Psoriasis or lichen planus: Intradermal triamcinolone acetonide suspension 2.5 mg/ml is injected into the nail matrix every two to four weeks to treat inflammatory nail dystrophy as a last resort.
  6. Onychocryptosis (ingrown nail)
    a) Pack under the free edge of the nail with a cotton wick or dental floss.
    b) If the nail is growing into the tissue, clip the nail and soak the finger or toe in warm saline water daily.
    c) Instruct the patient on clipping toenails straight across and to avoid tight-fitting shoes.
    d) Partial nail avulsion, lateral matricectomy, or surgical excision of nail matrix may be necessary for healing.
  7. Brittle nail disorder
    a) Hydrate nail with daily 15-minute soaks using emollients rich in phospholipids.
    b) Apply nail hardeners to strengthen nail plates.
    c) Daily intake of biotin 2.5 mg may be beneficial.
  8. Onychauxis: Periodic debridement may be necessary.
  9. Onychoclasis: Surgical removal of hyperkeratotic tissue or thickened nail may be necessary.
E. Correct nutritional and vitamin deficiencies PRN.

VII. Follow-up (Baran et al., 2014; Charles et al., 2016; Dunne et al., 2015; Matthews et al., 2020)
- A. Short term
  1. Follow up in one to two weeks and regularly to evaluate healing.
  2. Evaluate liver function test every four to six weeks for antifungal therapy.
- B. Long term: Monitor for development of secondary cutaneous neoplasms and subacute cutaneous lupus erythematosus as a result of chemotherapy, especially in those taking targeted EGFR inhibitors and multikinase inhibitors.

VIII. Referrals
- A. Dermatologist or podiatrist: For nail changes that do not heal with treatment or are suggestive of malignancy
- B. Surgeon: If debridement or excision is necessary
- C. Psychosocial, physical, occupational therapy: For effects on ADLs or QOL

The author would like to acknowledge Dawn Camp-Sorrell, MSN, FNP, AOCN®, for her contribution to this chapter that remains unchanged from the previous edition of this book.

References

Alessandrini, A., Starace, M., & Piraccini, B.M. (2017). Dermoscopy in the evaluation of nail disorders. *Skin Appendage Disorders, 3*(2), 70–82. https://doi.org/10.1159/000458728

Baran, R., Fouilloux, B., & Robert, C. (2014). Nail abnormalities in oncology practice. In M.E. Lacouture (Ed.), *Dermatologic principles and practice in oncology: Conditions of the skin, hair, and nails in cancer patients* (pp. 115–122). Wiley-Blackwell.

Charles, C., Bungener, C., Razavi, D., Mateus, C., Routier, E., Lanoy, E., … Dauchy, S. (2016). Impact of dermatologic adverse events induced by targeted therapies on quality of life. *Critical Reviews in Oncology/Hematology, 101,* 158–168. https://doi.org/10.1016/j.critrevonc.2016.03.003

Dunne, M., Liu, C.-M., & Lacouture, M. (2015). Skin and nail alterations. In C.G. Brown (Ed.), *A guide to oncology symptom management* (2nd ed., pp. 599–621). Oncology Nursing Society.

Gupta, A.K., & Stec, N. (2019). Emerging drugs for the treatment of onychomycosis. *Expert Opinion on Emerging Drugs, 24*(4), 213–220. https://doi.org/10.1080/14728214.2019.1685493

Lacouture, M., & Sibaud, V. (2018). Toxic side effects of targeted therapies and immunotherapies affecting the skin, oral mucosa, hair, and nails. *American Journal of Clinical Dermatology, 19*(1), 31–39. https://doi.org/10.1007/s40257-018-0384-3

Leggit, J.C. (2017). Acute and chronic paronychia. *American Family Physician, 96*(1), 44–51. https://www.aafp.org/afp/2017/0701/p44.html

Lipner, S.R., Hancock, J.E., & Fleischer, A.B. (2021). The ambulatory care burden of nail conditions in the United States. *Journal of Dermatological Treatment, 32*(5), 517–520. https://doi.org/10.1080/09546634.2019.1679337

Maddy, A.J., & Tosti, A. (2018). Hair and nail diseases in the mature patient. *Clinical Dermatology, 36*(2), 159–166. https://doi.org/10.1016/j.clindermatol.2017.10.007

Matthews, N.H., Moustafa, F., Kaskas, N.M., Robinson-Bostom, L., & Pappas-Taffer, L. (2020). Dermatologic toxicities of anticancer therapy. In J.E. Niederhuber, J.O. Armitage, M.B. Kastan, J.H. Doroshow, & J.E. Tepper (Eds.), *Abeloff's clinical oncology* (6th ed., pp. 621–648). Elsevier.

Mayeaux, E.J., Jr., Carter, C., & Murphy, T.E. (2019). Ingrown toenail management. *American Family Physician, 100*(3), 158–164. https://www.aafp.org/afp/2019/0801/p158.html

McFarlane, T., Rehman, N., Wang, K., Lee, J., & Carter, C. (2020). Cutaneous toxicities of new targeted cancer therapies: Must know for diagnosis, management, and patient-proxy empowerment. *Annals of Palliative Medicine, 9*(3), 1296–1306. https://doi.org/10.21037/apm.2019.08.05

Murdan, S. (2016). Nail disorders in older people, and aspects of their pharmaceutical treatment. *International Journal of Pharmaceutics, 512*(2), 405–411. https://doi.org/10.1016/j.ijpharm.2016.05.022

Robert, C., Sibaud, V., Mateus, C., Verschoore, M., Charles, C., Lanoy, E., & Baran, R. (2015). Nail toxicities induced by systemic anticancer treatments. *Lancet Oncology, 16*(4), e181–e189. https://doi.org/10.1016/S1470-2045(14)71133-7

Sibaud, V. (2018). Dermatologic reactions to immune checkpoint inhibitors: Skin toxicities and immunotherapy. *American Journal of Clinical Dermatology, 19*(3), 345–361. https://doi.org/10.1007/s40257-017-0336-3

Zawar, V., Bondarde, S., Pawar, M., & Sankalecha, S. (2019). Nail changes due to chemotherapy: A prospective observational study of 129 patients. *Journal of the European Academy of Dermatology and Venereology, 33*(7), 1398–1404. https://doi.org/10.1111/jdv.15508

CHAPTER 15

Pressure Injuries (Pressure Ulcers/Sores)

Tracy C. Wyant, DNP, AOCN®, CHPN, GERO-BC, CPPS, EBP-C

I. Definition: Localized injury to the skin or soft tissue, usually over a bony prominence, resulting from prolonged pressure or pressure in combination with friction and/or shear (Bulfone et al., 2018; Joint Commission, 2016; Porter-Armstrong et al., 2018; Ratliff et al., 2016)
   A. The interchangeable terms *pressure sore* or *pressure injury* are used for this injury.
   B. Terminology originates from *decubitus ulcer*, derived from the Latin *decumbere* (to lie down or recline). In 1747, the French used the term synonymously with "bedsore," erroneously suggesting bed rest as the sole etiology.

II. Physiology/Pathophysiology (Beers, 2019; Bulfone et al., 2018; European Pressure Ulcer Advisory Panel, National Pressure Injury Advisory Panel, & Pan Pacific Pressure Injury Alliance, 2019; Garza, 2019; Hajhosseini et al., 2020; Joint Commission, 2016, 2020; Ratliff et al., 2016; Ricci et al., 2017)
   A. Normal: Skin has three layers and provides an elastic, rugged, self-regenerating, protective covering for the body.
      1. Epidermis: Outermost layer; acts as a barrier for immune surveillance; protects against substances and infections; restricts water loss
      2. Dermis: Middle layer; separates epidermis from cutaneous adipose tissue; interacts with vascular connective tissue and nervous system; provides collagen to support skin structure
      3. Hypodermis: Deepest subcutaneous layer; consists of loose connective tissue and adipose tissue; plays a role in immune surveillance and energy balance
   B. Pathophysiology: The exact mechanism of how pressure and shear result in a pressure injury is not fully understood. Pressure injuries are the manifestation of local tissue damage or death, primarily caused by inadequate blood perfusion.
      1. Cellular metabolism is compromised by vascular occlusion and the effects of shear that lead to impaired perfusion to the area.
      2. Cells are denied nutrients for viability and growth, and waste products accumulate.
      3. Skin failure may be an associated complication of multisystem failure (e.g., Kennedy terminal ulcer).
      4. Pressure injuries can happen in any area that experiences prolonged pressure and shear. The most common sites tend to be the sacrum and heels. These injuries are staged according to an assessment system based on the depth of tissue damage. Once accurately staged, the wound can improve but does not progress to a reverse stage,

as the tensile strength of the tissue is forever altered. Lost muscle and subcutaneous tissue of a stage III or IV pressure injury is replaced by granulation tissue composed of endothelial cells, fibroblasts, collagen, and extracellular matrix. Healing pressure injuries are indicated by a decrease in wound measures; changes in exudate volume, or character; and absence of necrotic tissue.

5. Mucosal tissue (e.g., nares, oral cavity, lining of GI tract) can be affected due to pressure from medical devices, such as oxygen cannula or endotracheal or NG tubes. Mucosal tissue is histologically different from skin and cannot be staged. Damage to the mucous membranes related to pressure should be documented simply as mucosal pressure injuries.

III. Clinical features: Development of pressure injuries can be insidious, influenced by a number of interacting intrinsic and extrinsic factors. Typically, injuries occur over a bony prominence but can develop in soft tissue from prolonged pressure. Consequences of pressure-induced skin injury range from nonblanchable erythema of intact skin to deep injuries extending to the bone (Beers, 2019; Bulfone et al., 2018; European Pressure Ulcer Advisory Panel, National Pressure Injury Advisory Panel, & Pan Pacific Pressure Injury Alliance, 2019; Hajhosseini et al., 2020; Joint Commission, 2016, 2020; Lai et al., 2019; Ratliff et al., 2016; Ricci et al., 2017).

A. Risk factors: A number of factors contribute to pressure injury development, starting with the overall health of the patient. A validated skin risk assessment tool should be used with initial patient evaluation and at regular intervals throughout the course of treatment. However, clinicians should not solely rely on a risk assessment tool without assessing pressure injury risk.

1. Sensory perception: Diminished ability to respond to sustained pressure and related discomfort (e.g., paralysis, coma)

2. Prolonged skin exposure to moisture: Urine, perspiration, wound drainage

3. Diminished physical activity or mobility: Paralysis, stroke, arthritis

4. Inadequate fluid and/or nutritional intake based on history and hematologic measurement: Hypoalbuminemia, hypoproteinemia, vitamin deficiency (particularly vitamins A, C, and E)

5. Friction and shear: Created by two surfaces moving across one another in parallel but opposite directions; frequently occurs with repositioning
   a) Friction injury causes epidermal denuding related to direct mechanical trauma.
   b) Shearing results in deep tissue damage due to stretching and pulling of the tissues beneath the skin.

6. Advancing age: Cellular and structural changes of the skin associated with aging include flattening of the dermal–epidermal junction, resulting in reduced shearing/blistering thresholds and diminished microcirculation to the epidermis; reduction in sebaceous gland secretion and intracellular lipid layers, leading to decreased skin hydration and pruritus; and diminished keratinocyte proliferation and epidermal turnover, causing diminished capacity for wound healing.

7. Additional miscellaneous intrinsic and extrinsic factors
   a) Smoking: Associated with nicotine-induced peripheral vasoconstriction and resultant tissue hypoxia
   b) Hyperthermia: Elevates metabolic rates and oxygen consumption, exacerbating the effects of ischemia
   c) Hypotension: Results in diminished perfusion to the skin as blood is shunted to vital body organs; deep tissues may be particularly at risk because of their high vascularity.

     d) Stress: Causes release of cortisol, a glucocorticoid that triggers structural changes in connective tissue and affects cellular metabolism, which lowers tissue tolerance to pressure and delays healing

     e) Special settings: Pressure injury risk is higher in those undergoing vascular, cardiac, thoracic, orthopedic, or any lengthy surgical procedure. Visual skin changes related to operative procedures may appear immediately or up to 72 hours after surgery, commonly on the sacrum, flank, back, cheekbone, and elbow. Radiology, dialysis, or emergency department settings may present risks of pressure injury when high-acuity patients recline for an extended period on support surfaces with inadequate pressure reduction.

B. Etiology of pressure injuries

  1. Pressure: Approximately 32 mm Hg is a recognized threshold for capillary closing pressure; the tremendous variability in tissue tolerance is dependent on the patient's overall physical condition.

  2. Intensity: Amount of force or pressure exerted on a given area

  3. Duration: Length of time the force or pressure is applied

  4. Tolerance: Ability of the skin and supporting structures to endure pressure without adverse sequelae

C. History

  1. History of cancer and cancer treatment

  2. Current medications: Prescribed, over the counter, supplements

  3. History of pressure injuries: Precipitating factors, onset, location, duration, successful and unsuccessful treatment modalities, recurrence

  4. Changes in ADLs: Weakness and paralysis, effects on QOL

  5. Past medical history: Particularly conditions affecting tissue perfusion, such as cancer, diabetes, peripheral vascular disease, renal failure, COPD, or traumatic injuries

  6. Past surgical history: Prosthesis, implants, previous flaps, grafts

  7. Risk assessment: Use a structured risk assessment tool for all patients within eight hours of admission or at each outpatient visit, being sure to integrate clinical judgment and consideration of relevant risk factors.

D. Signs and symptoms

  1. Pain at pressure points: Patients often are unaware of the discomfort related to unrelieved pressure, especially if experiencing cognitive decline, when receiving significant doses of pain medications, or if neuropathies are present.

  2. Weight loss or generalized anasarca

  3. Fever or warmth of skin in a specific area

  4. Areas of edematous, erythematous, or darkened skin: Inflammatory response may be diminished in older adult, immunocompromised, or diabetic patients.

  5. Abrasions, bleeding, and exudate from disrupted skin integrity

E. Physical examination

  1. Vital signs: Fever, hypotension

  2. Integument: Use data from risk assessment. Describe objective findings from a comprehensive assessment, including pressure injury staging.

     a) Extent of erythema or hyperemia (blanchable erythema): Presents as an ill-defined erythematous area at the point of pressure on intact skin, varying in color from pale pink to bright red; digital compression produces total blanching, and erythema may reappear promptly when fingers are lifted.

     b) Include skin temperature, edema, and change in tissue consistency compared to surrounding areas.

     c) Pressure injury staging

(1) Stage I (nonblanchable erythema): Skin is intact with nonblanchable erythema of a localized area, usually over a bony prominence. Darkly pigmented skin may not have visible blanching but color may differ from surrounding area. The area may be painful, firm, soft, warmer, or cooler compared to adjacent tissue.

(2) Stage II (partial-thickness skin loss): This stage includes partial loss of dermis, presenting as a shallow open ulcer with a red or pink wound bed without slough. It may present as an intact or open/ruptured, serum-filled blister. This stage should not be used to describe excoriation, maceration, perineal dermatitis, skin tears, or stripping due to tape removal. Underlying bruising is an indication of deep tissue injury.

(3) Stage III (full-thickness skin loss): Subcutaneous fat may be visible, but bone, tendon, and muscle are not exposed. Slough may be present but does not obscure the depth of tissue loss. Undermining and tunneling may be present. The depth of a stage III pressure injury varies by anatomic location. The bridge of the nose, ear, occiput, and malleolus do not have subcutaneous tissue, and stage III injuries can be shallow. Areas of significant adipose tissue can develop extremely deep stage III pressure injuries.

(4) Stage IV (full-thickness tissue loss): Exposed bone, tendon, or muscle may be present. Slough or eschar may also be present on some parts of the wound bed. This stage may often include undermining and tunneling. Depth of a stage IV pressure injury varies by anatomic location. Stage IV injuries can extend into muscle and/or supporting structures (e.g., fascia, tendon or joint capsule), making osteomyelitis possible.

(5) Unstageable (depth unknown): Full-thickness tissue loss occurs, in which the base of the ulcer is covered by slough (yellow, tan, gray, green, or brown) and/or eschar (tan, brown, or black) in the wound bed. Until enough slough and/or eschar is removed to expose the base of the wound, the true depth, and therefore stage, cannot be determined. Stable (dry, adherent, intact without erythema or fluctuance) eschar on the heels serves as the body's natural (biologic) cover and should not be removed.

(6) Suspected deep tissue injury (depth unknown): Purple or maroon localized area of discolored intact skin or blood-filled blister is present because of damage of underlying soft tissue from pressure and/or shear. The area may be preceded by tissue that is painful, firm, mushy, boggy, warmer, or cooler compared to adjacent tissue. Deep tissue injury may be difficult to detect in individuals with dark skin tones. Presentation may include a thin blister over a dark wound bed. The wound may further evolve and become covered by thin eschar.

d) Wound assessment

(1) Anatomic location

(2) Size in centimeters (e.g., length, width, depth)

(3) Tunneling or undermining: Indicate measurement in centimeters, circumferential from wound using clock face descriptor.

(4) Color of the wound (e.g., pink, black, yellow)

(5) Stage: Used only for pressure injuries

(6) Drainage (e.g., volume, color, odor)

(7) Periwound skin status (e.g., intact, inflamed, macerated)

IV. Diagnostic tests (Bulfone et al., 2018; European Pressure Ulcer Advisory Panel, National Pressure Injury Advisory Panel, & Pan Pacific Pressure Injury Alliance, 2019; Joint Commission, 2016, 2020; Ratliff et al., 2016)
- A. Laboratory: Assess nutritional status and/or presence of clinical infection.
    1. Serum transferrin and prealbumin to measure visceral protein stores
    2. Creatinine to estimate skeletal muscle mass
    3. Hgb and ferritin level to detect iron-deficiency anemia
    4. WBC count to evaluate for wound infection
    5. Total lymphocyte count to evaluate visceral protein status and cellular immune function
    6. Blood cultures if systemic infection suspected
    7. Vitamin levels, such as B, C, and D, to evaluate deficiencies
    8. Wound culture, if indicated
- B. Radiology: Evaluate for osteomyelitis.
    1. Plain x-rays and MRI do not permit definitive diagnosis of osteomyelitis, as the presence of inflammation visualized is nonspecific.
    2. A triple-phase bone scan in the presence of an elevated WBC count may support associated findings of osteomyelitis.
- C. Other
    1. Tissue biopsy: Punch biopsy can identify clinical infection in the wound. Swab cultures often reflect surface contaminants despite cleansing/irrigation prior to culture. Chronic pressure injuries may be colonized with bacteria that do not impede wound healing.
    2. Wound biopsies can facilitate differential diagnosis if concerns about alternative etiologies exist.

V. Differential diagnosis (Bulfone et al., 2018; European Pressure Ulcer Advisory Panel, National Pressure Injury Advisory Panel, & Pan Pacific Pressure Injury Alliance, 2019; Joint Commission, 2016, 2020; Ratliff et al., 2016)
- A. Extravasation
- B. Tumor erosion
- C. Physical abuse
- D. Pyoderma gangrenosum
- E. Arterial or venous insufficiency (see Chapter 51)
- F. Diabetic neuropathic ulcer (see Chapter 151)
- G. Abscess
- H. Skin cancer

VI. Treatment (Agency for Healthcare Research and Quality, 2014; Beers, 2019; Bulfone et al., 2018; Eglseer et al., 2019; European Pressure Ulcer Advisory Panel, National Pressure Injury Advisory Panel, & Pan Pacific Pressure Injury Alliance, 2019; Furuya-Kanamori et al., 2019; Hajhosseini et al., 2020; Joint Commission, 2016, 2020; Lim et al., 2019; McInnes et al., 2018; Moore & Webster, 2018; Porter-Armstrong et al., 2018; Ratliff et al., 2016; Ricci et al., 2017)
- A. Prediction and prevention
    1. All patients should be assessed for pressure injury risk using a validated, structured skin risk assessment scale, such as the Braden scale. Clinical judgment should be used and risk factors considered when using the tool. An individualized plan of care should link risk assessment findings to specific preventive interventions.
    2. Head-to-toe skin inspection should be documented on initial contact with patient and at follow-up visits.

3. Removal of medical devices (e.g., stocking, splints) should be performed two times a day for skin hygiene, hydration, and inspection. Devices that cannot be removed (e.g., indwelling tubes or catheters) should be stabilized and repositioned for daily skin inspection.
4. The patient, primary caregiver, and/or family members should be educated about skin risk factors, assessment parameters, and pressure injury prevention measures. Patient handouts should include information about skin status and pressure injury risk, along with current off-loading device requirements.
5. Patients should be encouraged to maximize mobility/activity levels.
   a) Turn and reposition based on factors such as skin condition, whether a pressure redistribution support surface is in use, the patient's level of activity and tolerance of movement, and overall treatment goals.
   b) Use pillows or foam wedges to facilitate postural alignment and cushion bony prominences.
   c) Use pressure-relieving devices for heel suspension.
   d) Avoid positioning directly on the trochanter.
   e) Elevate the head of the bed less than 30° if possible.
   f) Use lifting devices to transfer and reposition whenever possible, rather than dragging against the bed linens.
   g) Use a reactive support surface or pressure redistribution mattress. Avoid use of sheepskin, which can cause heat and maceration. Foam overlays should be labeled as high specification to reduce pressure.
6. Patients should be educated on effective skin hygiene.
   a) Use tepid water and a pH-balanced skin cleanser for bathing.
   b) Apply moisturizers to promote skin hydration.
   c) Maintain environmental air humidification at greater than or equal to 40%.
7. Consistent incontinence care should be provided.
   a) Assess and treat urinary and fecal incontinence.
   b) If continence cannot be attained, use absorptive underpads that keep moisture away from the skin. Use briefs only when out of bed/ambulatory to limit associated heat and maceration.
   c) Cleanse the affected area with incontinence cleanser and tepid water at time of soiling.
   d) Apply a topical skin barrier.
8. Hydration/nutrition deficits should be identified and managed.
   a) Screen and assess nutritional status for each individual with a pressure injury with each condition change and/or when progress toward pressure injury closure is not observed.
   b) Assess weight status for each individual to determine weight history and significant weight loss from usual body weight (5% or greater change in 30 days or 10% or greater in 180 days).
   c) Assess ability to eat independently.
   d) Assess adequacy of total food and fluid intake.
   e) Provide sufficient calories (0–35 calories/kg body weight) for individuals at risk for a pressure injury or malnutrition, or for those who have a pressure injury. Adjust formula based on weight loss, weight gain, or level of obesity.
   f) Provide foods and/or oral nutritional supplements between meals if needed. Consider nutritional support (enteral or parenteral nutrition) when oral intake is inadequate.

B. Treatment
    1. Cleansing: Removal of surface debris and contaminants
        a) Cleanse the wound and periwound with each dressing change, using potable tap water, distilled water, cooled boiled water, or saline.
        b) Consider antiseptics for wounds not expected to heal or those with chronic colonization.
    2. Debridement: Removal of necrotic tissue to promote granulation and reepithelialization
        a) Surgical: A surgeon uses a scalpel, scissors, or laser to remove macroscopically identified necrotic tissue from the wound bed. Consider treatment goals and patient condition.
        b) Mechanical: Necrotic tissue is removed by applying a mechanical force (pulsatile lavage) or is loosened from the wound bed with wet-to-moist dressings.
        c) Chemical: Protein matter of necrotic tissue is denatured by an enzymatic agent, such as collagenase.
        d) Autolytic: The body's enzymes are used to digest devitalized tissue. Autolytic debridement may be facilitated with use of occlusive dressings.
    3. Dressings: The primary purpose of a dressing is to maintain a wound environment supportive of moist wound healing and to contain exudate, along with protecting the peri-ulcer skin. See Table 15-1 for a summary of wound dressings.
    4. Management of bacterial colonization and infection
        a) Effective wound cleansing and prompt debridement of necrotic tissue minimizes pressure injury colonization and enhances wound healing.
        b) Topical antibiotics may be used. Advanced wound care technology provides noncytotoxic, silver-impregnated dressings in a variety of applications.

TABLE 15-1	Wound Care Products		
Category	**Indications**	**Features**	**Considerations**
Alginates	Wounds with moderate to high exudate; peritracheotomy and drain sites	Highly absorptive; should be converted to gel when combined with wound exudate	May dry wound base if inadequate exudate; irrigating prior to removing may ease removal.
Cadexomer iodine dressing	Wounds with moderate to high exudate	Antiseptic properties	Do not use in those with impaired renal function, history of thyroid disorders, or iodine sensitivity.
Enzymatic debriding agents	Wounds with necrotic tissue	Can be applied alone with cover dressing or with saline-moistened gauze if dry wound base	Expect increased exudate as necrotic tissue denatures.
Foams	Wounds with moderate to high exudate; peritracheotomy and drain sites	Highly absorptive; provide cushion; may be impregnated with silver for antimicrobial action or charcoal for odor control	May require alternative contact layer dressing for irregular wound surface

(Continued on next page)

TABLE 15-1	Wound Care Products *(Continued)*		
Category	Indications	Features	Considerations
Hydrocolloids	Wounds of scant to moderate exudate; may be used to protect peri-wound skin from wound exudate or prevent skin stripping from tape	Support moist wound healing of partial-thickness, pink wounds; autolytic debridement of slough or eschar; protect wounds from incontinence and friction injury	Extended wear promotes patient comfort and saves caregiver time; expect odor and tan exudate on removal; contraindicated on infected or tunneled wounds; avoid excessively warm areas and areas where dressing may roll.
Hydrogels	Wounds with scant to moderate exudate; superficial to deep, tunneled, or undermined sites when used with appropriate wound contact layer or cover dressing	Provide moist healing environment; minimal absorptive capacity; conform to irregular wound surfaces; promote patient comfort	May cause transient localized burning in some patients
Silicone dressing	Wounds that need a contact layer and atraumatic dressing change	Can be used on fragile skin	Consider for patients needing limited trauma during dressing changes.
Silver-impregnated dressing	Infected, at risk for infection, or heavily colonized wounds	Antiseptic properties	Discontinue when infection is controlled; do not use if sensitive to silver.
Transparent films	Wounds with little or no exudate; may be used as secondary dressing for incontinence protection	Low moisture vapor transmission; waterproof; occlusive; minimize localized friction and discomfort	Avoid use on fragile skin; apply skin sealant beneath dressing; do not use as cover over debriding agents, gels, or ointments.
Wet-to-moist gauze	Wounds of significant size or depth with tunneling or undermining	Cost-effective treatment; may provide mechanical debridement or delivery of adjunct topical therapy	Wound healing may be disrupted if dressing is dry when removed; consider administration of analgesics before dressing changes as needed.

Note. Based on information from Bulfone et al., 2018; Furuya-Kanamori et al., 2019; McInnes et al., 2018; Moore & Webster, 2018; Ricci et al., 2017.

    c) Wounds resulting in soft tissue infections and/or osteomyelitis require systemic antibiotics (see Appendix C).

5. Pain management during wound care
   a) Patients who are cognitively impaired, have an altered mental status, or are otherwise unable to communicate about their pain should be assessed using nonverbal skills.
   b) Appropriate pharmacologic agents for analgesia should be provided prior to wound treatments for maximal effectiveness.
6. Consider other adjunctive therapies, such as platelet-derived growth factor, electrical stimulation, and negative pressure wound therapy.

VII. Follow-up (Bulfone et al., 2018; European Pressure Ulcer Advisory Panel, National Pressure Injury Advisory Panel, & Pan Pacific Pressure Injury Alliance, 2019; Joint Commission, 2016, 2020; Porter-Armstrong et al., 2018; Ratliff et al., 2016)
  A. Short term
    1. Reassess wound and use structured risk assessment at regular intervals, noting healing, progression, and changes in risk factors.
    2. Modify interventions PRN and consistent with overall plan of care.
  B. Long term
    1. Implement measures to prevent additional pressure injury formation.
    2. Continue periodic skin risk assessment; intervene to minimize risks.

VIII. Referrals
  A. Physical/occupational therapist: To identify daily exercise routines and positioning techniques for maximal mobility and activity, and to aid in the selection of appropriate seat cushion for off-loading, which may include the use of pressure mapping devices
  B. Registered dietitian: To identify optimal interventions for hydration and nutrition
  C. Wound, ostomy, and continence RN or advanced practice nurse: To design an individualized preventive skin care and wound management program
  D. Surgeon: To debride necrotic pressure injuries PRN and to evaluate for flap/graft placement
  E. Infectious disease specialist: To manage infected wounds or osteomyelitis

The author would like to acknowledge Kathleen Wright, RN, MSN, CWOCN, ACHRN, for her contribution to this chapter that remains unchanged from the previous edition of this book.

References

Agency for Healthcare Research and Quality. (2014). *Preventing pressure ulcers in hospitals: Section 7. Tools and resources.* https://www.ahrq.gov/patient-safety/settings/hospital/resource/pressureulcer/tool/pu7.html

Beers, E.H. (2019). Palliative wound care: Less is more. *Surgical Clinics of North America, 99*(5), 899–919. https://doi.org/10.1016/j.suc.2019.06.008

Bulfone, G., Bressan, V., Morandini, A., & Stevanin, S. (2018). Perioperative pressure injuries: A systematic literature review. *Advances in Skin and Wound Care, 31*(12), 556–564. https://doi.org/10.1097/01.ASW.0000544613.10878.ed

Eglseer, D., Hodl, M., & Lohrmann, C. (2019). Nutritional management of older hospitalised patients with pressure injuries. *International Wound Journal, 16*(1), 226–232. https://doi.org/10.1111/iwj.13016

European Pressure Ulcer Advisory Panel, National Pressure Injury Advisory Panel, & Pan Pacific Pressure Injury Alliance. (2019). Prevention and treatment of pressure ulcers: Quick reference guide: 2019. http://www.internationalguideline.com

Furuya-Kanamori, L., Walker, R.M., Gillespie, B.M., Clark, J., Doi, S.A.R., & Thalib, L. (2019). Effectiveness of different topical treatments in the healing of pressure injuries: A network meta-analysis. *Journal of the American Medical Directors Association, 20*(4), 399–407. https://doi.org/10.1016/j.jamda.2018.10.010

Garza, L. (2019). Developmental biology of the skin. In S. Kang, M. Amagai, A.L. Bruckner, A.H. Enk, D.J. Margolis, A.J. McMichael, & J.S. Orringer (Eds.), *Fitzpatrick's dermatology* (9th ed., pp. 49–61). McGraw-Hill Education.

Hajhosseini, B., Longaker, M.T., & Gurtner, G.C. (2020). Pressure injury. *Annals of Surgery, 271*(4), 671–679. https://doi.org/10.1097/SLA.0000000000003567

Joint Commission. (2016, July). Preventing pressure injuries. https://www.jointcommission.org/assets/1/23/Quick_Safety_Issue_25_July_20161.PDF

Joint Commission. (2020). *National Patient Safety Goals effective July 2020 for the Nursing Care Center Program.* https://www.jointcommission.org/-/media/tjc/documents/standards/national-patient-safety-goals/2020/npsg_chapter_ncc_jul2020.pdf

Lai, T.T.-K., Yip, O.-M., & Sham, M.M.K. (2019). Clinical parameters of wound healing in patients with advanced illness. *Annals of Palliative Medicine, 8*(Suppl. 1), S5–S14. https://doi.org/10.21037/apm.2019.01.05

Lim, E., Mordiffi, Z., Chew, H.S.J., & Lopez, V. (2019). Using the Braden subscales to assess risk of pressure injuries in adult patients: A retrospective case-control study. *International Wound Journal, 16*(3), 665–673. https://doi.org/10.1111/iwj.13078

McInnes, E., Jammali-Blasi, A., Bell-Syer, S.E.M., & Leung, V. (2018). Support surfaces for treating pressure ulcers. *Cochrane Database of Systematic Reviews, 2018*(10). https://doi.org/10.1002/14651858.CD009490.pub2

Moore, Z.E.H., & Webster, J. (2018). Dressings and topical agents for preventing pressure ulcers. *Cochrane Database of Systematic Reviews, 2018*(12). https://doi.org/10.1002/14651858.CD009362.pub3

Porter-Armstrong, A.P., Moore, Z.E.H., Bradbury, I., & McDonough, S. (2018). Education of healthcare professionals for preventing pressure ulcers. *Cochrane Database of Systematic Reviews, 2018*(5). https://doi.org/10.1002/14651858.CD011620.pub2

Ratliff, C.R., Droste, L.R., Bonham, P., Crestodina, L., Johnson, J.J., Kelechi, T., & Varnado, M.F. (2016). WOCN 2016 guideline for prevention and management of pressure injuries (ulcers): An executive summary. *Journal of Wound, Ostomy, and Continence Nursing, 44*(3), 241–246. https://doi.org/10.1097/WON.0000000000000321

Ricci, J.A., Bayer, L.R., & Orgill, D.P. (2017). Evidence-based medicine: The evaluation and treatment of pressure injuries. *Plastic and Reconstructive Surgery, 139*(1), 275e–286e. https://doi.org/10.1097/PRS.0000000000002850

CHAPTER 16

Pruritus

Kristine Dukart-Harrington, DNP, RN, AGNP-C, ACHPN

I. Definition: A cutaneous sensation or itch that provokes the urge to scratch or rub the skin (Anzelc & Burkhart, 2019; Kremer, 2019; Smith et al., 2019; Yang & Kim, 2019)
   A. Acute: Lasting less than six weeks
   B. Chronic: Symptoms lasting more than six weeks and often difficult to manage

II. Physiology/Pathophysiology (Anzelc & Burkhart, 2019; Hashimoto & Yosipovitch, 2019; Nakashima et al., 2019; Rinaldi, 2019; Song et al., 2018; Yang & Kim, 2019)
   A. Normal: Arises from sensory, unmyelinated, unspecialized free nerve endings of the skin located between cells of the epidermis, found near the dermal–epidermal junction, and associated with clinical presentation of the patient
   B. Pathophysiology: The neurologic pathways that lead to itch are not fully understood.
      1. Transmission of the sensation of itch occurs along unmyelinated, histamine-sensitive peripheral nerve C fibers, which are distinct from the nerve C fibers that transmit pain.
      2. Nonhistamine nerve fibers may be involved in the transmission of itch, which may account for poor response to oral histamines.
      3. Itch transmission in nerves may be stimulated by the action of a variety of neural mediators on sensory nerve endings in the epidermis, dermal–epidermal junction, and other sites.
      4. Dermal mast cells interact with nerve fibers and contain substances that act as direct and indirect mediators of itch.
      5. Peripheral mediators related to the pathophysiology of pruritus include histamine, neuropeptides, vasoactive peptides and proteases, arachidonic acid transformation products, and platelet-activating factor.
      6. Targeted nociceptors of slow-conducting unmyelinated C fibers
         a) Histamine receptors (H_1, H_3, H_4)
         b) Proteinase-activated receptor 2 (PAR-2)
         c) Transient receptor potential vanilloid 1 (TRPV1)
         d) Cannabinoid receptor 1 and 2 (CB1, CB2)
         e) Mu-opioid receptor (MOR)
      7. Itch-transmitting primary afferent C neurons synapse with secondary transmission neurons that cross over the contralateral spinothalamic tract and ascend to the thalamus. The stimulus travels to the cerebral cortex to multiple areas in the brain where it is activated.

III. Clinical features: Pruritis is a common symptom occurring in a variety of skin diseases and numerous systemic, neurologic, and psychiatric diseases. In severe or chronic cases, pruritus can be incapacitating. Chronic itch is common in older adult patients and is caused by a variety of conditions. Chronic pruritus is a symptom of various internal disorders and diseases (Anzelc & Burkhart, 2019; Fourzali & Yosipovitch, 2019; Hashimoto & Yosipovitch, 2019; Kremer, 2019; Kremer & Mettang, 2019; Pereira et al., 2016; Reich & Szepietowski, 2016; Smith et al., 2019).

A. Clinical manifestations
   1. Group 1: Pruritus on diseased (inflamed) skin
   2. Group 2: Pruritus on nondiseased skin
   3. Group 3: Pruritus presenting with severe, chronic scratchy lesions
B. Etiology: Diversity of underlying causes
   1. It may be localized or generalized, with or without skin lesions.
   2. It may represent an underlying disease or a prognostic variable of an identified disease such as Hodgkin lymphoma.
   3. Factors modulating itching include psychological factors, inflammation, dry skin, vasodilation, warmth, and coldness.
C. History: Age, preexisting diseases, severity of pruritus, impact on QOL, and attention to underlying origin
   1. History of cancer and cancer treatment
   2. Current medications: Prescribed, over the counter
   3. History of presenting symptoms: Precipitating factors, onset, location, duration
   4. Changes in ADLs: Levels of stress
   5. History of exposure to chemicals, plants, animals, and topical irritants (e.g., soaps, creams, perfumes)
   6. Past medical history: Chronic renal disease, hepatobiliary disease, hematologic disease, psychologic condition
D. Signs and symptoms
   1. Skin changes: Scaling, rash, pustules, macules, hives/wheals, dryness, cracking, excoriation
   2. Color changes: Erythema, jaundice
E. Physical examination: Focus on integument examination.
   1. Complete skin inspection: Assess the affected area and overall skin surface for scaling, dryness, xerosis, inflammation, scratch marks, breaks, excoriations, lichenification, lice, scabies, stasis dermatitis, jaundice, and distribution (localized or generalized).
   2. Pruritus is a systemic condition that requires a complete physical examination.
      a) Hepatomegaly, splenomegaly, and symptoms suggestive of liver disease
      b) Scleral icterus indicating liver disease
      c) Lymphadenopathy indicating infection or lymphoma

IV. Diagnostic tests: If no obvious abnormalities indicate an etiology, obtain in order of importance (Pereira et al., 2016; Reich & Szepietowski, 2016).
   A. Laboratory
      1. CBC with differential to evaluate for infection, anemia, or polycythemia
      2. ESR to evaluate for inflammatory process
      3. Chemical profile to evaluate for renal or hepatic disease, hyperglycemia, hypoglycemia, effects of drugs, pancreatic disorders, endocrine disorders, dietary imbalances, cholestasis, or malignancies
      4. Thyroid function studies to evaluate thyroid disorders
      5. Serum iron to evaluate iron deficiency
      6. SPEP or immunoelectrophoresis to evaluate protein gammopathies or malignancies

      7. Antinuclear antibody, rheumatoid factor to evaluate for autoimmune deficiency

      8. Skin scraping to confirm scabies

  B. Radiology: If laboratory studies are inconclusive, chest x-ray to evaluate adenopathy, malignancies, infection, or inflammation

  C. Other tests, as indicated: Skin biopsy with special stains and/or skin scrapings to determine presence of autoimmune diseases, malignancies, circulatory disorders, parasites, infections, or inflammation

V. Differential diagnosis (Hashimoto & Yosipovitch, 2019; Huang et al., 2019; Kremer, 2019; Kremer & Mettang, 2019; Pereira et al., 2016; Reich & Szepietowski, 2016)

  A. Localized pruritus: Primary dermatologic condition secondary to infection or infestation

  B. Generalized pruritus: A systemic condition or psychogenic etiology

  C. Targeted diagnosis based on neurophysiologic basis to peripheral mediators or targeted nociceptors

      1. TRPM8 (CMR1), ANKTM1: Reduction of pruritus of any kind for short time

      2. Vanilloid receptor subtype 1 (TRPV1): Localized forms of pain/pruritus, including notalgia paresthetica, PUVA (psoralen and ultraviolet A)-induced itch/pain, postherpetic neuralgia (see Chapter 22), brachioradial pruritus, aquagenic pruritus, lichen planus/lichen sclerosus, prurigo nodularis, chronic irritative hand dermatitis, rosacea, GVHD, genitoanal pruritus, and atopic dermatitis (see Chapter 18)

      3. Cannabinoid receptors (CB1, CB2): Uremic pruritus, pruritus of unknown origin, lichen simplex, prurigo nodularis, localized pruritus

      4. H_1 receptors: Urticaria, mastocytosis, urticarial drug reaction, pruritus of multifactorial origin in older adult patients, prurigo nodularis, renal pruritus, atopic dermatitis (see Chapter 18)

      5. H_2 receptors: Severe forms of polycythemia vera (see Chapter 128), Hodgkin lymphoma

      6. Leukotriene D_4 receptor: Urticaria, urticaria factitia, aquagenic pruritus

      7. Suppression of IL-1: Prurigo nodularis

      8. Nerve membrane stabilization: Brachioradial pruritus, notalgia paresthetica, meralgia paresthetica, small fiber neuropathy, hydroxyethyl starch–induced pruritus, renal pruritus, diabetic pruritus

      9. Mu-opioid receptor on spinal cord neurons: Cholestasis pruritus, chronic urticaria, atopic dermatitis, prurigo nodularis, pruritic mycosis fungoides

     10. Interference with presynaptic reuptake of neurotransmitters: Prurigo nodularis, chronic pruritus of unknown origin

  D. Drug induced: Heparin, trimethoprim/sulfamethoxazole, calcium channel blockers

VI. Treatment: Pruritus treatment is dependent on resolution of etiologic factors, as well as localized, symptomatic relief. If considered to be medication induced, medication should be discontinued. A wide variety of therapies have been used; however, limited data are available on efficacy (Besner Morin & Misery, 2019; Fourzali & Yosipovitch, 2019; Kremer, 2019; Mercadante, 2019; Metz, 2019; Sheriff et al., 2020; Song et al., 2018).

  A. Nonpharmacologic treatment

      1. Skin moisturization: Emollient soaps or lotions, tepid/cold baths, or soothing lotions with menthol may relieve local symptoms.

      2. Cool environment: Lightweight clothing, an air-conditioned environment, air humidification, and use of tepid baths or showers instead of hot water are recommended. Preparations such as calamine lotion can be drying; they are most effective on weeping pustules and provide a cooling sensation to the skin.

3. Avoidance of skin irritants: Use of oatmeal baths and mild nonperfumed soaps is recommended.
4. Stress reduction
5. Physical interventions: Trimmed fingernails, soft clothing, and occlusive dressings may help to discourage scratching an area that itches.

B. Topical treatment: Use of topical corticosteroids can be beneficial in treating inflammatory skin disease (see Appendix K).

C. Systemic: Antihistamines (see Appendix H), sedatives, ASA, or tricyclic antidepressants (see Appendix L) can relieve systemic symptoms. Other drugs may be systemically taken depending on the etiology and underlying disease process.

D. Targeted therapies based on nociceptors of slow-conducting unmyelinated C-fibers in the papillary dermis and epidermis
   1. TRPM8 (CMR1), ANKTM1: Topical therapies with cold, menthol 1%–3% cream or lotion
   2. Vanilloid receptor subtype 1 (VR1/TRPV1): Topical therapies specific to symptoms; capsaicin cream 0.025%–0.1%, applied three to six times a day
   3. Cannabinoid receptors (CB1, CB2): Palmidrol-containing cream applied two times a day; calcineurin inhibitors pimecrolimus 1%, or tacrolimus 0.1%, applied two to three times a day
   4. H_1 receptors: Systemic therapy with H_1 antihistamines (see Appendix H)
   5. H_2 receptors: H_2 blocker such as famotidine 20–40 mg PO two times a day
   6. Leukotriene D_4 receptor: Zafirlukast 20 mg two times a day, or montelukast 10 mg PO daily
   7. IL-2 suppression: Cyclosporine A, azathioprine, and mycophenolate have demonstrated antipruritic effects.
   8. Nerve membrane stabilization by blocking calcium channels: Gabapentin 300 mg PO at bedtime or pregabalin 75 mg PO two times a day
   9. Mu-opioid receptor
      a) Initiate low-dose continuous infusion of naltrexone for opioid-induced pruritus (starting at 0.002 mcg/kg/min), gradually titrating until control of pruritus is achieved and no opioid withdrawal-related symptoms are evident.
      b) Naloxone infusion can be rotated to PO therapy with opioid antagonists, such as naltrexone 25–50 mg PO daily (can divide into twice-a-day dosing).
   10. Interference with presynaptic reuptake of neurotransmitters (e.g., serotonin, noradrenaline): Amitriptyline 25–100 mg PO at bedtime, clomipramine 25 mg PO at bedtime, doxepin 75 mg PO at bedtime, mirtazapine 15 mg PO at bedtime, paroxetine 20 mg PO daily

E. Opioid-induced pruritus: Incidence is low for systemic administration but increases with spinal opioids.
   1. Preferred management: Rotate to an equianalgesic dose of a different opioid (e.g., morphine to hydromorphone) to relieve pruritus.
   2. Opioid antagonists: Initiate low-dose continuous infusion of naltrexone for opioid-induced pruritus, followed by PO naltrexone if needed. This is rare and used in specific situations in which interventions would be necessary.
   3. Inhibition of serotonin receptors (opioids may produce part of analgesic effect through the release of serotonin): $5\text{-}HT_3$ antagonists, such as ondansetron, may reduce pruritus.
   4. Antihistamines have limited benefit/efficacy for pruritus related to opioids.

F. Chronic pruritus: Tricyclic antidepressants (see Appendix L)

VII. Follow-up
   A. Short term: Within 48 hours of initial contact, verify partial or complete resolution of symptoms. Many cases of pruritus spontaneously resolve.
   B. Long term: Follow-up is dependent on the etiology and causative factors.

VIII. Referrals
   A. Patients who do not improve or resolve after 48 hours, show progression of symptoms, or present with newly diagnosed underlying disease processes require referral to a dermatologist.
   B. Patients with underlying psychogenic causes or exacerbated distress require referral to the appropriate specialist.

The author would like to acknowledge Joanne Lester, PhD, CNP, AOCN®, for her contribution to this chapter that remains unchanged from the previous edition of this book.

References

Anzelc, M., & Burkhart, C.G. (2019). Pain and pruritus: A study of their similarities and differences. *International Journal of Dermatology, 59*(2), 159–164. https://doi.org/10.1111/ijd.14678

Besner Morin, C., & Misery, L. (2019). Emerging treatments and novel pathways in pruritus. *Journal of Cutaneous Medicine and Surgery, 23*(5), 528–536. https://doi.org/10.1177/1203475419852050

Fourzali, K.M., & Yosipovitch, G. (2019). Management of itch in the elderly: A review. *Dermatology and Therapy, 9*(4), 639–653. https://doi.org/10.1007/s13555-019-00326-1

Hashimoto, T., & Yosipovitch, G. (2019). Itching as a systemic disease. *Journal of Allergy and Clinical Immunology, 144*(2), 375–380. https://doi.org/10.1016/j.jaci.2019.04.005

Huang, A.H., Kaffenberger, B.H., Reich, A., Szepietowski, J.C., Ständer, S., & Kwatra, S.G. (2019). Pruritus associated with commonly prescribed medications in a tertiary care center. *Medicines, 6*(3), 84. https://doi.org/10.3390/medicines6030084

Kremer, A.E. (2019). What are new treatment concepts in systemic itch? *Experimental Dermatology, 28*(12), 1485–1492. https://doi.org/10.1111/exd.14024

Kremer, A.E., & Mettang, T. (2019). Pruritus in systemic diseases: Common and rare etiologies. *Der Internist, 60*(8), 814–820. https://doi.org/10.1007/s00108-019-0637-0

Mercadante, S. (2019). Opioid analgesics adverse effects: The other side of the coin. *Current Pharmaceutical Design, 25*(30), 3197–3202. https://doi.org/10.2174/1381612825666190717152226

Metz, M. (2019). Treatments for chronic pruritus outside the box. *Experimental Dermatology, 28*(12), 1476–1481. https://doi.org/10.1111/exd.14007

Nakashima, C., Ishida, Y., Kitoh, A., Otsuka, A., & Kabashima, K. (2019). Interaction of peripheral nerves and mast cells, eosinophils, and basophils in the development of pruritus. *Experimental Dermatology, 28*(12), 1405–1411. https://doi.org/10.1111/exd.14014

Pereira, M.P., Kremer, A.E., Mettang, T., & Ständer, S. (2016). Chronic pruritus in the absence of skin disease: Pathophysiology, diagnosis and treatment. *American Journal of Clinical Dermatology, 17*(4), 337–348. https://doi.org/10.1007/s40257-016-0198-0

Reich, A., & Szepietowski, J.C. (2016). Diagnostic procedures of itch. In J.C. Szepietowski & E. Weisshaar (Eds.), *Current problems in dermatology: Vol. 50. Itch—Management in clinical practice* (pp. 24–28). Karger. https://doi.org/10.1159/000446013

Rinaldi, G. (2019). The itch-scratch cycle: A review of the mechanisms. *Dermatology Practical and Conceptual, 9*(2), 90–97. https://doi.org/10.5826/dpc.0902a03

Sheriff, T., Lin, M.J., Dubin, D., & Khorasani, H. (2020). The potential role of cannabinoids in dermatology. *Journal of Dermatological Treatment, 31*(8), 839–845. https://doi.org/10.1080/09546634.2019.1675854

Smith, M.P., Ly, K., Thibodeaux, Q., Weerasinghe, T., Wu, J.J., Yosipovitch, G., … Liao, W. (2019). Emerging methods to objectively assess pruritus in atopic dermatitis. *Dermatology and Therapy, 9*(3), 407–420. https://doi.org/10.1007/s13555-019-0312-3

Song, J., Xian, D., Yang, L., Xiong, X., Lai, R., & Zhong, J. (2018). Pruritus: Progress toward pathogenesis and treatment. *BioMed Research International, 2018,* 9625936. https://doi.org/10.1155/2018/9625936

Yang, T.-L.B., & Kim, B.S. (2019). Pruritus in allergy and immunology. *Journal of Allergy and Clinical Immunology, 144*(2), 353–360. https://doi.org/10.1016/j.jaci.2019.06.016

CHAPTER 17

Rash

Marlene SanFilippo, MSN, ARNP, FNP-C, AOCNP®

I. Definition: A general term referring to a skin eruption (McCann et al., 2017)

II. Physiology/Pathophysiology
   A. Normal (Habif, 2016; McCann et al., 2017; Rote, 2017; Sun & Li, 2019)
      1. Skin is the largest body organ and primarily functions as a protective barrier against loss of body fluids, microorganisms, and ultraviolet light.
      2. Skin regulates body temperature, plays a role in vitamin D synthesis, and is involved in immune surveillance.
      3. Skin contains microorganisms to protect against pathologic bacteria.
      4. Skin consists of several layers.
         a) Epidermis: Thin outer layer where keratin and melanin are synthesized
         b) Dermis: Deeper connective tissue layer containing blood vessels, lymphatic vessels, and nerve supply; also contains sensory receptors, sweat glands, mast cells, and hair follicles
         c) Hypodermis: Subcutaneous, deepest layer of connective tissue containing fat cells, nerves, blood vessels, and hair follicles; connects dermis to the muscle
   B. Pathophysiology
      1. Many rashes result from cell-mediated or delayed hypersensitivity.
      2. A variety of allergens, such as mechanical irritants, microorganisms, chemicals, or medications, can act as a sensitizing agent.
      3. The epidermal Langerhans cells (specialized dendritic cells) present the antigen to lymphocytic T cells, which proliferate and enter circulation.
      4. Sensitization occurs with the first exposure to the antigen.
      5. Repeat exposure causes T lymphocytes to release inflammatory mediators, such as histamine, resulting in vasodilation, vascular permeability, cellular infiltration, and stimulation of nerve endings. As a result, skin changes may occur, including erythema, warmth, edema, pus, pain, and pruritus.

III. Clinical features
   A. Etiology: A large number of conditions manifest as generalized or localized rashes (Goodheart & Gonzalez, 2016; Habif, 2016; McCann et al., 2017; Muzumdar et al., 2019; Santistevan et al., 2017; Sun & Li, 2019; Wolff et al., 2017; Yun et al., 2020).
      1. Allergic reaction
      2. Autoimmune
      3. Environmental: Exposure to elements or physical agents
      4. Idiopathic
      5. Infectious: Bacterial, viral, fungal

      6. Malignancy associated

      7. Medication induced: Secondary to allergic reaction, drug accumulation, mast-cell mediators, overdosage, phototoxic dermatitis, intolerance, or adverse effects; increased risk in immunocompromised patients

      8. Psychiatric: Stress, anxiety, psychosis

      9. Systemic disease: SLE, diabetes mellitus, psoriasis

     10. Treatment related: Chemotherapy, immunotherapy, radiation therapy

B. History

      1. History of cancer and cancer treatment

      2. Current medications: Prescribed, over the counter; especially any new medications or recent changes within the past six weeks

      3. History of presenting symptoms: Precipitating factors, onset, location, duration, pattern of evolution, spread

      4. Changes in ADLs

      5. Past medical history: Asthma, eczema, hay fever, autoimmune disorders, systemic diseases (e.g., diabetes, SLE, psoriasis)

      6. Family history: Psoriasis, atopy, melanoma, skin cancer

      7. Recent travel, occupational exposure, chemical exposure, insect and plant exposure, contact with ill individuals

C. Signs and symptoms

      1. Fatigue, malaise

      2. Fever, chills, night sweats

      3. Joint swelling or discomfort

      4. Muscle aches

      5. Pain

      6. Paresthesia in extremities

      7. Pruritus

      8. Redness, warmth

      9. Weight loss, anorexia

D. Physical examination: Focus on integument.

      1. Assess entire skin, including the nails, scalp, palms, soles, and oral cavity.

        a) Evaluate consistency and the feel of lesion on palpation.

        b) Use magnification with hand lens to examine fine detail, if necessary.

        c) Oblique lighting in a darkened room may increase ability to detect change in elevation or depression.

        d) Subdued lighting enhances contrast between pigmentation of lesions and normal skin.

        e) Diascopy: Firmly press microscopic slide or glass spatula over rash lesion. If red macule or papule does not blanche, color is caused by extravasation of blood (purpura or petechiae) rather than true erythema from capillary dilation.

        f) Scratch test: Write "hives" on skin with tongue blade and observe for dermographism.

      2. Type of lesions/rash (see Table 17-1)

        a) Atrophy: Thinning of skin surface and loss of skin markings with translucency of the epidermis

        b) Bulla (large blister): Circumscribed, elevated, fluid-filled lesion greater than 0.5 cm in diameter

        c) Burrow: Narrow, raised, irregular channel

        d) Comedo: Plug of sebaceous material in the opening of a hair follicle; open comedo has dilated orifice and is known as a blackhead; closed comedo has narrowed opening and is known as a whitehead.

TABLE 17-1	Common Rash Presentations[a]	
Presentation	**Localized**	**Generalized**
Nonpruritic Small lesions: < 1 cm	Acne Actinic keratosis Candidiasis Fixed drug eruption Folliculitis Herpes simplex Herpes zoster Idiopathic thrombocytopenic pur- pura Keratosis pilaris Polymorphous light eruption Rosacea Solar lentigines Tinea versicolor	Dermatomyositis Drug eruption Erythema infectiosum Erythema multiforme Folliculitis Keratosis pilaris Pityriasis rosea Rocky Mountain spotted fever Rubella Rubeola (measles) Scarlet fever Tinea versicolor Viral exanthem
Nonpruritic Large lesions: > 1 cm	Candidiasis Cellulitis Cutaneous lupus erythematosus Erythema nodosum Fixed drug eruption Mycosis fungoides Seborrheic dermatitis Solar lentigines Systemic lupus erythematosus Tinea versicolor	Dermatomyositis Drug eruption Erythema infectiosum Erythema multiforme Lyme disease Pityriasis rosea Seborrheic dermatitis Tinea Tinea versicolor Viral exanthem
Pruritic Small lesions: < 1 cm	Candidiasis Fixed drug eruption Folliculitis Herpes simplex Herpes zoster Impetigo Lichen planus *Molluscum contagiosum* Perioral dermatitis Polymorphous light eruption Scabies Tinea	Atopic dermatitis Contact dermatitis Drug eruption Erythema multiforme Folliculitis Lichen planus Pityriasis rosea Scabies Urticaria Varicella Viral exanthem
Pruritic Large lesions: > 1 cm	Candidiasis Fixed drug eruption Mycosis fungoides Psoriasis Tinea	Atopic dermatitis Contact dermatitis Drug eruption Erythema multiforme Pityriasis rosea Tinea Urticaria Viral exanthem

[a] Rashes with variable presentation may be in more than one category.

Note. Based on information from Goodheart & Gonzalez, 2016; Habif, 2016; Wolff et al., 2017.

e) Crust: Scabs formed by dried blood, serum, or exudate
f) Cyst: Cutaneous lesion containing fluid or semisolid material
g) Erosion: Shallow loss of tissue involving only the epidermis
h) Excoriation: Erosions often caused by scratching, picking, or digging

    i) Fissure: Linear ulcers or cracks in the skin

    j) Lichenification: Rough, thickened epidermis secondary to persistent rubbing or skin irritation

    k) Macule: Small, nonpalpable lesion of any size or color

    l) Morbilliform: eruption with both macules and papules ("measles-like")

    m) Nodule: Firm, solid, palpable lesion greater than 0.5 cm in diameter

    n) Papule: Raised, palpable lesion up to 0.5 cm in diameter

    o) Patch: Flat, nonpalpable, irregularly shaped macule greater than 1 cm in diameter

    p) Petechiae: Circumscribed deposit of blood less than 0.5 cm in diameter

    q) Plaque: Elevated plateau-like lesion less than 0.5 cm in diameter; may be formed by confluence of papules

    r) Purpura: Circumscribed deposit of blood less than 0.5 cm in diameter

    s) Pustule: Circumscribed, superficial lesion containing purulent material

    t) Scale: Visible shedding or flaking of the epidermis; desquamation is scaling in sheets.

    u) Telangiectasia: Dilated, superficial blood vessels

    v) Ulcer: Loss of skin that extends into the dermis or deeper; heals with scarring

    w) Vesicle (small blister): Circumscribed, elevated, fluid-filled lesion measuring up to 0.5 cm in diameter

    x) Wheal (hive): Transient, raised, flesh-colored or erythematous papule or plaque that disappears within 24–48 hours

3. Shape of lesions

    a) Annular: Ring shaped

    b) Arciform: In the shape of an arc

    c) Linear: Following a line

    d) Nummular: Coin shaped

    e) Reticulated: Net shaped

4. Distribution of rash

    a) Extent: Localized or generalized

    b) Pattern

        (1) Central distribution

        (2) Dermatomal

        (3) Disseminated

        (4) Exposed/unexposed areas

        (5) Extensor surfaces

        (6) Follicular localization

        (7) Grouped (clustered)

        (8) Pressure site areas

        (9) Random

        (10) Symmetric

5. Associated findings: Erythema, edema, drainage, pigmentation changes

6. Lymph node examination: Regional lymphadenopathy (see Appendix D)

IV. Diagnostic tests: Typically, not necessary to diagnose the majority of rashes (Habif, 2016; Wolff et al., 2017)

  A. Laboratory

    1. Biopsy for suspected malignancy or to establish definitive diagnosis such as GVHD

    2. CBC: Increased WBCs may be associated with systemic disease and some drug reactions. Increased eosinophils may occur in acute allergic reactions. Anemia may be associated with chronic disease, whereas thrombocytopenia may coincide with petechiae.

    3. ESR to evaluate possible increase with systemic illness

    4. Gram stain to evaluate for suspected bacterial or yeast infection

    5. Patch testing to determine causative agent for allergic dermatitis

    6. KOH (potassium hydroxide) preparation of skin scraping: Rod-shaped hyphae and branching consistent with fungal infection

    7. Prick testing to determine allergen

    8. Wood's lamp test to evaluate for tinea

    9. Tzanck test to evaluate for herpes simplex, varicella, or HZV

  B. Radiology: Not indicated

V. Differential diagnosis (Alcedo et al., 2020; Backer, 2020; Bray et al., 2016; Goodheart & Gonzalez, 2016; Habif, 2016; Karthik et al., 2017; Muzumdar et al., 2019; Narayanan et al., 2017; NCCN, 2021; Rodrigues et al., 2018; Santistevan et al., 2017; Sivaganeshan & Vimalachandran, 2020; Sun & Li, 2019; Tsai et al., 2015; Wolff et al., 2017; Yun et al., 2020; see Table 17-1)

  A. Allergic reaction

    1. Atopic dermatitis (see Chapter 18)

    2. Contact dermatitis (see Chapter 20)

    3. Keratosis pilaris: Small, rough, follicular papules most often found on the upper arms, thighs, or buttocks

    4. Medication allergies: See medication differential.

    5. Urticaria: Erythematous or white, small to large wheals

  B. Autoimmune

    1. Cutaneous lupus erythematosus: Annular, erythematous, hyperkeratotic plaques on the face, trunk, arms, and hands after exposure to sunlight; limited to the skin (see Chapter 110)

    2. Dermatomyositis: Flat-topped, scaly, violaceous, and erythematous papules or plaques most often noted along the neck, shoulders, and dorsal aspects of the hands (including joints) with associated proximal muscle weakness

    3. ITP: Petechial hemorrhages or purpura (see Chapter 124)

    4. Psoriasis: Sharply marginated, erythematous papules and plaques with a silvery-white scale most commonly found on elbows, knees, scalp, sacrum, and groin

    5. SLE: Red to violaceous nonpruritic papules and plaques on sun-exposed areas (sparing the joints) with butterfly rash and photosensitivity; systemic symptoms often present (see Chapter 110)

  C. Environmental

    1. Actinic keratosis (solar keratosis): Small, less than 1 cm, rough, scaly macules, papules, and plaques most often found on sun-exposed areas

    2. Polymorphous light eruption: Erythematous papules, plaques, and vesicles most commonly on the face, "V" area of neck, and arms appearing within hours of sun exposure

    3. Solar lentigines (liver spots): Tan to dark brown, macular, scattered lesions with irregular borders varying in size and appearing on sun-exposed areas

    4. Xerosis (dry skin): Exaggerated skin markings with possible scaling and pruritus

  D. Idiopathic

    1. Erythema nodosum: Multiple, bilateral, tender, erythematous, subcutaneous nodules occurring most commonly on shins; may be associated with autoimmune disorders, infections, medications, and malignancy

    2. Lichen planus: Flat-topped, violaceous, 1–10 mm, shiny papules and plaques occurring in various shapes and sizes and leaving darkly pigmented macules with healing

3. Livedo reticularis: Mottled bluish-purple discoloration that appears in a net-like pattern; may be physiologic occurring with exposure to cold or secondary to systemic disorders, such as antiphospholipid syndrome
4. Nummular eczema: Sharply defined, coin-shaped, erythematous, scaled lesions
5. Perioral dermatitis: Small, erythematous papules and pustules circling the mouth but sparing the vermilion border of the lips
6. Pityriasis rosea: 1–2 cm, salmon-colored or light brown papules and oval plaques with fine scaling presenting in a Christmas tree pattern along the trunk; often preceded by a larger (2–5 cm) herald patch located on the trunk or proximal extremity
7. Rosacea: Chronic facial flushing, erythema, papules and pustules, and/or telangiectasia
8. Seborrheic dermatitis: Macules or papules with overlying dry, whitish, or greasy orange-yellow scale on red inflamed skin most often appearing on the scalp, face, body folds, or behind the ears

E. Infectious
1. Acne: Comedones, papules, pustules, nodules, cysts
2. Cellulitis (see Chapter 19)
3. Cutaneous candidiasis: Initial pustules become well-demarcated erythematous patches with satellite pustules and papules possible. Erythematous base may be beefy red and have scales. It may be pruritic or painful and is commonly found in occluded sites (e.g., inframammary, axillae, groin, perineal, abdominal panniculus, intergluteal).
4. Erythema infectiosum (fifth disease): Erythematous plaques appearing on cheeks, (slapped cheeks) followed by a lacy, reticular eruption on the trunk and extremities; constitutional symptoms may be present.
5. Erythema multiforme: Bilateral and symmetric dusky red macules and papules evolving to target lesions; most commonly on extremities
6. Folliculitis: Multiple small papules and pustules on an erythematous base
7. Herpes simplex: Uniformly sized painful vesicles grouped on an erythematous base
8. HZV (see Chapter 22)
9. Impetigo: Papules, vesicles, bullae, or small erosions typically on the face and with honey-colored crusting
10. Lyme disease: Initial red macule or papule at the site of a tick bite progressing to annular, erythematous lesion (erythema migrans) measuring 4–7 cm (see Chapter 104)
11. Measles (rubeola): Erythematous macules and papules initially presenting on face and neck becoming confluent and spreading to trunk and arms
12. Molluscum contagiosum: Small, pearly white or flesh-colored umbilicated, dome-shaped papules with waxy appearance and often in a grouped pattern
13. Rocky Mountain spotted fever: Pink, blanchable macules progressing to deep red papules that become hemorrhagic beginning on ankles and wrists and spreading centrally; systemic symptoms often occur prior to rash.
14. Rubella: Pink to red macules and papules that begin on the neck and face, quickly spreading to trunk and extremities
15. Scabies: Inflammatory, erythematous, intensely pruritic papules most often located on wrists, elbows, axillae, buttocks, genitalia, feet, ankles, or between fingers; burrows may be evident.
16. Scarlet fever: Fine papular erythematous rash with a sandpaper appearance often occurring on trunk and extremities following a streptococcal infection

17. Tinea (ringworm): Well-demarcated erythematous plaques with small papules on the margin and fine white scaling
    a) Tinea capitis: Involving scalp and hair
    b) Tinea corporis: Involving trunk, arms, and legs
    c) Tinea cruris: Involving inguinal region
    d) Tinea pedis: Involving feet
18. Tinea versicolor: Sharply marginated round or oval macules with fine scaling, varying in size; lesions are hypopigmented on tanned skin, and brown on untanned or naturally brown-black skin.
19. Varicella (chicken pox): Fluid-filled vesicles progressing to pustules then crusted lesions; initially on the face and scalp and extending inferiorly to trunk and extremities
20. Viral exanthema: Generalized, blanching, erythematous macules and papules with systemic symptoms; may include vesicles or petechiae

F. Malignancy associated
    1. Basal cell carcinoma: Pearly papule or nodule with a rolled border and telangiectasia; may have eroded center
    2. Cutaneous T-cell lymphoma (most often mycoses fungoides): Randomly distributed red to brown patches and plaques that are scaly in appearance and may mimic eczema, psoriasis, or dermatophytosis; nodules may be present.
    3. Glucagonoma syndrome: Erythema with superficial pustules and erosions involving the face, intertriginous skin, and extremities; associated with alpha cell tumor of the pancreas
    4. Kaposi sarcoma: Palpable, nonpruritic, red, purple, or brown papules and macules progressing to nodules and plaques
    5. Leukemia cutis: Tan, pink, or skin-colored papules found most often in patients with acute myeloid leukemia
    6. Melanoma: Evolving lesion (most often a mole) with varied pigmentation, asymmetry, and irregular border
    7. Paraneoplastic syndrome (see Appendix M)
    8. Squamous cell carcinoma: Solitary or multiple erythematous nodules, papules, or plaques; may be scaly or ulcerated and have a thick hyperkeratotic surface
    9. Sister Mary Joseph nodule: Firm, indurated nodule near the umbilical area with possible ulceration and hyperpigmentation; associated with abdominal and pelvic malignancy
    10. Sweet syndrome: Reddish-blue or violet papules, plaques, or nodules with or without pustules; may have fever, arthralgia, neutrophilia, oral ulcers, or conjunctivitis; approximately 20% incidence associated with malignancy

G. Medication induced
    1. Acneiform: Pustular lesions distinguished from true acne by lack of comedones
    2. Eczematous eruptions: Pruritic, scale-like, erythematous lesions most often found on flexor surfaces
    3. Exanthematous drug reaction: Confluent, erythematous macules and papules with pruritus; occurs 7–21 days after medication ingestion
    4. Fixed drug eruption: Single or multiple, round, sharply demarcated plaques with residual macular hyperpigmentation after healing
    5. Photosensitivity reaction: Exaggerated sunburn; may be painful or pruritic
    6. Acute generalized exanthematous pustulosis: Nonfollicular sterile pustules on a diffuse, edematous, erythemic base
    7. Stevens-Johnson syndrome/toxic epidermal necrolysis: Flat, atypical target lesions and erythematous macules that are generalized; may have bullae, erosions, and necrosis

H. Psychiatric
   1. Factitial dermatitis: Self-inflicted, bizarrely shaped blisters, plaques, and ulcers uncharacteristic of other etiology
   2. Lichen simplex chronicus: Large, oval plaques self-inflicted by scratching and rubbing
   3. Neurotic excoriations: Linear excoriations or hypopigmented macules located only in easily accessible regions; spares the mid-back
I. Systemic
   1. Diabetes: Diffuse velvety hyperpigmentation with thickening along the neck, axillae, and skin folds (acanthosis nigricans) (see Chapter 151)
   2. Hyperthyroidism: Pretibial flesh-colored, waxy, translucent plaques (see Chapter 157)
   3. Lipid abnormalities: Multiple dome-shaped red papules transforming to yellow centers with a red halo
   4. Nutritional deficiency: Patches and plaques with dry, scaly eczematous dermatitis (zinc deficiency); dermatitis on dorsal area of hands, face, and neck (niacin or tryptophan deficiency)
J. Treatment related
   1. Chemotherapy and targeted therapies (e.g., checkpoint inhibitors): Acral erythema (e.g., palmar-plantar erythrodysesthesia), erythema, edema, tenderness of palms and soles
   2. Radiation (see Figure 17-1, Figure 17-2, and Table 17-2)
      a) Recall dermatitis: Macular and papular eruption on erythemic base with possible vesicle formation, scaling, and desquamation; occurs at previously irradiated sites following administration of chemotherapy agents, most commonly anthracyclines, taxanes, antimetabolites, immunotherapies, and molecular or targeted agents; antibiotics, antilipidemics, and other medications also implicated
      b) Radiation dermatitis: Ranges from mild erythema to moist desquamation and ulceration; may occur acutely within one to four weeks after initiation of radiation, or months to years after completion of treatment
   3. Immunotherapy (e.g., monoclonal antibodies, cytokines, retinoids): May manifest with maculopapular rash or with flushing and erythema
   4. GVHD
      a) Acute: Most often occurring 10–100 days after HSCT; initial presentation of erythematous macules and papules with violaceous hue and fine scaling; progresses to erythema and bulla formation with erosion
      b) Chronic: Most commonly occurring more than 100 days after HSCT; flat-topped violaceous papules (lichen planus-like) and dermal sclerosis with scaling (sclerodermoid-like)
   5. EGFR inhibitors: Papules and pustules (acneiform) often on an erythematous base typically manifesting one to three weeks after initiating treatment
   6. Pruritus (e.g., checkpoint inhibitors)

FIGURE 17-1   **Factors Affecting Development of Skin Changes**

- Advanced age
- Combined-modality treatment
- Comorbid conditions
- General skin condition
- Nutritional status
- Prior sun damage
- Radiation type, dose, and fractionation regimen
- Tobacco use

Note. Based on information from Bray et al., 2016; Wolff et al., 2017.

FIGURE 17-2   **Treatment of Radiation Dermatitis**

- Avoid sun exposure. Use sunscreen with at least SPF 15.
- For dry desquamation: Use hydrophilic moisturizers. Use low- to mid-potency topical steroids to decrease disease progression, burning, itching, and irritation. Wear loose-fitting clothing to prevent friction and irritation.
- For moist desquamation: Use hydrogels and hydrocolloid dressings and nonadherent dressings.
- Lotions: Use plain, unscented, lanolin-free moisturizer on intact skin only.
- Washing: Washing or bathing should not be restricted. Gentle cleansing with mild soap and water is encouraged.

Note. Based on information from Bray et al., 2016; Wolff et al., 2017.

VI. Treatment: Directed at providing symptomatic relief and eliminating causative factors (Habif, 2016; NCCN, 2021; Rodrigues et al., 2018; Wolff et al., 2017)
   A. Topical treatment (see Table 17-3 and Appendix K)
   B. Systemic treatment must be specific to symptoms and etiology of rash.
      1. Antibiotic, antifungal, and antiviral agents based on infectious etiology (see Appendices C and J)
      2. Antihistamines for pruritus and/or allergic reaction (see Appendix H)

TABLE 17-2   **Radiation Therapy–Induced Skin Changes**

Adverse Skin Presentation	Description	Comment
Atrophy	Thinning of skin surface with loss of skin markings; loss of dermal appendages (e.g., hair follicles, sweat glands)	Involves epidermis and dermis; may result in permanent alopecia and absent or reduced sweating
Dry desquamation	Dryness, flaking, and peeling; may be pruritic	Occurs with 20–25 Gy of radiation with an onset of 3–4 weeks
Erythema	Faint to bright redness; may be warm to touch and have associated edema	Typically occurs within 1–4 weeks from start of radiation and with doses of 2–10 Gy
Hyperpigmentation	Tanned appearance	Occurs following 2–3 weeks of radiation and/or 12–20 Gy; may resolve or become chronic
Hypopigmentation	Loss of skin color	May resolve or become chronic
Moist desquamation	Intense erythema with skin sloughing and serous exudate; pain secondary to exposure of nerve endings	Occurs with 30–40 Gy of radiation with onset > 4 weeks
Telangiectasia	Fine, irregular red lines resulting from capillary dilation	May result from boost dosing, acute radiation injury, and moist desquamation
Ulceration and tissue necrosis	Nonhealing wound of the skin; usually painful; may have a leathery yellow appearance	Rare; most often occurs with high doses of radiation at frequent intervals; may require debridement

Note. Based on information from Bray et al., 2016; Wolff et al., 2017.

TABLE 17-3	Topical Treatment of Rash	
Treatment	**Base**	**Purpose**
Antibiotics	Varies	Often indicated to treat pustular lesions; especially indicated to treat inflammatory pustules secondary to EGFR inhibitors
Antifungals	Varies	Indicated to treat fungal infections such as candidiasis and tinea; may be combined with steroids for inflamed fungal infections
Antiparasitics/scabicides	Varies Lotion or cream based	Indicated for the treatment of scabies
Corticosteroids	See Appendix K.	Especially helpful for inflammatory lesions
Creams	Semisolid mixture of oil and water; usually contains a preservative	May function as a barrier; may cause drying with continued use; more potent than lotions and less potent than ointments
Emollients	Complex mixtures that may contain urea or lactic acid	Promotes hydration; removes excess keratin; typically, in the form of creams or lotions; most effective if applied to moist skin, such as after bathing
Foams	May contain alcohol base unless it is an emollient foam	May be drying; easy to spread in hairy areas.
Gels	Contains propylene glycol and water; may contain alcohol	Greaseless; transparent; useful for scalp area
Lotions	May contain water and alcohol; if it contains propylene glycol, may have a drying effect	Moisturizer; clear or milky in appearance; useful for scalp lesions because of ability to penetrate past hair
Ointments	Oil base, such as petroleum jelly, with little or no water; usually preservative free	Greater penetration than creams secondary to semiocclusive nature; not for exudative inflammation or intertriginous areas
Solutions	Water or nonaqueous base, such as propylene glycol or alcohol	Often used in combination with a dressing or in bath soaks
Wet compresses	Water Acetic acid 1%–2.5% solution Aluminum acetate solution Silver nitrate	Used to treat wet lesions; the cycles of wet to dry will dry out the lesion. Once dry, the wet compress should be discontinued, and creams and lotions should be applied.

Points to Remember
- If it is dry, wet it; if it is wet, dry it.
- When topical medications are prescribed, apply a thin layer of the medium. More is not necessarily better. Only the thin layer in contact with the skin is absorbed; the rest is rubbed off.
- Use of occlusion by placing medication under a nonbreathing dressing will increase absorption.
- Reduce risk of adverse effects (e.g., atrophy, acneiform eruptions, and formation of telangiectasias) from topical corticosteroid use by prescribing the least potent that will be effective, for shortest amount of time.

Amount to Prescribe
An area the size of the adult hand requires 0.25 g of ointment for adequate application; an area equal to four hands requires 1 g of ointment. For example, to prescribe medication to cover an area equal to four hands twice a day for 1 week, a 15 g tube would be prescribed (2 g daily for 7 days).

Note. Based on information from Goodheart & Gonzalez, 2016; Habif, 2016.

      3. Biologics for rashes caused by specific autoimmune disorders; prescribed by a qualified specialist

      4. Glucocorticoids for significant allergic reactions or severe inflammation (see Appendix K)

      5. Immunosuppressive agent for rashes secondary to autoimmune responses: Autoimmune-mediated systemic disease, GVHD

      6. NSAIDs to reduce mild to moderate inflammation (see Appendix E)

      7. Immune checkpoint inhibitor induced

         a) Maculopapular rash: Use topical emollient and oral antihistamine for pruritus.

           (1) Mild: Treat with moderate potency topical steroids (see Appendix K).

           (2) Moderate to severe: Initiate prednisone 0.5–1 mg/kg PO daily and treat until symptoms improve; taper over at least four to six weeks.

           (3) Persistent to severe: Hold therapy and increase prednisone dose up to 2 mg/kg PO daily and treat until symptoms improve; taper over at least four to six weeks.

         b) Bullous dermatitis

           (1) Mild: Hold therapy and use high-potency topical steroids (see Appendix K).

           (2) Moderate: Hold therapy. Initiate prednisone 0.5–1 mg/kg PO daily and treat until symptoms improve; taper over four to six weeks. If no improvement after three days, consider adding rituximab.

           (3) Severe: Permanently discontinue therapy. Initiate prednisone 1–2 mg/kg PO daily and treat until symptoms improve; taper over four to six weeks. If no improvement after three days, consider adding rituximab or IVIg.

VII. Follow-up

    A. Short term: Within one to two weeks to evaluate response to treatment and resolution of rash

    B. Long term: Dictated by etiology and severity of rash

VIII. Referrals

    A. Dermatologist: To establish diagnosis in complex cases or for failure of rash to resolve with treatment

    B. Internist, nephrologist, rheumatologist, infectious disease specialist, or endocrinologist: For management of rashes secondary to underlying disease

    C. Psychiatrist or counselor: For rashes secondary to psychiatric disorder

    D. Surgeon or dermatologist: For patients who require biopsy for definitive diagnosis

References

Alcedo, P.E., Petitto, G.S., & Rojas-Hernandez, C. (2020). Immune thrombocytopenia (ITP). In F.J. Domino, R.A. Baldor, J. Golding, & M.B. Stephens (Eds.), *The 5-minute clinical consult 2020* (28th ed., pp. 525–529). Wolters Kluwer.

Backer, E.L. (2020). Tinea (capitis, corporis, cruris). In F.J. Domino, R.A. Baldor, J. Golding, & M.B. Stephens (Eds.), *The 5-minute clinical consult 2020* (28th ed., pp. 988–989). Wolters Kluwer.

Bray, F.N., Simmons, B.J., Wolfson, A.H., & Nouri, K. (2016). Acute and chronic cutaneous reactions to ionizing radiation therapy. *Dermatology and Therapy, 6*(2), 185–206. https://doi.org/10.1007/s13555-016-0120-y

Goodheart, H.P., & Gonzalez, M.E. (2016). *Goodheart's photoguide to common pediatric and adult skin disorders* (4th ed.). Wolters Kluwer Health.

Habif, T.P. (2016). *Clinical dermatology: A color guide to diagnosis and therapy* (6th ed). Elsevier.

Karthik, R., Mohan, N., Kumar, R., & Fenn, S.M. (2017). Cutaneous manifestations of internal malignancy. *International Journal of Contemporary Medical Research, 4*(4), 935–939. https://www.ijcmr.com/uploads/7/7/4/6/77464738/ijcmr _1410_may_20.pdf

McCann, S.A., Nicol, N.H., & Huether, S.E. (2017). Structure, function, and disorders of the integument. In S.E. Huether & K.L. McCance (Eds.), *Understanding pathophysiology* (6th ed., pp. 1053–1083). Elsevier.

Muzumdar, S., Rothe, M.J., & Grant-Kels, J.M. (2019). The rash with maculopapules and fever in adults. *Clinical Dermatology, 37*(2), 109–118. https://doi.org/10.1016/j.clindermatol.2018.12.004

Narayanan, S., Mujtaba, B., Koay, J.E., Elshikh, M., Madewell, J.E., & Varadhachary, G.R. (2017). Radiation recall masquerading as an infectious process. *International Journal of Radiology and Radiation Therapy, 2*(6), 161–163. https://doi .org/10.15406/ijrrt.2017.02.00047

National Comprehensive Cancer Network. (2021). *NCCN Clinical Practice Guidelines in Oncology (NCCN Guidelines®): Management of immunotherapy-related toxicities* [v.3.2021]. https://www.nccn.org/professionals/physician_gls/pdf /immunotherapy.pdf

Rodrigues, K.S., Oliveira-Ribeiro, C., de Abreu Fiuza Gomes, S., & Knobler, R. (2018). Cutaneous graft-versus-host disease: Diagnosis and treatment. *American Journal of Clinical Dermatology, 19*(1), 33–50. https://doi.org/10.1007 /s40257-017-0306-9

Rote, N.S. (2017). Innate immunity: Inflammation and wound healing. In S.E. Huether & K.L. McCance (Eds.), *Understanding pathophysiology* (6th ed., pp. 134–157). Elsevier.

Santistevan, J., Long, B., & Koyfman, A. (2017). Rash decisions: An approach to dangerous rashes based on morphology. *Journal of Emergency Medicine, 52*(4), 457–471. https://doi.org/10.1016/j.jemermed.2016.10.027

Sivaganeshan, L., & Vimalachandran, P.P. (2020). Erythema multiforme. In F.J. Domino, R.A. Baldor, J. Golding, & M.B. Stephens (Eds.), *The 5-minute clinical consult 2020* (28th ed., pp. 342–343). Wolters Kluwer.

Sun, W., & Li, J. (2019). Skin toxicities with epidermal growth factor receptor tyrosine kinase inhibitors in cancer patients: A meta-analysis of randomized controlled trials. *Cancer Investigation, 37*(6), 253–264. https://doi.org/10.1080 /07357907.2019.1634089

Tsai, C.C., Hsieh, C.F., Hung, C.C., Chao, C.M., & Lai, C.C. (2015). Sister Mary Joseph nodule. *QJM: An International Journal of Medicine, 108*(12), 983. https://doi.org/10.1093/qjmed/hcv135

Wolff, K., Johnson, R.A., Saavedra, A.P., & Roh, E.K. (2017). *Fitzpatrick's color atlas and synopsis of clinical dermatology* (8th ed.). McGraw-Hill Education.

Yun, D.H., Novotney, J.M., & Wang, S. (2020). Cutaneous drug reactions. In F.J. Domino, R.A. Baldor, J. Golding, & M.B. Stephens (Eds.), *The 5-minute clinical consult 2020* (28th ed., pp. 236–237). Wolters Kluwer.

CHAPTER 18

Atopic Dermatitis

Tracy C. Wyant, DNP, AOCN®, CHPN, GERO-BC, CPPS, EBP-C

I. Definition: Eczema is a chronic, relapsing, pruritic, superficial inflammatory skin condition. This term is used interchangeably with *dermatitis* (Eichenfield et al., 2014; Peters & Peters, 2019; Simpson et al., 2019).

II. Physiology/Pathophysiology (Alhusayen et al., 2014; Bonamonte et al., 2019; Boothe et al., 2017; Garza, 2019; Hale et al., 2019; Kalamaha et al., 2019; Matthews et al., 2020; Peters & Peters, 2019; Simpson et al., 2019; Souto et al., 2019)

   A. Normal: Skin provides an elastic, rugged, self-regenerating, protective covering for the body and has three layers.

   1. Epidermis: Thin outer layer that acts as a barrier for immune surveillance, protects against substances and infections, restricts water loss

   2. Dermis: Middle layer that separates epidermis from cutaneous adipose tissue, interacts with vascular connective tissue and nervous system, and provides collagen to support skin structure

   3. Hypodermis: Deepest subcutaneous layer that consists of loose connective tissue and adipose tissue and plays a role in immune surveillance and energy balance

   B. Pathophysiology

   1. Atopic dermatitis is attributed to skin barrier defects, primarily in the *FLG* gene, combined with environmental exposures and changes in various components of immune response.

   2. Dermatitis demonstrates increased capillary permeability, allowing easier movement of lymphocytes out of capillaries.

   a) Atopic skin inflammation is orchestrated by the local expression of proinflammatory cytokines and chemokines.

   b) T lymphocytes, stimulated by IL-1, will produce IL-2, which then acts as an autocrine stimulant of T-lymphocyte proliferation.

   c) The developing inflammatory process proceeds by attracting "innocent bystanders," usually T lymphocytes.

   3. Immunologic abnormalities are common, including elevated IgE levels and alterations in cell-mediated immune responses, cytokine modulation, and neutrophil and monocyte chemotaxis. The role of IgE is unclear; however, epidermal Langerhans cells possess high-affinity IgE receptors that can mediate dermatitis reactions.

   4. Atopic dermatitis is familiarly transmitted with a strong maternal influence. Environmental factors may provoke alterations in immunologic responses in T cells, antigen processing, inflammatory cytokines, host defense proteins, allergen sensitivity, and infection.

III. Clinical features: The hallmark feature of atopic dermatitis is pruritus. Atopic dermatitis usually begins in childhood, varying with acute, subacute, and chronic phases through adolescence. Symptoms may lessen with age; complete resolution in adulthood is common but may persist into adulthood or suddenly reappear after a long remission (Alhusayen et al., 2014; Boothe et al., 2017; Charles et al., 2016; Hale et al., 2019; Peters & Peters, 2019; Phillips et al., 2018; Simpson et al., 2019; Souto et al., 2019).

A. Risk factors
1. Demographics: Studies suggest lower prevalence in rural areas as compared to urban areas, with higher prevalence in those with higher incomes and education regardless of ethnicity.
2. Risk may be associated with climatic factors, obesity, frequent antibiotic use, exposure to air pollution, and hard water use.
3. Exacerbations are common during periods of physical and emotional stress and with exposure to food and airborne allergens.

B. Etiology
1. Personal or family history of the atopic triad: Dermatitis, asthma, allergic rhinitis
2. Xerosis or dysfunction of skin barrier
3. IgE reactivity

C. History
1. History of cancer and cancer treatment
2. Current medications: Prescribed, over the counter, supplements
3. History of presenting symptoms: Precipitating factors, onset, location, frequency, duration, associated symptoms (e.g., pruritus, dry skin)
4. Changes in ADLs: Effects on sleep, impact on QOL
5. Past medical history: Eczema, asthma, allergic rhinitis, dermatitis, recurrence
6. Family medical history: Asthma, allergic rhinitis, dermatitis

D. Signs and symptoms
1. Pruritis: Severe, easily triggered itching, especially at night
2. Red to brownish-gray colored patches
3. Thickened, cracked, or scaly skin
4. Raw, sensitive skin from scratching
5. Tough, thick skin from constant scratching (i.e., lichenification)
6. Other common findings: Dryness, serous oozing, crusting, facial pallor, darkening beneath the eyes, hyperlinearity of palms and soles

E. Physical examination: Complete integument examination
1. Flexural involvement: Presence of lesions on back of neck, antecubital fossae, around wrists, behind knees, and around ankles
2. Generalized dry skin
3. Local signs of irritation and/or scratching
4. Dry papules, excoriations, and/or lichenification in affected areas
5. Follicular reactions in dark-skinned patients
6. Prominent lower eyelid folds (Dennie-Morgan folds) that give appearance of being older than chronologic age
7. Cutaneous vasculature responding abnormally to stimulation: Instead of normal "wheal and flare" response, firm skin rubbing elicits white dermographism, a simple white linear streak along the site of pressure with no erythema.
8. Race: African Americans often present with discrete follicular papules involving all hair follicles of the involved site.

IV. Diagnostic tests: Based on personal and family history, as well as presence of chronic, recurrent pruritic skin eruptions in classic locations (Alhusayen et al., 2014; Simpson et al., 2019)
   A. Laboratory: Usually not indicated but may be helpful
      1. Elevated IgE in about 80% of patients: Levels vary widely among individuals, so results are considered to be inconclusive.
      2. CBC: Peripheral blood eosinophilia (common)
      3. Allergy skin testing: Not especially helpful in diagnosis, except to rule out other types of dermatitis
      4. Skin biopsy: Indicated if area does not respond to treatment
      5. Bacterial culture of pustules
   B. Radiology: Not indicated

V. Differential diagnosis (Barrett & Luu, 2017)
   A. Drug reactions: Targeted anticancer therapies (e.g., EGFR inhibitors, kinase inhibitors, BRAF inhibitors, mitogen-activated protein kinase (MEK) inhibitors, immunomodulators)
   B. Immunodeficiency syndromes: Omenn, IPEX (immune dysregulation, polyendocrinopathy enteropathy, X-linked), Wiskott-Aldrich
   C. Psoriasis
   D. Scabies
   E. Allergic contact dermatitis (see Chapter 20)
   F. Cutaneous T-cell lymphoma (mycosis fungoides)
   G. HZV (see Chapter 22)
   H. Dermatophytosis (ringworm)
   I. Seborrheic dermatitis
   J. Dyshidrotic dermatitis
   K. Nummular dermatitis
   L. Drug reactions
   M. Photosensitivity disorders
   N. Nutritional deficiencies (see Chapter 66)

VI. Treatment (Alhusayen et al., 2014; Boothe et al., 2017; Chiarella, 2019; Katoh et al., 2019; Matthews et al., 2020; Peters & Peters, 2019; Simpson et al., 2019; Souto et al., 2019; Wernham et al., 2019)
   A. Goal is to individualize care and education, decrease trigger factors, control pruritus, suppress inflammation, hydrate/lubricate the skin, and manage QOL issues.
      1. First-line care is prevention of flare-ups with hygiene and skin care practices.
      2. If symptoms worsen, obtain a history of past treatment and effectiveness.
   B. Preventive measures
      1. Eliminate factors that exacerbate factors, including keeping environmental temperature constant and avoiding excess humidity or extreme dryness. Consider humidifying indoor air, especially in dry climates or during winter months.
      2. Wear absorbent, nonirritating cotton clothing and avoid potentially irritating fabrics (e.g., wool).
      3. Use mild cleansers and warm water for bathing and avoid friction when drying by patting the skin dry.
         a) Vanicream™ cleansing bar
         b) Unscented Dove® bath bar
         c) Unscented Neutrogena® cleansing bar
         d) Aveeno® oatmeal soap

    4. Lubricate the body daily, immediately after bathing, to trap water in the skin. Use fragrance-free, lanolin-free moisturizers.

      a) Lubriderm®

      b) Nutraderm®

      c) Eucerin® or Eucerin Plus

      d) Moisturel®

    5. Wash clothing and towels in bland or hypoallergenic soap; thoroughly rinse.

C. Pharmacologic management

    1. Nonsteroidal immunomodulators

      a) Tacrolimus ointment: Apply thin layer of 0.03% or 0.1% to affected skin areas two times a day. Rub in gently and completely. Continue for one week after atopic dermatitis clears.

      b) Pimecrolimus 1%: Apply thin layer to affected skin two times a day. Rub in gently and completely. Reevaluate if symptoms persist beyond six weeks.

    2. Crisaborole 2%: This boron-based topical ointment is classified as a phosphodiesterase 4 (PDE4) inhibitor and is approved to treat mild to moderate atopic dermatitis. In addition, it likely decreases production of proinflammatory cytokines.

    3. Topical corticosteroids: Initiate treatment with a high-potency steroid to quickly reduce symptoms, and then use to the lowest potency to control symptoms.

      a) Ointments are harder to apply but provide better biologic activity than creams or lotions.

      b) Lotions have higher water content than creams, are easier to apply, and provide a protective, drying, and cooling effect.

      c) Topical corticosteroids should be applied to moist skin after bathing (see Appendix K).

        (1) Moderate disease (thicker or unresponsive areas): Medium-potency topical corticosteroid preparations to control symptoms

          (a) Triamcinolone: 0.1% cream or ointment two to three times a day

          (b) Mometasone furoate: 0.1% cream daily

        (2) Mild disease: Low-potency topical corticosteroid preparations

          (a) Hydrocortisone: 1%–2.5% cream

          (b) Desonide: 0.05% cream

        (3) Isolated lichenified lesions: Betamethasone dipropionate 0.05% cream or ointment two times a day for two to three weeks

    4. Oral corticosteroids (see Appendix K)

      a) Systemic steroids provide rapid relief in many cases; however, frequent use can lead to steroid dependence or rebound effect when discontinued. Systemic steroids should be limited to severe, acute episodes.

      b) Dosage is determined by severity of the episode. Prednisone 0.5–1 mg/kg PO daily for a maximum of 7–10 days is typically used.

    5. Antibiotics: Lesions often are colonized with *Staphylococcus aureus*.

      a) Antibiotic therapy may be helpful for persistent lesions or those with secondary infection. Treat with oral antibiotics effective against *S. aureus* (see Appendix C).

        (1) Cephalexin: 500 mg PO every six hours for 7–14 days

        (2) Dicloxacillin: 500 mg PO every six hours for 7–14 days

      b) For limited involvement, topical antibiotics may be beneficial in place of oral agents. Use mupirocin 2% ointment three times a day for 10 days. Caution against other topical antimicrobial use that can lead to resistance.

    6. Antiviral agents: Treat herpes infections aggressively because of predisposition to more severe and disseminated infections (see Chapter 22).

         a) Herpes simplex: Acyclovir 400 mg PO three times a day for 10 days or 200 mg four times a day for 10 days

         b) Varicella zoster: Valacyclovir 1,000 mg PO two times a day for seven days or famciclovir 500 mg PO three times a day for seven days

  D. Nonpharmacologic therapies

    1. Drying agents: Aluminum acetate (Burow) solution compresses should be applied for 20 minutes four to six times a day.

    2. Soothing baths: Oatmeal baths may be soothing and help reduce dryness. Mix one cup of oatmeal bath and two cups of cold tap water, shake, and pour into tub one-half full of lukewarm water. Remain in tub for 30 minutes.

    3. Cool environment and compresses: Cold, wet cloths may be soothing.

  E. Pruritus control (see Chapter 16)

    1. Use of topical corticosteroids and NSAIDs helps reduce inflammation and dryness, which can subsequently reduce pruritus.

    2. Oral antihistamines may offer relief at night (see Appendix H).

         a) Hydroxyzine hydrochloride 10–50 mg PO every six hours PRN

         b) Cyproheptadine hydrochloride: 4 mg PO three times a day, increasing the dosage to relieve symptoms but not to exceed 0.5 mg/kg daily

         c) Diphenhydramine hydrochloride: 25–50 mg PO every four to six hours PRN

    3. Other topical agents

         a) Pramoxine hydrochloride: May be purchased over the counter; follow label directions; may be used in addition to topical steroids

         b) Doxepin cream 5% for short-term use (i.e., less than eight days): May be applied four times a day PRN in addition to topical steroids; may cause drowsiness

    4. Severe atopic dermatitis: Phototherapy using ultraviolet light therapy or systemic immunosuppressants and targeted therapies (e.g., dupilumab, methotrexate, cyclosporine, IFN-γ) under the care of a dermatologist

VII. Follow-up (Alhusayen et al., 2014; Charles et al., 2016; Matthews et al., 2020; Simpson et al., 2019)

  A. Short term: Monitor patient for relief of symptoms; adjust therapies PRN.

  B. Long term: Evaluate exacerbation PRN. Assess for effect on QOL.

  C. Patient fact sheets are available from the National Eczema Association (https://national eczema.org/eczema/patient-fact-sheet).

VIII. Referral

  A. Dermatologist: For comprehensive differential diagnosis, treatment plan, and severe cases

  B. Psychosocial support: Counseling for sleep, ADLs, or QOL issues

The author would like to acknowledge Janet S. Fulton, PhD, RN, ACNS-BC, FAAN, for her contribution to this chapter that remains unchanged from the previous edition of this book.

References

Alhusayen, R.O., Knowles, S.R., & Shear, N.H. (2014). Types of dermatologic reactions. In M.E. Lacouture (Ed.), *Dermatologic principles and practice in oncology: Conditions of the skin, hair, and nails in cancer patients* (pp. 33–46). Wiley-Blackwell.

Barrett, M., & Luu, M. (2017). Differential diagnosis of atopic dermatitis. *Immunology and Allergy Clinics of North America, 37*(1), 11–34. https://doi.org/10.1016/j.iac.2016.08.009

Bonamonte, D., Filoni, A., Vestita, M., Romita, P., Foti, C., & Angelini, G. (2019). The role of the environmental risk factors in the pathogenesis and clinical outcome of atopic dermatitis. *BioMed Research International, 2019,* 2450605. https://doi.org/10.1155/2019/2450605

Boothe, D., Tarbox, J.A., & Tarbox, M.B. (2017). Atopic dermatitis: Pathophysiology. In E.A. Fortson, S.R. Feldman, & L.C. Strowd (Eds.), *Advances in experimental medicine and biology: Vol. 1027. Management of atopic dermatitis: Methods and challenges* (pp. 21–37). Springer. https://doi.org/10.1007/978-3-319-64804-0_3

Charles, C., Bungener, C., Razavi, D., Mateus, C., Routier, E., Lanoy, E., ... Dauchy, S. (2016). Impact of dermatologic adverse events induced by targeted therapies on quality of life. *Critical Reviews in Oncology/Hematology, 101,* 158–168. https://doi.org/10.1016/j.critrevonc.2016.03.003

Chiarella, S.E. (2019). Immunobiologic treatments for severe asthma, atopic dermatitis, and chronic urticaria. *Allergy and Asthma Proceedings, 40*(6), 485–489. https://doi.org/10.2500/aap.2019.40.4277

Eichenfield, L.F., Tom, W.L., Chamlin, S.L., Feldman, S.R., Hanifin, J.M., Simpson, E.L., ... Sidbury, R. (2014). Guidelines of care for the management of atopic dermatitis: Section 1. Diagnosis and assessment of atopic dermatitis. *Journal of the American Academy of Dermatology, 70*(2), 338–351. https://doi.org/10.1016/j.jaad.2013.10.010

Garza, L. (2019). Developmental biology of the skin. In S. Kang, M. Amagai, A.L. Bruckner, A.H. Enk, D.J. Margolis, A.J. McMichael, & J.S. Orringer (Eds.), *Fitzpatrick's dermatology* (9th ed., pp. 49–61). McGraw-Hill Education.

Hale, G., Davies, E., Grindlay, D.J.C., Rogers, N.K., & Harman, K.E. (2019). What's new in atopic eczema? An analysis of systematic reviews published in 2017. Part 2: Epidemiology, aetiology and risk factors. *Clinical and Experimental Dermatology, 44*(8), 868–873. https://doi.org/10.1111/ced.14075

Kalamaha, K., Reis, E., Newton, S., Roche, C., Julson, J., Fernandes, H., & Rodrigues, J. (2019). Atopic dermatitis: A review of evolving targeted therapies. *Expert Reviews of Clinical Immunology, 15*(3), 275–288. https://doi.org/10.1080/1744666X.2019.1560267

Katoh, N., Ohya, Y., Ikeda, M., Ebihara, T., Katayama, I., Saeki, H., ... Yamamoto-Hanada, K. (2019). Clinical practice guidelines for the management of atopic dermatitis 2018. *Journal of Dermatology, 46*(12), 1053–1101. https://doi.org/10.1111/1346-8138.15090

Matthews, N.H., Moustafa, F., Kaskas, N.M., Robinson-Bostom, L., & Pappas-Taffer, L. (2020). Dermatologic toxicities of anticancer therapy. In J.E. Niederhuber, J.O. Armitage, M.B. Kastan, J.H. Doroshow, & J.E. Tepper (Eds.), *Abeloff's clinical oncology* (6th ed., pp. 621–648). Elsevier.

Peters, N., & Peters, A.T. (2019). Atopic dermatitis. *Allergy and Asthma Proceedings, 40*(6), 433–436. https://doi.org/10.2500/aap.2019.40.4265

Phillips, G.S., Freites-Martinez, A., Hsu, M., Lucas, A.S., Barrios, D.M., Ciccolini, K., ... Lacouture, M.E. (2018). Inflammatory dermatoses, infections, and drug eruptions are the most common skin conditions in hospitalized cancer patients. *Journal of the American Academy of Dermatology, 78*(6), 1102–1109. https://doi.org/10.1016/j.jaad.2017.12.031

Simpson, E.L., Leung, D.Y.M., Eichenfield, L.F., & Boguniewicz, M. (2019). Atopic dermatitis. In S. Kang, M. Amagai, A.L. Bruckner, A.H. Enk, D.J. Margolis, A.J. McMichael, & J.S. Orringer (Eds.), *Fitzpatrick's dermatology* (9th ed., pp. 363–385). McGraw-Hill Education.

Souto, E.B., Dias-Ferreira, J., Oliveira, J., Sanchez-Lopez, E., Lopez-Machado, A., Espina, M., ..., Silva, A.M. (2019). Trends in atopic dermatitis—From standard pharmacotherapy to novel drug delivery systems. *International Journal of Molecular Sciences, 20*(22), 5659. https://doi.org/10.3390/ijms20225659

Wernham, A.G.H., Veitch, D., Grindlay, D.J.C., Rogers, N.K., & Harman, K.E. (2019). What's new in atopic eczema? An analysis of systematic reviews published in 2017. Part 1: Treatment and prevention. *Clinical and Experimental Dermatology, 44*(8), 861–867. https://doi.org/10.1111/ced.14044

CHAPTER 19

Cellulitis

Tracy C. Wyant, DNP, AOCN®, CHPN, GERO-BC, CPPS, EBP-C

I. Definition: A common, deep bacterial infection of the skin and subcutaneous tissue caused by a breach in the physical skin barrier with concurrent immunosuppression; characterized as purulent or nonpurulent (Cranendonk et al., 2017; Pearson & Margolis, 2019; Stevens et al., 2014)

II. Physiology/Pathophysiology (Balagula et al., 2014; Cranendonk et al., 2017; Garza, 2019; Matthews et al., 2020; Pearson & Margolis, 2019; Stevens et al., 2014)
   A. Normal: Skin provides an elastic, rugged, self-regenerating, protective covering for the body and has three layers.
      1. Epidermis: Thin outer layer that acts as a barrier for immune surveillance, protects against substances and infections, restricts water loss
      2. Dermis: Middle layer that separates epidermis from cutaneous adipose tissue, interacts with vascular connective tissue and nervous system, and provides collagen to support skin structure
      3. Hypodermis: Deepest subcutaneous layer that consists of loose connective tissue and adipose tissue and plays a role in immune surveillance and energy balance
   B. Pathophysiology
      1. An opportunistic organism enters the dermis through a cut, abrasion, or preexisting dermatologic disorder, such as an open ulcer, or it may be seeded by the hematogenous route from another source of infection in the body, such as a surgical wound.
         a) Tissue edema predisposes the skin to bacterial proliferation, producing a host of extracellular enzymes, including alpha- and beta-hemolysin, leukocidin, coagulase, hyaluronidase, and lipases. Anaerobic bacteria can produce the enzymes and act synergistically with aerobic bacteria.
            (1) Nonpurulent: Typically superficial, widespread, and rapidly spreading; the number of organisms in the affected area usually is low with difficulty obtaining specimen for cultures.
            (2) Purulent: Commonly involve smaller, contained area (e.g., sebaceous cyst, abscess, carbuncle, furuncle), allowing easier access to obtain culture specimen
         b) Damage to local lymphatics can result in residual lymphedema and predispose the patient to recurrent infections.
      2. Opportunistic organisms may multiply in conditions of reduced lymphatic drainage or reduced capillary perfusion.

III. Clinical features: Cellulitis and abscess are among the most common skin and soft tissue infections. Cellulitis is a frequently encountered condition but remains a challenging clinical entity (Balagula et al., 2014; Charles et al., 2016; Clebak & Malone, 2018; Cranendonk et al., 2017; Featherstone et al., 2019; Matthews et al., 2020; Neill et al., 2019; Pearson & Margolis, 2019; Phillips et al., 2018; Stevens et al., 2014; Sullivan & de Barra, 2018).

A. Risk factors
1. Diabetes mellitus
2. Alcoholism
3. Compromised lymphovascular, immune, hepatic, or renal function
4. Impaired skin integrity
5. Lymphedema
6. Radiation therapy
7. Exposure to opportunistic organisms by skin contaminations (e.g., animals)
8. Cellulitis of the central face that may extend to the cavernous sinus
9. Obesity
10. Insect bites or scratches by household pets and other animals
11. Recent surgical or IV procedure
12. Any reported risk factor for MRSA: Previous hospitalization, residence in a long-term care facility, hemodialysis, recent antibiotic use, crowded living arrangements

B. Etiology
1. Nonpurulent: Usual organisms are staphylococci groups A, B, C, and G beta-hemolytic streptococci and, less often, methicillin-susceptible *Staphylococcus aureus* (MSSA).
2. Purulent: It commonly is involved in smaller, contained area (e.g., sebaceous cyst, abscess, carbuncle, furuncle); common organisms include both MSSA and MRSA.
3. Cellulitis can occasionally be caused by other aerobic and anaerobic bacteria, as well as deep fungi, such as *Cryptococcus neoformans,* particularly in immunosuppressed patients.
4. Enteric aerobic and anaerobic bacteria can cause cellulitis of the perineum.
5. Mucosal surface injuries predispose one to anaerobic organisms, such as traumatic or extravasation wounds.
6. Infection spreads along the fascial planes if connective tissue is involved.
7. Variants of cellulitis
   a) Erysipelas: Common sites include the face, lower legs, and areas of preexisting lymphedema. It is predominantly caused by group A beta-hemolytic streptococci, is superficial, and involves lymphatics. Margins of lesions are raised, sharply demarcated from adjacent normal skin, and often painful. The surface has an "orange peel" (peau d'orange) appearance.
   b) Erysipeloid: It can be located on the hands, especially fingers, after handling saltwater fish, shellfish, meat, hides, or poultry. It is caused by *Erysipelothrix rhusiopathiae.* Systemic symptoms usually are not present.
   c) Ecthyma gangrenosum: It is usually located in the lower extremities. It is caused by *Pseudomonas aeruginosa.* The limb becomes ulcerated with necrosis.
   d) Cryptococcal cellulitis: It usually occurs on an extremity and in immunocompromised patients and presents with erythematous, hot, tender, edematous plaque. It rarely involves multiple noncontiguous sites.
   e) Infectious gangrene (gangrenous cellulitis): It is rapidly progressive and associated with extensive necrosis of subcutaneous tissue and overlying skin. It is usually caused by *Clostridium* species. Prognosis is guarded.
8. Local fibrosis: Ischemia after surgery, lymphatic and capillary sclerosis from radiation therapy, and stagnant lymph flow following node dissection are likely factors in long-term predisposition to cellulitis.

     9. Cellulitis following breast cancer surgery may occur years after treatment. Source of infection may be endogenous flora introduced through the ductal system and residing in the parenchyma, serving as a nidus for overt infection.

  C. History

    1. History of cancer and cancer treatment

    2. Current medications: Prescribed, over the counter, supplements

    3. History of presenting symptoms: Precipitating factors, onset, location, frequency, duration

    4. Changes in ADLs: Effects on sleep, impact on QOL

    5. Past medical history: Phlebitis, varicose veins, claudication, pretibial nodularity, diabetes, heart failure, peripheral vascular disease, lymphedema

  D. Signs and symptoms: Dependent on type, infectious organism, and location

    1. Classic nonpurulent: Diffuse warm, painful, erythematous rash

    2. Purulent: Bulla formation with localized area of hot, swollen, tender, erythematous skin

    3. Fever, chills, and rigor inconsistently present

    4. Diffuse myalgia, headache, malaise

    5. Peau d'orange appearance with lymphatic involvement, along with linear streaking and lymphadenopathy

    6. Inflammation, edema, hemorrhage

    7. Pain and crepitus with mobility or ambulation

  E. Physical examination

    1. Vital signs: Assess for fever.

    2. Integument

      a) Affected skin area is warm, swollen, tender, erythematous, and localized or diffuse; bulla may be present; edges are not well demarcated.

      b) Palpate for crepitus, indicating gas production and suggesting anaerobic involvement; note any foul odor.

      c) Note any skin breaks, ulceration, or atrophy.

    3. Lymph node examination (see Appendix D)

      a) If affected, regional lymph nodes usually are palpable and tender.

      b) After lymph node dissection or radiation therapy (e.g., breast cancer), the breast may be swollen, tender, erythematous, and warm to touch. Lymph node dissection with or without radiation is prone to cellulitis.

      c) Linear red streaking extending proximally with tender lymph nodes indicates lymphangitis.

IV. Diagnostic tests (Balagula et al., 2014; Cranendonk et al., 2017; Grada & Phillips, 2017; Neill et al., 2019; Pearson & Margolis, 2019; Stevens et al., 2014)

  A. Laboratory

    1. Wound culture

      a) Nonpurulent: Obtain culture and aspirate or biopsy at the leading edge of inflammation, if possible. Cultures often are inconclusive and not performed because organisms are diffuse.

      b) Purulent: Obtain culture from bulla and/or surrounding area.

      c) For aspiration method, inject 0.5–1 ml of nonbacteriostatic saline, then aspirate and send for a Gram stain and culture.

    2. Obtain blood cultures if patient has rigors, fever, or chills.

      a) If patient has a vascular access device, obtain cultures from the device and peripherally.

   b) Bacteremia is not common in cellulitis, and positive blood cultures are rarely noted; therefore, blood cultures are not routinely necessary.
  3. CBC with differential: WBC count may be elevated.
  4. ESR may be elevated.
  5. Possible necrotizing fasciitis requires immediate deep biopsy and frozen section for histopathology.
 B. Radiology
  1. Initiate plain x-ray of affected area if crepitus is present, as gas production may indicate gangrene.
  2. CT may show deep fascial thickening or associated deep tissue abscesses.
  3. MRI is useful in distinguishing cellulitis and necrotizing fasciitis.
 C. Other: Surgical intervention is the only way to definitively diagnose necrotizing soft tissue infections.

V. Differential diagnosis (Balagula et al., 2014; Grada & Phillips, 2017; Matthews et al., 2020; Neill et al., 2019; Pearson & Margolis, 2019; Phillips et al., 2018; Stevens et al., 2014)
 A. DVT (see Chapter 43), superficial hematoma, thrombophlebitis (see Chapter 164)
 B. Early contact dermatitis (see Chapters 18 and 20)
 C. Acute urticarial plaque from bee stings and insect bites
 D. Prevesicular HZV (see Chapter 22)
 E. Necrotizing fasciitis and synergistic gangrene
 F. Diabetes mellitus (see Chapter 151)
 G. Allergic reactions
 H. Peripheral vascular disease (see Chapter 51)
 I. Erythema nodosum
 J. Acute gout: Significant cutaneous inflammation beyond the involved joint (see Chapter 103)
 K. Osteomyelitis
 L. Erythema migrans
 M. Skin abscess
 N. Septic arthritis

VI. Treatment (Almulhim & Alotaibi, 2018; Balagula et al., 2014; Brindle et al., 2019; Clebak & Malone, 2018; Cranendonk et al., 2017; Dalal et al., 2017; Featherstone et al., 2019; Matthews et al., 2020; Pearson & Margolis, 2019; Stevens et al., 2014; Sullivan & de Barra, 2018)
 A. Overall goal is infection resolution with minimal tissue damage.
 B. Consider hospitalizing immunocompromised patients because decompensation can occur quickly.
 C. Supportive care includes rest, immobilization and elevation of limbs, and analgesia.
 D. Warm, moist compresses can be applied to the affected area for 20 minutes three to four times a day. To prevent burns and further tissue damage, do not use a heating pad or other electric heating device.
 E. For cellulitis prior to radiation therapy, postpone therapy until infection resolves.
 F. Antibiotics: Recommendations vary depending on presence of purulence and clinical evaluation for other symptoms; treatment decision depends on the causative organism, sensitivity to the antibiotic, and overall patient response (see Appendix C).
  1. If organism is not known, therapy should cover both group A beta-hemolytic streptococci and *S. aureus.*
  2. Studies have not demonstrated optimal type, dosing, and length of treatment; reassessment for response to therapy is essential, along with assessment of

cost-effectiveness. The Infectious Diseases Society of America recommends the following.

    a) 5–10 days for uncomplicated types

    b) 7–14 days for uncomplicated types in immunosuppressed patients

    c) Longer treatment courses for severe or systemic infections

    d) Prophylactic antibiotics considered if three to four recurrences per year

3. Nonpurulent

    a) Treat uncomplicated nonpurulent type with beta-lactam or non–beta-lactam agents. Clindamycin or trimethoprim/sulfamethoxazole may be added; use oral or parenteral depending on situation.

    b) For suspected systemic infection, consider cefazolin, ceftriaxone, or penicillin G; vancomycin if known MRSA; or broad-spectrum parenteral antibiotics for severe infections or in immunocompromised patients.

4. Purulent

    a) Until organism is identified, use oral antistaphylococcal agents.

    b) Consider treatment based on clinical assessment of suspected MSSA (e.g., cephalexin, dicloxacillin) or MRSA (e.g., clindamycin, tetracyclines, trimethoprim/sulfamethoxazole).

    c) For systemic infection or failed outpatient treatment, use parenteral antibiotics (with possible hospitalization) such as oxacillin, nafcillin, cefazolin, or clindamycin for MSSA and vancomycin, clindamycin, or linezolid for MRSA. Use broad-spectrum agents if organism is not yet known.

5. Fluoroquinolones for gram-negative cellulitis: Use with caution.

6. Necrotizing fasciitis and gangrene: Prompt surgical debridement and broad-spectrum IV antibiotics with hospitalization for monitoring therapy response are crucial for survival.

  G. Patients with drainable abscess should undergo incision and drainage procedure.

VII. Follow-up (Charles et al., 2016; Dalal et al., 2017; Matthews et al., 2020; Pearson & Margolis, 2019; Stevens et al., 2014)

  A. For oral outpatient therapy, follow-up should occur after one to two days to assess response to the antibiotic choice and determine need for additional supportive therapy.

  B. Hospitalization is indicated if the patient is not healing or has fevers, rigors, lymphangitis, or involvement of the face, orbit, or perineum.

  C. Regular follow-up is dependent on patient history and comorbidities.

VIII. Referrals: If cellulitis is suspected, refer to physician for complete evaluation.

  A. Infectious disease or surgical consult: May be needed for definitive diagnosis

  B. Pharmacologist: May be helpful in selecting and monitoring antibiotics

  C. Surgeon: For debridement of necrotizing fasciitis and gangrene

  D. Psychosocial support: Counseling for sleep, ADLs, or QOL issues

The author would like to acknowledge Janet S. Fulton, PhD, RN, ACNS-BC, FAAN, for her contribution to this chapter that remains unchanged from the previous edition of this book.

References

Almulhim, A.S., & Alotaibi, F.M. (2018). Comparison of broad-spectrum antibiotics and narrow-spectrum antibiotics in the treatment of lower extremity cellulitis. *International Journal of Health Sciences, 12*(6), 3–7.

Balagula, Y., Lacouture, M.E., & Ito, J.I. (2014). Dermatologic infections. In M.E. Lacouture (Ed.), *Dermatologic princi-ples and practice in oncology: Conditions of the skin, hair, and nails in cancer patients* (pp. 319–336). Wiley-Blackwell.

Brindle, R., Williams, O.M., Barton, E., & Featherstone, P. (2019). Assessment of antibiotic treatment of cellulitis and erysipelas: A systematic review and meta-analysis. *JAMA Dermatology, 155*(9), 1033–1040. https://doi.org/10.1001/jamadermatol.2019.0884

Charles, C., Bungener, C., Razavi, D., Mateus, C., Routier, E., Lanoy, E., ... Dauchy, S. (2016). Impact of dermatologic ad-verse events induced by targeted therapies on quality of life. *Critical Reviews in Oncology/Hematology, 101,* 158–168. https://doi.org/10.1016/j.critrevonc.2016.03.003

Clebak, K.T., & Malone, M.A. (2018). Skin infections. *Primary Care: Clinics in Office Practice, 45*(3), 433–454. https://doi.org/10.1016/j.pop.2018.05.004

Cranendonk, D.R., Lavrijsen, A.P.M., Prins, J.M., & Wiersinga, W.J. (2017). Cellulitis: Current insights into pathophysi-ology and clinical management. *Netherlands Journal of Medicine, 75*(9), 366–378. http://www.njmonline.nl/article_ft.php?a=1907&d=1260&i=210

Dalal, A., Eskin-Schwartz, M., Mimouni, D., Ray, S., Days, W., Hodak, E., ... Paul, M. (2017). Interventions for the preven-tion of recurrent erysipelas and cellulitis. *Cochrane Database of Systematic Reviews, 2017*(6). https://doi.org/10.1002/14651858.CD009758.pub2

Featherstone, P., Brindle, R., & Williams, O.M. (2019). Acute management of cellulitis: A review. *Acute Medicine, 18*(2). 112–119.

Garza, L. (2019). Developmental biology of the skin. In S. Kang, M. Amagai, A.L. Bruckner, A.H. Enk, D.J. Margolis, A.J. McMichael, & J.S. Orringer (Eds.), *Fitzpatrick's dermatology* (9th ed., pp. 49–61). McGraw-Hill Education.

Grada, A.A., & Phillips, T.J. (2017). Lymphedema: Diagnostic workup and management. *Journal of the American Academy of Dermatology, 77*(6), 995–1006. https://doi.org/10.1016/j.jaad.2017.03.021

Matthews, N.H., Moustafa, F., Kaskas, N.M., Robinson-Bostom, L., & Pappas-Taffer, L. (2020). Dermatologic toxicities of anticancer therapy. In J.E. Niederhuber, J.O. Armitage, M.B. Kastan, J.H. Doroshow, & J.E. Tepper (Eds.), *Abeloff's clin-ical oncology* (6th ed., pp. 621–648). Elsevier.

Neill, B.C., Stoecker, W.V., Hassouneh, R., Rajpara, A., & Aires, D.J. (2019). CELLULITIS: A mnemonic to increase accura-cy of cellulitis diagnosis. *Dermatology Online Journal, 25*(1), 14. https://escholarship.org/uc/item/9mt4b2kc

Pearson, D.R., & Margolis, D.J. (2019). Cellulitis and erysipelas. In S. Kang, M. Amagai, A.L. Bruckner, A.H. Enk, D.J. Mar-golis, A.J. McMichael, & J.S. Orringer (Eds.), *Fitzpatrick's dermatology* (9th ed., pp. 2746–2756). McGraw-Hill Edu-cation.

Phillips, G.S., Freites-Martinez, A., Hsu, M., Lucas, A.S., Barrios, D.M., Ciccolini, K., ... Lacouture, M.E. (2018). Inflam-matory dermatoses, infections, and drug eruptions are the most common skin conditions in hospitalized cancer pa-tients. *Journal of the American Academy of Dermatology, 78*(6), 1102–1109. https://doi.org/10.1016/j.jaad.2017.12.031

Stevens, D.L., Bisno, A.L., Chambers, H.F., Dellinger, E.P., Goldstein, E.J.C., Gorbach, S.L., ... Wade, J.C. (2014). Practice guidelines for the diagnosis and management of skin and soft tissue infections: 2014 update by the Infectious Diseases Society of America. *Clinical Infectious Diseases, 59*(2), e10–e52. https://doi.org/10.1093/cid/ciu296

Sullivan, T., & de Barra, E. (2018). Diagnosis and management of cellulitis. *Clinical Medicine Journal, 18*(2), 160–163. https://doi.org/10.7861/clinmedicine.18-2-160

CHAPTER 20

Contact Dermatitis

Tracy C. Wyant, DNP, AOCN®, CHPN, GERO-BC, CPPS, EBP-C

I. Definition: Dermatitis is an inflammatory response of the skin resulting from exposure to an environmental substance. Contact dermatitis is divided into two types (Garza, 2019; Nedorost, 2019; Milam & Cohen, 2019; Turrentine et al., 2019).
  A. Irritant: Nonimmunologic-mediated inflammation of the skin
  B. Allergic: T-cell–mediated delayed hypersensitivity

II. Physiology/Pathophysiology (Alhusayen et al., 2014; Brys et al., 2020; Kränke & Schuster, 2015; Matthews et al., 2020; Phillips et al., 2018; Turrentine et al., 2019)
  A. Normal: Skin provides an elastic, rugged, self-regenerating, protective covering for the body and has three layers.
    1. Epidermis: Thin outer layer that acts as a barrier for immune surveillance, protects against substances and infections, restricts water loss
    2. Dermis: Middle layer that separates epidermis from cutaneous adipose tissue, interacts with vascular connective tissue and nervous system, and provides collagen to support skin structure
    3. Hypodermis: Deepest subcutaneous layer that consists of loose connective tissue and adipose tissue and plays a role in immune surveillance and energy balance
  B. Pathophysiology: Multiple factors determine the response that leads to impaired barrier function of the skin and increased water loss.
    1. Irritant contact dermatitis: A nonallergic response from immune signaling occurs after exposure to irritating substances and causes physical epidermal damage. It is often affected by climate and specific irritant properties and can lead to or predispose a person to allergic contact and atopic dermatitis, as well as scarring if severe.
      a) Most common irritants are chemicals. Physical and biologic agents are less frequently irritants.
        (1) Mild to moderate: Substances that require repeated or prolonged exposure to produce inflammation (e.g., chapped/cracked skin)
        (2) Severe: Substances that injure skin immediately on contact (e.g., corrosive acids, alkalis)
      b) Irritants penetrate and disrupt the stratum corneum, injuring the epidermis and resulting in an inflammatory reaction.
      c) Hardening (symptom disappearance) can occur with continued exposure; reduced frequency and duration of contact may diminish symptoms.
    2. Allergic contact dermatitis: A delayed hypersensitivity response occurs from exposure to contact allergens. Prior sensitization precedes manifestation. Completely avoiding contact diminishes symptoms.

a) Simple chemicals bind to an epidermal protein to form a complete antigen, which then reacts with sensitized T lymphocytes.

b) These lymphocytes then release mediators that attract an inflammatory infiltrate and produce an eczematous response. Responses can be acute (short lived and mild) to chronic (persistent and more severe).

III. Clinical features: Common contact allergens are nickel, the preservative thimerosal, and fragrance ingredients. The *Asteraceae* or *Compositae* family of plants (e.g., aster, daisy, sunflower) and the *Toxicodendron* species (e.g., poison ivy, oak, sumac) can also be significant allergens. Irritant contact dermatitis is the most common type of contact dermatitis (Alhusayen et al., 2014; Esser et al., 2019; Holness, 2019; Kränke & Schuster, 2015; Matthews et al., 2020; Milam & Cohen, 2019; Phillips et al., 2018; Sung et al., 2019; Turrentine et al., 2019).

A. Risk factors

1. Increasing sensitivity to certain allergens occurs with aging. Women are often more sensitized to certain allergens than men. Caucasians report reactions more frequently than African Americans.

2. Solutions containing iodine and adhesive compounds on tapes and dressing materials can cause localized dermatitis consistent with the exposure area.

3. Latex allergies may manifest as contact dermatitis.

4. Contributing factors include genetic predisposition, duration of exposure, cutaneous permeability, and immune tolerance.

5. Tendency for flare-ups occurs in hot, humid climates.

6. Friction, pressure, occlusion, maceration, and temperature may intensify reaction.

B. Etiology

1. Allergies

2. Dermatitis

3. Infection

C. History

1. History of cancer and cancer treatment

2. Current medications: Prescribed, over the counter, supplements

3. History of presenting symptoms: Precipitating factors, onset, location, frequency, duration

4. Changes in ADLs: Effects on sleep, impact on QOL

5. Past medical history: Atopic dermatitis; exposure to known allergens or potential irritants, such as household cleaners, hair dyes, paint remover, or other chemical compounds; previous skin reactions to selected agents

6. Social history: Workplace environment

D. Signs and symptoms: Will vary; may be immediate after exposure or delayed

1. Localized stiff-feeling skin: Initial exposure induces increase in transepidermal water loss. Repeated exposure decreases water loss, leading to functional adaptation of hardening and reduced function of the skin barrier.

2. Discomfort related to dryness, chapping, cracked skin

3. Severe itching secondary to inflammation

4. Pain related to fissures, blisters, or ulcers

5. Allergic: Intense pruritic rash

a) Papular erythematous dermatitis with indistinct margins

b) Acute eczematous reaction with linear lesions with plant or leaf contact

E. Physical examination: Complete integument examination

1. Erythema and possibly edema can occur in a circumscribed area. Vesicle formation and oozing occur with stronger allergens.

2. Dry, thickened, fissured skin results from continued exposure to the irritant.

3. Findings may include tense vesicles, blisters, and edema, including swelling of facial, periorbital, and genital areas.

4. Affected area typically has a definite pattern with sharp margins (e.g., a "square" from a transparent adherent dressing, "stripes" from tape, "spots" from monitor leads). Lesions do not spread beyond the site of contact.

5. Chronic reactions can lead to scaling, fissures, and epidermal thickening.

6. Both irritant and allergic dermatitis occur with abdominal stomas, with higher rates among patients with ileostomies compared to colostomies. Substances in ostomy appliances can cause allergic dermatitis; if left untreated, it is associated with higher mortality.

IV. Diagnostic tests: Dependent on history of exposure (Fonacier et al., 2015; Kränke & Schuster, 2015; Matthews et al., 2020; Nedorost, 2019; Turrentine et al., 2019)

  A. Laboratory

  1. Patch testing is the gold standard for determining causative allergen. If irritant dermatitis is suspected, patch testing can exclude contact dermatitis. Test results are graded as positive, negative, questionable, or irritant. Allergen identification requires two criteria: positive test finding with a nonirritant concentration of a contact allergen, and a positive exposure history.

  2. Older adults have been found to have slower onset of reactivity, less intense reactions, and prolonged recovery with patch testing.

  3. The transepidermal water loss is being studied in clinical trials for irritant dermatitis and assesses the skin's ability to maintain homeostasis.

  B. Radiology: Not indicated

V. Differential diagnosis: Often dependent on timing, location, and distribution (Charles et al., 2016; Fonacier et al., 2015; Matthews et al., 2020; Nedorost, 2019; Turrentine et al., 2019)

  A. Drug reactions, including targeted anticancer therapies: EGFR inhibitors, kinase inhibitors, BRAF inhibitors, mitogen-activated protein kinase (MEK) inhibitors, immunomodulators

  B. Occupational type allergy: Latex, rubber

  C. Atopic dermatitis (see Chapter 18)

  D. Hand dermatitis

  E. Nummular dermatitis: Lower legs

  F. Scabies: Anogenital, hands

  G. Eczema

  H. Psoriasis: Scalp, upper extremities, trunk

  I. Paget disease: Breast

  J. SLE: Face, trunk, extremities (see Chapter 110)

VI. Treatment: The goal is to eliminate contact with irritants or allergens, alleviate symptoms, and promote healing (Alhusayen et al., 2014; Fonacier et al., 2015; Matthews et al., 2020; Nedorost, 2019; Phillips et al., 2018; Sung et al., 2019; Turrentine et al., 2019).

  A. Preventive measures

  1. Primary irritant dermatitis

  a) Decrease exposure to primary irritants (e.g., soaps, detergents, solutions, adhesives, topical agents).

  b) Avoid using abrasive soaps and cleansing agents; use of solvents to cleanse the skin is one of the most frequent predisposing factors.

  c) Barrier cream may be helpful to prevent further irritation.

        d) Lubricate with a high-lipid emollient or mild cream or lotion such as Lubriderm®, Nutraderm®, Eucerin® or Eucerin Plus, or Moisturel®.

        e) Topical immunomodulators may be beneficial in some cases.

    2. Allergic contact dermatitis

        a) Avoid contact with known allergens whenever possible.

        b) Wash the area with mild soap and water after exposure to allergens.

        c) Acute flare-ups due to unintentional exposure can be treated with topical corticosteroids. Patients may benefit from concurrent oral corticosteroid dosing.

  B. Pruritus management (see Chapter 16)

    1. Pharmacologic management

        a) Over-the-counter topical antipruritic lotions: Follow label directions.

        b) Oral antihistamines (see Appendix H)

           (1) Hydroxyzine hydrochloride: 10–50 mg PO every six hours PRN

           (2) Diphenhydramine hydrochloride: 25–50 mg PO every four to six hours PRN

           (3) Cyproheptadine hydrochloride: 4 mg PO three times a day, increasing for symptoms but not to exceed 0.5 mg/kg daily

        c) Topical and intralesional corticosteroids: Treatment is useful with limited involvement. It is best to apply after bathing. Begin with high-potency steroid to quickly reduce symptoms, then use lowest potency for symptom control. Ointments are harder to apply but provide better biologic support than creams. Lotions have higher water content than creams and are easier to apply (see Appendix K).

           (1) Betamethasone dipropionate: 0.05% cream two times a day (high potency)

           (2) Triamcinolone: 0.1% cream or ointment two to three times a day (medium potency)

           (3) Hydrocortisone: 1%–2.5% cream or ointment (low potency)

        d) Oral corticosteroids (see Appendix K): Reserve for generalized allergic contact dermatitis (e.g., poison ivy) or cases when itching cannot be controlled with local measures. Oral corticosteroids are inappropriate for use as chronic therapy. Dose is determined by severity; suggest prednisone 0.5–1 mg/kg daily tapered over two to three weeks.

        e) Pruritus management: Doxepin 10–15 mg PO at night PRN to control itching during sleep (see Chapter 16)

    2. Nonpharmacologic therapies

        a) Drying agents: Aluminum acetate (Burow) solution compresses may be applied for 20 minutes four to six times a day.

        b) Soothing baths: Oatmeal baths may be soothing and help reduce dryness. Mix one cup of oatmeal bath and two cups of cold tap water, shake, and pour into tub one-half full of lukewarm water. Remain in tub for 30 minutes.

        c) Cool environment and compresses: Cold, wet cloths may be soothing.

VII. Follow-up (Charles et al., 2016; Fonacier et al., 2015; Matthews et al., 2020; Nedorost, 2019; Phillips et al., 2018)

  A. Short term: Identify and eliminate the irritant. Monitor for relief of symptoms. Adjust therapies PRN.

  B. Long term: Evaluate for contact dermatitis recurrence and impact on QOL.

VIII. Referral

  A. Dermatologist: To determine irritants, long-term planning, and patch testing

  B. Psychosocial support: Counseling for sleep, ADLs, or QOL issues

The author would like to acknowledge Janet S. Fulton, PhD, RN, ACNS-BC, FAAN, for her contribution to this chapter that remains unchanged from the previous edition of this book.

References

Alhusayen, R.O., Knowles, S.R., & Shear, N.H. (2014). Types of dermatologic reactions. In M.E. Lacouture (Ed.), *Dermatologic principles and practice in oncology: Conditions of the skin, hair, and nails in cancer patients* (pp. 33–46). Wiley-Blackwell.

Brys, A.K., Rodriguez-Homs, L.G., Suwanpradid, J., Atwater, A.R., & MacLeod, A.S. (2020). Shifting paradigms in allergic contact dermatitis: The role of innate immunity. *Journal of Investigative Dermatology, 140*(1), 21–28. https://doi.org/10.1016/j.jid.2019.03.1133

Charles, C., Bungener, C., Razavi, D., Mateus, C., Routier, E., Lanoy, E., ... Dauchy, S. (2016). Impact of dermatologic adverse events induced by targeted therapies on quality of life. *Critical Reviews in Oncology/Hematology, 101,* 158–168. https://doi.org/10.1016/j.critrevonc.2016.03.003

Esser, P.R., Mueller, S., & Martin, S.F. (2019). Plant allergen-induced contact dermatitis. *Planta Medica, 85*(7), 528–534. https://doi.org/10.1055/a-0873-1494

Fonacier, L., Bernstein, D.I., Pacheco, K., Holness, D.L., Blessing-Moore, J., Khan, D., ... Wallace, D. (2015). Contact dermatitis: A practice parameter—Update 2015. *Journal of Allergy and Clinical Immunology Practice, 3*(Suppl. 3), S1–S39. https://doi.org/10.1016/j.jaip.2015.02.009

Garza, L. (2019). Developmental biology of the skin. In S. Kang, M. Amagai, A.L. Bruckner, A.H. Enk, D.J. Margolis, A.J. McMichael, & J.S. Orringer (Eds.), *Fitzpatrick's dermatology* (9th ed., pp. 49–61). McGraw-Hill Education.

Holness, D.L. (2019). Occupational dermatosis. *Current Allergy and Asthma Reports, 19*(9), 42. https://doi.org/10.1007/s11882-019-0870-6

Kränke, B., & Schuster, C. (2015). Contact dermatitis: Relevant differential diagnoses, simulators, and variants. *Journal der Deutschen Dermatologischen Gesellschaft, 13*(11), 1073–1089. https://doi.org/10.1111/ddg.12803

Matthews, N.H., Moustafa, F., Kaskas, N.M., Robinson-Bostom, L., & Pappas-Taffer, L. (2020). Dermatologic toxicities of anticancer therapy. In J.E. Niederhuber, J.O. Armitage, J.H. Doroshow, M.B. Kastan, & J.E. Tepper (Eds.), *Abeloff's clinical oncology* (6th ed., pp. 621–648). Elsevier.

Milam, E.C., & Cohen, D.E. (2019). Contact dermatitis: Emerging trends. *Dermatologic Clinics, 37*(1), 21–28. https://doi.org/10.1016/j.det.2018.07.005

Nedorost, S.T. (2019). Irritant dermatitis. In S. Kang, M. Amagai, A.L. Bruckner, A.H. Enk, D.J. Margolis, A.J. McMichael, & J.S. Orringer (Eds.), *Fitzpatrick's dermatology* (9th ed., pp. 414–427). McGraw-Hill Education.

Phillips, G.S., Freites-Martinez, A., Hsu, M., Lucas, A.S., Barrios, D.M., Ciccolini, K., ... Lacouture, M.E. (2018). Inflammatory dermatoses, infections, and drug eruptions are the most common skin conditions in hospitalized cancer patients. *Journal of the American Academy of Dermatology, 78*(6), 1102–1109. https://doi.org/10.1016/j.jaad.2017.12.031

Sung, C.T., McGowan, M.A., Machler, B.C., & Jacob, S.E. (2019). Systemic treatments for allergic contact dermatitis. *Dermatitis, 30*(1), 46–53. https://doi.org/10.1097/DER.0000000000000435

Turrentine, J.E., Sheehan, M.P., & Cruz, P.D., Jr. (2019). Allergic contact dermatitis. In S. Kang, M. Amagai, A.L. Bruckner, A.H. Enk, D.J. Margolis, A.J. McMichael, & J.S. Orringer (Eds.), *Fitzpatrick's dermatology* (9th ed., pp. 395–413). McGraw-Hill Education.

CHAPTER 21

Furuncle

Marlene SanFilippo, MSN, ARNP, FNP-C, AOCNP®

I. Definition: A furuncle is an acute, inflamed, painful, firm, walled-off collection of pus involving a hair follicle and extending through the dermis into the subcutaneous layer. It is also known as a *boil*. A coalescence of multiple furuncles is referred to as a *carbuncle* (Dinulos, 2021; Nowicka & Grywalska, 2019; Wolff et al., 2017).

II. Physiology/Pathophysiology (Dinulos, 2021; McCann et al., 2017; Wolff et al., 2017)
   A. Normal
      1. The primary function of the skin is to serve as a protective barrier.
      2. Normal skin flora may include *Staphylococcus aureus*, which has the potential to become pathologic.
      3. The skin consists of three layers: epidermis, dermis, and subcutaneous.
      4. Hair follicles begin at the bulb, deep in the dermis, and extend from the dermis at an angle.
         a) Follicles have an erector pili muscle attached near the mid-dermis that straightens the follicle when contracted, causing the hair to stand up.
         b) Hair growth begins in the bulb and progresses up the follicle to the skin surface.
   B. Pathophysiology
      1. A break in the integrity of the skin creates a portal of entry for bacteria into the hair follicle.
      2. Inflammation occurs by the release of chemotactic factors and enzymes produced by the bacteria.
      3. Abscess formation occurs and extends through the follicular wall into the dermis and eventually into the subcutaneous layers.

III. Clinical features: Furuncle commonly affects adolescents and young adults. It can occur at any site that contains hair follicle (Dinulos, 2021; Goodheart & Gonzalez, 2016; Ibler & Kromann, 2014; Natsis & Cohen, 2019; Nowicka & Grywalska, 2019; Trizna, 2020; Wolff et al., 2017).
   A. Risk factors
      1. Alcoholism
      2. Atopic dermatitis
      3. Chronic *S. aureus* carrier state, commonly in nares, axillae, and perineum
      4. Diabetes mellitus
      5. Immunodeficiency states: Common variable immunodeficiency, HIV/AIDS, cancer, therapeutic immunosuppression
      6. Malnutrition
      7. Obesity

        8. Poor hygiene

        9. Positive family history of furuncles

    B. Etiology

        1. Furuncle is a suppurative sequela of folliculitis.

        2. *S. aureus* is the most common pathogen, although other bacteria may cause furuncles (e.g., *Escherichia coli, Pseudomonas aeruginosa, Enterococcus faecalis, Bacteroides, Lactobacillus, Peptococcus, Peptostreptococcus, Mycobacteria*).

        3. The increasing incidence of furunculosis is secondary to community-acquired MRSA.

        4. A small percentage of furuncles (approximately 5%) are sterile and occur in response to a foreign body (e.g., splinter, inclusion cyst, injection site).

    C. History

        1. History of cancer and cancer treatment

        2. Current medications: Prescribed, over the counter

        3. History of presenting symptoms: Precipitating factors, onset, location, duration

        4. Changes in ADLs

        5. Past medical history: Prior furuncles or folliculitis, recent infection with MRSA or physical contact with person with known MRSA, diabetes, HIV infection, renal disease, recurrent skin disease

        6. Family history

    D. Signs and symptoms

        1. Furuncles are located on hair-bearing sites, especially those prone to friction and perspiration (e.g., belt line, anterior thighs, nape of neck, groin, axillae, buttocks).

        2. There may be an absence of initial systemic symptoms of fever. Malaise and fever may occur as infection progresses.

        3. Firm, tender, red papules can occur that rapidly evolve into a deep, painful nodule.

        4. Nodule may become fluctuant with abscess formation.

        5. Throbbing pain intensifies as purulent material accumulates.

        6. Central pustule is often present.

        7. Spontaneous drainage may occur.

    E. Physical examination

        1. Vital signs: Elevated temperature

        2. Integument: Assessment with concentration on hair-bearing areas

            a) Appearance of lesion

                (1) Deep-seated, painful, firm, erythematous nodule with central pustule

                (2) Potential fluctuant mass

                (3) Typically ranges in size from 1–5 cm

                (4) Presence of purulent drainage

            b) Number of lesions: Solitary or multiple clustered lesions

            c) Surrounding erythema and inflammation

        3. Lymph node: Presence of lymphadenopathy corresponding to infected site (see Appendix D)

IV. Diagnostic tests (Goodheart & Gonzalez, 2016; Ibler & Kromann, 2014; Wolff et al., 2017)

    A. Laboratory: Not indicated for all patients; obtained for failure to respond to treatment, significant comorbid conditions, immunocompromised state, and/or systemic symptoms (e.g., fever)

        1. Culture and sensitivities of purulent drainage

        2. Gram stain: Usually reveals gram-positive cocci

    3. Culture of anterior nares, axillae, and perineum if suspected colonization with MRSA: Repeat nares culture three months after treatment.

  B. Radiology: None routinely indicated

V. Differential diagnosis (Dinulos, 2021; Goodheart & Gonzalez, 2016; Ibler & Kromann, 2014; Wolff et al., 2017)

  A. Arthropod bite reaction

  B. Carbuncle

  C. Folliculitis

  D. Hidradenitis suppurativa

  E. Ruptured epidermoid or pilar cyst

VI. Treatment: The overall goal of treatment is to eliminate the pathogen to allow healing (Dinulos, 2021; Goodheart & Gonzalez, 2016; Ibler & Kromann, 2014; Natsis & Cohen, 2019; Nowicka & Grywalska, 2019; Stevens et al., 2014; Trizna, 2020; Wolff et al., 2017).

  A. Nonpharmacologic measures

    1. Moist heat: Application of warm, moist compresses for 30 minutes four times a day provides comfort and promotes localization/consolidation to aid early spontaneous drainage.

    2. Incision and drainage: Furuncles that fail to adequately drain and heal spontaneously require incision and drainage.

  B. Pharmacologic measures

    1. Indications for antibiotics (see Appendix C)

      a) Immunocompromised state

      b) Associated comorbidities

      c) Lesions in areas difficult to drain (e.g., hand, face, genitalia)

      d) Presence of multiple furuncles

      e) Significant surrounding inflammation

      f) Accompanying cellulitis

      g) Presence of systemic symptoms (e.g., fever)

      h) Failure of furuncle to resolve with incision and drainage

    2. The progression of the abscess may be halted if antibiotics are given at the first sign of a developing furuncle in patients with recurrent furunculosis.

    3. Systemic antibiotics: Directed at methicillin-susceptible *S. aureus*

      a) Oral antibiotics

        (1) Dicloxacillin: 500 mg PO every six hours for 10–14 days

        (2) Cephalexin: 500 mg PO every six hours for 10–14 days

        (3) Clindamycin: 300–450 mg PO three or four times a day for 10–14 days

        (4) If MRSA is suspected: Trimethoprim/sulfamethoxazole 1–2 double-strength tablets PO two times a day for 10–14 days

      b) IV antibiotics

        (1) Oxacillin: 2 g IV every four hours

        (2) Cefazolin: 1 g IV every eight hours

        (3) Vancomycin: 15–20 mg IV every 12 hours if MRSA suspected; goal trough: 15–20 mcg/ml

    4. Recurrent infection: Defined by three or more infections within a 12-month period; may require treatment for colonization

      a) Topical treatment

        (1) Nares: Apply mupirocin ointment inside nares two times a day for 5–10 days of every month until reevaluation with repeat culture at three months.

      (2) Skin: Wash skin and fingernails daily for 5–14 days with 2%–4% chlorhexidine. Alternatively, use dilute bleach bath of one teaspoon bleach per one gallon of water for 15 minutes two times per week for three months.

  b) Educate patients to reduce the risk of reinfection.

      (1) Change and wash towels, washcloths, and sheets daily.

      (2) Clean shaving instruments daily.

      (3) Do not share personal hygiene items with other household members.

      (4) Keep wounds covered and change dressings frequently.

  c) If recurrent furunculosis occurs and attempts at topical eradication have not been successful, a combination oral antibiotic regimen containing rifampin may be considered.

      (1) Doxycycline: 100 mg PO two times a day with rifampin 600 mg PO daily for 7–10 days

      (2) Trimethoprim/sulfamethoxazole: 1–2 double-strength tablets PO two times a day with rifampin 600 mg PO daily for 7–10 days

VII. Follow-up

  A. Follow up frequently (every one to three weeks) until resolution of lesion.

  B. Follow up at three months with repeat cultures for patients treated with decolonization measures.

VIII. Referrals

  A. Dermatologist or surgeon: For incision and drainage, if required

  B. Infectious disease specialist: For consultation for patients with recurrent furunculosis after failure to achieve eradication of colonization with topical therapy

References

Dinulos, J.G.H. (2021). *Habif's clinical dermatology: A color guide to diagnosis and therapy* (7th ed.). Elsevier.

Goodheart, H.P., & Gonzalez, M.E. (2016). *Goodheart's photoguide to common skin disorders* (4th ed.). Wolters Kluwer Health.

Ibler, K.S., & Kromann, C.B. (2014). Recurrent furunculosis—Challenges and management: A review. *Clinical, Cosmetic and Investigational Dermatology, 7*, 59–64. https://doi.org/10.2147/CCID.S35302

McCann, S.A., Nicol, N.H., & Huether, S.E. (2017). Structure, function, and disorders of the integument. In S.E. Huether & K.L. McCance (Eds.), *Understanding pathophysiology* (6th ed., pp. 1053–1083). Elsevier.

Natsis, N.E., & Cohen, P.R. (2019). Coagulase-negative Staphylococcus skin and soft tissue infections. *American Journal of Clinical Dermatology, 19*(5), 671–677. https://doi.org/10.1007/s40257-018-0362-9

Nowicka, D., & Grywalska, E. (2019). *Staphylococcus aureus* and host immunity in recurrent furunculosis. *Dermatology, 235*(4), 295–305. https://doi.org/10.1159/000499184

Stevens, D.L., Bisno, A.L., Chambers, H.F., Dellinger, E.P., Goldstein, E.J.C., Gorbach, S,L, ... Wade, J.C. (2014). Executive summary: Practice guidelines for the diagnosis and management of skin and soft tissue infections: 2014 update by the Infectious Diseases Society of America. *Clinical Infectious Diseases, 59*(2), 147–159. https://doi.org/10.1093/cid/ciu444

Trizna, Z. (2020). Furunculosis. In F.J. Domino, R.A. Baldor, J. Golding, & M.B. Stephens (Eds.), *The 5-minute clinical consult 2020* (28th ed., pp. 372–373). Wolters Kluwer.

Wolff, K., Johnson, R.A., Saavedra, A.P., & Roh, E.K. (2017). *Fitzpatrick's color atlas and synopsis of clinical dermatology* (8th ed.). McGraw-Hill Education.

CHAPTER 22

Herpes Zoster

Marlene SanFilippo, MSN, ARNP, FNP-C, AOCNP®

I. Definitions (Choi et al., 2020; Conway & Gleich, 2020; Dinulos, 2021; Goodheart & Gonzalez, 2016; Newman & Jhaveri, 2019; Vrcek et al., 2017)
   A. Herpes zoster virus (HZV), otherwise known as *shingles*, is a painful, cutaneous viral infection usually involving the skin of a single dermatome that results from reactivation of VZV.
   B. Herpes zoster ophthalmicus (HZO) occurs in 10%–20% of HZV cases when the VZV affects the ophthalmic division of the trigeminal nerve.
   C. Zoster sine herpete is the rare occurrence of symptoms of pain, allodynia (altered sensitivity to touch), itching, and burning along a dermatome without characteristic eruption.
   D. Ramsay Hunt syndrome is painful peripheral facial nerve palsy with vesicular rash in the ear (zoster oticus) or mouth occurring when VZV infects the facial nerve.
   E. Disseminated HZV is the occurrence of 20 or more lesions beyond the primary dermatome and is usually associated with an immunocompromised state.

II. Physiology/Pathophysiology (Bharucha et al., 2019; Choi et al., 2020; Dinulos, 2021; Goodheart & Gonzalez, 2016; Kerr et al., 2017; Levin et al., 2016; Mallick-Searle et al., 2016; McCann et al., 2017; Wolff et al., 2017)
   A. Normal
      1. The PNS is composed of cranial and spinal nerves and their associated branches and ganglia. Spinal nerves contain sensory neurons.
      2. Sensation is initiated by stimulation of sensory receptors located in the skin, muscles, tendons, and viscera.
      3. An impulse generated by one of the receptors travels along a sensory nerve fiber toward the spinal cord.
      4. Sensation travels along areas of cutaneous innervation at the dermatomes, or segments of the spinal cord (see Appendix B).
   B. Pathophysiology
      1. VZV infection results in varicella (chicken pox) and occurs through inhalation of infectious droplets or through contact from skin lesions. It predominantly infects T cells and causes infection of organs and seeds the skin, resulting in vesicles.
      2. VZV in vesicles access termini of sensory neurons and ascend in the sensory nerves to the dorsal root ganglia, where it remains latent.
      3. If the level of VZV T-cell–mediated immunity is depressed, VZV may propagate and cause infection of ganglions, resulting in neuropathic pain that precedes the rash of HZV.
      4. Pain occurs in the distribution of skin innervated by the sensory nerve (dermatome).
      5. Infection of the ganglion is followed by VZV descending in the sensory nerve to the skin innervated by that nerve, resulting in local inflammation and vesicle formation along the affected dermatome.

      6. Postherpetic neuralgia (PHN)

        a) Pain is secondary to damage to the peripheral and central neurons.

        b) Damage to neurons causes a lower threshold for action potential, spontaneous discharge, and exaggerated response to stimuli, resulting in peripheral sensitivity and pain without painful stimuli.

III. Clinical features: The lifetime risk of HZV is approximately 30% in the general population. The incidence of a second episode occurring is approximately 5%. More than two-thirds of cases occur in patients aged 50 years and older. HZV manifests as burning, itching, or paresthesia four to five days prior to eruption of erythematous and maculopapular rash, which evolves into grouped vesicles usually in one dermatome. Successive vesicles continue to appear for seven days before becoming umbilicated, pustular, and/or hemorrhagic in three to four days. Lesions typically crust and heal in four weeks. PHN results in chronic, often debilitating pain lasting at least three months to years after HZV rash resolution. It occurs in 18% of adult patients and more than 33% of older patients aged 79 years or older (Bharucha et al., 2019; Choi et al., 2020; Conway & Gleich, 2020; Dinulos, 2021; Goodheart & Gonzalez, 2016; Kawai & Yawn, 2017; Levin et al., 2016; Newman & Jhaveri, 2019; Park et al., 2016; Qian et al., 2018; Saguil et al., 2017; Vrcek et al., 2017; Wolff et al., 2017).

  A. Risk factors

    1. Age: Adults aged 60 years or older are 8–10 times more likely to develop HZV, largely from the decline in VZV-specific, T-cell–mediated immunity that occurs with aging.

    2. Cancer related

      a) Increased risk with hematologic malignancy: Risk may occur two years preceding diagnosis and treatment. The greatest risk is within the first year after the diagnosis.

      b) Increased risk from chemotherapy: Solid tumor

      c) Increased risk with HSCT

    3. Comorbidities

      a) Asthma

      b) COPD

      c) Depression

      d) Diabetes

    4. Exposure to active varicella or zoster: Rare

    5. Immunocompromised state

      a) HIV

      b) Organ transplantation

      c) Immunosuppressive medications: Steroids, chemotherapy, transplant-related immunosuppressive medications

    6. Physical trauma

    7. Spinal cord trauma or injury

  B. Etiology: Reactivation of latent VZV that gained access to sensory ganglia during varicella zoster infection

  C. History

    1. History of cancer and cancer treatment

    2. Current medications: Prescribed, over the counter

    3. History of presenting symptoms: Precipitating factors, onset, location, duration, associated symptoms (e.g., pain over nerve involvement described as tingling and painful)

    4. Changes in ADLs

    5. Past medical history: Past varicella zoster prior to HZV, recent exposure to active VZV

D. Signs and symptoms
   1. Three clinical phases
      a) Prodrome lasts four to five days and is characterized by pain, tenderness, itching, and/or paresthesia along dermatome. Flu-like symptoms may occur with fever, headache, malaise, and photophobia.
      b) The eruptive phase may last 7–21 days, with healing typically by day 28. It gives the appearance of rash and is associated with acute pain described as sharp, burning, or aching. Pain may be evoked by superficial touch (superficial layer of epidermis) or have flu-like symptoms.
      c) PHN is ongoing pain and heightened sensitivity to mild stimuli (allodynia). It may last months to years.
   2. Urinary hesitancy or urgency: Neurogenic bladder may be present if involvement of dermatome S2, S3, or S4 (see Appendix B).
   3. Motor weakness
E. Physical examination: Examine entire skin for characteristic lesions and distribution.
   1. Vital signs: Fever
   2. HEENT: Rash involving periocular skin (e.g., eyelid), medial canthal area, and tip of nose (Hutchison sign)
      a) Eyes
         (1) Conjunctival injection and chemosis (boggy edema of the conjunctiva)
         (2) Decreased visual acuity
         (3) Keratitis, corneal epithelial defects
         (4) Decreased corneal sensation
      b) Ears: Otoscopic examination for presence of vesicles within the canal and on the tympanic membrane—Ramsay Hunt syndrome
      c) Oral: Lesions or ulcers—Ramsay Hunt syndrome
   3. Integument
      a) Initial erythematous and maculopapular rash progress to grouped vesicles ranging in size 3–5 mm and usually following one dermatome, most commonly the thoracic, trigeminal, lumbosacral, or cervical.
      b) It may extend to 2–3 adjacent dermatomes (see Appendix B).
      c) Occasionally, a few vesicles appear across the midline.
      d) Vesicles may appear pustular, umbilicated, hemorrhagic, or crusting if they have been present for more than four days.
      e) Approximately 20–30 vesicles scattered outside the dermatome suggests viremia.
   4. Neurologic
      a) Hyperesthesia in dermatomal distribution with increased sensitivity with light touch
      b) If lesions in ear or mouth, assessment for peripheral facial palsy with weakness
      c) Cranial nerves for involvement for Ramsay Hunt syndrome or HZO (see Appendix A)
      d) Focal weakness of extremities, which may occur two to three weeks after appearance of rash and may persist for several weeks; referred to as segmental zoster paresis
   5. Lymph node: Regional lymphadenopathy (see Appendix D)

IV. Diagnostic tests: Diagnosis is typically clinical. Consider testing in patients with recurring lesions, atypical presentations, such as disseminated lesions, or to differentiate another dermatosis (Bharucha et al., 2019; Choi et al., 2020; Saguil et al., 2017).

A. Laboratory
   1. Tzanck smear: Cannot distinguish HZV from herpes simplex
   2. Viral culture of lesion
   3. Immunofluorescent antibody staining of vesicular lesion, sensitivity limited by the quality of specimen
   4. Polymerase chain reaction testing of vesicle or other body fluid: Most sensitive testing to diagnose HZV with rapid turnaround (typically one day) for results
   5. Varicella zoster–specific IgM
B. Radiology: Not routinely indicated

V. Differential diagnosis (Saguil et al., 2017)
   A. Acute abdomen
   B. Cellulitis (see Chapter 19)
   C. Contact dermatitis (see Chapter 20)
   D. Coxsackievirus
   E. Renal colic
   F. Herpes simplex
   G. Impetigo
   H. MI (see Chapter 49)
   I. Pleurisy
   J. Poison ivy
   K. Superficial pyoderma
   L. Vertebral disease

VI. Treatment: Goals of treatment are to accelerate healing, shorten duration and severity of pain, and reduce the risk of complications such as PHN. All immunocompromised individuals should receive pharmacologic treatment (Bharucha et al., 2019; Choi et al., 2020; Dinulos, 2021; Goodheart & Gonzalez, 2016; Mallick-Searle et al., 2016; Newman & Jhaveri, 2019; Saguil et al., 2017; Vrcek et al., 2017; Wolff et al., 2017).
   A. Nonpharmacologic measures
      1. Acute HZV phase: Consider a sterile, nonocclusive, nonadherent dressing over the site to decrease stimulation from clothing and reduce transmission of VZV to susceptible people.
      2. Pain management
         a) Nerve blocks should occur during acute phase to lessen severe pain. Epidural blocks should occur for PHN.
         b) Transcutaneous electrical stimulation and acupuncture may provide benefit, though this has not been proven in clinical trials.
         c) Wet compresses should be applied for 20 minutes twice per day to remove crust and suppress bacterial grown.
         d) Colloidal oatmeal may improve itching and burning.
   B. Pharmacologic measures: Pharmacologic antiviral therapy is primarily recommended for patients aged 50 years or older with severe rash or pain, involvement of face or eye, or other complications. It should be initiated within 72 hours of rash onset or radicular pain. All immunocompromised individuals should be treated with antiviral therapy immediately upon presentation, regardless of time frame (see Appendix J).
      1. Antiviral therapy in immunocompetent patients: Therapy is continued for at least seven days or until lesions have healed.
         a) Acyclovir: 800 mg PO five times a day

  b) Famciclovir: 500 mg PO three times a day

  c) Valacyclovir: 1,000 mg PO three times a day

 2. Antiviral therapy for patients who are immunocompromised, have severe HZO, or disseminated disease: Duration is dependent on individual circumstances and institutional guidelines. Therapy is typically for at least seven days or until lesions have healed.

  a) Acyclovir: 10 mg/kg IV every eight hours

  b) Oral agents with acyclovir, valacyclovir, and famciclovir at standard dosage: May be used with extension to 10 days for mildly immunocompromised patients

  c) Foscarnet (viral DNA polymerase inhibitor): 40 mg/kg IV every eight hours for 10 days or until resolution can be used in the setting of acyclovir resistance

C. Acute and neuropathic pain: Early treatment of pain may reduce the risk of PHN by preventing sensitization of the CNS.

 1. NSAIDs and opioid analgesics may be required (see Appendices E and F).

 2. Short course of steroids in combination with oral antivirals is controversial, though some experts have suggested it may be helpful in acute neuritis.

 3. Anticonvulsants may reduce the symptoms of neuropathic pain.

  a) Gabapentin: Starting dose of 100–300 mg PO daily, increased gradually by 100–300 mg three times a day every one to seven days to a maximum dose of 3,600 mg daily in divided doses

  b) Pregabalin: Starting dose of 150 mg PO daily in divided doses, increased to 300 mg PO daily in divided doses after three to seven days to a maximum dose of 600 mg PO daily in divided doses

 4. Tricyclic antidepressants

  a) Amitriptyline: 10–25 mg PO at bedtime, increased gradually up to 150 mg PO daily

  b) Nortriptyline: 25 mg PO at bedtime, increased by 25 mg every two to three days to a maximum dose of 150 mg daily

 5. Topical treatments: Skin must be completely healed.

  a) Capsaicin cream: 0.025%–0.075% four times a day; may cause burning with initial applications; available without prescription

  b) Capsaicin 8% patch: Up to four patches for one hour every three months applied by a trained professional or healthcare provider only; topical anesthetic applied one hour prior to patch

  c) Lidocaine 5% patch: Up to three patches to painful area for 12 hours on and 12 hours off once every 24 hours

VII. Follow-up (Choi et al., 2020)

A. Short term: Depending on severity of illness, three to seven days for patients with severe disease, immunocompromised state, or HZO

B. Long term: If failure to heal after 21–28 days or signs of complications

 1. Acute retinal necrosis

 2. Cranial or nerve palsy

 3. Disseminated disease

 4. Hepatitis

 5. Meningitis

 6. Myelitis

 7. PHN

 8. Pneumonitis

 9. Secondary or superinfection of skin lesions

VIII. Referrals
   A. Ophthalmologist: For immediate referral for complete ophthalmic examination for suspected HZO
   B. Pain management specialist: For uncontrolled PHN pain

The author would like to acknowledge Patricia A. Spencer-Cisek, MS, APN-BC, AOCN®, for her contribution to this chapter that remains unchanged from the previous edition of this book.

References

Bharucha, T., Houlihan, C.F., & Breuer, J. (2019). Herpesvirus infections of the central nervous system. *Seminars in Neurology, 39*(3), 369–382. https://doi.org/10.1055/s-0039-1687837

Choi, E.Y., Choi, L.S., & Larson, S.I. (2020). Herpes zoster (shingles). In F.J. Domino, R.A. Baldor, J. Golding, & M.B. Stephens (Eds.), *The 5-minute clinical consult 2020* (28th ed., pp. 462–463). Wolters Kluwer.

Conway, S.L., & Gleich, G. (2020). Herpes eye infections. In F.J. Domino, R.A. Baldor, J. Golding, & M.B. Stephens (Eds.), *The 5-minute clinical consult 2020* (28th ed., pp. 458–459). Wolters Kluwer.

Dinulos, J.G.H. (2021). *Habif's clinical dermatology: A color guide to diagnosis and therapy* (7th ed.). Elsevier.

Goodheart, H.P., & Gonzalez, M.E. (2016). *Goodheart's photoguide to common pediatric and adult skin disorders* (4th ed.). Wolters Kluwer Health.

Kawai, K., & Yawn, B.P. (2017). Risk factors for herpes zoster: A systematic review and meta-analysis. *Mayo Clinic Proceedings, 92*(12), 1806–1821. https://doi.org/10.1016/j.mayocp.2017.10.009

Kerr, L.M., Huether, S.E., & Sugerman, R.A. (2017). Structure and function of the neurologic system. In S.E. Huether & K.L. McCance (Eds.), *Understanding pathophysiology* (6th ed., pp. 307–335). Elsevier.

Levin, M.J., Weinberg, A., & Schmid, D.S. (2016). Herpes simplex virus and varicella-zoster virus. *Microbiology Spectrum, 4*(3), DMIH2-0017-2015. https://doi.org/10.1128/microbiolspec.DMIH2-0017-2015

Mallick-Searle, T., Snodgrass, B., & Brant, J.M. (2016). Postherpetic neuralgia: Epidemiology, pathophysiology, and pain management pharmacology. *Journal of Multidisciplinary Healthcare, 9,* 447–454. https://doi.org/10.2147/JMDH.S106340

McCann, S.A., Nicol, N.H., & Huether, S.E. (2017). Structure, function, and disorders of the integument. In S.E. Huether & K.L. McCance (Eds.), *Understanding pathophysiology* (6th ed., pp. 1053–1083). Elsevier.

Newman, A.M., & Jhaveri, R. (2019). Myths and misconceptions: Varicella-zoster virus exposure, infection risks, complications, and treatments. *Clinical Therapeutics, 41*(9), 1816–1822. https://doi.org/10.1016/j.clinthera.2019.06.009

Park, S.-E., Ganji, P., Ji, J.-H., & Park, S.H. (2016). Transient motor paresis caused by herpes zoster. *Journal of Shoulder and Elbow Surgery, 25*(10), e309–e312. https://doi.org/10.1016/j.jse.2016.07.023

Qian, J., Haywood, A.E., Karki, S., Banks, E., Macartney, K., Chantrill, L., & Liu, B. (2018). Risk of herpes zoster prior to and following cancer diagnosis and treatment: A population-based prospective cohort study. *Journal of Infectious Disease, 220*(1), 3–11. https://doi.org/10.1093/infdis/jiy625

Saguil, A., Kane, S., Mercado, M., & Lauters, R. (2017). Herpes zoster and postherpetic neuralgia: Prevention and management. *American Family Physician, 96*(10), 656–663. https://www.aafp.org/afp/2017/1115/p656.html

Vrcek, I., Choudhury, E., & Durairaj, V. (2017). Herpes zoster ophthalmicus: A review for the internist. *American Journal of Medicine, 130*(1), 21–26. https://doi.org/10.1016/j.amjmed.2016.08.039

Wolff, K., Johnson, R.A., Saavedra, A.P., & Roh, E.K. (2017). *Fitzpatrick's color atlas and synopsis of clinical dermatology* (8th ed.). McGraw-Hill Education.

Respiratory

CHAPTER 23

Cough

Victoria Sherry, DNP, CRNP, AOCNP®

I. Definition: An essential defensive reflex that safeguards the lungs from inhalation of harmful agents and clears the airways of unwanted secretions (Gibson & Vertigan, 2015; Jiang et al., 2016; McGarvey & Gibson, 2019; Wang et al., 2017)
   A. Acute: Less than three weeks duration
   B. Subacute: Three to eight weeks duration
   C. Chronic: More than eight weeks duration

II. Physiology/Pathophysiology (Keller et al., 2017; Mazzone & Undem, 2016; McGarvey & Gibson, 2019)
   A. Normal: Cough is a normal response to airway irritation and protects the airway and preserves airway patency. It can be voluntary (consciously generated) or reflexive (caused by a stimulus) and occurs as a triphasic event.
      1. Inspiratory: Gas is inhaled into the lungs.
      2. Compressive: Forced expiratory effort against a closed glottis creates a rise in intrathoracic pressure.
      3. Expulsive: The glottis opens because of rapid expiratory airflow, creating the coughing sound.
   B. Pathophysiology: Airway sensory fibers located within the nasopharynx, larynx, trachea, and bronchial tree initiate the cough reflex.
      1. Stimuli that activate the cough receptors are either chemical or mechanical irritation.
      2. Impulses are conducted along afferent pathways via cranial nerves IX and X, terminating at the cough center in the medulla oblongata.
      3. The cough reflex occurs through efferent pathways that cause forceful contraction of the diaphragm and other expiratory muscles.

III. Clinical features: Cough is the most prevalent symptom for which people seek medical care. It significantly impacts QOL and is associated with financial, physical, and psychological distress (Dicpinigaitis, 2015; Smith & Woodcock, 2016; Wang et al., 2017; Young-Wolff et al., 2018).
   A. Etiology
      1. Acute cough is usually caused by a viral URI (common cold) and is self-limiting.
      2. Subacute cough is usually caused by prolonged postviral/postinfectious cough or *Bordetella pertussis* (whooping cough).
      3. A chronic cough is most commonly caused by upper airway cough syndrome (UACS) in patients who do not smoke, do not have an active pulmonary process followed radiographically (e.g., lung cancer), or have not received an ACE inhibitor medication.
         a) UACS embodies a variety of rhinosinusitis conditions (e.g., postnasal drip, rhinitis).

        b) Other etiologies include GERD, asthma, nonasthmatic eosinophilic bronchitis, acid reflux, nonacid reflux, or occupational/environmental factors.

    4. *Cough hypersensitivity syndrome* is an umbrella term for an idiopathic, refractory, and unexplained cough.

B. History
1. History of cancer and cancer treatment
2. Current medications: Prescribed, over the counter
3. History of presenting symptoms: Onset, location, duration, characteristics (e.g., trigger factors, whether cough is daytime or nocturnal, sound of cough), associated symptoms, relieving and aggravating factors, severity
4. Changes in ADLs
5. Past medical history: COPD, GERD, allergies, recent illness, postnasal drip, asthma
6. Social history: Tobacco use, vaping, marijuana use, exposure to occupational or environmental irritants

C. Signs and symptoms
1. Fever
2. Presence or absence of sputum production
3. Dyspnea
4. Wheezing
5. Fatigue
6. Congestion
7. Hemoptysis
8. Weight loss

D. Physical examination
1. Vital signs: Increased temperature and respiratory rate
2. Integument: Skin temperature, color, peripheral edema, and clubbing of nails indicating infection, cardiac disease, or lung disease
3. Nasal: Presence of obstruction and/or discharge indicating infection
4. Oropharynx: Presence of mucus, erythema, or a "cobblestone" appearance to the mucosa suggestive of postnasal drip
5. Ear: Assessment for cerumen or foreign bodies (ear is innervated by vagal nerve) in auditory canal or tympanic membrane
6. Pulmonary
    a) Inspection for accessory muscle use
    b) Inspiratory stridor on auscultation suggestive of upper airway disease
    c) Rhonchi or expiratory wheezing on auscultation suggestive of lower airway disease
    d) Inspiratory crackles on auscultation suggestive of a process involving the pulmonary parenchyma, such as interstitial lung disease, alveolitis, pneumonia, or pulmonary edema
    e) Wet crackles in the lung bases suggestive of CHF
7. Cardiac: Jugular vein distention and S_3 gallop suggestive of CHF

IV. Diagnostic tests (Irwin et al., 2018; Kaplan, 2019; Mahashur, 2015)
A. Laboratory
1. CBC with differential: May be normal or show leukocytosis suggestive of infection
2. Sputum for cytology or gram and acid-fast stains: Should be used in any patient with a smoking history and an unexplained cough
    a) Cytology may be positive in the presence of malignancy.
    b) Gram and acid-fast stains may reveal an infectious pathogen.

    B. Radiology
        1. Chest radiograph if indicated to evaluate for lung disease
        2. CT scan if chest x-ray suspicious for parenchymal lung disease
    C. Other
        1. Pulmonary function tests if COPD is suspected
        2. Bronchoscopy if chest x-ray/CT scan is suspicious of mass or interstitial disease
        3. EGD to evaluate for reflux disease
        4. Sinus radiograph to evaluate for sinus infection or blockage
        5. Methacholine challenge to evaluate for asthma; often used with PFTs
        6. Esophageal pH monitoring to evaluate for reflux disease

V. Differential diagnosis: Determining the length of time cough has been present is the first step in identifying a differential diagnosis (Irwin et al., 2018; Kaplan, 2019).
    A. Medication induced: ACE inhibitors; beginning one week after initiating treatment
    B. Diseases
        1. Postnasal drainage/UACS: Most common cause of persistent cough
        2. Asthma: Second leading cause of unrelieved cough (see Chapter 28)
        3. GERD: Third most common cause of persistent cough (see Chapter 71)
        4. Infections
           a) Pneumonia (see Chapter 30)
           b) Bronchitis (see Chapter 28)
           c) Sinusitis (see Chapter 11)
           d) Lung abscess
           e) TB (see Chapter 36)
           f) Nonasthmatic eosinophilic bronchitis
           g) *Mycoplasma*
           h) *B. pertussis*
           i) *Chlamydia pneumoniae*
           j) Aspiration pneumonia
        5. CHF (see Chapter 42)
        6. Tumors of the lung
        7. Lymphangitis
        8. Carcinomatosis: Widespread dissemination of carcinoma in the body
        9. Pleural effusion (see Chapter 29)
       10. Hypersensitivity pneumonitis
       11. Radiation pneumonitis
       12. Pericardial effusion (see Chapter 50)
       13. Vocal cord paralysis and spastic (spasmodic) dysphonia
       14. Motor neuron diseases: Multiple sclerosis, stroke (see Chapter 146)
       15. Interstitial lung disease
       16. Aortic aneurysm
       17. Paraneoplastic syndrome: Rare (see Appendix M)
       18. Sarcoidosis
       19. Vasculitis
       20. Laryngopharyngeal reflux
       21. Bronchiectasis
    C. Exposure to chemical or environmental irritants
    D. Chemical aspiration
    E. Rare causes
        1. Premature ventricular contractions

    2. Holmes-Adie syndrome

    3. Chronic tonsillar enlargement

    4. Laryngeal sensory neuropathy

    5. Arteriovenous malformations

    6. Impacted cerumen

    7. Psychogenic or "habit cough"

VI. Treatment: Therapeutic intervention is based on an algorithm aimed at identifying the underlying cause and focusing treatment as indicated (Chamberlain et al., 2016; Gibson & Vertigan, 2015; Gibson et al., 2016; Robertson et al., 2016; Smith & Woodcock, 2016; Wang et al., 2017; Young-Wolff et al., 2018).

    A. Elimination of exogenous causative agents, such as cigarette smoke, vaping, and ACE inhibitors

    B. Control of endogenous causative agents, such as postnasal drip (see Chapter 11) and gastroesophageal reflux (see Chapter 71)

    C. Treatment of specific respiratory tract infections (see Chapter 37)

    D. Bronchodilators for reversible airflow obstruction with bronchiectasis (see Chapter 28)

    E. Treatment of lung tumors with surgery, radiation, chemotherapy, targeted therapy, or immunotherapy

    F. Treatment of interstitial lung disease with bronchial dilators and steroids, such as prednisone

    G. Medication management to suppress the cough once serious underlying cardiopulmonary pathology has been excluded (see Table 23-1)

        1. Inhaled corticosteroids

        2. Neuromodulatory therapy

        3. Nonpharmacologic

        4. Other therapies

VII. Follow-up: Dependent on definitive diagnosis and treatment plan (Irwin et al., 2018)

    A. Short term: Diagnosis determines specific follow-up.

    B. Long term: For chronic cough, follow-up should occur every four to nine weeks.

VIII. Referrals: For a refractory cough, consult a specialist cough clinic.

References

Chamberlain, S.A.F., Garrod, R., Clark, L., Douiri, A., Parker, S.M., Ellis, … Birring, S.S. (2016). Physiotherapy, and speech and language therapy intervention for patients with refractory chronic cough: A multicentre randomised control trial. *Thorax, 72*(2), 129–136. https://doi.org/10.1136/thoraxjnl-2016-208843

Dicpinigaitis, P.V. (2015). Clinical perspective—Cough: An unmet need. *Current Opinion in Pharmacology, 22,* 24–28. https://doi.org/10.1016/j.coph.2015.03.001

Gibson, P.G., & Vertigan, A.E. (2015). Management of chronic refractory cough. *BMJ, 351,* h5590. https://doi.org/10.1136/bmj.h5590

Gibson, P.G., Wang, G., McGarvey, L., Vertigan, A.E., Altman, K.W., & Birring, S.S. (2016). Treatment of unexplained chronic cough: CHEST guideline and expert panel report. *Chest, 149*(1), 27–44. https://doi.org/10.1016/j.chest.2017.10.016

Irwin, R.S., French, C.L., Chang, A.B., & Altman, K.W. (2018). Classification of cough as a symptom in adults and management algorithms: CHEST guideline and expert panel report. *Chest, 153*(1), 196 209. https://doi.org/10.1016/j.chest.2017.10.016

Jiang, M., Guan, W.-J., Fang, Z.-F., Xie, Y.-Q., Xie, J.-X., Chen, H., … Zhong, N.-S. (2016). A critical review of the quality of cough clinical practice guidelines. *Chest, 150*(4), 777–788. https://doi.org/10.1016/j.chest.2016.04.028

TABLE 23-1	Treatment Options for Cough
Treatment	**Adult Dose (12 Years and Older)**
Inhaled Corticosteroids	
Beclomethasone	500 mg three times a day
Mometasone	400 mg daily
Neuromodulators	
Amitriptyline	10 mg PO at night
Gabapentin	300 mg PO daily, titrated up to a maximum tolerable dose of 1,800 mg daily
Morphine sulfate	10 mg PO two times a day
Nonpharmacologic	
Physiotherapy	Physiotherapist for chest physiotherapy or pulmonary rehabilitation
Speech therapy	Speech pathologist to teach methods to help suppress the urge to cough
Other Treatments	
Albuterol or ipratropium (bronchodilators)	2 puffs every 4 hours as needed
Antihistamine + decongestant	25–50 mg PO every 4 hours as needed
Benzonatate	100–200 mg PO three times daily; should not be chewed
Dextromethorphan	10–20 mg PO every 4–8 hours or 30 mg every 6–8 hours; maximum of 120 mg every 24 hours; lozenges or elixir
Diphenhydramine + pseudoephedrine	30–60 mg PO every 6 hours as needed
Herbal agents	Menthol vapor rub, high-dose zinc; started within 24 hours of symptoms
Leukotriene antagonist	10 mg PO daily

Note. Based on information from Gibson et al., 2016; Irwin et al., 2018; Robertson et al., 2016.

Kaplan, A.G. (2019). Chronic cough in adults: Make the diagnosis and make a difference. *Pulmonary Therapy, 5*(1), 11–21. https://doi.org/10.1007/s41030-019-0089-7

Keller, J.A., McGovern, A.E., & Mazzone, S.B. (2017). Translating cough mechanisms into better cough suppressants. *Chest, 152*(4), 833–841. https://doi.org/10.1016/j.chest.2017.05.016

Mahashur, A. (2015). Chronic dry cough: Diagnostic and management approaches. *Lung India, 32*(1), 44–49. https://doi.org/10.4103/0970-2113.148450

Mazzone, S.B., & Undem, B.J. (2016). Vagal afferent innervation of the airways in health and disease. *Physiological Reviews, 96*(3), 975–1024. https://doi.org/10.1152/physrev.00039.2015

McGarvey, L., & Gibson, P.G. (2019). What is chronic cough? Terminology. *Journal of Allergy and Clinical Immunology: In Practice, 7*(6), 1711–1714. https://doi.org/10.1016/j.jaip.2019.04.012

Robertson, S., Robinson, M., Schultz, A., & Villella, R. (2016). Do over-the-counter remedies relieve cough in acute upper respiratory infections? *Evidence-Based Practice, 19*(9), 1–2. https://journals.lww.com/ebp/Abstract/2016/09000/Do_over_the_counter_remedies_relieve_cough_in.1.aspx

Smith, J., & Woodcock, A. (2016). Chronic cough. *New England Journal of Medicine, 375*(16), 1544–1551. https://doi.org/10.1056/NEJMc1615067

Wang, K., Milojevic, N., Sheinman, B., & Usmani, O.S. (2017). Cough management in primary, secondary and tertiary settings. *Pulmonary Pharmacology and Therapeutics, 47,* 93–98. https://doi.org/10.1016/j.pupt.2017.05.001

Young-Wolff, K.C., Klebaner, D., Folck, B., Carter-Harris, L., Solloum, R.G., Prochaska, J.J., ... Tan, A.S.L. (2018). Do you vape? Leveraging electronic health records to assess clinician documentation of electronic nicotine delivery system use among adolescents and adults. *Preventative Medicine, 105,* 32–36. https://doi.org/10.1016/j.ypmed.2017.08.009

CHAPTER 24

Dyspnea

Leslie Matthews, MS, ANP-BC, AOCNP®

I. Definition: A subjective experience of breathing discomfort that consists of qualitatively distinct sensations that vary in intensity; has multiple physiologic, psychologic, social, and environmental factors that may induce secondary physiologic and behavioral responses (Campbell, 2017; Coccia et al., 2016)

II. Physiology/Pathophysiology (Campbell, 2017; Coccia et al., 2016; Mahler, 2017)
   A. Normal
      1. Respiration makes oxygen available to tissues for metabolism and removes carbon dioxide, the main byproduct of metabolism.
      2. This gas exchange is accomplished by simple diffusion as inspired air moves in close proximity to the pulmonary capillary bed.
      3. Breathing is automatic and unconsciously controlled by the respiratory center in the brain.
   B. Pathophysiology
      1. Dyspnea has multiple causes and occurs when individual workload exceeds normal ventilation abilities.
      2. The sensation of dyspnea is the discrepancy or mismatch between outgoing central respiratory motor activity and incoming information from both central and peripheral chemoreceptors and mechanoreceptors in the airways, lung, and chest wall structures.

III. Clinical features: Dyspnea can present as a stable or unstable clinical status. Urgent evaluation is required for unstable patients. Dyspnea can be an acute or chronic event (Johnson et al., 2014; Mahler, 2017; Rietbroek et al., 2018).
   A. Etiology (see Figure 24-1)
      1. Dyspnea is most commonly caused by respiratory or cardiac disorders.
      2. Any disease resulting in impairment of the cardiovascular, respiratory, metabolic, neurologic, or hematologic system can cause dyspnea.
   B. History
      1. History of cancer and cancer treatment
      2. Current medications: Prescribed, over the counter
      3. History of presenting symptoms: Precipitating factors, onset, location, duration, associated symptoms (e.g., quality of breathing sensation, timing [episodic or constant, occurrence at rest or with exertion], chest pain, palpitations, cough, fever, sputum production, indigestion or dysphagia, anxiety, perioral paresthesia, paresthesia of fingers)
      4. Changes in ADLs: Exercise tolerance or activity limitation related to dyspnea such as stair climbing, walking, washing, dressing, or speaking; number of pillows used for sleep, recent immobilization

| FIGURE 24-1 | Causes of Dyspnea in Patients With Cancer |

Dyspnea as a Result of Cancer	Dyspnea as an Indirect Result of Cancer	Dyspnea as a Result of Cancer Treatment	Dyspnea Unrelated to Cancer
• Hepatomegaly • Lymphangitic carcinomatosis • Multiple tumors • Paraneoplastic syndromes • Pericardial effusion • Pleural tumor • Primary or metastatic cancer to the lung • Pulmonary leukostasis • Superior vena cava syndrome	• Anemia • Ascites • Cachexia • Electrolyte imbalances • Pneumonia • Pulmonary emboli	• Chemotherapy-induced pulmonary toxicity: Bleomycin, carmustine, mitomycin, busulfan, cyclophosphamide, methotrexate, gefitinib, erlotinib • Immunotherapy induced • Radiation therapy induced • Surgery	• Aspiration • Asthma • Chronic obstructive pulmonary disease • Congestive heart failure • Goiter • Infection (e.g., tuberculosis) • Obesity • Pneumothorax • Pulmonary hypertension

Note. Based on information from Brahmer et al., 2018; Coccia et al., 2016; Rietbroek et al., 2018.

5. Past medical history: Asthma, bronchitis, pneumonia, heart disease, anemia
6. Social history: Allergies, tobacco use (pack-years), exposure to secondhand smoke, recent long-distance travel, occupational or agricultural exposure to dust, radon, or asbestos
7. Family history: Clotting, DVT, PE, hypercoagulable state

C. Signs and symptoms: Dyspnea can be described as air hunger or the inability to get enough air.
   1. Orthopnea: Dyspnea while in a supine posture; common indicator of CHF, obesity, or asthma
   2. Paroxysmal nocturnal dyspnea: Awakens person at night and is relieved when he or she sits up; suggests CHF, asthma, or COPD
   3. Sudden and unexpected dyspnea without exertion: May be suggestive of PE, spontaneous pneumothorax, myocardial ischemia, bronchospasm, or anxiety
   4. Dyspnea only with exertion: Suggests anemia or deconditioning
   5. Chest tightness
   6. Constriction or choking sensation

D. Physical examination
   1. General appearance: Distress, decreased ability to speak in complete sentences
   2. Vital signs: Weight status (obesity contributes to dyspnea); fast, slow, or normal respiratory rate; fever indicating infection
   3. Integument
      a) Pallor indicating anemia
      b) Cyanosis with a pulmonary origin
      c) Diaphoresis from extreme sympathetic stimulation, such as PE or MI
   4. Neck
      a) JVD suggestive of heart failure
      b) Carotid bruits suggestive of stenosis
      c) Enlarged thyroid suggestive of goiter
      d) Deviated trachea from mass or enlarged thyroid
   5. Cardiac
      a) Tachycardia, irregular rhythm
      b) S_3 gallop suggestive of CHF

        c) Murmur suggestive of CHF, endocarditis, or pulmonary edema

        d) Distant or muffled heart sounds suggestive of CHF or effusion

        e) Displaced point of maximal impulse suggestive of CHF or effusion

        f) Pulsus paradoxus suggestive of tamponade, pericarditis, or COPD

    6. Pulmonary/thorax

        a) Intercostal retraction or use of accessory muscles indicating increased work of breathing

        b) Digital clubbing indicative of severe chronic hypoxia

        c) Increased anterior–posterior diameter (barrel-shaped chest) indicating COPD

        d) Diminished or adventitious breath sounds (e.g., wheezes, stridor, rales, and rhonchi, indicating pneumonia), CHF, pulmonary edema

        e) Prolonged expiration suggestive of COPD

        f) Hyperresonance to percussion suggestive of COPD

        g) Dullness to percussion over an effusion

    7. Peripheral vascular

        a) Peripheral edema and quality of pulses indicating cardiac origin

        b) Capillary refill indicative of oxygen perfusion

        c) Unilateral palpable cord, positive Homan sign, edema, erythema suggestive of DVT

    8. Mental status: Memory or concentration problems, confusion, or restlessness suggestive of hypoxia

    9. Psychosocial: Anxiety, fear, distress

IV. Diagnostic tests: Guided by stage of disease, patient stability, usefulness of information for therapeutic intervention, and acute onset of symptoms (Rietbroek et al., 2018)

    A. Laboratory

        1. CBC to evaluate for infection, neutropenia, anemia, and thrombocytopenia

        2. Metabolic panel to evaluate for change in acid-base balance

        3. TSH to detect thyroid abnormality presenting as dyspnea

        4. ABGs to document presence of hypoxemia or hypercapnia, to characterize acid-base status, and to detect significant carboxyhemoglobin

        5. Cardiac biomarkers, such as BNP, to evaluate for cardiac ischemia or CHF

        6. D-dimer to evaluate for PE

        7. Glucose, as indicated, to measure in diabetics

    B. Radiology

        1. Chest x-ray to evaluate for infiltrates, atelectasis, hyperinflation, mass lesion, pleural effusion, pneumothorax, and cardiac enlargement

        2. Echocardiogram to assess right and left ventricular function or the presence of valvular heart disease

        3. Spiral CT scan of chest to evaluate for obstruction, effusions, pneumonitis, and PE

        4. Ventilation/perfusion scan: Demonstrates 100% sensitivity for PE; if ventilation/perfusion scan is normal, PE is not present.

    C. Other

        1. ECG to evaluate for evidence of cardiac ischemia, infarction, or ventricular hypertrophy

        2. Pulmonary function tests

            a) Serve as a baseline parameter in illness

            b) Establish presence and severity of obstructive or restrictive lung disease or reduced diffusing capacity

            c) Evaluate reversibility of airway obstruction and results of therapy

3. Pulse oximetry: A rapid, widely available assessment; oxygen saturation less than 94% represents clinically significant hypoxemia.

4. Treadmill or cardiopulmonary exercise testing: Useful in select cases to target myocardial ischemia as cause of dyspnea

5. Sleep study to evaluate for sleep apnea

V. Differential diagnosis (see Figure 24-1; Brahmer et al., 2018; Rietbroek et al., 2018)

A. Pulmonary
1. Asthma, bronchitis (see Chapter 28)
2. Pneumothorax (see Chapter 31)
3. PE (see Chapter 33)
4. Pneumonia (see Chapter 30)
5. Pleural effusion (see Chapter 29)
6. Interstitial lung disease
7. COPD (see Chapter 28)
8. Upper airway obstruction
9. Pneumonitis

B. Cardiac
1. Pericardial effusion (see Chapter 50)
2. CHF (see Chapter 42)
3. CAD
4. Dysrhythmia (see Chapter 45)
5. Valvular heart disease
6. Cardiac tamponade (see Chapter 50)

C. Other diseases
1. Anaphylaxis/angioedema
2. Electrolyte imbalances (see Chapters 152–156)
3. Severe anemia (see Chapters 113–119)
4. Acute blood loss or hemolysis
5. Cachexia (see Chapter 66)
6. Psychogenic causes: Anxiety (see Chapter 161)
7. Obesity
8. Neuromuscular disorders
9. Foreign object in upper or lower respiratory tract
10. Hyperthyroidism (see Chapter 157)

D. Cancer related
1. Tumors: Primary or metastatic
2. Paraneoplastic syndromes (see Appendix M)
3. Surgery: Pneumonectomy
4. Radiation- or chemotherapy/immunotherapy-induced pulmonary or cardiac disease

VI. Treatment: Optimal treatment of dyspnea includes using specific therapies to reverse the cause as indicated. Palliative therapies can be used to treat irreversible causes for symptomatic relief (Baldwin & Cox, 2016; Haywood et al., 2019; NCCN, 2021; Shreves & Pour, 2018).

A. Treat and correct underlying etiology, as appropriate.
1. Asthma, bronchitis (see Chapter 28)
2. Pneumothorax (see Chapter 31) and pleural effusion (see Chapter 29) relieved by thoracentesis procedure and oxygen therapy
3. PE (see Chapter 33)
4. Pneumonia (see Chapter 30)

     5. CHF (see Chapter 42)

     6. Pericardial effusion (see Chapter 50)

     7. SVC syndrome

     8. COPD (see Chapter 28)

     9. Electrolyte imbalances (see Chapters 152–156)

     10. Anemia (see Chapters 113–119)

     11. Cachexia (see Chapter 66)

     12. Cancer treatment for paraneoplastic syndromes: Combination of these modalities (see Appendix M)

     13. Interstitial lung disease

     14. Anxiety (see Chapter 161)

     15. Dysrhythmia (see Chapter 45)

     16. Cardiac tamponade (see Chapter 50)

     17. Diabetic ketoacidosis (see Chapter 151)

B. Blood loss or hemolysis

     1. Transfuse blood products, as appropriate.

     2. Determine cause and treat.

C. Airway obstruction due to tumor

     1. Radiation therapy: External beam, brachytherapy

     2. Airway stenting with or without laser ablation

D. General guidelines for supportive care

     1. Administer supplemental oxygen therapy, 0.5–4 L/min for hypoxia unless hypercapnia is present or strongly suspected.

     2. Patient assumes position of choice for respiratory comfort.

     3. Administer immediate-release oral or parenteral opioids (see Appendix F).

     4. Consider corticosteroids orally or inhaled; controversial benefit for dyspnea exists.

     5. Cooler environment and/or ambient airflow (fan or open window) directed across cheek or through nose to stimulate trigeminal nerve receptors may be effective.

     6. Chest wall vibration and neuroelectric muscle stimulation are likely to be helpful in some situations.

     7. Walking aid to decrease exertion may be beneficial in reducing dyspnea.

     8. Breathing training exercises may be helpful to some patients.

     9. Encourage smoking cessation.

VII. Follow-up: Based upon the diagnosis and treatment plan

    A. Acute dyspnea may require hospitalization for diagnostic studies and interventions.

    B. Less acute dyspnea may be followed up in an ambulatory setting within 24–48 hours.

VIII. Referral: Refer to pulmonologist or appropriate subspecialist as indicated if symptoms do not resolve.

The author would like to acknowledge Margaret Joyce, PhD, ANP-BC, AOCN®, for her contribution to this chapter that remains unchanged from the previous edition of this book.

References

Baldwin, J., & Cox, J. (2016). Treating dyspnea: Is oxygen therapy the best option for all patients. *Medical Clinics of North America, 100*(5), 1123–1130. https://doi.org/10.1016/j.mcna.2016.04.018

Brahmer, J.R., Lacchetti, C., Schneider, B.J., Atkins, M.B., Brassil, K.J., Caterino, J.M., ... Thompson, J.A. (2018). Management of immune-related adverse events in patients treated with immune checkpoint inhibitor therapy: American Society of Clinical Oncology clinical practice guideline. *Journal of Clinical Oncology, 36*(17), 1714–1768. https://doi.org/10.1200/JCO.2017.77.6385

Campbell, M.L. (2017). Dyspnea. *Critical Care Nursing Clinics of North America, 29*(4), 461–470. https://doi.org/10.1016/j.cnc.2017.08.006

Coccia, C.B.I., Palkowski, G.H., Schweitzer, B., Motshohi, T., & Ntusi, N.A.B. (2016). Dyspnoea: Pathophysiology and a clinical approach. *South African Medical Journal, 106*(1), 32–36. https://doi.org/10.7196/SAMJ.2016.v106i1.10324

Haywood, A., Duc, J., Good, P., Khan, S., Rickett, K., Vayne-Bossert, P., & Hardy, J.R. (2019). Systemic corticosteroids for the management of cancer-related breathlessness (dyspnea) in adults. *Cochrane Database of Systematic Reviews, 2019*(2). https://doi.org/10.1002/14651858.CD012704.pub2

Johnson, M.J., Currow, D.C., & Booth, S. (2014). Prevalence and assessment of breathlessness in the clinical setting. *Expert Review of Respiratory Medicine, 8*(2), 151–161. https://doi.org/10.1586/17476348.2014.879530

Mahler, D.A. (2017). Evaluation of dyspnea in the elderly. *Clinics in Geriatric Medicine, 33*(4), 503–521. https://doi.org/10.1016/j.cger.2017.06.004

National Comprehensive Cancer Network. (2021). *NCCN Clinical Practice Guidelines in Oncology (NCCN Guidelines®): Palliative care* [v.3.2021]. http://www.nccn.org/professionals/physician_gls/pdf/palliative.pdf

Rietbroek, M.V., Slats, A.M., Kiès, P., de Grooth, G.J., Chavannes, N.H., Taube, C., & Bonten, T.N. (2018). The integrated dyspnea clinic: An evaluation of efficiency. *International Journal of Integrated Care, 18*(4), 15. https://doi.org/10.5334/ijic.3983

Shreves, A., & Pour, T.R. (2018). Emergency department management of dyspnea in the dying patient. *Emergency Medicine Practice, 20*(7), 1–20. https://www.ebmedicine.net/topics/ethics/dyspnea-in-dying

CHAPTER 25

Hemoptysis

Victoria Sherry, DNP, CRNP, AOCNP®

I. Definitions: Expectoration of blood originating from the lungs or bronchioles (Choi et al., 2018; Davidson & Shojaee, 2020; Radchenko et al., 2017; Xia et al., 2015)
   A. Characterized as mild, moderate, or massive
      1. Mild hemoptysis (less than 30 ml in 24 hours) and moderate hemoptysis (30–200 ml in 24 hours): Hemoptysis of this degree is usually self-limited and has a good prognosis with conservative management.
      2. Massive (or major) hemoptysis: No universal volume definition exists; however, 200–300 ml is a common cutoff. Massive hemoptysis can be life threatening, causing exsanguination and death.
   B. Cryptogenic or idiopathic hemoptysis: No cause identified
   C. Pseudohemoptysis: Source of blood from upper respiratory tract (i.e., nasopharynx or oropharynx)

II. Physiology/Pathophysiology (Ittrich et al., 2017)
   A. Normal: Often divided into the upper and lower respiratory tracts
      1. The upper respiratory tract includes the nose, paranasal sinuses, and pharynx.
         a) Nasal mucosa: Responsible for warming and humidifying the incoming air and filtering out any particles; contains olfactory sensory cells
         b) Paranasal sinus: Connects with the nasal cavity and is lined by the nasal mucosa
         c) Pharynx: Extends from the posterior position of the nose to the esophagus and larynx and is divided into the nasopharynx (behind the nose), oropharynx (behind the mouth), and laryngopharynx (behind the larynx); normally, pharyngeal openings are relaxed for respiration and closed off by a complex reflex during swallowing or vomiting.
      2. The lower respiratory tract includes the larynx, the trachea, the bronchial tree, and the lungs.
         a) Larynx: A strong cartilaginous tube that forms the upper end of the trachea; vocal cords are the primary structures responsible for sound, and the epiglottis tips over the larynx to prevent aspiration.
         b) Trachea: Tube that keeps the airway open and branches into the bronchi
         c) Bronchi: Branches into the right and left and further divides into secondary and tertiary bronchi and bronchioles
         d) Bronchioles: Divide into smaller tubes to the alveoli, which form the major portion of the lungs
         e) Lung: Elastic tissue used for air exchange
      3. The lung has a dual blood supply consisting of the bronchial and pulmonary vessels.

        a) The bronchial arteries provide the main vascular supply to the airways as a systemic circulatory pressure that supplies the supporting structures of the lung, including the pleura, intrapulmonary lymphoid tissue, large branches of the pulmonary vessels, and nerves.

        b) The pulmonary arteries supply the pulmonary parenchymal tissue, which is low pressure, and the alveoli.

  B. Pathophysiology: Hemoptysis arises from inflammatory diseases, bronchial carcinoma and metastasis, tumor, bronchiectasis, cardiovascular disease, or anticoagulation causing irritation to the lung tissue.

III. Clinical features: Approximately 70%–90% of cases are caused by bronchitis, bronchiectasis, TB, and necrotizing pneumonia. Features range from nonalarming blood to a life-threatening condition associated with an immediate risk of airway obstruction and death (Cardenas-Garcia & Feller-Kopman, 2018; Cordovilla et al., 2016; Davidson & Shojaee, 2020; Earwood & Thompson, 2015; Gagnon et al., 2017; Ittrich et al., 2017; Mondoni et al., 2019; Ong et al., 2016; Radchenko et al., 2017).

  A. Risk factors

    1. 60:40 male predominance

    2. Occurs in all age groups

    3. Smoking history: High risk for neoplasm with greater than 40 pack-year smoking history

    4. HIV infection

    5. Use of immunosuppressants

    6. Exposure to TB

    7. Recent immobilization or surgery

    8. Known cancer

    9. Prior or family history of clotting

    10. Pregnancy

    11. Use of estrogen-containing drugs

    12. Long-distance travel/air travel: PE

  B. Etiology

    1. Pulmonary disease

        a) Airway infections: TB

        b) Bronchial carcinoma

        c) Bronchiectasis/cystic fibrosis

        d) Pulmonary edema

        e) Invasive aspergillosis

        f) Benign bronchial tumors

        g) Vasculitis: Behçet disease, granulomatosis with polyangiitis, Goodpasture syndrome

    2. Cardiovascular

        a) PE

        b) Vascular malformations

        c) Idiopathic pulmonary hemosiderosis

        d) Septic embolism

        e) PH

    3. Other

        a) Iatrogenic: Lung biopsy, right heart catheterization, anticoagulation treatment

        b) Trauma/lung contusion

        c) Foreign body

      d) Hematologic : Thrombocytopenia, coagulopathy

      e) Tuberous sclerosis

      f) Drugs and toxins: Solvents, crack cocaine, bevacizumab, nitrofurantoin, penicillamine

      g) Lung transplantation

      h) Endometriosis

C. History

  1. History of cancer and cancer treatment

  2. Current medications: Prescribed, over the counter, anticoagulants

  3. History of presenting symptoms: Precipitating factors, onset, location, duration (e.g., abrupt onset, cyclical recurrence), characteristics (e.g., approximate volume of blood, color of blood), associated symptoms (e.g., fever, nosebleeds, night sweats, easy bruising, recent weight loss), aggravating factors (e.g., allergen exposure, cold exertion, or supine position), severity

  4. Change in ADLs

  5. Past medical history: DVT, PE, TB, valvular heart disease, bleeding disorders, trauma, pulmonary disease, respiratory infections

  6. Social history: Tobacco use, vaping, recent travel

  7. Family history: Hypercoagulable state, clotting history, vascular autoimmune disease

D. Signs and symptoms

  1. Dyspnea

  2. Pleuritic chest pain

  3. Warm sensation or gurgling in the chest

  4. Cough

  5. Bloody sputum

  6. Anxiety

E. Physical examination: Usually unreliable in locating source of bleeding

  1. Vital signs: Fever, tachycardia, tachypnea, and low oxygen saturation suggestive of a pulmonary, cardiac, or infectious cause; constitutional signs (e.g., weight loss, level of patient distress)

  2. Integument

      a) Assessment for petechiae, ecchymoses, and telangiectasia

      b) Clubbing present in smokers

  3. HEENT: Oropharynx for bleeding and/or gingivitis

  4. Pulmonary

      a) Thorax for signs of blunt trauma

      b) Breath sounds: Symmetry, stridor, wheezing, crackles, or diminished breath sounds indicative of possible obstruction or CHF

      c) Dullness to percussion and egophony indicative of possible collapse or consolidation

      d) Absent or distant breath sounds indicative of obstruction or collapse

      e) Crackles indicative of pneumonia of infectious or inflammatory process or volume overload in heart failure

      f) Pleural friction rub indicative of PE

      g) Normal breath sounds: Common

  5. Cardiac

      a) S_4 or diastolic murmur consistent with heart failure

      b) JVD consistent with heart failure

      c) Peripheral edema consistent with heart failure or valve disease

      6. Lymph node: Enlarged nodes indicative of infection or malignancy (see Appendix D)

      7. Abdominal: Signs of hepatic congestion or masses suggestive of cancer or hematemesis from potential esophageal varices

IV. Diagnostic tests (Cardenas-Garcia & Feller-Kopman, 2018; Cordovilla et al., 2016; Earwood & Thompson, 2015; Gagnon et al., 2017; Ittrich et al., 2017; Mondoni et al., 2019; Ong et al., 2016)

  A. Laboratory

    1. CBC to assess for anemia and presence of thrombocytopenia

    2. Coagulation studies to assess for prolonged values if coagulopathy or hypercoagulable state suspected

    3. Basic chemistry panel to evaluate baseline values and renal function

    4. Type and crossmatch for RBCs, if indicated

    5. Immunologic workup: Cytoplasmic antineutrophilic cytoplasmic antibody (c-ANCA); perinuclear antineutrophilic cytoplasmic antibody (p-ANCA); antinuclear antibody (ANA); and antibody against double-stranded deoxyribonucleic acid (ds-DNA-AB) to evaluate for immune-mediated disorders (e.g., SLE, antiphospholipid syndrome, vasculitis)

  B. Radiology

    1. Lateral and anterior–posterior chest x-ray

      a) Apical cavitary lesions suggestive of TB

      b) Diffuse infiltrates suggestive of blood aspiration or microvascular bleeding

      c) Atelectasis with COPD

      d) Masses indicative of cancer

      e) Fine reticulonodular pattern suggestive of intra-alveolar bleeds or pneumonia

      f) Focal consolidation suggestive of pneumonia

      g) Normal chest x-ray: Does not determine source of bleeding is outside the thorax

    2. CT angiography of chest with contrast: Perform if chest x-ray is abnormal to assess for pattern or distribution of diffuse lung disease or origin of bleeding. This method is superior for identifying peripheral site of bleeding that bronchoscopy cannot reach.

  C. Other

    1. ABGs to evaluate ventilation and circulation for respiratory compromise noted with hypoxemia and hypercapnia

    2. Pulse oximetry to evaluate oxygen saturation

    3. Sputum culture for bacteria, fungi, and mycobacteria as indicated

    4. Bronchoscopy: Most useful technique to evaluate massive hemoptysis and small, central endobronchial lesions for direct visualization of central airways

V. Differential diagnosis (Cardenas-Garcia & Feller-Kopman, 2018; Gagnon et al., 2017; Ong et al., 2016)

  A. Airway disorders

    1. Bronchitis/bronchiectasis (see Chapter 28)

    2. Fistula formation

    3. Airway trauma

    4. Pulmonary malignancy

    5. Foreign body

    6. Dieulafoy lesion: Submucosal vessel that causes bleeding in the airway and GI tract

    7. Pulmonary fungal infection (e.g., *Aspergillus*)

    8. Sarcoidosis

B. Pulmonary parenchymal diseases
1. Infection: TB (most common worldwide) (see Chapter 36)
2. Lung abscess
3. Pneumonia (see Chapter 30)
4. Mycetoma
5. Miscellaneous
   a) Drug induced: Cocaine, bevacizumab
   b) Pulmonary endometriosis
   c) Nitrogen dioxide exposure: Indoor ice arenas
C. Rheumatic and immune disorders
1. Goodpasture syndrome
2. Lupus pneumonitis (see Chapter 110)
3. Wegener granulomatosis with polyangiitis
4. Behçet disease
5. Idiopathic pulmonary hemosiderosis
D. Genetic disorders: Ehlers-Danlos syndrome
E. Coagulopathies: Thrombocytopenia and anticoagulants (see Chapters 122 and 129)
F. Iatrogenic: Percutaneous or transbronchial lung biopsy
G. Pulmonary vascular diseases
1. PE (see Chapter 33)
2. Arteriovenous malformations: Osler-Weber-Rendu syndrome
3. Elevated pulmonary capillary pressure
4. Hughes-Stovin syndrome
5. Pulmonary artery pseudoaneurysms
6. Perforation from a Swan-Ganz catheter
H. Idiopathic: Up to 30% of patients have no identifiable cause.

VI. Treatment: The three goals of therapy are to maintain airway patency, stop the bleeding, and treat the cause of bleeding using an interprofessional team (e.g., pulmonologists, intensivists, thoracic surgeons, interventional radiologists) (Cardenas-Garcia & Feller-Kopman, 2018; Cordovilla et al., 2016; Davidson & Shojaee, 2020; Earwood & Thompson, 2015; Gagnon et al., 2017; Ittrich et al., 2017; Ong et al., 2016; Radchenko et al., 2017).
A. Massive bleeds: Admit to ICU for management.
1. Provide oxygen and frequent suction to the airway.
2. Secure airway with large-diameter endotracheal tube (8 mm or larger to allow for bronchoscopy).
3. Monitor pulse oximetry and ABGs PRN.
4. Start IV infusion of fluids, begin replacing lost blood with packed RBCs, and correct coagulopathies with fresh frozen plasma and/or platelets.
5. Perform invasive procedures to control bleeding.
   a) Bronchial artery embolization: If the patient is stable, an angiogram is performed to visualize the bleeding site, and the area is embolized.
   b) Bronchoscopy-guided topical hemostatic tamponade: After bleeding site is visualized, a hemostatic agent is applied to aid in the formation of a clot.
   c) Bronchoscopy with cold saline lavage
B. Moderate bleeds
1. Provide oxygen and monitor.
2. Administer fluids and blood PRN.
3. Encourage bed rest with semi-sitting position.
4. Continue evaluation for etiology.

    C. Minor bleeds: Observe and continue workup for etiology. If chest radiograph is normal and patient is younger than 40 years old with no smoking history, treat for bronchitis with a mild cough suppressant and an oral broad-spectrum antibiotic (e.g., levofloxacin 750 mg daily). Follow up in one to two weeks to evaluate for resolution.

    D. Inhaled bronchodilators (see Chapter 28), antitussives (see Table 23-1 in Chapter 23): May be useful for comfort measures

    E. Cancer treatment for sensitive tumors with chemotherapy or radiation

    F. Cryosurgery: Performed through a bronchoscope. Can be used to destroy obstructive tumors

    G. Surgery: Bleeding caused by necrotizing tumor, cavernous TB, or aspergilloma

VII. Follow-up (Depuydt & Soares, 2015)

    A. After antibiotics to ensure symptoms have subsided

    B. At intervals during cancer treatment to evaluate whether treatment is improving disease or controlling hemoptysis

VIII. Referrals (Depuydt & Soares, 2015)

    A. Thoracic surgeon: For possible surgery for arteriovenous malformations, chest injuries, or leaking aortic aneurysm

    B. Pulmonologist: For bronchoscopy

    C. Infectious disease specialist: For management of infection

    D. Medical or radiation oncologist: For treatment of cancer

References

Cardenas-Garcia, J., & Feller-Kopman, D. (2018). Point: Should all initial episodes of hemoptysis be evaluated by bronchoscopy? Yes. *Chest, 153*(2), 302–305. https://doi.org/10.1016/j.chest.2017.09.036

Choi, J., Baik, J.H., Kim, C.H., Song, S.H., Kim, S.K., Kim, M., & Yun, S. (2018). Long-term outcomes and prognostic factors in patients with mild hemoptysis. *American Journal of Emergency Medicine, 36*(7), 1160–1165. https://doi.org/10.1016/j.ajem.2017.11.053

Cordovilla, R., Bollo de Miguel, E., Nuñez Ares, A., Cosano Povedano, F.J., Herráez Ortega, I., & Jiménez Merchán, R. (2016). Diagnosis and treatment of hemoptysis. *Archivos de Bronconeumología, 52*(7), 368–377. https://doi.org/10.1016/j.arbr.2016.05.010

Davidson, K., & Shojaee, S. (2020). Managing massive hemoptysis. *Chest, 157*(1), 77–88. https://doi.org/10.1016/j.chest.2019.07.012

Depuydt, P., & Soares, M. (2015). A bleeding problem in lung cancer patients. *European Respiratory Journal, 45*(3), 601–603. https://doi.org/10.1183/09031936.00199914

Earwood, J.S., & Thompson, T.D. (2015). Hemoptysis: Evaluation and management. *American Family Physician, 91*(4), 243–249. https://www.aafp.org/afp/2015/0215/p243.html

Gagnon, S., Quigley, N., Dutau, H., Delage, A., & Fortin, M. (2017). Approach to hemoptysis in the modern era. *Canadian Respiratory Journal, 2017*, 1565030. https://doi.org/10.1155/2017/1565030

Ittrich, H., Bockhorn, M., Klose, H., & Simon, M. (2017). The diagnosis and treatment of hemoptysis. *Deutches Ärzteblatt International, 114*(21), 371–381. https://doi.org/10.3238/arztebl.2017.0371

Mondoni, M., Carlucci, P., Cipolla, G., Fois, A., Gasparini, S., Marani, S., ... Sotgiu, G. (2019). Bronchoscopy to assess patients with hemoptysis: Which is the optimal timing? *BMC Pulmonary Medicine, 19*, 36. https://doi.org/10.1186/s12890-019-0795-9

Ong, Z.Y.T., Chai, H.Z., How, C.H., Koh, J., & Low, T.B. (2016). A simplified approach to haemoptysis. *Singapore Medical Journal, 57*(8), 415–418. https://doi.org/10.11622/smedj.2016130

Radchenko, C., Alraiyes, A.H., & Shojaee, S. (2017). A systematic approach to the management of massive hemoptysis. *Journal of Thoracic Disease, 9*(Suppl. 10), S1069–S1086. https://doi.org/10.21037/jtd.2017.06.41

Xia, X.-D., Ye, L.-P., Zhang, W.-X., Wu, C.-Y., Yan, S.-S., Weng, H.-X., ... Dong, L. (2015). Massive cryptogenic hemoptysis undergoing pulmonary resection: Clinical and pathological characteristics and management. *International Journal of Clinical and Experimental Medicine, 8*(10), 18130–18136.

CHAPTER 26

Orthopnea

Victoria Sherry, DNP, CRNP, AOCNP®

I. Definition (Tana et al., 2017; Thibodeau & Drazner, 2018)
   A. Respiratory difficulty (dyspnea) that develops or is increased by lying supine
   B. Paroxysmal nocturnal dyspnea: Orthopnea that causes the patient to suddenly awaken one to two hours after sleep with the sensation of air hunger and choking, with relief achieved upon sitting up

II. Physiology/Pathophysiology (Meysman, & Droogmans, 2018; Perino et al., 2016; Tana et al., 2017)
   A. Normal
      1. Neuromuscular coordination of thoracic and abdominal muscles results in an organized respiratory cycle and inflation/deflation of compliant lungs with effective gas exchange.
      2. Pulmonary blood flow is maintained and supported by the cardiovascular system through compliant and toned vasculature.
   B. Pathophysiology
      1. When one or more systems are damaged or compromised (e.g., neurologic, muscular, cardiovascular, pulmonary), inspiratory/expiratory effort and/or pulmonary blood flow and volume may be altered with a resulting sensation of dyspnea.
      2. When the individual is supine, dyspnea may develop or increase (orthopnea) because of alterations in the mechanics of breathing, increased work of breathing, change in pulmonary blood volume, or inability of the heart to handle increased venous return when supine.

III. Clinical features: Orthopnea is commonly seen as a late manifestation of heart failure, abdominal obesity, or pulmonary disease. In neuromuscular diseases, orthopnea is a sign of diaphragmatic weakness (Long et al., 2019; Perino et al., 2016; Tana et al., 2017; Thibodeau & Drazner, 2018).
   A. Etiology
      1. Pulmonary
         a) COPD: Asthma, emphysema
         b) Tumor invasion
         c) Pleural effusion: Malignant or otherwise
         d) Atelectasis
         e) Pulmonary edema
         f) PH
         g) Pneumonia
         h) Diaphragmatic weakness/paralysis

   i) Lymphangitic spread of cancer

   j) Pulmonary veno-occlusive disease

   k) Radiation pulmonary fibrosis

   l) Acute PE

   m) Chemotherapy drugs: Bleomycin, mitomycin, and carmustine cause greatest risk.

  2. Cardiac

   a) CHF

   b) Cardiomyopathy

   c) Cor pulmonale

   d) Left/right heart failure

   e) Increased left ventricular filling pressure

   f) Pericardial effusion

   g) Valvular disorder: Stenosis, insufficiency

   h) Tumor invasion

   i) Endomyocardial fibrosis

   j) Cardiotoxicity from chemotherapy or immunotherapy agents: Doxorubicin, daunorubicin, epirubicin, 5-fluorouracil, mitoxantrone, trastuzumab

  3. Mechanical defect/other

   a) Obesity

   b) Neuromuscular weakness

   c) Anemia

   d) Hypercapnia

   e) Renal insufficiency

   f) Mediastinal tumor

   g) SVC syndrome

   h) Compressive pulmonary/cardiac growths and/or tumors

   i) Ascites

B. History

  1. History of cancer and cancer treatment

  2. Current medications: Prescribed, over the counter

  3. History of presenting symptoms: Precipitating factors, onset, location, duration, severity, associated symptoms (e.g., GERD, fever, chills, sputum production, wheezing, edema, chest pain, palpitations, pleural pain with inspiration, dysphagia, facial/upper torso swelling)

  4. Changes in ADLs

  5. Past medical history: Heart disease, pulmonary disease, GI status (e.g., GERD, aspiration, hiatal hernia)

  6. Social history: Tobacco use, alcohol use, environmental exposures (e.g., asbestos, inhaled toxins), nutritional status over time (e.g., obesity, cachexia), sleep habits, number of pillows used

  7. Past surgical history: Chest wall, lung, cardiac/pericardial, surgical sites proximate to diaphragm, phrenic nerve, abdominal

C. Signs and symptoms

  1. Unable to rest or sleep in supine position without elevation on multiple pillows

  2. Sleep interruptions: Wakes patient, needs to move out of bed and ambulate to relieve symptoms

  3. Signs of increased respiratory effort

   a) Fast breathing

   b) Inability to complete sentence because of dyspnea

   c) Nasal flaring

      d) Pursed-lip breathing

      e) Shallow respiratory pattern, exacerbated when supine

   4. Feeling of inability to "fill lungs" with air, unable to take deep breath

   5. Cough

   6. Pleuritic chest pain

   7. Anxiety/panic attacks related to breathlessness, feeling of suffocation

   8. Clubbing from chronic hypoxia

D. Physical examination

   1. Vital signs: Increased respirations and change in quality, respiratory rate/depth

   2. HEENT

      a) Facial edema indicative of SVC syndrome

      b) Nasal flaring with difficulty breathing

      c) Pursed-lip breathing

   3. Pulmonary

      a) Deep breathing with prolonged expiratory phase or increased rate with shallow depth; variable with position change

      b) Uneven expansion/diaphragmatic movement with muscle weakness or paralysis

      c) Wheeze: Fluid overload, bronchoconstriction/reactive airway disease, COPD

      d) Rales: Pulmonary edema, CHF; may be absent if chronic because of compensation by pulmonary lymphatic system

      e) Absence of breath sounds: Atelectasis, plugging, compression of lobes by pleural effusion

      f) Rub noted with pleural effusion, especially if uremic/inflammatory

      g) Accessory muscle use: Intercostal, abdominal, paradoxical rocking abdominal–thoracic motion throughout cycle

   4. Cardiac

      a) Pulses, warmth of extremities, edema indicating peripheral vascular disease or CHF

      b) Heart sounds

         (1) S_3, S_4 with CHF: Change in S_3 over time suggestive of increased filling pressure

         (2) Murmurs of specific or general valvular dysfunction/stenosis

         (3) Distant heart sounds with pericardial effusion

         (4) Rub noted with pericardial effusion if uremic/inflammatory

      c) JVD: Cardiomyopathy, CHF, fluid overload, SVC syndrome

      d) Point of maximum intensity: Displacement associated with ventricular hypertrophy

      e) Hepatojugular reflux: CHF (see Appendix D)

      f) Pulsus alternans: Regular pulse with alternating strong and weak beats suggestive of left ventricular systolic impairment

      g) Precordial palpation for thrills (palpable murmur) and heaves (suggestive of hypertrophy)

   5. Integument: Clubbing suggestive of chronic hypoxia

IV. Diagnostic testing (Keelan et al., 2017; Long et al., 2019; Meysman & Droogmans, 2018; Oelsner et al., 2015; Tana et al., 2017; Young et al., 2017)

  A. Laboratory

   1. CBC to evaluate for anemia and leukocytosis

   2. Chemistry

      a) Renal function

   b) Electrolyte imbalances associated with muscle weakness: Hypocalcemia and hypercalcemia, hypophosphatemia-induced diaphragm weakness

  3. BNP and N-terminal prohormone BNP: Elevated in cardiac dysfunction; either primary or secondary

  4. ABGs to evaluate for hypoxia

  5. D-dimer typically normal: PE

 B. Radiology

  1. Chest x-ray to evaluate for pleural effusion, pneumonia, infiltrates

  2. CT angiogram of chest to evaluate for PE: High-resolution CT scan of chest is more sensitive for detecting ground glass opacities.

  3. Angiography to evaluate cardiac symptoms

  4. Ventilation/perfusion scan to evaluate for PE

 C. Other

  1. Pulse oximetry at rest and with ambulation to evaluate oxygen saturation

  2. Spirometry pre- and postinhaled bronchodilator or full pulmonary function tests to evaluate lung capacity

   a) FVC, FEV_1, total lung capacity, diffusing capacity of the lung for carbon monoxide (DLCO)

    (1) Tests may be performed sitting, standing, and supine to identify differences in functional status with position change.

    (2) FVC decrease of 30% when supine is consistent with diaphragmatic paralysis.

   b) Transdiaphragmatic pressure gradient may be measured to evaluate diaphragm strength and mobility.

   c) Peak expiratory flow is used for asthma evaluation

  3. ECG to evaluate for dysrhythmias, if indicated

  4. Echocardiogram

   a) Cardiac wall motion abnormalities, chamber filling, chamber size, flow disturbances

   b) PH evaluation

   c) Valvular evaluation

  5. Multigated acquisition scan to evaluate cardiac function

  6. Radionuclide ventriculography to evaluate left ventricular systolic function: Used in obese patients and those with advanced COPD

  7. Sleep studies to evaluate for sleep apnea

  8. Cardiopulmonary exercise test and invasive cardiopulmonary exercise test: Useful in the screening of PH, this test evaluates if decreased tolerance to exercise or shortness of breath with activity is caused by cardiac or pulmonary disease.

V. Differential diagnosis (Tana et al., 2017)

 A. Anterior mediastinal mass: Most common tumor is thymoma.

 B. COPD/COPD exacerbation (see Chapter 28)

 C. Asthma (see Chapter 28)

 D. Pneumonia (see Chapter 30)

 E. Pulmonary edema (see Chapter 32)

 F. PH (see Chapter 52)

 G. PE (see Chapter 33)

 H. Pleural effusion (see Chapter 29)

 I. Cardiomyopathy (see Chapter 41)

 J. Constrictive pericarditis (see Chapter 50)

 K. Pericardial effusion/tamponade (see Chapter 50)

L. Radiation-/chemotherapy-induced heart disease

M. SVC syndrome

N. Obesity

O. Ascites (see Chapter 54)

P. Sleep apnea (see Chapter 34)

Q. Sarcoidosis

R. Depression (see Chapter 162)

S. Drug side effect

VI. Treatment (Baysal et al., 2018)

A. Immediate interventions

1. Place patient in a seated position with the arms supported by pillows or the arm rest of a chair, leaning forward over a bedside table or chair back.

2. Promote diaphragmatic excursion.

   a) Remove tight clothing.

   b) Reverse Trendelenburg in bed if increased abdominal pressure; consider dangling legs off bed.

3. Provide oxygen therapy if oxygen saturation is less than 91%–93%, depending on patient's baseline saturation and if dyspnea was preceded by or in conjunction with hypoxemia.

4. Noninvasive positive pressure ventilation can be used.

5. Helium/oxygen (HeO_2, heliox) is used for patients with partial airway obstruction or impaired ability to generate inspiratory pressure.

B. Nonpharmacologic interventions

1. Relaxation techniques

2. Slow, deeper breaths to increase ventilation and lung volume

3. Cool room temperature; use of fan to move air across face to decrease sensation of dyspnea

4. Cool cloth on face

5. Pulmonary rehabilitation and respiratory therapy: Diaphragmatic and pursed-lip breathing

6. Acupuncture

C. Pharmacologic interventions

1. Consider opioid agents to relieve dyspnea. Morphine is the most widely used, but codeine, dihydrocodeine, hydromorphone, and diamorphine have been shown to be effective.

2. Consider bronchodilator therapy by nebulizer or multidose inhaler if evidence of wheezing. This therapy may provide symptomatic relief in patients without audible wheezing but with feeling of inability to fully expand lungs.

3. Consider use of benzodiazepines as second-line therapy for treatment of orthopnea, as an adjunct to therapy when anxiety is significant.

4. Consider administration of loop diuretic for treatment of acute fluid overload.

5. Consider use of promethazine (histamine H_1 antagonist) in combination with opioids as a second-line agent.

6. Consider use of glucocorticoids, which is not used to treat dyspnea as a symptom but to treat underlying causes of dyspnea.

7. Consider palliative sedation (use of nonopioid drug to reduce patient's awareness of symptoms) at the end of life.

D. Treatment for underlying causes

1. Chemotherapy, targeted therapy, immunotherapy, and/or radiation therapy as appropriate for malignant disease, or stop if they are the precipitating factor

2. Pulmonary: Refer to disease-specific chapters for more detailed treatment of asthma, COPD (Chapter 28), emphysema (see Chapter 28), pneumonia (Chapter 30), PH (Chapter 52), pulmonary edema (Chapter 32), and pleural effusion (Chapter 29).
   a) Pulmonary edema (see Chapter 32)
      (1) Diuresis
      (2) Oxygen therapy to maintain oxygen saturation 91%–93% or greater
      (3) Noninvasive ventilation: Most effective if pulmonary disorder is a result of CHF or COPD exacerbation
      (4) Intubation and mechanical ventilation
   b) Pleural effusion (see Chapter 29)
      (1) Thoracentesis for short-term and potentially long-term relief, diagnostics
      (2) Chest tube placement for extended drainage
      (3) Heimlich valve for prolonged drainage
      (4) Pleurodesis, decortication
   c) Asthma exacerbation (see Chapter 28)
      (1) Beta-2 agonist and anticholinergic therapy
      (2) Glucocorticoid dosing.
      (3) Epinephrine dosing, IV magnesium, and methylxanthines
      (4) Need for admission and intubation
   d) Central airway obstruction: Airway debulking and stents
   e) Develop and design inpatient and outpatient treatment plans in conjunction with pulmonary/critical care consultant.
3. Cardiac: Refer to disease-specific chapters for more detailed treatment of CHF (Chapter 42), heart failure, pericardial effusion/tamponade (Chapter 50), dysrhythmias (Chapter 45).
   a) Volume overload
      (1) Diuresis using loop or thiazide diuretics
      (2) Diuresis using synthetic BNP
      (3) Dialysis (intermittent or continuous) if unable to diurese
      (4) Family and patient education regarding diet and sodium load
   b) Pump failure
      (1) Control of atrial and ventricular dysrhythmias, as required
      (2) Inotropic support: Dobutamine, norepinephrine, milrinone
      (3) Vasodilator therapy
      (4) Decrease in PH
      (5) Need for balloon-pump therapy
      (6) Need for ventricular assist devices
   c) Constrictive/restrictive pericardial disease (see Chapter 50)
      (1) Pericardial stripping: May be required for fibrotic banding resulting in cardiac compromise
      (2) Pericardiocentesis for pericardial effusions/tamponade
      (3) Pericardial sclerosis, pericardial window, or stripping for recurrent pericardial effusions/tamponade
      (4) In acute tamponade, rapid IV infusion to fill chambers sufficiently to overcome tamponade
      (5) Need for ventricular assist devices
   d) Develop and design inpatient and outpatient treatment plans in conjunction with cardiac/critical care consultant.
4. Anemia: Consider RBC transfusion and growth factors to maintain Hgb at 7–9 mg/dl.

5. Sleep apnea: Treat with continuous positive airway pressure and bilevel positive airway pressure, as indicated (see Chapter 34).

VII. Follow-up: Dependent on etiology and overall prognosis (e.g., curative, palliative, hospice)

VIII. Referrals: Refer to pulmonologist, cardiologist, and critical care for collaborative management.

References

Baysal, E., Sağkal Midilli, T., & Ergin, E. (2018). Effects of different position changes on hemodynamic parameters and dyspnea severity in patients with dyspnea. *Clinical and Experimental Health Sciences, 8,* 261–267. https://doi.org/10.5152/clinexphealthsci.2017.751

Keelan, E., Kidney, J., & Judge, E.P. (2017). An unusual case of orthopnea. *Clinical Medicine Journal, 17*(3), 245–247. https://doi.org/10.7861/clinmedicine.17-3-245

Long, B., Koyfman, A., & Gottlieb, M. (2019). Diagnosis of acute heart failure in the emergency department: An evidence-based review. *Western Journal of Emergency Medicine, 20*(6), 875–884. https://doi.org/10.5811/westjem.2019.9.43732

Meysman, M., & Droogmans, S. (2018). Orthopnea and pulmonary hypertension. Treat the underlying disease. *Respiratory Medicine Case Reports, 24,* 105–107. https://doi.org/10.1016/j.rmcr.2018.05.004

Oelsner, E.C., Lima, J.A.C., Kawut, S.M., Burkat, K.M., Enright, P.L., Ahmed, F.S., & Barr, R.G. (2015). Noninvasive tests for the diagnostic evaluation of dyspnea among outpatients: The Multi-Ethnic Study of Atherosclerosis lung study. *American Journal of Medicine, 128*(2), 171–180.e5. https://doi.org/10.1016/j.amjmed.2014.09.023

Perino, E., Nesme, P., Germain, M., & Guérin, C. (2016). Mechanisms of orthopnea in stable obese subjects. *Respiratory Care, 61*(8), 1015–1022. https://doi.org/10.4187/respcare.04146

Tana, C., di Carlo, S., Silingardi, M., Giamberardino, M.A., Cipollone, F., & Meschi, T. (2017). Orthopnea and fever in an elderly woman. *Italian Journal of Medicine, 11*(4), 399–402. https://doi.org/10.4081/itjm.2017.922

Thibodeau, T., & Drazner, H. (2018). The role of the clinical examination in patients with heart failure. *JACC: Heart Failure, 6*(7), 543–551. https://doi.org/10.1016/j.jchf.2018.04.005

Young, M., Dumont, T., & Singh, A. (2017). It's not the lung! When a neuromuscular disease presented as recurrent episodes of shortness of breath. *Chest, 152*(4 Suppl.), 917A. https://doi.org/10.1016/j.chest.2017.08.952

CHAPTER 27

Wheezing

Leslie Matthews, MS, ANP-BC, AOCNP®

I. Definition: A high-pitched, prolonged, musical respiratory sound (Quirt et al., 2018)

II. Physiology/Pathophysiology (Bush, 2019; Reynolds & Cullinan, 2014)
   A. Normal: Lungs are spongy and highly elastic with three right lobes and two left lobes. The tracheobronchial tree is a tubular system that provides a pathway for air to move from the upper airway to the alveoli.
   B. Pathophysiology: Wheezes are generated by the vibration of the bronchial wall resulting from narrowing of the lumen of a respiratory pathway and causing airflow limitation; this may be from inflammation, edema, or obstruction.

III. Clinical features: Wheezing is most commonly associated with asthma; however, other conditions, such as COPD, can produce a similar presentation and may coexist with asthma (Enilari & Sinha, 2019; Global Initiative for Asthma [GINA], 2019; Melbye et al., 2016; Menon & Patel, 2019; Reynolds & Cullinan, 2014; Quirt et al., 2018; Yawn & Han, 2017).
   A. Etiology
      1. Bronchospasm, bronchoconstriction
      2. Airway edema or collapse
      3. Intraluminal obstruction by neoplasm or secretions
      4. Asthma
      5. Croup
      6. Allergies, anaphylaxis
      7. Diffuse parenchymal lung disease
      8. Pleural effusion
      9. Cardiac: Left ventricular failure, mitral stenosis
      10. Goiter
   B. History
      1. History of cancer and cancer treatment
      2. Current medications: Prescribed, over the counter
      3. History of presenting symptoms: Precipitating factors, onset, duration, associated symptoms (e.g., dyspnea, orthopnea)
      4. Changes in ADLs
      5. Past medical history: Bronchitis, pneumonia, URIs
      6. Social history: Tobacco use, vaping, occupation, chemical or agricultural exposure
   C. Signs and symptoms
      1. Nocturnal wheezing
      2. Wheezing triggered by irritants, allergens, or exercise
      3. Stridor indicating obstruction

        4. Anxiety or restlessness

        5. Hemoptysis

        6. Pleuritic pain

        7. Dyspnea and cough

        8. Fever, sore throat

D. Physical examination

    1. HEENT: Ears, pharynx, sinuses, and teeth to evaluate for local infection

      a) Ears: Erythema, edema, drainage

      b) Pharynx: Erythema, nasal posterior drainage

      c) Sinus: Tenderness to percussion

      d) Teeth: Erythema of gums, decay

      e) Face/tongue: Swelling, angioedema of clinical concern

    2. Lymph node: Adenopathy signifying infection (see Appendix D)

    3. Pulmonary

      a) Wheezes generally are more prominent during expiration than inspiration on auscultation.

        (1) Localized areas of wheezing raise the suspicion of airway obstruction, possibly by tumor or foreign body.

        (2) Wheezing that is loudest in the laryngeal area is more indicative of upper airway obstruction.

        (3) Expiratory wheeze is neither sensitive nor specific for asthma.

        (4) Inspiratory wheeze is neither sensitive nor specific for extrathoracic upper airway disease or obstruction.

      b) Barrel chest is seen more commonly in patients with emphysema than with asthma.

      c) Accessory muscle use indicates increased work of breathing.

    4. Integument

      a) Clubbing of the fingers indicating fibrotic lung disease (e.g., cystic fibrosis, interstitial lung disease), chronic hypoxia

      b) Nail beds assessment for cyanosis indicating poor oxygenation

    5. Vital signs

      a) Fever, tachycardia, tachypnea indicating infection

      b) Decreased oxygen saturation suggestive of hypoxia

IV. Diagnostic tests (Bush, 2019; Drazen & Harrington, 2018; GINA, 2019; Menon & Patel, 2019; Reynolds & Cullinan, 2014; Yawn & Han, 2017)

  A. Laboratory

    1. ABGs to evaluate hypoxemia indicated by reduced partial pressure of oxygen (less than 80 mm Hg) in asthma and COPD

    2. CBC to assess for anemia or leukocytosis indicative of infection

    3. Complete metabolic panel to evaluate baseline renal function and electrolytes

    4. BNP to evaluate for cardiac dysfunction

    5. Blood cultures to evaluate fever, as indicated

  B. Radiology

    1. Chest x-ray to evaluate for obstruction, infiltrates

    2. High-resolution CT scan of chest if bronchiectasis or mass is suspected

  C. Other

    1. Spirometry before and after the patient uses an inhaled bronchodilator: FEV_1/FVC ratio less than 0.70 indicates airflow obstruction.

    2. Allergen testing: Consider after diagnosis of asthma is confirmed.

3. Fiber-optic nasolaryngoscopy examination if vocal cord dysfunction is suspected
4. Bronchoscopy if central airway obstruction is suspected
5. Pulmonary function tests to measure lung capacity

V. Differential diagnosis (Yawn & Han, 2017)
   A. Asthma (see Chapter 28)
   B. Vocal cord dysfunction
   C. Bronchiectasis
   D. Upper or central airway obstruction by laryngeal edema, bronchial stenosis, foreign body aspiration, or tumor
   E. Bronchitis (see Chapter 28)
   F. Lung cancer
   G. Sarcoidosis
   H. Emphysema (see Chapter 28)
   I. Allergic reaction
   J. Drug-induced bronchospasm secondary to etoposide, paclitaxel, or docetaxel

VI. Treatment: Treatment is dependent on determining the underlying disease process and initiating appropriate therapy (Drazen & Harrington, 2018; Enilari & Sinha, 2019; GINA, 2019; Menon & Patel, 2019; Reynolds & Cullinan, 2014; Quirt et al., 2018; Yawn & Han, 2017).
   A. Vocal cord dysfunction: Patient education regarding disorder should occur. Speech therapy is primary intervention.
   B. Bronchiectasis: Treatment is dependent on cause of bronchiectasis. Causes include Ig deficiencies, recurrent aspiration, immotile cilia syndrome (Kartagener syndrome), and postinfection conditions.
   C. Upper or central airway obstruction by laryngeal edema, bronchial stenosis, foreign body aspiration, or tumor: Treatment is dependent on etiology.
   D. Treat underlying COPD (acute asthma) (see Chapter 28).

VII. Follow-up: Determined by the rapidity, severity, and cause of the wheezing

VIII. Referrals: Refer to pulmonologist; cardiologist; ear, nose, and throat specialist; or allergist based on etiology.

The author would like to acknowledge Robert G. Hanks, PhD, FNP-C, RNC, for his contribution to this chapter that remains unchanged from the previous edition of this book.

References

Bush, A. (2019). Pathophysiological mechanisms of asthma. *Frontiers in Pediatrics, 7,* 68. https://doi.org/10.3389/fped.2019.00068

Drazen, J.M., & Harrington, D. (2018). New biologics for asthma. *New England Journal of Medicine, 378*(26), 2533–2534. https://doi.org/10.1056/NEJMe1806037

Enilari, O., & Sinha, S. (2019). The global impact of asthma in adult populations. *Annals in Global Health, 85*(1), 2. https://doi.org/10.5334/aogh.2412

Global Initiative for Asthma. (2019). *Asthma management and prevention for adults and children older than 5 years: A pocket guide for health professionals; Updated 2019.* https://ginasthma.org/wp-content/uploads/2019/04/GINA-2019-main-Pocket-Guide-wms.pdf

Melbye, H., Garcia-Marcos, L., Brand, P., Everard, M., Priftis, K., & Pasterkamp, H. (2016). Wheezes, crackles and rhonchi: Simplifying description of lung sounds increases the agreement on their classification: A study of 12 physicians' classification of lung sounds from video recordings. *BMJ Open Respiratory Research, 3*(1), e000136. https://doi.org/10.1136/bmjresp-2016-000136

Menon, D.P., & Patel, N.M. (2019). 65-year-old woman with a wheeze. *Mayo Clinic Proceedings, 94*(3), e39–e44. https://doi.org/10.1016/j.mayocp.2018.04.035

Quirt, J., Hildebrand, K.J., Mazza, J., Noya, F., & Kim, H. (2018). Asthma. *Allergy, Asthma and Clinical Immunology, 14*(Suppl. 2), 50. https://doi.org/10.1186/s13223-018-0279-0

Reynolds, C., & Cullinan, P. (2014). Wheeze. *British Journal of Hospital Medicine, 75*(Suppl. 9), c137–c140. https://doi.org/10.12968/hmed.2014.75.9.C137

Yawn, B.P., & Han, M.K. (2017). Practical considerations for the diagnosis and management of asthma in older adults. *Mayo Clinic Proceedings, 92*(11), 1697–1705. https://doi.org/10.1016/j.mayocp.2017.08.005

CHAPTER 28

Chronic Obstructive Pulmonary Disease

Leslie Matthews, MS, ANP-BC, AOCNP®

I. Definition (Banfield & Murphy, 2019; Global Initiative for Chronic Obstructive Lung Disease [GOLD], 2020; Riley & Sciurba, 2019; Tantucci & Pini, 2015)
   A. COPD is a disease process that interferes with ventilation characterized by persistent respiratory symptoms and progressive airflow limitation that is not fully reversible and is associated with an enhanced abnormal inflammatory response of the lung to noxious particles or gases.
   B. The chronic airflow limitation characteristic of COPD is caused by small airway disease (obstructive bronchiolitis) and parenchymal destruction (emphysema), although the current definition of COPD no longer includes these as subcategories.
   C. Emphysema is a pathologic diagnosis that denotes abnormal permanent enlargement and destruction of the gas-exchanging surfaces of the lung (alveoli). It is one of several abnormalities found in COPD.
   D. Chronic bronchitis is a clinical condition in which patients produce excessive secretion of bronchial mucus and is manifested by daily productive cough for a duration of three months or longer in at least two consecutive years.
   E. Asthma is an episodic and chronic disease characterized by airway inflammation that can coexist with COPD; the airway inflammation is pathologically very different in the two diseases, although it may not be easy to clinically distinguish asthma from COPD.

II. Physiology/Pathophysiology (Gentry & Gentry, 2017; GOLD, 2020; Ko et al., 2016; Riley & Sciurba, 2019)
   A. Normal
      1. Neuromuscular coordination of thoracic and abdominal muscles results in an organized respiratory cycle and inflation/deflation of compliant lungs with effective gas exchange.
      2. The respiratory system maintains the homeostasis of carbon dioxide and oxygen by adjusting the ventilation of the pulmonary alveoli to maintain a constant concentration of carbon dioxide in the arterial blood.
      3. The level of ventilation maintains the homeostasis of oxygen normally required for Hgb to become saturated with oxygen.
      4. The lower respiratory system performs the functions of gas exchange and ventilation.
   B. Pathophysiology: COPD results in poorly reversible structural changes to the lung resulting in mucus hypersecretion, severe airflow limitation and air trapping (lead-

ing to hyperinflation), gas exchange abnormalities, and cor pulmonale (right-sided heart failure).

1. Chronic inflammation caused by inhaled cigarette smoke and other noxious particles is an important component of the pathogenesis of COPD.
2. Chronic inflammation in people with COPD may represent a genetically determined amplified inflammatory response of the respiratory tract.
   a) Chronic inflammation activates an increased number of inflammatory cell types and inflammatory mediators that induce structural lung changes.
   b) Structural lung changes are also induced by repeated injury and normal repair processes resulting in small airway fibrosis.
3. Oxidative stress exists. An imbalance of the oxidant–antioxidant system occurs in which cigarette smoke directly depletes antioxidants, thereby shifting the balance toward oxidant burden.
   a) A reduction in endogenous antioxidants may result because of a reduction in transcription factor that regulates antioxidant genes.
   b) Oxidative stress is further increased in COPD exacerbations.
4. Increased numbers of inflammatory leukocytes and alveolar macrophages contribute to the increased pro-oxidant environment in the pulmonary tissue.
   a) Protease–antiprotease imbalance exists.
   b) An imbalance between proteases that break down lung connective tissue and antiproteases that protect against breakdown occurs such that proteases and destruction are increased.
   c) Protease destruction of elastin in lung connective tissue is believed to be a feature of emphysema.
5. In severe COPD, respiratory muscle dysfunction can occur as a result of deconditioning, malnutrition, skeletal muscle myopathy, and low levels of circulating anabolic hormones.

III. Clinical features: COPD is a major and increasing (due to an aging population) worldwide health problem that is the fourth most common cause of death in the United States. Although COPD is a common disease, it is a frequently underrecognized diagnosis. CHF frequently coexists with COPD in clinical practice, as both illnesses share the same risk factors. Other chronic comorbidities seen with COPD include hypertension, diabetes, osteoporosis, and depression. COPD progression can be stopped or slowed by smoking cessation, especially in the early stages. The three goals of COPD assessment are to define the level of airflow limitation, evaluate effect of COPD on health status, and evaluate the risk of future events, including exacerbations, hospitalizations, or death. COPD assessment now separates lung function measures from respiratory symptom scores, as lung function has been found to be weakly correlated to symptoms and health status impairment (see Figure 28-1; Agrawal et al., 2019; Banfield & Murphy, 2019; Duffy & Criner, 2019; Gentry & Gentry, 2017; GOLD, 2020; Hillas et al., 2020; Matarese et al., 2019; Riley & Sciurba, 2019; Weiss et al., 2020).

A. Risk factors
   1. Genetic predisposition or susceptibility
   2. Cigarette smoking: Most commonly encountered risk factor
   3. Indoor air pollution: Especially from burning biomass fuels in confined space
   4. Occupational dusts and chemicals: Vapors, irritants, fumes
   5. Recurrent or chronic respiratory infection: Bacterial, viral, and atypical pathogens
   6. Passive exposure to cigarette smoke: Environmental tobacco smoke
   7. Outdoor air pollution: Small risk compared to cigarette smoking
   8. Age: Most common in fifth decade of life

FIGURE 28-1	Clinical Features of Chronic Obstructive Pulmonary Disease

Asthma
- Airway hyperresponsiveness
- Airway inflammation
- Chest tightness
- Dyspnea
- Possible exercise component
- Possible presence of allergy
- Reversibility or partial reversibility
- Widespread airway obstruction
- Wheezing

Chronic Bronchitis
- Chronic cough with sputum production (for at least 3 months for 2 successive years)
- Frequent respiratory infections
- Hemoptysis
- History of tobacco use
- Post-tussive syncope
- Severe obstruction, although not consistent

Emphysema
- Barrel chest
- Digital clubbing
- Exertional dyspnea
- History of tobacco use
- Possibly secondary to polycythemia
- Pursed-lip breathing

Note. Based on information from Global Initiative for Chronic Obstructive Lung Disease, 2020.

B. Etiology
1. Chronic inflammation from tobacco smoke and other noxious particles
2. Genetic factors: Alpha-1 antitrypsin deficiency
3. Exacerbation by viruses or bacterial colonization
    a) *Streptococcus pneumoniae*
    b) *Haemophilus influenzae*
    c) *Moraxella catarrhalis*
C. History
1. History of cancer and cancer treatment
2. Current medications: Prescribed, over the counter
3. History of presenting symptoms: Precipitating factors, onset, location, duration, associated symptoms (e.g., cough, sputum production, dyspnea)
4. Changes in ADLs: Difficulty speaking or performing tasks
5. Past medical history: CHF, osteoporosis, frequent URIs, colds, influenza
6. Social history: Tobacco use with number of pack-year history (number of packs of cigarettes smoked a day multiplied by the number of years the individual has smoked), occupation, exposure to chemicals
D. Signs and symptoms: Usually nonspecific
1. Dyspnea: Persistent, progressive, worse with exercise; may occur with rest in end-stage disease
2. Chronic cough
3. Chronic sputum production
4. Decrease in exercise tolerance, interference with ADLs
5. Chest tightness
6. Wheezing
7. Fatigue
8. Depressed/anxious affect
9. In severe disease, extrapulmonary or systemic effects
    a) Anorexia
    b) Weight loss
    c) Nutritional deficits
    d) Loss of skeletal muscle mass
    e) Skeletal muscle weakness
E. Physical examination
1. Vital signs: Weight loss, tachypnea, tachycardia, hypertension

2. Pulmonary
   a) Auscultation of wheezing, particularly end-expiratory wheeze
   b) Retraction of intercostal and sternocleidomastoid muscles: Observation of increased work of breathing with use of accessory muscles
   c) Decreased respiratory expansion
   d) Diminished or distant breath sounds in advanced disease
   e) Hyperresonance to percussion
   f) Possible pursed-lip breathing pattern observed in late stages
   g) Increased anteroposterior diameter of the thorax resulting from hyperinflation of the lungs, dorsal kyphosis, prominent anterior chest, elevated ribs, and widening of costal angle, giving the chest a barrel-shaped appearance
   h) Decreased tactile fremitus
   i) Decreased diaphragmatic excursion
   j) End-expiratory crackles
3. Cardiac
   a) Distant heart sounds with heart failure
   b) Murmur with hypertrophy
   c) Gallop with hypertrophy or CHF
4. Musculoskeletal: Loss of muscle mass, especially in lower extremities
5. Peripheral vascular
   a) Clubbing of the fingers: Sign of prolonged peripheral hypoxia
   b) Pedal or lower extremity edema: Sign of right-sided heart failure

IV. Diagnostic tests (Gentry & Gentry, 2017; GOLD, 2020; Kim et al., 2020; Matarese et al., 2019; Riley & Sciurba, 2019; Takei et al., 2019)
   A. Laboratory
   1. CBC: Polycythemia vera can occur with elevated hematocrit.
   2. Pulse oximetry to evaluate peripheral oxygen saturation: If less than 92%, ABGs should be assessed.
   3. ABGs: Typically normal early in the disease; it is indicated when acid-base disturbance, hypoxemia, or hypercapnia is suspected.
      a) Hypoxemia (reduced arterial partial pressure of oxygen) is the most common abnormality.
         (1) Normal partial pressure of oxygen levels range from 70–100 mm Hg.
         (2) Partial pressure of oxygen level less than 70 mm Hg indicates hypoxemia.
      b) Hypercapnia (elevated partial pressure of carbon dioxide) may become chronically elevated and/or may show an acute rise during an infection or other medical complications.
         (1) Normal partial pressure of carbon dioxide levels range from 35–45 mm Hg.
         (2) A partial pressure of carbon dioxide level greater than 45 mm Hg indicates hypercapnia.
   4. Serum alpha-1 antitrypsin deficiency screening: A value approximately 15%–20% below normal suggests deficiency. Higher serum levels are associated with worse systemic inflammation and higher mortality.
   5. BNP, if indicated: BNP is elevated with CHF.
   6. Sputum culture with frequent exacerbations to evaluate bacteria sensitivity
   7. Vitamin D level: Increased vitamin D level is a higher risk for deficiency.
   B. Radiology
   1. Chest x ray: An x-ray may be normal early in disease and has poor sensitivity for detecting COPD.

    a) With advanced disease, reveals flattened diaphragm and an increase in volume of the retrosternal space; apparent hyperinflation

    b) Possible parenchymal bullae or subpleural blebs indicative of lung tissue destruction

  2. High-resolution CT scan of chest

    a) Greater sensitivity and specificity than standard chest x-ray for detection of emphysema but not chronic bronchitis or asthma

    b) To evaluate for other pulmonary manifestations and determine possible suitability for lung volume reduction surgical procedure (part of lung is resected to reduce hyperinflation and improve expiratory flow rate)

  3. DEXA scan, if indicated: Prolonged use of oral corticosteroids can induce osteoporosis.

C. Other

  1. Pulmonary function tests to assess ventilation, diffusion, and mechanical properties (see Table 28-1)

    a) Spirometry remains the gold standard for diagnosing COPD and monitoring its progression.

    b) Spirometry measures the volume of air exhaled forcibly from point of maximal inspiration (FVC) and the volume of air exhaled during the first second of this maneuver (FEV_1).

    c) The ratio of these two measures is calculated FEV_1/FVC.

    d) Postbronchodilator FEV_1/FVC ratio is recommended for the diagnosis and assessment of severity of COPD.

    e) A postbronchodilator FEV_1/FVC ratio less than 0.70 confirms the presence of airflow limitation that is not fully reversible.

    f) FEV_1 is used as an index to airflow obstruction and evaluates the prognosis in emphysema

  2. Diffusing capacity of the lung for carbon monoxide (DLCO) is the measurement of a single breath's diffusing capacity for carbon monoxide.

    a) Reflects the ability of the lung to transfer gas across the alveolar and capillary interface

    b) Normal or reduced diffusing capacity

TABLE 28-1	Spirometric Classification of Airflow Limitation

Increasing spirometric grade (GOLD 1–4) corresponds to more severe airflow limitation measured by reduced FEV_1

GOLD Stage	Obstruction	Spirometric Assessment
1	Mild	FEV_1/FVC ratio < 0.70, FEV_1 ≥ 80% predicted, with or without symptoms
2	Moderate	FEV_1/FVC ratio < 0.70, FEV_1 50%–80% predicted, with chronic symptoms, shortness of breath on exertion
3	Severe	FEV_1/FVC ratio < 0.70, FEV_1 ≥ 30% or < 50% predicted, with dyspnea, reduced exercise tolerance, and exacerbations affecting quality of life
4	Very severe	FEV_1/FVC ratio < 0.70, FEV_1 < 30% predicted, or FEV_1 < 50% predicted plus chronic respiratory failure

FEV_1—forced expiratory volume in one second; FVC—forced vital capacity; GOLD—Global Initiative for Chronic Obstructive Lung Disease

Note. Based on information from Banfield & Murphy 2019; Global Initiative for Chronic Obstructive Lung Disease, 2020.

        c) ECG, if indicated: May show sinus tachycardia, supraventricular tachycardia, ventricular irritability, P wave changes, and axis deviation reflective of right atrial and right ventricular hypertrophy

    3. ECG: Increased risk for sinus tachycardia and atrial fibrillation

    4. Echocardiogram: Evaluation of PH, if indicated

  D. Diagnostic criteria

    1. Diagnostic criteria of COPD includes history of progressive dyspnea (usually worse with exercise), chronic cough or sputum production, and/or a history of exposure to risk factors for the disease.

    2. Spirometry testing confirming airflow limitation that is not fully reversible is required to make the diagnosis.

V. Differential diagnosis (Gentry & Gentry, 2017)

  A. Asthma

  B. CHF (see Chapter 42)

  C. Bronchiectasis

  D. TB (see Chapter 36)

  E. Obliterative bronchiolitis

  F. PE (see Chapter 33)

  G. Pneumonia (see Chapter 30)

  H. Pneumothorax (see Chapter 31)

  I. URI (see Chapter 37)

  J. Hypersensitivity pneumonitis

  K. Cystic fibrosis

  L. Allergic reactions

  M. Polycythemia vera (see Chapter 128)

VI. Treatment: Management is based on stage of disease and diagnosis of stable COPD disease or acute COPD exacerbation. Although disease prevention is the ultimate goal, once COPD is diagnosed, effective management goals aim to improve survival, relieve symptoms, and decrease risk of exacerbations (Agrawal et al., 2019; Araujo et al., 2019; Banfield & Murphy, 2019; Duffy & Criner, 2019; Gentry & Gentry, 2017; GOLD, 2020; Hillas et al., 2020; Pérez Valdés et al., 2017; Riley & Sciurba, 2019; Tantucci & Pini, 2015; U.S. Department of Health and Human Services, 2014; Weiss et al., 2020; Williams & Rubin, 2018).

  A. Smoking cessation therapies: Quitting smoking can prevent or delay the development of airflow limitation and reduce the progression of COPD. All smokers should be offered the most intensive intervention feasible.

    1. Brief smoking cessation counseling should take place at every contact with healthcare provider using the 5 A's model: **A**sk about tobacco use, **A**dvise to quit, **A**ssess willingness to make quit attempt, **A**ssist in quit attempt, and **A**rrange follow-up.

    2. Nicotine replacement therapies: Gums, inhalers, nasal sprays, transdermal patches, sublingual tablets, lozenges

    3. Bupropion: 150 mg PO (sustained release) once a day for three days initially, followed by 150 mg two times a day for eight weeks, starting one to two weeks before quit date

    4. Varenicline: 0.5 mg PO once a day for three days initially, followed by 0.5 mg two times a day for four days, followed by 1 mg two times a day for 12–24 weeks, starting one week before quit date

    5. Social support groups

  B. Bronchodilators: These drugs alter airway smooth muscle tone, improve expiratory airflow, and reduce hyperinflation. Administration methods include metered-dose inhalers with or without a spacer, handheld or mask nebulizers, dry powder inhalers, or oral agents (e.g., tablet, lozenge).

   1. Beta-2 agonists: Short-acting
      a) Short-acting inhaler
         (1) Fenoterol 100–200 mcg via metered dose inhaler or 1 mg/ml solution for nebulizer every four to six hours
         (2) Levalbuterol (45 mcg/dose inhaler) 45–90 mcg (one puff every four hours or two puffs every four to six hours)
         (3) Salbutamol (albuterol, 90 mcg/dose inhaler) 90–180 mcg (one to two puffs every four to six hours)
         (4) Terbutaline 2.5–5 mg PO three times a day
      b) Provides faster action but for shorter duration (four to six hours)
      c) On a regular or as-needed basis
   2. Beta-2 agonists: Long acting
      a) Long-acting inhaler
         (1) Formoterol (12 mcg/dose inhaler) 12 mcg (one puff) every 12 hours
         (2) Indacaterol (75 mcg/cap dry powder inhaler) one cap every 24 hours
         (3) Salmeterol (50 mcg/dose inhaler) 50 mcg (one puff) two times a day
      b) Shows 12-hour duration effect except for indacaterol
   3. Anticholinergics
      a) Ipratropium inhaled (17 mcg/dose inhaler) 34 mcg (two puffs) up to four times a day
      b) Long acting: Tiotropium inhaled (18 mcg/dose inhaler) 18 mcg (one puff) once a day
      c) Slow onset but long duration of action (eight hours for ipratropium, 24 hours for tiotropium)
      d) Can be administered with saline as nebulized aerosol
   4. Combination short-acting beta-agonist plus anticholinergic
      a) Fenoterol/ipratropium 200 mcg/80 mcg per dose inhaler
      b) Salbutamol/ipratropium 75 mcg/15 mcg per dose inhaler (two to four puffs every 12 hours)
      c) Faster action
      d) Long duration
   5. Methylxanthines
      a) Aminophylline (administered IV; dose dependent on acute versus maintenance therapy and patient characteristics)
      b) Theophylline 10 mg/kg PO immediate-release preparation every six to eight hours initially (maximum 300 mg per day)
      c) Narrow therapeutic window (10–20 mg/ml) with significant toxicity
      d) Monitoring of serum levels required
   6. Phosphodiesterase type 4 inhibitor
      a) Roflumilast 500 mcg PO a day
      b) Not a bronchodilator; reduces inflammation through selectively inhibiting phosphodiesterase type 4, leading to increased intracellular cyclic adenosine monophosphate (referred to as cAMP)

C. Corticosteroids: Oral or inhaled
   1. Systemic corticosteroids: Prednisone 5–60 mg PO a day; or methylprednisolone 40–60 mg PO a day or in two divided doses
      a) This treatment is beneficial in the management of acute exacerbations and has shown to shorten recovery time and improve lung function (FEV_1) and hypoxemia.

       b) Long-term therapy is not supported by evidence. A side effect of long-term therapy is steroid myopathy, which contributes to muscle weakness and decreased functionality.

   2. Inhaled corticosteroids

      a) Types

         (1) Beclomethasone (40 or 80 mcg/dose inhaler) 80–240 mcg a day given in two divided doses

         (2) Budesonide (90, 100, 180, 200, or 400 mcg/dose inhaler) 180–600 mcg a day given in two divided doses

         (3) Fluticasone propionate (44, 110, or 220 mcg/dose inhaler) 88–440 mcg a day given in two divided doses

      b) No evidence to support trial of oral corticosteroids to predict response to inhaled route

      c) Recommended for patients with severe (stage 3) and very severe (stage 4) COPD and those with repeated exacerbations

      d) Adverse effects: Associated with high prevalence of oral candidiasis and possibly increased risk of pneumonia

D. Oxygen therapy

   1. Long-term oxygen administration (more than 15 hours a day) for stage 4 COPD has been shown to improve survival in hypoxemia and cor pulmonale. It should be initiated if oxygen saturation is less than 89%.

   2. Oxygen delivery during exercise can increase duration of exercise and/or reduce end-exercise breathlessness whether or not patient is hypoxic at rest.

E. Antibiotics for acute exacerbation

   1. Prophylactic, continuous use of antibiotic has been shown to have no effect on the frequency of exacerbations.

   2. Antibiotics can shorten recovery time, reduce risk of early relapse and treatment failure, and shorten length of hospital stay.

   3. The choice of antibiotic therapy should be based on local bacterial resistance pattern. Usual initial empirical treatment is amoxicillin with clavulanate 500 mg PO every eight hours or 875 mg PO every 12 hours; a macrolide, such as azithromycin 500 mg PO on day 1 followed by 250 mg once a day on days 2–5; or tetracycline 250–500 mg PO four times a day or alternatively doxycycline 100 mg PO two times a day. Recommended length of therapy is 5–10 days.

   4. In patients with frequent exacerbations and/or requiring mechanical ventilation, a sputum culture should be obtained to evaluate bacterial sensitivity to antibiotic.

F. Pulmonary rehabilitation

   1. Exercise training to increase exercise tolerance: Walking, upper limb exercises, pursed-lip breathing, inspiratory muscle training

   2. Nutritional counseling

   3. Education about importance of adherence to treatment plan

G. Lung transplantation can be considered in patients with reasonably stable health with severe COPD with FEV$_1$ less than 35%.

H. Lung volume reduction surgery to reduce hyperinflation has both symptom and mortality benefits in select patients with upper lobe disease with predominantly emphysema.

I. Vitamin D supplementation should be taken as indicated.

VII. Follow-up

A. Pneumococcal vaccination every five years to reduce risk of COPD exacerbation and prevent pneumococcal infections

B. Yearly influenza vaccine
C. Frequent visits to monitor smoking status, symptoms, exacerbation history, and disease progression

VIII. Referrals (Duffy & Criner, 2019; Weiss et al., 2020)
A. Pulmonary rehabilitation: To educate about general exercise conditioning
1. Graded aerobic physical exercise program such as walking three times a week for 20 minutes
2. Helps to prevent deterioration of physical condition
B. Home health or medical supply company: For oxygen
C. Pulmonologist: For diagnosis and initial treatment plan
D. Hospitalization: For acute exacerbations
E. Thoracic surgeon: For possible surgery
F. Palliative care: For assistance with symptom management

References

Agrawal, R., Moghtader, S., Ayyala, U., Bandi, V., & Sharafkhaneh, A. (2019). Update on management of stable chronic obstructive pulmonary disease. *Journal of Thoracic Disease, 11*(Suppl. 14), S1800–S1809. https://doi.org/10.21037/jtd.2019.06.12

Araujo, Z.T.S., Mendonça, K.M.P., Souza, B.M.M., Santos, T.Z.M., Chaves, G.S.S., Andriolo, B.N.G., & Nogueira, P.A.M.S. (2019). Pulmonary rehabilitation for people with chronic obstructive pulmonary disease: A protocol for an overview of Cochrane reviews. *Medicine, 93*(38), e17129. https://doi.org/10.1097/MD.00000000000017129

Banfield, J., & Murphy, K.R. (2019). Highlights of the 2019 update to Global Initiative for Chronic Obstructive Lung Disease (GOLD) report and their application to practice. *Clinician Reviews, 29*(1 Suppl.) https://www.mdedge.com/content/cr-copd-newsletter

Duffy, S.P., & Criner, G.J. (2019). Chronic obstructive pulmonary disease: Evaluation and management. *Medical Clinics of North America, 103*(3), 453–461. https://doi.org/10.1016/j.mcna.2018.12.005

Gentry, S., & Gentry, B. (2017). Chronic obstructive pulmonary disease: Diagnosis and management. *American Family Physician, 95*(7), 433–441. https://www.aafp.org/afp/2017/0401/p433.html

Global Initiative for Chronic Obstructive Lung Disease. (2020). *Global strategy for the diagnosis, management, and prevention of chronic obstructive pulmonary disease: 2020 Report.* https://goldcopd.org/wp-content/uploads/2019/12/GOLD-2020-FINAL-ver1.2-03Dec19_WMV.pdf

Hillas, G., Papaporfyriou, A., Dimakou, K., & Papaioannou, A.I. (2020). Pharmacological treatment of stable COPD: Need for a simplified approach. *Postgraduate Medicine, 132*(2), 126–131. https://doi.org/10.1080/00325481.2019.1706996

Kim, C., Ko, Y., Jung, J.Y., Lee, J.S., Rhee, C.K., Lee, J.H., ... Park, Y.B. (2020). Severe vitamin D deficiency is associated with emphysema progression in male patients with COPD. *Respiratory Medicine, 163,* 105890. https://doi.org/10.1016/j.rmed.2020.105890

Ko, F.W., Chan, K.P., Hui, D.S., Goddard, J.R., Shaw, J.G., Reid, D.W., & Yang, I.A. (2016). Acute exacerbation of COPD. *Respirology, 21*(7), 1152–1165. https://doi.org/10.1111/resp.12780

Matarese, A., Sardu, C., Shu, J., & Santulli, G. (2019). Why is chronic obstructive pulmonary disease linked to atrial fibrillation? A systematic overview of the underlying mechanisms. *International Journal of Cardiology, 276,* 149–151. https://doi.org/10.1016/j.ijcard.2018.10.075

Pérez Valdés, C.R., Lenoir, A., & Nicod, L. (2017). COPD exacerbation and prevention. *Cardiovascular Medicine, 20*(2), 38–45. https://doi.org/10.4414/cvm.2017.00461

Riley, C.M., & Sciurba, F.C. (2019). Diagnosis and outpatient management of chronic obstructive pulmonary disease: A review. *JAMA, 321*(8), 786–797. https://doi.org/10.1001/jama.2019.0131

Takei, N., Suzuki, M., Makita, H., Konno, S., Shimizu, K., Kimura, H., ... Nishimura, M. (2019). Serum alpha-1 antitrypsin levels and the clinical course of chronic obstructive pulmonary disease. *International Journal of Chronic Obstructive Pulmonary Disease, 14,* 2885–2893. https://doi.org/10.2147/COPD.S225365

Tantucci, C., & Pini, L. (2015). COPD: It is time to change! *International Journal of Chronic Obstructive Pulmonary Disease, 10,* 2451–2457. https://doi.org/10.2147/COPD.S87696

U.S. Department of Health and Human Services. (2014). *The health consequences of smoking—50 years of progress: A report of the Surgeon General.* https://www.ncbi.nlm.nih.gov/books/NBK179276/pdf/Bookshelf_NBK179276.pdf

Weiss, A., Porter, S., Rozenberg, D., O'Connor, E., Lee, T., Balter, M., & Wentlandt, K. (2020). Chronic obstructive pulmonary disease: A palliative medicine review of the disease, its therapies, and drug interactions. *Journal of Pain and Symptom Management, 60*(1), 135–150. https://doi.org/10.1016/j.jpainsymman.2020.01.009

Williams, D.M., & Rubin, B.K. (2018). Clinical pharmacology of bronchodilator medications. *Respiratory Care, 63*(6), 641–654. https://doi.org/10.4187/respcare.06051

CHAPTER 29

Pleural Effusion

Enza Esposito Nguyen, DNP, RN, ANP-BC, AOCNP®

I. Definition: Accumulation of fluid in the pleural space in excess of the average amount of 15 ml (Aboudara & Maldonado, 2019; Ferreiro et al., 2017)

II. Physiology/Pathophysiology (Aboudara & Maldonado, 2019; Ferreiro et al., 2017)
   A. Normal
      1. The lungs are lined by the visceral pleura, which folds back upon itself to form the parietal pleura (lining the chest wall, mediastinum, and diaphragm).
      2. The pocket created between the layers is known as the pleural space.
      3. The pleurae are made of epithelial cells (mesothelium), which produce lubricating fluid that allows for free movement of the lungs during respiration.
      4. Approximately 10–20 ml of fluid is present in the space. The fluid is released into the pleural space predominantly by the capillaries on the parietal surface and reabsorbed on the visceral surface by the pulmonary vessels and lymphatic system. The rate of fluid absorption by the lymphatic system can increase significantly before effusions begin to accumulate.
   B. Pathophysiology
      1. Pleural effusions develop when disequilibrium exists between the amount of fluid entering and leaving the pleural space.
      2. Mechanisms include increased capillary permeability of the pleural membrane, increased hydrostatic capillary pressure (systemic or pulmonary), decreased negative intrapleural pressure, decreased colloid osmotic pressure, obstructed lymphatic drainage, and diaphragmatic defects.
      3. Pleural effusions restrict the lung's ability to expand, impairing gas exchange and leading to hypoxia.
      4. Prolonged effusions lead to a fibrinopurulent phase, which impedes pleural fluid drainage.
      5. Malignant effusions develop as a result of impaired lymphatic drainage, direct extension of the tumor on the pleura, or enlargement of lymph nodes. Seeding of pleura with cancer cells can increase fluid formation.

III. Clinical features: Malignant pleural effusions are a common complication of advanced malignancy with an estimated incidence of more than 1.5 million yearly in the United States. Approximately one-half of all patients with metastatic disease will develop a malignant effusion (Aboudara & Maldonado, 2019; Bhatnagar & Maskell, 2015; Lim & Ryu, 2019; Rami-Porta & Eberhardt, 2018).
   A. Etiology and classification
      1. Exudate: Typically caused by local influences resulting in the escape of protein-rich fluid that results from an increase in capillary permeability with or without changes

in hydrostatic and colloid osmotic pressure; results primarily from pleural and lung inflammation or from impaired lymphatic drainage and is the most common cause of malignant effusion

  a) Neoplasm: Bronchogenic carcinoma (30%–40%), breast cancer (20%–25%), lymphoma (10%–15%), leukemia (5%–10%), ovarian carcinoma, multiple myeloma
  b) Paraneoplastic: Obstruction of lymph nodes, bronchial obstruction, SVC syndrome
  c) Infection and parapneumonic: Viral pneumonia, bacterial pneumonia, *Mycoplasma*, TB, fungal disease, parasitic disease, abscess, empyema, hepatic abscess, splenic abscess, hepatitis
  d) Lymphatic abnormalities: Lymphangiectasis, chylothorax, pseudochylothorax, yellow nail syndrome, malignancies
  e) Collagen vascular diseases: SLE, RA, scleroderma, Wegener granulomatosis, amyloidosis
  f) Other: PE, acute respiratory distress syndrome, pancreatitis, postcardiotomy, coronary artery bypass surgery, Dressler syndrome, post-abdominal surgery, ruptured esophagus, chronic effusion due to CHF
  g) Chronic peritoneal dialysis with uremia
  h) Iatrogenic: Enteral feeding tube in pleural space, radiofrequency ablation of pulmonary neoplasm, radiation therapy
  i) Drug induced: TKIs (protein discordance)
2. Transudate: Typically systemic etiology; increased systemic or pulmonary capillary hydrostatic pressure and/or decreased osmotic pressure in circulation with capillary permeability remaining normal; rarely a cause of malignant effusions
  a) CHF
  b) Hepatic cirrhosis with ascites
  c) Nephrotic syndrome
  d) Atelectasis
  e) Peritoneal dialysis
  f) PE
  g) Constrictive pericarditis
  h) Mediastinal fibrosis (after chest irradiation)
  i) SVC obstruction
  j) Meigs syndrome
  k) Urinothorax
  l) Hypothyroidism
  m) Iatrogenic: Misplaced IV catheter into pleural space
  n) Drug induced: Cyclophosphamide, taxanes, methotrexate
  o) CSF leak into pleural space
B. History
  1. History of cancer and cancer treatment
  2. Current medications: Prescribed (e.g., amiodarone, phenytoin, nitrofurantoin), over the counter, supplements
  3. History of presenting symptoms: Precipitating factors, onset, location, duration, associated symptoms, alleviating factors
  4. Changes in ADLs
  5. Past medical history: CHF, liver disease, kidney disease, renal failure, arthritis, trauma
  6. Social history: Occupational or environmental exposures (e.g., asbestos, tobacco use, drug use)

C. Signs and symptoms: May be asymptomatic
1. Dyspnea
2. Dry cough
3. Orthopnea
4. Chest discomfort, pressure, or pain
5. Reduced activity levels
6. Weight loss/weight gain
7. Anorexia
8. Hemoptysis
9. Night sweats
10. Malaise
11. Peripheral edema
D. Physical examination
1. Vital signs: Tachypnea; tachycardia; weak, thready pulse; hypotension; low-grade fever present with infection
2. General: Presence of anxiety or altered mental status
3. Neck examination: Assessment for use of accessory muscles on inspiration, tracheal deviation (with large effusions), neck vein distension
4. Pulmonary
   a) Inspiratory intercostal retractions on inspiration: Asymmetric expansion of thoracic cage with decreased expansion on affected side
   b) Decreased tactile fremitus on palpation over effusion
   c) Dullness on percussion over effusion
   d) Auscultation: Absent breath sounds, increased vocal fremitus, pleural friction rub, egophony and bronchophony over effusion
5. Cardiac
   a) JVD indicative of heart failure
   b) Poor or sluggish capillary refill with poor perfusion
   c) Displaced heart sounds with large effusion
6. Abdominal: Organomegaly, ascites, tenderness on palpation
7. Integument: Cyanotic; cool temperature with poor tissue perfusion

IV. Diagnostic tests (Aboudara & Maldonado, 2019; Bhatnagar & Maskell, 2015; Ferreiro et al., 2017; Jany & Welte, 2019; Lim & Ryu, 2019; Saguil et al., 2014; Shen et al., 2017)
A. Laboratory
1. CBC: Elevation of WBC may indicate infection.
2. Comprehensive metabolic panel to assess kidney and liver function and to evaluate for abnormalities (e.g., elevated transaminase noted in cirrhosis; electrolyte imbalances noted in nephrotic syndrome)
3. N-terminal prohormone BNP: If greater than 1,500 pg/ml, suggests an effusion due to heart failure (transudate); may assess levels in pleural fluid
4. Pleural fluid analysis (see Table 29-1)
5. Blood cultures to identify potential cause of infection, as indicated
B. Radiology
1. Thoracic ultrasound: Level 1 recommendation
   a) Higher sensitivity: Can detect 5 ml of fluid
   b) Detection of cellular debris indicative of malignant effusion
   c) Solid pleural abnormalities associated with malignancy
2. Chest x-ray: To include posteroanterior, lateral, and decubitus films
   a) Decubitus film can detect 100 ml of free-flowing fluid.

TABLE 29-1	Pleural Fluid Analysis

Summary	Transudate	Exudate
Albumin[a]	> 1.2 g/dl	< 1.2 g/dl
Cholesterol	–	> 450 mg/L
LDH ratio[b]	< 0.6	> 0.6
LDH (serum)	–	> 67% ULN
LDH fluid	< 200 IU	> 200 IU
pH	7.4–7.55	7.3–7.45
Protein	–	> 30 mg/L
Protein ratio	< 0.5	> 0.5
Red blood cell count	< 10,000/mm^3	> 10,000/mm^3
Specific gravity	< 1.015	> 1.015
White blood cell count	< 100/mm^3	> 1,000/mm^3

[a] Albumin gradient difference is between serum and pleural fluid values.
[b] Ratio is measurement of pleural fluid and serum.
LDH—lactate dehydrogenase; ULN—upper limit of normal
Note. Based on information from Heffner, 2010; Saguil et al., 2014.

b) Lateral view can detect 50 ml of fluid with blunting of posterior costophrenic recess.
c) Posteroanterior view can detect 200 ml by obscuring the lateral recess.
d) Assess for evidence of elevated hemidiaphragm.
3. CT scan of chest with contrast
a) Ability to detect loculated fluid pockets
b) Irregular or thickened pleura suggestive of inflammation or malignancy
c) May identify primary malignancy
4. PET scan: Increased fludeoxyglucose uptake suggestive of malignant effusion
5. MRI of chest: Excellent visualization of soft tissues; usually reserved for more complex cases
C. Other
1. Bronchoscopy is used only if abnormality is noted on chest x-ray or CT scan.
2. Thoracentesis: Bedside procedure to remove fluid for diagnostic and therapeutic purposes
a) Maximum recommended drainage: Approximately 1.5 L
b) Fluid inspection
(1) Straw colored: Normal pleural fluid
(2) Blood tinged: Suggestive of malignancy, PE, trauma, benign asbestos pleural effusion, Dressler syndrome
(3) Pus: Empyema and anaerobic infection
(4) Milky: Chylothorax or cholesterol effusion
(5) Brown: Long-standing bloody effusion
(6) Black: *Aspergillus*

        (7) Debris: Malignancy, rheumatoid pleurisy
        (8) Food particles: Esophageal rupture
        (9) Odorous: Empyema
     c) Fluid analysis: Typically includes cell count, pH, protein, and LDH (see Table 29-1)
        (1) Comparison of fluid to serum: If at least one of the criteria is present, fluid is considered exudate (Light criteria).
        (2) Pleural fluid protein/serum protein ratio greater than 0.5
        (3) Pleural fluid LDH/serum LDH ratio greater than 0.6
        (4) Pleural fluid LDH greater than 67% ULN of the laboratory normal serum LDH
     d) Fluid analysis: No serum for comparison
        (1) Pleural fluid cholesterol greater than 45 mg/dl
        (2) Pleural fluid LDH 0.45 × ULN of laboratory normal serum LDH
        (3) Pleural fluid protein greater than 2.9 g/dl (29 g/L)
     e) Cytology: If no primary malignancy is identified, may require repeat cytology for results or genetic analysis
        (1) Gene expression tests may help to identify gene mutations (e.g., EGFR) and differentiate between cancers.
        (2) Consider flow cytometry (100 ml for diagnostic yield).
     f) Additional tests: Tumor markers (carcinoembryonic antigen, cancer antigen (CA)-125, CA 15-3), cholesterol, amylase, antinuclear antibody, rheumatoid factor, CRP for underlying etiology
  3. Pleural biopsy
     a) Pleuroscopy (medical thoracoscopy): CT or ultrasound guided; patient moderately sedated with spontaneous breathing, using one to two ports; limited visualization and small biopsy sample sizes
     b) Video-assisted thoracoscopy: Procedure performed in operating room with patient ventilated, using two to four ports; provides wide visualization of pleura and ability to obtain multiple biopsies
     c) Endobronchial ultrasound: Less-invasive procedure
  4. Pulse oximetry: Provides noninvasive means of measuring delivery of oxygen from the atmosphere to the pulmonary capillaries
  5. Spirometry: Measures FVC, FEV_1, FEV_1/FCV ratio; FVC reduced and ratio elevated in pleural effusion

V. Differential diagnosis (He & Oh, 2018; Jany & Welte, 2019)
  A. CHF (see Chapter 42)
  B. Pneumonia (see Chapter 30)
  C. PE (see Chapter 33)
  D. Malignancy
  E. Atelectasis
  F. Carcinomatosis
  G. Pleuritis
  H. Infection (see Chapter 37)
  I. Trauma
  J. SLE (see Chapter 110)
  K. RA (see Chapter 108)
  L. Empyema
  M. Esophageal rupture

    N. Chylothorax

    O. Hemothorax

VI. Treatment: Based on underlying cause, rate of accumulation, stability of patient, prognosis, and patient performance status (Aboudara & Maldonado, 2019; Bhatnagar & Maskell, 2015; Clive et al., 2016; Heffner, 2010; Jany & Welte, 2019; Shen et al., 2017).

    A. Uncomplicated or asymptomatic: Treatment is not needed if effusion is stable and patient asymptomatic. It may resolve spontaneously or with conservative therapy.

    B. Complicated: Effusion does not resolve without drainage. Drainage contributes the following.

       1. Provides symptom relief

       2. Promotes reexpansion of the lung

       3. Prevents long-term pleural fibrosis

    C. Thoracentesis: Ultrasound guidance is recommended.

       1. Drainage of fluid is performed for diagnostic testing.

       2. Thoracentesis is repeated for slowly reaccumulating effusions (longer than one month) or for patients who are not able to tolerate pleurodesis. If rapid accumulation, consider catheter placement for long-term management.

       3. Maximum drainage should not exceed 1.5 L to avoid reexpansion pulmonary edema.

       4. Thoracentesis is commonly performed for patients with shorter life expectancies (less than three months).

       5. An increased risk exists of vasovagal response, pneumothorax, empyema, and pleural fluid loculations.

    D. Chest tube thoracotomy: Short-term, large-bore tube is placed.

       1. It requires water seal suction for drainage and hospitalization.

       2. Pleurodesis is attempted after lung reexpansion.

    E. Fibrinolytic therapy for management of multiloculated effusions

       1. Fibrin sheets may develop, preventing adequate drainage of fluid or reexpansion of the lung.

       2. Fibrinolytics (e.g., streptokinase, urokinase, tissue plasminogen activator) are instilled via chest tube into the pleural space. The tube is clamped for two hours and then drained. It may require repeat instillations.

    F. Pleurodesis: This procedure promotes inflammation and fibrosis of pleural lining to prevent reaccumulation of fluid. It usually requires hospitalization for several days.

       1. Chemical pleurodesis: Installation of sclerosing agent (e.g., talc, doxycycline, bleomycin) via thoracoscopy, video-assisted thoracoscopy, or chest tube

       2. Mechanical pleurodesis: Pleural abrasion during thoracoscopy or thoracotomy to promote inflammation and fibrosis; mechanism to lyse adhesions and remediate loculations that may interfere with pleurodesis

       3. Recommended for patients with longer life expectancies (more than two to three months)

       4. Not recommended for patients with trapped lung or multiple loculated effusions

       5. Complications: Pneumothorax, cough, pain, empyema

    G. Tunneled indwelling pleural catheter: For long-term management of malignant pleural effusions

       1. Catheter allows for cost-effective outpatient placement for short life expectancies.

       2. Catheter is tunneled under skin and placed with CT or ultrasound guidance to ensure positioning. Attached to the catheter is a polyester cuff meant to be embedded under the skin during insertion to maintain stability of catheter and establish barrier between the pleural lining and the external skin to minimize infection.

3. This allows for intermittent outpatient drainage by patient and family using a disposable vacuum bottle system.
4. Drainage should not exceed 1,000 ml every eight hours.
5. Catheter may promote spontaneous pleurodesis. It can be removed after successive drainages with little output.
6. Risk of painful drainage procedure, blockages, and cellulitis is increased.
H. Pleuroperitoneal shunt: Procedure is reserved for patients with large recurrent effusions who have failed other therapies. It requires frequent shunt pumping and is associated with high risk of occlusion, with complications occurring in 15% of patients.
I. Pleurectomy: Radical total or subtotal pleurectomy (resection of the visceral and parietal pleura) and decortication (removal of fibrous pleural rind) are performed for failed pleurodesis. It is the primary therapeutic modality for malignant pleural mesothelioma effusions and should only be considered in patients with prolonged life expectancy.
J. Antitumor therapy: Rarely adequate
   1. Chemotherapy: Treatment of choice for chemosensitive tumors (e.g., breast cancer, small cell lung cancer, lymphoma)
   2. Radiation therapy: Directed at primary tumor, particularly if mediastinal disease involvement
K. Supportive care: Oral or IV opioids (see Appendix F) and oxygen may be appropriate in patients with end-stage disease.
L. Antibiotics: For associated infections

VII. Follow-up
A. Short term
   1. Monitor for complications of pleural effusion, such as PE, hemodynamic instability, reexpansion pulmonary edema, and infection.
   2. Monitor for complications of effusion treatment, such as pneumothorax following thoracentesis, pneumonitis after radiation therapy, or trapped lung.
B. Long term: Perform chest x-ray to monitor for recurrence of effusion or other complications.

VIII. Referrals
A. Thoracic surgeon: For biopsy, pleurectomy
B. Interventional pulmonologist: For thoracentesis, placement of tunneled catheter
C. Medical/radiation oncologist: For treatment of underlying malignancy, palliative care
D. Other (e.g., cardiologist, pulmonologist, rheumatologist): For management of other causes of effusion

The author would like to acknowledge Marianne Davies, RN, MSN, CNS-BC, ACNP-BC, AOCNP®, for her contribution to this chapter that remains unchanged from the previous edition of this book.

References

Aboudara, M., & Maldonado, F. (2019). Update in the management of pleural effusions. *Medical Clinics of North America, 103*(3), 475–485. https://doi.org/10.1016/j.mcna.2018.12.007
Bhatnagar, R., & Maskell, N. (2015). The modern diagnosis and management of pleural effusions. *British Medical Journal, 351,* h4520. https://doi.org/10.1136/bmj.h4520
Clive, A.O., Jones, H.E., Bhatnagar, R., Preston, N.J., & Maskell, N. (2016). Interventions for the management of malignant pleural effusions: A network meta-analysis. *Cochrane Database of Systematic Reviews, 2016*(5). https://doi.org/10.1002/14651858.CD010529.pub2

Ferreiro, L., Porcel, J.M., & Valdés, L. (2017). Diagnosis and management of pleural transudates. *Archivos Bronconeumologia, 53*(11), 629–636. https://doi.org/10.1016/j.arbres.2017.04.018

He, T., & Oh, S. (2018). Diagnostic approach to pleural effusions. *AME Medical Journal, 3,* 116. https://doi.org/10.21037/amj.2018.12.02

Heffner, J.E. (2010). Management of the patient with malignant pleural effusion. *Seminars in Respiratory and Critical Care Medicine, 31*(6), 723–733. https://doi.org/10.1055/s-0030-1269831

Jany, B., & Welte, T. (2019). Pleural effusion in adults—etiology, diagnosis, and treatment. *Deutsches Ärzteblatt International, 116*(21), 377–386. https://doi.org/10.3238/arztebl.2019.0377

Lim, J.H., & Ryu, J.-S. (2019). Current perspective on the diagnosis of malignant pleural effusion. *Journal of Thoracic Disease, 11*(Suppl. 9), S1234–S1236. https://doi.org/10.21037/jtd.2019.02.64

Rami-Porta, R., & Eberhardt, W.E.E. (2018). Clinical implications of the innovations in the primary tumour and metastasis of the 8th edition of the TNM classification for lung cancer. *Journal of Thoracic Disease, 10*(Suppl. 22), S2682–S2685. https://doi.org/10.21037/jtd.2018.03.100

Saguil, A., Wyrick, K., & Hallgren, J. (2014). Diagnostic approach to pleural effusion. *American Family Physician, 90*(2), 99–104. https://www.aafp.org/afp/2014/0715/p99.html

Shen, K.R., Bribriesco, A., Crabtree, T., Denlinger, C., Eby, J., Eiken, P., … Kozower, B. (2017). The American Association for Thoracic Surgery consensus guidelines for the management of empyema. *Journal of Thoracic Cardiovascular Surgery, 153*(6), e129–e146. https://doi.org/10.1016/j.jtcvs.2017.01.030

CHAPTER 30

Pneumonia

Victoria Sherry, DNP, CRNP, AOCNP®

I. Definition (Mandell & Niederman, 2019; Prina et al., 2015)
   A. Inflammatory response in the lung that involves the pulmonary parenchyma caused by an infectious agent
   B. Subclassifications
      1. Community-acquired pneumonia (CAP): Not acquired in a hospital or long-term care facility
      2. Ambulatory CAP: Occurs in young adults
      3. Nosocomial pneumonia: Acute infection of the pulmonary parenchyma
         a) Hospital-acquired pneumonia (HAP): Occurs at least 48 hours after admission; that which was not incubating at the time of admission
         b) Ventilator-associated pneumonia (VAP): Occurs more than 48 hours after intubation
      4. Aspiration pneumonia: Develops after the inhalation of oropharyngeal secretions and colonized organisms; not a separate entity but includes CAP and HAP

II. Physiology/Pathophysiology (Cillóniz et al., 2018)
   A. Normal
      1. The lower respiratory tract is made up of the larynx, trachea, bronchial tree, and lungs.
      2. The right lung has three lobes; the left has two.
      3. The lung tissue is very elastic, and the lungs are always stretched to fill the thoracic cavity on both sides of the mediastinum. This creates a negative pressure in the intrathoracic space.
      4. Neuromuscular coordination of thoracic and abdominal muscles results in an organized respiratory cycle with effective exchange of oxygen and carbon dioxide gases.
      5. Host immune defenses recognize potentially problematic pathogens and prevent infection of the lower respiratory tract. Those defenses are mechanical (ciliated epithelium and mucus production/coverage), humoral (antibody and complement mediated), and cellular (polymorphonucleocytes, macrophages, lymphocytes, and cytokines).
   B. Pathophysiology
      1. Pneumonia occurs when normal host defenses of the lung are unable to prevent pathogens from invading and persisting in the lower respiratory tract.
      2. Pathogens can access the pulmonary parenchyma by hematogenous, inhalation, or microaspiration.
         a) Hematogenous: Originates from a distant source and reaches the lungs via the bloodstream

    b) Inhalation: Via organisms that bypass normal respiratory defense mechanisms or via inhalation of aerobic gram-negative organisms that may colonize the upper respiratory tract or respiratory support equipment

    c) Microaspiration: Most common; aspiration of colonized upper respiratory tract secretions

III. Clinical features: CAP affects more than 5 million adults each year in the United States, 80% of whom receive outpatient treatment. Acute respiratory tract infection is the most common reason for antibiotic prescription in adults (Arumugam et al., 2018; Ho & Ip, 2019; Magill et al., 2018; Mandell & Niederman, 2019; Musher et al., 2017; Ramirez et al., 2017).

  A. Etiology and risk factors

    1. CAP

      a) Principal cause of morbidity and mortality worldwide

      b) *Streptococcus pneumoniae*: Most common organism

      c) No pathogen found in more than one-half of cases

      d) Risk factors: Older adult (age greater than 65 years), underlying comorbidities (e.g., COPD), cigarette smoking, alcoholism, opioid use, living circumstances (e.g., extended-care facility, prison, homeless shelter), toxins (e.g., gasoline, paint)

    2. HAP

      a) Most common nosocomial infection in the United States

      b) Major pathogen responsible: Aerobic gram-negative bacilli (e.g., *Escherichia coli, Klebsiella pneumonia, Pseudomonas aeruginosa*)

      c) Associated with high morbidity and mortality (33%–50%)

      d) Increases hospital stay by seven to nine days and can increase hospital costs by an average of $40,000 per patient

      e) Risk factors: Mechanical ventilation (most significant risk factor), aspiration, thoracic surgery, immunosuppression, chronic lung disease, older adult, depression, previous antibiotic use, opioids, trauma, central venous catheter, muscle relaxants

    3. VAP

      a) Most common pathogens: *Staphylococcus aureus, P. aeruginosa, Klebsiella* species, *Enterobacter* species, *Acinetobacter baumannii, E. coli*

      b) Four-fold increase of VAP in trauma patients

      c) Risk factors: Recent exposure to antibiotics or other medications, severity of underlying illness, prior surgery, reintubation, invasive respiratory devices and equipment

    4. Aspiration pneumonia

      a) Three classifications

        (1) Chemical pneumonitis: Aspiration of toxic substances (e.g., gastric acid)

        (2) Bacterial: Mainly anaerobic bacteria

        (3) Airway obstruction: Aspiration of nontoxic fluids (e.g., saline, barium, water)

      b) Risk factors predisposing patients

        (1) Disorders of the esophagus (e.g., GERD, esophageal stricture) or conditions associated with altered or reduced consciousness (e.g., alcoholism, drug overdose, seizures, stroke, head trauma, general anesthesia, intracranial mass lesion)

        (2) Esophageal conditions: Dysphagia, strictures, neoplasm, diverticula, GERD, tracheoesophageal fistula

        (3) Neurologic disorders: Multiple sclerosis, Parkinson disease, myasthenia gravis, pseudobulbar palsy, dementia

(4) Other associated conditions: Protracted vomiting, supine/prone position, deconditioning, critical illness

5. Epidemiologic variables
   a) Time of onset
      (1) HAP/VAP occurring within the first four days usually has better prognosis; bacteria are more likely to be sensitive to antibiotic.
      (2) Late onset of HAP/VAP (five days or later) has increased morbidity/mortality and is more likely to be caused by multidrug-resistant pathogens.
   b) Multidrug-resistant organisms
      (1) If the patient has been exposed to antibiotics prior to development of pneumonia or has been hospitalized within 90 days of development, organism is likely to be multidrug resistant.
      (2) Pathogens vary within and among institutions and across time.
      (3) Multidrug resistance varies by patient population, exposure to antibiotics, and type of ICU admission (e.g., trauma, sepsis, surgical).
      (4) Risk factors
         (a) Antimicrobial therapy within 90 days before diagnosis
         (b) Current hospitalization for five days or longer
         (c) Acute respiratory distress syndrome
         (d) Septic shock
   c) Older adult patients
      (1) Patients in long-term care facilities: Different exposure risks
      (2) Pathogens similar to late-onset HAP/VAP
      (3) Decreased lung elasticity
      (4) Decreased immune function
   d) Immunocompromised patients
      (1) Increased risk of pneumonia exists from *Legionella pneumophila* and *P. aeruginosa* from a tainted water or air supply.
      (2) Increased risk exists of viral pneumonia (e.g., CMV), yeast infections (e.g., *Cryptococcus*), unusual infections (e.g., *Nocardia*, nontuberculous *Mycobacteria*), fungal infections (e.g., *Candida, Aspergillus fumigatus*), and/or encapsulated bacteria (e.g., *S. pneumoniae*).
      (3) Multiple infections (e.g., *Pneumocystis jirovecii* pneumonia, CMV) and sequential infections (viral prior to bacterial or fungal) are common.
      (4) An increased risk for HAP exists with intubation, mechanical ventilation, lung injury (e.g., COPD), and aspiration.
      (5) Septic emboli in the lungs in conjunction with bacteremia or fungemia is often caused by central venous devices.
      (6) Reactivation of dormant infections (e.g., CMV, strongyloidiasis, cryptococcosis, toxoplasmosis, mycobacterial infection) may occur.

B. History
   1. History of cancer and cancer treatment
   2. Current medications: Prescribed, over the counter, herbal medications
   3. History of presenting symptoms: Precipitating factors, onset, location, duration, characteristics, aggravating and alleviating factors, severity
   4. Changes in ADLs
   5. Past medical history: COPD, asthma, diabetes, CHF, HIV, renal/cardiac compromise or failure, dementia, aspiration history, cystic fibrosis, bronchiectasis, immunosuppression, neutropenia

6. Past surgical history: Chest wall, lung, cardiac/pericardial, surgical sites proximate to diaphragm, phrenic nerve, or abdomen
7. Social history: Nutrition; alcohol, tobacco, or illicit drug use; vaping; exposure to bird droppings, rabbits, rodents, construction sites, or farms; incarceration

C. Signs and symptoms: Classical symptoms of CAP include sudden chills, fever, pleuritic pain, and productive cough.
   1. Productive or nonproductive cough
   2. Dyspnea
   3. Pleuritic chest pain
   4. Malaise
   5. Fever, chills
   6. Cyanosis
   7. Wheezing
   8. Mental status change
   9. GI symptoms: Nausea, vomiting, diarrhea
   10. Rhinorrhea with viral infection
   11. Hemoptysis
   12. Anorexia
   13. Fatigue
   14. Diaphoresis

D. Physical examination
   1. General
      a) Vital signs: Tachypnea, tachycardia, hypotension, fever (occurs in 80% of people and can be absent in older adults)
      b) Slight weight loss
      c) Ill appearance
   2. Pulmonary
      a) Increased and shallow respiratory rate/depth
      b) Wheeze, rales, and rhonchi on auscultation of lungs
      c) Dullness to percussion or increased tactile fremitus and egophony to the involved lobes on lung palpation
   3. Neurologic: Altered mental status with hypoxia or sepsis

IV. Diagnostic testing (Kaysin & Viera, 2016; Metlay et al., 2019; Ramirez et al., 2017)
   A. Laboratory
      1. CBC with differential to evaluate for left shift
      2. BUN and creatinine to assess fluid status
      3. ABGs to check for respiratory alkalosis
      4. May see a rise in inflammatory markers: ESR, CRP, procalcitonin
      5. Testing for unusual infectious agents, as indicated: *Legionella* species, influenza virus, coronaviruses (e.g., MERS-CoV, COVID-19)
      6. Blood cultures
         a) Two sets: Obtain before antibiotic treatment is initiated whenever possible.
         b) May not grow responsible organism (low sensitivity)
      7. Influenza season is November through March; send nasopharyngeal aspirate for antigen test and culture.
      8. Rapid antigen detection for virus
   B. Radiology
      1. Chest x-ray: Gold standard
         a) Perform posterior–anterior and lateral if possible; anterior–posterior otherwise.

    b) Assess for lobes involved and adenopathy (hilar and mediastinal).
  2. Lung ultrasound: Excellent tool if unable to obtain chest x-ray or if chest x-ray is poor quality
  3. CT scan of chest: Not recommended for CAP, as data are inadequate, cost is high, and research does not support improved patient outcomes
 C. Other
  1. Microbiologic examination of purulent sputum
   a) Obtain a gram stain and culture of sputum production.
   b) Tracheal colonization is common but unimportant unless clinical signs of infection are present.
  2. Fiber-optic bronchoscopy to evaluate lungs and obtain cultures, as indicated
  3. Thoracentesis (diagnostic) to evaluate for empyema or parapneumonic effusion (a pleural effusion that arises as a result of pneumonia)
  4. *Legionella* and pneumococcus urinary antigen tests for ICU patients
  5. Nasopharyngeal polymerase chain reaction to detect *Chlamydia pneumoniae* and *Mycoplasma pneumoniae*, as well as 14 respiratory tract viruses
  6. Pulse oximetry to assess need for oxygen support

V. Differential diagnosis
 A. COPD/COPD exacerbation (see Chapter 28)
 B. Asthma (see Chapter 28)
 C. Pulmonary edema (see Chapter 32)
 D. PH (see Chapter 52)
 E. PE (see Chapter 33)
 F. Pleural effusion (see Chapter 29)
 G. Radiation/chemotherapy-induced pulmonary disease
 H. Lung contusion
 I. Pulmonary hemorrhage
 J. Lung abscess
 K. CHF (see Chapter 42)
 L. Acute respiratory distress syndrome
 M. TB (see Chapter 36)
 N. Altitude illness: Pulmonary syndrome
 O. Septic shock (see Chapter 160)
 P. Lung carcinoma
 Q. Adult epiglottitis

VI. Treatment (CDC, 2020; Ho & Ip, 2019; Kalil et al., 2016; Kaysin & Viera, 2016; Metlay et al., 2019; Tansarli & Mylonakis, 2018; see Table 30-1 and Appendix C)
 A. CAP/aspiration pneumonia
  1. Initiate antibiotic as soon as diagnosis is confirmed.
  2. IV administration is favored for hospitalized patients.
  3. Clinical improvement should be noticeable in 24–48 hours.
  4. Note that radiographic improvement is delayed compared to clinical response.
  5. A switch to oral therapy may occur once a clinical response is observed. Treat for a minimum of five days; patient must be afebrile for 48–72 hours before discontinuing an antibiotic.
  6. Longer antibiotic duration may be required for some patient conditions.
   a) Infection outside of the lungs (meningitis)
   b) *P. aeruginosa, Burkholderia pseudomallei,* fungal pneumonia

| TABLE 30-1 | Antibiotic Recommendations for Treatment of Bacterial Pneumonia |

Likely Pathogen	Recommended Antibiotic(s)
Community-acquired pneumonia • *Chlamydophila pneumoniae* • Gram-negative rods • *Haemophilus influenzae* • Influenza • *Legionella pneumophila* • *Mycoplasma pneumoniae* • *Staphylococcus aureus* • *Streptococcus pneumoniae*	Outpatient, no antibiotic exposure within 90 days • Macrolide (e.g., erythromycin, azithromycin, clarithromycin) or doxycycline Outpatient, with antibiotic exposure within 90 days or with significant comorbidities (prescribe antibiotic from different class than prior exposure) • Respiratory fluoroquinolone monotherapy (e.g., moxifloxacin, levofloxacin, gemifloxacin), or • Beta-lactam (e.g., high-dose amoxicillin or amoxicillin/clavulanate; alternative agents: ceftriaxone, cefpodoxime, or cefuroxime) plus a macrolide (e.g., azithromycin, clarithromycin, erythromycin) Nursing home residents, outpatient treatment • Respiratory fluoroquinolone, or • Combination of amoxicillin/clavulanate and an advanced macrolide Inpatient therapy (non–intensive care unit) • Respiratory fluoroquinolone monotherapy, or • Combination advanced macrolide and antipneumococcal beta-lactam (e.g., cefotaxime, ceftriaxone, ampicillin/sulbactam, ertapenem) plus macrolide (e.g., azithromycin, clarithromycin, erythromycin) Intensive care unit therapy • An antipneumococcal beta-lactam (e.g., cefotaxime, ceftriaxone, ampicillin/sulbactam) plus azithromycin, or • An antipneumococcal beta-lactam (e.g., cefotaxime, ceftriaxone, ampicillin/sulbactam) plus a respiratory fluoroquinolone (e.g., moxifloxacin, gemifloxacin, levofloxacin), or • For penicillin-allergic patients, a respiratory fluoroquinolone (e.g., moxifloxacin, gemifloxacin, levofloxacin) plus aztreonam If *Pseudomonas aeruginosa* is a possible diagnosis • An antipneumococcal, antipseudomonal beta-lactam (e.g., piperacillin/tazobactam, cefepime, imipenem, meropenem) plus either ciprofloxacin or levofloxacin, or • The above beta-lactam plus an aminoglycoside plus azithromycin, or • The above beta-lactam plus an aminoglycoside plus a respiratory fluoroquinolone (e.g., moxifloxacin, gemifloxacin, levofloxacin [750 mg]); for penicillin-allergic patients, substitute aztreonam for above beta-lactam. If community-acquired methicillin-sensitive *S. aureus* (MRSA) is a possible diagnosis • Vancomycin or linezolid Community-acquired pneumonia with aspiration • Ampicillin/sulbactam (1.5–3 g IV every 6 hours for those with normal renal function) • For patients who can tolerate oral therapy, amoxicillin/clavulanate (immediate release 875 mg PO two times a day or extended release 2 g PO two times a day) Other regimens • Metronidazole (500 mg PO or IV three times a day) plus either amoxicillin (500 mg PO three times a day) or penicillin G (1–2 million units IV every 4–6 hours)

(Continued on next page)

TABLE 30-1	Antibiotic Recommendations for Treatment of Bacterial Pneumonia *(Continued)*
Likely Pathogen	**Recommended Antibiotic(s)**

Hospital-acquired pneumonia/ventilator-associated pneumonia, multidrug resistant not suspected, early onset
• Antibiotic-sensitive enteric gram-negative bacilli
  – *Enterobacter* species
  – *Escherichia coli*
  – *Klebsiella pneumoniae*
  – *Proteus* species
  – *Serratia marcescens*
• *H. influenzae*
• MRSA
• *S. pneumoniae*
	• Penicillin: Piperacillin/tazobactam 4.5 g IV every 6 hours, or
	• Cephalosporin: Cefepime 2 g IV every 8 hours, or
	• Quinolone: Levofloxacin 750 mg IV every 24 hours
	
	If no risk factors and in an intensive care unit in which ≤ 10% of gram-negative isolates are resistant to an agent being considered for monotherapy but > 20% of *S. aureus* isolates in the unit are methicillin resistant or the local MRSA prevalence is unknown, the patient should receive one agent with activity against *P. aeruginosa* and one agent with activity against MRSA.
	• Piperacillin/tazobactam 4.5 g IV every 6 hours, or
	• Cefepime 2 g IV every 8 hours, or
	• Ceftazidime 2 g IV every 8 hours, or
	• Levofloxacin 750 mg IV daily (when the patient is clinically improved and able to take oral medications, levofloxacin may be administered orally at the same dose as that used for IV administration), or
	• Ciprofloxacin 400 mg IV every 8 hours (when the patient is clinically improved and able to take oral medication, ciprofloxacin may be administered orally at 750 mg two times a day), or
	• Aztreonam 2 g IV every 8 hours
	
	Plus one of the following
	• Vancomycin 1.5 mg/kg IV (max 2 g per dose) every 8–12 hours with goal to target 15–20 mcg/ml trough level, or
	• Linezolid 600 mg IV every 12 hours, or
	• Telavancin 10 mg/kg IV every 24 hours

Hospital-acquired pneumonia/ventilator-associated pneumonia, multidrug resistant suspected, late onset • As above, plus multidrug resistant pathogens • *P. aeruginosa* • *K. pneumoniae* (extended-spectrum beta-lactamase)[a] • *Acinetobacter* • MRSA • *L. pneumophila*[b]	• Piperacillin/tazobactam 4.5 g IV every 6 hours, or • Cefepime 2 g IV every 8 hours, or • Ceftazidime 2 g IV every 8 hours, or • Imipenem 500 mg IV every 6 hours, or • Meropenem 1 g IV every 8 hours, or • Aztreonam 2 g IV every 8 hours Plus one of the following • Amikacin 15–20 mg/kg IV daily, or • Gentamicin 5–7 mg/kg IV daily, or • Tobramycin 5–7 mg/kg IV daily Plus one of the following • Vancomycin 1.5 mg/kg IV (max 2 g per dose) every 8–12 hours with goal to target 15–20 mcg/ml trough level, or • Linezolid 600 mg IV every 12 hours, or • Telavancin 10 mg/kg IV every 24 hours

[a] If extended-spectrum beta-lactamase strain is suspected, carbapenems are recommended.

[b] If *Legionella pneumophila* is suspected, the combination regimen should include a macrolide, or a fluoroquinolone should be used instead of aminoglycoside.

Note. Based on information from Kalil et al., 2016; Kaysin & Viera, 2016.

       c) Necrotizing pneumonia, lung abscess, or empyema

       d) Parapneumonic effusions

B. Empiric antibiotic initiation in patients suspected of having HAP and VAP with or without a known multidrug resistance

    1. When suspected clinically, obtain diagnostic specimens as soon as possible and initiate antimicrobial therapy.

    2. A delay in initiation of antibiotics is associated with increased mortality.

    3. Antibiotic selection is determined by risk factors for specific pathogens, unit/hospital culture data, and pattern of resistant organisms; if recent antibiotic use (within two weeks), initiate coverage from a different class of antibiotics.

    4. Treat for a minimum of seven days.

    5. Monitor procalcitonin levels sequentially to determine when to discontinue antibiotics. A low or declining procalcitonin level (e.g., less than 0.25 ng/ml, greater than or equal to 80% decrease from peak) indicates it is safe to discontinue antibiotic therapy.

C. Aspiration

    1. Chemical

       a) Maintenance of the airway

       b) Clearance of secretions with suction

       c) Oxygen supplementation and ventilation as required (early use of positive end-expiratory pressure)

       d) Support with IV fluids

       e) Antibiotics usually not required

    2. Bacterial (see Table 30-1)

    3. Airway obstruction

       a) Remove obstruction through Heimlich maneuver, tracheal suction, and/or bronchoscopy.

       b) Place in semi-upright or upright position.

       c) Evaluate for development of negative pressure pulmonary edema.

D. Viral

    1. Supportive care

    2. Empiric antiviral therapy for severe symptoms refractory to initial antimicrobial agents, for immunocompromised patients, or if influenza is suspected

       a) Influenza: Oseltamivir 75 mg PO two times a day; zanamivir 10 mg (two inhalations) two times a day; peramivir 600 mg IV as a single dose; baloxavir 40 mg PO as a single dose for patients 40–80 kg in weight and 80 mg as a single dose for patients greater than 80 kg in weight

       b) HSV: Acyclovir 800 mg PO every 12 hours; valacyclovir 500 mg PO every 12 hours

       c) VZV: Acyclovir 200 or 400 mg PO five times a day; famciclovir 750 mg PO two times a day for one day or 1,500 mg PO as a single dose; valacyclovir 2 g PO two times a day for one day

       d) Measles: For patients older than one year, vitamin A 200,000 IU once a day; ribavirin 15–20 mg/kg PO daily in two doses

       e) CMV: Ganciclovir 5 mg/kg IV every 12 hours, foscarnet 90 mg/kg IV every 12 hours for two weeks; valganciclovir 900 mg PO every 12 hours; cidofovir 5 mg/kg IV every two weeks

       f) Hantavirus: Supportive care and ribavirin

E. Fungus

    1. Fungi are rare but may occur in organ transplant recipients and patients who are immunocompromised or neutropenic.

2. *Aspergillus* species can be treated with agents such as triazoles (e.g., voriconazole, posaconazole, itraconazole, fluconazole), amphotericin B (e.g., liposomal amphotericin B, amphotericin B lipid complex), and echinocandins (e.g., caspofungin, micafungin, anidulafungin).

3. *Candida albicans* and other species in endotracheal aspirates are common but usually represent colonization and rarely require treatment in immunocompetent patients.

4. Yeast in a blood culture should not be considered a contaminant; empiric therapy is required until specification of source.

F. Neutropenic/Immunocompromised patients (see Chapter 127)

1. Treat per guidelines as described previously and in Table 30-1, with recognition that empiric dosing of antifungal medications may be required for patients not showing signs of improvement as expected.

2. Tailor antibiotics to unit-based, institution-based, and population-based susceptibility profiles.

VII. Follow-up

A. If resolution of symptoms, a follow-up chest x-ray is not needed. Patients older than 50 years need a follow-up chest x-ray 7–12 weeks following treatment.

B. Patients should follow up with primary care provider or pulmonologist one week after completion of treatment.

VIII. Referrals

A. Pulmonary rehabilitation: To increase pulmonary endurance

B. Pulmonologist: For residual effects related to pneumonia (e.g., asthma, bronchitis, decreased pulmonary endurance)

References

Arumugam, S.K., Mudali, I., Strandvik, G., El-Menyar, A., Al-Hassani, A., & Al-Thani, H. (2018). Risk factors for ventilator-associated pneumonia in trauma patients: A descriptive analysis. *World Journal of Emergency Medicine, 9*(3), 203–210. https://doi.org/10.5847/wjem.j.1920–8642.2018.03.007

Centers for Disease Control and Prevention. (2020, August 31). Influenza antiviral medications: Summary for clinicians. https://www.cdc.gov/flu/professionals/antivirals/summary-clinicians.htm

Cillóniz, C., Cardozo, C., & García-Vidal, C. (2018). Epidemiology, pathophysiology, and microbiology of community-acquired pneumonia. *Annals of Research Hospitals, 2*(1), 1. https://doi.org/10.21037/arh.2017.12.03

Ho, J., & Ip, M. (2019). Antibiotic-resistant community-acquired bacterial pneumonia. *Infectious Disease Clinics of North America, 33*(4), 1087–1103. https://doi.org/10.1016/j.idc.2019.07.002

Kalil, A.C., Metersky, M.L., Klompas, M., Muscedere, J., Sweeney, D.A., Palmer, L., ... Brozek, J.L. (2016). Management of adults with hospital-acquired and ventilator-associated pneumonia: 2016 clinical practice guidelines by the Infectious Diseases Society of America and the American Thoracic Society. *Clinical Infectious Diseases, 63*(5), e61–e111. https://doi.org/10.1093/cid/ciw353

Kaysin, A., & Viera, A.J. (2016). Community-acquired pneumonia in adults: Diagnosis and management. *American Family Physician, 94*(9), 698–706. https://www.aafp.org/afp/2016/1101/p698.html

Magill, S.S., O'Leary, E., Janelle, S.J., Thompson, D.L., Dumyati, G., Nadle, J., ... Edwards, J.R. (2018). Changes in prevalence of health care–associated infections in U.S. hospitals. *New England Journal of Medicine, 379*(18), 1732–1744. https://doi.org/10.1056/NEJMoa1801550

Mandell, L.A., & Niederman, M.S. (2019). Aspiration pneumonia. *New England Journal of Medicine, 380*(7), 651–663. https://doi.org/10.1056/NEJMra1714562

Metlay, J.P., Waterer, G.W., Long, A.C., Anzueto, A., Brozek, J., Crothers, K., ... Whitney, C.G. (2019). Diagnosis and treatment of adults with community-acquired pneumonia. An official clinical practice guideline of the American Thoracic Society and Infectious Diseases Society of America. *American Journal of Respiratory and Critical Care Medicine, 200*(7), e45–e67. https://doi.org/10.1164/rccm.201908-1581st

Musher, D.M., Abers, M.S., & Bartlett, J.G. (2017). Evolving understanding of the causes of pneumonia in adults, with special attention to the role of pneumococcus. *Clinical Infectious Diseases, 65*(10), 1736–1744. https://doi.org/10.1093/cid/cix549

Prina, E., Ranzani, O.T., & Torres, A. (2015) Community-acquired pneumonia. *Lancet, 386*(9998), 1097–1108. https://doi.org/10.1016/S0140-6736(15)60733-4

Ramirez, J.A., Wiemken, T.L., Peyrani, P., Arnold, F.W., Kelley, R., Mattingly, W.A., … Carrico, R.M. (2017). Adults hospitalized with pneumonia in the United States: Incidence, epidemiology, and mortality. *Clinical Infectious Diseases, 65*(11), 1806–1812. https://doi.org/10.1093/cid/cix647

Tansarli, G.S., & Mylonakis, E. (2018). Systematic review and meta-analysis of the efficacy of short-course antibiotic treatments for community-acquired pneumonia in adults. *Antimicrobial Agents and Chemotherapy, 62*(9), e00635–18. https://doi.org/10.1128/AAC.00635-18

CHAPTER 31

Pneumothorax

Victoria Sherry, DNP, CRNP, AOCNP®

I. Definition: Gas or air in the pleural space (Bobbio et al., 2015; Helgeson et al., 2019; Roberts et al., 2015; Tsai et al., 2017)
   A. Traumatic pneumothorax: Results from direct or indirect injury, such as blunt trauma or penetrating trauma
   B. Iatrogenic pneumothorax: Secondary to diagnostic or therapeutic medical intervention
   C. Spontaneous (idiopathic): Occurs in absence of thoracic trauma
      1. Primary spontaneous pneumothorax: Affects patients without pulmonary diseases; occurs without an obvious preceding event
      2. Secondary spontaneous pneumothorax: Occurs in patients with pulmonary disease, usually COPD
   D. Tension pneumothorax: Life-threatening condition that occurs when air pressure in the pleural space becomes greater than atmospheric pressure; can develop from traumatic, iatrogenic, or spontaneous pneumothorax

II. Physiology/Pathophysiology (Plojoux et al., 2019)
   A. Normal
      1. Visceral pleura covers the entire surface of each lung.
      2. The parietal pleura separates the lungs from the mediastinum, lines the inside wall of the thorax, and covers the surface of the diaphragm.
      3. The pericardium lies on top of the epicardium of the heart.
      4. Many of these tissues are pressed flat against each other and are separated only by a thin layer of fluid.
      5. The fluid-filled region between the visceral and parietal pleura is the pleural space (normally 10–20 ml of fluid).
   B. Pathophysiology: Collapse of lung caused by disruption of the visceral pleura with subsequent air entering the pleural space
      1. The lung falls away from the inner chest wall and collapses. The lung cannot fully expand because of the compression.
         a) Open pneumothorax: Air moves freely into and out of the pleural space.
         b) Closed pneumothorax: Air is trapped in the pleural space.
      2. Buildup of air pressure causes the lung, heart, and other structures to be shifted away from the pneumothorax.
      3. Blood flow into the thorax usually is impaired, cardiac output falls, and cardiopulmonary failure can occur from large pneumothorax.
      4. Ventilation of the collapsed lung becomes markedly reduced while the ventilation of the opposite lung is increased.

5. When the area between the pleural space and the atmosphere is sealed, the trapped air eventually reabsorbs, resulting in gradual reestablishment of subatmospheric pressure and reexpansion of the lung.

III. Clinical features: Incidence of pneumothorax is 20% after thoracentesis and pleural biopsy, 3% after transbronchial biopsy, and 50% after transthoracic needle lung biopsy. Primary spontaneous pneumothorax commonly occurs between ages 10 and 30 years, especially in patients with known lung disorders. Secondary spontaneous pneumothorax occurs more often between ages 60–64 years. Smoking increases the risk of pneumothorax by more than 20-fold in men and 10-fold in women. Male to female ratio is 6:1 (Onuki et al., 2017; Stodghill et al., 2019).

A. Etiology
   1. Traumatic, iatrogenic, or tension pneumothorax
      a) Blunt trauma: Car accident, physical assault
      b) Penetrating trauma: Gunshot wound, knife
      c) Barotrauma
      d) Lung biopsy
      e) Acupuncture of chest
      f) Pneumoperitoneum
      g) Bochdalek hernia with trauma
      h) Displaced thoracic spine fractures
   2. Primary spontaneous pneumonia
      a) Subpleural bullae that rupture into the pleural space
      b) Smoking: Cigarette (tobacco), cannabis
      c) Genetic predisposition
   3. Secondary spontaneous pneumonia
      a) COPD
      b) Cystic fibrosis
      c) Lung malignancy: Primary, metastatic
      d) Necrotizing lung infections
         (1) HIV-related *Pneumocystis* pneumonia
         (2) Bacterial pneumonia
         (3) Fungal pneumonia
         (4) Cystic lung disorders: Lymphangioleiomyomatosis, diffuse Langerhans cell histiocytosis, lymphocytic interstitial pneumonitis (e.g., Sjögren syndrome), Birt-Hogg-Dubé syndrome
         (5) Catamenial: Associated with menses and endometriosis
         (6) Abnormalities of pleural membrane
            (a) Marfan syndrome
            (b) Homocystinuria
            (c) Ehlers-Danlos syndrome
         (7) Other
            (a) Ankylosing spondylitis
            (b) Asthma
            (c) Interstitial lung disease: Idiopathic pulmonary fibrosis
            (d) Granulomatous lung diseases: Sarcoidosis
B. History
   1. History of cancer and cancer treatment
   2. Current medications: Prescribed, over the counter
   3. History of presenting symptoms: Precipitating factors, onset, location, duration, severity

      4. Changes in ADLs

      5. Past medical history: COPD, trauma, lung disease, acupuncture procedure

      6. Social history: Tobacco use, vaping

  C. Signs and symptoms: Symptoms may present slowly and increase gradually or may develop acutely and abruptly.

      1. Pleuritic chest pain: More severe with inspiration and localized at the site of the pneumothorax

      2. Shortness of breath/dyspnea

      3. Anxiety

      4. Tension pneumothorax: Diaphoresis, cyanosis, weakness, hypotension, cardiovascular collapse

  D. Physical examination: Abnormal findings may not be present.

      1. Vital signs: Rapid pulse and hypotension

      2. Neck

        a) Deviation of trachea (deviates away from the affected lung) from large pneumothorax

        b) Subcutaneous crepitus (air lying under the skin from the pneumothorax) with neck and shoulder palpitation

        c) Neck vein distention

      3. Pulmonary

        a) Decreased or absent breath sounds over the collapsed lung

        b) Resonant percussion over affected hemithorax

        c) Asymmetric chest wall movement

        d) Diminished or absent tactile fremitus

IV. Diagnostic tests (Stodghill et al., 2019)

  A. Laboratory

      1. ABG analysis to evaluate oxygen saturation (e.g., hypoxia, occasional hypocapnia with hyperventilation)

      2. CBC: May show leukocytosis without left shift

      3. Creatine kinase-MB and troponin: Elevations indicate MI as the cause of chest pain.

  B. Radiology

      1. Pleural ultrasonography to evaluate pleural cavity for pneumothorax at bedside for unstable patients

      2. Chest x-ray to reveal air in the pleural cavity

        a) Visceral pleural line will be identified.

        b) Entire lung will appear to have detached from the chest wall in large pneumothorax.

        c) Absence of vascular markings and increased density of the lung aid in pneumothorax detection.

        d) Pleural cavity air is reported as a percentage of lung collapse on the chest x-ray.

      3. CT scan of chest if chest x-ray does not visualize pneumothorax: Usually reserved for patients with an uncertain diagnosis

  C. Other

      1. Pulse oximetry to evaluate oxygen saturation for hypoxia

      2. ECG: May show axis deviations, nonspecific ST segment changes, and T-wave inversion

V. Differential diagnosis (Unlu et al., 2016)

  A. Pleural effusion (see Chapter 29)

B. Pulmonary fibrosis
C. Pleural adhesions
D. Treatment induced
1. Thoracentesis
2. Pleural biopsy
3. Percutaneous or transbronchial lung biopsy
4. Vascular access device
5. Chest or neck surgery
6. Post-tracheostomy
E. Emphysema with pleural bullae (see Chapter 28)
F. COPD exacerbation (see Chapter 28)
G. Pericarditis (see Chapter 50)
H. Trauma: Rib fracture
I. Viral pleuritis
J. Pneumonia (see Chapter 30)
K. Costochondritis
L. PE (see Chapter 33)
M. Empyema
N. TB (see Chapter 36)

VI. Treatment (Hallifax & Janssen, 2019; Plojoux et al., 2019; Stodghill et al., 2019)
   A. Spontaneous pneumothorax can be managed with supplemental oxygen, observation, and/or aspiration.
      1. Oxygen: Use high-flow oxygen of 10 L/min; use caution in patients diagnosed with COPD to avoid hypercarbia.
      2. Observation: Stable asymptomatic patients with a small pneumothorax (less than 2–3 cm between the lung and chest wall on a chest x-ray) should be observed for three to six hours. If no progression of the pneumothorax by chest x-ray, the patient can be sent home with careful instructions.
      3. Aspiration: A small catheter is inserted into the pleural space to remove the air and catheter is removed immediately.
   B. Treatment for large pneumothorax (greater than 3 cm rim of air on chest x-ray) includes placement of a small-bore tube to reexpand lung.
      1. Indications for tube insertion: Chest pain, shortness of breath, decreased oxygenation
         a) Pneumothorax greater than 25% of volume of hemithorax
         b) Tension pneumothorax
      2. Vast majority resolve within 24–72 hours following tube insertion. Failure to resolve is because of catheter malposition or large air leak.
      3. Placement of chest tube can be performed under fluoroscopic or CT guidance.
      4. Chest tube placement with water seal device may be required if lung fails to expand or for persistent air leak.
         a) Air leaks (alveolar–pleural fistulas) are a common complication after elective pulmonary resection and video-assisted thoracoscopy procedure.
         b) Water seal is used with chest tube to manage air leaks.
      5. If patients are unstable with a large pneumothorax, insertion of a chest tube attached to a water seal device with or without suction is necessary to reexpand the lung.
      6. Air leaks can be treated by placing a Heimlich valve in the chest cavity, which vents the pleural cavity. It is often used for patients who are discharged home.
   C. Chemical sclerosing with doxycycline or talc may be used for persistent or recurrent pneumothorax. Up to 50% of patients suffer from recurrence.

    D. Surgical options include treatment with a parietal pleurectomy, bullectomy, or parietal pleural abrasion.

    E. Encourage smoking cessation, which may help to prevent recurrent pneumothorax.

VII. Follow-up (Chaturvedi et al., 2016)

    A. Chest x-ray within 12 hours to two days for spontaneous pneumothorax treated with observation to document resolution

    B. Chest x-ray to monitor reexpansion of lung following removal of air PRN or when patient is symptomatic

VIII. Referrals

    A. Surgeon: For placement of chest tube or catheter or pleurodesis

    B. Pulmonologist: For management of pulmonary disease

    C. Smoking cessation counselor

References

Bobbio, A., Dechartres, A., Bouam, S., Damotte, D., Rabbat, A., Régnard, J.-F., ... Alifano, M. (2015). Epidemiology of spontaneous pneumothorax: Gender-related differences. *Thorax, 70*(7), 653–658. https://doi.org/10.1136/thoraxjnl-2014-206577

Chaturvedi, A., Lee, S., Klionsky, N., & Chaturvedi, A. (2016). Demystifying the persistent pneumothorax: Role of imaging. *Insights Into Imaging, 7*(3), 411–429. https://doi.org/10.1007/s13244-016-0486-5

Hallifax, R., & Janssen, J.P. (2019). Pneumothorax—Time for new guidelines? *Seminars in Respiratory and Critical Care Medicine, 40*(3), 314–322. https://doi.org/10.1055/s-0039-1693499

Helgeson, S.A., Fritz, A.V., Tatari, M.M., Daniels, C.E., & Diaz-Gomez, J.L. (2019). Reducing iatrogenic pneumothoraces: Using real-time ultrasound guidance for pleural procedures. *Critical Care Medicine, 47*(7), 903–909. https://doi.org/10.1097/CCM.0000000000003761

Onuki, T., Ueda, S., Yamaoka, M., Sekiya, Y., Yamada, H., Kawakami, N., ... Matsumiya, N. (2017). Primary and secondary spontaneous pneumothorax: Prevalence, clinical features, and in-hospital mortality. *Canadian Respiratory Journal, 2017,* 6014967. https://doi.org/10.1155/2017/6014967

Plojoux, J., Froudarakis, M., Janssens, J.-P., Soccal, P.M., & Tschopp, J.-M. (2019). New insights and improved strategies for the management of primary spontaneous pneumothorax. *Clinical Respiratory Journal, 13*(4), 195–201. https://doi.org/10.1111/crj.12990

Roberts, D.J., Leigh-Smith, S., Faris, P.D., Blackmore, C., Ball, C.G., Robertson, H.L., ... Stelfox, H.T. (2015) Clinical presentation of patients with tension pneumothorax: A systematic review. *Annals of Surgery, 261*(6), 1068–1078. https://doi.org/10.1097/SLA.0000000000001073

Stodghill, J.D., Collins, D.T., Mahajan, A.K., & Khandhar, S.J. (2019). Primary spontaneous pneumothorax: A pathway to practice. *AME Medical Journal, 4,* 8. https://doi.org/10.21037/amj.2018.11.05

Tsai, T.-M., Lin, M.-W., Li, Y.-J., Chang, C.-H., Liao, H.-C., Liu, C.-Y., ... Chen, J.-S. (2017). The size of spontaneous pneumothorax is a predictor of unsuccessful catheter drainage. *Scientific Reports, 7,* 181. https://doi.org/10.1038/s41598-017-00284-8

Unlu, E.N., Annakkaya, A.N., Balbay, E.G., Aydın, L.Y., Safcı, S., Boran, M.,& Guclu, D. (2016). An unusual cause of recurrent spontaneous pneumothorax: The Mounier-Kuhn syndrome. *American Journal of Emergency Medicine, 34*(1), 122. E1–122.E2. https://doi.org/10.1016/j.ajem.2015.05.050

CHAPTER 32

Pulmonary Edema

Victoria Sherry, DNP, CRNP, AOCNP®

I. Definition: Excessive accumulation of fluid in the extravascular space of the lungs (Chioncel et al., 2016)

II. Physiology/Pathophysiology (Casey et al., 2019; Dobbe et al., 2019; Finsterer, 2019; Powell et al., 2016; Simko & Culleiton, 2019)
   A. Normal
      1. Lungs are highly elastic, spongy tissue consisting of three right lobes and two left lobes.
      2. According to Starling's law, the flow of fluid from the pulmonary capillaries to the lungs equals the removal of fluid by pulmonary lymphatics.
      3. To prevent pulmonary edema, an active process of sodium (Na^+) transport by an osmotic process removes fluid from the alveoli as a protective mechanism.
   B. Pathophysiology
      1. Cardiogenic pulmonary edema may occur because of an increase in the hydrostatic pressure gradient associated with an altered hemodynamic status, such as in CHF. An elevated pulmonary capillary wedge pressure occurs because of left ventricular dysfunction.
      2. Noncardiogenic pulmonary edema is caused by leakage of fluid from pulmonary capillaries with a decrease in plasma oncotic pressure and elevation of capillary pressure, producing interstitial and intra-alveolar edema.
         a) This type of pulmonary edema may be caused by several clinical conditions that result in fluid and protein accumulation in the alveoli.
         b) This edema usually begins more abruptly and is more severe than cardiogenic form.
      3. Neurogenic pulmonary edema is characterized by acute respiratory distress triggered by acute, serve compromise of the CNS.
      4. Decreased lung and small airway compliance may result in altered ventilation, hypoxia, and respiratory failure.
      5. Hypoxia reduces the ability to actively transport sodium, leading to alveolar edema.

III. Clinical features: In pulmonary edema, fluid collects in the numerous air sacs in the lungs, making breathing difficult. In most cases, heart problems cause pulmonary edema (Assaad et al., 2018; Busl & Bleck, 2015; Casey et al., 2019; Dobbe et al., 2019; Finsterer, 2019; Nanjappa et al., 2016).
   A. Etiology (see Table 32-1)
   B. History
      1. History of cancer and cancer treatment
      2. Current medications: Prescribed, over the counter

TABLE 32-1	Types of Pulmonary Edema

Type	Etiology	Clinical Features	Hemodynamic Parameters	Diagnostic Studies
Cardiogenic	Episode of acute heart failure Myocardial infarction Minor ischemia Hypertensive crisis Cardiomyopathy Severe dysrhythmias Renal artery stenosis Cold immersion History of heart failure History of valvular or ischemic heart disease Left atrial tumor Thrombosis of prosthetic valve	Harsh heart murmurs Severe respiratory distress Oxygen saturation < 90% on room air	Increased PCWP Increased BNP plasma levels Increased LV pressures Reduced LV contractility Increased SVR Increased troponin and creatinine kinase	Chest x-ray—enlarged heart ECG—abnormal
Neurogenic	Head injury Intracranial hemorrhage Subarachnoid hemorrhage Seizures Tumors Hydrocephalus Neurosurgical procedures	Highly variable	Increased SVR Decreased LV contractility Increased alveolar capillary leakage	–
Noncardiogenic	ARDS Infection Shock Toxic damage Postoperative (reperfusion pulmonary edema) Pregnancy related Transfusion associated Excess fluid accumulation Opioid overdose (heroin and methadone) Salicylate toxicity High altitudes Drowning Pulmonary embolism Pneumothorax (reexpansion pulmonary edema) Pulmonary veno-occlusive disease Lung transplantation Viral infections (hantavirus, dengue virus, coronavirus)	Hypoxia Severe respiratory distress	Increased PCWP	Chest x-ray—bilateral consolidative pattern, interstitial edema, diffuse infiltrates

ARDS—acute respiratory distress syndrome; BNP—B-type natriuretic peptide; ECG—electrocardiogram; LV—left ventricle; PCWP—pulmonary capillary wedge pressure; SVR—systemic vascular resistance

Note. Based on information from Assaad et al., 2018; Busl & Bleck, 2015; Nanjappa et al., 2016.

3. History of presenting symptoms: Precipitating factors, onset, location, duration, severity

4. Changes in ADLs

5. Past medical history: Seizures, hypertension, MI, CHF

C. Signs and symptoms

1. Dyspnea, orthopnea (late sign)

2. Anxiety or feeling of impending doom

3. Frothy-pink or salmon-colored sputum

4. Cough

5. Cyanosis, pallor

6. Diaphoresis

7. Unable to lie flat

D. Physical examination

1. Vital signs: Tachypnea, tachycardia, hypotension

2. Integument examination: Skin pallor, cyanosis, diaphoresis, livedo reticularis (skin discoloration with mottled appearance)

3. Pulmonary

   a) Observation of abnormal breathing pattern with the use of accessory muscles

   b) Auscultation revealing inspiratory crackles usually at the bases but sometimes throughout both lungs

   c) Rhonchi and wheezing

4. Cardiac

   a) Pulsus alternans, alternating weak and strong pulse possibly signaling left ventricular failure in CHF (see Appendix D)

   b) Narrow pulse pressures assessed in heart failure or cardiac tamponade

   c) Heart sounds with presence of S_3 gallop indicating left ventricular end-diastolic pressure and left ventricular dysfunction associated with cardiogenic etiology

   d) JVD indicating heart failure

   e) Peripheral edema of extremities

5. Abdominal: Possible hepatomegaly with vascular congestion

6. Poor prognostic physical findings

   a) Hypoxia

   b) High or low blood pressure

   c) High heart rate

   d) High respiratory rate

IV. Diagnostic tests (Assaad et al., 2018; Chioncel et al., 2016; Dobbe et al., 2019; see Table 32-1)

A. Laboratory

1. CBC to evaluate for infection and anemia

2. ABGs

   a) Hypoxia (oxygen saturation less than 90% and partial pressure of oxygen less than 60 mm Hg)

   b) Hypercapnia (partial pressure of carbon dioxide greater than 45–55 mm Hg)

   c) Acidosis (pH less than 7.35): Early findings of pulmonary edema may include respiratory alkalosis because of hyperventilation.

3. Serum albumin: May be low (normal 3.6–5 g/dl)

4. BUN and creatinine to evaluate kidney function to ensure that renal perfusion is occurring

5. Liver function tests to evaluate hepatic function: Elevations in ALT, aspartate aminotransferase, and bilirubin are seen with right ventricular failure and hepatic congestion.

      6. Hyponatremia suggesting severe heart failure

      7. Plasma BNP levels: May be increased in cardiovascular pulmonary edema

      8. BNP and N-terminal prohormone BNP: Used to distinguish severe heart failure

  B. Radiography: Chest x-ray

      1. Noncardiogenic: Bilateral consolidative pattern, interstitial edema

      2. Cardiogenic: Diffuse bilateral infiltrates, cardiomegaly

  C. Other: Hemodynamic monitoring

      1. Pulmonary arterial pressure measurements with elevated pulmonary capillary wedge pressure (normal 6–12 mm Hg)

      2. Systemic vascular resistance elevation (normal 800–1,200 dynes/s/m^2)

      3. Increased pulmonary capillary wedge pressure, which is a poor prognostic sign

      4. ECG to determine whether ventricular function and hemodynamics are consistent with heart failure: Evaluation for dysrhythmia

V. Differential diagnosis: Table 32-1 lists common causes of pulmonary edema.

  A. CHF (see Chapter 42)

  B. Capillary leak syndrome (see Chapter 35)

  C. Acute respiratory distress syndrome

  D. Early phase of septic shock (see Chapters 160)

  E. Diffuse alveolar hemorrhage

  F. Cancer: Cancer, lymphoma, leukemia, lymphangitic spread of solid tumors or acute toxicity from chemotherapy

  G. Cardiac tamponade (see Chapter 50)

  H. Ischemic stroke (see Chapter 146)

  I. Brain injury

VI. Treatment: No known measures currently exist to correct permeability abnormalities. Management involves treatment of underlying disease by decreasing pulmonary venous and capillary pressure, improving cardiac output, and correcting underlying pathology while waiting for the acute lung injury to resolve. The patient is hospitalized for management (Bellani et al., 2016; Casey et al., 2019; Dobbe et al., 2019; Finsterer, 2019; Kor et al., 2016; Powell et al., 2016; Simko & Culleiton, 2019).

  A. Drug therapy

      1. Use of loop diuretics (e.g., furosemide, bumetanide, torsemide) causes vasodilation and decreases pulmonary congestion.

      2. Restrict fluids to 1.5–2 L daily.

      3. Vasodilators (e.g., nitric oxide, prostacyclin) cause vasodilation, thereby decreasing pulmonary vascular pressure.

  B. Oxygen therapy

      1. Oxygen therapy often is used, and dose is titrated to patient response. Patients receive 100% oxygen by nonrebreather mask while in the upright position. Intubation and mechanical ventilation may be necessary.

      2. If hypoxia is severe, bilevel positive airway pressure has been found to be superior to oxygen therapy in decreasing the need for mechanical ventilation.

      3. If the patient has carbon dioxide retention or is obtunded, then tracheal intubation and assisted ventilation are required.

  C. Pulmonary arterial catheter may be placed to evaluate the cause of pulmonary edema.

  D. Position the patient in semi-Fowler position.

  E. Obtain daily weight to monitor fluid status and frequent intake and output measurements.

F. Treatment is determined by the course of the neurologic disorder and not the neurogenic pulmonary edema. Treatment should focus on the neurologic damage while neurogenic pulmonary edema is managed supportively.

G. For high-altitude pulmonary edema, limiting exertion, descending to a lower altitude, receiving oxygen, getting rest, and staying warm are key to survival.

    1. Other treatments include hyperbaric therapy, expiratory positive airway pressure, or breathing through pursed lips.

    2. Drug therapy includes nifedipine 30 mg PO every 12 hours, tadalafil 10 mg PO every 12 hours, and sildenafil 50 mg PO every eight hours.

    3. High-risk patients should prophylactically take nifedipine starting the day prior to ascent and continue for five days at altitude or until descent below 2,500 m (8,200 ft) is completed; or sildenafil 50–100 mg once prior to acute ascent; or tadalafil 10 mg PO every 12 hours.

    4. Patients who are in high altitude for two to six days should take sildenafil 40 mg PO three times a day.

H. Reperfusion pulmonary edema may appear 72 hours after surgery, ranging from mild to fatal. Treatment may require venovenous extracorporeal life support.

I. Reexpansion pulmonary edema treatment is supportive and self-limited.

J. Opioid overdose should be treated with assisted ventilation and administration of naloxone.

K. Salicylate overdose should be treated with volume resuscitation and sodium bicarbonate administration.

VII. Follow-up

A. Daily physical assessment and evaluation of response to treatment is necessary.

B. Diagnostic studies such as chest x-ray and ABGs may be completed to evaluate patient condition.

VIII. Referrals

A. Pulmonologist: To evaluate lung status and assist with medical management

B. Respiratory therapist: May be needed for oxygen therapy, ventilatory management, percussion, or respiratory treatments

C. Neurologists: To assist with medical management of neurologic pulmonary edema

References

Assaad, S., Kratzert, W.B., Shelley, B., Friedman, M.B., & Perrino, A., Jr. (2018). Assessment of pulmonary edema: Principles and practice. *Journal of Cardiothoracic Vascular Anesthesia, 32*(2), 901–914. https://doi.org/10.1053/j.jvca.2017.08.028

Bellani, G., Laffey, J.G., Pham, T., Fan, E., Brochard, L., Esteban, A., ... Pesenti, A. (2016). Epidemiology, patterns of care, and mortality for patients with acute respiratory distress syndrome in intensive care units in 50 countries. *JAMA, 315*(8), 788–800. https://doi.org/10.1001/jama.2016.0291

Busl, K.M., & Bleck, T.P. (2015). Neurogenic pulmonary edema. *Critical Care Medicine, 43*(8), 1710–1715. https://doi.org/10.1097/CCM.0000000000001101

Casey, J.D., Semler, M.W., & Rice, T.W. (2019). Fluid management in acute respiratory distress syndrome. *Seminars in Respiratory and Critical Care Medicine, 40*(1), 57–65. https://doi.org/10.1055/s-0039-1685206

Chioncel, O., Ambrosy, A.P., Bubenek, S., Filipescu, D., Vinereanu, D., Petris, A., ... Collins, S.P. (2016). Epidemiology, pathophysiology, and in-hospital management of pulmonary edema: Data from the Romanian acute heart failure syndromes registry. *Journal of Cardiovascular Medicine, 17*(2), 92–104. https://doi.org/10.2459/JCM.0000000000000192

Dobbe, L., Rahman, R., Elmassry, M., Paz, P., & Nugent, K. (2019). Cardiogenic pulmonary edema. *American Journal of the Medical Sciences, 358*(6), 389–397. https://doi.org/10.1016/j.amjms.2019.09.011

Finsterer, J. (2019). Neurological perspectives of neurogenic pulmonary edema. *European Neurology, 81*(1-2), 94–102. https://doi.org/10.1159/000500139

Kor, D.J., Carter, R.E., Park, P.K., Festic, E., Banner-Goodspeed, V.M., Hinds, R., … Gong, M.N. (2016). Effect of aspirin on development of ARDS in at-risk patients presenting to the emergency department: The LIPS-A randomized clinical trial. *JAMA, 315*(22), 2406–2414. https://doi.org/10.1001/jama.2016.6330

Nanjappa, S., Jeong, D.K., Muddaraju, M., Jeong, K., Hill, E.D., & Greene, J.N. (2016). Diffuse alveolar hemorrhage in acute myeloid leukemia. *Cancer Control, 23*(3), 272–277. https://doi.org/10.1177/107327481602300310

Powell, J., Graham, D., O'Reilly, S., & Punton, G. (2016). Acute pulmonary oedema. *Nursing Standard, 30*(23), 51–60. https://doi.org/10.7748/ns.30.23.51.s47

Simko, L.C., & Culleiton, A.L. (2019). Uncommon causes of noncardiogenic pulmonary edema. *Nursing Critical Care, 14*(2), 22–29. https://doi.org/10.1097/01.CCN.0000553077.26034.e1

CHAPTER 33

Pulmonary Embolism

Beth Sandy, MSN, CRNP

I. Definition: Obstruction of the pulmonary artery or one of its branches by a thrombus (Schwartz, 2017)

II. Physiology/Pathophysiology (Giordano et al., 2017; Konstantinides et al., 2020)
   A. Normal
      1. Oxygen-depleted blood is returned to the right heart via the IVC and SVC.
      2. Blood is pumped through the right and left pulmonary arteries to the lungs.
      3. Arteries are further divided into smaller arteries and capillaries, carrying blood to the alveoli.
      4. Carbon dioxide is exchanged, and oxygen is absorbed by the blood.
      5. Oxygenated blood leaves the lungs via the pulmonary veins and returns to the left heart for systemic distribution.
   B. Pathophysiology
      1. Thrombus formation is promoted by venous stasis, hypercoagulability, and endothelial vessel injury (Virchow triad) with vessel inflammation.
      2. Venous stasis disrupts blood flow, increasing platelet contact with the vascular endothelium.
      3. A hypercoagulable state results from inherited or acquired alteration of the normal balance of procoagulant factors, anticoagulant proteins, and fibrinolytic enzymes.
      4. Endothelial injury activates the coagulation cascade and platelet adhesion and aggregation, leading to emboli formation.
      5. Most pulmonary emboli arise from thrombi originating in the deep veins of the lower extremities (iliac, femoral, and popliteal veins).
      6. Thrombi may form in renal, pelvic, or upper extremity veins; right heart; vascular access devices; or filters in the IVC.
      7. Thrombi that dislodge create an embolus. Emboli circulate to the right side of the heart and to the lungs via the pulmonary artery. Large emboli may lodge at the bifurcation of the main pulmonary artery of the lower branches, leading to hemodynamic compromise. This phenomenon is often referred to as a *saddle embolus*. Smaller thrombi continue traveling to smaller branches distally, causing occlusion.
      8. Emboli are most common; however, alternatives may be a fat globule, air, or foreign body.
      9. Pathophysiologic results include hypoxemia, increased pulmonary vascular resistance, impaired gas exchange, alveolar hyperventilation, increased airway resistance, and decreased pulmonary compliance.
      10. Hemodynamic instability leads to PH and right ventricular failure.

11. Cancer and cancer treatments promote a thrombotic state.
    a) Malignant cells, cytokines from tumor cells, and chemotherapy promote endothelial damage.
    b) Tumors may produce circulating procoagulant that results in hypercoagulability.
    c) Venous compression by direct extension of tumor or associated lymphadenopathy leads to venous stasis.
12. PE presentation may be acute or chronic.
    a) Massive PE with hemodynamic instability
    b) Submassive PE with right ventricular strain without hemodynamic compromise
    c) Nonmassive PE marked by lack of right ventricular strain and normal hemodynamics

III. Clinical features: High-risk PE and hemodynamic instability are associated with 40% mortality within 90 days. PE is the third most common cause of cardiovascular death. The Wells' Score or the Geneva Score (revised) for PE are scoring tables that predict risk for PE based on clinical presentation factors (Corrigan et al., 2016; Essien et al., 2019; Font et al., 2017; Giordano et al., 2017; Konstantinides et al., 2020).

A. Etiology and risk factors
   1. Virchow triad: Hypercoagulability, hemodynamic changes, endothelial injury/dysfunction
   2. Immobility
   3. Surgery within past 30 days
   4. Vascular access devices, implanted pacemakers, and defibrillators
   5. Age older than 60 years
   6. Prior venous thromboembolism
   7. Heparin-induced thrombocytopenia
   8. Obesity
   9. Medical conditions: PH, chronic lung disease, cerebral vascular accident, nephrotic syndrome, malignancy; history of cancer in remission is not associated with increased risk.
   10. Blood disorders: Inherited thrombophilia, factor V Leiden mutation, prothrombin gene mutation, defects in fibrinolysis and hyperhomocysteinemia, protein C and S deficiency, antiphospholipid antibodies, polycythemia vera, sickle cell disease
   11. Recent pregnancy
   12. Oral contraceptive use (three- to four-fold increased risk) or hormone replacement therapy
   13. Varicose veins
   14. Recent trauma to lower extremities within past 30 days
   15. Prolonged air travel
   16. Cigarette smoking

B. History
   1. Cancer and cancer treatment
   2. Current medications: Prescribed (e.g., oral contraceptives, estrogen or hormone replacement therapy, exposure to heparin), over the counter
   3. History of presenting symptoms: Precipitating factors, onset, location, duration
   4. Past medical history: Prior venous thromboembolism, CHF, chronic lung disease, cerebrovascular accident, hypercoagulable state
   5. Social history: Tobacco use, recent air travel
   6. Family history: Inherited coagulopathy or blood disorders

C. Signs and symptoms: Associated symptoms range from asymptomatic to nonspecific to dramatic compromise. Intensity of symptoms is dependent on the size of the clot and location.
1. Chest pain/tightness, crushing, nonradiating, stabbing pain; increased with inspiration
2. Pleuritic pain: Associated with breathing
3. Dyspnea: Usually sudden onset
4. Orthopnea
5. Cough: Acute onset
6. Hemoptysis
7. Hypoxemia
8. Wheezing
9. Fever
10. Diaphoresis
11. Anxiety/restlessness
12. Shock

D. Physical examination
1. Vital signs: Possible tachycardia, tachypnea, hypotension, fever
2. General: Anxiety, mental status (e.g., alert, oriented)
3. Pulmonary
   a) Chest tenderness on affected side
   b) Pleural friction rub
   c) Crackles/rales
   d) Use of accessory muscles
4. Cardiac examination: Right-sided gallop indicating CHF, S_4, loud S_2
5. Extremities: Positive Homan sign (painful calf), palpable cord, erythema, edema (usually unilateral, indicative of DVT)
6. Integument: Cyanosis present with occlusion

IV. Diagnostic tests: Clinical suspicion is highly predictive of PE; several clinical prediction models have been developed that can predict the likelihood of PE and drive diagnostic tests. Data used in each model vary; therefore, these models cannot be used interchangeably (Corrigan et al., 2016; Essien et al., 2019; Konstantinides et al., 2020; Ma & Wen, 2017).
A. Laboratory data
1. CBC to evaluate for anemia or infection
2. Blood cultures, if indicated
3. ABGs: Respiratory alkalosis and hypocapnia
4. PT, INR: Increased risk for PE with ineffective anticoagulation
5. Enzyme-linked immunosorbent assay (ELISA): Measures degradation of fibrin indicating recent activity in the coagulation system; sensitive and high negative predictive value (less than 500 ng/ml normal)
   a) D-dimer test, using an age-adjusted cutoff or adapted to clinical probability, should be considered as an alternative to the fixed cutoff level.
   b) D-dimer levels are elevated in PE with a high negative predictor value, in that if the D-dimer level is normal, it is unlikely patient has PE or DVT.
   c) Elevated D-dimer can be indicative of other medical conditions (e.g., DIC, intravascular coagulation) and should not be used alone to diagnose PE.
6. BNP: Prognostic marker, not diagnostic (greater than 90 pg/ml poor prognostic indicator)
7. Troponin: Indicative of acute right heart strain; elevations are a poor prognostic factor (greater than 0.07 ng/ml).

       8. Growth differentiation factor-15: Upregulated with PE; poor prognostic marker

       9. Sodium: Hyponatremia associated with increased mortality

     10. Inherited disorders

        a) Protein C and protein S levels to assess for deficiency

        b) Antithrombin III

        c) Prothrombin mutation

        d) Homocysteine levels

        e) Factor V Leiden mutation

        f) Anticardiolipin antibodies Igs (e.g., IgG, IgM, IgA)

  B. Radiology

     1. A chest x-ray may be normal. It is not a sufficient test to detect PE.

     2. CT chest angiography/PE protocol is the gold standard.

        a) This test is highly sensitive and specific.

        b) It has the capability of diagnosing small emboli, using thin slices and extra cuts.

        c) History of contrast allergy or renal insufficiency may preclude use because of the necessity of using IV contrast.

     3. CT chest with contrast is the standard protocol and can detect emboli in the sub-segmental branches and lung bases, usually incidentally. It does not have the fine cuts that CT chest angiography exhibits.

     4. Ventilation/perfusion scan (lung scintigraphy) is a two-stage scan with poor sensitivity. It is reported as normal, high probability, and nondiagnostic.

        a) Ventilation scan: Demonstrates movement of air in the lungs

        b) Perfusion: Demonstrates blood supply to affected area of the lung

        c) High probability: Represented by multiple segmental or larger defects with normal ventilation in at least one area of abnormal perfusion; known as "mismatch"

        d) Alternative to angiography in patients with contrast allergies or renal insufficiency

        e) Not a reliable test to detect PE in patients who have preexisting poor lung function.

     5. Pulmonary angiography is rarely performed because it is invasive, nonspecific, and expensive. Risks include arrhythmias, anaphylaxis, nephrotoxicity, and death. It is necessary if embolectomy is considered.

     6. Doppler ultrasound is used to evaluate for DVT. A negative scan does not rule out PE because this test is performed on the extremities and cannot detect thrombus in the lungs.

     7. An echocardiogram is a poor diagnostic tool and is primarily used for prognosis. A transthoracic echocardiogram can identify right ventricular hypokinesis and right ventricular hypertrophy and overload from the PE, predicting poor prognosis.

     8. Pulmonary magnetic resonance angiography has low sensitivity to detect PE, high proportion of inconclusive results, and low availability in emergency settings, making it an undesirable choice.

  C. Other

     1. Pulse oximetry: Provides noninvasive means of measuring delivery of oxygen from the atmosphere to the pulmonary capillaries

     2. ECG: Potential evidence of right heart strain (e.g., T-wave inversion, new right bundle branch block, tachycardia, atrial fibrillation)

V. Differential diagnosis: PE may present in conjunction with the following conditions, complicating diagnosis (Capel & Broderick, 2018; Palm et al., 2019).

  A. MI (see Chapter 49)

  B. Pneumonitis/interstitial lung disease

  C. Endocarditis (see Chapter 46)

D. Myocarditis

E. Pericarditis (see Chapter 50)

F. CHF (see Chapter 42)

G. Pericardial tamponade (see Chapter 50)

H. Dissecting aortic aneurysm

I. Pneumonia (see Chapter 30)

J. Pneumothorax (see Chapter 31)

K. Pleuritis

L. COPD flare (see Chapter 28)

M. Anxiety disorder with hyperventilation (see Chapter 161)

N. GI abnormalities: Esophageal rupture, peptic ulcer disease, gastritis (see Chapters 72 and 78)

O. Progressive cancer in the lungs

VI. Treatment: The pulmonary embolism severity index (PESI) or other scales may be used as an adjunct to classify patients as low risk or high risk to drive treatment approach. The simplified PESI assigns a risk value of one point to six variables (age older than 80 years, history of cancer, chronic cardiopulmonary disease, pulse greater than 110 bpm, systolic blood pressure less than 100 mm Hg, oxyhemoglobin saturation levels). Patients with one point or higher are considered high-risk patients. Patients who are asymptomatic and hemodynamically stable may be managed as outpatients (Agnelli et al., 2015; Essien et al., 2019; Jiménez et al., 2010; Key et al., 2019; Konstantinides et al., 2020; Lyman et al., 2015; Raskob et al., 2018; Schwartz, 2017; Schwartz, 2019; Son et al., 2017; Wang et al., 2018; Young et al., 2018).

A. Prevention

1. Identification of high-risk patients

2. Management of underlying disorders

B. Supportive

1. Oxygen: Mechanical ventilation for hypoxia

2. Hemodynamic support: IV fluids, vasopressors

C. Anticoagulation: Anticoagulation is the main therapy with the goal of treating the current PE and preventing recurrent PEs. It blocks the clotting cascade, stabilizes the existing clot, and allows the endogenous thrombolytic system to dissolve preexisting thrombi. It also prevents further thrombus formation from occurring.

1. Direct-acting oral anticoagulant therapy: This current gold standard of anticoagulation for PE has benefit of using the oral route, as opposed to injection, without the need for routine blood testing to assess for therapeutic index. It is associated with low risk of bleeding as compared to other anticoagulant therapies.

   a) Rivaroxiban: 15 mg PO two times a day with food for the first 21 days, followed by 20 mg PO daily with food

   b) Apixaban: 10 mg PO two times a day for seven days, followed by 5 mg two times a day

   c) Edoxaban: After five days of a LMWH lead-in, 60 mg PO daily or 30 mg PO daily for patients with creatinine clearance of 15–50 ml/min or body weight less than 60 kg or patients who use certain P-glycoprotein inhibitors (e.g., PPIs)

2. LMWH: It is an attractive option due to very short half-life. Anticoagulation effect is reversible as soon as the last dose has been completed. Traditionally, a lack of need exists for laboratory monitoring, prevention of recurrence, and lower bleeding rates.

   a) Use with caution in patients with renal insufficiency.

   b) Monitoring of anti-Xa levels is reserved for patients with morbid obesity, cachexia, anasarca, or persistent clotting while on LMWH.

      c) Prolonged use (longer than 6–12 months) carries an increased risk of osteoporosis.

      d) Examples

          (1) Dalteparin: 200 units/kg subcutaneous daily for 30 days, then dose reduced to 150 units/kg daily

          (2) Enoxaparin: 1.5 mg/kg subcutaneous daily or 1 mg/kg subcutaneous two times a day (preferred with large clot burden or body weight greater than 100 kg)

3. Unfractionated heparin: It is used if the patient is hemodynamically or unstable at increased risk for bleeding, or if there is concern about subcutaneous absorption (significant cachexia or obesity) or with renal insufficiency (creatinine clearance less than 30 ml/min). Unfractionated heparin has the shortest half-life, and its effect can be reversed if bleeding occurs.

      a) IV: 80 units/kg bolus followed by continuous infusion of 18 units/kg/hr

      b) Rate titrated every four to six hours to therapeutic aPTT, 1.5–2.5 times the control aPTT (heparin levels of 0.3–0.7 IU/ml anti-Xa activity)

      c) Subcutaneous: 333 units/kg, followed by 250 units/kg every 12 hours

      d) Risk of heparin-induced thrombocytopenia

4. Warfarin (vitamin K antagonist): This oral agent is not the preferred anticoagulation method and is considered third-line therapy if LMWH or direct oral anticoagulants are contraindicated.

      a) Daily dosing is required and initiated with parenteral treatment for acute PE. It should overlap for a minimum of five days or until INR is between 2–3 for at least 24 hours. Initiation dose is 5 mg for first two days then adjusted to INR.

      b) Higher initiation dose (7.5 mg PO): Weight greater than 85 kg, African American patient, hypothyroidism, concomitant medications that decrease warfarin effect

      c) Lower initiation dose (2.5 mg PO): Older adult, Asian patient, hepatic insufficiency, malnutrition, hyperthyroidism, concomitant medications that increase warfarin effect

          (1) Frequent monitoring of INR level (range 2–3 therapeutic) should occur daily while in hospital and at least monthly thereafter.

          (2) Multiple drug–drug and food–drug interactions interfere with therapeutic treatment. Foods high in vitamin K content, such as green, leafy vegetables, will decrease absorption of warfarin.

5. Parenteral factor Xa inhibitor

      a) Inhibits fibrin formation, promotes factor Xa inactivation by antithrombin without inhibiting thrombin; no antidote for reversal of anticoagulation

      b) Fondaparinux: 5–10 mg subcutaneous daily; dosing based on body weight: 5 mg if less than 50 kg; 7.5 mg for 50–100 kg; 10 mg for greater than 100 kg

      c) Long half-life: Contraindicated in patients with renal insufficiency

6. Duration of anticoagulation therapy is dependent on location of thrombosis, type of thrombosis, and risk of recurrence (malignancy diagnosis); typically, a minimum of six months is required.

      a) In patients with metastatic cancer, duration is indefinite with active disease and/or while on treatment.

      b) If due to atrial fibrillation from surgical procedure and patient does not have active cancer, anticoagulation may be a shorter course.

7. Contraindications for anticoagulation include active bleeding, recent brain surgery, recent spinal surgery, and recent hemorrhagic stroke.

D. Systemic thrombolysis: It is a potentially life-saving intervention in hemodynamically unstable patients (e.g., hypotensive, hypoperfusion, right ventricular failure, or cardiac arrest). Systemic thrombolysis accelerates lysis of acute PEs.
  1. Tissue plasminogen activator: 100 mg infusion over two hours, followed by IV unfractionated heparin
  2. Tissue plasminogen activator: 100 mg bolus with cardiac arrest
  3. Urokinase: 4,400 IU/kg loading dose over 10 minutes followed by 4,400 IU/kg/hr for 12 hours; heparin infusion given concurrently

E. Surgical
  1. Vena cava filter placement includes mechanical obstruction of IVC with a screen to prevent the migration of DVT. It is recommended for patients with recurrent veno-thromboembolism, contraindication for anticoagulation, or those with the inability to adequately anticoagulate.
  2. Risks include filter misplacement or migration, infection, vessel perforation, or IVC obstruction due to filter thrombosis.
  3. Current literature suggests that IVC filters be retrieved after threat of PE has resolved, due to potential complications of an indwelling device; however, filter removal can have complications. Risks and benefits must be considered when deciding to retrieve.

F. Pulmonary embolectomy: Surgical removal of embolus is reserved for patients who have a large PE with resultant shock, failed anticoagulation, or a contraindication to thrombolytics.

VII. Follow-up (Konstantinides et al., 2020)
  A. Monitoring of PT and INR for patients on vitamin K antagonist
  B. Monitoring of hemodynamic status
  C. Monitoring for bleeding
  D. Monitoring for compliance of orals or injectables
  E. Monitoring for financial difficulties: Many recommended therapies are expensive.
  F. Discharge planning for patients and families if admission to hospital required
    1. Education regarding maintenance medication and monitoring
    2. Visiting nurse monitoring, if necessary

VIII. Referrals
  A. Anticoagulation clinic: For long-term management
    1. Especially for early-stage patients with cancer who may not require frequent follow-up with oncology
    2. For patients who are prescribed warfarin; includes routine blood monitoring and frequent dose adjustments
  B. Hematologist: For management of hematologic coagulation disorders
  C. Surgery or interventional radiology: For placement or retrieval of IVC filter or embolectomy

The author would like to acknowledge Marianne Davies, RN, MSN, CNS-BC, ACNP-BC, AOCNP®, for her contribution to this chapter that remains unchanged from the previous edition of this book.

References

Agnelli, G., Buller, H.R., Cohen, A., Gallus, A.S., Lee, T.C., Pak, R., ... Yamabe, T. (2015). Oral apixaban for the treatment of venous thromboembolism in cancer patients: Results from the AMPLIFY trial. *Journal of Thrombosis and Haemostasis, 13*(12), 2187–2191. https://doi.org/10.1111/jth.13153

Capel, K.W., & Broderick, L.S. (2018). PE or no PE? Alternative diagnoses on CTA. *Applied Radiology, 47*(3), 8–13. https://www.appliedradiology.com/articles/pe-or-no-pe-alternative-diagnoses-on-cta

Corrigan, D., Prucnal, C., & Kabrhel, C. (2016). Pulmonary embolism: The diagnosis, risk-stratification, treatment and disposition of emergency department patients. *Clinical and Experimental Emergency Medicine, 3*(3), 117–125. https://doi.org/10.15441/ceem.16.146

Essien, E.-O., Rali, P., & Mathai, S.C. (2019). Pulmonary embolism. *Medical Clinics of North America, 103*(3), 549–564. https://doi.org/10.1016/j.mcna.2018.12.013

Font, C., Carmona-Bayonas, A., Beato, C., Reig, Ò., Sáez, A., Jiménez-Fonseca, P., ... Otero, R. (2017). Clinical features and short-term outcomes of cancer patients with suspected and unsuspected pulmonary embolism: The EPIPHANY study. *European Respiratory Journal, 49*(1), 1600282. https://doi.org/10.1183/13993003.00282-2016

Giordano, N.J., Jansson, P.S., Young, M.N., Hagan, K.A., & Kabrhel, C. (2017). Epidemiology, pathophysiology, stratification, and natural history of pulmonary embolism. *Techniques in Vascular and Interventional Radiology, 20*(3), 135–140. https://doi.org/10.1053/j.tvir.2017.07.002

Jiménez, D., Aujesky, D., Moores, L., Gómez, V., Lobo, J.L., Uresandi, F., ... Yusen, R.D. (2010). Simplification of the pulmonary embolism severity index for prognostication in patients with acute symptomatic pulmonary embolism. *Archives of Internal Medicine, 170*(15), 1383–1389. https://doi.org/10.1001/archinternmed.2010.199

Key, N.S., Khorana, A.A., Kuderer, N.M., Bohlke, K., Lee, A.Y.Y., Arcelus, J.I., ... Falanga, A. (2019). Venous thromboembolism prophylaxis and treatment in patients with cancer: ASCO clinical practice guideline update. *Journal of Clinical Oncology, 38*(5), 496–520. https://doi.org/10.1200/JCO.19.01461

Konstantinides, S.V., Meyer, G., Becattini, C., Bueno, H., Geersing, G.-J., Harjola, V.-P., ... Zamorano, J.L. (2020). 2019 ESC guidelines for the diagnosis and management of acute pulmonary embolism developed in collaboration with the European Respiratory Society (ERS): The task force for the diagnosis and management of acute pulmonary embolism of the European Society of Cardiology (ESC). *European Heart Journal, 41*(4), 543–603, https://doi.org/10.1093/eurheartj/ehz405

Lyman, G.H., Bohlke, K., Khorana, A.A., Kuderer, N.M., Lee, A.Y., Arcelus, J.I., ... Falanga, A. (2015). Venous thromboembolism prophylaxis and treatment in patients with cancer: American Society of Clinical Oncology clinical practice guideline update 2014. *Journal of Clinical Oncology, 33*(6), 654–656. https://doi.org/10.1200/JCO.2014.59.7351

Ma, L., & Wen, Z. (2017). Risk factors and prognosis of pulmonary embolism in patients with lung cancer. *Medicine, 96*(16), e6638. https://doi.org/10.1097/MD.0000000000006638

Palm, V., Rengier, F., Rajiah, P., Heussel, C.P., & Partovi, S. (2019). Acute pulmonary embolism: Imaging techniques, findings, endovascular treatment and differential diagnoses. *RöFo, 191*(5). https://doi.org/10.1055/a-0900-4200

Raskob, G.E., van Es, N., Verhamme, P., Carrier, M., Di Nisio, M., Garcia, D., ... Segers, A. (2018). Edoxaban for the treatment of cancer-associated venous thromboembolism. *New England Journal of Medicine, 378*(7), 615–624. https://doi.org/10.1056/NEJMoa1711948

Schwartz, R.N. (2017). Management of venous thromboembolism for patients with hematologic malignancies. *Journal of the Advanced Practitioner in Oncology, 8*(3), 297–302. https://doi.org/10.6004/jadpro.2017.8.3.14

Schwartz, R.N. (2019). Treating venous thrombosis in oncology. *Journal of the Advanced Practitioner in Oncology, 10*(3), 230–232. https://doi.org/10.6004/jadpro.2019.10.3.5

Son, J., Bae, M., Chung, S.W., Lee, C.W., Huh, U., & Song, S. (2017). Should we remove the retrievable cook celect inferior vena cava filter? Eight years of experience at a single center. *Korean Journal of Thoracic and Cardiovascular Surgery, 50*(6), 443–447. https://doi.org/10.5090/kjtcs.2017.50.6.443

Wang, T.-F., Li, A., & Garcia, D. (2018). Managing thrombosis in cancer patients. *Research and Practice in Thrombosis and Haemostasis, 2*(3), 429–438. https://doi.org/10.1002/rth2.12102

Young, A.M., Marshall, A., Thirlwall, J., Chapman, O., Lokare, A., & Hill, C., ... Levine, M. (2018). Comparison of an oral factor Xa inhibitor with low molecular weight heparin in patients with cancer with venous thromboembolism: Results of a randomized trial (SELECT-D). *Journal of Clinical Oncology, 36*(20), 2017–2023. https://doi.org/10.1200/JCO.2018.78.8034

CHAPTER 34

Sleep Apnea (Sleep Disorder Breathing)

Enza Esposito Nguyen, DNP, RN, ANP-BC, AOCNP®

I. Definition (Cowie, 2017; Javaheri et al., 2017; Patel, 2019)
   A. Apnea is the absence of inspiratory airflow for at least 10 seconds and is associated with hypoxemia, sleep disturbances, and hemodynamic changes. There are two types of sleep apnea, or sleep disorder breathing.
      1. Central: Episodic loss of drive to breathe
      2. Obstructive: Intermittent collapse/obstruction of airway
   B. Sleep apnea is a periodic reduction (hypopnea) or cessation (apnea) of breathing during sleep.

II. Physiology/Pathophysiology (Badr & Javaheri, 2019; Cowie, 2017; Javaheri et al., 2017; Pham & Schwartz, 2015; Tadic et al., 2021)
   A. Normal
      1. Central respiratory chemosensitivity is regulated by chemoreceptor neurons throughout the brain stem. They detect proximal carbon dioxide and regulate breathing in a classic feedback loop.
      2. Coordinated interactions of more than 20 skeletal muscles stent open the oropharynx and allow normal thoracic muscular work of breathing and alveolar gas exchange.
      3. Activity from medullary neurons and electromyogram responses from the diaphragm, in combination with abductor muscles from the upper airway, demonstrate a decrease in airway width when transitioning from an awake to a sleep state in healthy humans.
   B. Pathophysiology: The sequela caused by untreated sleep disorder breathing, whether central, obstructive, or both, is largely a result of repetitive hypoxia, intermittent hypercapnia, activation of the sympathetic nervous system, and hemodynamic alterations resulting in sleep disruption.
      1. Several processes of compensation that vary from person to person result in cyclical apnea.
      2. Retropalatal section of oropharynx is the most common site of airway collapse. Exact location of closure also varies depending on excess weight and/or anatomical variations.
      3. Increased tissue thickness of the tongue structures and soft tissues in the pharyngeal cavity decreases the passageway for air to the trachea, resulting in apnea.
      4. As a direct result of catecholamine release, the effect causes vasodilation of the heart and brain and constriction in other organs, resulting in atrial fibrillation. These

responses happen repeatedly during the night, leading to prolonged inflammation and stress on the body.

III. Clinical features: Sleep apnea is the most common sleep disorder and is often misdiagnosed. Some types of sleep apnea are sporadic hypoxemias that often result in transient arousal from sleep throughout the night and compensatory sequela from the autonomic nervous system. Sleep apnea is associated with nocturnal cardiac dysrhythmia and chronic and acute cardiac events. During sleep, apnea is worsened by supine sleeping position. The incidence of sleep apnea in the morbidly obese population is 38%–88% (Badr & Javaheri, 2019; Cowie, 2017; Farrell & Richards, 2017; Javaheri et al., 2017; Liu et al., 2015; Patel, 2019; Posadas et al., 2020; Semelka et al., 2016; Tadic et al., 2021).
   A. Risk factors
      1. Excess body weight
      2. Age (40–70 years)
      3. Family history of obstructive sleep apnea
      4. Male sex
      5. Postmenopausal women not taking hormone therapy
      6. Cranial/facial structure variations
      7. Alcohol ingestion resulting in decreased airway muscle tone within the first two hours after ingestion
      8. Hypertension
   B. Etiology (see Figure 34-1)
      1. Obesity
      2. Upper airway obstruction
      3. Respiratory control center instability
      4. Nasomaxillary abnormalities that may lead to the following
         a) Intermittent hypoxemia
         b) Intermittent hypercapnia
         c) Increased negative intrathoracic pressure alterations
         d) Increased arousal from sleep
      5. Sleep depravation
      6. Sympathetic nervous system activation from anxiety
      7. Metabolic dysregulation: Obesity, insulin resistance, dyslipidemia
      8. Oxidative stress: Tiredness, muscle cramps, pain, headache
      9. Inflammation caused by acute or chronic conditions: Trauma, RA, FMS
      10. Vascular endothelial dysfunction: Smoking, diabetes, hypertension
   C. History
      1. History of cancer and cancer treatment
      2. Current medications: Prescribed, over the counter
      3. History of presenting symptoms: Precipitating factors, onset, location, duration, associated symptoms (e.g., daytime sleepiness, loud snoring, fatigue, irritability, depression, morning headache)
      4. Changes in ADLs: Decreased cognitive abilities
      5. Past medical history: Diabetes, obesity, hypertension, frequent URIs
      6. Past surgical history: Nasopharyngeal or facial surgery
      7. Social history: Sleep pattern, alcohol consumption, illicit drug use, tobacco use
      8. Family history: Obstructive sleep apnea
   D. Signs and symptoms
      1. Irregular heartbeat or palpitations
      2. Depression

FIGURE 34-1 **Factors Causing Sleep Apnea**

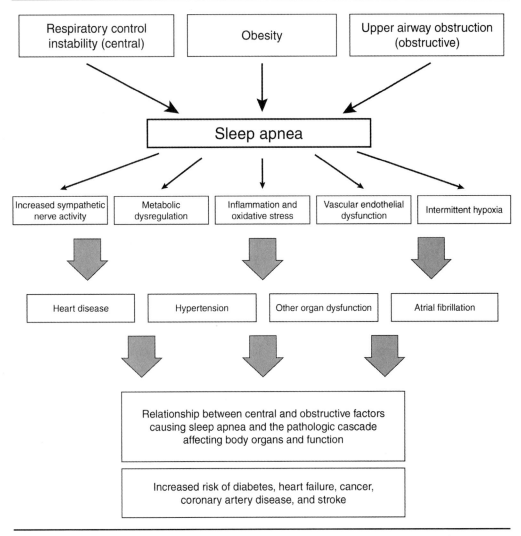

Note. Based on information from Badr & Javaheri, 2019; Cowie, 2017; Patel, 2019; Pham & Schwartz, 2015; Semelka et al., 2016.

3. Excessive daytime sleepiness
4. Fatigue
5. Irritability
6. Decreased cognitive abilities
7. Morning headaches
8. Erectile dysfunction
9. Dizziness

E. Physical examination
   1. Vital signs
      a) Possible elevated blood pressure; hypertension as a risk factor for sleep apnea
      b) Irregular heart rate with the presence of dysrhythmia
      c) Weight assessment; sleep apnea in obese individuals (common)

2. HEENT: Structures blocking the airway
   a) Oral: Abnormalities in mouth
   b) Posterior oropharynx: Presence and size of adenoids and tonsils
   c) Tongue: Macroglossia
   d) Uvula: Elongation and enlargement
   e) Face: Abnormal position of the maxilla or mandible in relation to the face and soft tissues, such as severe overbite
   f) Nasal: Septal deviation, nasal polyps
   g) Neck: Thyroid enlargement or nodules suggestive of thyroid disorders
3. Extremities: Edema suggestive of cardiac etiology

IV. Diagnostic test: Based on a comprehensive sleep apnea diagnostic evaluation in conjunction with a comprehensive sleep assessment; typically not helpful in confirmation or exclusion of sleep apnea (Javaheri et al., 2017; Kapur et al., 2017; Patel, 2019; Semelka et al., 2016; Tadic et al., 2021)
   A. Laboratory
      1. CBC: Anemia or blood dyscrasia that can affect oxygenation contributing to apnea
      2. Metabolic panel: Glucose level for hyperglycemia indicating diabetes; liver and kidney function to evaluate at baseline
      3. Lipid panel: Dyslipidemia
      4. TSH, T_3, T_4: Thyroid function for hyper/hypothyroidism
      5. Carbon dioxide: Elevation
   B. Radiology
      1. Chest x-ray: Respiratory problems that could affect breathing at night
      2. Nasal or oropharynx MRI: Abnormal anatomy that could block airway
      3. Echocardiogram: Cardiac output and ventricular function; sleep apnea as a result of cardiac etiology
      4. ECG: Heart rhythm; increased incidence of atrial fibrillation with sleep apnea
   C. Other
      1. Polysomnography is the standard diagnostic test for sleep apnea. The study records brain waves, oxygen level, breathing rate and quality, heart rate, as well as eye and leg movement during sleep.
      2. Assess the risk of sleep apnea using questionnaires, such as the Berlin Questionnaire and STOP-Bang Questionnaire.
      3. Assess daytime sleepiness using scales, such as the Epworth Sleepiness Scale.
      4. Consider a psychology evaluation for depression, anxiety, or irritability, which are increased in risk with sleep apnea.

V. Differential diagnosis (Badr & Javaheri, 2019; Patel, 2019; Semelka et al., 2016; Tadic et al., 2021)
   A. COPD (see Chapter 28)
   B. Depression (see Chapter 162)
   C. Anxiety disorders (see Chapter 161)
   D. CHF (see Chapter 42)
   E. Dysrhythmias: Atrial fibrillation, ventricular tachycardia (see Chapter 45)
   F. Nocturia secondary to BPH (see Chapter 87), prostate cancer
   G. Neuromuscular disease
   H. GERD (see Chapter 71)
   I. Narcolepsy
   J. Restless legs syndrome (see Chapter 107)

K. PH (see Chapter 52)

L. Substance abuse

M. Tonsillar hypertrophy

VI. Treatment: The goal of treatment is to increase QOL and decrease or manage factors that interfere with proper oxygenation during sleep, diminishing morbidity and mortality. The combination of several of these therapies is often recommended (Badr & Javaheri, 2019; Cowie, 2017; Farrell & Richards, 2017; Jonas et al., 2017; Patel, 2019; Posadas et al., 2020; Semelka et al., 2016; Sutherland & Cistulli, 2019; Tadic et al., 2021; Weaver, 2019).

A. Nonpharmacologic measure: Lifestyle changes

1. Weight loss, as indicated

2. Regular exercise to aid in maintaining weight

3. Smoking cessation, as indicated

4. Drinking alcohol moderately and avoiding alcohol before bedtime

5. Position therapy: Education on using cushions/pillows/sleeping aids to change sleep position from supine to lateral

B. Medical management of comorbid conditions (e.g., diabetes; see Chapter 151), thyroid disease (see Chapters 157 and 158), and hypertension (see Chapter 47)

C. Oral appliances: Used for mild or moderate sleep apnea

1. Requires dental examination

2. Custom made oral appliances to improve airway and/or decrease airway collapse

3. Tongue retaining device to hold the tongue in a forward position without mandibular repositioning

4. Devices that keep airway open by bringing the lower jaw forward, which can relieve snoring and obstruction

D. Surgery

1. Bariatric surgery consideration to aid in weight loss

2. Upper airway or craniofacial surgery to correct facial or oral pharyngeal structures that open airway

a) Uvulopalatopharyngoplasty: Removal of tissue from the back of mouth and top of throat to increase airway opening

b) Tonsil or adenoid removal for persistent enlargement causing obstruction of airway

3. Maxillomandibular adjustment procedure to move upper and lower jaw forward away from facial bone, enlarging space behind the tongue and soft palate

4. Nasal surgery to remove polyps or correct deviated septum

E. Continuous positive airway pressure (CPAP) given through nasal or nasal/oral device

1. Noninvasive mechanism to keep airway open, push tongue forward, and deliver oxygen

2. Recommended to use during naps and sleep

F. Bilevel positive airway pressure (BiPAP): Used when a patient cannot tolerate the continuous pressure of a CPAP or if higher pressure settings are required through a mask

1. Device is used mainly in obstructive sleep apnea or COPD.

2. Pressure flexes with patient breath cycle make it easier to exhale and give BiPAP a more diverse range of use than CPAP.

G. Upper airway stimulation: Approved for moderate to severe sleep apnea

1. Hypoglossal nerve stimulator implanted under the skin on upper chest

2. Detects breathing patterns, stimulating the glossal nerve to move tongue away from airway during obstruction

VII. Follow-up (Sutherland & Cistulli, 2019; Weaver, 2019)
  A. Perform long-term follow-up with an interprofessional team, including pulmonary, cardiology, and sleep medicine.
  B. Monitor adherence with therapy selection.
  C. Educate on cleaning CPAP or BiPAP machine to lessen likelihood of incurring URIs.

VIII. Referrals (Patel, 2019; Sutherland & Cistulli, 2019)
  A. Dietitian: For education on healthy diet and weight loss measures
  B. Physical therapy: For orofacial therapy to improve tongue positioning and strengthen muscles that control the lips, tongue, soft palate, lateral pharyngeal wall, and face
  C. Sleep medicine/pulmonologist: To adjust CPAP and BiPAP machines
  D. Cardiologist: To manage cardiac disorders, as indicated
  E. Surgeon: For evaluation and surgical procedures, as indicated
  F. Dental: For evaluation and oral appliance development and adjustments, as indicated

References

Badr, M.S., & Javaheri, S. (2019). Central sleep apnea: A brief review. *Current Pulmonology Reports, 8*(1), 14–21. https://doi.org/10.1007/s13665-019-0221-z

Cowie, M.R. (2017). Sleep apnea: State of the art. *Trends in Cardiovascular Medicine, 27*(4), 280–289. https://doi.org/10.1016/j.tcm.2016.12.005

Farrell, P.C., & Richards, G. (2017). Recognition and treatment of sleep-disordered breathing: An important component of chronic disease management. *Journal of Translational Medicine, 15,* 114. https://doi.org/10.1186/s12967-017-1211-y

Javaheri, S., Barbe, F., Campos-Rodriguez, F., Dempsey, J.A., Khayat, R., Javaheri, S., ... Somers, V.K. (2017). Sleep apnea: Types, mechanisms, and clinical cardiovascular consequences. *Journal of the American College of Cardiology, 69*(7), 841–858. https://doi.org/10.1016/j.jacc.2016.11.069

Jonas, D.E., Amick, H.R., Feltner, C., Weber, R.P., Arvanitis, M., Stine, A., ... Harris, R.P. (2017). Screening for obstructive sleep apnea in adults: Evidence report and systematic review for the US Preventive Services Task Force. *JAMA, 317*(4), 415–433. https://doi.org/10.1001/jama.2016.19635

Kapur, V.K., Auckley, D.H., Chowdhuri, S., Kuhlmann, D.C., Mehra, R., Ramar, K., & Harrod, C.G. (2017). Clinical practice guideline for diagnostic testing for adult obstructive sleep apnea: An American Academy of Sleep Medicine clinical practice guideline. *Journal of Clinical Sleep Medicine, 13*(3), 479–504. https://doi.org/10.5664/jcsm.6506

Liu, L., Kang, R., Zhao, S., Zhang, T., Zhu, W., Li, E., ... Zhao, Z. (2015). Sexual dysfunction in patients with obstructive sleep apnea: A systematic review and meta-analysis. *Journal of Sexual Medicine, 12*(10), 1992–2003. https://doi.org/10.1111/jsm.12983

Patel, S.R. (2019). Obstructive sleep apnea. *Annals of Internal Medicine, 171*(11), ITC81–ITC96. https://doi.org/10.7326/AITC201912030

Pham, L.V., & Schwartz, A.R. (2015). The pathogenesis of obstructive sleep apnea. *Journal of Thoracic Disease, 7*(8), 1358–1372. https://doi.org/10.3978/j.issn.2072-1439.2015.07.28

Posadas, T., Oscullo, G., Zaldivar, E., Garcia-Ortega, A., Gomez-Olivas, J.D., Monteagudo, M., & Martinez-Garcia, M.A. (2020). Treatment with CPAP in elderly patients with obstructive sleep apnoea. *Journal of Clinical Medicine, 9*(2), 546. https://doi.org/10.3390/jcm9020546

Semelka, M., Wilson, J., & Floyd, R. (2016). Diagnosis and treatment of obstructive sleep apnea in adults. *American Family Physician, 94*(5), 355–360. https://www.aafp.org/afp/2016/0901/p355.html

Sutherland, K., & Cistulli, P.A. (2019). Oral appliance therapy for obstructive sleep apnoea: State of the art. *Journal of Clinical Medicine, 8*(12), 2121. https://doi.org/10.3390/jcm8122121

Tadic, M., Cuspidi, C., Grassi, G., & Mancia, G. (2021). Obstructive sleep apnea and cardiac mechanics: How strain could help us? *Heart Failure Reviews, 26*(4), 937–945. https://doi.org/10.1007/s10741-020-09924-0

Weaver, T.E. (2019). Novel aspects of CPAP treatment and interventions to improve CPAP adherence. *Journal of Clinical Medicine, 8*(12), 2220. https://doi.org/10.3390/jcm8122220

CHAPTER 35

Systemic Capillary Leak Syndrome

Enza Esposito Nguyen, DNP, RN, ANP-BC, AOCNP®

I. Definition: Increased capillary permeability, which causes accumulation of fluids and plasma into interstitial and extravascular spaces; fluid leak can lead to hypovolemic shock and death (Jeong et al., 2019; Raith et al., 2018; Xie et al., 2014; Xie et al., 2019).

II. Physiology/Pathophysiology (Jeong et al., 2019; Raith et al., 2018; Xie et al., 2014; Xie et al., 2019)
   A. Normal
      1. Small blood vessels carry blood and form the capillary system. Capillaries connect the smallest arteries (arterioles) with the smallest veins (venules).
      2. The vascular endothelium is a semipermeable barrier that controls the passage of fluid and macromolecules between the intravascular and interstitial spaces.
   B. Pathophysiology: The mechanism that leads to the increase in capillary permeability is not yet completely understood; however, several hypotheses have been suggested.
      1. Endothelial damage caused by cytokines, such as IL-2, IL-6, IFN-γ, TNF-α, and anti–IL-1β, and cluster of differentiation 8–positive lymphocytes is present and may have a role in triggering capillary leak syndrome.
      2. Endothelial cell damage may occur because of endotoxin exposure, ischemia, vessel injury with platelet deposition, or mechanical injury.
      3. Platelet-activating factor and vascular endothelial growth factor increase vascular permeability.
      4. Leukotriene B4, an inflammatory mediator, has been shown by in vivo studies to increase capillary permeability, but its role has yet to be determined.
      5. Inflammatory reactions cause microvascular permeability, capillary leak, loss of albumin, tissue edema, and hypoalbuminemia.
      6. A shift of fluid and albumin into body tissues occurs.
      7. An associated decrease in peripheral vascular resistance and intravascular volume and hypotension compound the fluid shift.
      8. Compartment syndrome, a complication of capillary leak syndrome, can occur with leakage of fluid into the muscular compartment, which increases the pressure inside that compartment.

III. Clinical features: Capillary leak syndrome was first described in 1960 and classified in the National Organization for Rare Disorders database in 2007. Often, it is diagnosed as anaphylaxis or septic shock, also known as *Clarkson disease* (Baloch et al., 2018; Druey & Parikh,

2017; Gottlieb et al., 2019; Jeong et al., 2019; National Organization for Rare Disorders, 2020; Raith et al., 2018; Siddall et al., 2017; Xie et al., 2014; Xie et al., 2019).

A. Classification
   1. Idiopathic: Unexpected, recurrent, nonseptic, related episodes of increased capillary permeability with large fluid and protein shifts and subsequent hypovolemic shock
      a) During the attacks, profound derangement of vascular endothelium results in leakage of plasma and proteins into interstitial tissue.
      b) Idiopathic episodes occur at regular intervals that span days and follow an inciting event, such as intense physical activity, allergies, or menstruation.
   2. Skin disease: Associated with erythroderma and pustular psoriasis
   3. Drug induced: Associated with retinoids, chemotherapy agents, immunotherapy, and G-CSFs
B. Etiology
   1. Demographic
      a) Idiopathic capillary leak syndrome is most prevalent during the fourth or fifth decade of life.
      b) It affects both sexes equally without geographic prevalence.
   2. HSCT
      a) During preparative regimen from high-dose chemotherapy and total body irradiation
      b) During time of engraftment, along with abnormalities in liver and renal function
      c) During rapid steroid tapers
      d) During infection (flu) or GVHD
      e) During infusion of donor WBCs
      f) During infusion of marrow/blood stem cells
      g) HLA-mismatched bone marrow transplant recipient
   3. Oxygen toxicity, decompression sickness when diving
   4. Kidney transplantation
   5. Liver transplantation
   6. Immunotherapy (e.g., IFN, IL-2): Most patients with IL-2 infusion develop symptoms within 24–72 hours with pruritus, orbital edema, and skin eruptions.
   7. Chemotherapy, especially gemcitabine
   8. Diagnosis of MGUS
   9. Infection or sepsis, including dengue shock syndrome
   10. POEMS syndrome (polyneuropathy, organomegaly, endocrinopathy, monoclonal protein, and skin changes): Rare paraneoplastic disorder associated with an underlying plasma cell dyscrasia
   11. Exposure to colony-stimulating growth factors
   12. Hereditary angioedema: Deficiency of C1 esterase
   13. Systemic mastocytosis
   14. Carbon monoxide poisoning
   15. Pustular psoriasis
C. History
   1. History of cancer and cancer treatment
   2. Current medications: Prescribed, over the counter
   3. History of presenting symptoms: Precipitating factors, onset, location, duration
   4. Changes in ADLs
   5. Past medical history: Recent viral or bacterial infection
   6. Family history: Hereditary angioedema
D. Signs and symptoms
   1. Fever

    2. Lethargy, malaise, obtundation

    3. Weight gain

    4. Chest pain

    5. Shortness of breath

    6. Productive or nonproductive cough

    7. Tachypnea

    8. Decreased urine output

    9. Ascites

    10. Edema and/or anasarca: Generalized total body edema

    11. Confusion, restlessness

    12. Cyanosis and pallor of skin, lips, and nail beds

    13. Flushing

    14. Hypothermia

    15. Findings are characterized in three phases.

       a) Prodromal phase: Flu-like symptoms, fever, irritability, abdominal pain, nausea, myalgia, polydipsia, weight gain (can last one to four days)

       b) Extravasation phase (leak): One to four days after prodromal phase with massive third spacing, leading to hypotension and generalized edema (one to three days)

       c) Recovery phase: Shift of fluid back into intravascular space with symptoms of fluid overload, such as dyspnea, tachycardia, cough, and anxiety

  E. Physical examination

    1. Vital signs: Weight (signs of gain), blood pressure (hypotension), pulse (tachycardia), fever

    2. Pulmonary: Presence of rales and rhonchi on auscultation; dullness on percussion over consolidated areas; absent over pleural effusion

    3. Cardiac: Presence of S_3, S_4, murmur, or gallop; tachycardia; peripheral edema; grades to evaluate degree of capillary leak syndrome are the following.

       a) Grade 1: Minimal ankle edema, minimal pitting

       b) Grade 2: Ankle edema with greater than 10-pound weight gain

       c) Grade 3: Peripheral edema, weight gain of greater than or equal to 10 pounds, pulmonary effusion compensated without need for treatment intervention

       d) Grade 4: Anasarca, ascites, pleural effusion with pulmonary deficits, generalized body edema

       e) Grade 5: Respiratory failure requiring artificial ventilation, marked hypotension requiring vasopressors

    4. Abdominal: Ascites, tenderness, distention, softness or firmness; hepatomegaly; splenomegaly; presence or absence of bowel sounds

    5. Integument: Presence of purpuric lesions, flesh-colored or erythematous lesions, livedo, rash in sun-exposed areas, erythematous papules

    6. Extremities: Compartment syndrome, pressure-induced muscle damage (e.g., excessive pain, palpable tightness of the extremity, progressive local paresthesia)

IV. Diagnostic tests (Gottlieb et al., 2019)

  A. Laboratory

    1. CBC with differential

       a) Elevated WBC count may increase suspicion of infection.

       b) Hemoconcentration may occur with an increased WBC count and hematocrit. This is often mistaken for sepsis or polycythemia vera, as hematocrit and leukocytosis may increase 60% from baseline.

    2. CRP: Elevated with sepsis, infection, or inflammation

        3. Procalcitonin: Elevated with sepsis or infection

        4. Urinalysis

           a) Presence of leukocytes may be caused by infection.

           b) Presence of protein or casts may indicate renal failure or disease.

        5. LFTs, including total and direct bilirubin, to evaluate for hepatobiliary disease

        6. Renal function tests, including urea and creatinine, to evaluate renal function; rhabdomyolysis resulting from compartment syndrome will increase creatinine.

        7. Serum albumin: May be decreased, leading to decreased oncotic pressure and edema

        8. Blood and urine culture to evaluate for causative organisms

        9. Serum tryptase to evaluate for possible anaphylaxis

       10. Serum immunofixation or protein electrophoresis (immunoelectrophoresis, SPEP) and possible bone marrow biopsy to determine MGUS paraprotein and evaluate for multiple myeloma

   B. Radiology

        1. Chest x-ray to evaluate noncardiogenic pulmonary edema, pleural effusion, pulmonary venous hypertension, interstitial infiltrates, and pericardial effusions

        2. CT scan of the chest, abdomen, and pelvis to evaluate for masses, effusions, or ascites

   C. Other

        1. Bronchoscopy, with or without lung biopsy, to rule out infection, hemorrhage, or other causes of respiratory distress

        2. ABGs to show hypoxia and carbon dioxide retention

        3. Pulmonary function tests to reveal decreased pulmonary compliance

        4. Hemodynamic monitoring including pulmonary capillary wedge pressure (PCWP) and cardiac output to measure fluid status (normal PCWP = 6–12 mm Hg; normal cardiac output = 4–8 L/min)

           a) Decreased PCWP may indicate hypovolemia.

           b) Increased PCWP may indicate left ventricular failure or cardiac insufficiency.

           c) Cardiac output may be increased early in capillary leak syndrome and decreased later in the syndrome.

        5. Skin biopsy: Mild perivascular, nonspecific dermal mononuclear infiltrates; mucinous deposits; mild lymphocytic infiltration

        6. Transpulmonary thermodilution and pulse contour analysis: Hemodynamic monitoring

        7. IM pressure measurements of the peripheral extremity to monitor for rhabdomyolysis in the presence of compartment syndrome

        8. ECG/echocardiogram to assess cardiac function and for heart failure

V. Differential diagnosis (Baloch et al., 2018; Druey & Parikh, 2017)

   A. Paraproteinemia or diseases/conditions with low protein levels

   B. Lymphoma and/or mast cell disease/MGUS

   C. Psoriasis

   D. Drug induced

        1. IV cyclosporine

        2. Amphotericin B

        3. Chemotherapy

        4. Immunotherapy

   E. Viral syndrome

        1. CMV, dengue

        2. GI viral disease

   F. Malaria

   G. Pneumonitis

H. Sepsis/toxic shock syndrome

I. DIC (see Chapter 120)

J. Anaphylaxis: Classical laryngeal edema and urticaria are absent; will not respond to epinephrine (see Chapter 150)

K. Polycythemia vera (see Chapter 128)

L. Gleich syndrome

M. Adrenal insufficiency

N. Primary amyloidosis

O. Carcinoid syndrome

P. Chronic illness including autoimmune disorders: SLE (see Chapter 110), multiple sclerosis, Sjögren syndrome

Q. Chronic heart or renal failure (see Chapters 42 and 86)

R. Cirrhosis (see Chapter 69)

S. Nephrotic syndrome (see Chapter 91)

T. CAR T cells

U. Compartment syndrome

VI. Treatment: Largely empiric and dependent on stage of presentation, with availability of transfer to an ICU setting (Baloch et al., 2018; Druey & Parikh, 2017; Gottlieb et al., 2019; Hajare et al., 2018)

A. Treat the underlying cause.

B. Anti-inflammatory therapies, such as Ig and IV theophylline, terbutaline, steroids, indomethacin, spironolactone, cyclosporine, plasmapheresis, and prostacyclin, may be used to help control symptoms such as hypotension, edema, and hypoperfusion.

C. Provide IV fluid replacement.

1. Inspect for jugular vein filling (intravascular space).

2. Assess for presence or absence of leg edema (interstitial space).

3. Evaluate for ascites or pleural effusion (third space).

4. Infusion of colloids, such as blood or albumin, is preferred to crystalloids.

5. Administration of diuretics is controversial because intravascular hypovolemia is present, and AKI may develop.

6. Restrict oral fluids to 500–1,000 ml daily. Gradually increase fluids as condition improves. Limit oral intake to electrolyte-concentrated fluids.

7. Monitor urine electrolytes and renal function for acute tubular necrosis; hemodialysis may be necessary for AKI.

D. Mechanical ventilation may be indicated if respiratory distress or failure occurs.

E. Prophylactic antibiotics may promote growth of organisms and are not recommended.

F. Sedating antihistamines can relieve itching and reduce anxiety (see Appendix H).

G. Administer vasopressors such as dopamine PRN for management of hypotension (see Chapter 48).

H. Provide nutritional support such as enteral or total parenteral nutrition to maintain high caloric intake because of increased energy expenditure.

I. IVIg infusion has shown promise in case reports of idiopathic capillary leak syndrome; role remains unknown.

J. Provide DVT prophylaxis in the presence of elevated clotting factors (see Chapter 43).

VII. Follow-up

A. Inpatient hospitalization is necessary to manage the signs, symptoms, and complications of capillary leak syndrome.

B. Perform daily monitoring of intake, output, weight, and renal and liver function.

C. Perform frequent chest radiographs to monitor pulmonary edema.

VIII. Referrals

A. Nephrologist: To evaluate for AKI and recommend management

B. Pulmonologist: To evaluate lung function, perform bronchoscopy, and recommend management

C. Orthopedist: For advanced compartment syndrome for possible fasciotomy, muscle debridement, and wound closure/care

D. Hematologist/oncologist: To evaluate serum electrophoresis/bone marrow biopsy and to provide recommendations and management for MGUS or oncology-related syndromes

E. Cardiologist: To evaluate heart function, interpret cardiac testing, and recommend management

F. Infectious disease specialist: To evaluate and recommend infection management

The author would like to acknowledge Dana L. Viviano, RN, BS, for her contribution to this chapter that remains unchanged from the previous edition of this book.

References

Baloch, N.U.-A., Bikak, M., Rehman, A., & Rahman, O. (2018). Recognition and management of idiopathic systemic capillary leak syndrome: An evidence-based review. *Expert Review of Cardiovascular Therapy, 16*(5), 331–340. https://doi.org/10.1080/14779072.2018.1456920

Druey, K.M., & Parikh, S.M. (2017). Idiopathic systemic capillary leak syndrome (Clarkson disease). *Journal of Allergy and Clinical Immunology, 140*(3), 663–670. https://doi.org/10.1016/j.jaci.2016.10.042

Gottlieb, M., Koyfman, A., & Long, B. (2019). Evaluation and management of abdominal compartment syndrome in the emergency room. *Journal of Emergency Medicine, 58*(1), 43–53. https://doi.org/10.1016/j.jemermed.2019.09.046

Hajare, K.R, Patil, P., & Bansode, J. (2018). Idiopathic systemic capillary leak syndrome. *Indian Journal of Critical Care Medicine, 22*(5), 369–371. https://doi.org/10.4103/ijccm.IJCCM_464_17

Jeong, G.H., Lee, K.H., Lee, I.R., Oh, J.H., Kim, D.W., Shin, J.W., ... Shin, J.I. (2019). Incidence of capillary leak syndrome as an adverse effect of drugs in cancer patients: A systematic review and meta-analysis. *Journal of Clinical Medicine, 8*(2), 143. https://doi.org/10.3390/jcm8020143

National Organization for Rare Disorders. (2020). Systemic capillary leak syndrome. http://www.rarediseases.org/rare-disease-information/rare-diseases/byID/1106/viewFullReport

Raith, E.P., Ihle, J.F., Jamieson, J., Kalff, A., & Bosco, J. (2018). Idiopathic systemic capillary leak syndrome presenting as septic shock: A case report. *Heart and Lung, 47*(4), 425–428. https://doi.org/10.1016/j.hrtlng.2018.04.008

Siddall, E., Khatri, M., & Radhakrishnan, J. (2017). Capillary leak syndrome: Etiologies, pathophysiology, and management. *Kidney International, 92*(1), 37–46. https://doi.org/10.1016/j.kint.2016.11.029

Xie, Z., Chan, E., Yin, Y., Ghosh, C.C., Wisch, L., Nelson, C., ... Druey, K.M. (2014). Inflammatory markers of the systemic capillary leak syndrome (Clarkson disease). *Journal of Clinical and Cellular Immunology, 5*, 213. https://doi.org/10.4172/2155-9899.1000213

Xie, Z., Kuhns, D.B., Gu, X., Otu, H.H., Libermann, T.A., Gallin, J.I., ... Druey, K.M. (2019). Neutrophil activation in systemic capillary leak syndrome (Clarkson disease). *Journal of Cellular and Molecular Medicine, 23*(8), 5119–5127. https://doi.org/10.1111/jcmm.14381

CHAPTER 36

Tuberculosis

Karen L. Pitman, RN, MSN, ARNP, NP-C

I. Definition: An airborne bacterial infection caused by *Mycobacterium tuberculosis*, an acid-fast bacillus characterized by the growth of nodules (tubercles) in the tissues, especially the lungs (Pai et al., 2016)

II. Physiology/Pathophysiology (Dheda et al., 2019; Furin et al., 2019; Pai et al., 2016)
   A. Normal
      1. The lungs are highly elastic, spongy tissue consisting of three right lobes and two left lobes.
      2. The bronchotracheal tree is a tubular system that provides a pathway for air to move from the upper airway to the alveoli of the lungs.
      3. The main bronchus is divided into three branches on the right and two on the left. The branches further divide into bronchioles.
      4. The bronchi transport air and, to some extent, trap noxious foreign particles in the mucus of their cavities and sweep the particles toward the pharynx via cilia.
   B. Pathophysiology: TB may occur in three stages: primary, latent, and active infection.
      1. When a person inhales droplet nuclei 1–5 microns in diameter, expelled by a person with TB disease, most of the larger particles become lodged in the upper respiratory tract and infection is unlikely to develop; however, if the droplet nuclei reach the alveoli, infection may occur.
      2. Small numbers of bacilli may spread through lymphatic channels to lymph nodes and through the bloodstream to more distant tissue and organs.
         a) The immune system responds by sending leukocytes, lymphocytes, and macrophages to surround the bacilli.
         b) Local lymph nodes swell and become inflamed.
         c) If the encapsulated bacilli (tubercles) and the inflamed nodes rupture, the infection contaminates the surrounding tissue and may spread through the blood and lymphatic system to distant sites.
      3. Two to 10 weeks after exposure and subsequent infection, the immune system usually is effective in preventing replication of the bacteria and development of disease.
      4. TB infection progresses to TB disease when the tubercle bacilli overcome the immune system and begin to multiply.
      5. TB disease is characterized by pulmonary infiltrates and formation of granulomas (chronic infection causes small tissue mass) with caseation (dead tissue decayed into a mass), fibrosis (thick scarring of connective tissue), and cavitation (collapse of body tissue, leading to cavities).

III. Clinical features: TB can develop in the lungs (85%), CNS, bones, and joints, or may be rapidly disseminated (miliary TB). Some people develop TB within weeks after infection, as their immune system is not able to contain the TB bacillus. Others may not develop TB until years after exposure, when their immune system is weakened. People infected with latent TB have a 5%–15% lifetime risk of becoming ill with active TB. More than 95% of all deaths reported due to TB are from developing countries. A total of 8,916 TB cases (2.7 cases per 100,000, representing a 1.6% decrease in number of cases) were reported in the United States in 2019, representing the country's lowest case count on record (Schwartz et al., 2020).

A. Risk factors for people recently infected with *M. tuberculosis*
1. Close contact with a person with TB disease
2. People who have emigrated from areas of the world with high rates of TB
3. Children younger than five years of age who have a positive TB test
4. Groups with high rates of transmission, such as homeless people, injection drug users, and people with HIV
5. People who work or reside with people who are at high risk for TB in facilities or institutions such as hospitals, homeless shelters, prisons, nursing homes, and residential homes for those with HIV

B. Risk factors for people with medical conditions that weaken the immune system
1. HIV infection is the strongest known risk factor for progressing from latent TB infection to TB disease. TB is a leading killer of HIV-positive individuals.
2. Substance abuse
3. Silicosis
4. Diabetes mellitus
5. Severe kidney disease
6. Low body weight
7. Organ transplantation
8. Head and neck cancer
9. Medical treatments with corticosteroids
10. Specialized treatment for RA or Crohn disease

C. Etiology
1. Latent TB
   a) People with latent TB infection have *M. tuberculosis* in their bodies but do not have TB disease and cannot spread the infection to other people. A person with latent TB infection is not regarded as having a case of TB disease and is not infectious.
   b) Approximately 5%–10% of infected people who do not receive treatment for latent TB infection will develop TB disease at some time in their lives. For people whose immune systems are weakened, the risk of developing TB disease is higher.
2. Active TB infection: TB occurs in every part of the world, but the majority of new active cases reported occur in Southeast Asia/Western Pacific (62%) and African (25%) regions.

D. History
1. History of cancer and cancer treatment
2. Current medications: Prescribed, over the counter
3. History of presenting symptoms: Precipitating factors, onset, location, duration, associated symptoms (e.g., cough, weight loss, night sweats)
4. Changes in ADLs

E. Signs and symptoms: More than 90% of individuals are asymptomatic at the time of primary infection and have a positive TB test.

1. Cough lasting three or more weeks, with or without sputum production; possible bloody sputum
2. Fatigue
3. Fever
4. Nights sweats
5. Unexplained weight loss less than 10 pounds in six months
6. Pleuritic or chest pain
7. Hemoptysis: Result of small vessel rupture in a cavity
8. Hoarseness: Associated with laryngeal TB

F. Physical examination: A physical examination cannot be used to confirm or rule out TB. Physical findings are absent in mild to moderate disease.
   1. Vital signs
      a) Elevated temperature
      b) Weight decreased to normal
   2. Pulmonary
      a) Dullness with decreased fremitus indicating pleural thickening or effusion
      b) Rales throughout inspiration or heard after a cough (post-tussive rales)
      c) Positive whispered pectoriloquy or tubular breath sounds in large areas of consolidation
   3. Extremities: Digital clubbing, particularly in people native to African countries; may be associated with severe destructive disease
   4. Lymph node: Cervical and axillary nodes, which may be enlarged (see Appendix D)

IV. Diagnostic tests (Bibbins-Domingo et al., 2016; Dodd & Schlesinger, 2017; Lewinsohn et al., 2017; Nachiappan et al., 2017; Sosa et al., 2019)
   A. Laboratory (see Table 36-1)
      1. Tuberculin skin testing (TST), known as purified protein derivative (PPD) testing or Mantoux testing, is helpful in identifying those who may be infected with *M.*

TABLE 36-1   Interpretation of Mantoux Skin Test

Reaction Size (mm)	Result	Group
< 5	Negative reaction	–
≥ 5	Positive reaction	• Suspected or known HIV infection • Recent contact with infectious case of tuberculosis • People with fibrotic changes on chest radiograph consistent with previous tuberculosis disease • People who are immunosuppressed
≥ 10	Positive reaction	• People who are recent arrivals (< 5 years) from high-prevalence countries • People who inject drugs • Residents of prisons, institutions, homeless shelters, and long-term care facilities • People with high-risk medical conditions (e.g., silicosis, diabetes, chronic renal failure, gastrectomy, carcinoma of the head or neck)
≥ 15	Positive reaction	• All people with no known risk factors for tuberculosis

Note. Based on information from Centers for Disease Control and Prevention, 2016.

tuberculosis. A newer detection test, IFN-γ release assay (IGRA), is positive within two to six weeks.

- a) It can take two to eight weeks after the initial TB infection for the immune system to react to TST and for the infection to be detected by TST.
- b) Those with a positive skin test who do not have TB disease are not considered to be infectious.
- c) Once an individual has been infected and has a true-positive TST or IGRA, usually the test will remain positive. Some people will lose reactivity with time.
- d) Indications and/or recommendations for applying TB skin tests
  - (1) Signs and symptoms of TB
  - (2) Recent close contact with known TB case
  - (3) Abnormal chest x-ray
  - (4) High risk of TB
  - (5) HIV infection
  - (6) Immigrants from Africa, Asia, South America, and Oceania; inner-city populations; healthcare workers; residents in nursing homes, prisons, or homeless shelters
- e) A negative test does not exclude the possibility of TB. Up to 25% of individuals with active TB have negative skin tests because of T-cell immunodeficiency.
- f) Booster effect
  - (1) Some people with TB infection may have a negative skin test reaction when tested many years after infection.
  - (2) The initial skin test may stimulate (boost) their ability to react to tuberculin. Positive reactions to subsequent tests may be misinterpreted as a new infection.
  - (3) Two-step testing is used to distinguish boosted reactions and reactions caused by a new infection.
  - (4) If the reaction to the first test is classified as negative, a second test should be performed one to three weeks later.
  - (5) A positive reaction to the second test represents a boosted reaction, and the person is classified as previously infected and treated accordingly (not a skin test conversion).
  - (6) Boosting has been reported in people who have received the bacillus Calmette-Guérin (BCG) vaccine.

2. PPD administration
   - a) Approximately 0.1 ml of five tuberculin units (PPD) is administered intradermally into dorsal surface of the forearm. A 6–10 mm wheal should develop.
   - b) Reactions are read 48–72 hours after administration. The transverse diameter of induration is measured by inspection and palpation. Erythema of the skin is not significant.
   - c) Interpretation of PPD: Three different cut points exist for individuals with varying risk factors for TB (see Table 36-1).
   - d) Multiple puncture (tine) tests are not recommended.

3. IGRA testing: QuantiFERON®-TB Gold or T-Spot®.TB
   - a) IGRA testing measures the release of IFN by T lymphocytes in response to stimulation with TB-specific antigens.
   - b) It is a highly specific test, even with previous BCG administration, and is at least as sensitive as skin testing in detecting latent TB and TB disease.
   - c) Neither TST nor IGRA testing differentiates latent TB from TB disease.

    d) IGRA testing is recommended over TST in the United States; IGRA is not recommended for use in combination with TST.

4. Skin tests for anergy (controls, mumps, *Candida*, tetanus) are no longer recommended, even for high-risk individuals.

    a) In immunosuppressed individuals, delayed-type hypersensitivity responses (TB skin tests) may decrease or disappear (anergy).

    b) Anergy may be caused by HIV infection, overwhelming miliary or pulmonary TB, severe or febrile illness, viral infections, Hodgkin lymphoma, sarcoidosis, live-virus vaccination, corticosteroids, or immunosuppressive drugs.

5. Sputum specimen collection for acid-fast bacillus

    a) At least three specimens should be examined by smear and culture.

    b) Sputum specimens should be collected at least eight hours apart, and at least one specimen should be collected in the early morning.

    c) Healthcare workers should supervise the first specimen collection and instruct the patient to do the following.

        (1) Clean and thoroughly rinse mouth with water. Breathe slowly and deeply three times.

        (2) After third breath, cough hard and try to bring up sputum (not saliva from the nasal passages or throat) and expectorate sputum (at least one teaspoon) into sterile container.

        (3) Stay in the room with door closed until coughing stops.

        (4) Aerosol induction may be necessary for patients having difficulty expectorating. While using a mist, breathe normally for 15 minutes and then cough hard.

    d) Smears positive for acid-fast bacillus may indicate active TB. Results may take up to 24 hours.

    e) Nucleic acid amplification tests can rapidly identify *M. tuberculosis* in hours, yielding earlier confirmation of disease, earlier treatment initiation, and decreased transmission risk.

    f) Routine smears positive for acid-fast bacillus may grow other atypical acid-fast bacillus.

    g) A culture that is positive and identified as *M. tuberculosis* confirms the diagnosis of TB. Results may take 10–14 days or up to four to six weeks. Culture remains the gold standard for laboratory confirmation of TB disease, and growing bacteria are required to perform drug-susceptibility testing and genotyping.

6. CBC to assess for anemia

7. LFTs for baseline of hepatic function prior to initiating therapy

8. HIV testing, as indicated

9. Renal panel to evaluate renal status prior to initiating therapy

B. Radiology: Chest x-ray, typically posterior–anterior and/or lateral view; CT scan may be necessary.

1. Results in people with TB may include abnormalities in the apex or posterior segments of the upper lobes or in the superior segments of the lower lobes, including infiltrates, mediastinal, or hilar lymphadenopathy, and cavitation. In addition, pleural effusions or solitary nodules may be present.

2. Unusual radiographic changes may occur in HIV-infected individuals with pulmonary TB.

3. Radiologic tests are useful in ruling out TB in individuals with a positive skin test and no symptoms; however, they cannot confirm TB.

C. Other
    1. Bronchoscopy
        a) Procedure is useful when person is unable to cough up sputum.
        b) Bronchial washings, brushings, and biopsies may be obtained.
        c) A bronchoscopy should never be substituted for sputum collection and testing but used as an additional diagnostic tool.
    2. Gastric aspiration
        a) Aspiration is useful when unable to obtain sputum by another method.
        b) Gastric acid is toxic to mycobacterium and must be processed immediately.
    3. Tissue biopsy is necessary for extrapulmonary disease because sputum and gastric samples are usually negative.

V. Differential diagnosis (Nachiappan et al., 2017)
    A. HIV infection
    B. Pneumonia (see Chapter 30)
    C. COPD (see Chapter 28)
    D. Cancer of the lung
    E. URI (see Chapter 37)

VI. Treatment (Borisov et al., 2018; CDC, 2018, 2020; Furin et al., 2019; Metersky & Schluger, 2017; Nachiappan et al., 2017; Nahid et al., 2016; Pai et al., 2016; Pettit et al., 2018; Sosa et al., 2019; Talwar et al., 2019)
    A. Prevention for healthcare workers coming into contact with patients with suspected or confirmed diagnosis
        1. Airborne isolation precautions, including negative pressure rooms with doors closed, should be initiated for a patient with confirmed or suspected TB disease.
        2. The patient should wear a tight-fitting surgical mask when in the healthcare facility if it does not have negative air ventilation. This stopgap measure should only be used while transfer to an appropriate facility is being arranged.
        3. Healthcare workers should wear an N95 respirator mask when the patient is in a negative air room or when the patient is outside of the room and is unable to wear a surgical mask. A HEPA-filter or positive air purifier respirator also is acceptable.
        4. Isolation precautions should be enforced until the patient has been deemed noninfectious by meeting all of the following criteria.
            a) Adequate therapy received for two to three weeks
            b) Favorable clinical response to therapy
            c) Three consecutive negative sputum smear results from sputum collected on different days
    B. Preventive pharmacologic therapy (see Figure 36-1)
        1. Isoniazid for six to nine months, 5 mg/kg PO daily (up to 300 mg daily) or 15 mg/kg PO two times a week (up to 900 mg weekly); for latent TB, 300 mg PO daily
            a) Used for people with latent TB infection (positive skin test) who do not have active disease
            b) Reduces the incidence of active disease by up to 90% in adherent individuals
            c) Use of pyridoxine supplementation to prevent isoniazid-induced neuropathy
        2. Monitor at least monthly for adverse reactions and compliance to prescribed therapy. Monitor LFTs for hepatotoxicity. Monitor for peripheral neuropathy.
        3. Review for contraindications, including pregnancy, liver disease, and previous drug reactions.

FIGURE 36-1	High-Priority Candidates for Tuberculosis Preventive Therapy

People in these groups should be given high priority for preventive therapy if they have a positive skin test reaction, **regardless of their age:**
- People with HIV infection
- Close contacts of people with infectious tuberculosis disease
- People whose skin test reaction converted from negative to positive within the past 2 years
- People with chest x-ray findings suggestive of previous tuberculosis disease
- People who inject illicit drugs
- People with medical conditions that appear to increase the risk for tuberculosis disease

People in these groups should be given high priority for preventive therapy if they have a positive skin test reaction and they are **younger than 35 years old:**
- People born in areas of the world where tuberculosis is common (e.g., Asia, Africa, Latin America)
- Low-income groups with poor access to health care
- People who live in residential facilities (e.g., nursing homes, prisons)
- Children younger than 4 years old
- People in other groups as identified by local public health officials

Note. Based on information from Centers for Disease Control and Prevention, 2018.

C. Treatment of active disease: TB medications are provided free of charge through state or local health departments.
　　1. Four regimens are recommended for treating patients with TB caused by drug-susceptible organisms. Each regimen has an initial phase of two months followed by a choice of several options for the continuation phase of either four or seven months.
　　2. Regimens usually includes four drugs.
　　　　a) Isoniazid: 5 mg/kg PO daily (up to 300 mg daily) or 15 mg/kg PO two times a week (up to 900 mg weekly)
　　　　b) Rifampin: 10 mg/kg PO daily (up to 600 mg)
　　　　c) Pyrazinamide: 15–30 mg/kg PO daily or 50–70 mg/kg two times a week
　　　　d) Ethambutol: 15–25 mg/kg PO daily; streptomycin: 15 mg/kg IM or IV daily (up to 1 g) or 25–30 mg/kg IM two times a week; or fluoroquinolone (levofloxacin): 750 mg PO daily
　　3. Three drugs may be adequate for initial regimen once resistance in the community is established.
　　4. Isoniazid and rifampin for nine months is acceptable for people who are unable to or should not take pyrazinamide.
　　5. Noncompliance is a major problem. Direct observation therapy may be necessary.
　　6. Drug susceptibility tests should be repeated after three months of treatment in patients who have had positive cultures.
　　7. Following four months of treatment, patients with positive cultures should be considered as having failed treatment and managed accordingly.
　　8. Rifampin is associated with many drug interactions and could reduce the efficacy of cytochrome P450 (CYP)3A4, CYP2C9, and CYP2C19 substrates (e.g., warfarin, azole antifungals, diltiazem, benzodiazepines, TKIs).

VII. Follow-up (CDC, 2020)
　　A. Short term after initial diagnosis
　　　　1. Report positive TB test promptly to the local health department.
　　　　2. Provide evaluation of close contacts, including TB tests.

    3. Educate the patient and household contacts on transmission of disease, importance of therapy and compliance, and the necessity of reporting noncompliance to health department.

    4. Provide a surgical mask for the patient to use when in the healthcare system.

B. For monitoring individuals on therapy

    1. Adhere to the prescribed protocol, including the counting of medications and periodic urine tests.

    2. Observe for signs and symptoms of hepatitis and neurotoxicity and assess CBC and LFTs every six to eight weeks while on treatment.

    3. Response to treatment

        a) For individuals with previously positive sputum cultures, obtain specimens for culture at least monthly until two consecutive cultures are reported as negative.

        b) When sputum is no longer positive for *M. tuberculosis* after two months of treatment, obtain one additional sputum culture.

    4. Chest x-ray

        a) For patients with positive cultures, consider chest x-ray at two months, and repeat chest x-ray at completion of therapy for future baseline.

        b) For patients with initial negative sputum cultures, obtain chest x-ray after two months of treatment to assist with a presumptive diagnosis and repeat chest x-ray at completion of treatment.

C. Long term

    1. Evaluate the patient at regular intervals for medication compliance and toxicity.

    2. Obtain sputum smears/cultures at two months, five months, and completion of treatment.

    3. Assess for response to treatment.

    4. Assess for complications such as bronchopleural fistulas, pleural effusion, and pneumonia.

    5. Monitor for long-term side effects of medications.

        a) Isoniazid: Hepatotoxicity, agranulocytosis, neuropathy

        b) Ethambutol: Hepatotoxicity, optic neuritis

        c) Rifampin: Hepatotoxicity, purpura, myelosuppression

VIII. Referrals

A. Infectious disease specialist: For management of drug therapy

B. Pulmonologist: For evaluation and treatment management

C. Local health department: For disease reporting, case follow-up, and supply of medications

The author would like to acknowledge Gayle K. Gilmore, RN, MA, MIS, for her contribution to this chapter that remains unchanged from the previous edition of this book.

References

Bibbins-Domingo, K., Grossman, D.C., Curry, S.J., Bauman, L., Davidson, K.W., Epling, J.W., Jr., … Pignone, M.P. (2016). Screening for latent tuberculosis infection in adults: US Preventive Services Task Force recommendation statement. *JAMA, 316*(9), 962–969. https://doi.org/10.1001/jama.2016.11046

Borisov, A.S., Morris, S.B., Njie, G.J., Winston, C.A., Burton, D., Goldberg, S., … Vernon, A. (2018). Update of recommendations for use of once-weekly isoniazid-rifapentine regimen to treat latent *Mycobacterium tuberculosis* infection. *Morbidity and Mortality Weekly Report, 67*(25), 723–726. https://doi.org/10.15585/mmwr.mm6725a5

Centers for Disease Control and Prevention. (2016). Tuberculin skin testing. https://www.cdc.gov/tb/publications/factsheets/testing/skintesting.htm

Centers for Disease Control and Prevention. (2018). Deciding when to treat latent TB infection. https://www.cdc.gov/tb/topic/treatment/decideltbi.htm

Center for Disease Control and Prevention. (2020). Treatment regimens for latent TB infections (LTBI). https://www.cdc.gov/tb/topic/treatment/ltbi.htm

Dheda, K., Gumbo, T., Maartens, G., Dooley, K.E., Murray, M., Furin, J., ... Warren, R.M. (2019). *The Lancet Respiratory Medicine* Commission: 2019 update: Epidemiology, pathogenesis, transmission, diagnosis, and management of multidrug-resistant and incurable tuberculosis. *Lancet Respiratory Medicine, 7*(9), 820–826. https://doi.org/10.1016/S2213-2600(19)30263-2

Dodd, C.E., & Schlesinger, L.S. (2017). New concepts in understanding latent tuberculosis. *Current Opinion in Infectious Disease, 30*(3), 316–321. https://doi.org/10.1097/QCO.0000000000000367

Furin, J., Cox, H., & Pai, M. (2019). Tuberculosis. *Lancet, 393*(10181), 1642–1656. https://doi.org/10.1016/S0140-6736(19)30308-3

Lewinsohn, D.M., Leonard, M.K., LoBue, P.A., Cohn, D.L., Daley, C.L., Desmond, E., ... Woods, G.L. (2017). Official American Thoracic Society/Infectious Diseases Society of America/Centers for Disease Control and Prevention clinical practice guidelines: Diagnosis of tuberculosis in adults and children. *Clinical Infectious Disease, 64*(2), 111–115. https://doi.org/10.1093/cid/ciw778

Metersky, M.L., & Schluger, N.W. (2017). New guidelines for the treatment of drug-susceptible tuberculosis from the American Thoracic Society, Center for Disease Control and Prevention, and the Infectious Diseases Society of America. Now comes the hard part. *American Journal of Respiratory and Critical Care Medicine, 194*(7), 791–793. https://doi.org/10.1164/rccm.201607-1419ED

Nachiappan, A.C., Rahbar, K., Shi, X., Guy, E.S., Barbosa, E.J.M., Jr., Shroff, G.S., ... Hammer, M.M. (2017). Pulmonary tuberculosis: Role of radiology in diagnosis and management. *RadioGraphics, 37*(1), 52–72. https://doi.org/10.1148/rg.2017160032

Nahid, P., Dorman, S.E., Alipanah, N., Barry, P.M., Brozek, J.L., Cattamanchi, A., ... Vernon, A. (2016). Official American Thoracic Society/Centers for Disease Control and Prevention/Infectious Diseases Society of America clinical practice guidelines: Treatment of drug-susceptible tuberculosis. *Clinical Infectious Disease, 63*(7), e147–e195. https://doi.org/10.1093/cid/ciw376

Pai, M., Behr, M.A., Dowdy, D., Dheda, K., Divangahi, M., Boehme, C.C., ... Raviglione, M. (2016). Tuberculosis. *Nature Reviews Disease Primers, 2,* 16076. https://doi.org/10.1038/nrdp.2016.76

Pettit, A.C., Shepherd, B.E., & Sterling, T.R. (2018). Treatment of drug-susceptible tuberculosis among people living with human immunodeficiency virus infection: An update. *Current Opinion in HIV and AIDS, 13*(6), 469–477. https://doi.org/10.1097/COH.0000000000000506

Schwartz, N.G., Price, S.F., Pratt, R.H., & Langer, A.J. (2020). Tuberculosis—United States, 2019. *Morbidity and Mortality Weekly Report, 69*(11), 269–289. https://doi.org/10.15585/mmwr.mm6911a3

Sosa, L.E., Njie, G.J., Lobato, M.N., Morris, B.S., Buchta, W., Casey, M.L., ... Belknap, R. (2019). Tuberculosis screening, testing, and treatment of U.S. health care personnel: Recommendations from the National Tuberculosis Controllers Association and CDC, 2019. *Morbidity and Mortality Weekly Report, 68*(19), 439–443. https://doi.org/10.15585/mmwr.mm6819a3

Talwar, A., Tsang, C.A., Price, S.F., Pratt, R.H., Walker, W.L., Schmit, K.M., & Langer, A.J. (2019). Tuberculosis—United States, 2018. *Morbidity and Mortality Weekly Report, 68*(11), 257–262. https://doi.org/10.15585/mmwr.mm6811a2

CHAPTER 37

Upper Respiratory Infection

Leslie Matthews, MS, ANP-BC, AOCNP®

I. Definition: Illnesses caused by an acute infection that involves the upper respiratory tract—the nose, sinuses, pharynx, or larynx (Kardos & Malek, 2017)

II. Physiology/Pathophysiology (Hakansson et al., 2018; Kincade & Long, 2016)
   A. Normal: The head and neck form an anatomically complex region that includes the nose, paranasal sinuses, ears and mastoids, oral cavity, pharynx, and larynx.
      1. Functions
         a) Exchange and filtering of air
         b) The intake and separation of foods and liquids from the airway
         c) Functions of speech, taste, smell, and hearing
      2. Respiratory ciliated epithelium lines the areas involved in air exchange.
      3. Squamous cells line the oral cavity, tongue, and oropharynx.
   B. Pathophysiology
      1. A variety of pathogens may cause inflammation of the pharynx, larynx, and nasal mucosa or lymph tissue.
      2. Inflammation of the mucosal membranes of the nose usually is accompanied by edema or nasal discharge resulting in obstruction of the sinus ostia.
      3. Transmission occurs by way of droplets or surface-to-surface contact in the common cold.

III. Clinical features: URIs are the most common acute illnesses in the United States and the industrialized world. The common cold, pharyngitis, laryngitis, rhinitis, sinusitis, OE, and OM are the most frequent infections that fall under the broader category of URIs (Degeorge et al., 2019; Kardos & Malek, 2017; Kinkade & Long, 2016; London & Ramanathan, 2018).
   A. Etiologies: Usually viral in nature
      1. Common cold: Caused by a variety of viruses including rhinoviruses (more commonly seen in early fall and mid to late spring), coronaviruses (occurring more in midwinter), influenza, parainfluenza, respiratory syncytial virus, and adenoviruses
      2. Pharyngitis
         a) Most often occurs as part of common colds caused by rhinovirus, coronavirus, or parainfluenza virus
         b) May be caused by infectious mononucleosis, herpangina, or group A *Streptococcus*

3. Laryngitis
   a) Most commonly associated with rhinovirus, influenza virus, parainfluenza virus, and adenovirus
   b) Occasionally associated with group A *Streptococcus*, *Moraxella catarrhalis*, and *Candida*
4. Rhinosinusitis
   a) May be allergic or nonallergic
   b) May be triggered by seasonal pollens, molds, or mildew
5. Tonsillitis
6. OM

B. History
   1. History of cancer and cancer treatment
   2. Current medications: Prescribed, over the counter
   3. History of presenting symptoms: Precipitating factors, onset, location, duration
   4. Changes in ADLs
   5. History of recent infections
   6. Past medical history of immune disorders

C. Signs and symptoms
   1. Common cold
      a) Malaise
      b) Rhinorrhea
      c) Sneezing
      d) Cough
      e) Sore throat
      f) Hoarseness
      g) Nasal congestion
      h) Enlarged cervical lymph nodes
   2. Pharyngitis
      a) Malaise
      b) Cough
      c) Sore throat
      d) Nasal congestion
      e) Inflamed pharynx
      f) Fever
      g) Enlarged cervical lymph nodes
   3. Laryngitis
      a) Sore throat
      b) Hoarseness
   4. Rhinitis
      a) Rhinorrhea
      b) Sneezing
      c) Cough
      d) Sore throat
      e) Nasal congestion
      f) Itchy eyes
      g) Enlarged cervical lymph nodes

D. Physical examination
   1. Common cold
      a) Vital signs: Absence of fever

      b) HEENT: Examination of the pharynx, nasal cavity, ears, and sinuses is usually negative. Occasionally, erythema or swollen nasal mucous membranes are noted.

      c) Lymph node: Possible enlarged cervical lymph nodes (see Appendix D)

      d) Pulmonary: Lungs typically clear

  2. Pharyngitis

      a) Vital signs: Possible fever

      b) HEENT

          (1) Possible herpangina: Small oral vesicles or ulcers on tonsils, pharynx, or posterior buccal mucosa

          (2) Erythema of tonsils and pharynx

          (3) Exudate in tonsillar area

      c) Lymph: Enlarged and tender anterior cervical lymph nodes (see Appendix D)

      d) Pulmonary: Lungs typically clear

  3. Laryngitis: Focus on HEENT examination.

      a) Hoarseness or loss of voice

      b) Presence of oral *Candida* in immunosuppressed patients appear as raised white patches

  4. Rhinosinusitis

      a) HEENT

          (1) Pale, boggy nasal mucosa with purulent discharge indicating infectious rhinitis or sinusitis

          (2) Clear, thin secretions indicating allergic and vasomotor rhinitis

          (3) Enlarged inferior nasal turbinates

          (4) Dark discoloration beneath both eyes ("allergic shiners")

          (5) Occasional enlarged tonsils or adenoids, sore throat, and palatal petechiae

          (6) Facial or sinus tenderness indicating rhinitis or sinusitis

      b) Pulmonary: Normal lung sounds

IV. Diagnostic tests: For the majority of URIs, no diagnostic tests are required (London & Ramanathan, 2018).

  A. Laboratory

    1. Rapid strep test to evaluate for *Streptococcus* infection

    2. Throat culture to evaluate for *Streptococcus, Neisseria gonorrhoeae, Neisseria meningitis, Neisseria lactamica, Arcanobacterium haemolyticum, Mycoplasma pneumoniae,* and *Chlamydia trachomatis*

    3. Mononucleosis spot test

    4. CBC with differential: Elevated WBC count in bacterial infections

    5. Cultures for any exudate or drainage, especially in neutropenic patients

  B. Radiology: Sinus x-rays; fluid-filled sinus cavities on x-ray indicate sinusitis.

  C. Other: Skin testing for allergies should be considered, if indicated.

V. Differential diagnosis: Immunocompromised patients are at increased risk for developing URIs (Rosenfield et al., 2015; Syke et al., 2018).

  A. Pharyngitis (see Chapter 4)

    1. Stomatitis (see Chapter 12)

    2. Rhinitis (see Chapter 11)

    3. Sinusitis (see Chapter 11)

    4. Epiglottitis

    5. Mononucleosis

  B. Laryngitis

       1. Oral candidiasis

       2. Pharyngitis (see Chapter 4)

       3. Esophagitis

   C. Rhinitis

       1. Sinusitis (see Chapter 11)

       2. OM (see Chapter 10)

       3. Deviated nasal septum

       4. Nasal polyps or foreign body in nasal passage

       5. Hypothyroidism (see Chapter 158)

VI. Treatment: Treatment is dependent on identifying the underlying diagnosis, determining the causative agent, and then initiating appropriate therapy. Numerous over-the-counter drugs are available to treat URI symptoms (Cots et al., 2015; Degeorge et al., 2019; Franck & Zehtabchi, 2019; Harris et al., 2016; Lemiengre et al., 2018; Lin & Kacker, 2019; London & Ramanathan, 2018; McKay et al., 2016; Rosenfield et al., 2015; Sedaghat, 2017; Syke et al., 2018).

   A. Common cold: Symptomatic treatment

       1. Fever

          a) NSAIDs: Avoid if history of bleeding ulcers, receiving anticoagulant therapy, and/or thrombocytopenic (see Appendix E).

          b) Acetaminophen: Caution patients to avoid taking greater than 4,000 mg of acetaminophen in 24 hours.

       2. Congestion/runny nose

          a) Steam or cool mist to help to liquefy secretions

          b) Antihistamines (see Appendix H)

          c) Oral decongestants (see Table 37-1)

          d) Oral antihistamine/decongestant combinations (see Appendix N)

          e) Topical decongestants (see Table 37-1)

          f) No evidence that expectorants are of benefit in URIs

          g) Saline nasal spray for congestion

       3. Cough

          a) Ipratropium bromide 1–2 inhalations four times a day

          b) Cromolyn available in a solution for nebulized treatments as indicated

TABLE 37-1	**Oral and Topical Decongestants for Symptom Treatment**
Agent	**Recommended Dose**
Oral decongestants	
• Phenylephrine	10–20 mg PO every 4 hours as needed
• Pseudoephedrine	Immediate release: 30–60 mg PO every 4–6 hours as needed Sustained release: 120 mg PO every 12 hours as needed Maximum daily dose: 240 mg
Topical decongestants	
• Oxymetazoline hydrochloride nasal solution	2–3 sprays in each nostril every 10–12 hours (usually in the morning and evening), not to exceed twice in 24 hours, limited to 3 days
• Phenylephrine hydrochloride	1–3 sprays of 1% solution may be repeated in 4 hours as needed for no longer than 3 days

Note. Based on information from Degeorge et al., 2019; Van Driel et al., 2018.

   c) Dextromethorphan: 10–30 mg PO every 4–6 hours PRN or 60 mg PO every 12 hours not to exceed 120 mg PO in 24 hours

 B. Pharyngitis (*Streptococcus*; see Chapter 4 and Appendix C)

  1. Penicillin V: 500 mg PO three times a day for 10 days

  2. Amoxicillin: 500 mg PO three times a day or 875 mg two times a day for 10 days

  3. Benzathine penicillin G: Single dose of 1.2 million units IM

  4. Cephalexin: 500 mg PO two times a day for 10 days

  5. Azithromycin: 500 mg PO on day 1 followed by 250 mg on days 2–5 (for patients with a penicillin or cephalosporin allergy)

 C. Laryngitis

  1. Pain

   a) Acetaminophen: Caution patients to avoid taking more than 4,000 mg of acetaminophen in 24 hours.

   b) NSAIDs: Avoid if history of bleeding ulcers, receiving anticoagulant therapy, and/or thrombocytopenic.

  2. Group A *Streptococcus*: See recommendations for pharyngitis (see Chapter 4).

  3. *M. catarrhalis*

   a) Amoxicillin/clavulanate: 500 mg PO every eight hours for 10 days

   b) Trimethoprim/sulfamethoxazole double-strength: 1 tablet PO two times a day for 10 days

   c) Erythromycin: 250 mg PO four times a day for 10 days

   d) Other alternatives: Azithromycin, clarithromycin, second- and third-generation cephalosporins

 D. Rhinitis: Combination of decongestant and antihistamines (see Appendices H, I, and N)

 E. Tonsillitis (see Chapter 4)

 F. OM (See Chapter 10)

VII. Follow-up

 A. Symptoms generally last 3–14 days; if lasting longer, consider alternative diagnosis, such as sinusitis, allergy, pneumonia, and bronchitis.

 B. Patients who are suspected of having acute bacterial or fungal infections should be seen in 24–48 hours if no significant improvement is noted.

 C. In patients whose symptoms improve, schedule return visit in 10–14 days.

VIII. Referrals: Not indicated unless symptoms do not resolve or are recurrent; referral to otolaryngologist or an allergist may be indicated.

The author would like to acknowledge Robert G. Hanks, PhD, FNP-C, RNC, for his contribution to this chapter that remains unchanged from the previous edition of this book.

References

Cots, J.M., Alós, J.-I., Bárcena, M., Boleda, X., Cañada, J.L., Gómez, N., … Llor, C. (2015). Recommendations for management of acute pharyngitis in adults. *Acta Otorrinolaringológica Española, 66*(3), 159–170. https://doi.org/10.1016/j.otorri.2015.01.001

Degeorge, K.C., Ring, D.J., & Dalrymple, S.N. (2019). Treatment of the common cold. *American Family Physician, 100*(5), 281–289. https://www.aafp.org/afp/2019/0901/p281.html

Franck, N., & Zehtabchi, S. (2019). Antibiotics for acute rhinosinusitis in adults. *American Family Physician, 100*(7). https://www.aafp.org/afp/2019/1001/od1.html

Hakansson, A.P., Orihuela, C.J., & Bogaert, D. (2018). Bacterial-host interactions: Physiology and pathophysiology of respiratory infection. *Physiological Reviews, 98*(2), 781–811. https://doi.org/10.1152/physrev.00040.2016

Harris, A.M., Hicks, L.A., & Qaseem, A. (2016). Appropriate antibiotic use for acute respiratory tract infection in adults: Advice for high value care from the American College of Physicians and the Centers for Disease Control and Prevention. *Annals of Internal Medicine, 164*(6), 425–434. https://doi.org/10.7326/M15-1840

Kardos, P., & Malek, F.A. (2017). Common cold—An umbrella term for acute infections of nose, throat, larynx and bronchi. *Pneumologie, 71*(4), 221–226. https://doi.org/10.1055/s-0042-116112

Kinkade, S., & Long, N.A. (2016). Acute bronchitis. *American Family Physician, 94*(7), 560–565. https://www.aafp.org/afp/2016/1001/p560.html

Lemiengre, M.B., van Driel, M.L., Merenstein, D., Liira, H., Mäkelä, M., & De Sutter, A.I.M. (2018). Antibiotics for acute rhinosinusitis in adults. *Cochrane Database of Systematic Reviews, 2018*(9). https://doi.org/10.1002/14651858.CD006089.pub5

Lin, J., & Kacker, A. (2019). Management strategies for recurrent acute rhinosinusitis. *Laryngoscope Investigative Otolaryngology, 4*(4), 379–382. https://doi.org/10.1002/lio2.294

London, N.R., Jr., & Ramanathan, M., Jr. (2018). Sinuses and common rhinologic conditions. *Medical Clinics of North America, 102*(6), 993–1000. https://doi.org/10.1016/j.mcna.2018.06.003

McKay, R., Mah, A., Law, M.R., McGrail, K., & Patrick, D.M. (2016). Systematic review of factors associated with antibiotic prescribing for respiratory tract infections. *Antimicrobial Agents and Chemotherapy, 60*(7), 4106–4118. https://doi.org/10.1128/AAC.00209-16

Rosenfield, R.M., Piccirillo, J.F., Chandrasekhar, S.S., Brook, I., Kumar, K.A., Kramper, M., … Corrigan, M.D. (2015) Clinical practice guideline (update): Adult sinusitis. *Otolaryngology—Head and Neck Surgery, 152*(Suppl. 2), s1–s39. https://doi.org/10.1177/0194599815572097

Sedaghat, A.R. (2017). Chronic rhinosinusitis. *American Family Physician, 98*(8), 500–506. https://www.aafp.org/afp/2017/1015/p500.html

Syke, E.P., Harrison, R.V., Terrell, J.E., & Zao, D.H. (2018). *Guidelines for clinical care ambulatory: Acute rhinosinusitis in adults.* University of Michigan. https://www.med.umich.edu/1info/FHP/practiceguides/Rhino/rhino.pdf

Van Driel, M.L., Scheire, S., Deckx, L., Gevaert, P., & De Sutter, A. (2018). What treatments are effective for common cold in adults and children? *BMJ, 363*, k3786. https://doi.org/10.1136/bmj.k3786

Cardiovascular

CHAPTER 38

Palpitations

Brenda K. Shelton, DNP, APRN-CNS, RN, CCRN, AOCN®

I. Definition (Clementy et al., 2018; Gale & Camm, 2016; Giada & Raviele, 2018)
   A. Subjective sensation described as heart skipping, fluttering, pounding, or racing
   B. Uncomfortable awareness of one's own heartbeat
   C. Disagreeable sensation of throbbing or movement in the chest or adjacent area
   D. Any rhythm that is not normal sinus rhythm with normal AV conduction

II. Physiology/Pathophysiology (Gale & Camm, 2016; Giada & Raviele, 2018; Wells & Tonkin, 2016; Wexler et al., 2017; Wilken, 2016)
   A. Normal: An electrical conduction system coordinates the muscular contractions of the cardiac cycle.
      1. An electrical impulse originating in the sinoatrial node of the right atrium stimulates each muscle contraction.
      2. The impulse travels through the atria to the AV node in the atrial septum down to the bundle of His and its branches, then Purkinje fibers, stimulating ventricular contraction.
      3. During sinus rhythm, the heart rate is in the normal range, the P waves are normal on ECG, and the rate is stable.
   B. Pathophysiology (see Table 38-1)

III. Clinical features: Clinical significance of palpitations is dependent on whether they are related to actual changes in cardiac function or an altered sensation of heartbeats with approximately 1% mortality. Up to 15%–22% of complaints never reach a confirmatory diagnosis because of intermittent nature. Palpitations are one of the most common problems of outpatients who seek medical attention. Usually benign, palpitations can occasionally be a manifestation of potentially life-threatening arrhythmia. Cardiac origin is present in 34%–43% of cases (Clementy et al., 2018; Gale & Camm, 2016; Giada & Raviele, 2018; Harskamp et al., 2017; Inayat et al., 2017; Matura et al., 2016; Miranda et al., 2018; Ruzieh et al., 2018; Tokuda et al., 2017; van der Wardt et al., 2017; Wexler et al., 2017; Wilken, 2016; Zhang et al., 2017).
   A. Etiology (see Table 38-1)
      1. Cardiac dysrhythmias causing palpitations occur as primary clinical conditions (e.g., Wolff-Parkinson-White syndrome) or secondary, induced by stressors on the heart (e.g., hypoxia, acidosis). Older adult patients are at greater risk of developing dysrhythmias and consequently palpitations.
         a) Rapid heart rates exceeding 150 bpm indicate dysrhythmias, such as sinus tachycardia, atrial flutter, atrial fibrillation, supraventricular tachycardia, or ventricular tachycardia. The sensation of palpitations may be related to the high heart rate or irregularity of the rhythm.

| TABLE 38-1 | Pathophysiology and Etiology of Palpitations |

Pathophysiologic Mechanism	Etiology Examples
Autonomic dysregulation with altered blood flow and syncope/near syncope	Hypertension Musculoskeletal deformities (e.g., pectus excavatum, kyphosis) Orthostatic hypotension: neurologic disease, fibromyalgia, calcium channel blockers, withdrawn hypertensive Pheochromocytoma Retroperitoneal or pelvic disorders (e.g., endometriosis, hematoma, polycystic ovary syndrome) Temporal lobe seizures with orthostatic tachycardia Vasomotor syndrome
Direct cardiac stimulation	Cardiac injury/contusion, tumor involvement Fluid and electrolyte imbalances Hyperthyroidism Stimulant medications/drugs, alcohol, anticholinergics, amphetamines, cocaine, nicotine, caffeine Thiamine deficiency
Extra-cardiac stimulation of the vagus nerve	Acidosis Beta-blocker withdrawal Constipation Extreme nausea/vomiting
Hyperdynamic circulation or increased blood volume	Hypercapnia Hyperthermia Hyperthyroidism Paget disease Pregnancy Renal failure Valvular incompetence
Simulation of atrial irritability	Lung cancer Pleural effusions Pneumonia
Sudden changes in heart rate or rhythm or cardiac movement in the thorax	Atrial fibrillation Ectopic heartbeats; premature contractions (e.g., atrial, junctional, ventricular) Exercise Intermittent heart block/bradycardia, ventricular tachycardia
Sympathetic stimulation (adrenergic surge) with increased automaticity and contractility	Anemia Anxiety Heart failure Hypoglycemia Hypoxemia Panic attack Stimulant medications/recreational drugs

Note. Based on information from Gale & Camm, 2016; Giada & Raviele, 2018; Wells & Tonkin, 2016; Wexler et al., 2017; Wilken, 2016.

b) Bradycardic dysrhythmias, such as sinus bradycardia or heart block, cause compensatory hyperdynamic cardiac performance and palpitations. Although not exclusively associated with bradycardia, prolonged QT syndrome (congenital or disease or medication induced) can cause both bradycardia and irregular beats with palpitations.

c) Intermittent irregular heartbeats, such as premature atrial, junctional, or ventricular beats, and blocked beats, produce irregular cardiac output that can be sensed as palpitations. Slow ventricular response atrial fibrillation also has been associated with palpitations, likely due to its irregularity.

2. Structural heart abnormalities and acquired heart pathologies produce turbulent blood flow through the heart, causing the sensation of palpitations.
   a) Inflammatory/infectious heart disorders: Endocarditis, myocarditis
   b) Valvular disorders: Mitral valve (most common)
   c) Displaced devices or sensing wires: Pacemakers, implantable defibrillators
   d) Cardiomyopathy with or without accompanying dysrhythmias; more common with hypertrophic cardiomyopathy
   e) Malignancy involving the heart: Lymphoma, myxoma, sarcomas (e.g., angiosarcoma, Kaposi sarcoma, synovial sarcoma), hepatocellular cancer
   f) Rheumatoid conditions involving the heart: SLE, systemic scleroderma, amyloidosis, relapsing chondritis, advanced Sjögren syndrome
   g) PH

3. Blood volume variations
   a) Hypervolemia produces hyperdynamic cardiac performance that can cause palpitations, such as with heart failure, renal failure, SIADH, and pregnancy.
   b) Hypovolemia causes compensatory increased cardiac contractility that can cause palpitations, such as with adrenal insufficiency, nausea and vomiting, hyperglycemia, and hypercalcemia.

4. Autonomic dysregulation occurring as a result of a neurologic condition (e.g., neurologic orthostasis) or loss of vascular tone (e.g., sepsis) can cause a near-syncopal syndrome associated with palpitations.

5. Sleep deprivation causes heart rate variability that can be felt as palpitations.

6. Etiologies with poorly defined mechanisms
   a) Lactose or other food intolerances
   b) Narcolepsy
   c) Athletics: More common in older individuals practicing endurance sports
   d) Postconcussion orthostatic tachycardia

B. History: Palpitations may be the first or only manifestation of dysrhythmias. A thorough health history can reflect strong risk factors or other previously overlooked signs or symptoms.

1. History of cancer and cancer treatment

2. Current medications: Prescribed (e.g., antidepressant, weight loss medications, antiparkinsonism), over the counter (e.g., allergy/cold medications containing antihistamines), herbals/nutraceuticals

3. History of presenting symptoms: Precipitating factors, onset, location, duration, prodromal or associated symptoms (e.g., dizziness, diaphoresis, nausea), alleviating factors (ask patient if coughing or Valsalva maneuver stops symptoms); symptoms lasting more than five minutes likely have a cardiac origin.

4. Changes in ADLs: Interfering with self-care, influencing perception of QOL

5. Past medical history: Heart defects, mitral valve prolapse, dysrhythmias, implanted cardiac devices, altered blood pressure, angina, MI, palpitations, rheumatic fever, endocarditis, anxiety or panic disorder, syncope, vertigo, seizures, anemia, nutritional changes, infection, electrolyte imbalances, endocrine dysfunction

6. Family history: Heart disease, anemia, orthostasis

7. Social history: Nicotine consumption (e.g., cigarettes, chewing tobacco, pipe smoking), illicit drug use (e.g., amphetamines, marijuana), caffeine intake, energy drink consumption

C. Signs and symptoms
   1. Sensations and awareness of heart beating, fluttering, skipping, or pounding
   2. Chest tightness or discomfort
   3. Shortness of breath
   4. Presyncope: Nausea, chest discomfort, headache, diaphoresis, palpitations, dyspnea, and paresthesias more likely associated with dysrhythmias
   5. Dizziness, vertigo
   6. Tinnitus
   7. Weakness
   8. Anxiety
   9. Pounding in neck
D. Physical examination: Focus on neurocardiac examination. Typically, the patient is not experiencing palpitations during the examination. An examination is useful in defining potential cardiovascular abnormalities and indications of dysrhythmia.
   1. Cardiac
      a) Apical heart rate: Fast or irregular
      b) Pulse deficit: Difference in the rate between the apical and radial pulse (radial lower); more indicative of premature beats than a rapid pulse
      c) Pulsus alternans or other irregularity: Variable peripheral pulses indicative of low or inconsistent cardiac output; may indicate heart failure
      d) Heart sounds: Possible gallops or murmurs present in valvular conditions, septal defects, heart failure, MI, pregnancy, or hyperthyroidism
      e) JVD/pulsations: Evidence of heart failure with venous congestion
      f) Peripheral pulse: Increased or decreased heart rate, irregular heart rhythm
      g) Orthostatic heart rate or blood pressure: Heart rate greater than 20 bpm higher value when sitting than when lying down; blood pressure greater than 20 mm Hg lower value when sitting than when lying down
   2. Neurologic: Sensory perceptual difficulties exacerbated when sitting or standing (e.g., vertigo, dizziness, tinnitus, presyncope)
      a) Observe patient standing up straight after bending over. This may elicit sensation if related to dysrhythmia.
      b) Observe patient lying down. Sensation may end if related to dysrhythmia.

IV. Diagnostic tests (Abi Khalil et al., 2017; Giada & Raviele, 2018; Quan, 2019; Reed et al., 2019; Sakhi et al., 2019; Wexler et al., 2017)
   A. Laboratory
      1. CBC to identify anemia and assess blood volume
      2. Blood chemistry
         a) Electrolytes to evaluate fluid and electrolyte imbalances that can cause dysrhythmias and to assess blood volume status
         b) BUN and creatinine to assess for kidney disease, risk for fluid excess
      3. Thyroid function tests: Free T_4 (thyroxin) and TSH to assess for thyroid disorders
      4. Cosyntropin test to evaluate for adrenal insufficiency
      5. Blood cultures to assess for sepsis, as indicated
      6. Blood levels of medications known to affect heart rate and rhythm, as indicated
   B. Radiology: Usually not indicated
   C. Other
      1. ECG rhythm strip in leads II, aVF, V_1, and 12-lead ECG: Clearly defines a particular portion of the P, QRS, and T waves, intervals, and their directional deflection

that helps to discern one rhythm disturbance from another; usually initial test to assess for clear cardiac pathology

    a) Prolonged QT increases risk for lethal ventricular dysrhythmia.

    b) Shortened PR suggests risk for re-entrant tachycardia.

    c) If the rhythm is not always present, an exercise stress test may be performed in an attempt to trigger the rhythm disturbance. If triggered by exercise, this test has increased value.

2. Echocardiogram may be used to identify clinical effects of a dysrhythmia, presence of valvular disease, presence of cardiomyopathy, or heart failure.

3. 24-hour Holter monitor provides 24 hours of continuous rhythm monitoring, which is particularly helpful if rhythm disturbance is intermittent. The patient also keeps a diary that will aid in identifying clinical symptoms directly related to rhythm disturbance. This test is used when patients describe palpitations and cardiac rhythm disturbances cannot be confirmed.

4. Event monitoring may be used with Holter monitoring to reduce the amount of tape that must be processed. Event monitoring only records when certain cardiac rhythm criteria are met or when the patient triggers a record button. Some event monitoring is linked to a central monitoring facility that can prompt emergency interventions PRN. Newer smartphone-operated single lead rhythm documentation may be a valuable first assessment.

5. Implantable loop recorders have proven helpful in diagnosing the etiology of intermittent dysrhythmias when Holter monitoring has not been definitive. Implanted recorders can run for extended periods, enhancing the potential for dysrhythmia detection.

6. Electrophysiologic testing is used for life-threatening dysrhythmias and enables the physician to map the source of dysrhythmia. It also provides an avenue for direct destruction of the dysfunctional cell pathway.

    a) Testing can be helpful for establishing the origin, signs, and symptoms when the patient has multiple dysrhythmias.

    b) Ablative therapy (e.g., laser, electrocautery, cryotherapy) can provide an alternative to medications.

7. Tilt table test is performed when palpitations are accompanied by dizziness or syncope. This test is a more accurate method of diagnosing orthostasis than bedside evaluation (see Appendix D).

V. Differential diagnosis (Aşkın et al., 2017; Wilken, 2016)

  A. Adrenal disease

  B. Aortic dissection type A, aneurysm

  C. Cardiac valve disease

  D. CAD: Angina, unstable angina, MI (see Chapters 40 and 49)

  E. Cardiomyopathy: Dilated, hypertrophic (Chapter 41)

  F. Endocarditis (see Chapter 46)

  G. FMS (see Chapter 101)

  H. Fluid overload

  I. Heart tumors

  J. Hypertensive urgency

  K. Hypoxia/respiratory failure

  L. Malignancy involving heart: Myxoma, hemangioma, lymphoma

  M. Rheumatoid condition involving heart: Autoimmune myocarditis, sarcoid, scleroderma, SLE

  N. Congenital conduction abnormalities: Wolff-Parkinson-White syndrome, Brugada syndrome

  O. PE (see Chapter 33)

P. Hyperthyroidism (see Chapter 157)

Q. Electrolyte imbalances (see Chapters 152–156)

VI. Treatment: Dependent on the etiologic factors, patient's tolerance, and planned treatment goals (Barley & Lawson, 2016; Giada & Raviele, 2018; Wells & Tonkin, 2016; Wexler et al., 2017; Wilken, 2016)

A. Do not treat palpitations if all of the following are true.
1. The cause of rhythm is known and treatable.
2. Significant clinical symptoms are absent, signaling cardiac instability.
3. Rhythm is unlikely to disintegrate into a life-threatening and unstable rhythm.

B. Low-risk features to treat and evaluate may occur over time.
1. Isolated infrequent palpitations not associated with exercise or waking from sleep
2. Absence of syncope
3. Normal ECG

C. Emergency management of palpitations
1. Provide supplemental oxygen and IV fluids if not contraindicated. Many etiologies of palpitations respond well to one of these general therapies.
2. Determine the patient's cardiac instability and need for emergency medical care (e.g., chest pain, hypotension, dyspnea, hypoxemia, mental status changes).
3. If associated with rapid pulse and heart rate, have patient perform a vagal maneuver.

D. Correct underlying etiology or risk factors, if known.
1. Implant devices such as pacemakers to assess function or control dysrhythmia.
2. Discontinue medications that may increase risk of dysrhythmias.
3. Eliminate nicotine. Alcohol and caffeine should be consumed in moderation.
4. Regulate metabolic rate. Control fevers and other factors that increase metabolic rate (e.g., stress, pain).
5. Correct vascular volume disturbances. Administer fluids or diuretics.
6. Correct electrolyte imbalances (see Chapters 152–156) or nutritional deficits.
7. Supportive therapy for orthostatic hypotension may include increased salt intake or compression wrapping of the lower legs.
8. Treat dysrhythmias according to defined standards (see Chapter 45).
9. Treat endocarditis (see Chapter 46) or primary cardiac diseases, such as hypertension (see Chapter 47), MI (see Chapter 49), cardiomyopathy (see Chapter 41), and heart failure (see Chapter 42), according to defined standards.

E. Evidence-based principles for care
1. Recommendations are all consensus based.
2. All patients are evaluated for ischemic etiology.
3. Nonspecific ECG abnormalities should not be considered normal and warrant investigation.
4. Syncope or autonomic dysfunction warrants tilt-table testing.
5. Evidence of heart failure or structural disease warrants echocardiogram evaluation.

F. Supportive care
1. Assist the patient in identifying triggers for symptoms and altering lifestyle (e.g., rest patterns; consumption of alcohol, caffeine, or nicotine) to reduce risk.
2. Provide patient education regarding orthostasis management or administration of antidysrhythmic medications.
3. Herbal agents are believed to abrogate palpitations (e.g., thiamine, coenzyme Q).
4. Perform safety assessment of the patient and living circumstances based on severity of symptoms and probable etiology or risk of serious adverse effects. Act on this safety assessment to modify living conditions or supervision of ADLs.

VII. Follow-up (Gale & Camm, 2016)
   A. Patients with untreated palpitations that resolve spontaneously may not need formalized follow-up.
   B. Patients should avoid cardiac stimulants (e.g., caffeine, alcohol, tobacco, antihistamines) indefinitely.
   C. Patients with high-risk features associated with syncope should be evaluated promptly by a cardiologist.
   D. Patients requiring medical treatment for dysrhythmias may have routine laboratory and specific cardiac tests performed on a periodic basis depending on the type and etiology of the dysrhythmia.
      1. Management of the dysrhythmias may require an electrophysiologist or cardiologist.
      2. Antiarrhythmic medication serum levels may need to be monitored.
      3. Electrolyte levels should be maintained at high-normal when the patient has experienced palpitations or is at risk for dysrhythmias (e.g., potassium greater than 4 mEq/L, magnesium greater than 2 mEq/L).

VIII. Referrals (Barley & Lawson, 2016; Owens et al., 2016)
   A. Cardiologist: For evaluation of dysrhythmias of unknown origin or when refractory to treatment; symptoms and specific diagnosis will determine whether to consult a dysrhythmia specialist or interventional cardiologist.
   B. Neurologist: For assessment and management of syncope or orthostasis
   C. Pharmacist: To advise patients on the correct administration of antidysrhythmics; many of these agents have altered absorption with food, pH levels, or other concomitant medications.
   D. Dietitian: To assist the patient with revising eating habits to decrease the risk of dysrhythmias (e.g., avoiding caffeine), supplementing electrolytes, or altering salt intake (more if orthostasis, less if hypervolemic)
   E. Psychologist or psychology support professional: For cognitive behavioral approaches to symptom distress management, which have been effective for treatment of nonemergent etiologies of palpitations
   F. Tobacco cessation or alcohol rehabilitation programs, if appropriate

References

Abi Khalil, C., Haddad, F., & Al Suwaidi, J. (2017). Investigating palpitations: The role of Holter monitoring and loop recorders. *BMJ, 358,* j3123. https://doi.org/10.1136/bmj.j3123

Aşkın, A., Güvendi, E., Özkan, A., Şimşek, E.Ç., Kocabaş, U., & Tosun, A. (2017). Prevalence of fibromyalgia syndrome and its correlations with arrhythmia in patients with palpitations. *Acta Medica, 60*(4), 146–151. https://doi.org/10.14712/18059694.2018.10

Barley, E., & Lawson, V. (2016). Using health psychology techniques to manage chronic physical symptoms. *British Journal of Nursing, 25*(22), 1258–1262. https://doi.org/10.12968/bjon.2016.25.22.1258

Clementy, N., Fourquet, A., Andre, C., Bisson, A., Pierre, B., Fauchier, L., … Angoulvant, D. (2018). Benefits of an early management of palpitations. *Medicine, 97*(28), e11466. https://doi.org/10.1097/MD.0000000000011466

Gale, C.P., & Camm, A.J. (2016). Assessment of palpitations. *BMJ, 352,* h5649. https://doi.org/10.1136/bmj.h5649

Giada, F., & Raviele, A. (2018). Clinical approach to patients with palpitations. *Cardiac Electrophysiology Clinics, 10*(2), 387–396. https://doi.org/10.1016/j.ccep.2018.02.010

Harskamp, R.E., Thole, O.B., & Moggré, I. (2017). Palpitations: When you hear hoof beats don't forget to think zebras. *Practitioner, 261*(1803), 23–25.

Inayat, K., Danish, N., & Hassan, L. (2017). Symptoms of menopause in peri and postmenopausal women and their attitude towards them. *Journal of Ayub Medical College, Abbottabad, Pakistan, 29*(3), 477–480.

Matura, L.A., McDonough, A., & Carroll, D.L. (2016). Symptom prevalence, symptom severity, and health-related quality of life among young, middle, and older adults with pulmonary hypertension. *American Journal of Hospice and Palliative Medicine, 33*(3), 214–221. https://doi.org/10.1177/1049909114554079

Miranda, N.A., Boris, J.R., Kouvel, K.M., & Stiles, L. (2018). Activity and exercise intolerance after concussion: Identification and management of postural orthostatic tachycardiac syndrome. *Journal of Neurologic Physical Therapy, 42*(3), 163–171. https://doi.org/10.1097/NPT.0000000000000231

Owens, J.E., Schorling, J., Plews-Ogan, M., Goodman, M., Moorman, R., Zaklin, R., & Dent, J. (2016). A randomized controlled trial evaluating mindfulness-based stress reduction (MBSR) for the treatment of palpitations: A pilot study. *International Journal of Cardiology, 223,* 25–27. https://doi.org/10.1016/j.ijcard.2016.08.183

Quan, K.J. (2019). Palpitation: Extended electrocardiogram monitoring: Which tests to use and when. *Medical Clinics of North America, 103*(5), 785–791. https://doi.org/10.1016/j.mcna.2019.05.005

Reed, M.J., Grubb, N.R., Lang, C.C., O'Brien, R., Simpson, K., Padarenga, M., … Coats, T. (2019). Multi-centre randomized controlled trial of a smart phone-based event recorder alongside standard care versus standard care for patients presenting to the emergency department with palpitation and pre-syncope: The IPED (Investigation of Palpitations in the ED) study. *EClinicalMedicine, 3*(8), 37–46. https://doi.org/10.1016/j.eclinm.2019.02.005

Ruzieh, M., Moustafa, A., Sabbagh, E., Karim, M.M., & Karim, S. (2018). Challenges in treatment of inappropriate sinus tachycardia. *Current Cardiology Reviews, 14*(1), 42–44. https://doi.org/10.2174/1573403X13666171129183826

Sakhi, R., Theuns, D.A.M.J., Szili-Torok, T., & Yap, S.-C. (2019). Insertable cardiac monitors: Current indications and devices. *Expert Review of Medical Devices, 16*(1), 45–55. https://doi.org/10.1080/17434440.2018.1557046

Tokuda, H., Nakago, S., Kato, H., Oishi, T., & Kotsuji, F. (2017). Bleeding in the retroperitoneal space under the broad ligament as a result of uterine perforation after dilatation and curettage: Report of a case. *Journal of Obstetrics and Gynaecology Research, 43*(4), 779–782. https://doi.org/10.1111/jog.13252

van der Wardt, V., Harrison, J.K., Welsh, T., Conroy, S., & Gladman, J. (2017). Withdrawal of antihypertensive medication: A systematic review. *Journal of Hypertension, 35*(9), 1742–1749. https://doi.org/10.1097/HJH.0000000000001405

Wells, R., & Tonkin, A. (2016). Clinical approach to autonomic dysfunction. *Internal Medicine Journal, 46*(10), 1134–1139. https://doi.org/10.1111/imj.13216

Wexler, R.K., Pleister, A., & Raman, S.V. (2017). Palpitations: Evaluation in the primary care setting. *American Family Physician, 96*(12), 784–789. https://www.aafp.org/afp/2017/1215/p784.html

Wilken, J. (2016). Evidence-based recommendations for the evaluation of palpitations in the primary care setting. *Medical Clinics of North America, 100*(5), 981–989. https://doi.org/10.1016/j.mcna.2016.04.006

Zhang, R., Gupta, D., & Albert, S.G. (2017). Pheochromocytoma as a reversible cause of cardiomyopathy: Analysis and review of the literature. *International Journal of Cardiology, 249,* 319–3223. https://doi.org/10.1016/j.ijcard.2017.07.014

CHAPTER 39

Peripheral Edema

Wendy H. Vogel, MSN, FNP, AOCNP®

I. Definition: Palpable swelling due to accumulation of fluid within the interstitial spaces localized to the peripheries; may occur in the upper as well as the lower extremities (Trayes et al., 2013)

II. Physiology/Pathophysiology (Trayes et al., 2013)
   A. Normal
      1. Body fluids are essential to the internal and external environment of a healthy cell.
      2. Body fluids contain water and dissolved substances called *electrolytes*.
      3. Body fluids consist mainly of water, which is 60% of body weight. Body fluid is contained in two compartments separated by semipermeable membranes.
         a) Intracellular refers to inside the cell.
         b) Extracellular refers to outside the cell.
      4. The balance of hemodynamic forces along the capillary wall and the proper functioning of lymphatic vessels prevent edema.
      5. Fluid is usually removed from interstitial spaces by vascular return from the capillary bed or lymphatic drainage.
   B. Pathophysiology (Kumarasinghe & Carroll, 2015; Trayes et al., 2013)
      1. Edema is caused by an imbalance in capillary hemodynamics between the forces containing fluid within the vasculature and those forcing fluid through the vascular wall to interstitial spaces where pressure is lower (increased capillary hydrostatic pressure, decreased capillary oncotic pressure, and/or increased capillary permeability).
         a) In heart failure, endothelin is released, which causes arterial vasoconstriction.
         b) Albumin causes retention of fluid in the vascular bed. When albumin is decreased, fluid leaks into the interstitial spaces.
         c) Increased capillary permeability may be caused by endotoxins and cellular mediators.
      2. Extrinsic sodium and water retention by the kidneys caused by renal failure, reduction of cardiac output (as in heart failure), or systemic vascular resistance (as in cirrhosis) can cause edema. Stimulation of the renin–angiotensin system causes an increase in pressure in the vascular bed, thus forcing fluid into interstitial spaces.
      3. Edema can be caused by lymphatic or venous obstruction forcing fluid to move through the blood vessel wall into the tissue.

III. Clinical features: Peripheral edema is often a nonspecific finding common to many diseases that range from benign to life threatening. Edema is a problem of fluid distribution and does not always indicate fluid excess. For example, renal sodium and water retention is an appropriate compensatory response to restore tissue perfusion. When interstitial volume increases by 2.5–3 L, edema becomes clinically apparent. Peripheral edema can be pitting or nonpitting. The presence of tissue depression applied to the area for at least five seconds is considered pitting (Breznik et al., 2018; Friedman et al., 2017; Frison et al., 2015; Kumarasinghe & Carroll, 2015; Simon, 2014; Trayes et al., 2013; Veizi et al., 2016; Yang et al., 2017; Yeo et al., 2016; Zimmerman & Davis, 2018).

A. Etiology
1. The most common causes of peripheral edema are heart failure (right or left ventricular failure), cirrhosis, nephrotic syndrome (or other renal disease), and edema related to menses or pregnancy.
2. Some drugs may cause peripheral edema due to vasodilation, vasoconstriction, or an adverse drug reaction.
   a) Thiazolidinediones
   b) Calcium channel blockers
   c) NSAIDs (see Appendix E)
   d) Estrogens
   e) Chemotherapy agents: Docetaxel, pemetrexed
   f) Immunotherapy agents: Mitogen-activated protein kinase (MEK) inhibitors
   g) Opioids
   h) Drugs that cause peripheral edema (see Figure 39-1)
   i) Drug-induced peripheral edema usually occurs in the lower extremities within a few weeks after drug initiation and usually is dose dependent.
3. Unilateral extremity edema indicates a local inflammatory or obstructive response.
4. Unilateral upper extremity edema is rare and usually is the result of obstruction of the subclavian vein or innominate vein by a malignancy or thrombosis, as well as lymphedema, cellulitis, or a catheter-induced event.

FIGURE 39-1   Medications That May Cause Peripheral Edema[a]

- Antidepressants: Selective serotonin reuptake inhibitors, monoamine oxidase inhibitors
- Antidiabetics, thiazolidinediones class: Rosiglitazone, pioglitazone
- Antifungals
- Antihypertensives: Clonidine, methyldopa, reserpine
- Antineoplastics: Docetaxel, gemcitabine, lenalidomide, thalidomide
- Beta-blockers
- Calcium channel blockers, dihydropyridines class: Nicardipine, nifedipine
- Corticosteroids: Long-term intake
- Direct vasodilators: Nitrates
- Estrogen/progesterones
- Hormonal agents: Testosterone
- Hormonal antineoplastics: Megestrol, leuprolide
- Immunotherapy such as mitogen-activated protein kinase (MEK) inhibitors
- Insulin
- Interferons
- Monoclonal antibodies: Cetuximab, rituximab
- Morphine sulfate and other opioids
- Neurologic agents: Pregabalin, gabapentin
- Nonsteroidal anti-inflammatory drugs
- Selective and nonselective cyclooxygenase inhibitors
- Temsirolimus

---

[a] Listing is not all-inclusive.

Note. Based on information from Simon, 2014; Trayes et al., 2013; Veizi et al., 2016; Yang et al., 2017; Yeo et al., 2016.

    5. Bilateral upper extremity edema is rare and usually is the result of obstruction of the SVC by a malignancy or thrombosis.

    6. Decreased physical activity decreases the ability of calf muscles to pump fluid, thus decreasing venous return, increasing venous stasis, and resulting in edema.

    7. Malnutrition, such as decreased protein intake, causes decreased colloid osmotic–oncotic pressure, resulting in leakage of fluid into the interstitial space.

    8. Muscle strain causes tearing or twisting to the extremity.

B. History

    1. History of cancer and cancer treatment

    2. Current medications: Prescribed, over the counter, supplements, alternative treatments

    3. History of presenting symptoms: Precipitating factors, onset, location, duration, characteristics of edema (e.g., persistent or intermittent, pitting or nonpitting), associated symptoms (e.g., pain, numbness, tingling, swelling, or cramping of extremities; shortness of breath at rest and with activity; chest discomfort at rest and with activity; constipation; cold intolerance; warmth of extremity; discolored lower extremities)

    4. Changes in ADLs

    5. Past medical history: Heart disease, DVT, diabetes, hypertension, heart murmur, alcohol abuse

    6. Past surgical history: Lymph node dissection, placement of vascular access device

C. Signs and symptoms

    1. Edematous extremities: Bilateral or unilateral

    2. Pitting or nonpitting edema

    3. Difficulty walking or using upper extremities

    4. Presence of other signs of edema, including periorbital edema or ascites

    5. Associated symptoms may assist in determining etiology of peripheral edema.

        a) Pulmonary edema: Shortness of breath, orthopnea, chest pain, fatigue

        b) Heart failure: Swelling in abdomen, dyspnea on exertion, orthopnea, paroxysmal nocturnal dyspnea, sudden weight gain, fatigue

        c) Cirrhosis: Swelling in abdomen, change in skin color, itching, feelings of fullness or right upper quadrant pain, anorexia, fatigue, nausea, flatulence, change in bowel habits, easy bruising or bleeding

        d) Thrombosis: Unilateral edema, pain, warmth or redness of extremity, poor response to diuretics, history of venous catheter, feeling of fullness in fingers or feet, low-grade fevers

        e) Lymphedema: History of surgery with lymph node dissection, unilateral edema, changes in skin texture

        f) Nephrotic syndrome: Frequent urination

D. Physical examination: Assists in establishing diagnosis, noting distribution of edema, signs of increased central venous pressure, and signs of pulmonary edema

    1. Vital signs

        a) Weight loss or gain; peripheral edema may not be clinically apparent until there is approximately a 10% weight increase.

        b) Tachycardia and hypertension with heart disease

        c) Possible decreased or absent pulses in heart disease and peripheral vascular disease

    2. HEENT: JVD suggestive of heart disease and heart failure; periorbital edema noted in nephrotic syndrome; edema of face, face plethora, and neck suggestive of SVC syndrome

    3. Integument

        a) Alterations of skin integrity such as cellulitis

        b) Hemosiderin staining because of RBC breakdown and deposits in the skin *c)* Peripheral vascular changes such as mottled appearance

      d) Signs of infection or trauma

4. Respiratory: Presence of lung crackles, tachypnea, diaphoresis, rales suggestive of pulmonary edema

5. Cardiac: Heart murmur, gallop, displaced point of maximal intensity suggestive of heart disease

6. Abdominal

      a) Presence of ascites (e.g., abdominal distention, dullness to percussion, fluid wave with percussion), positive hepatojugular reflux indicative of heart failure or cirrhosis (see Appendix D)

      b) Distended abdominal wall veins, spider telangiectasias, splenomegaly, hepatomegaly noted in cirrhosis

7. Extremities

      a) Assess for pitting, and document clinical grade (1+ to 4+). Ankle circumference measurement is a reliable method of assessment.

      b) Pitting edema is noted when applying pressure to edematous limb for at least five seconds and noting a dent in the tissue surface due to the movement of excess interstitial water in response to pressure. It is noted in the lower extremities of ambulatory patients and over the sacrum in nonambulatory patients.

      c) Nonpitting edema may indicate lymphatic obstruction or hypothyroidism.

      d) Severe edema may precipitate skin breakdown, as with pressure ulcers.

      e) Thrombosis/obstruction: Unilateral edema, warmth, erythema, palpable cord, positive Homan sign, dilation of collateral veins in chest/neck, edema of face, neck, and upper chest

      f) Lymphedema: Unilateral edema with history of surgery on ipsilateral extremity, nonpitting edema, cutaneous and subcutaneous thickening, positive Stemmer sign (inability to tent skin at base of digits on affected extremity)

      g) Upper extremity edema can be suggestive of SVC syndrome.

IV. Diagnostic tests (Kumarasinghe & Carroll, 2015; Trayes et al., 2013)

  A. Laboratory

    1. Nephrotic syndrome indications

      a) Serum albumin: Decreased; less than 3 g/dl

      b) Total protein: Decreased; less than 6 g/dl

      c) Urine protein excretion: greater than 3.5 g/24 hours

      d) Serum creatinine and BUN: Increased

    2. Cholesterol: Fasting cholesterol greater than 200 g/dl

    3. Serum creatinine: Increased in nephrotic syndrome

    4. Antinuclear antibody: Increase possibly indicative of SLE-inducing nephrotic syndrome

    5. LFTs: Elevated AST and alanine transaminase, alkaline phosphatase, and bilirubin indicating liver-induced condition

    6. PT: Prolonged indicative of liver-induced condition

    7. SPEP: Serum protein levels decreased in liver disease

    8. TSH to evaluate thyroid-related edema (myxedema)

    9. Urinalysis: Red cell casts possibly signifying active renal disease

    10. BNP: A cellular mediator released in CHF that increases capillary permeability

  B. Radiology

    1. Chest x-ray: Kerley B lines (increased interstitial edema), cardiac enlargement indicating heart failure

2. Echocardiogram: Decreased left ventricular ejection fraction, valvular disease, hypertrophy, chamber size suggestive of heart failure

3. Duplex ultrasonography to evaluate thrombophlebitis or DVT

C. Other

1. Renal or liver biopsy to make a definitive diagnosis, if needed

2. Paracentesis to make a definitive diagnosis or for comfort measures, if needed

3. Pulmonary capillary wedge pressure: Value of greater than 18 mm Hg indicative of pulmonary edema due to heart disease or primary renal sodium retention

4. ECG to assess for heart disease

V. Differential diagnosis (Kumarasinghe & Carroll, 2015; Trayes et al., 2013)

A. Unilateral lower extremity edema: Indicates a local inflammatory response or obstruction

1. Lymphedema (see Chapter 112)

2. Venous insufficiency

3. Thrombophlebitis (see Chapter 164)

4. Cellulitis (see Chapter 19)

5. Ruptured Baker cyst

6. Gynecologic cancer with obstruction

7. DVT (see Chapter 43)

8. Trauma

B. Bilateral lower extremity edema

1. CHF (see Chapter 42)

2. Nephrotic syndrome (see Chapter 91)

3. Liver failure/cirrhosis (see Chapter 69)

4. Acute glomerulonephritis

5. Dependent edema

6. Medications (see Figure 39-1)

7. Venous insufficiency

8. Pregnancy

9. Idiopathic

C. Unilateral upper extremity edema

1. Lymphedema (see Chapter 112)

2. Obstruction of innominate or subclavian vein

3. Trauma

D. Bilateral upper extremity edema: SVC obstruction

VI. Treatment: Dependent on the underlying etiology of the edema (Kumarasinghe & Carroll, 2015; Simon, 2014; Trayes et al., 2013)

A. General management includes dietary sodium restriction (2–3 g daily), fluid restriction (2 L daily), and diuretic therapy, carefully considering how quickly edema must be controlled and potential consequences of removal of fluid.

B. CHF (see Chapter 42)

C. Nephrotic syndrome (see Chapter 91)

D. Liver failure/cirrhosis (see Chapter 69)

E. Venous insufficiency

1. Bed rest with leg(s) elevated

2. Intermittent elevation of legs during day

3. Avoidance of prolonged standing

4. Support hose/compression stockings or layered compression wraps; caution if weeping edema is present

     5. Diuretic therapy: May lead to volume depletion; should be used with caution in these patients

F. Thrombophlebitis (see Chapter 164)

G. Lymphedema (see Chapter 112)

H. DVT (see Chapter 43)

I. Other general treatments

     1. Elevation of extremity above heart level should be encouraged, especially at night and for one to two hours during the day.

     2. Pedal-push exercises can be performed to build calf pumping ability; encourage walking.

     3. For weeping edema, absorbent materials should be placed under extremity in order to avoid skin maceration and breakdown. Avoid plastic-backed pads that do not wick away moisture.

     4. Sequential compression devices may be used.

     5. Protection and cleansing of skin surface is important.

VII. Follow-up: As indicated by the underlying disease process (Simon, 2014; Trayes et al., 2013)

A. Daily skin assessment for acutely ill patients to assess for skin breakdown

B. Periodic weight recording: Instruct patients to report a gain of 2–3 lbs in two to three days.

C. Serial ankle circumference assessment

D. Assessment for complications of peripheral edema, such as cellulitis, nonhealing wounds, pain, gait disturbance, and alterations in self-image

VIII. Referrals (Simon, 2014; Trayes et al., 2013)

A. Cardiologist: For CHF, MI, valvular heart disease, or long-standing or poorly controlled hypertension

B. Vascular surgeon: For venous insufficiency or peripheral vascular disease

C. Dietitian: For dietary interventions (e.g., low-fat, low-cholesterol, low-sodium diet)

D. Gynecologist: If unilateral painless lower extremity edema is present to rule out pelvic tumor causing obstruction (in women)

E. Renal specialist: For nephrotic syndrome

F. Gastroenterologist: For liver failure

G. Radiation oncologist: For SVC syndrome

H. Physical therapist: For lymphedema or reconditioning

References

Breznik, V., Dai, K., & Marovt, M. (2018). Chronic peripheral edema in a patient with rheumatoid arthritis. *Acta Dermatovenerologica, 27*(1), 37–39. https://doi.org/10.15570/actaapa.2018.9

Friedman, T., Quencer, K.B., Kishore, S., Winokur, R.S., & Madoff, D.C. (2017). Malignant venous obstruction: Superior vena cava syndrome and beyond. *Seminars in Interventional Radiology, 34*(4), 398–408. https://doi.org/10.1055/s-0037-1608863

Frison, S., Checchi, F., & Kerac, M. (2015). Omitting edema measurement: How much acute malnutrition are we missing? *American Journal of Clinical Nutrition, 102*(5), 1176–1181. https://doi.org/10.3945/ajcn.115.108282

Kumarasinghe, G., & Carroll, G. (2015). A guide to peripheral oedema. *Medicine Today, 16*(6), 26–34. https://medicinetoday.com.au/2015/june/feature-article/guide-peripheral-oedema

Simon, E. (2014). Leg edema assessment and management. *Medsurg Nursing, 23*(1), 44–53.

Trayes, K.P., Studdiford, J.S., Pickle, S., & Tully, A.S. (2013). Edema: Diagnosis and management. *American Family Physician, 88*(2), 102–110. https://www.aafp.org/afp/2013/0715/p102.html

Veizi, E., Tornero-Bold, M., & Hayek, S.M. (2016). Resolution of intrathecal hydromorphone or morphine-induced peripheral edema by opioid rotation to fentanyl: A case series. *Pain Practice, 16*(6), E94–E98. https://doi.org/10.1111/papr.12443

Yang, Y., Liu, Y.-H., Sun, X., Yu, M.-W., Yang, L., Cheng, P.-Y., … Wang, X.-M. (2017). Risk of peripheral edema in cancer patients treated with MEK inhibitors: A systematic review and meta-analysis of clinical trials. *Current Medical Research and Opinion, 33*(9), 1663–1675. https://doi.org/10.1080/03007995.2017.1349657

Yeo, P.M., Koh, W.L., & Lim, S.P.R. (2016). Tramadol-induced peripheral oedema. *Clinical and Experimental Dermatology, 41*(5), 557–558. https://doi.org/10.1111/ced.12822

Zimmerman, S., & Davis, M. (2018). Rapid fire: Superior vena cava syndrome. *Emergency Medicine Clinics of North America, 36*(3), 577–584. https://doi.org/10.1016/j.emc.2018.04.011

CHAPTER 40

Stable Angina

Renee Genther, MSN, ANP-C, AOCNP®,

and Deborah Kirk, DNP, FNP-BC, NP-C, AOCN®, FAANP

I. Definition: Angina pectoris is described as a smothering sensation or tightness across the front of the chest. Stable angina is arbitrarily defined as when episodes are stable over a period of three to six months (Ferrari et al., 2018, 2019).

II. Physiology/Pathophysiology (Ferrari et al., 2018, 2019; Ford et al., 2018; Han et al., 2017; Herrmann et al., 2016; Rousan & Thadani, 2018)
   A. Normal
      1. Adequate delivery of oxygen to vital organ systems and coronary autoregulation require a balance between myocardial oxygen demand (MOD) and myocardial oxygen supply (MOS).
      2. Demand is dependent on heart rate, systolic blood pressure (afterload), myocardial wall tension, and myocardial contractility.
      3. Supply is influenced by coronary artery diameter and tone, collateral blood flow, perfusion pressure (difference in aortic diastolic pressure and right arterial diastolic pressure), and heart rate.
      4. In response to increased cardiac metabolic demand, the coronary arteries will increase coronary flow reserve.
   B. Pathophysiology
      1. Angina develops when MOD exceeds MOS. Myocardial cells switch from aerobic to anaerobic metabolism with progressive impairment of metabolic, mechanical, and electrical functions.
         a) In the presence of ischemia, there is decreased formation of ATP, loss of the normal ATP sodium–potassium pump, altered myocardial membrane integrity, and acidosis, which leads to the release of chemical substances and mechanical stimulation of sensory afferent nerve endings in the coronary vessels and myocardium.
            (1) Substances released include lactate, serotonin, bradykinin, histamine, reactive oxygen species, and adenosine (downregulated from ATP during ischemia).
            (2) Evidence suggests that adenosine is the primary chemical mediator of angina and acts by stimulating the A1 receptors in cardiac afferent nerve endings.
         b) Other substances that may be responsible for ischemia as a result of platelet release are thromboxane A2 and 5-HT.
      2. Angina is caused by a transient reduction of oxygen supply from coronary artery constriction and previously narrowed vessels unable to supply adequate oxygen during increased oxygen demands.

3. Angina related to dysfunction of the small coronary arteries and arterioles is known as microvascular angina. Impaired endothelial function, increased release of local vasoconstrictors, and reduced nitric oxide production are thought to play a role in microvascular angina.

4. Ischemia can result from extravascular forces or factors that lead to altered blood composition.
   a) Left ventricular hypertrophy
   b) Severe anemia (Hgb less than 8 g/dl) resulting in decreased oxygen carrying capacity of the blood
   c) Carbon monoxide buildup usually related to long-term smoking
   d) Compression from cardiac and noncardiac tumors, such as mediastinal lymphomas or thymomas

5. Postprandial angina may occur after eating, as blood is shifted away from territories supplied by stenosed arteries to those areas supplied by less diseased or normal arteries. This is known as steal phenomenon.

6. Angina decubitus is a variant of angina pectoris that occurs at night while the patient is recumbent. Some have suggested that it is induced by an increase in MOD caused by expansion of the blood volume with increased venous return during recumbency.

7. Cancer treatment–related angina
   a) Vascular reactivity and alteration in smooth muscle signaling leading to vasoconstriction, such as with 5-flurouracil or, more commonly, taxanes
   b) Injured endothelium and altered vasoreactivity, such as with cisplatin combined with bleomycin or vinca alkaloids
   c) Endothelial dysfunction causing alteration in the nitric oxide synthase activity with targeted therapies, such as vascular endothelial growth factor inhibitors
   d) Accelerated atherosclerosis formation leading to occlusions from long-term exposure to TKIs (e.g., sorafenib)

III. Clinical features: Stable angina affects a significant number of patients with CAD, impairing their QOL. Comorbid conditions are frequently encountered, affecting prognosis and making the diagnosis and management of angina more challenging. Normally, angina is precipitated by exertion, eating, exposure to cold, or emotional stress (Balla et al., 2018; Farmakis et al., 2019; Ferrari et al., 2018; Ford et al., 2018; Herrmann et al., 2016).

A. Risk factors
   1. Modifiable: Smoking, obesity, inactivity, dyslipidemia, alcohol consumption, illicit drug use, diet, hypertension, diabetes
   2. Nonmodifiable: Increasing age, gender, family history, genetic makeup; angina is more often the presenting symptom in men than in women.

B. Etiology
   1. Atherosclerosis: Most common
   2. Altered MOD secondary to vigorous exercise, mental stress, tachycardia, hypothermia, hypertension, explosive anger, fever, hyperthyroidism, sexual activity, or chemotherapy exposures
   3. Altered MOS secondary to coronary lesions, vasospasm, embolism, arteritis, or fibrosis
   4. Postprandial angina
   5. Angina decubitus

C. History
   1. History of cancer and cancer treatment
   2. Current medications: Prescribed, over the counter, herbal supplements

3. History of presenting symptoms: Quality, severity, provoking factors, onset, timing, location, radiation, duration, relieving factors, associated symptoms (e.g., diaphoresis, nausea and vomiting, indigestion, belching, dyspnea, palpitations, back pain, fatigue, anxiety)
4. Changes in ADLs: Functional limitations
5. Dietary history: High fat, high cholesterol, increased salt consumption
6. Past medical history: Atherosclerosis, dyslipidemia, diabetes mellitus, angina, MI, metabolic syndrome, hypertension, elevated homocysteine level, obesity, thyroid disease, tachycardia, sleep apnea, COPD, psychiatric disorders, GERD
7. Family history: Cardiac disease, diabetes
8. Social history: Tobacco use, illicit drug use, occupational factors, exercise patterns

D. Signs and symptoms
1. Typical episode begins as retrosternal chest discomfort rather than frank pain.
2. Pain is described as a pressure, heaviness, squeezing, heartburn, knot in the center of the chest, lump in the throat, ache, elephant sitting on the chest, like a bra that is too tight, or choking.
    a) Some patients have difficulty qualifying the pain and place their fist in the center of their chest, known as Levine sign.
    b) Pain described as dull, knife-like, stabbing, or pins and needles is generally not angina.
    c) Duration is approximately one to five minutes, and the pain is typically relieved by rest or nitroglycerin.
    d) Atypical symptoms are more frequent in women, such as dyspnea, indigestion, nausea and vomiting, weakness, and back pain.
3. Substernal or retrosternal pain: Radiation down the ulnar surface of the left arm, jaw, and right arm is atypical with angina. Pain above the neck or below the epigastrium is not commonly associated with angina.
4. Dyspnea
5. Dizziness
6. Fatigue
7. Belching/dyspepsia
8. Diaphoresis

E. Physical examination: Often normal
1. Vital signs: Blood pressure in both arms, widening pulse pressure
2. Weight: Overweight or obesity
3. HEENT
    a) Xanthelasma: Appears as a sharply demarcated yellow deposit of fat underneath the skin and is usually found near the inner canthus of the eyelid
    b) Arcus senilis: Typically in older adults; a gray to white opaque ring around the cornea indicating hyperlipidemia
    c) Funduscopic examination
        (1) Retinal exudates seen as bright reflective white or cream-colored lesions indicating hyperlipidemia
        (2) AV nicking with constriction of vein indicative of possible arteriosclerosis
4. Pulmonary: Pulmonary etiology (e.g., pneumonia) on auscultation
5. Cardiovascular
    a) Presence of S_3/S_4 possibly indicative of left ventricular systolic or diastolic dysfunction; murmur possibly due to mitral regurgitation associated with papillary muscle dysfunction or anemia
    b) Presence of a pericardial friction rub indicative of pericarditis or early tamponade

      c) Distant or muffled heart tones indicative of pericardial effusion or tamponade

      d) Rapid or irregular heart rate/rhythm indicative of atrial fibrillation or runs of ventricular tachycardia

      e) Evaluation of JVD, a reliable indicator of right atrial function, for right-sided heart failure

      f) Palpation of peripheral pulses to assess vascular sufficiency; diminished in peripheral vascular disease

   6. Musculoskeletal: Palpation of cervical and upper thoracic spine to evaluate for musculoskeletal origin

   7. Abdominal: Auscultation of abdomen for presence of bruit; palpation for hepatomegaly

IV. Diagnostic tests (Balla et al., 2018; Farmakis et al., 2019; Ferrari et al., 2018; Joseph et al., 2018; Wee et al., 2015)

  A. Laboratory studies

    1. CBC to evaluate anemia: Elevated WBC count suggests pneumonia.

    2. Cardiac biomarkers (troponins/creatine kinase-MB): Elevations indicate myocardial necrosis and not stable angina.

    3. BNP: Not the most reliable marker for stable angina, it can reflect diastolic dysfunction or fluid overload and can be normal despite poor heart function.

    4. Lipid panel: Low HDL, high LDL, and elevated triglyceride levels are common findings in atherosclerosis.

    5. Fasting glucose or Hgb A1c: Check for presence of diabetes mellitus.

    6. Thyroid function: Elevated levels can cause atrial fibrillation, and hyperthyroidism increases MOD.

    7. Homocysteine (intermediary amino acid in protein metabolism): Elevated level is a vascular risk factor.

    8. CRP: It is elevated in the presence of inflammation. Increased levels are associated with risk for cardiovascular disease.

  B. Radiology: Chest radiograph is normal in most cases but may reveal cardiomegaly or coronary artery calcification.

  C. Other

    1. Twelve-lead ECG: Perform on every patient with suspected angina. A normal ECG (in 50% of cases) does not exclude pathology. New ST-segment deviation greater than or equal to 0.5 mm, T-wave inversion greater than or equal to 2 mm, new left bundle branch block, or ventricular arrhythmia suggests necrosis.

    2. Exercise ECG testing: This is the test of choice in the presence of symptoms and a normal ECG.

    3. Myocardial perfusion imaging with thallium or technetium sestamibi: Imaging is useful when the resting ECG is abnormal, in those who cannot exercise because of other comorbidities, or in the presence of generalized deconditioning.

      a) Pharmacologic challenge is performed using dipyridamole, adenosine, or dobutamine. Dipyridamole is not used in asthmatics, and adenosine is avoided in patients with sick sinus syndrome or high-grade AV block.

      b) Patients with two or more perfusion defects and ventricular dysfunction should be referred for consideration of angiography.

    4. CT measurement of coronary artery calcium: Coronary calcium score is a strong predictor of CAD and provides predictive information beyond standard risk factors.

    5. Echocardiography: It is noninvasive and provides information on cardiac blood flow, chamber size, ejection fraction, and valve function.

      6. Coronary angiography: It is the gold standard for diagnosis of CAD and indicated in patients experiencing angina with a markedly positive stress test.

V. Differential diagnosis (Farmakis et al., 2019; Herrmann et al., 2016; Katz, 2017)
    A. Cardiac origin
        1. MI (see Chapter 49)
        2. Aortic dissection
        3. Acute pericarditis (see Chapter 50)
        4. Prolapsed mitral valve/mitral regurgitation
        5. Atherosclerotic disease
        6. Coronary vasospasm
        7. Aortic stenosis
        8. Radiation-induced valvular stenosis
        9. Cardiomyopathy (see Chapter 41)
      10. Pericardial effusion (see Chapter 50)
      11. Cardiac contusion
    B. GI origin
        1. Gastroesophageal reflux (see Chapter 71)
        2. Esophageal motility disorders/spasm
        3. Peptic ulcer disease (see Chapter 78)
        4. Cholecystitis/cholelithiasis (see Chapter 68)
        5. Pancreatic disease (see Chapter 77)
        6. Gastritis (see Chapter 72)
        7. Hiatal hernia
    C. Pulmonary origin
        1. Pneumonia (see Chapter 30)
        2. Bronchitis (see Chapter 28)
        3. Pleurisy
        4. Pneumothorax (see Chapter 31)
        5. PE (see Chapter 33)
        6. Pleural effusion (see Chapter 29)
        7. Severe PH (see Chapter 52)
    D. Musculoskeletal origin
        1. Cervical radiculopathy
        2. Costochondritis
        3. OA (see Chapter 105)
    E. Other
        1. Anemia (see Chapters 113–119)
        2. Hyperventilation/anxiety (see Chapter 161)
        3. HZV, left chest (see Chapter 22)
        4. Drug abuse
        5. Hyperthyroidism (see Chapter 157)
        6. SLE (see Chapter 110)
        7. Hyperviscosity syndrome
        8. Cancer treatment induced

VI. Treatment: Treatment includes identification and management of risk factors and the source of angina (Barbero et al., 2016; Han et al., 2017; Herrmann et al., 2016; Wee et al., 2015).
    A. Identify and treat underlying disease, such as anemia or drug abuse.
    B. Smoking cessation

     1. Encourage patient and family to stop smoking.

     2. Provide referral to special programs with follow-up. For most, pharmacotherapy is recommended (including nicotine replacement).

     3. A stepwise strategy for smoking cessation is best (ask about tobacco use, advise to quit, assess willingness to make quit attempt, assist in quit attempt, arrange follow-up).

C. Weight management: Target BMI is 18.5–24.9 kg/m². If waist circumference is greater than or equal to 40 inches (102 cm) in men and greater than or equal to 35 inches (89 cm) in women, initiate lifestyle changes.

     1. Initial goal is to gradually reduce body weight by 10% from baseline.

     2. Diet should consist of lean meat and fish, vegetables, fruits, legumes, nuts, seeds, unrefined whole grains, no salt, 1% or less dairy products, and moderate alcohol intake.

D. Physical activity: Use exercise testing to guide treatment. Physical activity of 30–60 minutes, seven days per week (minimum five) is recommended.

     1. Refer for medically supervised cardiac rehabilitation when indicated.

     2. As tolerated, expand physical program to include resistance training two days per week.

E. Blood pressure control: Target is less than or equal to 140/90 mm Hg. If the patient has diabetes or CKD, then goal is less than 130/80 mm Hg. For patients with hypertension and CAD, it is useful to add medication, treating initially with beta-blockers and/or ACE inhibitors (see Chapter 47).

F. Lipid management: Assess with fasting lipid profile (see Chapter 44).

G. Pharmacologic therapy

     1. Beta-blockers are antianginal, antiarrhythmic, and antihypertensive; they selectively antagonize beta-1 adrenergic receptors and decrease heart rate, contractility, and MOD. Because of their chronotropic effect, they prolong diastole, raise coronary artery blood flow, and increase myocardial perfusion. Some beta-blockers have alpha-1 adrenergic blocking effects, causing vasodilatation (e.g., labetalol, carvedilol).

        a) Beta-blockers are indicated for angina caused by coronary atherosclerosis and to manage stress-related angina, syncope, and palpitations.

        b) They are contraindicated in Prinzmetal angina, AV block, severe bradycardia, sick sinus syndrome, high-grade left ventricular failure, asthma, peripheral vascular disease, cocaine-induced coronary vasoconstriction, and clinical depression.

        c) Use cautiously in patients with type 1 diabetes mellitus, renal impairment, myasthenia gravis, bronchospastic disease, or hepatic dysfunction. Avoid abrupt withdrawal.

        d) Start and continue indefinitely in patients who have had MI, acute coronary syndrome, or left ventricular dysfunction without heart failure symptoms.

        e) Side effects include bradycardia, bronchoconstriction, activity intolerance, fatigue, insomnia, accelerated claudication, impotence, depression, and nightmares.

        f) Examples

           (1) Metoprolol succinate: 25–200 mg PO two times a day

           (2) Atenolol: 25–200 mg PO daily

           (3) Nadolol: 40–80 mg PO daily

           (4) Labetalol: 200–600 mg PO two times a day

           (5) Carvedilol: 3.125–25 mg PO two times a day

     2. Nitrates act by relaxing arterial smooth muscle and stimulating intracellular cyclic guanosine monophosphate production, resulting in dilation of epicardial coronary

arteries, even partially stenosed ones, and reduction in blood pressure. Reduced MOD results from a reduction of left ventricular and arterial pressure, primarily by preload reduction.

   a) Short-acting nitrates have an onset of one to five minutes and are indicated for relief of effort or rest angina. They can be used for prophylaxis to avoid ischemic episodes when taken five minutes before planned exercise. Long-acting nitrates have an onset of action of 20–60 minutes and are used for the prevention of recurrent angina.

   b) Nitrates are relatively contraindicated in patients with severe anemia, orthostatic hypotension, mitral stenosis, closed-angle glaucoma, increased ICP, and aortic stenosis.

   c) Avoid the use of nitrates (e.g., sildenafil, tadalafil, vardenafil) within a 24-hour period because of the risk of severe hypotension.

   d) Dose interruption of an 8–12-hour nitrate-free interval is necessary with long-acting nitrates (including transdermal) to prevent nitrate tolerance.

   e) Side effects include headache, hypotension, flushing, and dizziness.

   f) Examples

      (1) Sublingual nitroglycerin: Tablets 0.3–0.6 mg every five minutes, maximum three per 15 minutes; sublingual spray 0.4 mg per spray, 1–2 sprays every five minutes, maximum three per 15 minutes; notify emergency medical system if pain has not improved after first dose.

      (2) Isosorbide mononitrate (sustained release): 30–240 mg PO daily; drug interactions with propranolol and sildenafil are possible.

      (3) Nitroglycerin transdermal: 0.2–0.8 mg/hr/day; avoid alcohol.

3. Calcium channel blockers are antianginal and antihypertensive.

   a) They are indicated for angina caused by coronary artery spasm and chronic stable angina. They inhibit movement of calcium ions across membranes of cardiac and arterial muscle cells by exerting a negative inotropic effect, resulting in coronary and peripheral vasodilatation, reduced contractility, and improved blood flow. Nondihydropyridine calcium channel blockers (verapamil and diltiazem) also slow sinoatrial and AV node conduction.

   b) They are contraindicated in sick sinus syndrome, heart block, and ventricular dysfunction because they slow the velocity of cardiac impulse conduction and depress myocardial contractility and dilation of coronary arteries.

   c) Multiple potential drug interactions exist. Calcium channel blockers are contraindicated with ophthalmic beta-blockers, pimozide, and niacin/simvastatin. Avoid use with cimetidine or grapefruit juice.

   d) Side effects include suppressed cardiac function, hypotension, headache, flushing, constipation, peripheral edema, increased aminotransferases, and dizziness. Short-acting nifedipine has been linked to an increased risk of MI in those with unstable angina.

   e) Examples

      (1) Verapamil: 80–120 mg PO every eight hours (maximum 480 mg daily; available in extended-release formulation)

      (2) Diltiazem: 30–90 mg PO every six hours (maximum 360 mg daily; available in extended-release formulation)

      (3) Amlodipine: 5–10 mg PO daily (maximum 10 mg daily)

      (4) Nifedipine (extended release): 30–60 mg PO daily (maximum dose 120 mg daily)

4. Antiplatelet therapy

a) ASA should be initiated at 81 mg PO daily in all patients unless contraindicated. It acts by selectively and irreversibly inhibiting cyclooxygenase and synthesis of platelet thromboxane A2 or by reducing blood concentrations of thrombin, collagen, and platelet-activating factors.

b) Avoid combination ASA with NSAIDs, which may reduce ASA effectiveness.

c) Side effects include bruising, GI irritation, bleeding, tinnitus, rash, hyperuricemia, and thrombocytopenia.

5. PPIs or H_2 blockers, antacids, or antibiotics for esophageal pain and biliary colic (see Chapter 71)

6. Chronic angina: Ranolazine, a late sodium channel blocker, is dosed at 500–1,000 mg two times a day. Common side effects include dizziness, constipation, dry mouth, headache, peripheral edema, and dyspnea. It is contraindicated in cirrhosis. A number of drug interactions exist, including ketoconazole, diltiazem, paroxetine, simvastatin, and digoxin.

7. Invasive therapy in patients for whom other therapy fails

a) Coronary angiography and revascularization is performed in patients with symptoms and lesions for which revascularization has benefit. It is also indicated when medical therapy fails if risks are acceptable.

b) Coronary artery bypass grafting is usually well tolerated in older adults.

VII. Follow-up (Barbero et al., 2016; Pollack et al., 2014; Wee et al., 2015)

A. Follow-up smoking cessation visits should include documentation of patient progress.

B. Frequent follow-up should occur to monitor and address diabetes, hypertension, dyslipidemia, obesity, and cardiac stability.

C. Survivorship care planning and coordination should occur to evaluate cardiac functioning.

D. Stable patients should be seen every three to six months.

VIII. Referrals (Pollack et al., 2014)

A. Cardiologist

1. When basic therapies are ineffective (refractory angina)
2. Unstable angina/ST-elevation MI
3. Prior history of MI or coronary artery bypass grafting

B. Dietitian: For diet modification (essential component)

C. Cardiac rehabilitation: For those with stable angina who have difficulty in planning and conducting effective exercise routine or who would benefit from increased support

D. Smoking cessation: For support and prevention of relapse

The authors would like to acknowledge Kelley Duncan Mayden, MSN, FNP, AOCNP®, for her contribution to this chapter that remains unchanged from the previous edition of this book.

References

Balla, C., Pavasini, R., & Ferrari, R. (2018). Treatment of angina: Where are we? *Cardiology, 140*(1), 52–67. https://doi.org/10.1159/000487936

Barbero, U., D'Ascenzo, F., Nijhoff, F., Moretti, C., Biondi-Zoccai, B., Mennuni, M., ... Gaita, F. (2016). Assessing risk in patients with stable coronary disease: When should we intensify care and follow-up? Results from a meta-analysis of observational studies of the COURAGE and FAME era. *Scientifica, 2016*, 3769152. https://doi.org/10.1155/2016/3769152

Farmakis, D., Andrikopoulos, G., Giamouzis, G., Giannakoulas, G., Poulimenos, L., Skalidis, E., ... Parissis, J. (2019). Practical recommendations for the diagnosis and medical management of stable angina: An expert panel consensus. *Journal of Cardiovascular Pharmacology, 74*(4), 308–314. https://doi.org/10.1097/FJC.0000000000000716

Ferrari, R., Caimic, P.G., Crea, F., Danchin, N., Fox, K., Maggioni, A.P., ... Lopez-Sendon, J.L. (2018). A 'diamond' approach to personalized treatment of angina. *Nature Reviews Cardiology, 15*(2), 120–132. https://doi.org/10.1038/nrcardio.2017.131

Ferrari, R., Pavasini, R., & Balla, C. (2019). The multifaceted angina. *European Heart Journal Supplements, 21*(Suppl. C), C1–C5. https://doi.org/10.1093/eurheartj/suz035

Ford, T.J., Corcoran, D., & Berry, C. (2018). Stable coronary syndromes: Pathophysiology, diagnostic advances and therapeutic need. *Heart, 104*(4), 284–292. https://heart.bmj.com/content/104/4/284

Han, X., Zhou, Y., & Liu, W. (2017). Precision cardio-oncology: Understanding the cardiotoxicity of cancer therapy. *NPJ Precision Oncology, 1,* 31. https://doi.org/10.1038/s41698-017-0034-x

Herrmann, J., Yang, E.H., Iliescu, C.A., Cilingiroglu, M., Charitakas, K., Hakeem, A., ... Marmagkiolis, K. (2016). Vascular toxicities of cancer therapies: The old and the new—An evolving avenue. *Circulation, 133*(13), 1272–1289. https://doi.org/10.1161/circulationaha.115.018347

Joseph, J., Velasco, A., Hage, F.G., & Reyes, E. (2018). Guidelines in review: Comparison of ESC and ACC/AHA guidelines for the diagnosis and management of patients with stable coronary artery disease. *Journal of Nuclear Cardiology, 25*(5), 509–515. https://doi.org/10.1007/s12350-017-1055-0

Katz, J. (2017). Stable angina; chest pain; angina pectoris. *Cancer Therapy Advisor.* https://www.cancertherapyadvisor.com/home/decision-support-in-medicine/critical-care-medicine/stable-angina-chest-pain-angina-pectoris

Pollack, C.E., Frick, K.D., Herbert, R.J., Blackford, A.L., Neville, B.A., Wolff, A.C., ... Snyder, C.F. (2014). It's who you know: Patient-sharing, quality, and cost of cancer survivorship care. *Journal of Cancer Survivorship, 8*(2), 156–166. https://doi.org/10.1007/s11764-014-0349-3

Rousan, T.A., & Thadani, U. (2018). Stable angina medical therapy guidelines: A critical review of guidelines from the European Society of Cardiology and National Institute of Health and Care Excellence. *European Cardiology Review, 14*(1), 18–22. https://doi.org/10.15420/ecr.2018.26.1

Wee, Y., Burns, K., & Bett, N. (2015). Medical management of chronic stable angina. *Australian Prescriber, 38*(4), 131–136. https://doi.org/10.18773/austprescr.2015.042

CHAPTER 41

Cardiomyopathy

Deborah Kirk, DNP, FNP-BC, NP-C, AOCN®, FAANP

I. Definition: The structural and/or functional dysfunction of the myocardium, which eventually leads to cardiac failure (McKenna et al., 2017; Ponikowski et al., 2016; Weintraub et al., 2017)
   A. Primary cardiomyopathies mostly involve the myocardium and are divided based on whether they are genetic, mixed, or acquired.
      1. Genetic: Arrhythmogenic right ventricular cardiomyopathy, hypertrophic cardiomyopathy
      2. Acquired: Myocarditis, peripartum, stress cardiomyopathy
      3. Mixed: Dilated cardiomyopathy, restrictive cardiomyopathy
   B. Secondary cardiomyopathy describes heart muscle disease that is associated with other organ systems, disorders, or exposures, such as, but not limited to, inflammatory reactions, neurologic disorders, toxic reactions, autoimmune disorders, endocrine disorders, radiation, or infiltrative disorders.

II. Physiology/Pathophysiology (McKenna et al., 2017; Sisakian, 2014; Weintraub et al., 2017)
   A. Normal
      1. The myocardium (heart muscle) receives its blood supply from the right and left coronary arteries, which branch from the aorta just behind the aortic and pulmonary valves.
      2. The myocardium requires sequential depolarization, normal myocardial contractility during systole and relaxation during diastole, normal intracardiac volume before contraction (preload), and limited resistance to the flow of blood out of the heart (afterload) for normal function.
      3. The muscle fibers of the atria and ventricles interconnect by the AV node.
   B. Pathophysiology: The heart becomes abnormally enlarged, thickened, or stiffened, resulting in the heart muscle's inability to pump.
      1. Dilated cardiomyopathy: The heart muscle is enlarged and weakened and cannot pump blood adequately to the body, resulting in decreased ventricular contractility.
         a) Decreased contractility leads to decreased ejection fraction, decreased stroke volume, and increased end-diastolic and residual volumes.
         b) Cardiac cellular membrane damage, calcium overload, and energy depletion occur.
         c) Compensatory adrenergic mechanisms from heart failure cause further heart muscle damage.
         d) Increases in cardiac wall tension and wall stress produce cellular hypertrophy and fibrosis in a dilated heart.
         e) Tricuspid and mitral valve regurgitation are common because of chamber dilation.
         f) Embolic events caused by ventricular and atrial thrombi may occur.

2. Hypertrophic cardiomyopathy: An abnormal growth of muscle fibers occurs in the heart muscle (thickened septum) and is caused by a variety of mutations, usually affecting the left ventricle.

   a) Thickened muscle fibers prevent the chamber from relaxing completely after diastole, causing diastolic dysfunction.

   b) Increased septal thickness may misalign the papillary muscles so that the septum and mitral valve obstruct blood flow from the left ventricle into the aorta during ventricular contraction.

   c) Left ventricular outflow tract obstruction, mitral regurgitation, diastolic dysfunction, and myocardial ischemia lead to changes in preload, afterload, and contractility.

   d) This genetic cardiac disorder is caused by a missense mutation in one of at least 10 genes that encode the proteins of the cardiac sarcomere. Genetic mutations involve the beta-myosin heavy chain, troponin T, alpha-tropomyosin, and myosin-binding protein C genes.

3. Restrictive cardiomyopathy: The heart muscle is unable to adequately relax after contraction and thus is unable to fill completely with blood because the ventricle walls are stiff and rigid.

   a) It is characterized by abnormal diastolic filling with reduced or normal biventricular volumes and normal or mildly abnormal biventricular systolic function.

   b) Restriction can be isolated to one or both ventricles.

4. Arrhythmogenic right ventricular dysplasia, also referred to as arrhythmogenic right ventricular cardiomyopathy (ARVC): This genetically determined disease is characterized by fat infiltration of the right ventricle associated with fibrosis.

   a) This very rare cardiomyopathy is associated with an increased risk of sudden death by dysrhythmia.

   b) Distinctive features are ventricular myocardial atrophy with fat fibrosis.

   c) It is considered an inherited cardiomyopathy most consistent with an autosomal dominant pattern of Mendelian inheritance.

5. Unclassified cardiomyopathies: These less common, progressive diseases tend to occur in young people; most are idiopathic, causing buildup of fat and proteins in the myocardium.

III. Clinical features: Dilated cardiomyopathy is the most common form of cardiomyopathy and the most frequent reason for heart transplantation. The most common cause of sudden death among young athletes is hypertrophic (Brieler et al., 2017; Elliott et al., 2014; Ponikowski et al., 2016; Sisakian, 2014; Weintraub et al., 2017).

A. Etiology (see Figure 41-1)

B. History

1. History of cancer and cancer treatment

2. Current medications: Prescribed, over the counter

3. History of presenting symptoms: Precipitating factors, onset, location, duration, associated symptoms (e.g., shortness of breath at rest, when active, or both; orthopnea; palpitations; chest discomfort)

4. Changes in ADLs

5. Past medical history: Valve disorders, MI, CAD, sarcoidosis, amyloidosis, and hemochromatosis; previous chemotherapy treatment, radiation therapy, infections, endocrine disorders, autoimmune disorders

6. Family history: Cardiac disease, sudden death, familial tendencies of hemochromatosis or troponin I mutation

7. Social history: Alcohol use

FIGURE 41-1	**Cardiomyopathy Etiologies**

Dilated
- Alcoholism (e.g., chronic, excessive)
- Autoimmune and system disorders
- Coronary artery disease, ischemic disease
- Drug induced (e.g., trastuzumab, anthracyclines)
- Endocrine disorders (e.g., thyroid dysfunction, pheochromocytoma)
- Genetic factors (mostly autosomal dominant)
- Hypertension
- Idiopathic myocarditis
- Infections (e.g., viral, bacterial, fungal, mycobacterial, parasitic)
- Neuromuscular diseases (e.g., muscular dystrophy)
- Nutritional deficiencies (e.g., Celiac disease; thiamine, selenium, and L-carnitine deficiencies)
- Toxins (e.g., metals, cocaine)
- Valvular disease

Hypertrophic
- Genetic disease
- Glycogen storage disease
- Metabolic myopathies
- Systemic diseases in older patients (e.g., Friedreich ataxia, pheochromocytoma, neurofibromatosis, lentiginosis, tuberous sclerosis)

Restrictive
- Chemotherapy
- Familial (often autosomal dominant—troponin I mutations)
- Fibroelastosis
- Hemochromatosis
- Hypereosinophilic syndromes
- Idiopathic
- Mediastinal irradiation
- Myocardial fibrosis (scarring of the heart following heart attack or open-heart surgery)
- Systemic disorders (e.g., amyloidosis, sarcoidosis, carcinoid heart disease, scleroderma)
- Thrombosis

Miscellaneous
- Obesity
- Pheochromocytoma

Note. Based on information from Brieler et al., 2017; Elliott et al., 2014; McKenna et al., 2017; Ponikowski et al., 2016; Sisakian, 2014; Yancy et al., 2016, 2017.

    C. Signs and symptoms
        1. Could be asymptomatic
        2. Dyspnea, orthopnea, or paroxysmal nocturnal dyspnea
        3. Syncope: Unexplained; is a marker for sudden death risk
        4. Angina
        5. Chest pain during exertion: May be atypical chest pain (ARVC)
        6. Palpitations
        7. Dry cough
        8. Dizziness
        9. Fatigue
        10. Peripheral edema
        11. Cutaneous effects: Extremely curly hair; seen only in ARVC
    D. Physical examination
        1. Vital signs

        a) Pulse: Rate, rhythm, character, tachycardia

        b) Weight: Close monitoring for increase

        c) Blood pressure: Systolic, diastolic; hypertension indicative of cause for cardiomyopathy

        d) Temperature: Fever present with infection

  2. General: Assessment of alertness

  3. Cardiac

        a) Heart sounds: Apex often displaced

           (1) Dilated: Possible parasternal lift; third heart sound (gallop) and systolic murmur are greater at the apex or tricuspid area.

           (2) Hypertrophic: Systolic ejection murmur that becomes increasingly loud during maneuvers that decrease preload (such as a change in the patient's position from squatting to standing) and murmur along the left sternal border, S_4

           (3) Restrictive: S_4 in most cases, often no murmur

        b) Assessment for peripheral and sacral edema

        c) JVD indicating raised venous pressure

  4. Pulmonary: Respiratory rate for basal rales indicating pulmonary congestion and possible pleural effusion

  5. Abdominal: In severe cases, hepatomegaly and ascites

IV. Diagnostic tests (Dennis et al., 2020; Elliott et al., 2014; Hoss et al., 2020; Ponikowski et al., 2016; Sisakian, 2014; Weintraub et al., 2017)

  A. Laboratory

    1. BNP level increased in heart failure and cardiomyopathy

    2. Baseline chemistry for electrolytes, renal function, and liver function

    3. CBC to evaluate WBC count for infection and Hgb for anemia

    4. Genetic testing for mutations for hypertrophic cardiomyopathy

    5. Glucose and Hgb A1c to monitor blood glucose; cardiovascular disease increases with diabetes.

    6. Lipid profile for baseline or to monitor with cardiac disease

    7. Thyroid function for hyperthyroidism indicative of cardiomyopathy

    8. Iron studies to evaluate for iron overload such as hemochromatosis

  B. Radiology

    1. Chest x-ray: Enlarged heart usually present

        a) Pulmonary edema

        b) Dilated: Pleural effusion (common)

    2. MRI of heart: Useful alternative to complement echocardiogram and in characterization of the myocardium without the need for invasive biopsy; beneficial in inherited cardiomyopathies

  C. Other

    1. Echocardiogram

        a) Dilated: Dilated ventricles with mural thrombus is possible.

        b) Hypertrophic: Hypertrophy of the ventricle usually is asymmetric with septal thickness greater than the thickness of the free wall; mitral regurgitation is possible.

        c) Restrictive: Mitral and tricuspid regurgitation is present. Tricuspid regurgitation may arise from underlying PH. Left ventricular diastolic pressure is significantly increased. Classical finding is the restrictive pattern, bilateral atrial enlargement.

       d) ARVC: Anomalies in myocardial contractility can be seen. Images are limited because they appear to be similar to the surrounding tissue.

   2. Twenty-four-hour Holter monitoring to detect associated dysrhythmias

   3. ECG

       a) Dilated: Sinus tachycardia, low-voltage QRS, ST segment depression, inverted T waves, left bundle branch block

       b) Hypertrophic: Left ventricular hypertrophy, pathologic Q waves, left anterior hemiblock or left bundle branch block, premature ventricular complexes, ventricular tachycardia, supraventricular tachyarrhythmias, negative T waves (apical form)

       c) Restrictive: Depolarization and repolarization changes mostly localized to right precordial leads; ventricular dysrhythmia of right ventricular origin

       d) Arrhythmogenic right ventricular: Sinus rhythm with QRS duration, long T-wave inversion, sharp spike in the ST segment

   4. Transesophageal echocardiography: To evaluate the chamber structures when patient is hemodynamically unstable

   5. Cardiac catheterization

       a) To demonstrate diffusely dilated cardiac chambers

       b) Restricted: Increased left ventricular and right ventricular diastolic pressures; biopsy of right ventricle is useful in detecting infiltrative disease.

V. Differential diagnosis (Brieler et al., 2017; McGregor & Husain, 2015)

  A. Endocarditis (see Chapter 46)

  B. Pericarditis (see Chapter 50)

  C. SLE (see Chapter 110)

  D. Valvular disorder

  E. Hypertension (see Chapter 47)

  F. Amyloidosis

  G. PH (see Chapter 52)

  H. Hypereosinophilic syndrome

  I. CAD

  J. Hyperthyroidism (see Chapter 157)

  K. Congenital heart disease

VI. Treatment (Brieler et al., 2017; Elliott et al., 2014; Ponikowski et al., 2016; Sisakian, 2014; Yancy et al., 2016, 2017)

  A. Nonpharmacologic

   1. Treatment of underlying cause and comorbidities

   2. Lifestyle changes including weight loss, reduced alcohol intake, low-intensity exercise, smoking cessation, and low-sodium diet

  B. Pharmacologic: Treatment should be tailored to the individual based on symptoms and stage of heart failure associated with the cardiomyopathy (see Table 41-1).

   1. Dilated cardiomyopathy

       a) ACE inhibitor, ARB, or angiotensin receptor/neprilysin inhibitor

       b) Vasodilators

       c) Beta-blockers: Metoprolol, carvedilol, and bisoprolol are recommended. Isosorbide dinitrate/hydralazine is recommended in African Americans.

       d) Diuretics: Loop or potassium sparing

       e) Digoxin: 0.125–0.25 mg PO daily indicated with systolic function impairment or atrial dysrhythmias; requires periodic therapeutic drug monitoring

TABLE 41-1   Pharmacologic Treatment of Cardiomyopathies With Associated Heart Failure

Category	Indications	Contraindications	Monitoring	Example of Dosing	Adverse Effects
Aldosterone antagonists	Patients with moderate to severe systems (class III–IV heart failure) LVEF ≤ 35% Taking a beta-blocker and ACEI or ARB	Serum K > 5 mEq/L Serum Cr > 2.5 mg/dl Taking K supplements Taking combination of ACEI and ARB	BUN/Cr Electrolytes Recheck lab at weeks 1 and 4 after starting.	Spironolactone 12.5–25 mg PO daily + ACEI or ARB Titrate up after 4–8 weeks if needed. **Use caution with ACEI/ ARB combination.**	Increased K Increased BUN/Cr Breast tenderness or enlargement
ACEI	Patients with symptoms LVEF ≤ 40%	Serum K > 5 mEq/L Serum Cr > 2.5 mg/dl Severe aortic stenosis History of angioedema	BUN/Cr Electrolytes Check lab in 1–2 weeks after starting medication. Recheck lab after dose adjustments.	Captopril 6.25 mg PO three times a day Titrate up after 2–4 weeks.	Increased K Increased BUN/Cr Decreased BP Cough
Angiotensin receptor/neprilysin inhibitor	Patients with heart failure with reduced ejection fraction	History of angioedema with ACEI or ARB therapy Do not use with ACEI. Do not use with aliskiren in patients with diabetes.	BUN/Cr Electrolytes BP	Sacubitril/valsartan 49 mg/51 mg PO two times a day Titrate up after 2–4 weeks.	Increased K Decreased BP Cough Dizziness Renal failure
ARBs	Patients with symptoms taking ACEI and beta-blockers	If taking aldosterone antagonist Serum K > 5 mEq/L Serum Cr > 2.5 mg/dl If taking ACEI and aldosterone antagonist	BUN/Cr Electrolytes Recheck in 1 week after starting medication.	Candesartan 4–8 mg PO daily; valsartan 40 mg PO twice a day Titrate up after 2–4 weeks if needed.	Increased K Increased BUN/Cr Decreased BP
Anticoagulants	Patients with heart failure with atrial fibrillation Prevention of thromboembolism	Bleeding disorders Severe liver disease	PT and INR—goal for INR between 2–3	Warfarin oral dose varies and should be given based on INR.	Bleeding

(Continued on next page)

TABLE 41-1 Pharmacologic Treatment of Cardiomyopathies With Associated Heart Failure (Continued)

Category	Indications	Contraindications	Monitoring	Example of Dosing	Adverse Effects
Beta-blockers	Patients with mild to severe symptoms LVEF ≤ 40%	Asthma Second- or third-degree heart block Sick sinus syndrome	BP Heart rate	Bisoprolol 1.25 mg PO daily Carvedilol 3.125–6.25 mg two times a day Metoprolol controlled/extended release 12.5–25 mg PO daily	Decreased BP Worsening heart failure Bradycardia
Digoxin	Patients with heart failure with atrial fibrillation Atrial fibrillation with LVEF < 40%	Second- and third-degree heart blocks; digoxin intolerance; preexcitation syndromes	Heart rate and rhythm	0.25 mg PO daily In older adults: 0.125 or 0.0625 mg PO daily	Toxicity Atrial and ventricular arrhythmias Sinoatrial and atrioventricular block
Diuretics	For relief of symptoms of pulmonary and venous congestion	Renal failure	BUN/Cr Electrolytes BP	Use with ACEI/ARB. Start low and adjust as needed. Furosemide 20–40 mg PO daily	Renal failure Decreased BP Decreased electrolytes Dehydration
Hydralazine and isosorbide dinitrate (drug of choice for patients of African American descent)	Alternative to ACEIs/ARBs	Low BP Systemic lupus erythematosus Renal failure	BUN/Cr BP	Hydralazine 37.5 mg PO three times a day Isosorbide dinitrate 20 mg PO three times a day Titrate after 2–4 weeks.	Decreased BP Arthralgias Joint pain/swelling Rash

ACEI—angiotensin-converting enzyme inhibitor; ARB—angiotensin II receptor blocker; BP—blood pressure; BUN—blood urea nitrogen; Cr—creatinine; INR—international normalized ratio; K—potassium; LVEF—left ventricular ejection fraction; PT—prothrombin time

Note. Based on information from Elliott et al., 2014; Ponikowski et al., 2016; Yancy et al., 2016, 2017.

f) Other: Cardiac resynchronization therapy; implantation of cardioverter defibrillator in patients at risk for sudden death; transplantation, if needed

2. Hypertrophic cardiomyopathy: Avoid strenuous exercise; avoid volume depletion.

    a) Beta-blockers can be helpful in relieving symptoms (angina or dyspnea). Start with low doses and titrate PRN to keep heart rate at 60–65 bpm.

    b) Calcium channel blockers can be used for those who do not respond to or tolerate beta-blockers. Start with low doses of verapamil and titrate up to 480 mg PO daily.

    c) Disopyramide should be added to beta-blockers or verapamil if no response is shown to single-agent treatment. It should not be used as a single agent and should be avoided with class 1A or class 1C antiarrhythmics or propranolol because the combination may excessively prolong conduction, particularly in patients with cardiac decomposition.

    d) Diuretics should be used with caution.

    e) Other treatments

        (1) Surgical septal myectomy is used in patients who continue to have dyspnea or angina that limits daily activity.

        (2) Alcohol-induced septal ablation produces a controlled MI, resulting in a decrease in obstruction.

        (3) Implantation of a dual-chamber pacemaker helps to reduce the outflow gradient.

        (4) Implantable cardioverter defibrillator may be used to prevent sudden death in patients with a high-risk profile, such as a history of syncope or ventricular tachyarrhythmia.

3. Restrictive cardiomyopathy

    a) Diuretics: Loop or potassium sparing; low to medium doses

    b) Vasodilators: Hydralazine and/or isosorbide dinitrate

    c) Digoxin: 0.125–0.25 mg PO daily indicated with systolic function impairment or atrial dysrhythmias

    d) Verapamil: Initiated at 240 mg PO daily

    e) Beta-blocker: Extended-release metoprolol 12.5–25 mg PO daily

    f) ACE inhibitor: Lisinopril 5–20 mg PO daily; ARB: Losartan 25–100 mg PO daily

4. Arrhythmogenic: Treatment is aimed at suppression of recurrent ventricular tachyarrhythmias and prevention of sudden death; the patient should avoid competitive sports.

    a) Sotalol 80 mg PO two times a day or amiodarone 400–800 mg PO daily

    b) Implantation of cardioverter defibrillator

    c) Catheter ablation using conventional or electroanatomic mapping techniques to eliminate targeted dysrhythmia

    d) Cardiac transplantation for refractory disease

5. Anticoagulation

    a) Patients with atrial fibrillation, left ventricular hypertrophy, or with very low ejection fraction (less than 25%) should be considered for anticoagulation due to the higher incidence of stroke.

    b) Anticoagulation agents include ASA, warfarin, or nonwarfarin oral anticoagulants.

6. Dysrhythmic agents (see Chapter 45): Treat according to dysrhythmia and monitor closely to adjust doses according to ECG results.

7. Surgeries

a) Heart transplantation can be used for restrictive cardiomyopathy that is no longer responding to medication.

b) Coronary artery bypass graft surgery may also be considered.

VII. Follow-up: Ongoing evaluation and management of anticoagulation therapy
  A. Short term
      1. Measure electrolyte levels when using diuretics.
      2. Monitor weight and status of fluid retention.
      3. Monitor for complications, such as atrial fibrillation, infective endocarditis, and end-stage heart failure.
      4. Monitor for complications of implanted cardioverter defibrillator.
  B. Long term
      1. Monitor for heart failure progression.
      2. Perform serial imaging studies, such as echocardiogram or ECG.

VIII. Referrals
  A. Cardiologist: For evaluation and treatment plan
  B. Electrophysiologist: If evaluation for resynchronization or implantable defibrillator is indicated
  C. Genetic counselor: For cardiac evaluation of family members and genetic counseling.
  D. Primary health practitioner: Current recommendations are to screen every five years for cardiac disease.

References

Brieler, J., Breeden, M.A., & Tucker, J. (2017). Cardiomyopathy: An overview. *American Family Physician, 96*(10), 640–646. https://www.aafp.org/afp/2017/1115/p640.html

Dennis, M., Ugander, M., Kozor, R., & Puranik, R. (2020). Cardiovascular magnetic resonance imaging of inherited heart conditions. *Heart, Lung and Circulation, 29*(4), 584–593. https://doi.org/10.1016/j.hlc.2019.12.008

Elliott, P.M., Anastaskakis, A., Borger, M.A., Borggrefe, M., Cecchi, F., Charron, P., ... Watkins, H. (2014). 2014 ESC guidelines on diagnosis and management of hypertrophic cardiomyopathy: The Task Force for the Diagnosis and Management of Hypertrophic Cardiomyopathy of the European Society of Cardiology (ESC). *European Heart Journal, 35*(39), 2733–2779. https://doi.org/10.1093/eurheartj/ehu284

Hoss, S., Habib, M., Silver, J., Care, M., Chan, R.H., Hanneman, K., ... Adler, A. (2020). Genetic testing for diagnosis of hypertrophic cardiomyopathy mimics: Yield and clinical significance. *Circulation: Genomic and Precision Medicine, 13*(2), e002748. https://doi.org/10.1161/CIRCGEN.119.002748

McGregor, S.M., & Husain, A.N. (2015). A brief review and update of the clinicopathologic diagnosis of arrhythmogenic cardiomyopathy. *Archives of Pathology and Laboratory Medicine, 139*(9), 1181–1186. https://doi.org/10.5858/arpa.2014-0114-RS

McKenna, W.J., Maron, B.J., & Thiene, G. (2017). Classification, epidemiology, and global burden of cardiomyopathies. *Circulation Research, 121*(7), 722–730. https://doi.org/10.1161/CIRCRESAHA.117.309711

Ponikowski, P., Voors, A.A., Anker, S.D., Bueno, H., Cleland, J.G.F., Coats, A.J.S., ... van der Meer, P. (2016). 2016 ESC guidelines for the diagnosis and treatment of acute and chronic heart failure: The task force for the diagnosis and treatment of acute and chronic heart failure of the European Society of Cardiology (ESC); Developed with the special contribution of the Heart Failure Association (HFA) of the ESC. *European Heart Journal, 37*(27), 2129–2200. https://doi.org/10.1093/eurheartj/ehw128

Sisakian, H. (2014). Cardiomyopathies: Evolution of pathogenesis concepts and potential for new therapies. *World Journal of Cardiology, 6*(6), 478–494. https://doi.org/10.4330/wjc.v6.i6.478

Weintraub, R.G., Semsarian, C., & Macdonald, P. (2017). Dilated cardiomyopathy. *Lancet, 390*(10092), 400–414. https://doi.org/10.1016/S0140-6736(16)31713-5

Yancy, C.W., Jessup, M., Bozkurt, B., Butler, J., Casey, D.E., Jr., Colvin, M.M., ... Westlake, C. (2016). 2016 ACC/AHA/HFSA focused updated on new pharmacological therapy for heart failure: An update of the 2013 ACCF/AHA guideline for the management of heart failure: A report of the American College of Cardiology/American Heart Association

Task Force on Clinical Practice Guidelines and the Heart Failure Society of America. *Journal of the American College of Cardiology, 68*(13), 1476–1488. https://doi.org/10.1016/j.jacc.2016.05.011

Yancy, C.W., Jessup, M., Bozkurt, B., Butler, J., Casey, D.E., Jr., Colvin, M.M., ... Westlake, C. (2017). 2017 ACC/AHA/HFSA focused update of the 2013 ACCF/AHA guideline for the management of heart failure: A report of the American College of Cardiology/American Heart Association Task Force on Clinical Practice Guidelines and the Heart Failure Society of America. *Journal of the American College of Cardiology, 70*(6), 776–803. https://doi.org/10.1016/j.jacc.2017.04.025

CHAPTER 42

Congestive Heart Failure

Renee Genther, MSN, ANP-C, AOCNP®,

and Deborah Kirk, DNP, FNP-BC, NP-C, AOCN®, FAANP

I. Definition: A condition characterized by signs and symptoms of intravascular and interstitial volume overload when the heart is unable to generate a cardiac output sufficient to meet the body's metabolic needs due to altered heart function (Arrigio et al., 2016; Azad & Lemay, 2014)

II. Physiology/Pathophysiology (Inamdar & Inamdar, 2016; Thibodeau & Drazner, 2018; Wright & Thomas, 2018)
   A. Normal
      1. In the healthy individual, the cardiovascular system adjusts the total cardiac output to meet the metabolic demands of the peripheral tissues.
         a) These adjustments include alterations in ventricular rate and stroke volume.
         b) The product of these two parameters results in the cardiac output.
      2. The autonomic nervous system primarily controls the ventricular rate.
         a) The parasympathetic system reduces the heart rate through cholinergic mechanisms mediated by the vagus nerve.
         b) The sympathetic nervous system increases the heart rate by local and humoral release of catecholamines.
      3. Stroke volume is a function of innate cardiac contractility as well as the end-diastolic pressure or preload and the impedance to flow or afterload.
         a) According to the Frank-Starling Curve, the preload is increased by increasing cardiac filling, resulting in an increased stroke volume.
         b) Decreasing afterload increases stroke volume.
         c) Increasing contractility increases cardiac stroke volume.
   B. Pathophysiology
      1. The initial event in the development of heart failure is myocyte damage or overload caused by increased pressure or volume. These two factors result in increased wall tension resulting in pulmonary vascular congestion and reduced cardiac output.
      2. Ischemia results in decreased compliance secondary to scarring, asynchronous left ventricular relaxation, and remodeling.
      3. Heart failure can be the result of systolic dysfunction (pump failure) and/or diastolic dysfunction (increased resistance to filling and reduced compliance).

III. Clinical features: CHF is a serious and common condition affecting an estimated 6.2 million Americans. It is characterized by high mortality, frequent hospitalization, poor QOL, multiple comorbidities, and a complex therapeutic treatment regimen. Approximately 550,000 new cases and 287,000 deaths from heart failure occur each year. More than one-half of those who develop CHF die within five years of diagnosis. The total annual cost of health care, medications, and lost productivity exceeds $39.2 billion (Arrigio et al., 2016; Azad & Lemay, 2014; Benjamin et al., 2019; Fernandez, 2017; Fishbein, 2017; Inamdar & Inamdar, 2016; Voigt et al., 2014; Wright & Thomas, 2018).

A. Etiology
   1. CAD: Underlying cause (MI or ischemia)
      a) Systolic dysfunction generally results from CAD.
      b) Diastolic dysfunction results from uncontrolled or poorly controlled hypertension.
   2. Uncontrolled or poorly controlled hypertension
   3. Cardiomyopathy: Idiopathic, alcohol induced, illicit drug use (especially cocaine), myocarditis, infiltrative processes, some chemotherapy agents
   4. Valvular heart disease from mitral regurgitation and aortic stenosis
   5. Congenital heart disease: Accounts for only a small portion of cases
   6. Aging process
   7. Connective tissue disease
   8. Left ventricular dysfunction indicative of impending/existing heart failure
B. History
   1. History of cancer and cancer treatment
   2. Current medications: Prescribed, over the counter
   3. History of presenting symptoms: Precipitating factors, onset, location, duration, associated symptoms (e.g., shortness of breath, fatigue, chest discomfort, extremity edema, orthopnea, syncope, paroxysmal nocturnal dyspnea)
   4. Changes in ability to perform ADLs
   5. Past medical history/family history of heart disease
   6. Social history: Smoking, illicit drug use
C. Signs and symptoms
   1. Many patients with significantly impaired left ventricular function have no symptoms of heart failure.
   2. Approximately 20% of patients with left ventricular ejection fraction (LVEF) less than 40% (normal LVEF is greater than or equal to 55%) meet none of the clinical criteria for heart failure.
   3. Approximately 40% of patients with LVEF less than 30% have dyspnea on exertion.
   4. Systolic dysfunction: Impaired pumping ability
      a) Paroxysmal nocturnal dyspnea
      b) Orthopnea
      c) Dyspnea on exertion that is progressive
      d) Bilateral lower extremity edema or sacral edema if bedridden (dependent edema)
      e) Decreased exercise tolerance; easy fatigability
      f) Unexplained confusion, altered mental status, or fatigue in an older adult patient
      g) Abdominal symptoms associated with ascites/hepatic engorgement
         (1) Distended abdomen
         (2) Nausea and vomiting
   5. Diastolic dysfunction
      a) Dyspnea on exertion
      b) Orthopnea
      c) Paroxysmal nocturnal dyspnea
      d) Weight gain: Rapid over short period of time (e.g., three to four pounds in one to three days)
D. Physical examination: Focus on cardiac and pulmonary examinations.
   1. Vital signs

        a) Hypotension: May occur later in disease process

        b) Tachycardia: May occur later in disease process

    2. Systolic dysfunction

        a) Elevated JVD

        b) S_3

            (1) Most sensitive finding

            (2) Found in approximately 65% of patients with LVEF less than 30%

        c) Laterally displaced apical impulse

        d) The previously listed physical signs (a–c) are the most specific and are virtually diagnostic in a patient with compatible symptoms (e.g., dyspnea on exertion, paroxysmal nocturnal dyspnea, orthopnea).

        e) Pulmonary rales that do not clear with cough

        f) Peripheral edema not caused by venous insufficiency

        g) Hepatojugular reflux to evaluate the jugular veins (see Appendix D)

        h) Possible abdominal swelling with fluid retention or hepatic congestion

    3. Diastolic dysfunction: As many as 30%–40% of patients with heart failure have normal systolic function; however, all patients with systolic dysfunction have some degree of diastolic dysfunction.

        a) Minimally displaced, forceful point of maximal impulse without an S_3

        b) S_4: Indicates normal left atrial pressure, a decreased rate of relaxation, and early filling; may be present for years before symptoms develop

        c) Diastolic blood pressure greater than 105 mm Hg and the absence of elevated JVD

IV. Diagnostic tests (Fishbein, 2017; Inamdar & Inamdar, 2016)

  A. Laboratory

    1. CBC to evaluate for anemia as contributing factor or ACD

    2. Electrolytes to evaluate for imbalances

    3. BUN and creatinine to evaluate for evidence of impaired renal perfusion

    4. Urinalysis: Evidence of target organ disease (proteinuria)

    5. LFTs: Elevated liver enzymes in the absence of other causes indicative of possible hepatic congestion

    6. PT: Prolonged indicative of hepatic congestion

    7. Thyroid function tests: T_4, TSH to evaluate for hyperthyroidism

    8. BNP

        a) A cardiac peptide hormone released by stretching of the atria and ventricular hypertrophy

        b) Elevated in primary PH, pulmonary emboli, and renal failure

        c) Most often used in the emergency department setting but can be ordered in the office setting to assist in diagnosis

        d) Correlates with long-term morbidity and mortality

        e) Levels greater than 100 pg/ml (picograms per milliliter) generally indicative of CHF

        f) Levels greater than 700 pg/ml diagnostic of acute decompensated heart failure

  B. Radiography: Chest x-ray to evaluate for cardiomegaly, left ventricular hypertrophy, pulmonary edema, PH, and pleural effusion

  C. Other

    1. ECG

        a) Left ventricular hypertrophy evidence by abnormal Q waves, premature ventricular contraction, and ventricular tachycardia

  b) Evidence of ischemia/infarction with ST changes
2. Echocardiography: Evaluate left ventricular size and function, ejection fraction, rate of contraction, and changes in wall thickness to assist in confirming diagnosis. This is the most useful diagnostic test.
3. Radionuclide ventriculogram: The majority of patients with heart failure have moderate to severe left ventricular dysfunction and LVEF less than 35%–40%.
4. Stress testing to evaluate ischemia as possible cause for CHF
5. Cardiac catheterization
  a) Evidence of PH
  b) Valvular disease
  c) CAD
  d) Presence of elevated pulmonary capillary wedge pressure
6. Dysrhythmia screening
  a) Ventricular dysrhythmias are common in patients with heart failure, and sudden death as a result of these dysrhythmias occurs in approximately 50% of patients.
  b) Atrial fibrillation is present in 10%–15% of patients and may occur in up to 50% of patients with class III–IV heart failure.

D. Functional classifications of heart disease: New York Heart Association classification
1. Class I: No limitation of physical activity is noted; normal activity does not cause increased fatigue, dyspnea, or anginal pain.
2. Class II: Slight limitation of physical activity is experienced; normal physical activity causes symptoms.
3. Class III: Marked limitation of physical activity is noted; patients are comfortable at rest, but less than normal activity results in symptoms.
4. Class IV: Patients are unable to participate in any physical activity without discomfort; symptoms may be present at rest.
5. Severity staging and interventions
  a) Stage A: At high risk for CHF but asymptomatic without structural disorders; treat with lifestyle changes and ACE inhibitors.
  b) Stage B: Structural disorder but no symptoms, such as left ventricular hypertrophy; treat as for stage A. Addition of beta-blockers may be appropriate for some patients.
  c) Stage C: Current or past symptoms of CHF with underlying structural heart disease; treat as for stage A plus beta-blockers and possibly digoxin.
  d) Stage D: End-stage disease; treat as for stage A, B, or C plus inotropes, mechanical assistance, transplant, or hospice, as appropriate.

V. Differential diagnosis (Cuomo et al., 2019; Fadol, 2018; Fernandez, 2017; Inamdar & Inamdar, 2016; Tawil & Gelzinis, 2016)
A. COPD (see Chapter 28)
B. Valvular heart disease
C. Hyperthyroidism (see Chapter 157)
D. Angina (see Chapter 40)
E. Renal disease (see Chapter 86)
F. Liver disease (see Chapters 69 and 75)
G. Venous insufficiency
H. Medications: This listing is noninclusive.
1. Prolonged use of diuretics with recent noncompliance with medications
2. NSAID- and cyclooxygenase-2 inhibitor–induced fluid retention (see Appendix E)
3. Oncologic agents

        a) Chemotherapy induced
- (1) Anthracyclines
- (2) High-dose cyclophosphamide
- (3) 5-Fluorouracil
- (4) Paclitaxel
- (5) Bleomycin
- (6) Estramustine
- (7) Docetaxel

        b) Immunotherapy induced: Cytokines
- (1) IFN-α
- (2) IL

        c) Vascular endothelial growth factor
- (1) Alemtuzumab
- (2) Bevacizumab
- (3) Sunitinib
- (4) Sorafenib

        d) HER2 targeted
- (1) Trastuzumab
- (2) Lapatinib

        e) BCR-ABL targeted
- (1) Imatinib
- (2) Dasatinib
- (3) Nilotinib

  I. Malnutrition: Thiamine deficiency
  J. Pelvic tumors
  K. Radiation induced, especially mediastinal irradiation
  L. Myocardial and pericardial metastases

VI. Treatment (Arrigio et al., 2016; Azad & Lemay, 2014; Briasoulis et al., 2019; Fishbein, 2017; Galdo et al., 2013; Inamdar & Inamdar, 2016; Kim et al., 2017; Owens et al., 2016; Sarsam et al., 2020; Udelson & Stevenson, 2016)

  A. Determine and treat underlying etiology of CHF.

  B. Systolic dysfunction

    1. Nonpharmacologic: Patient and family education/counseling on nature of disease process, signs and symptoms, treatment plan, dietary restrictions (e.g., sodium 1–2 g/day), risk factor reduction, smoking cessation, cardiac rehabilitation, compliance issues, activity recommendations, and prognosis

    2. Pharmacologic

        a) ACE inhibitors: Use the maximum dose tolerated by the patient, but start slowly and titrate upward.

- (1) Patients with heart failure caused by left ventricular systolic dysfunction should begin taking an ACE inhibitor unless specific contraindications exist, such as history of intolerance or adverse reactions, serum potassium greater than 5.5 mEq/L refractory to reduction, and symptomatic hypotension (systolic blood pressure less than 90 mm Hg).
- (2) If used in patients with serum creatinine greater than 3 mg/dl, use one-half of the usual dose, as hyperkalemia is more likely in patients with some degree of renal insufficiency.
- (3) Administration of ACE inhibitors reduces blood pressure and systemic vascular resistance and significantly reduces left and right atrial pressures.

This is accompanied by a modest increase in cardiac output, increased exercise tolerance, and improved well-being and QOL.

(4) Watch for worsening of chronic renal failure. Discontinue if indicated.

(5) Examples

    (*a*) Ramipril 1.25–10 mg PO daily

    (*b*) Captopril 6.25–50 mg PO three times a day

    (*c*) Enalapril 2.5–10 mg PO two times a day

    (*d*) Lisinopril 12.5–25 mg PO daily

b) Aldosterone inhibitors

  (1) Spironolactone: Nonselective

    (*a*) Used for New York Heart Association classes III and IV

    (*b*) May cause hyperkalemia, especially in the setting of chronic renal insufficiency

    (*c*) Dose: 25–200 mg PO daily

  (2) Eplerenone: More selective

    (*a*) Approved for CHF post-MI

    (*b*) May cause hyperkalemia

    (*c*) Dose: 25–50 mg PO daily

c) Anticoagulation: Routine anticoagulation is not recommended unless the patient has a history of systemic embolism or PE, atrial fibrillation, PH, or a mobile left ventricular thrombus (see Chapters 33, 43, 45, and 52).

d) ARBs

  (1) ARBs inhibit the rate-limiting enzyme, which controls the conversion of angiotensin I to angiotensin II.

  (2) Do not initiate in a dehydrated patient.

  (3) Examples approved for those who are ACE-inhibitor intolerant include the following.

    (*a*) Candesartan: 4–32 mg PO daily

    (*b*) Losartan: 25–50 mg PO daily; maximum of 100 mg daily

    (*c*) Valsartan: 80–160 mg PO daily; maximum of 320 mg daily in divided doses

    (*d*) Olmesartan: 40 mg PO daily

  (4) Stop potassium supplementation or monitor frequently because of increased risk of hyperkalemia.

e) Beta-blockers

  (1) Examples

    (*a*) Carvedilol 6.25–50 mg PO twice a day and metoprolol 100–200 mg PO daily are approved and frequently used beta-blockers for CHF. Carvedilol has alpha-blocking properties and may be the most advantageous.

    (*b*) Bisoprolol has extensive evidence of effectiveness with doses of 5–10 mg PO daily.

  (2) Beta-blockers impede catecholamine-induced progressive cardiomyopathy. They also decrease preload and afterload by causing vasodilation and decreasing peripheral vascular resistance. Studies show decreased mortality rates.

  (3) Beta-blockers are indicated in all patients with CHF.

  (4) A low starting dose should be advanced slowly.

  (5) Initial worsening may be seen during uptitration of doses.

  (6) Beta-blockers are contraindicated in patients with asthma, severe liver dysfunction, symptomatic bradycardia, and second- and third-degree

block. Use with caution in patients with COPD, diabetes, or peripheral vascular disease.

f) Diuretics

   (1) Patients presenting with signs or symptoms of significant volume overload should be treated immediately with a loop diuretic.

   (2) Moderate to severe overload should be treated with loop diuretics. Initiate at a low dose (e.g., furosemide 20 mg PO daily).

   (3) Mild overload can be treated with thiazide diuretics. Initiate at a low dose (e.g., hydrochlorothiazide 25 mg PO daily).

   (4) Diuretics reduce the chance of disease progression and improve exercise capacity.

g) Inotropic agents

   (1) Digoxin: 0.125–0.25 mg PO daily; requires periodic therapeutic drug monitoring

      (a) It is effective for patients with atrial fibrillation with a rapid ventricular response not responsive to beta-blockers.

      (b) Drug can prevent clinical deterioration and improve symptoms.

      (c) Digoxin should be added for patients with persistent symptoms after optimal management with ACE inhibitors/ARBs, beta-blockers, and diuretics.

   (2) Dobutamine and milrinone

      (a) Treatment should be reserved for patients who no longer benefit from other inotropic agents.

      (b) Combination should not be used in the outpatient setting because it requires cardiac monitoring and can increase mortality.

h) Vasodilators: Arteriolar vasodilators (e.g., hydralazine)

   (1) A major component of heart failure is an excess increase in systemic vascular resistance; hydralazine decreases systemic vascular resistance and increases cardiac output. Dose is 75–300 mg PO daily in two to four divided doses. It is used as first-line therapy.

   (2) Cardiac output increases approximately 50% along with a similar degree of reduction of systemic vascular resistance.

i) Vasodilators

   (1) Nitrates reduce atrial pressures by dilating peripheral veins and redistributing blood so that more is present in the peripheral veins and less is in the chest.

   (2) Nitrates also increase exercise tolerance.

   (3) Arteriolar vasodilators increase cardiac output, and vasodilators decrease filling pressures.

   (4) Isosorbide dinitrate: 30–240 mg PO daily

j) Special considerations for systolic dysfunction

   (1) For patients with systolic dysfunction and angina who are not candidates for revascularization, nitrates and ASA are the drugs of choice.

   (2) As a result of their negative inotropic effect, calcium channel blockers generally are not recommended. Amlodipine has been shown to *not* increase mortality.

   (3) The combination of ACE inhibitors and ARBs is not approved but also not contraindicated.

   (4) Eliminate NSAIDs and cyclooxygenase-2 inhibitors (see Appendix E).

   (5) An increased risk of decompensation exists with the use of plasma volume expanders (e.g., glucocorticoids, NSAIDs), negative inotropes (e.g.,

propafenone, disopyramide, calcium channel blockers/antagonists), and resistance to ACE inhibitors.

C. Diastolic dysfunction

1. Control heart rate and maintain normal sinus rhythm. Tachycardia will reduce cardiac output by decreasing filling time and will increase ischemic episodes. Beta-blockers and calcium channel blockers are the drugs of choice for diastolic dysfunction, as they decrease oxygen consumption and ischemia, thereby improving relaxation.

2. Inotropic agents (e.g., digoxin) may worsen diastolic dysfunction by increasing oxygen consumption and decreasing the filling time.

3. Prevent/reduce left ventricular hypertrophy. Treat the underlying condition (e.g., antihypertensive, valve replacement).

4. Prevent ischemia. Use beta-blockers, calcium channel blockers, nitrates, and revascularization.

5. Relieve venous congestion. Vigorous diuresis will result in decreased filling pressures and is not tolerated in patients with diastolic dysfunction because they require higher filling pressures. Use diuretics with caution.

6. Diastolic CHF is best treated by volume control with carefully administered diuretic therapy.

D. Interventional cardiology

1. Device-based arrhythmic therapy

   a) Implantable cardiac defibrillator

      (1) It is utilized for the prevention of sudden cardiac death for both ischemic and nonischemic disease.

      (2) Usage guidelines are not established.

   b) Cardiac resynchronization therapy: Biventricular pacing

      (1) Promising studies have shown increased cardiac output and decreased remodeling.

      (2) Usage guidelines are not established.

2. Angioplasty and stent placement for single- or multiple-vessel disease

E. Surgical interventions

1. Revascularization for those with multiple-vessel disease

2. Mitral and/or aortic valve replacement

3. Dynamic cardiomyoplasty: For New York Heart Association classes III/IV with an ejection fraction less than 40% but greater than 15%; latissimus dorsi muscle wrapped around weakened heart muscle and synchronously paced

4. Transmyocardial revascularization: Ejection fraction must be greater than 35%. A laser is used to create channels in viable myocardium, promoting angiogenesis and new collateral circulation.

5. Batista procedure: Partial left ventriculectomy; experimental for end-stage disease

6. Cardiac transplantation

F. Emerging therapy

1. Sinus node inhibition with medication: Ivabradine

2. Immunotherapy: T-cell therapy

3. Immunomodulation therapy

4. Neurohormones and antagonists

   a) Vasopressin receptor antagonists

   b) Adrenomedullin

   c) Sildenafil

   d) Relaxin

      5. Inspiratory muscle training

      6. Mechanical ultrafiltration

  G. Acute decompensated heart failure

      1. Acute decompensated heart failure is a common cause of acute respiratory distress syndrome/pulmonary edema, and when it occurs with dramatic and rapid onset, it is referred to as *flash pulmonary edema.*

        a) It occurs as a result of increased transudation (movement) of protein-poor fluid into the pulmonary interstitium and alveolar spaces.

        b) Compensatory mechanisms result in tachycardia and elevation of systemic vascular resistance (increased afterload).

        c) It should not be confused with noncardiogenic pulmonary edema, which does not increase pulmonary capillary wedge pressure.

      2. Acute decompensated heart failure may be precipitated by myocardial ischemia with or without MI, acute aortic regurgitation, stress-induced cardiomyopathy, papillary muscle rupture, or volume overload. The presence of renovascular hypertension increases risk of occurrence.

VII. Follow-up (Inamdar & Inamdar, 2016)

  A. Telephone or return clinic visit: Within 24 hours of initiating treatment

  B. Return clinic appointment: Within two weeks until patient's weight is stable, when symptoms resolve, and then every three to six months

  C. Laboratory follow-up: Dependent on therapy

      1. Potassium levels: For patients started on diuretics and ACE inhibitors; weekly during titration

      2. Serum creatinine: For patients started on diuretics and ACE inhibitors

      3. Digoxin levels: 7–10 days after treatment is initiated and, if stable, every three to six months

        a) Repeat levels for worsening heart failure.

        b) Repeat levels if deterioration in renal function.

        c) Repeat levels if signs of toxicity (e.g., confusion, nausea, visual disturbances) are present.

        d) Concomitant use of digoxin can alter the plasma level of numerous drugs (e.g., quinidine, verapamil, amiodarone, antibiotics, calcium channel blockers, erythromycin, phenobarbital, anticholinergic agents); check digoxin levels one week after initiation of any of these medications.

      4. During exacerbation: Monitoring of PT because of increased incidence of bleeding

  D. Patient education: Signs and symptoms requiring immediate attention

VIII. Referrals

  A. Emergency department and cardiologist: Immediately refer for the following.

      1. Cardiogenic shock

        a) Most commonly seen post-MI

        b) Other causes: Acute mitral regurgitation, myocarditis, dilated cardiomyopathy, dysrhythmia, pericardial tamponade

      2. Pulmonary edema

  B. Internist/cardiologist

      1. Newly diagnosed patients

      2. Patients with heart failure with complicating conditions (e.g., renal failure, liver failure)

3. Patients with signs or symptoms of dysrhythmias
4. Patients who deteriorate after stabilization
C. Home-health referral: For homebound patients

The authors would like to acknowledge Kathy Sharp, MSN, FNP-BC, AOCNP®, CCD, for her contribution to this chapter that remains unchanged from the previous edition of this book.

References

Arrigio, M., Parissis, J.T., Akiyama, E., & Mebazaa, A. (2016). Understanding acute heart failure: Pathophysiology and diagnosis. *European Heart Journal Supplements, 18*(Suppl. G), G11–G18. https://doi.org/10.1093/eurheartj/suw044

Azad, M., & Lemay, G. (2014). Management of chronic heart failure in the older patient. *Journal of Geriatric Cardiology, 11*(4), 329–337. https://doi.org/10.11909/j.issn.1671-5411.2014.04.008

Benjamin, E.J., Muntner, P., Alonso, A., Bittencourt, M.S., Callaway, C.W., Carson, A.P., ... Virani, S.S. (2019). Heart disease and stroke statistics—2019 update: A report from the American Heart Association. *Circulation, 139*(10), e56–e528. https://doi.org/10.1161/CIR.0000000000000659

Briasoulis, A., Inampudi, C., Hatzis, G., & Asleh, R. (2019). Management of patients with heart failure: Focus on new pharmaceutical and device options. *Current Medicinal Chemistry, 27*(27), 4522–4535 https://doi.org/10.2174/0929867326666190523083747

Cuomo, A., Rodolico, A., Galdieri, A., Russo, M., Campi, G., Franco, R., ... Mercurio, V. (2019). Heart failure and cancer: Mechanisms of old and new cardiotoxic drugs in cancer patients. *Cardiac Failure Review, 5*(2), 112–118. https://doi.org/10.15420/cfr.2018.32.2

Fadol, A.P. (2018). Management of chemotherapy-induced left ventricular dysfunction and heart failure in patients with cancer while undergoing cancer treatment: The MD Anderson practice. *Frontiers in Cardiovascular Medicine, 5,* 24. https://doi.org/10.3389/fcvm.2018.00024

Fernandez, A.E. (2017). Chemotherapy-induced dysfunction. *e-Journal of Cardiology Practice, 14*(40). https://www.escardio.org/Journals/E-Journal-of-Cardiology-Practice/Volume-14/Chemotherapy-induced-dysfunction

Fishbein, D. (2017). Acute decompensated heart failure: Presentation, physical examination, and laboratory evaluation. In Eisen, H. (Ed.), *Heart failure: A comprehensive guide to pathophysiology and clinical care* (pp. 171–193). Springer. https://doi.org/10.1007/978-1-4471-4219-5_9

Galdo, J.A., Riggs, A.R., & Morris, A.L. (2013). Acute decompensated heart failure. *U.S. Pharmacist, 38*(2), HS2–HS8. https://www.uspharmacist.com/article/acute-decompensated-heart-failure-39145

Inamdar, A.A., & Inamdar, A.C. (2016). Heart failure: Diagnosis, management and utilization. *Journal of Clinical Medicine, 5*(7), 62. https://doi.org/10.3390/jcm5070062

Kim, D.H., Chien, F.-J., & Eisen, H.J. (2017). Pharmacologic management for heart failure and emerging therapies. *Current Cardiology Reports, 19*(10), 94. https://doi.org/10.1007/s11886-017-0899-x

Owens, A.T., Brozena, S.C., & Jessup, M. (2016). New management strategies in heart failure. *Circulation Research, 118*(3), 480–495. https://doi.org/10.1161/CIRCRESAHA.115.306567

Sarsam, L., Malik, M.B., & Bashir, K. (2020). Ultrafiltration in acute decompensated heart failure. In *StatPearls.* https://www.ncbi.nlm.nih.gov/books/NBK499823

Tawil, J., & Gelzinis, T.A. (2016). Differential diagnosis and clinical management of diastolic heart failure: Current best practice. *Research Reports in Clinical Cardiology, 9,* 117–136. https://doi.org/10.2147/RRCC.S80291

Thibodeau, J.T., & Drazner, M.H. (2018). The role of clinical examination in patients with heart failure. *JACC: Heart Failure, 6*(7), 543–551. https://doi.org/10.1016/j.jchf.2018.04.005

Udelson, J.E., & Stevenson, L.W. (2016). The future of heart failure diagnosis, therapy, and management. *Circulation, 133*(25), 2671–2686. https://doi.org/10.1161/CIRCULATIONAHA.116.023518

Voigt, J., John, M.S., Taylor, A., Krucoff, M., Reynolds, M.R., & Gibson, M. (2014). A reevaluation of the costs of heart failure and its implication for the allocation of health resources in America. *Clinical Cardiology, 37*(5), 312–321. https://doi.org/10.1002/clc.22260

Wright, P., & Thomas, M. (2018). Pathophysiology and management of heart failure. *Clinical Pharmacist, 10*(12). https://doi.org/10.1211/CP.2018.20205742

CHAPTER 43

Deep Venous Thrombosis

Beth Faiman, PhD, MSN, APRN-BC, AOCN®, FAAN,
and Mailey Wilks, DNP, MSN, APRN, NP-C

I. Definition: A blood clot in the deep vascular system that impedes blood flow and may produce emboli (Di Nisio et al., 2016; NCCN, 2021; Ye et al., 2019)
   A. Symptomatic: Presence of symptoms leading to imaging confirmation
   B. Asymptomatic: Incidental finding on imaging without symptoms

II. Physiology/Pathophysiology (Di Nisio et al., 2016; NCCN, 2021; Ye et al., 2019)
   A. Normal: Veins are endothelial-lined blood vessels that carry unoxygenated blood to the heart. Veins differ from arteries in that veins have thinner walls and contain valves. These valves keep blood flowing in one direction—away from the heart.
   B. Pathophysiology
      1. A thrombus starts as a clot nidus in the setting of stasis, endothelial injury, and a hypercoagulable state (Virchow triad).
      2. The clot nidus, composed of RBCs, fibrin, and platelets, propagates to fill the vein lumen, causing partial or complete obstruction of blood flow, or it may shed emboli.
      3. The thrombus may float freely in the blood vessel, leading to embolization.
      4. Cancer cells activate the clotting system and stimulate platelets, endothelial cells, and leukocytes to express procoagulant activity.
      5. DVT develops most often in the legs but can also develop in the deep veins of the arms, the splanchnic veins, and the cerebral veins.

III. Clinical features (Di Nisio et al., 2016; Douce et al., 2019; Farge et al., 2019; Heit, 2015; Khorana, 2018; Khorana & Connolly, 2009; Khorana et al., 2008; NCCN, 2021; Park & Khorana, 2019; Song et al., 2019; Sourdon et al., 2017; Ye et al., 2019)
   A. Risk factors
      1. Risk assessment scores in cancer predict patients at high risk of developing cancer-associated thrombosis.
         a) The Khorana Risk Score (see Table 43-1) provides five patient characteristics to determine score: primary site of cancer, prechemotherapy platelet count, Hgb level, prechemotherapy leukocyte count, and BMI.
         b) Patient risk categories are low (0), intermediate (1–2), and high (3 or more).
      2. Risk factors for DVT
         a) High-risk cancer types
            (1) Solid tumor types at a high risk for developing venous thromboembolism are pancreas (8.1%), ovary (5.6%), kidney (5.6%), lung (5.1%), stomach (4.9%), and brain (4.7%).

TABLE 43-1	Khorana Risk Score	
Patient Characteristic		**Risk Score**
Site of cancer		
• Very high risk (e.g., stomach, pancreas)		2
• High risk (e.g., lung, lymphoma, gynecologic, bladder, testicular)[a]		1
Prechemotherapy platelet count ≥ 350,000/mm^3		1
Hemoglobin level < 10 g/dl or use of red cell growth factors		1
Body mass index ≥ 35 kg/m^2		1

[a] High risk is defined as score of greater than or equal to 3.

Note. Based on information from Douce et al., 2019; Khorana, 2018; Khorana et al., 2008; National Comprehensive Cancer Network, 2021.

>   (2) Hematologic malignancies (e.g., lymphoma, leukemia, myeloma) are considered to be high risk of venous thromboembolism.
>
>   *b)* Sepsis
>   *c)* Presence of a vascular access device
>   *d)* Cardiac disease: CHF, hypertension, hyperlipidemia
>   *e)* Obesity
>   *f)* Presence of coagulopathies: Antithrombin III deficiency, protein S and protein C deficiency, activated protein C resistance (factor V Leiden), antiphospholipid antibody
>   *g)* Dysfibrinogenemia
>   *h)* SLE
>   *i)* Polycythemia vera/ET
>   *j)* Recent surgery or trauma, especially orthopedic
>   *k)* Paralysis or recent casting of a lower limb
>   *l)* Recently bedridden for more than three days, prolonged immobilization
>   *m)* Recent long-distance travel
>   *n)* Family history of DVT
>   *o)* Chemotherapy
>   (1) Agents considered risk factors include tamoxifen, raloxifene, EPO-stimulating growth factors, thalidomide, lenalidomide, pomalidomide, bortezomib, and vascular endothelial growth factor inhibitors (e.g., bevacizumab, ramucirumab, sunitinib).
>   (2) In a cohort study assessing 16,000 ambulatory patients with cancer receiving chemotherapy, 7.3% developed venous thromboembolic events 3.5 months after chemotherapy.
>   *p)* Prior superficial vein thrombosis
>   *q)* Liver disease
>   *r)* Nephrotic syndrome
>   *s)* Inflammatory bowel disease
>   *t)* Pregnancy, oral contraceptives, hormone replacement therapy
>   *u)* Paroxysmal nocturnal hemoglobinuria
>   *v)* Increased WBC count
>   *w)* Increased platelet count
>   *x)* African American heritage
>   *y)* Female gender
>   *z)* Smoking

      3. Upper extremity DVT risk factors differ from lower extremity DVT and include the following.
- *a)* Presence of a vascular access device
- *b)* Presence of a pacemaker
- *c)* History of cancer
- *d)* Age older than 67 years
- *e)* BMI greater than 25 kg/m^2
- *f)* Hospitalization

B. Etiology
1. Numerous factors contribute to development of DVT. These may be acquired (e.g., medication, illness, immobility) or congenital (e.g., anatomic variant, enzyme deficiency, mutation).
2. Diagnosis based on clinical findings alone is accurate less than 50% of the time. A statistically significant correlation exists between idiopathic DVT and later symptomatic development of cancer.

C. History
1. History of cancer and cancer treatment
2. Current medications: Prescribed, over the counter
3. History of presenting symptoms: Precipitating factors, onset, location, duration, associated symptoms (e.g., chest pain, shortness of breath, edema)
4. Changes in ADLs
5. Past medical history: DVT, cardiac disease, liver disease, nephrotic syndrome,, risk factors for DVT
6. Family history: DVT, PE, hypercoagulable state

D. Signs and symptoms
1. Unilateral swelling, erythema, and warmth of the involved extremity
2. A dull ache, tight feeling, or frank pain in the calf or upper extremity, especially with walking
3. Distention of the superficial venous collateral vessels
4. Slight fever possible
5. Tenderness over the involved vein
6. Most common sites: Anterior and posterior tibial veins, perineal veins, popliteal veins, superficial and deep femoral veins

E. Physical examination
1. Vital signs: Fever and tachycardia
2. Integument
- *a)* Skin cyanotic: If severe obstruction
- *b)* Skin pale and cool: If reflex arterial spasm is superimposed
3. Extremities
- *a)* Unilateral edema in the involved extremity; may not have obvious swelling if early
- *b)* Warmth and erythema of involved extremity
- *c)* Thigh or calf tenderness to palpation
- *d)* Tender palpable venous cord of involved vein
- *e)* Homan sign: Calf pain produced with dorsiflexion of the foot (see Appendix D); positive in less than 50% of cases and has high incidence of false positives
4. Head/neck: Swelling in face, neck, or supraclavicular space in upper extremity DVT

IV. Diagnostic tests (Moya Mateo & Muñoz Rivas, 2019; NCCN, 2021; Ye et al., 2019)
A. Laboratory
1. CBC, PT, aPTT, chemistry panel for baseline measurements

2. D-dimer testing: A negative enzyme-linked immunosorbent assay (ELISA) has a high negative predictive value for excluding DVT.
   a) Bedside testing using whole blood is less sensitive than ELISA but has the advantage of rapid results that are less labor intensive.
   b) D-dimer testing is less accurate in older adults, people with cancer, and patients with prior DVT/PE.
   c) If the D-dimer is negative and there is a low degree of suspicion for acute DVT, no further testing is recommended. If the D-dimer is positive, evaluation with Doppler ultrasonography is recommended.
3. Evaluation for hypercoagulable states, such as protein C deficiency, protein S deficiency, antithrombin III deficiency, factor V Leiden mutation, prothrombin gene mutation, homocysteine elevation, and presence of antiphospholipid antibodies

B. Radiology
1. Doppler ultrasonography: It measures venous patency by detecting the movement of RBCs through the vein.
   a) The primary diagnostic tool for proximal DVT, with a sensitivity of 97%
   b) Noninvasive and inexpensive
   c) Less sensitive for calf DVT or asymptomatic proximal or distal DVT
   d) Useful for upper extremity DVT
   e) Repeat testing in one week if symptoms persist and initial test was negative
2. Impedance plethysmography: Technique assesses the change in blood flow after compression of the calf; it is less accurate than Doppler ultrasound, and most institutions no longer have the equipment to perform this test.
3. Contrast venography: It has been considered the gold standard for diagnosis of DVT but is not recommended as first-line evaluation because of its invasive nature and patient discomfort.
4. CT or magnetic resonance venography: Technique may be indicated if ultrasound is negative and a high degree of suspicion remains.
   a) It is the preferred testing modality for suspected DVT of the intra-abdominal vessels, proximal subclavian vein, brachiocephalic vein, or the SVC.
   b) The ability to evaluate adjacent structures may lead to alternate diagnoses.

V. Differential diagnosis (Moya Mateo & Muñoz Rivas, 2019)
A. Calf muscle strain or tear
B. IM hematoma
C. Cellulitis (see Chapter 19)
D. Superficial phlebitis (see Chapter 164)
E. Obstruction of lymphatics by tumor or from irradiation or lymph node dissection
F. Acute arterial occlusion
G. Ruptured Baker cyst
H. Chronic venous insufficiency
I. Lymphangitis/fibrositis
J. Kidney, liver, or heart disease: Usually has bilateral edema
K. Hypoalbuminemia

VI. Treatment (Farge et al., 2019; Gould et al., 2012; Hutchinson et al., 2019; Kahn et al., 2012; Kearon et al., 2012; Key et al., 2019; Khorana et al., 2019; NCCN, 2021; Park & Khorana, 2019; Song et al., 2019; Wells et al., 2014)
A. Prevention of DVT in high-risk patients
1. Most hospitalized patients have one or more risk factors for DVT.

2. Without prophylaxis, the incidence of hospital-acquired DVT is 10%–40% among medical or general surgery patients and 40%–60% after major orthopedic surgery.

3. Prophylaxis against DVT based on group-specific risk factors is the most appropriate strategy to reduce incidence and long-term complications (see Table 43-1).

4. Mechanical methods of prophylaxis should be used in patients at high risk for bleeding or as an adjunct to anticoagulation. Proper fit, use, and compliance are important.

   a) Elevate the foot of the bed 15°–20° with slight knee flexion.

   b) Perform frequent leg exercises to improve venous flow   every two hours if bedridden.

   c) Use graduated compression stockings and intermittent pneumatic venous compression devices. Use with caution in patients with arterial insufficiency.

5. ASA alone is not recommended as prophylaxis for DVT in any patient group.

6. The routine use of prophylaxis to prevent thrombosis in patients with long-term indwelling central venous catheters has shown no decrease in development of DVT and is not recommended.

7. In outpatients with cancer with no additional risk for DVT, routine prophylaxis is not recommended most of the time. For patients with solid tumors, additional risk factors, and low risk of bleeding, consider prophylaxis with LMWH or low-dose unfractionated heparin (UFH). Two recent randomized controlled trials using direct oral anticoagulants (DOACs) provide support for prevention of DVT in patients with cancer: AVERT with apixaban (DOAC) and CASSINI with rivaroxaban. Guidelines are being updated to include this new data in providing recommendations for outpatient prophylaxis.

B. Initial treatment of acute DVT of the leg

1. Subcutaneous LMWH, DOACs, or fondaparinux are recommended as initial treatment over IV UFH for outpatients, if possible. Patients must be hemodynamically stable, have adequate renal function, and be at low risk for bleeding.

   a) Enoxaparin sodium: 1 mg/kg subcutaneous two times a day, or 1.5 mg/kg subcutaneous daily; caution in patients with creatinine clearance less than 30 ml/min

   b) Direct oral anticoagulants such as rivaroxaban, a direct factor Xa inhibitor, are approved for the treatment and prevention of DVT. Treatment dose of rivaroxaban is 15 mg PO two times a day for 21 days followed by 20 mg PO daily (see Table 43-2).

   c) Dalteparin sodium: 200 IU/kg subcutaneous daily month 1, then 150 IU/kg subcutaneous daily thereafter

   d) Fondaparinux: 5 mg subcutaneous daily for weight less than 50 kg; 7.5 mg subcutaneous daily for weight 50–100 kg; 10 mg subcutaneous daily for weight greater than 100 kg

2. In patients with cancer, DOACs are now frequently used as first-line therapy.

   a) Bleeding risk was higher in all types of GI cancers (i.e., esophageal, gastric, colorectal, hepatobiliary, and pancreatic) and in patients with both resected and unresected tumors. Careful consideration of DOAC use in this patient population is warranted. LMWH is preferred.

   b) Poor renal function (GFR less than 30 mg/min) would warrant careful consideration of DOAC use, as these medications are cleared through the kidneys and could increase bleeding risks.

3. In patients with severe renal failure, IV UFH should be used instead of subcutaneous LMWH or DOACs.

4. If IV UFH is used, it should be administered by continuous infusion with dose adjustment to achieve and maintain an aPTT level that corresponds to plasma heparin levels.

TABLE 43-2	Direct-Acting Oral Anticoagulant Comparisons and Dosages				
Direct Oral Anticoagulants	Enzyme Target	Renal Clearance (%)	Half-Life	Approval	Dose
Apixaban	Xa	27	8–12 hrs	Deep venous thrombosis/pulmonary embolism	10 mg twice a day for 7 days, then 5 mg 2 times a day
Dabigatran	Thrombin	80	14–17 hrs	Deep venous thrombosis/pulmonary embolism	150 mg twice a day after 5–10 days of parenteral anticoagulants
Edoxaban	Xa	50	8–10 hrs	Deep venous thrombosis/pulmonary embolism	60 mg daily after 5–10 days of heparin
Rivaroxaban	Xa	36	7–11 hrs	Deep venous thrombosis/pulmonary embolism	15 mg twice a day for 21 days, then 20 mg daily

Note. Based on information from National Comprehensive Cancer Network, 2021; Park & Khorana, 2019; Wells et al., 2014.

    a) Weight-adjusted regimen of 80 U/kg bolus followed by 18 U/kg/hr is used. The preferred administration method from the American College of Chest Physicians guidelines is as follows.

    b) Check aPTT every six hours and adjust dose until at therapeutic level (plasma heparin levels of 0.3–0.7 IU/ml anti-Xa activity by the amidolytic assay), then check aPTT daily.

    c) It is common for health systems to use nurse-managed heparin protocols to guide rate titration to therapeutic range based on aPTT or anti-Xa results.

    d) Check Hgb, hematocrit, and platelet count every two to three days for the first 14 days, then every two weeks.

5. Subcutaneous UFH can be used as an adequate alternative to IV UFH.

    a) Monitored subcutaneous UFH: Initial dose is 17,500 U/kg or a weight-based dose of 250 U/kg two times a day. Adjust dose to achieve aPTT level that corresponds to plasma heparin levels of 0.3–0.7 IU/ml anti-Xa activity measured six hours after injection.

    b) Fixed-dose unmonitored subcutaneous UFH: Initial dose is 333 U/kg, followed by 250 U/kg two times a day.

6. Recurrence or progression of DVT is 15 times more frequent when therapeutic aPTT level is not reached within the first 48 hours of treatment.

7. Initial treatment with an injectable anticoagulant (e.g., LMWH, UFH) should be given for at least five days.

8. In patients with a high degree of clinical suspicion for DVT, treatment should be initiated while awaiting test results, particularly if results will be delayed by more than four hours.

9. Guidelines recommend using anticoagulation the first three to six months of therapy in patients with DVT and cancer. Subsequent anticoagulation should be continued until the cancer is resolved.

10. If a decision is made to use a vitamin K antagonist (e.g., warfarin), it should be started on day 1 of treatment with LMWH or UFH.

    a) Obtain baseline INR.

    b) Give 5–10 mg PO the first day.

    c) In older adults or patients who are debilitated, malnourished, or who have CHF or liver disease, the initial dose should not exceed 5 mg daily.

    d) Repeat INR the next day; give the same dose if the level is unchanged.

    e) Obtain daily INR and adjust dose until a value of 2–3 is achieved, usually in three to five days.

    f) Once a therapeutic dose has been achieved and maintained for at least two days, stop LMWH or UFH, and check INR two or three times weekly for one or two weeks, then less often depending on stability of the results.

    g) Fluctuations in INR may occur because of inaccuracy of testing, changes in vitamin K intake or absorption, changes in warfarin metabolism, drug or food interactions, or patient noncompliance.

    h) Management of a patient with a prolonged INR is controversial, as most treatments have not been tested. If the INR elevation is minimal, decreasing the dose, holding a dose, or monitoring more frequently with the expectation that the level will decrease are all acceptable options (see Table 43-3).

    i) Check aPTT every six hours and adjust dose until at therapeutic level (plasma heparin levels of 0.3–0.7 IU/ml anti-Xa activity by the amidolytic assay), then check aPTT daily.

    j) Check Hgb, hematocrit, and platelet count every 2–3 days for the first 14 days, then every two weeks.

  11. Anticoagulation is contraindicated in the following conditions.

    a) Underlying coagulopathy: Hemophilia, von Willebrand disease, vitamin K deficiency

    b) Recent major surgical procedures at high risk of bleeding

    c) Thrombocytopenia (platelets less than 50,000/mm^3) or severe platelet dysfunction

    d) Trauma

    e) Recent CNS bleed, intracranial or spinal lesion at high risk for bleeding

    f) High risk for falls

    g) Active bleeding, more than 2 units transfused in 24 hours, or chronic, clinically significant measurable bleeding for more than 48 hours

    h) Heparin allergy

  12. If the patient has acute distal DVT and no additional risk factors, no additional treatment is necessary, but testing should be repeated in one week. If additional risk factors are present, treatment should be initiated as per proximal DVT.

C. Long-term treatment of acute DVT of the leg

  1. Long-term treatment with warfarin, DOACs, LMWH, and fondaparinux is effective in preventing recurrent DVT.

  2. An INR of 2–3 is the preferred intensity of anticoagulation.

  3. For patients on a stable dose of warfarin, INR monitoring should occur approximately every four to six weeks. If INR fluctuates, monitoring frequency should be increased.

  4. Duration of treatment varies based on clinical factors (see Table 43-4).

D. For most patients with DVT, it is not recommended to routinely use a vena cava filter to prevent PE. Filters have not been shown to reduce mortality and are associated with an increased incidence of recurrent DVT. Consider their use if anticoagulation is not possible because of risk of bleeding.

E. IV thrombolytics, catheter-directed thrombolysis, and venous thrombectomy are not recommended as routine treatment of acute DVT but may be applicable in patients with iliofemoral DVT, symptoms for less than 14 days, good functional status, and life expectancy longer than one year.

F. Treatment of acute upper extremity DVT

TABLE 43-3	Reversal of Anticoagulation

Anticoagulant	Reversal
Unfractionated heparin (half-life 1 hour)	Give protamine 1 mg/100 units of heparin slow IV infusion. Follow aPTT closely. Maximum dose is 50 mg per administration.
Low-molecular-weight heparin (half-life 3–7 hours)	Give protamine 1 mg/mg IV of enoxaparin or protamine 1 mg/100 units of dalteparin if given within 8 hours of dose. Give protamine 0.5 mg/mg IV of enoxaparin, or protamine 0.5 mg/100 units of dalteparin, or protamine 0.5 mg/100 units if given > 8 hours prior. If > 12 hours since dose, consider clinical scenario before treating. Give slow IV infusion; maximum dose is 50 mg per administration.
Warfarin (half-life 20–60 hours) • INR < 5, no bleeding	Hold dose.
• INR 5–9, no bleeding	Hold dose; consider low-dose oral vitamin K_1 1–2.5 mg if high risk of bleeding.[a] Monitor INR closely; resume at lower dose.
• INR > 9, no bleeding	Hold dose; consider low-dose oral vitamin K_1 2.5 mg if high risk of bleeding.[a] Monitor INR closely; resume at lower dose.
• Serious or life-threatening bleeding at any INR	Hold dose; give vitamin K_1 10 mg by slow IV infusion.[b] Give three-factor PCC 25–50 units/kg plus FFP 2–3 units, or FFP 15 ml/kg if no PCC available, or rhFVIIa 10–90 mcg/kg IV. Vitamin K_1 can be repeated every 12 hours.
Fondaparinux (half-life 17–21 hours)	No specific antidote is available. Give rhFVIIa 90 mcg/kg IV.[c]
Rivaroxaban (half-life 9–12 hours) Apixaban (half-life 12 hours)	Andexanet alfa • Low dose (400 mg bolus [target 30 mg/min] followed by 500 mg infusion over 125 minutes [or 4 mg/min for up to 120 minutes]) • High dose (800 mg IV bolus [target 30 mg/min]) followed by 1,000 mg over 125 minutes (or 8 mg/min for up to 120 minutes) • Low- vs. high-dose regimen depends on amount of time that has passed since last anticoagulant dose and dose (in mg) that was previously administered.[d]

[a] Vitamin K_1 should not be given subcutaneously because of erratic and delayed absorption.
[b] Rapid infusion of IV vitamin K_1 has a high risk of anaphylaxis.
[c] PCC and rhFVIIa have been associated with thrombotic events.
[d] Low- and high-dose regimens are rounded to the nearest vial size and are indicated only for patients who have life-threatening or uncontrolled bleeding with rivaroxaban or apixaban. This regimen has not been shown to be effective for, and is not indicated for, the treatment of bleeding related to any factor Xa inhibitors other than apixaban or rivaroxaban.

aPTT—activated partial thromboplastin time; FFP—fresh frozen plasma; INR—international normalized ratio; PCC—prothrombin complex concentrate; rhFVIIa—recombinant human activated factor VII

Note. Based on information from Momin & Hughes, 2019; National Comprehensive Cancer Network, 2021.

1. Subcutaneous LMWH, DOACs, fondaparinux, and UFH can be used for initial treatment of acute upper extremity DVT in the same dosing fashion as DVT of the leg.
2. A short course of thrombolytic therapy may be used in patients with a high risk for bleeding from LMWH or UFH.
3. Surgical embolectomy and placement of a vena cava filter may be indicated in patients who fail anticoagulant or thrombolytic therapy.
4. If associated with catheter use, anticoagulate as long as catheter is in place. Do not remove the catheter if it is functional and there is an ongoing need. Consider catheter removal if symptoms persist, and consider catheter-directed thrombolysis in appropriate candidates. Anticoagulate for a minimum of three months.

TABLE 43-4	Recommended Length of Anticoagulation Therapy Based on Clinical Factors

Clinical Factor	Length of Treatment
First episode of DVT because of reversal factor	3 months
First episode of idiopathic DVT	6–12 months
DVT and cancer	Indefinite, or until cancer is resolved
First episode of DVT and antiphospholipid antibodies, or two or more thrombophilic conditions	12 months
First episode of DVT and one or more thrombophilic conditions	6–12 months
Two or more episodes of DVT	Indefinite
Venous access device related	3 months, or as long as catheter in place

DVT—deep venous thrombosis

Note. Based on information from Kearon et al., 2012; National Comprehensive Cancer Network, 2021.

   G. Elastic compression stockings with an ankle pressure gradient of 30–40 mm Hg should be started as soon as feasible and continued for a minimum of two years, longer if patients have postphlebitic syndrome.

VII. Follow-up (Key et al., 2019; Park & Khorana, 2019; Song et al., 2019)
   A. Short term
      1. Frequent dose adjustments of warfarin may be necessary; adjust dose by 5%–10% of total weekly dose and check PT and INR every one to two weeks until stable. When stable dose has been achieved, PT and INR may be checked every four to six weeks.
      2. Monitor for the serious complication of heparin-induced thrombocytopenia.
         a) Suspected if the platelet count falls by more than 50%
         b) Typically develops at a median of 10 days (ranges 3–15 days) after exposure to heparin but may occur earlier in patients who have been previously sensitized to heparin
   B. Long term
      1. A postphlebitic syndrome characterized by some combination of chronic vascular insufficiency, chronic pain, venous stasis, recurrent cellulitis, and ulceration can occur in up to 50% of people with DVT. It may be disabling in a minority of patients. The use of below-knee elastic compression stockings for two years post-DVT can decrease the incidence by up to 50%.
      2. Recurrence of DVT is common; instruct patients to immediately report signs and symptoms of recurrence.
      3. Consider long-term heparin therapy if the patient cannot take oral medications, if the thrombus is refractory to warfarin (paraneoplastic syndrome), or with peptic ulcer disease, alcoholism, or hepatic disorders.
      4. Discontinue anticoagulants three to five days prior to invasive procedures.

VIII. Referral: Vascular surgeon for complicated cases or if chronic sequelae exist

The authors would like to acknowledge Kristine Turner Story, RN, MSN, APRN, BC, for her contribution to this chapter that remains unchanged from the previous edition of this book.

References

Di Nisio, M., van Es, N., & Buller, H. (2016). Deep vein thrombosis and pulmonary embolism. *Lancet, 388*(10063), 3060–3073. https://doi.org/10.1016/S0140-6736(16)30514-1

Douce, D.R., Holmes, C.E., Cushman, M., MacLean, C.D., Ades, S., & Zakai, N.A. (2019). Risk factors for cancer-associated venous thromboembolism: The venous thromboembolism prevention in the ambulatory cancer clinic (VTE-PACC) study. *Journal of Thrombosis and Haemostatsis, 17*(12), 2152–2159. https://doi.org/10.1111/jth.14614

Farge, D., Frere, C., Connors, J.M., Ay, C., Khorana, A.A., Munoz, A., ... Douketis, J. (2019). 2019 international clinical practice guidelines for the treatment and prophylaxis of venous thromboembolism in patients with cancer. *Lancet Oncology, 20*(10), e566–e581. https://doi.org/10.1016/S1470-2045(19)30336-5

Gould, M.K., Garcia, D.A., Wren, S.M., Karanicolas, P.J., Arcelus, J.I., Heit, J.A., & Samama, C.M. (2012). Prevention of VTE in nonorthopedic surgical patients: Antithrombotic therapy and prevention of thrombosis, 9th ed: American College of Chest Physicians evidence-based clinical practice guidelines. *Chest, 141*(2 Suppl.), e227S–e277S. https://doi.org/10.1378/chest.11-2297

Heit, J.A. (2015). Epidemiology of venous thromboembolism. *Nature Reviews Cardiology, 12*(8), 464–474. https://doi.org/10.1038/nrcardio.2015.83

Hutchinson, A., Rees, S., Young, A., Date, K., & Johnson, M.J. (2019). Oral anticoagulation is preferable to injected, but only if it is safe and effective: An interview study of patient and carer experience of oral and injected anticoagulant therapy for cancer-associated thrombosis in the select-d trial. *Palliative Medicine, 33*(5), 510–517. https://doi.org/10.1177/0269216318815377

Kahn, S.R., Lim, W., Dunn, A.S., Cushman, M., Dentali, F., Akl, E.A., ... Murad, M.H. (2012). Prevention of VTE in non-surgical patients: Antithrombotic therapy and prevention of thrombosis, 9th ed: American College of Chest Physicians evidence-based clinical practice guidelines. *Chest, 141*(2 Suppl.), e195S–e226S. https://doi.org/10.1378/chest.11-2296

Kearon, C., Akl, E.A., Comerota, A.J., Prandoni, P., Bounameaux, H., Goldhaber, S.Z., ... Kahn, S.R. (2012). Antithrombotic therapy for VTE disease: Antithrombotic therapy and prevention of thrombosis, 9th ed: American College of Chest Physicians evidence-based clinical practice guidelines. *Chest, 141*(2 Suppl.), e419S–e494S. https://doi.org/10.1378/chest.11-2301

Key, N.S., Khorana, A.A., Kuderer, N.M., Bohlke, K., Lee, A.Y.Y., Arcelus, J.L., ... Falanga, A. (2019). Venous thromboembolism prophylaxis and treatment in patients with cancer: ASCO clinical practice guideline update. *Journal of Clinical Oncology, 38*(5), 496–520. https://doi.org/10.1200/JCO.19.01461

Khorana, A. (2018). Simplicity versus complexity: An existential dilemma as risk tools evolve. *Lancet Haematology, 5*(7), e273–e274. https://doi.org/10.1016/S2352-3026(18)30067-X

Khorana, A.A., & Connolly, G.C. (2009). Assessing risk of venous thromboembolism in the patient with cancer. *Journal of Clinical Oncology, 27*(29), 4839–4847. https://doi.org/10.1200/JCO.2009.22.3271

Khorana, A.A., Kuderer, N.M., Culakova, E., Lyman, G.H., & Francis, C.W. (2008). Development and validation of a predictive model for chemotherapy-associated thrombosis. *Blood, 111*(10), 4902–4907. https://doi.org/10.1182/blood-2007-10-116327

Khorana, A.A., Soff, G.A., Kakkar, A.K., Vadhan-Raj, S., Riess, H., Wun, T., Streiff, M.B., ... Lyman, G.H. (2019). Rivaroxaban for thromboprophylaxis in high-risk ambulatory patients with cancer. *New England Journal of Medicine, 380*(8),720–728. https://doi.org/10.1056/NEJMoa1814630

Momin, J.H., & Hughes, G.J. (2019). Andexanet alfa (Andexxa®) for the reversal of direct oral anticoagulants. *Pharmacy and Therapeutics, 44*(9), 530–532, 549.

Moya Mateo, E., & Muñoz Rivas, N. (2019). Clinical ultrasonography in venous thromboembolism disease. *Revista Clínica Española, 220*(2), 126–134. https://doi.org/10.1016/J.rce.2019.05.014

National Comprehensive Cancer Network. (2021). *NCCN Clinical Practice Guidelines in Oncology (NCCN Guidelines®): Cancer-associated venous thromboembolic disease* [v.2.2021]. http://www.nccn.org/professionals/physician_gls/pdf/vte.pdf

Park, D.Y., & Khorana, A.A. (2019). Risks and benefits of anticoagulation in cancer and noncancer patients. *Seminars in Thrombosis and Hemostasis, 45*(6), 629–637. https://doi.org/10.1055/s-0039-1693474

Song, A.B., Rosovsky, R.P., Connors, J.M., & Al-Samkari, H. (2019). Direct oral anticoagulants for treatment and prevention of venous thromboembolism in cancer patients. *Vascular Health and Risk Management, 15,* 175–186. https://doi.org/10.2147/VHRM.S132556

Sourdon, J., Lager, F., Viel, T., Balvay, D., Moorhouse, R., Bennana, E., ... Tavitian, B. (2017). Cardiac metabolic deregulation induced by the tyrosine kinase receptor inhibitor sunitinib is rescued by endothelin receptor antagonism. *Theranostics, 7*(11), 2757–2774. https://doi.org/10.7150/thno.19551

Wells, P.S., Forgie, M.A., & Rodger, M.A. (2014). Treatment of venous thromboembolism. *JAMA, 311*(7), 717–728. https://doi.org/10.1001/jama.2014.65

Ye, F., Tekiner, H., Yale, E.S., Mazza, J.J., Stalvey, C., & Yale, S.H. (2019). Venothromboembolic signs and medical eponyms: Part 1. *Thrombosis Research, 182,* 194–204. https://doi.org/10.1016/j.thromres.2019.06.012

CHAPTER 44

Dyslipidemia

Allison Strider, MSN, AGNP-BC, AOCNP®,

and Deborah Kirk, DNP, FNP-BC, NP-C, AOCN®, FAANP

I. Definition: Disorders characterized by an elevation in serum cholesterol, LDL, or triglyceride concentrations, or a decrease in HDL (Grundy et al., 2019)

II. Physiology/Pathophysiology (Grundy et al., 2019)
   A. Normal: Serum cholesterol is a measure of normal body production of cholesterol plus dietary intake of cholesterol.
      1. Lipids, such as cholesterol and triglycerides, are complex proteins (i.e., lipoproteins) that circulate in the blood.
      2. Lipoprotein–protein components are known as apoproteins, which have structural and functional roles.
      3. The four major classes of lipoproteins are based on density.
         a) Chylomicrons: Transport dietary fat
            (1) They are low density.
            (2) Lipoprotein lipase removes dietary fat from the body.
            (3) The ability to contribute to atherosclerosis development is unknown.
         b) Very-low-density lipoproteins: Acted on by lipoprotein lipase
            (1) These lipoproteins function to carry triglycerides synthesized in the liver and intestines to capillary beds in adipose tissue and muscle, where they are hydrolyzed.
            (2) After triglyceride removal, they are further metabolized to LDLs.
            (3) These lipoproteins serve as receptors of cholesterol transferred from HDLs, which is mediated by the enzyme cholesterol ester transfer protein.
            (4) They also play a role in atherogenesis.
         c) LDLs: Major carriers of cholesterol
            (1) LDLs are most clearly implicated in atherogenesis.
            (2) When levels are greater than the normal range, they traverse the endothelial wall and become trapped in the arterial intima.
         d) HDLs: Believed to function in peripheral tissues as receptors of free cholesterol
            (1) Cholesterol is esterified and stored in the central core of the HDL.
            (2) They do not contribute to atherogenesis.
   B. Pathophysiology: High blood cholesterol levels result from hepatic dysfunction in the production of LDL receptors, which facilitate absorption of LDL and circulating cholesterol.

III. Clinical features: Dyslipidemia may be asymptomatic or may be associated with other disorders, such as atherosclerotic cardiovascular disease (ASCVD). Therefore, clinical manifestations may be present as a result of other symptom disorders (Alonso et al., 2020; American Heart Association, 2018; Dennison Himmelfarb & Coke, 2019; Grundy et al., 2019; Pencina et al., 2009).

A. Risk factors (see Figure 44-1)
   1. Increased dietary fat
   2. Genetic variations in lipoprotein structures, receptors, and metabolic enzymes
   3. Obesity
   4. Sedentary lifestyle
   5. Risk assessment: 10-year ASCVD risk estimation
      a) Identification of patients that necessitate intensive treatment
      b) Framingham scoring for those with multiple risk factors
         (1) Calculates total score for risk factors of age, total cholesterol, HDL cholesterol, blood pressure, and cigarette smoking
         (2) Classifies 10-year risk for ASCVD of greater than 20%, 10%–20%, and less than 10%
B. Etiology (see Figure 44-2)
C. History
   1. History of cancer and cancer treatment
   2. Current medications: Prescribed, over the counter
   3. History of presenting symptoms: Precipitating factors, onset, location, duration
   4. Changes in ADLs
   5. Past medical history: Hypertension, diabetes, menopause
   6. Family history: Heart disease, endocrine disorders, familial hypercholesterolemia
   7. Social history: Tobacco use, alcohol use, diet, stress
D. Signs and symptoms: Nonspecific
E. Physical examination
   1. Vital signs: Elevation of blood pressure can occur.
   2. Cardiac: Carotid or aortic bruits or cardiac murmurs may be present.

IV. Diagnostic tests (Grundy et al., 2019)
   A. Laboratory

FIGURE 44-1   **Coronary Heart Disease Risk Factors[a]**

Positive Risk Factors
- Men older than 40 years
- Women older than 40 years or postmenopausal without estrogen replacement therapy; premature menopause
- Family history of premature coronary heart disease: Myocardial infarction in father before age 55 years or in mother before age 65 years
- Cigarette smoking
- Hypertension: Blood pressure > 140/90 mm Hg or taking antihypertensive medications
- Diabetes mellitus
- Chronic kidney disease
- Metabolic syndrome
- Inflammatory diseases (e.g., rheumatoid arthritis, psoriasis, HIV)
- Ethnicity (i.e., South Asian ancestry)

Negative Risk Factors
- High high-density lipoprotein level: > 60 mg/dl

---

[a] Subtract one positive risk factor if negative risk factor is present.

Note. Based on information from Grundy et al., 2019.

FIGURE 44-2	Etiology of Secondary Dyslipidemia

Increased Low-Density Lipoprotein Level	Increased Triglyceride Level	Decreased High-Density Lipoprotein Level
• Beta-blockers	• Alcoholism	• Beta-blockers
• Diabetes mellitus	• Beta-blockers	• Cigarette smoking
• Hypothyroidism	• Diabetes mellitus	• Diabetes mellitus
• Nephrotic syndrome	• Diuretics	• Hypertriglyceridemia
• Obstructive liver disease	• Estrogens	• Menopause
• Progestin	• Hypothyroidism	• Obesity
• Protease inhibitors	• Obesity	• Progestins
• Steroids	• Renal insufficiency	• Steroids
• Thiazides	• Ticlopidine	• Uremia

Note. Based on information from Grundy et al., 2019.

1. Measure total cholesterol and HDL levels in a fasting state every five years beginning at age 20 years in patients without evidence of ASCVD or positive risk factors.
2. If cholesterol, HDL, or triglyceride concentrations are elevated in a patient without known ASCVD, perform a lipoprotein analysis (see Table 44-1).
3. Diagnosis is based on repeat measurements of lipids; a single measurement of cholesterol is insufficient.
4. Measure fasting blood glucose level, liver, thyroid, kidney, and endocrine function; complete urinalysis to evaluate secondary causes of dyslipidemia.

  B. Radiology: Not indicated

V. Differential diagnosis (Herrmann et al., 2016)
  A. Diabetes mellitus (see Chapter 151)
  B. Laboratory error
  C. Lipid infusion for nutrition
  D. Drug induced: Asparaginase, thiazide diuretics, letrozole, bexarotene, TKIs, mechanistic target of rapamycin (mTOR) inhibitors, androgen deprivation therapy, cisplatin with or without bleomycin, vinca alkaloids
  E. Hypothyroidism (see Chapter 158)
  F. Renal failure (see Chapter 86)
  G. Nephrotic syndrome (see Chapter 91)

TABLE 44-1	Lipoprotein Analysis

Classification	Total Cholesterol Level	Low-Density Lipoprotein Level	High-Density Lipoprotein Level	Triglycerides
Desirable	< 200 mg/dl	< 100 mg/dl	≥ 60 mg/dl	< 150 mg/dl
Near optimal/above optimal	–	100–129 mg/dl	–	–
Borderline high	200–239 mg/dl	130–159 mg/dl	40–59 mg/dl	150–199 mg/dl
High	≥ 240 mg/dl	160–189 mg/dl	< 40 mg/dl	200–499 mg/dl
Very high	–	≥ 190 mg/dl	–	≥ 500 mg/dl

Note. Based on information from Grundy et al., 2019.

    H. Nonalcoholic fatty liver disease

    I. Metabolic syndrome

    J. Cholangitis

VI. Treatment (Alonso et al., 2020; American Heart Association, 2018; Dennison Himmelfarb & Coke, 2019; Grundy et al., 2019; Morales-Palomo et al., 2020; Ray et al., 2016; U.S. Department of Health and Humans Services, 2016)

    A. Initiation of treatment is based on LDL level and the presence of ASCVD risk factors (see Table 44-2 and Figure 44-1).

    B. All ages should be assessed and encouraged to engage in a healthy lifestyle consisting of a balanced diet, physical activity, and healthy weight.

    C. Patients with risk enhancers should be engaged in a risk discussion.

    D. Diet recommendations (see Table 44-3): Trial of diet therapy for 6–12 weeks before drug therapy is initiated for primary prevention of ASCVD in low-risk individuals. A diet should be low calorie with decreased intake of saturated fat and dietary cholesterol and no consumption of trans fat.

    E. Regular physical activity program

        1. Individualized program

        2. Average of 30 minutes of moderate to vigorous exercise at least five days a week

    F. Weight reduction program with goal of ideal body weight

    G. Drug therapy

        1. Consider in patients with an elevated LDL level after three months of therapeutic lifestyle changes.

        2. Obtain baseline LFTs, as drug therapy can increase liver function enzymes.

            a) Statins: First-line therapy

                (1) Atorvastatin: 10–80 mg PO daily

                (2) Fluvastatin: 20–80 mg PO at bedtime

                (3) Rosuvastatin: 5–40 mg PO daily

                (4) Lovastatin: 20 mg, 40 mg, or 80 mg PO with evening meal

---

TABLE 44-2   **Treatment Initiation and Target Low-Density Lipoprotein Levels**

| | Low-Density Lipoprotein Initiation Levels | | |
Classification	Therapeutic Lifestyle Changes[a]	Drug Therapy	Target Levels
No atherosclerotic cardiovascular disease (ASCVD); less than 2 risk factors	> 190 mg/dl	160–189 mg/dl after 3 months of therapeutic lifestyle changes	< 160 mg/dl
No ASCVD; less than 2 risk factors	160–189 mg/dl	Optional	< 160 mg/dl
No ASCVD; more than 2 risk factors			
• 10-year risk > 20%	> 100 mg/dl	> 100 mg/dl	< 100 mg/dl
• 10-year risk: 10%–20%	≥ 130 mg/dl	≥ 130 mg/dl	< 130 mg/dl
• 10-year risk < 10%	≥ 130 mg/dl	≥ 160 mg/dl	< 130 mg/dl
ASCVD or other atherosclerotic disease	> 100 mg/dl	> 100 mg/dl	< 100 mg/dl

[a] Therapeutic lifestyle changes include diet modifications, increased physical activity, and weight reduction.

Note. Based on information from Grundy et al., 2019.

TABLE 44-3	Diet Recommendations for a Therapeutic Lifestyle Change
Component	**Recommendation**
Total fat	25%–35% of total calories
Saturated fats	Less than 7% of total calories
Dietary cholesterol	Less than 200 mg daily
Carbohydrate	50%–60% of total calories
Dietary fiber	20–30 g daily
Protein	Approximately 15% of total calories

Note. Based on information from U.S. Department of Health and Human Services, 2016.

      (5) Pravastatin: 10–80 mg PO at bedtime
      (6) Simvastatin: 10–40 mg PO at bedtime
      (7) Pitavastatin: 1–4 mg PO daily
   b) Proprotein convertase subtilisin/kexin type 9 (PCSK9) inhibitors
      (1) Alirocumab: 75–300 mg subcutaneous every two to four weeks
      (2) Evolocumab: 140 or 420 mg subcutaneous every two to four weeks
   c) Cholesterol absorption inhibitor: Ezetimibe 10 mg PO daily
   d) Bile acid sequestrants: Contraindicated if triglycerides greater than 300 mg/dl
      (1) Cholestyramine: 4 g PO two times a day (maximum 24 g daily)
      (2) Colestipol: 5–30 g PO two times a day
      (3) Colesevelam: 3.75 g PO daily
   e) Fibric acid derivatives. Contraindicated with severe hepatic or renal insufficiency; should be avoided in combination with statin, as can cause muscle damage
      (1) Gemfibrozil: 600 mg PO two times a day
      (2) Fenofibrate tablets: 48–145 mg PO daily
      (3) Clofibrate: 1,000 mg PO two times a day
   f) Nicotinic acid: 1.5–6 g PO daily in divided doses; may cause flushing and increase blood glucose
   g) Combination agents: Ezetimibe plus simvastatin 10 mg/10 mg to 10 mg/80 mg PO daily
   h) Omega-3 fatty acid capsules to lower triglycerides: 4 g daily or 2 g two times a day

VII. Follow-up (Grundy et al., 2019; Robinson, 2019)
   A. Measure LDL level and LFTs at four and 12 weeks after initiation of drug therapy.
   B. If the LDL target level is not reached after four to six weeks, intensify LDL-lowering therapy.
   C. If the LDL target level is not reached after 12 weeks, intensify drug therapy or refer to a cardiologist.
      1. If the LDL target level is reached, monitor follow-up levels every three to six months.
      2. Perform annual follow-up lipoprotein analysis for patients with ASCVD.
   D. Measure LFTs every six months.
   E. Monitor for myalgia or muscle weakness induced with statins.

VIII. Referral: Cardiologist if no reduction in LDL level after 12 weeks of drug therapy or if patient is classified as high risk

The authors would like to acknowledge Diane G. Cope, PhD, ARNP-BC, AOCNP®, for her contri-bution to this chapter that remains unchanged from the previous edition of this book.

References

Alonso, R., Perez de Isla, L., Muñiz-Grijalvo, O., & Mata, P. (2020). Barriers to early diagnosis and treatment of familial hy-percholesterolemia: Current perspectives on improving patient care. *Vascular Health and Risk Management, 16,* 11–25. https://doi.org/10.2147/VHRM.S192401

American Heart Association. (2018). *Cholesterol management guide for healthcare practitioners.* https://www.heart.org/-/media/files/health-topics/cholesterol/cholesterol-guide-for-hc-practitioners-english.pdf

Dennison Himmelfarb, C.R., & Coke, L. (2019). New 2018 cholesterol guideline: Enhanced risk estimation and therapeu-tic options drive shared decision making. *Journal of Cardiovascular Nursing, 34*(2), 103–105. https://doi.org/10.1097/JCN.0000000000000563

Grundy, S.M., Stone, N.J., Bailey, A.L., Beam, C., Birtcher, K.K., Blumenthal, R.S., ... Yeboah, J. (2019). 2018 AHA/ACC/AACVPR/AAPA/ABC/ACPM/ADA/AGS/APhA/ASPC/NLA/PCNA guideline on the management of blood choles-terol: A report of the American College of Cardiology/American Heart Association task force on clinical practice guidelines. *Circulation, 139*(25), e1082–e1143. https://doi.org/10.1161/CIR.0000000000000625

Herrmann, J., Yang, E.H., Iliescu, C.A., Cilingiroglu, M., Charitakis, K., Hakeem, A., ... Marmagkiolis, K. (2016). Vascular toxicities of cancer therapies: The old and the new—An evolving avenue. *Circulation, 133*(13), 1272–1289. https://doi.org/10.1161/CIRCULATIONAHA.115.018347

Morales-Palomo, F., Ramirez-Jimenez, M., Ortega, J.F., Moreno-Cabañas, A., & Mora-Rodriguez, R. (2020). Exercise training adaptations in metabolic syndrome individuals on chronic statin treatment. *Journal of Clinical Endocrinology and Metabolism, 105*(4), e1695–e1704. https://doi.org/10.1210/clinem/dgz304

Pencina, M.J., D'Agostino, R.B., Sr., Larson, M.G., Massaro, J.M., & Vasan, R.S. (2009). Predicting the 30-year risk of cardiovascular disease: The Framingham heart study. *Circulation, 119*(24), 3078–3084. https://doi.org/10.1161/CIRCULATIONAHA.108.816694

Ray, K.K., Ginsberg, H.N., Davidson, M.H., Pordy, R., Bessac, L., Minini, P., ... Cannon, C.P. (2016). Reductions in athero-genic lipids and major cardiovascular events: A pooled analysis of 10 ODYSSEY trials comparing alirocumab with con-trol. *Circulation, 134*(24), 1931–1943. https://doi.org/10.1161/CIRCULATIONAHA.116.024604

Robinson, J.G. (2019). New insights into managing symptoms during statin therapy. *Progress in Cardiovascular Diseases, 62*(5), 390–394. https://doi.org/10.1016/j.pcad.2019.10.005

U.S. Department of Health and Human Services. (2016). *For professionals: Recommendations at-a-glance: Dietary guidelines for Americans 2015–2020* (8th ed.). https://health.gov/dietaryguidelines/2015/resources/DGA_Recommendations-At-A-Glance.pdf

CHAPTER 45

Dysrhythmias

Brenda K. Shelton, DNP, APRN–CNS, RN, CCRN, AOCN®

I. Definition: Disturbance in the regular excitation of the heart (Padeletti & Bagliani, 2017)
   A. An abnormal rate or rhythm of the heart classified by the region of the heart in which it arises (e.g., sinus, atrial, AV junction [also called nodal, junctional, or ventricular])
   B. Also called *arrhythmias*, technically meaning "without rhythm"
   C. Subtypes classified by the area of the heart in which the dysrhythmia originates

II. Physiology/Pathophysiology (Padeletti & Bagliani, 2017; Tso et al., 2015)
   A. Normal: An electrical conduction system coordinates the sequence of muscular contractions during the cardiac cycle.
      1. An electrical impulse stimulates initiation of each contraction, which originates in the sinoatrial node, located in the right atrium.
      2. The impulse travels through both atria via intra-atrial pathways to the AV node in the atrial septum.
      3. A pause in the AV node allows for atrial contraction.
      4. The impulse continues into the ventricle through the bundle of His and its branches to the Purkinje fibers in the ventricles, ending with ventricle contraction.
   B. Pathophysiology (see Table 45-1)
      1. Disruptions in normal rhythm or rate cause compromised cardiac output via the following mechanisms.
         a) Decreased contractility leads to decreased cardiac output.
         b) Diminished cardiac filling time leads to reduced cardiac output.
         c) Asynchronous myocardial cell conduction results in lack of coordinated ejection.
         d) Delayed repolarization alters myocardial cell irritability.
      2. Reduced tissue perfusion occurs from loss of atrial contraction (one-third of cardiac output).
      3. Unstable dysrhythmia
         a) When cardiac output is reduced, the body will compensate by shunting blood to the major organs—the heart, lungs, and brain.
         b) Unstable cardiac rhythms demonstrate an inability to perfuse these major organs and result in symptoms of hypoxemia within these body systems.
      4. Abnormal rhythms with adequate perfusion to the major organs are considered stable dysrhythmia. Patients may exhibit symptoms but do not have hemodynamic or homeostatic compromise.
      5. The potential for the rhythm disturbance to disintegrate into a life-threatening rhythm exists in the following circumstances.
         a) Frequent sinus pauses
         b) Rapid supraventricular tachycardia

TABLE 45-1	Pathophysiologic Mechanisms of Specific Dysrhythmias	
Mechanism of Dysrhythmia	Examples of Resulting Dysrhythmias	Etiologies of Physiologic Alteration
Alternative conduction pathways	Supraventricular tachycardia	Congenital condition Wolff-Parkinson-White syndrome Mitral valve prolapse Atrial enlargement Pulmonary disease
Catecholamine dependence	Sinus tachycardia Supraventricular tachycardia Premature ventricular contractions Ventricular tachycardia	Catecholamine medications: Dopamine, levodopa, inhalant sympathomimetics Pheochromocytoma Prolonged stress or anxiety Fever
Conduction pathway blockage or slowing through the atrioventricular (AV) node; nerve damage	First-degree AV block Second-degree AV block (type I or type II) Third-degree AV block	Medications: Digoxin and derivatives, beta-blockers, calcium channel blockers Acidosis Cardiac exposure to radiation Myocardial ischemia Cardiothoracic surgery: Aortic valve (most common valve surgery), heart transplant, esophagectomy (may destroy innervation and require cardiac pacemaker implantation)
Myocardial irritability	Atrial flutter Premature ventricular contraction/beats Ventricular tachycardia Ventricular fibrillation	Hypoxemia Myocardial ischemia Electrolyte imbalances Pain Fear, anxiety Hypertension Severe heart failure Stress-induced heart failure/Takotsubo syndrome
Normal variants	Sinus arrhythmia	–
QT prolongation with prolonged refractory period	Ventricular tachycardia, torsades de pointes variant	Female gender Preexisting bradycardia Electrolyte imbalances: Hypokalemia, hypomagnesemia, hypocalcemia Genetic predisposition Antidysrhythmic medications: Amiodarone, dofetilide, sotalol Antineoplastic medications: Arsenic trioxide, immune checkpoint inhibitors, mechanistic target of rapamycin (mTOR) inhibitors, P13K-AKT inhibitors, protease inhibitors, tamoxifen, tyrosine kinase inhibitors Supportive care medications: Azole antifungals, fluoroquinolones, loperamide, macrolide antibiotics, methadone, opiates, phenothiazines, proton pump inhibitors, selective serotonin antagonist antidepressants, selective serotonin reuptake inhibitors, antiemetics

(Continued on next page)

TABLE 45-1	Pathophysiologic Mechanisms of Specific Dysrhythmias *(Continued)*

Mechanism of Dysrhythmia	Examples of Resulting Dysrhythmias	Etiologies of Physiologic Alteration
Vagal stimulation	Sinus bradycardia Sinus pauses Junctional rhythm Second-degree heart block, type I	Vomiting Intractable coughing Right coronary artery disease Hepatic disease

Note. Based on information from De Ponti et al., 2019; Herring et al., 2019; Leonelli et al., 2019a, 2019b; Padeletti & Bagliani, 2017; Porta-Sánchez et al., 2017.

> *c)* Ventricular tachycardia or ventricular fibrillation
> *d)* Heart blocks: Second-degree heart block II, third-degree heart block
> *e)* Cardiac arrest: Pulseless ventricular tachycardia or ventricular fibrillation, asystole, or pulseless electrical activity (any visible heart rhythm without a pulse)

III. Clinical features: Dysrhythmias vary among individuals based on their general health, compensatory mechanisms, and beginning cardiac reserve. Severity of the rhythm disturbance is determined by whether the patient is "stable" or "unstable" by symptomatology (American Heart Association [AHA], 2016; Chu et al., 2019; Costantini, 2019; Littmann et al., 2019).

A. Risk factors: Dysrhythmias are associated with specific physiologic disorders, medications, cancer therapies, and electrolyte imbalances (see Tables 45-2 and 45-3).

B. Etiology (see Tables 45-1, 45-2, and 45-3)

C. History
   1. History of cancer and cancer treatment
   2. Current medications: Prescribed, over the counter, herbal/vitamin supplements
   3. History of presenting symptoms: Precipitating factors, onset, location, duration
   4. Changes in ADLs
   5. Past medical history/family history: Cardiac disease, heart rhythm disturbances (e.g., Wolff-Parkinson-White syndrome, prolonged QT syndrome), syncope, sudden unexplained death, anemia, diabetes mellitus
   6. Surgical history: Thoracic, esophageal, or gastric surgeries may sever or injure the vagus nerve, causing an increased risk for tachydysrhythmias; heart transplantation results in absent vagus nerve and unresponsiveness to atropine.
   7. Social history: Illicit drug use, excessive daily caffeine consumption (more than three caffeinated drinks), smoking

D. Signs and symptoms: Symptoms considered indicative of cardiovascular "instability" resulting from the rhythm disturbance are marked with an asterisk (*).
   1. Palpitations
   2. Anxiety
   3. Chest discomfort*: May radiate to left arm, shoulder, or jaw
   4. Dyspnea*
   5. Headache
   6. Dizziness/syncope/near syncope: More pronounced when sitting or standing
   7. Tinnitus
   8. Mental status changes*
   9. Reduced urine output, infrequent urination/concentrated urine
   10. Anorexia

TABLE 45-2 **Risk Factors for Dysrhythmias**

Risk Factor/Concomitant Diseases	High-Risk Dysrhythmias	Etiology of Rhythm Disturbance
Amyloid of the heart	Tachycardia Atrial dysrhythmias Ventricular premature beats or nonsustained ventricular tachycardia	Oncologic disorders associated with development of amyloid include the following. • Benign monoclonal gammopathy • Multiple myeloma • Primary amyloidosis • Waldenström macroglobulinemia
Anemia	Tachycardia Atrial dysrhythmias Premature ventricular contractions	Tissue hypoxia causes myocardial irritability.
Diabetes mellitus	Tachycardia Atrial dysrhythmias	Autonomic neuropathies from high glucose levels decrease autonomic regulation capabilities of autonomic nerves such as the vagus nerves.
Fever	Sinus tachycardia Atrial dysrhythmias, especially with rapid ventricular response	Increased metabolic rate drives increased heart rate to meet demand. Vasodilation with fever causes autonomic response to perceived reduced vascular volume.
Hyperthyroidism	Tachycardia	Increased thyroid hormone levels lead to increased metabolic rate and sympathetic stimulation.
Hypothermia	Bradycardia Junctional rhythm Heart block	Decreased body temperature slows ion transfer across the myocyte cell membrane and slows conduction.
Hypothyroidism	Bradycardia Heart block	Reduced metabolic rate causes decreased cardiac conduction rate.
Increased intracranial pressure	Bradycardia Heart block	Pressure in the brain affects function of the autonomic regulatory center and leads to hypertension. Autoregulatory failure and compensatory mechanisms for hypertension lead to slow heart rate.
Ingestants	Bradycardia Tachycardia Prolonged QT/torsades de pointes	Licorice has stimulant effects causing tachycardia. Most QT-prolonging ingestants (e.g., grapefruit juice, mushrooms, toxic honey, liquid protein drinks) act in the cytochromes P450 pathway to slow conduction, causing QT prolongation or its related dysrhythmias.
Sleep disorders (i.e., obstructive sleep apnea and its variants)	Tachycardia Ventricular dysrhythmias	Disordered sleep can lead to tachycardia or ventricular irritability from hypertension, coronary artery disease, or heart failure.

(Continued on next page)

TABLE 45-2   Risk Factors for Dysrhythmias *(Continued)*

Risk Factor/Concomitant Diseases	High-Risk Dysrhythmias	Etiology of Rhythm Disturbance
Cancer-Related Therapy[a]		
Arsenic trioxide	Bradycardia Heart block Ventricular dysrhythmias	Prolonged repolarization leads to prolonged QT with initial bradycardia and increased risk for automaticity later.
Cetuximab, panitumumab	Sudden death from ventricular dysrhythmias	Exact mechanism is unknown.
Fluoropyrimidines (e.g., 5-fluorouracil, capecitabine)	Tachycardia Ventricular rhythms	Exact mechanism for increased ventricular irritability is unknown. The diarrhea produced by these agents depletes electrolytes and increases the risk of dysrhythmias.
Ibrutinib	Atrial fibrillation	It is thought to be related to inflammation.
Radiation to the chest region	Conduction disturbances with heart block	It occurs late (> 8 years) after exposure. It is likely due to radiation-induced fibrosis of the heart muscle that affects conduction pathways.
Targeted agents	Prolonged QT with risk for ventricular tachycardia/torsades de pointe variant	Variable mechanisms of altered electrolyte influx into the cells causes prolonged conduction and myocardial cell recovery and prolonged QT interval, predisposing to dysrhythmias.
Cancer Induced		
Heart involvement with cancer, primary or metastatic disease (e.g., atrial myxoma, lymphoma, sarcoma)	Atrial dysrhythmias Premature ventricular beats or ventricular tachycardia	Cancer infiltrates the myocardial muscle, causing increased irritability or alternative conduction pathways.
Pheochromocytoma	Tachycardia	Endogenous catecholamines are released in excessive amounts into the bloodstream.
Recent Surgery		
Gastrectomy, vagotomy, esophagectomy	Tachycardia	Destruction of the vagus nerve from surgery or tumor invasion causes reduced parasympathetic tone, permitting excessive sympathetic activity.
Pneumonectomy	Tachycardia	Severed autonomic nerves lead to decreased autoregulation.
Medications		
Anesthetic agents (e.g., local agents, inhaled anesthetics, thiopental)	Tachycardia Ventricular dysrhythmias Bradycardia/heart block Ischemia and myocardial infarction	It is more common with local anesthetics, which block sodium and potassium channels of neuromuscular tissue. Inhalant anesthetics cause myocardial depression and possible ischemia.

(Continued on next page)

TABLE 45-2	**Risk Factors for Dysrhythmias** *(Continued)*	
Risk Factor/Concomitant Diseases	**High-Risk Dysrhythmias**	**Etiology of Rhythm Disturbance**
Bronchodilators	Tachycardia Premature beats, especially ventricular	Most bronchodilators act by stimulating beta sympathetic receptors. Receptor stimulation causes increased sympathetic tone.
Haloperidol, droperidol	Bradycardia Ventricular dysrhythmias	Prolonged repolarization leads to prolonged QT with initial bradycardia and increased risk for automaticity later.
Methylxanthines	Tachycardia Premature beats, especially ventricular	Caffeine-like stimulation of the heart causes increased conduction rate.

[a] Antineoplastic agents causing direct dysrhythmias, not just a condition placing at risk such as QT prolongation

Note. Based on information from Chandrasekhar & Fradley, 2019; Chu et al., 2019; Herring et al., 2019; Leonelli et al., 2019b; Woosley et al., 2017.

    11. Nausea
    12. Abdominal cramping
    13. Undigested food in the stool
    14. Peripheral/dependent edema, effusions
    15. Unexplained fatigue
  E. Physical examination: Stable rhythms typically are without outward physical signs. Unstable rhythms have the potential to be life threatening and exhibit abnormal findings of the heart, lungs, and brain.
    1. Vital signs
      a) Blood pressure: Systolic blood pressure less than 90 mm Hg, mean blood pressure less than 60 mm Hg, or greater than 40 mm Hg drop from baseline systolic is indicative of hypotension.
      b) Pulse strength and equality: Evaluate several sites (e.g., apical, carotid, radial, femoral, pedal) and compare to normal; determine the apical/peripheral pulse deficit, evidence of weak or thready pulses at one site, or pulsus alternans (i.e., alternating strong and weak pulse). Weaker peripheral pulses indicate inadequate cardiac output from the rhythm disturbance.
      c) Irregular pulse, often acute onset: It may be preceded by premature contractions or a primary atrial rhythm that can cause an irregular pulse, making it difficult to ascertain when the rhythm converts from frequent premature atrial contractions to atrial fibrillation or flutter.
      d) Atrial flutter often presents with rapid escalation of the heart rate and rates of 180–200 bpm, which are higher than other narrow complex tachycardias.
      e) Respiratory rate and effort are increased when perfusion is inadequate.
    2. Integument
      a) Assessment for changes in skin color, temperature, and appearance
      b) Cyanosis, mottling, and cool/clammy skin indicative of poor perfusion
      c) Edema indicative of heart failure
    3. Cardiac
      a) Heart sounds: S_3, S_4, split heart sounds, and summation gallops, which may indicate cardiovascular incompetence

TABLE 45-3	Acid-Base and Electrolyte Imbalances and Electrocardiogram Rhythm Disturbances
Electrolyte Imbalance	**Dysrhythmia, Electrocardiogram Abnormality**
Acidosis: pH < 7.06 is most likely to cause dysrhythmias.	• Slowed conduction—bradycardia, junctional rhythm, heart block
Hypercalcemia: Corrected serum calcium > 12 mg/ml	• Shortened QT interval • Bradycardia, junctional rhythm, heart block
Hyperkalemia: Serum potassium values > 6.5–6.8 mEq/L are most likely to cause dysrhythmias.	• Increased irritability, premature beats • Ventricular fibrillation
Hypocalcemia: Ionized calcium < 1 mEq/L	• Increased irritability, premature beats • Heart block • Ventricular fibrillation • Prolonged QT intervals
Hypokalemia: Serum potassium values < 3.4 mEq/L can cause no specific low point, which increases risk.	• Increased irritability, premature beats • Flattening T wave or appearance of U wave
Hypomagnesemia: Serum magnesium < 2 mEq/L	• Increased irritability, premature beats • Increased conduction through atrioventricular node (tachycardia)

Note. Based on information from Leonelli et al., 2019a; Padeletti & Bagliani, 2017; Trenor et al., 2018.

      b) S_3 gallop: Slow or rapid heart rates and ventricular dysrhythmias causing heart failure that may present with this abnormal heart sound

      c) S_4 gallop: Indicates decreased compliance of the left ventricle, which can occur with PH, CAD, aortic stenosis, systemic hypertension, and pulmonic stenosis

      d) Summation gallop: S_3 and S_4 present during tachydysrhythmia

      e) Split S_2 heart sounds: Clinically significant in tachydysrhythmia

      f) Jugular venous pressure/JVD: Greater than 2 cm above the clavicle when cardiac output is compromised; more pronounced and appears as a large wave moving up the neck when ventricular tachycardia is present

      g) Capillary refill: Longer than three seconds considered indicative of compromised cardiac output when other obvious causes or peripheral vascular disease are not present

   4. Neurologic: Quick Mini-Mental Status Examination; wakefulness, orientation, appropriateness, and visual acuity to provide data to reflect brain perfusion

   5. Abdominal: Decreased bowel sounds with decreased perfusion

IV. Diagnostic tests (AHA, 2016; Chen et al., 2019; De Ponti et al., 2019; Haugaa et al., 2017; Hussain & Nabi, 2017; Leonelli et al., 2019a, 2019b; Littmann et al., 2019; Padeletti & Bagliani, 2017; Singh & Peter, 2016; Tso et al., 2015)

   A. Laboratory

      1. CBC to identify anemia as a potential cause of dysrhythmia

      2. Electrolytes to evaluate for imbalances: Magnesium, calcium, potassium

      3. Free T_4 and TSH to evaluate for hyperthyroidism and hypothyroidism

      4. Adrenal corticotropic stimulation test to evaluate for adrenal insufficiency

      5. ABGs, as indicated, to evaluate for hypoxemia

6. Cardiac enzymes and troponins to evaluate for cardiac ischemia/infarction

7. BNP to detect heart failure: Has been used to predict recurrence of atrial fibrillation

8. Drug levels if drug toxicity is suspected: Digoxin, phenytoin, tacrolimus

B. Radiology: Chest x-ray to rule out cardiomyopathy and CHF

C. ECG

1. ECG rhythm strip in leads II, aVF, and V_1 each clearly define a particular portion of the normal P, QRS, and T waves. Table 45-4 outlines differences among rhythm disturbances, and Table 45-5 lists common dysrhythmias and key clinical features. The recommended order for examining the rhythm is as follows.

   a) Determine rate—less than 60 bpm, 60–100 bpm, greater than 100 bpm.

   b) Determine regularity—regular, irregular with a pattern, grossly irregular.

   c) Determine if P waves precede every QRS or some QRS, or if no P waves.

   d) Measure PR interval if present; normal value is 0.12–0.20 seconds.

      (1) Note if PR interval varies with a pattern or is inconsistent or erratic.

      (2) Note early beats with or without a P wave, even if the QRS complex is unchanged.

   e) Measure QRS interval; normal value is 0.04–0.10 seconds.

      (1) Note all varied appearances of the QRS.

      (2) Measure each different QRS.

      (3) Determine if QRS complexes all go in the same direction and, if not, whether specific variants go in the opposite direction.

2. Twelve-lead ECG will better define the rhythm disturbance and determine whether accompanying ischemia is present.

   a) Fifteen- and 18-lead ECGs are more important for detection of MI than dysrhythmia interpretation.

   b) If the rhythm is not always present, an exercise stress test may be performed to trigger the rhythm disturbance.

3. A 24-, 48-, or 96-hour Holter monitor provides continuous rhythm monitoring and is helpful if the rhythm disturbance is intermittent. The patient keeps a diary to identify clinical symptoms related to the rhythm disturbance.

4. Event-triggered recorders may be used in place of Holter monitoring; however, the risk of missed events must be balanced with speed and comparative ease of interpretation.

5. Implanted loop recorders can detect dysrhythmias for an extended period of time and are useful to detect complex, multifactorial, and multiorigin dysrhythmia-related symptoms.

D. Other

1. Electrophysiologic testing: This test is used for life-threatening dysrhythmias to map the source of the dysrhythmia and provide an avenue for definitive treatment.

2. Echocardiogram: It is not used to diagnose dysrhythmias but provides information regarding the cause for the rhythm.

3. Cardiac radionuclide imaging: Imaging is helpful for identifying structural issues, ischemia, or myopathy contributing to dysrhythmia.

4. Pulse oximetry: Oxygen saturation is diminished when cardiac output is impaired.

V. Differential diagnosis (see Tables 45-4 and 45-5)

VI. Treatment: Treatment is dependent on etiologic factors, patient tolerance, and aggressiveness of planned support (Al-Khatib et al., 2018; Al Mahameed & Ziv, 2019; AHA, 2016; Brembilla-Perrot et al., 2018; Camm, 2017; Dahya & Taigen, 2019; Dan et al., 2018; De Ponti et al., 2019; Elbanhawy et al., 2019; January et al., 2019; Kachur & Morin, 2019; Lei et al., 2018; Leonelli

| TABLE 45-4 | Differentiating Electrocardiogram Rhythm Disturbances | | | | |

Electrocardiogram Rhythm[a]	Rate (bpm)	Regularity	P Waves	PR Interval	QRS Interval
Normal sinus rhythm	60–100	Regular	Normal	Constant	Normal
Normal sinus bradycardia	< 60	Regular	Normal	Constant	Normal
Sinus pauses/arrest	< 60 60–100	Irregular	Normal	Constant	Normal
Normal sinus tachycardia	> 100	Regular	Normal	Constant	Normal
Atrial fibrillation	< 60 60–100 > 100	Irregular	None	Not identifiable	Normal
Atrial flutter	< 60 60–100 > 100	Regularly irregular	None	Not identifiable	Normal
Supraventricular tachycardia	> 100	Regular	None	Not identifiable	Normal
Junctional (nodal) rhythm	< 60	Regular	None	None	Normal
Accelerated junctional (nodal) rhythm	60–100	Regular	None	None	Normal
Premature ventricular contractions	< 60 60–100 > 100	Regularly irregular	Normal	Constant	Wide
Ventricular tachycardia	> 100	Regular	None	None	Wide
Ventricular fibrillation	Not identifiable	None	None	None	None
Asystole	Not identifiable	None	None	None	None
First-degree atrioventricular block (1° AVB)	< 60 60–100	Regular	Normal	Constant	Normal
Second-degree atrioventricular block, type I (2° AVB-I)	< 60 60–100	Regularly irregular	Normal	Varies	Normal
Second-degree atrioventricular block, type II (2° AVB-II)	< 60 60–100	Irregular	Normal	Constant	Normal Wide
Third-degree atrioventricular block (3° AVB)	< 60	Regular	Normal	Varies	Wide

[a] Some categories vary with the rhythm (i.e., rate can be slow, normal, or rapid in atrial fibrillation); therefore, some rhythms may have more than one criteria within the same category.

Note. Based on information from Chen et al., 2019; Costantini, 2019; De Ponti et al., 2019; Leonelli et al., 2019a, 2019b; Padeletti & Bagliani, 2017; Singh & Peter, 2016.

TABLE 45-5	Key Features of Common Dysrhythmias	
Origin	**Dysrhythmia**	**Key Features**
Sinus node (rate)	Normal sinus rhythm	Normal intervals, normal rate
	Sinus tachycardia	Normal intervals, rate > 100 bpm
	Sinus bradycardia	Normal intervals, rate < 60 bpm
	Sinus arrhythmia	Variation of rate that coincides with respirations
Atria (P wave, PR)	Premature atrial contractions	Early beat with a P wave, normal QRS
	Atrial flutter	F waves (sawtooth), same upside down and right-side up, usually regular rate and normal QRS
	Atrial fibrillation	Irregular rate, normal QRS
	Paroxysmal atrial tachycardia	Sudden-onset tachycardia with indistinguishable Ps and Ts, narrow QRS
	Supraventricular tachycardia	Same as above, may have a less sudden onset
Atrioventricular node/ junction (PR)	Premature junctional contractions	Early beat without a P wave or inverted P wave, normal QRS
	Junctional rhythm	Absent, inverted or late P waves, regular rate 40–60 bpm
	Accelerated junctional rhythm	Same as above but with rate > 60 bpm
Ventricle (QRS)	Premature ventricular contractions	Early beat without a P wave, widened QRS
	Idioventricular rhythm	Regular rate 20–40 bpm, wide QRS
	Ventricular tachycardia	Wide QRS, rate > 140 bpm
	Ventricular fibrillation	Erratic activity, no discernible P or QRS
Atrioventricular node block (P/QRS relationship)	First-degree heart block	Regular rate, prolonged PR
	Second-degree heart block (type I/Wenckebach)	Progressively lengthening PR until QRS is dropped, then returning to baseline PR
	Second-degree heart block (type II)	Randomly dropped QRSs but consistent PR interval when QRS is present
	Third-degree heart block	Regular QRS with itself and regular P waves with themselves, but no consistent relationship to each other. Rate usually is slow, and QRS usually is wide.
No activity	Asystole	No electrical activity (if only P waves are present, may be called ventricular standstill)

Note. Based on information from Costantini, 2019; De Ponti et al., 2019; Leonelli et al., 2019a, 2019b; Padeletti & Bagliani, 2017; Singh & Peter, 2016.

et al., 2019a; Mahtani & Nair, 2019; Mankad & Kalahasty, 2019; Markman & Nazarian, 2019; Miften et al., 2019; Rhea et al., 2019; Shah et al., 2019; Steffen et al., 2019; Trenor et al., 2018).

A. Do not administer specific antiarrhythmic drugs if any of the following are true.
    1. Cause of rhythm is known and treatable.
    2. No symptoms of instability are present.
    3. The rhythm is unlikely to disintegrate into a life-threatening unstable rhythm.

B. Emergency management of dysrhythmia
    1. Determine patient tolerance.
    2. Correct underlying etiology.
    3. Regulate metabolic balance (e.g., electrolytes, hormones).

C. Nutraceuticals/herbs reported to "regulate heart rhythm" may be used to supplement other therapies or as a preventive measure in patients at risk for dysrhythmias.
    1. Selenium supplementation may prevent ventricular dysrhythmias. Foods rich in selenium include meat, poultry, whole grains, legumes, nuts, peas, brewer's yeast, wheat germ, broccoli, onions, tomatoes, and garlic.
    2. Thiamine (vitamin B_1) may reduce the incidence of all dysrhythmias. L-carnitine is a coenzyme similar in action to thiamine.
    3. Taurine is an essential amino acid thought to reduce sympathetic nervous system stimulation and associated tachydysrhythmias. It is found in meats, poultry, grains, and legumes.
    4. Omega-3 fatty acids are found in flaxseed, perilla, and fish oils and are reported to reduce dysrhythmias.
    5. Vitamin E at approximately 2,000 IU daily is reported to reduce atrial and ventricular fibrillation in high-risk individuals.
    6. Vitamin D has been proposed to reduce risk of cardiovascular disease in general, but studies have not established this benefit.
    7. Herbs/nutraceuticals that have effects similar to calcium channel–blocking agents include angelica, garlic, ginger, ginkgo biloba, grape seed, green tea, hawthorn, magnesium, and olive leaf.
    8. Herbs/nutraceuticals that have effects similar to beta-blockers include grape seed, green tea, hawthorn, and magnesium.
    9. Coenzyme Q10 is a well-known supplement taken at 120 mg daily and is thought to decrease the incidence of angina, dysrhythmias, and heart failure.

D. Definitive pharmacologic treatment, as indicated
    1. Antidysrhythmic medications act by various mechanisms, many of which are related to the inhibition of electrolyte transmission and creation of an electrical impulse. Sodium, potassium, and calcium channels have the ability to slow or speed cardiac conduction, producing dysrhythmias.
    2. Selection of a medication is based on the specific dysrhythmia, the mechanism of the dysrhythmia, the objective of treatment (e.g., conversion vs. rate control), and other patient-related variables.
    3. Combining medications from several classes may improve antidysrhythmic potential but can create cumulative adverse effects.
    4. When converting from IV to PO, many IV agents have a short half-life; subsequently, the first PO dose is administered immediately after discontinuing the IV drip.
    5. Therapeutic drug level monitoring is performed when appropriate.

E. Interventional strategies for all dysrhythmias
    1. Observation and no immediate treatment indicated
        a) Asymptomatic and not life threatening: Specific types of ventricular preexcitation syndromes, Wolff-Parkinson-White syndrome

    b) Low risk for complications: Slow, asymptomatic atrial fibrillation in older adults without ischemia or major risk factors for stroke

2. Dysrhythmias can be mapped electrically and "ablated" to remove irritable foci.
   a) Decision based on symptom severity/frequency and risk for sudden death
   b) Complications of ablation for dysrhythmias: Sudden cardiac arrest, postprocedure dysrhythmias, vascular injury, bleeding at insertion site, stroke, hemothorax/pneumothorax

3. Myocardial restructuring may employ AV pacing to coordinate muscular contraction and enhance cardiac output.

4. Implantable devices are multifunctional (e.g., pacemaker, defibrillator), which may require adjustment of settings. Recognition of specific features can help providers understand when the device is functioning normally or needs to be adjusted.
   a) Know whether single or multichamber (atrial, ventricular, both); ECG rhythm appearance will differ depending on these features.
   b) Rationale for insertion can include rescue for bradyarrhythmia or ventricular tachycardia/fibrillation or override for tachydysrhythmia; mechanisms for trigger and expected heart rate will differ.
   c) Intermittent pacing is more common if native rhythm has not been ablated.
   d) Know if heart rate is adjustable to demand. If not, the patient may require increased rate with increased metabolic demand such as fever.
   e) Device may allow multiple abnormal rhythms of short duration with single electrical impulses to convert before continuous pacing or defibrillation, so patients may exhibit symptoms and variable heart rates.
   f) All devices can be temporarily inactivated by placing a magnet on the chest over the pulse generator. Temporary inactivation may be desired during radiation treatments to minimize radiation exposure.
   g) Classify patients as high, medium, or low risk for adverse events if the device malfunctions, and select interventions appropriate for risk level.

F. Management of tachydysrhythmias (see Table 45-6)

1. Vagal maneuvers (e.g., coughing, bearing down as if to have a bowel movement, manual carotid massage) frequently will break paroxysmal supraventricular tachycardia.

2. Whether the patient is stable or unstable, administer adenosine if it is readily available. It has a short half-life and few adverse effects and may break the rhythm or identify flutter waves that definitively diagnose the rhythm.

3. Electrical therapy: Synchronized cardioversion
   a) Defibrillators have a "synchronous mode" that allows delivery of electricity on the R wave, reducing the risk for ventricular fibrillation or asystole with electrical delivery.
   b) Patients should be sedated and given an amnesic prior to synchronous cardioversion.
   c) Saline or gel pads reduce the risk of skin burns with defibrillation.
   d) New defibrillator using the biphasic electrical delivery is likely to produce myocardial damage with cardioversion than older biphasic models.

G. Management of atrial dysrhythmias

1. It is unclear whether rhythm conversion improves long-term outcomes better than rate control.

2. If the patient is thought to be having the rhythm for more than two weeks, anticoagulation is recommended prior to conversion so that any clot accumulation in the atria is resolved prior to regulation of atrial contraction.

TABLE 45-6	Antidysrhythmic Therapy for Supraventricular Tachycardia		
Drug	**Dose**	**Category**	**Miscellaneous**
Adenosine	6 mg IV rapid push followed by a fluid bolus; wait 1–2 minutes, and if no response, may administer 12 mg by rapid IV. push followed by a fluid bolus. Central line administration may be given at one-half the recommended dose.	Purine analog	It can cause several seconds of asystole. Patient may experience crushing chest pain. Supraventricular tachycardia will recur 50%–60% of the time. Half-life is < 5 seconds. Patients on theophylline may require larger doses, whereas dipyridamole potentiates its effects.
Amiodarone	In cases of stable ventricular or supraventricular tachycardia, the loading dose is 150 mg IV over 10 minutes, followed by 1 mg/min infusion over 6 hours (completing the load), and then 0.5 mg/min for 18 additional hours. Discontinuation or conversion to oral is recommended by that time.	Potassium channel inhibitor	Most common immediate adverse effect is hypotension, counteracted partly by infusion rather than IV push. Bolus dose is acceptable to administer in normal saline and via polyethylene bag, but infusion should be mixed with dextrose in a glass bottle or polyolefin bag. Long-term adverse effects that may be potentiated by other oncologic therapies include pulmonary fibrosis, hypothyroidism, hepatic transaminase elevations, and peripheral neuropathies. Long half-life of drug limits use in patients with high risk for heart block.
Digoxin	It is administered at 10–15 mcg/kg (lean body weight) IV or PO in a loading dose over 2–4 hours, followed by a daily dose of 0.125–0.50 mg PO daily.	Digitalis glycoside	Rate and conduction effect is seen within 5–30 minutes; peak effect is within 90 minutes and 3 hours. Correct hypokalemia, hypocalcemia, and hypomagnesemia to reduce risk of toxicity.
Diltiazem	Bolus dose of 0.25 mg/kg (average 20–25 mg) is given over 2 minutes; if not controlled after 15 minutes, may give an additional 0.35 mg/kg IV over 2–5 minutes. Follow with 5–15 mg/hr continuous infusion. *Most patients with cancer and many older adults are extremely sensitive to this agent and usually receive half the recommended dose.*	Calcium channel blocker	Less incidence of myocardial depression occurs than with verapamil.

(Continued on next page)

TABLE 45-6	Antidysrhythmic Therapy for Supraventricular Tachycardia *(Continued)*

Drug	Dose	Category	Miscellaneous
Dofetilide	A dose of 500 mg PO is given twice daily with adjustment for reduced creatinine clearance.	Potassium channel inhibitor	It is effective in cardiomyopathy-induced atrial fibrillation. It is less likely than other agents to worsen bradycardias or heart block. It can prolong the QT interval and cause ventricular dysrhythmias.
Esmolol	Load with 250–500 mcg/kg IV for 1 minute, followed by IV continuous infusion of 25–50 mcg/kg/min, titrated upward every 5–10 minutes until a maximum of 200 mcg/kg/min.	Beta selective blocker	It has a very rapid onset and short duration. Dose should be diluted to 10 mg/ml before administration. Do not use in patients with significant atrioventricular block or bradycardia.
Labetalol	A 20 mg IV dose is given over 2 minutes, followed by 40–80 mg IV at 10-minute intervals until the blood pressure drops; maximum dose is 2 mg/min or 300 mg total daily dose.	Alpha-beta blocker	Alpha and beta effects lead to blocking receptors in both heart and vasculature with decreased work on the heart, as well as direct cardiac effects.
Metoprolol	Administer 5 mg via IV push over 1–2 minutes. This dose may be repeated 2 additional times 5–15 minutes apart.	Beta selective blocker	Onset of action is approximately 5 minutes, and duration varies among individuals. No clear reversal agent exists, but some clinicians prescribe IV glucagon as an antidote in potential overdose. Effective beta blockade is determined by a heart rate ≤ 70 bpm without stress-related increases (e.g., exercise, fever).
Sotalol	A 75 mg dose via IV is given over 5 hours one to two times a day, with a maintenance dose of 75–300 mg PO once or twice daily. An 80 mg dose is given with potential dose adjustments every three days until a maximum of 240–320 mg PO daily.	Potassium channel inhibitor	Occasional higher doses are used in ventricular dysrhythmias. Drug has a long half-life, so dosing more than two times daily is not necessary. Check QT interval prior to and during therapy to reduce risk of proarrhythmic effects of agent. Renal dose adjustment is recommended.
Verapamil	5 mg IV push over 2 minutes, 5–10 mg IV after 15–30 minutes; maximum dose is 30 mg. *Most patients with cancer and many older adults are extremely sensitive to this agent and usually receive half the recommended dose.*	Calcium channel blocker	Observe blood pressure closely. Reverse effects with calcium chloride 0.5–1 g slowly for best absorption. Consider not using this agent in patients with Wolff-Parkinson-White syndrome.

Note. Based on information from American Heart Association, 2016; Camm, 2017; Dahya & Taigen, 2019; Dan et al., 2018; Lei et al., 2018; Mahtani & Nair, 2019; Mankad & Kalahasty, 2019.

3. It is recommended to use a risk scoring system to determine risk–benefit ratio for cardioversion of rhythm. Factors included in the CHA_2DS_2-VASc scoring system are presence of CHF, hypertension, diabetes, history of ischemic stroke, vascular disease, female gender, and age older than 65 years.

4. Medications to convert the rhythm include calcium channel blockers.

5. Electrical synchronized cardioversion may convert the rhythm to normal.
   a) Electrical cardioversion is most successful using the biphasic defibrillator.
   b) Electrical cardioversion requires sedation.
   c) Levels of electricity (joules) are lower than when converting ventricular dysrhythmias.

6. Medications to control rate include digitalis and beta-blockers.

7. Atrial rhythm disturbances not controlled by medications may be amenable to catheter ablation.

8. When the focus of dysrhythmia cannot be identified, myocardial remodeling with AV pacing may be helpful.

9. If it is determined to leave the patient in atrial rhythm (no attempt of conversion), anticoagulation for life is recommended.
   a) Anticoagulation has been shown to decrease incidence of stroke (see Chapter 146).
   b) Oral thrombin inhibitor anticoagulants (e.g., dabigatran 150 mg PO two times a day, rivaroxaban 20 mg PO daily) are indicated for chronic atrial fibrillation.

H. Management of bradydysrhythmias
   1. Asymptomatic/stable: Medical therapy
   2. Atropine 0.5 mg IV is the treatment of choice unless vagotomy has been performed previously.
   3. Dopamine infusion 4–20 mcg/kg/min may effectively increase heart rate.
   4. A pacemaker is the treatment of choice for persistent bradydysrhythmias (e.g., automatic external, temporary transvenous, permanent).

I. Management of ventricular dysrhythmias
   1. Asymptomatic/stable: Medical therapy
      a) Premature ventricular contractions (PVCs) with absent or few symptoms often are not treated. Current evidence suggests these rhythm disturbances increase the risk of cardiomyopathy, stroke, and sudden death.
      b) Amiodarone is most effective and most commonly used. It is given at 150 mg IV over 10 minutes, may be repeated, and then infused at 1 mg/min for six hours and 0.5 mg/min for 18 hours.
      c) Lidocaine at 50–75 mg/kg bolus, followed by infusion of 1–4 mg/min, has been used extensively, but no clinical trials have proved its efficacy.
   2. Unstable: Electrical therapy
      a) Synchronous cardioversion is preferred when time permits; however, unstable rhythms may require asynchronous defibrillation.
      b) Automatic implanted cardioverters/defibrillators deliver electricity spontaneously when a lethal dysrhythmia is detected and often contain a mechanism to pace the heart if it does not immediately return to a normal rhythm.
      c) Catheter-directed ablation may be used for patients unresponsive or intolerant of medication therapies.
   3. Prolonged QT interval and high risk for ventricular tachycardia of torsades de pointes variant (see Table 45-1)
      a) Measure QT interval periodically.
         (1) QT interval is corrected for heart rate. Slower heart rates are naturally associated with longer QT intervals, referred to as the *corrected QT interval*.

        (2) Corrected QT greater than 0.45 ms warrants evaluation and correction of avoidable causes.

        (3) Corrected QT greater than 0.50 ms increases risk for life-threatening ventricular dysrhythmias.

    b) Recognize patient-related risk factors for prolonged QT interval (e.g., increased age, preexisting heart failure, structural heart disease).

    c) Most medications used to treat dysrhythmias are also proarrhythmic based on mechanism of action. This is often the result of prolonged QT interval and is especially prevalent in the potent potassium channel inhibitors (e.g., amiodarone, dofetilide, sotalol).

    d) Recognize antineoplastic agents, concomitant medications, or clinical conditions that increase risk for prolonged QT interval (see Table 45-1).

    e) Maintain normal electrolytes (goal potassium greater than 4 mEq/L; goal magnesium greater than 2 mEq/L) to reduce extra risk for dysrhythmias (see Chapters 152–156).

    f) Consider implantable defibrillator if risks deemed high and cannot be abrogated.

  4. Ventricular tachycardia of torsades de pointes variant

    a) It is an unstable and irregular variation of ventricular tachycardia.

    b) It is often related to prolonged QT (see Table 45-1).

    c) Most effective treatment is magnesium sulfate 1–2 g IV push or short infusion.

    d) Defibrillation may be effective.

  5. Wearable defibrillator vests are used when patients have uncertain causes of ventricular fibrillation arrests or they have contraindications for implanting automatic devices.

VII. Follow-up (AHA, 2016; Chandrasekhar & Fradley, 2019; Porta-Sánchez et al., 2017)

  A. Patients may be discharged immediately to home after elective electrical cardioversion, but dysrhythmia recurrence rate may be up to 30%. Follow-up instructions and early return for physician evaluation are recommended.

  B. Holter monitor is performed periodically (usually once every year) as follow up to ascertain whether the antidysrhythmic treatment is effective.

  C. Twelve-lead ECG evaluation with QT measurement has variable recommendations for follow up based on individual risks, the continuation or overlapping prescription of known QT prolonging drugs, and known changes in the patient's QT interval.

  D. Medication blood levels should be monitored every dose change when regulating the appropriate dose, and then every three months if the patient's physical condition remains unchanged.

  E. Routine laboratory tests every six months, including CBC, serum chemistry, and hepatic profile for patients on antidysrhythmic pharmacologic therapy, should be performed to detect toxicities.

  F. Periodic assessment of electrolytes is obtained more frequently if levels are being replenished because low electrolytes predispose reemergence of dysrhythmias.

  G. Implanted pacemaker/defibrillator tests and battery changes are performed every one to three years.

  H. Cardiac imaging may be used to assess influence of rhythm disturbances on cardiac ischemia when recurrent rhythms have occurred.

VIII. Referrals

  A. Cardiologist: For evaluation of dysrhythmias of unknown origin or when patient is refractory to treatment; special considerations in selection of antidysrhythmic agents, given potential overlapping toxicities with antineoplastic agents

B. Electrophysiologist/interventional cardiologist: If dysrhythmias are persistent and presumed to be related to accessory pathway; allows electrical mapping of the heart and potential ablation therapy; may insert and monitor pacemakers or implanted defibrillators, as indicated

C. Pharmacist: To advise patients regarding correct administration of antidysrhythmic medications, as many of these agents have altered absorption with food, pH levels, or other concomitant medications; for use of over-the-counter medications that may interfere with antidysrhythmics or act as cardiac stimulants (e.g., cold and allergy remedies)

D. Dietitian: For patients who must monitor their intake of certain electrolytes; to advise on food substances that contain caffeine or other cardiac stimulants (e.g., cola, chocolate)

E. Tobacco cessation program: For patients who use tobacco, as nicotine replacement products are contraindicated in patients with dysrhythmias

References

Al-Khatib, S.M., Stevenson, W.G., Ackerman, M.J., Bryant, W.J., Callans, D.J., Curtis, A.B., ... Page, R.L. (2018). 2017 AHA/ACC/HRS guideline for management of patients with ventricular arrhythmias and the prevention of sudden cardiac death: A report of the American College of Cardiology/American Heart Association Task Force on Clinical Practice Guidelines and the Heart Rhythm Society. *Journal of the American College of Cardiology, 72*(14), e91–e220. https://doi.org/10.1016/j.jacc.2017.10.054

Al Mahameed, S.T., & Ziv, O. (2019). Ventricular arrhythmias. *Medical Clinics of North America, 103*(5), 881–895. https://doi.org/10.1016/j.mcna.2019.05.008

American Heart Association. (2016). *Advanced cardiovascular life support: Provider manual* (16th ed.). Author.

Brembilla-Perrot, B., Girerd, N., & Sellal, J.-M. (2018). Unresolved questions associated with the management of ventricular preexcitation syndrome. *Pacing and Clinical Electrophysiology, 41*(7), 839–844. https://doi.org/10.1111/pace.13367

Camm, A.J. (2017). Hopes and disappointments with antiarrhythmic drugs. *International Journal of Cardiology, 237,* 71–74. https://doi.org/10.1016/j.ijcard.2017.03.056

Chandrasekhar, S., & Fradley, M.G. (2019). QT interval prolongation associated with cytotoxic and targeted cancer therapeutics. *Current Treatment Options in Oncology, 20*(7), 55. https://doi.org/10.1007/s11864-019-0657-y

Chen, Q., Gasperetti, A., Della Rocca, D.G., Mohanty, S., Gedikli, O., Trivedi, C., ... Natale, A. (2019). The value of baseline and arrhythmic ECG in the interpretation of arrhythmic mechanisms. *Cardiac Electrophysiology Clinics, 11*(2), 219–238. https://doi.org/10.1016/j.ccep.2019.02.007

Chu, G., Versteeg, H.H., Verschoor, A.J., Trines, S.A., Hemels, M.E.W., Ay, C., ... Klok, F.A. (2019). Atrial fibrillation and cancer—An unexplored field in cardiovascular oncology. *Blood Reviews, 35,* 59–67. https://doi.org/10.1016/j.blre.2019.03.005

Costantini, O. (2019) Basic principles of cardiac electrophysiology. *Medical Clinics of North America, 103*(5), 767–774. https://doi.org/10.1016/j.mcna.2019.04.002

Dahya, V., & Taigen, T.L. (2019). Pharmacologic and nonpharmacologic management of atrial fibrillation. *Medical Clinics of North America, 103*(5), 835–846. https://doi.org/10.1016/j.mcna.2019.04.004

Dan, G.-A., Martinez-Rubio, A., Agewall, S., Boriani, G., Borggrefe, M., Gaita, F., ... Wolpert, C. (2018). Antiarrhythmic drugs—Clinical use and clinical decision-making: A consensus document from the European Heart Rhythm Association (EHRA) and European Society of Cardiology (ESC) Working Group on Cardiovascular Pharmacology, endorsed by the Heart Rhythm Society (HRS), Asia-Pacific Heart Rhythm Society (APHRS) and International Society of Cardiovascular Pharmacotherapy (ISCP). *EP Europace, 20*(5), 731–732an. https://doi.org/10.1093/europace/eux373

De Ponti, R., My, I., Vilotta, M., Caravati, F., Marazzato, J., Bagliani, G., & Leonelli, F.M. (2019). Advanced cardiac signal recording. *Cardiac Electrophysiology Clinics, 11*(2), 203–217. https://doi.org/10.1016/j.ccep.2019.01.005

Elbanhawy, N., Chalil, S., & Abozguia, K. (2019). Bradyarrhythmias for the internist. *Medical Clinics of North America, 103*(5), 897–912. https://doi.org/10.1016/j.mcna.2019.05.003

Haugaa, K.H., Basso, C., Badano, L.P., Bucciarelli-Ducci, C., Cardim, N., Gaemperli, O., ... & Edvardsen, T. (2017). Comprehensive multi-modality imaging approach in arrhythmogenic cardiomyopathy—An expert consensus document of the European Association of Cardiovascular Imaging. *European Heart Journal—Cardiovascular Imaging, 18*(3), 237–253. https://doi.org/10.1093/ehjci/jew229

Herring, N., Kalla, M., & Paterson, D.J. (2019). The autonomic nervous system and cardiac arrhythmias: Current concepts and emerging therapies. *Nature Reviews Cardiology, 16*(12), 707–726. https://doi.org/10.1038/s41569-019-0221-2

Hussain, M.A., & Nabi, F. (2017). Complex structural interventions: The role of computed tomography, fluoroscopy, and fusion imaging. *Methodist DeBakey Cardiovascular Journal, 13*(3), 98–105. https://doi.org/10.14797/mdcj-13-3-98

January, C.T., Wann, L.S., Calkins, H., Chen, L.Y., Cigarroa, J.E., Cleveland, J.C., Jr., … Yancy, C.W. (2019). 2019 AHA/ACC/HRS focused update of the 2014 AHA/ACC/HRS guideline for the management of patients with atrial fibrillation: A report of the American College of Cardiology/American Heart Association task force on clinical practice guidelines and the Heart Rhythm Society in collaboration with the Society of Thoracic Surgeons. *Circulation, 140*(2), e125–e151. https://doi.org/10.1161/CIR.0000000000000665

Kachur, S., & Morin, D.P. (2019). Who should receive a wearable defibrillator vest at hospital discharge? *Current Cardiology Reports, 21*(10), 125. https://doi.org/10.1007/s11886-019-1215-8

Lei, M., Wu, L., Terrar, D.A., & Huang, C.L.-H. (2018). Modernized classification of cardiac antiarrhythmic drugs. *Circulation, 138*(17), 1879–1896. https://doi.org/10.1161/CIRCULATIONAHA.118.035455

Leonelli, F.M., De Ponti, R., & Baglaini, G. (2019a). Challenges in bradicardias interpretation. *Cardiac Electrophysiology Clinics, 11*(2), 261–281. https://doi.org/10.1016/j.ccep.2019.02.002

Leonelli, F.M., De Ponti, R., & Baglaini, G. (2019b). Electrocardiographic approach to complex arrhythmias: P, QRS, and their relationships. *Cardiac Electrophysiology Clinics, 11*(2), 239–260. https://doi.org/10.1016/j.ccep.2019.02.001

Littmann, L., Olson, E.G., & Gibbs, M.A. (2019). Initial evaluation and management of wide-complex tachycardia: A simplified and practical approach. *American Journal of Emergency Medicine, 37*(7), 1340–1345. https://doi.org/10.1016/j.ajem.2019.04.027

Mahtani, A.U., & Nair, D.G. (2019). Supraventricular tachycardia. *Medical Clinics of North America, 103*(5), 863–879. https://doi.org/10.1016/j.mcna.2019.05.007

Mankad, P., & Kalahasty, G. (2019). Antiarrhythmic drugs: Risks and benefits. *Medical Clinics of North America, 103*(5), 821–834. https://doi.org/10.1016/j.mcna.2019.05.004

Markman, T.M., & Nazarian, S. (2019). Treatment of ventricular arrhythmias: What's new? *Trends in Cardiovascular Medicine, 29*(5), 249–261. https://doi.org/10.1016/j.tcm.2018.09.014

Miften, M., Mihailidis, D., Kry, S.F., Reft, C., Esquivel, C., Farr, J., … Wilkinson, J. (2019). Management of radiotherapy patients with implanted cardiac pacemakers and defibrillators: A report of the AAPM TG-203. *Medical Physics, 46*(12), e757–e788. https://doi.org/10.1002/mp.13838

Padeletti, L., & Bagliani, G. (2017). General introduction, classification, and electrocardiographic diagnosis of cardiac arrhythmias. *Cardiac Electrophysiology Clinics, 9*(3), 345–363. https://doi.org/10.1016/j.ccep.2017.05.009

Porta-Sánchez, A., Gilbert, C., Spears, D., Amir, E., Chan, J., Nanthakumar, K., & Thayendiranathan, P. (2017). Incidence, diagnosis, and management of QT prolongation induced by cancer therapies: A systematic review. *Journal of the American Heart Association, 6*(12), e007724. https://doi.org/10.1161/JAHA.117.007724

Rhea, I., Burgos, P.H., & Fradley, M.G. (2019). Arrhythmogenic anticancer drugs in cardio-oncology. *Cardiology Clinics, 37*(4), 459–468. https://doi.org/10.1016/j.ccl.2019.07.011

Shah, S.R., Park, K., & Alweis, R. (2019). Long QT syndrome: A comprehensive review of the literature and current evidence. *Current Problems in Cardiology, 44*(3), 92–106. https://doi.org/10.1016/j.cpcardiol.2018.04.002

Singh, D.K., & Peter, C.T. (2016). Use of the surface electrocardiogram to define the nature of challenging arrhythmias. *Cardiac Electrophysiology Clinics, 8*(1), 1–24. https://doi.org/10.1016/j.ccep.2015.10.021

Steffen, M.M., Osborn, J.S., & Cutler, M.J. (2019). Cardiac implantable electronic device therapy: Permanent pacemakers, implantable cardioverter defibrillators, and cardiac resynchronization devices. *Medical Clinics of North America, 103*(5), 931–943. https://doi.org/10.1016/j.mcna.2019.04.005

Trenor, B., Cardona, K., Romero, L., Gomez, J.F., Saiz, J., Raiamani, S., … Giles, W. (2018). Pro-arrhythmic effects of low plasma [K$^+$] in human ventricle: An illustrated review. *Trends in Cardiovascular Medicine, 28*(4), 233–242. https://doi.org/10.1016/j.tcm.2017.11.002

Tso, C., Currie, G.M., Gilmore, D., & Kiat, H. (2015). Electrocardiography: A technologist's guide to interpretation. *Journal of Nuclear Medicine Technology, 43*(4), 247–252. https://doi.org/10.2967/jnmt.115.163501

Woosley, R.L., Romero, K., Heise, C.W., Gallo, T., Tate, J., Woosley, R.D., & Ward, S. (2017). Adverse drug event causality analysis (ADECA): A process for evaluating evidence and assigning drugs to risk categories for sudden death. *Drug Safety, 40*(6), 465–474. https://doi.org/10.1007/s40264-017-0519-0

CHAPTER 46

Endocarditis

Brenda K. Shelton, DNP, APRN–CNS, RN, CCRN, AOCN®

I. Definition (Cahill et al., 2017; Tattevin & Mainardi, 2016)
   A. *Endocarditis* is a general term used to describe inflammation of the endocardial lining or valves of the heart.
   B. Other terms for nonbacterial endocarditis include *marantic endocarditis, Libman-Sacks endocarditis,* or *verrucous endocarditis.*

II. Physiology/Pathophysiology (Cahill et al., 2017; Liu & Frishman, 2016; Yang & Frazee, 2018)
   A. Normal: Endocardium is the innermost layer of the heart. It lines the inner chambers (atria and ventricles) of the heart and covers the heart valves and small muscles associated with the opening and closing of the valves.
   B. Pathophysiology
      1. Endocarditis is an inflammatory disorder that results from injury to the endocardial surface of the heart.
         a) Turbulent blood flow or the presence of pathogenic organisms is the most common cause of endothelial injury.
         b) This injury initiates thrombus formation to protect the injured site.
         c) In patients who are hypercoagulable, the degree of injury required to initiate a thrombus is less than in other patients, increasing the risk of "sterile thrombus" production or precipitation of nonbacterial thrombotic endocarditis.
         d) Vegetations in nonbacterial endocarditis are smaller, more friable, easily embolized, and more difficult to diagnose.
      2. In bacterial endocarditis, the pathogens adhere to the injured endocardial surface and are incorporated into the thrombus.
         a) The process of endocarditis starts with bacteria adhesion from the bloodstream to the endothelial wall.
         b) The growth of these pathogens produces "fern-like" deposits known as vegetations.
         c) Vegetations are most likely to be present on rough surfaces or in areas of turbulent, high-velocity blood flow (e.g., near the cardiac valves).
         d) Vegetations may be more common when viridans streptococci is the causative organism or when symptoms are present for fewer than 10 days.
         e) Vegetations may break off and travel to any area of the body, leading to variation in clinical signs and symptoms. Neurologic embolization is common, particularly in older adults or those with significant medical disease.
         f) Vegetations may affect valve integrity (e.g., leaky valves).
         g) Hypermetabolic states that increase heart rate and cardiac output may enhance the risk for embolization.

III. Clinical features: Endocarditis is classified by its acuity of presentation (acute vs. subacute) and whether it is infective or noninfective (see Table 46-1). Endocarditis is relatively prevalent in certain patient populations, affecting as many as 1 in 1,000 patients admitted to hospitals. Although previously associated with rheumatic or congenital heart disease, more than 25% of cases are diagnosed from other etiologies. Mortality rate is approximately 30% of cases despite advances in detection, stronger antimicrobial agents, and successful surgical treatment. Endocarditis is not commonly reported with malignancy; however, as many as 4% of autopsied patients with cancer had noninfective endocarditis. Most endocarditis is infectious, but occurrence of noninfectious endocarditis in patients with inflammatory disorders, such as autoimmune disease and malignancy, is higher than in other medical–surgical patients with endocarditis. Infectious endocarditis has a higher mortality rate than noninfectous (Cahill et al., 2017; Gala et al., 2019; Holubar et al., 2016; Liu & Frishman, 2016; Pasha et al., 2016; Samol et al., 2015; Tattevin & Mainardi, 2016; Ursi et al., 2019; VanEperen & Segreti, 2016; Vogkou et al., 2016; Yang & Frazee, 2018).

  A. Etiology: The most common source is noninfectious clots. Bacteremia is the second most common (see Table 46-2).

    1. Noninfectious: Most commonly affects mitral and aortic valves

      a) Arterial vascular disease with clot dislodgment from the vascular endothelium

      b) Atrial or ventricular clot dislodged with contraction of the heart chamber

      c) Vascular access device causing irritation and inflammation

      d) Embolization common in approximately 40% of patients

    2. Infectious etiologies by population group: Bacteremia can cause endocarditis, even in a normal, healthy, and intact endocardium. A specific precipitating event for the infection cannot be identified in many cases. Common infectious organisms associated with endocarditis are outlined in Table 46–2.

  B. Risk factors

    1. Most common risk factors in the general population: Structural heart disease with turbulent flow with or without valve irregularities (e.g., prosthetic heart valves, mitral valve prolapse, congenital heart disease, rheumatic heart disease, CHF)

    2. Autoimmune systemic illness

      a) SLE

      b) Scleroderma

TABLE 46-1	Clinical Presentation of Acute and Subacute Bacterial Endocarditis	
Clinical Feature	**Acute Endocarditis**	**Subacute Endocarditis**
Onset	Less than six weeks onset	Greater than six weeks onset
Organisms	*Staphylococcus aureus* Beta-hemolytic *Streptococcus*	Alpha-hemolytic *Streptococcus*
Valves involved	Tricuspid; pulmonic	Mitral
Valves presentation	Valve perforation common Large friable vegetations with high tendency to embolize	Valve perforation rare Smaller, thicker vegetations
Valvular status before disorder	Previously normal valves	Previously damaged valves
Virulence	Very virulent	Less virulent

Note. Based on information from Dong et al., 2015.

TABLE 46-2	Infectious Causes of Endocarditis
Risk Factor	**Microorganism**
Early after prosthetic valve replacement	*Staphylococcus* coagulase-positive or coagu-lase-negative: 50% Gram-negative: 20% Fungal: 10% Other: 20%
Later after prosthetic valve replacement	Alpha-hemolytic *Streptococcus*: 35% *Staphylococcus* coagulase-negative: 20% *Staphylococcus* coagulase-positive: 10% Gram-negative: 10% Other: 25%
IV drug abuse	*Staphylococcus* coagulase-positive: 50% *Streptococcus* (alpha and beta): 15% Other: 35%
Immunosuppressed patients (i.e., those who have undergone solid organ or hematopoietic stem cell transplantation, those who are HIV-positive but not IV drug users, those with autoimmune disease who are on corticosteroids)	*Staphylococcus* coagulase-positive or coagu-lase-negative: 50% *Streptococcus* (alpha and beta): 20% Fungal: 10% Opportunistic: 5% Other: 5%

Note. Based on information from Cahill et al., 2017; Holubar et al., 2016; Pasha et al., 2016; Samol et al., 2015; Tattevin & Mainardi, 2016; VanEperen & Segreti, 2016; Vogkou et al., 2016; Yang & Frazee, 2018.

  c) Antiphospholipid syndrome: Libman-Sacks lesions on valve leaflets are sterile fibrinous vegetations that can occur involving deposits of anticardiolipin/beta-2 glycoprotein 1 antibodies, usually on mitral valve.

3. IV drug use: Lifetime incidence is 0.5%–12%, and it usually affects right-sided valves.
4. Systemic infections: HIV, *Staphylococcus*, *Streptococcus*, *Pseudomonas*
5. Burn injury
6. Recent cardiac surgery: Coronary artery bypass, valvuloplasty, valve replacement
7. Male gender: Not supported in studies of patients with malignancy
8. Age older than 70 years: Double the risk in the absence of any other risk factors
9. Diabetic patients receiving hemodialysis
10. Long-term indwelling catheters: vascular access devices (most common)
  a) Tunneled and nontunneled
  b) Increased risk if tip is in the atria
11. Cardiac implanted devices: Implanted cardioverter–defibrillators, ventricular assist devices; usually indicates infection spread from a pocket infection and often affects right-sided valves
12. Cancers: Often cause nonbacterial endocarditis
  a) Intestinal tumors: Highly associated with colorectal cancer
  b) Gynecologic malignancies: Ovarian, endometrial
  c) Metastasis to heart: Cause endocarditis less than 2% of the time
  d) Tumor types identified as causing right-sided valvular disorders (e.g., tricuspid, pulmonic): Kidney, testes, thyroid, melanoma
  e) Tumor types identified as causing left-sided valvular lesions (e.g., mitral, aortic): Bronchogenic

    f) Leukemia and myeloproliferative disorders caused by eosinophilic infiltration cardiomyopathy: Loeffler endocarditis

  13. Nonbacterial thrombotic endocarditis: Cancer related

    a) Pancreatic cancer: 38%; most likely to cause vegetations

    b) Lymphoma: 26%

    c) Carcinoma of GI tract: 20%

    d) Carcinoma of lung: 16%

  14. HSCT: Incompetent immune system, most likely related to endothelial wall injury

  15. Intestinal disease: Crohn disease, ulcerative colitis, bowel ischemia

  16. Hypercoagulable conditions

    a) Trousseau syndrome

    b) Protein C deficiency

    c) Protein S deficiency

    d) Antithrombin III deficiency

    e) DIC

    f) Antiphospholipid syndrome

    g) Carcinoid syndrome, especially right-sided valves

C. History

  1. History of cancer and cancer treatment

  2. Current medications: Prescribed, over the counter (e.g., procoagulants, immunosuppressive agents, corticosteroids)

  3. History of presenting symptoms: Precipitating factors, onset, location, duration, associated symptoms (e.g., recent fever or chills, recent loss of appetite, weight loss, fatigue, chest pain, visual loss)

  4. Changes in ADLs

  5. Past medical history: Cardiac disease, hypercoagulable conditions

D. Signs and symptoms (see Table 46-1)

  1. Flu-like syndrome: Low-grade fever (most prevalent symptom, occurring in 90% of patients), chills

  2. Arthralgia: Joint and bone pain indicative of osteomyelitis

  3. Myalgia

  4. Weakness, fatigue

  5. Night sweats: Dependent on organism

  6. Respiratory symptoms: Dyspnea, orthopnea, persistent cough

    a) Septic PE with acute respiratory distress or pleuritic chest pain may occur with right-sided valve disease.

    b) Respiratory symptoms may also indicate heart failure.

  7. Cardiac dysfunction: Chest or back discomfort results from endocardial or valvular inflammation, reduced contractility, or embolization to coronary arteries.

  8. Mental status changes: Changes usually reflect stroke; CNS involvement in infective endocarditis occurs in 20%–40% of patients, usually with sudden onset.

    a) Focal (unilateral) symptoms if embolic stroke is suspected

    b) Generalized (less focal) if caused by hypoxemia/ischemia

  9. GI symptoms

    a) Abdominal pain: Occurs with decreased perfusion (cardiac dysfunction) but may signal embolization to the GI organs

    b) Anorexia, weight loss

    c) Nausea

    d) Constipation

  10. GU dysfunction: Oliguria; dark, concentrated urine

E. Physical examination: Patients with new onset of heart murmur in the face of risk factors and fever should always be evaluated for evidence of endocarditis.
   1. Vital signs and constitutional symptoms: Fever, hypotension, weight loss
   2. Integument
      a) Possible petechiae of skin, oral mucosa, or conjunctivae
      b) Osler nodes: Painful, red, tender, subcutaneous nodules in the finger pads
      c) Janeway lesions: Flat, small, painless, irregular, nontender red spots on the palms of hands and soles of feet
      d) Splinter hemorrhage of fingernails
   3. HEENT
      a) Roth spots: Retinal hemorrhages characterized by a white or yellow center surrounded by a red, irregular halo
      b) Possible conjunctival hemorrhage
      c) Visual field cuts: Noted by point discrimination testing; present after embolic stroke
      d) Decreased finger-to-nose testing in visual field (see Appendix D)
   4. Pulmonary
      a) Peripheral tissue hypoxemia indicated by presence of skin cyanosis and cool extremities
      b) Generalized hypoxemia with decreased oxygen saturation if cardiac dysfunction is present
      c) Central cyanosis indicated by presence of bluish inner eyelids and bluish oral mucosa
      d) Chronic hypoxemia indicated by presence of finger clubbing and dark spots on the skin
   5. Cardiac
      a) Pansystolic murmur heard best at the base of heart
      b) Full bounding point of maximal impulse
   6. Vascular
      a) Weak, thready peripheral pulses
      b) Weaker distal pulses
   7. Abdominal
      a) Splenomegaly: Tenderness present in an acute episode and previous embolic infarctions have not occurred; more common in subacute endocarditis
      b) Hepatomegaly: Tenderness present in an acute episode
      c) Diffuse abdominal pain to palpation: May be present as a result of bowel ischemia/infarction
   8. Neurologic
      a) Mental status changes, aphasia
      b) Paresis: Noted by bilateral strength testing; usually unilateral weakness

IV. Diagnostic tests (Bertrand et al., 2016; Cahill et al., 2017; Gomes et al., 2017; Liesman et al., 2017; Millar et al., 2019; Samol et al., 2015; Tattevin & Mainardi, 2016; Wong et al., 2016; Yang & Frazee, 2018)
   A. Laboratory
      1. CBC
         a) Normocytic, normochromic anemia
         b) Leukocytosis, often moderate to high elevations (15,000–25,000/mm^3): Higher WBC count at onset predicts for poor long-term outcomes.
         c) Increased number of granulocytes and bands with sudden onset
         d) Inflammatory markers: Increased ESR, CRP, or procalcitonin may be useful but inconclusive.

2. Blood cultures
   a) To identify bacteremia organism, three or more sets, each with at least 10 ml of blood, are recommended over at least one hour from multiple venipuncture sites to enhance yield between collections before organism is isolated.
   b) Approximately 2%–30% of patients have negative blood cultures, varying based on organism, culture technique, and other undefined variables.
   c) A person with culture-negative endocarditis may be more likely to present with heart failure, have right-sided valvular disease, have previously treated *Streptococcus* infection, or have a pacemaker.
   d) Tests of organ perfusion, such as lactate, are increased with hypoxia or low peripheral perfusion.
3. Molecular examination of valve biopsies to examine nucleic acids; gene amplification; polymerase chain reaction to delineate etiology
4. Serologic antigen or antibody assays to identify unusual infectious etiologies: *Coxiella burnetii, Bartonella, Chlamydophila, Legionella, Brucella*
5. Rheumatoid factor if suspected as etiology

B. Radiology
   1. Chest x-ray may show enlarged heart.
   2. PET-CT is useful for diagnosis of occult prosthetic valve–induced infective endocarditis.
   3. MRI superimposed with multislice CT scan of the heart traditionally has been used to diagnose complications such as aortic root abscesses or fistulae, but current expertise of radiologists who read these diagnostic tests is inconsistent and leads to unreliable interpretations. These tests have not replaced the value of transesophageal echocardiogram.
   4. MRI of the brain in patients with infective endocarditis is useful to evaluate for embolic lesions.

C. Other
   1. Echocardiogram
      a) This is the definitive diagnostic tool when endocarditis involves valve abnormalities (more than 90% of cases), yet it does not rule out endocarditis if negative.
      b) Limitations of echocardiogram include its inability to differentiate vegetation from clot and infective versus noninfective vegetations. It also may miss vegetations and periannular extensions in presence of prosthetic or intracardiac devices.
   2. Presence of valvular vegetations or perforation: Vegetations less than 3 mm cannot be detected on traditional echocardiogram and may require transesophageal echocardiogram.
      a) Transthoracic echocardiogram is considered the gold standard for initial diagnostic evaluation. Patients with blood culture positive for *Staphylococcus aureus* or *Candida* should have a transthoracic echocardiogram within 7–10 days of starting treatment or in the first 24 hours if strong suspicion of endocarditis.
      b) Some clinicians advocate for use of transesophageal echocardiogram exclusively in monitoring treatment response because small vegetations still require ongoing antimicrobial therapy but may not be detected by traditional echocardiogram. Sensitivity with this diagnostic modality is 90%–100%.
      c) Echocardiogram only detects 25% of vegetations less than 5 mm and 70% of vegetations 6–10 mm in size.
      d) It is the preferred method if patient has a prosthetic heart valve.

    e) Negative transesophageal echocardiogram in the face of clinical symptoms warrants repeat diagnostic test in approximately two to three days while treating for presumed endocarditis.

       (1) It assesses competence of valves.

       (2) Global myocardial hypokinesis may be seen in the absence of valvular abnormalities and can be used with blood culture results to confirm diagnosis of endocarditis.

   3. ECG: Conduction disturbances (e.g., heart block, bradycardia, prolonged PR interval, left bundle branch block)

  D. Diagnostic scoring system for infectious endocarditis: The Duke criteria with modifications combine pathologic and clinical criteria. Sensitivity and specificity is approximately 80%, with lower rates if related to prosthetic material (Gomes et al., 2017; Yang & Frazee, 2018).

   1. Pathologic criteria

    a) Positive culture or histology

    b) Evidence of endocardial involvement: Vegetations, abscesses

   2. Clinical criteria

    a) Two major criteria, or

    b) One major and three minor criteria, or

    c) Five minor criteria

   3. Definitions for major criteria

    a) Positive blood culture in two separate blood cultures or persistently positive culture

    b) Positive echocardiogram

    c) Moving "fern-like" intracardiac mass or abscess

    d) New partial valve separation (prosthetic valve) or incompetence of valves

   4. Definitions for minor criteria

    a) High-risk condition: Known prosthetic valve, rheumatic heart disease, IV drug use

    b) Vascular phenomena: Major arterial emboli, septic pulmonary, hepatic, or splenic infractions

    c) Fever

    d) Immunologic phenomena: Glomerulonephritis, new rheumatoid condition without other risk factors

    e) Positive blood culture but not meeting major criteria

    f) Abnormal echocardiogram but not meeting major criteria

V. Differential diagnosis (Cahill et al., 2017; Jiad et al., 2017; Liu & Frishman, 2016)

  A. Bacteremia/septicemia from other etiologic mechanisms

  B. CHF (see Chapter 42)

  C. Myocardial abscesses

  D. MI (see Chapter 49)

  E. Pericarditis (see Chapter 50)

  F. Pneumonia (see Chapter 30)

  G. New or primary cardiac valvular disorder

  H. Stroke from other etiologies (see Chapter 146)

VI. Treatment (Akashi et al., 2019; Cahill et al., 2017; Dayer & Thornhill, 2018; Gil-Navarro et al., 2018; Holubar et al., 2016; Jiad et al., 2017; Mihos et al., 2017; Murphy & Vikram, 2019; Pasha et al., 2016; Randhawa et al., 2016; Samol et al., 2015; Silver et al., 2016; VanEperen & Segreti, 2016; Yang & Frazee, 2018)

A. Prophylaxis against endocarditis with antimicrobials in high-risk groups
   1. Guidelines have changed in the past 10–15 years because of the development of resistant organisms; routine antimicrobial prophylaxis is no longer recommended for minor procedures with local anesthetic and nonsystemic infectious diseases.
   2. It is recommended only in patients who are at risk for endocarditis and are at high risk for fatal outcome if endocarditis occurs.
   3. Recommended procedures for prophylaxis consideration include dental procedures involving manipulation of the gingiva, perforation of the oral mucosa, or invasion of the upper respiratory tract mucosa including tonsils and adenoids.
   4. Body procedures in which prophylaxis is **not** routinely recommended are those involving skin and soft tissues, GI tract, or urogenital tract.
   5. Penicillin is the usual agent, such as amoxicillin 2 g PO or clindamycin 600 mg PO one to two hours prior to procedure. Exact timing is based on data from specific procedure risk for infection.
B. Antibiotic treatment: Based on most common organism or isolated organism from blood cultures (see Appendix C)
   1. Treatment must be given via IV for at least 14 days. Oral therapy is rarely used because of unclear efficacy.
   2. Antibiotic therapy is usually required for four to six weeks, with the possibility of several weeks of oral therapy after IV.
   3. If blood cultures are still positive after 21 days (or if the patient becomes more acutely ill), permanent indwelling catheter should be removed.
   4. Antimicrobial therapeutic treatment
       a) Aminoglycosides may be used in high-risk individuals for maximum antimicrobial effect, but benefits and risks should be considered.
       b) Newer antistaphylococcal agents (e.g., daptomycin, ceftaroline, linezolid) have been used in suspected resistant staphylococcal infections.
       c) Fungal infections are more prevalent in immunocompromised patients; *Candida* species is the most common pathogen, and the second most likely is *Aspergillus* species. Diagnosis of fungal endocarditis is challenging and therapy may be empirically initiated.
       d) Older adult patients are at greatest risk for severe disease with endocarditis and often have other chronic conditions predisposing them to complications. The potential for limited organ reserve predisposes the older adult population to added adverse effects from antimicrobial agents.
   5. Home antimicrobial IV therapy may be an option for patients who are stable and responding, have no symptoms of heart failure, are not candidates for surgery, and in the absence of extracardiac infectious sources.
C. Anticoagulation or thrombolytic therapy: To prevent embolization of vegetations (see Chapter 43)
   1. Controversial outcomes: It is not clear that vegetations are reduced or embolization risk is diminished. Therapy can aggravate risk for potentially fatal hemorrhage.
       a) Decision to anticoagulate is best based on underlying risk for endocarditis rather than presence of endocarditis.
       b) Anticoagulation is **not** recommended for *Staphylococcus*- or polycythemia vera–induced endocarditis because of increased frequency of ischemic stroke and intracranial hemorrhage.
   2. Weight-based heparin: To achieve PTT, 1.3–1.5 times control may be used in prosthetic valve endocarditis but is at least temporarily discontinued if cerebrovascular embolism occurs.

3. Conversion to oral anticoagulant: Conversion is performed after a clear echocardio-gram unless the patient has a known malignancy-associated hypercoagulable state.

D. Surgical interventions

1. Surgery is indicated when endocarditis is refractory to antibiotics after six weeks, heart failure persists, or embolization has occurred at least twice.

2. Early valvular surgical intervention in infective endocarditis with prosthetic valves may lead to improved long-term outcomes.

3. Surgery is required in 40%–50% of patients with prosthetic valve–related endo-carditis.

4. Valve replacement may be indicated in disease-free patients.

5. Valvular replacement surgery is more complex and requires significant cardiopul-monary bypass time. It is associated with more complications than coronary artery bypass surgery.

6. Valvuloplasty is not usually the surgical procedure of choice because of the need to prevent future valvular vegetations.

E. Heart transplantation: When infection is due to ventricular assist devices

F. Supportive care: For complications of embolization (stroke is most common), heart fail-ure from incompetent valves, or multiorgan failure

1. Cerebrovascular complications occur in approximately 25%–70% of patients.

2. Embolic stroke from endocarditis usually affects middle cerebral artery, causing parietal stroke (see Chapter 146).

3. Cerebral hemorrhages can occur from antithrombotic therapy adverse events and infected aneurysms of the cerebral vasculature.

4. Splenic abscesses and infarctions, renal infarction, prosthetic joint infections, and spinal/epidural infections have been reported.

VII. Follow-up (Cahill et al., 2017)

A. Prolonged antimicrobial therapy requires frequent medical follow-up with physical exam-ination, including heart sounds, heart failure symptoms, and skin assessment; follow-up assists in determining if selection of antimicrobial therapy is appropriate.

B. No specific guidelines exist for repeat echocardiography during therapy.

C. After one episode of endocarditis, prophylactic antimicrobial treatment is prescribed for certain procedures that pose risk for embolization (e.g., dental work, bladder catheter-ization, surgery of any type, vaginal delivery).

D. Patients undergoing valve surgery are likely to take long-term antiplatelet and/or anticoag-ulant medications and should be followed by a hematologist or anticoagulation specialist.

VIII. Referrals (Jiad et al., 2017; Samol et al., 2015)

A. Cardiologist: If endocarditis is complicated by multiple embolization episodes or if echo-cardiogram does not return to normal with therapy

B. Surgical heart valve specialists: Indicated for patients with left-sided valve endocar-ditis

C. Neurologist: For assessment of neurologic deficits and appropriate interventions

D. Infection control specialist: Should be involved for best antimicrobial prescribing practices

E. Pharmacist: To address antimicrobial and anticoagulation therapy plans

F. Anticoagulation clinic: For referral for monitoring and dose adjustments in some patients on long-term anticoagulation therapy

G. Palliative care: In cases of severe heart failure or multiorgan dysfunction to assist with symptom management

References

Akashi, M., Nanba, N., Kusumoto, J., & Komori, T. (2019). Perioperative intervention by oral medicine team in cardiovascular surgery patients. *General Thoracic and Cardiovascular Surgery, 67*(2), 197–202. https://doi.org/10.1007/s11748-018-1020-0

Bertrand, P.B., Levine, R.A., Isselbacher, E.M., & Vandervoort, P.M. (2016). Fact or artifact in two-dimensional echocardiography: Avoiding misdiagnosis and missed diagnosis. *Journal of the American Society of Echocardiography, 29*(5), 381–391. https://doi.org/10.1016/j.echo.2016.01.009

Cahill, T.J., Baddour, L.M., Habib, G., Hoen, B., Salaun, E., Pettersson, G.B., ... Prendergast, B.D. (2017). Challenges in infective endocarditis. *Journal of the American College of Cardiology, 69*(3), 325–344. https://doi.org/10.1016/j.jacc.2016.10.066

Dayer, M., & Thornhill, M. (2018). Is antibiotic prophylaxis to prevent infective endocarditis worthwhile? *Journal of Infection and Chemotherapy, 24*(1), 18–24. https://doi.org/10.1016/j.jiac.2017.10.006

Dong, Y., Huang, J., Li, G., Li, L., Li, W., Li, X., ... Zhou, X. (2015). Guidelines for the prevention, diagnosis, and treatment of infective endocarditis in adults: The task force for the prevention, diagnosis, and treatment of infective endocarditis in adults of Chinese Society of Cardiology of Chinese Medical Association, and of the editorial board of Chinese Journal of Cardiology. *European Heart Journal Supplements, 17*(Suppl. C), C1–C16. https://doi.org/10.1093/eurheartj/suv031

Galar, A., Weil, A.A., Dudzinski, D.M., Muñoz, P., & Siedner, M.J. (2019). Methicillin-resistant *Staphylococcus aureus* prosthetic valve endocarditis: Pathophysiology, epidemiology, clinical presentation, diagnosis, and management. *Clinical Microbiology Reviews, 32*(2), e00041-18. https://doi.org/10.1128/CMR.00041-18

Gil-Navarro, M.V., Lopez-Cortes, L.E., Luque-Marquez, R., Galvez-Acebal, J., & de Alarcon-Gonzalez, A. (2018). Outpatient parenteral antimicrobial therapy in *Enterococcus faecalis* infective endocarditis. *Journal of Clinical Pharmacy and Therapeutics, 43*(2), 220–223. https://doi.org/10.1111/jcpt.12635

Gomes, A., Glaudemans, A.W.J.M., Touw, D.J., van Melle, J.P., Willems, T.P., Maass, A.H., ... Sinha, B. (2017). Diagnostic value of imaging in infective endocarditis: A systematic review. *Lancet Infectious Diseases, 17*(1), e1–e14. https://doi.org/10.1016/S1473-3099(16)30141-4

Holubar, M., Meng, L., & Deresinski, S. (2016). Bacteremia due to methicillin-resistant *Staphylococcus aureus*: New therapeutic approaches. *Infectious Disease Clinics of North America, 30*(2), 491–507. https://doi.org/10.1016/j.idc.2016.02.009

Jiad, E., Gill, S.K., Krutikov, M., Turner, D., Parkinson, M.H., Curtis, C., & Werring, D.J. (2017). When the heart rules the head: Ischaemic stroke and intracerebral haemorrhage complicating infective endocarditis. *Practical Neurology, 17*(1), 28–34. https://doi.org/10.1136/practneurol-2016-001469

Liesman, R.M., Pritt, B.S., Maleszewski, J.J., & Patel, R. (2017). Laboratory diagnosis of infective endocarditis. *Journal of Clinical Microbiology, 55*(9), 2599–2608. https://doi.org/10.1128/JCM.00635-17

Liu, J., & Frishman, W.H. (2016). Nonbacterial thrombotic endocarditis: Pathogenesis, diagnosis, and management. *Cardiology in Review, 24*(5), 244–247. https://doi.org/10.1097/CRD.0000000000000106

Mihos, C.G., Capoulade, R., Yucel, E., Picard, M.H., & Santana, O. (2017). Surgical versus medical therapy for prosthetic valve endocarditis: A meta-analysis of 32 studies. *Annals of Thoracic Surgery, 103*(3), 991–1004. https://doi.org/10.1016/j.athoracsur.2016.09.083

Millar, B.C., Abegão de Camargo, R.A., Alavi, A., & Moore, J.E. (2019). PET/computed tomography evaluation of infection of the heart. *PET Clinics, 14*(2), 251–269. https://doi.org/10.1016/j.cpet.2018.12.006

Murphy, K.M., & Vikram, H.R. (2019). Heart transplantation for infective endocarditis: Viable option for a limited few? *Transplant Infectious Disease, 21*(1), e13006. https://doi.org/10.1111/tid.13006

Pasha, A.K., Lee, J.Z., Low, S.-W., Desai, H., Lee, K.S., & Al Mohaier, M. (2016). Fungal endocarditis: Update on diagnosis and management. *American Journal of Medicine, 129*(10), 1037–1043. https://doi.org/10.1016/j.amjmed.2016.05.012

Randhawa, M.S., Pile, J., & Gomes, M. (2016). Can patients with infectious endocarditis be safely anticoagulated? *Cleveland Clinic Journal of Medicine, 83*(3), 169–171. https://doi.org/10.3949/ccjm.83a.15027

Samol, A., Kaese, S., Bloch, J., Görlich, D., Peters, G., Waltenberger, J., ... Lebiedz, P. (2015). Infective endocarditis on ICU: risk factors, outcome and long-term follow-up. *Infection, 43*(3), 287–295. https://doi.org/10.1007/s15010-014-0715-0

Silver, B., Behrouz, R., & Silliman, S. (2016). Bacterial endocarditis and cerebrovascular disease. *Current Neurology and Neuroscience Reports, 16*(12), 104. https://doi.org/10.1007/s11910-016-0705-y

Tattevin, P., & Mainardi, J.-L. (2016). Analysis of the 2015 American and European guidelines for the management of infective endocarditis. *Médecine et Maladies Infectieuses, 46*(8), 406–410. https://doi.org/10.1016/j.medmal.2016.05.008

Ursi, M.P., Durante Mangoni, E., Rajani, R., Hancock, J., Chambers, J.B., & Prendergast, B. (2019). Infective endocarditis in the elderly: Diagnostic and treatment options. *Drugs and Aging, 36*(2), 115–124. https://doi.org/10.1007/s40266-018-0614-7

VanEperen, A.S., & Segreti, J. (2016). Empirical therapy in methicillin-resistant *Staphylococcus aureus* infections: An up-to-date approach. *Journal of Infection and Chemotherapy, 22*(6), 351–359. https://doi.org/10.1016/j.jiac.2016.02.012

Vogkou, C.T., Vlachogiannis, N.I., Palaiodimos, L., & Kousoulis, A.A. (2016). The causative agents in infective endocarditis: A systematic review comprising 33,214 cases. *European Journal of Clinical Microbiology and Infectious Diseases, 35*(8), 1227–1245. https://doi.org/10.1007/s10096-016-2660-6

Wong, D., Rubinshtein, R., & Keynan, Y. (2016). Alternative cardiac imaging modalities to echocardiography for the diagnosis of infective endocarditis. *American Journal of Cardiology, 118*(9), 1410–1418. https://doi.org/10.1016/j.amjcard.2016.07.053

Yang, E., & Frazee, B.W. (2018). Infective endocarditis. *Emergency Medicine Clinics of North America, 36*(4), 645–663. https://doi.org/10.1016/j.emc.2018.06.002

CHAPTER 47

Hypertension

Keri McLendon Hyde, DNP, MBA, FNP-C, AOCNP®,

and Deborah Kirk, DNP, FNP-BC, NP-C, AOCN®, FAANP

I. Definition: A systolic blood pressure greater than or equal to 140 mm Hg and/or a diastolic pressure greater than or equal to 90 mm Hg based on the average of two or more blood pressure readings (while seated) at two or more visits (Chobanian et al., 2004)

II. Physiology/Pathophysiology (James et al., 2014; Ohishi, 2018)
   A. Normal
      1. Blood pressure is maintained as a result of the continuous regulation of cardiac output and systemic vascular resistance. This regulation takes place at the site of the heart, pre- and postcapillary venules, and the kidneys.
      2. The overall regulation of these sites is stimulated or suppressed by the autonomic nervous system and humoral influences, such as the renin–angiotensin–aldosterone system.
         a) The juxtaglomerular apparatus secretes renin in response to a number of stimuli, including a decrease in intravascular volume, decreased perfusion pressure, beta-adrenergic stimulation, and hyperkalemia.
         b) Renin acts on angiotensinogen to form angiotensin I, which is converted in the lung to angiotensin II by ACE.
            (1) Angiotensin II is a potent vasoconstrictor that acts on the adrenal cortex to release aldosterone.
            (2) Aldosterone increases sodium and water reabsorption in the distal tubule of the nephron.
         c) Renin production is inversely proportional to effective blood volume. Stimuli that increase effective blood volume suppress renin; stimuli that decrease effective blood volume stimulate renin.
      3. Catecholamines affect blood pressure regulation centrally by the vasomotor centers in the brain and peripherally through the action of the sympathetic nervous system.
   B. Pathophysiology
      1. Essential hypertension is elevated peripheral vascular resistance, increased sympathetic neural activity with enhanced beta-adrenergic responsiveness, and angiotensin II activity and mineralocorticoid excess.
      2. Catecholamines elevate blood pressure by increasing peripheral resistance and increasing cardiac output (e.g., as in pheochromocytoma).
      3. Increased calcium appears to increase vascular tone, which can lead to increased blood pressure.

III. Clinical features: Hypertension is the most common primary diagnosis in the United States, yet control rates are still under the 50% goal. Control of hypertension is achieved by reaching a set blood pressure goal, which varies based on age and comorbid conditions. Hypertension, if uncontrolled or left untreated, can lead to significant cardiovascular events, including organ failure, stroke, and other life-threatening changes (Asher et al., 2017; Bhagani et al., 2018; Chobanian et al., 2004; Cohen et al., 2019; Hong et al., 2020; James et al., 2014; Lewek et al., 2020; Poulter et al., 2015; Whelton et al., 2018; Wojtaszek & Dang, 2014).

A. Risk factors
   1. Modifiable contributing factors to the development of primary hypertension
      a) Obesity, physical inactivity
      b) Excessive use of alcohol
      c) Cigarette smoking: Acutely raises blood pressure
      d) Polycythemia
      e) NSAIDs can raise blood pressure 5 mm Hg; hypertensive patients should avoid if possible (see Appendix E).
      f) Diet
         (1) Increased salt intake
            (a) Salt alone may not be enough to significantly raise normal blood pressure; however, a genetic predisposition to salt sensitivity often contributes to hypertension.
            (b) African Americans and older adults have a high prevalence of salt sensitivity.
         (2) Caffeine intake: Increased risk for development of hypertension
   2. Nonmodifiable risk factors for the development of primary hypertension
      a) Age: Men older than 55 years, women older than 65 years
      b) Gender: Men have a greater incidence of hypertension than premenopausal women.
      c) Race: In African Americans, incidence and earlier onset of hypertension are increased, and the severity of hypertension is greater with an increased incidence of target organ damage (TOD).
   3. Secondary hypertension
      a) Age, history, physical examination, severity of hypertension, or initial laboratory findings not consistent with essential hypertension (e.g., age younger than 30 years, blood pressure greater than 180/110 mm Hg at diagnosis, significant TOD at diagnosis)
      b) Blood pressure responding poorly to drug therapy
      c) Previously well-controlled hypertension and current increase in blood pressure
      d) Blood pressure accelerating or in those who have malignancy
      e) Presentation of sudden onset of hypertension
      f) Presentation of electrolyte imbalances, especially low potassium
      g) Family history of secondary hypertension or hypertension-related syndrome.
B. Classification: According to the Joint National Committee on Prevention, Detection, Evaluation, and Treatment of High Blood Pressure (JNC 8), the following guidelines are used.
   1. General for those older than age 60 years: Normal blood pressure less than 150 mm Hg systolic and less than 90 mm Hg diastolic
   2. General for those 60 years old or younger: Normal blood pressure less than 140 mm Hg systolic and less than 90 mm Hg diastolic
   3. Diabetes: Less than 140/90 mm Hg
   4. CKD: Less than 140/90 mm Hg
C. Etiology
   1. Primary hypertension is of unknown etiology. It is thought to arise from multiple genetic traits, along with environmental and lifestyle factors.

    2. Heredity predisposes individuals to hypertension.

    3. Secondary hypertension has an identifiable cause, including numerous conditions and diseases. This type of hypertension accounts for approximately 5%–10% of hypertensive patients.

D. History

    1. History of cancer and cancer treatment

    2. Current medications: Prescribed, over the counter, herbals and other supplements (may increase blood pressure or interfere with antihypertensive drug therapy; e.g., grapefruit, cranberry, black cohosh, kava, green tea extract, ginkgo, garlic, ginseng, goldenseal, licorice, coenzyme Q10, St. John's wort, saw palmetto, valerian, yohimbine)

    3. History of presenting symptoms: Precipitating factors, onset, duration, associated symptoms (e.g., being jittery, nervous, or sweaty for no reason; experiencing heart palpitations)

    4. Changes in ADLs

    5. Past medical history: Cardiovascular disease, cerebrovascular disease, renal disease, diabetes mellitus, dyslipidemia, gout, thyroid dysfunction

    6. Family history: Hypertension, premature CAD (e.g., MI before age 55 years in father, first-degree male relative, before age 65 years, mother or first-degree female relative), stroke, other cardiovascular diseases, diabetes mellitus, dyslipidemia

    7. Social history: Tobacco use, alcohol use, illicit drug use

    8. Diet history: Fat, cholesterol, sodium, and caffeine intake

E. Signs and symptoms

    1. Patients with mild to moderate primary hypertension generally are asymptomatic. They may experience headaches, epistaxis, lethargy, dizziness, or flushing.

    2. Patients with severe or poorly controlled hypertension may present with symptoms of TOD, such as peripheral edema, dyspnea, blurred vision, or loss of movement (e.g., CHF, nephropathy, retinopathy, stroke).

F. Physical examination: According to JNC 7 guidelines, assess for the involvement of TOD (e.g., heart, brain, kidneys, eyes, peripheral arteries) and for evidence of a secondary cause.

    1. Vital signs

       a) Hypertension should not be diagnosed based on a singular blood pressure measurement.

          (1) Confirm elevated readings on at least two subsequent visits during a period of one to several weeks (unless blood pressure is greater than or equal to 180 systolic and/or greater than or equal to 110 diastolic), with average levels of systolic readings greater than or equal to 140 mm Hg and/or diastolic readings averaging greater than or equal to 90 mm Hg.

          (2) Take blood pressure in both arms with the patient in the same position; document the higher reading. Always take blood pressure in the same manner to achieve accurate readings.

          (3) JNC 7 guidelines recommend taking blood pressures with the patient seated and arm free of clothing and supported at heart level. The patient should not have smoked or ingested caffeine within 30 minutes of measurement.

          (4) Select the proper cuff size; the bladder should encircle at least 80% of the arm.

          (5) Elevated pressure in arms and lower legs may indicate coarctation of the aorta.

       b) Height and weight to assess for overweight status

      c) Peripheral pulses: May be diminished with atherosclerosis; delay of femoral pulse compared to radial pulse indicative of possible coarctation of the aorta

  2. Integument

      a) Café-au-lait spots (patchy pigmentation of skin characteristic of neurofibroma) indicating pheochromocytoma

      b) Acanthosis nigricans (dark, velvety skin associated with diabetes) for overlap between hypertension and diabetes indicating possible metabolic syndrome

      c) Truncal obesity, striae, acne, thin skin, bruises, and hyperpigmentation evident in Cushing syndrome

  3. HEENT/funduscopic indicating retinal TOD

      a) Arteriolar narrowing

      b) Arteriovenous nicking

      c) Hemorrhages

      d) Exudate

      e) Papilledema

      f) Retinopathy

  4. Neck

      a) Carotid bruits indicating vascular disease

      b) Distended jugular veins indicating vascular disease

      c) Enlarged thyroid suggestive of hypo- or hyperthyroidism

  5. Cardiac: May indicate CAD, CHF, or cardiomyopathy, if present

      a) Increased rate

      b) Increased size by percussion

      c) Precordial heave

      d) Clicks

      e) Murmurs: Presence in the front and back of the chest indicative of coarctation of the aorta

      f) Irregular heart rate

      g) S_3 indicating CHF

      h) S_4 indicating cardiovascular damage

      i) Suspected pseudohypertension when TOD is absent despite hypertension; can be confirmed by Osler maneuver

  6. Pulmonary: Rales; coarse sounds indicating CHF

  7. Abdominal

      a) Bruits: Aortic; renal indicating possible vascular occlusion or atherosclerosis

      b) Enlarged kidneys indicative of possible polycystic kidney disease or hydronephrosis

      c) Masses indicative of possible polycystic kidney disease

      d) Abnormal aortic pulsation indicative of possible aneurysm

      e) Hepatomegaly with heart failure

  8. Extremities indicating peripheral vascular disease

      a) Diminished or absent pulses indicative of coarctation of aorta

      b) Bruits (femoral)

      c) Edema

      d) Proximal muscle weakness and atrophy evident in Cushing syndrome

IV. Diagnostic tests (Bhagani et al., 2018)

  A. Laboratory

    1. CBC to evaluate for anemia or polycythemia

    2. Urinalysis to evaluate for nephropathy (e.g., proteinuria)

    3. Fasting glucose to evaluate for diabetes mellitus (metabolic syndrome) and elevated in Cushing syndrome

    4. Serum electrolytes

      a) Potassium

        (1) Baseline value before initiating diuretic or ACE inhibitor

        (2) Hypokalemia: May elevate blood pressure or indicate secondary causes, such as atherosclerosis, renal vascular disease, or Cushing syndrome

      b) Calcium: Abnormalities are associated with an increased prevalence of hypertension in hypercalcemia.

      c) Sodium: Hypernatremia may lead to increased blood pressure and can be an indicator of secondary causes of hypertension, such as Cushing syndrome or diabetes mellitus. A 24-hour urine collection for electrolytes can estimate salt intake.

    5. Creatinine and BUN: Elevated in patients with TOD; estimated GFR to further evaluate renal function for CKD

    6. Uric acid: Frequently elevated in patients with hypertension and may reflect decreased renal blood flow

    7. Fasting cholesterol profile (total, HDL, LDL, triglycerides) to identify cardiovascular risk profile data

    8. Serum aldosterone, plasma renin activity, urine aldosterone, and renin activity to evaluate for primary aldosteronism

    9. Plasma-free metanephrines and 24-hour fractionated urinary metanephrines to evaluate for pheochromocytoma

    10. Twenty-four-hour urinary free cortisol: Levels greater than three times normal confirms Cushing syndrome.

    11. Urine or serum human chorionic gonadotropin, as indicated, for pregnancy-induced hypertension

  B. Radiology

    1. Chest x-ray

      a) Cardiac enlargement indicating heart failure

      b) Evidence of pulmonary edema/CHF

    2. Renal angiography to evaluate for atherosclerotic renal stenosis, fibromuscular dysplasia, and other renal vascular diseases

    3. Renal ultrasound to evaluate for secondary hypertension, such as reninoma, polycystic kidney disease

    4. Doppler of renal arteries to evaluate for renovascular diseases

    5. MRI or CT scan of chest to evaluate for coarctation of the aorta

    6. Cardiac MRI or transthoracic echocardiography to evaluate for left ventricular hypertrophy; has greater sensitivity and specificity

  C. Other

    1. Sleep study to evaluate for sleep apnea, which contributes to hypertension

    2. Echocardiogram: Not routinely performed unless evidence of TOD

    3. ECG to evaluate for electrical left ventricular hypertrophy, atrial fibrillation, history of MI, or ischemia

V. Differential diagnosis (Bhagani et al., 2018; Hong et al., 2020; Poulter et al., 2015)

  A. Diseases

    1. Paraneoplastic syndrome (see Appendix M)

    2. Secondary diseases

      a) Atherosclerotic renal stenosis

      b) Adrenal aldosteronism or Cushing syndrome

    c) Pheochromocytoma

    d) Coarctation of the aorta

    e) Renal parenchymal disease

    f) Thyroid disorders (see Chapters 157 and 158)

    g) Disorders of corticosteroid synthesis

    h) Acromegaly

    i) Obstructive sleep apnea (see Chapter 34)

    j) Autonomic failure

    k) Pregnancy

B. Medication induced

  1. Chemotherapy/immunotherapy agents

  2. EPO

  3. Steroids

  4. Oral contraceptives

  5. NSAIDs (see Appendix E)

  6. Cyclosporine

  7. Nasal decongestants (see Appendix I)

  8. Cough suppressants

  9. Tricyclic (and other) antidepressants (see Appendix L)

  10. Monoamine oxidase inhibitors

  11. Various herbal supplements

C. White coat hypertension

  1. Elevated blood pressure when in doctor's office

  2. May indicate hypertensive tendency; patients should have blood pressure checked outside of office for a period of 7–10 days and report levels if elevated.

D. Pseudohypertension

  1. Present in older adults

  2. Caused by rigid brachial arteries that do not compress by sphygmomanometer cuff; gives false high readings

  3. Can be caused by incorrect cuff size

VI. Treatment (Bhagani et al., 2018; Cohen et al., 2019; Hong et al., 2020; James et al., 2014; Lewek et al., 2020; Smith et al., 2020; Whelton et al., 2018)

A. Goals include reduction and prevention of morbidity and mortality and control of blood pressure by the least intrusive means.

B. Target the following blood pressures.

  1. Less than 140/90 for general, nonpregnant patients aged 8–59 years with hypertension

  2. Less than 150/90 for patients aged 60 or older with hypertension

  3. Less than 140/90 for patients with heart failure, diabetes, or renal disease

C. Therapies require lifelong commitments to lifestyle modification and, possibly, drug therapy.

  1. Tobacco avoidance

  2. Weight reduction: Reduce systolic blood pressure 5–20 mm Hg.

  3. Moderation of alcohol intake: Limit to no more than two drinks per day in men and no more than one drink per day in women.

  4. Physical activity: Regular activity can reduce systolic blood pressure by up to 10 mm Hg. Hypertension should be controlled before recommending an exercise program. Typical interventions shown to be effective for lowering BP include aerobic physical activity of, on average, at least 12 weeks duration, three to four sessions per

week, lasting on average 40 minutes per session, and involving moderate to vigorous intensity physical activity.

5. Moderation of dietary sodium intake: Intake of less than 2.4 g daily (2,400 mg) may reduce systolic blood pressure 5–20 mm Hg per 10 kg of loss. The DASH diet (Dietary Approaches to Stop Hypertension) consists of increasing intake of fruits, vegetables, and low-fat dairy products combined with a decrease in salt intake. The focus is on lowering fat, sodium, and cholesterol while increasing potassium and calcium in the diet.

   a) Increase calcium intake to recommended daily allowance (800–1,200 mg).

   b) Decrease fats to less than 30% of diet.

   c) Decrease caffeine intake.

D. Pharmacologic treatment (see Table 47-1)

1. Treatment is dependent on the patient's degree of hypertension, comorbidities, age, and race.

2. Initiate drug therapy after establishing a lifestyle modification program.

3. For patients with hypertension of African descent, including those with diabetes

TABLE 47-1   Oral Agents for Hypertension

Type[a]	Action	Special Considerations
ACE Inhibitors		
• Benazepril 10 mg daily • Captopril 25 mg divided dose • Enalapril[b] 5 mg daily • Fosinopril 10 mg daily • Lisinopril[b] 10 mg daily • Quinapril[b] 10 mg daily • Ramipril[b] 5 mg daily	Inhibits the formation of angiotensin II, resulting in direct decrease in arterial pressure and indirect decrease in venous pressure	Side effects: Absence of taste, cough, rash, hyperkalemia, neutropenia, renal failure May increase or decrease digoxin levels May be necessary to decrease or discontinue diuretics during titration of ACE inhibitor to prevent hypotension Decreased dose in patients with Cr > 2.5 mg/dl Monitor: Serum potassium, Cr, and BUN levels weekly during initiation/titration Can cause acute kidney injury in patients with bilateral renal artery stenosis or severe stenosis in a single artery
Aldosterone Antagonist (Minimum Daily Dose)		
• Eplerenone 50 mg daily	Blocks aldosterone in epithelial and nonepithelial tissues, decreasing blood pressure and sodium reabsorption	May increase potassium May increase BUN/Cr
Alpha-Blockers		
• Doxazosin 1 mg daily • Prazosin 2 mg divided dose • Terazosin 1 mg daily	Relaxes smooth muscle, thus dilating arterioles and veins and decreasing total peripheral resistance; mostly block alpha 1	Given at bedtime to reduce side effect of syncope

(Continued on next page)

TABLE 47-1	Oral Agents for Hypertension *(Continued)*	
Type[a]	Action	Special Considerations
Mixed Alpha/Beta-Blockers		
• Carvedilol 12.5 mg divided dose • Labetalol 200 mg divided dose	Similar to beta-blockers Vasodilation	May be more effective in African Americans than other beta-blockers May cause postural hypotension; base titration on standing blood pressure.
ARBs		
• Eprosartan 400 mg daily • Losartan 50 mg daily • Olmesartan 20 mg daily • Telmisartan 40 mg daily • Valsartan 80 mg daily	Blocks vasoconstriction	Increased risk for hyperkalemia when ACE and ARB used together Valsartan is less likely to be associated with side effects of cough and angioedema.
Beta-Blockers (Minimum Daily Dose)		
• Atenolol 25 mg daily • Metoprolol 50 mg daily • Nebivolol 5 mg daily • Propranolol 40 mg divided dose	Generally, relaxes smooth muscle Metoprolol: Selectively beta 1 Nebivolol: Lacks membrane-stabilizing activity and has beta 1 and 2 activity at higher doses Propranolol: Decreases automaticity of contractions	Ideal for those with mild to moderately severe left ventricular dysfunction or peripheral vascular disease
Calcium Channel Blockers		

• Nondihydropyridines
  – Diltiazem 120 mg daily
  – Verapamil 80 mg divided dose daily
	Blocks inward movement of calcium ions across cell membranes, resulting in smooth muscle relaxation	Blocks slow channels in the heart and can reduce sinus rate and produce heart block

• Dihydropyridines
  – Amlodipine[c] 2.5 mg daily
  – Felodipine[c] 2.5 mg daily
  – Nifedipine extended-release 30 mg daily
	Same as other calcium channel blockers	More potent peripheral vasodilators than diltiazem and may result in increased dizziness, headache, peripheral edema, and tachycardia

Cardiac Selective Beta-Blockers		
• Clonidine 0.1 mg daily	Reduces sympathetic outflow, resulting in decreased blood pressure	Side effects: Dry mouth, drowsiness, sedation, constipation, depression Should not be discontinued abruptly; may cause severe rebound hypertension May cause orthostatic hypotension

(Continued on next page)

TABLE 47-1   Oral Agents for Hypertension *(Continued)*

Type[a]	Action	Special Considerations
Direct Vasodilators		
• Hydralazine 25 mg daily to four times a day • Minoxidil 2.5 mg daily (indicated for severe hypertension that is not manageable with maximum therapeutic doses of a diuretic and two other antihypertensives)	Directs smooth muscle vasodilation	May exacerbate angina Should be used in combination with beta-blockers and diuretics because of fluid retention and reflex tachycardia
• Nitroglycerin	Causes arterial and venous dilation Decreases preload and afterload, which decreases myocardial oxygen demand	Can cause hypotension Not a typical first-, second-, or third-line choice for hypertension treatment
Diuretics		

• Thiazide
  – Chlorthalidone 12.5 mg daily
  – Hydrochlorothiazide 12.5 mg daily
  – Metolazone 2.5 mg daily
	Inhibits reabsorption of sodium and chloride at ascending loop of Henle and distal tubules
	Decreases plasma volume
	Decreases extravascular fluid volume
	Decreases cardiac output followed by decreased peripheral resistance with normalization of cardiac output
		More effective antihypertensive than loop diuretics
		Preferred diuretic
		May decrease potassium, sodium, chloride, and magnesium
		May increase calcium, uric acid, blood sugar, and triglycerides

• Loop
  – Bumetanide 0.5 mg daily
  – Ethacrynic acid 25 mg daily
  – Furosemide 20 mg daily
  – Torsemide 2.5 mg daily
	Inhibits reabsorption of sodium/chloride at loop of Henle
	Decreases plasma volume
	Decreases extravascular fluid volume
	Decreases cardiac output followed by decreased peripheral resistance with normalization of cardiac output
		Causes greater potassium loss, resulting in enhanced effect of digoxin
		Causes calcium loss

• Potassium-sparing
  – Amiloride 5 mg daily
  – Spironolactone 25 mg daily
  – Triamterene 100 mg two times a day when used alone
	Interferes with sodium reabsorption at the distal tubules
	Aldosterone antagonist
		Used in combination with other diuretics to avoid or reverse hypokalemia
		Weak diuretic when used alone

[a] This is not a complete list of all available medications, but rather a representative sample.
[b] Drug is also used in CHF.
[c] Worsening of CHF may be less with these agents.

ACE—angiotensin-converting enzyme; ARB—angiotensin II receptor blocker; BUN—blood urea nitrogen; CHF—congestive heart failure; Cr—serum creatinine

Note. Based on information from Bhagani et al., 2018; Chobanian et al., 2004; Cohen et al., 2019; James et al., 2014; Lewek et al., 2020; Smith et al., 2020; Whelton et al., 2018.

   a) Patients should begin pharmacologic therapy with either thiazide-type diuretic or calcium channel blocker.
   b) Each of these classes of drugs have been found to have comparable benefits related to overall mortality and cardiovascular, cerebrovascular, and renal effects.
   c) These drug classes have been shown to reduce risks for negative cerebrovascular and cardiovascular events (including heart failure) better than ACE inhibitors in this population.
4. For patients with hypertension and comorbid CKD, pharmacologic therapy with an ACE inhibitor or ARB is recommended, regardless of race or diabetic status.
5. It is important to note that beta-blockers are not recommended as initial drug therapy for any population according to JNC 8 guidelines.
   a) Recommendation is based on studies that show a decreased risk of cardiovascular events with the use of an ARB versus a beta-blocker.
   b) Beta-blockers may still be used in conjunction with other antihypertensives, especially with comorbid conditions which have demonstrated benefit from use of beta-blockers, such as atrial fibrillation and CAD.
6. If goal blood pressure cannot be achieved, reevaluate for secondary causes of hypertension and consult with a hypertension specialist.
7. Initial therapy should be monotherapy if less than 20 mm Hg systolic or less than 10 mm Hg diastolic above goal. If blood pressure remains elevated for two to four weeks after initiating monotherapy, consider the following.
   a) Substituting an agent from another class if no response
   b) Increasing the dose of the initial drug if partial response
   c) Adding a second agent from another class
8. Hypertensive urgencies are those situations (e.g., greater than or equal to 180/120) that require immediate blood pressure reduction within minutes. Hypertensive urgencies include severe elevations in blood pressure to prevent or limit TOD, such as hypertensive encephalopathy, intracerebral hemorrhage, acute MI, acute left ventricular failure with pulmonary edema, pulmonary edema, dissecting aortic aneurysm, or AKI.
9. ACE inhibitors are effective and generally well tolerated.
   a) Less effective but not ineffective for African Americans
   b) No adverse effects on plasma lipid concentration or glucose tolerance
   c) May prolong survival in patients with heart failure or left ventricular dysfunction after MI and preserve renal function in patients with diabetes mellitus
   d) Significantly reduce proteinuria and slow the rate of progressive loss of renal function
   e) May cause a rise in serum creatinine
   f) Excessive hypotensive responses possible in patients with high levels of plasma resin activity
   g) Possible hyperkalemia, especially in patients taking potassium supplements or potassium-sparing diuretics or those with reduced renal function
10. Aldosterone antagonist: Eplerenone
   a) Doses greater than 100 mg PO daily not recommended because of increased risk of hyperkalemia
   b) For heart failure post-MI
   c) Increases excretion of aldosterone, renin, and sodium via the kidney
   d) May prevent proteinuria, slow vascular lesions related to hypertension, and slow development of cardiac fibrosis and heart failure after MI

11. ARBs
    a) Interfere with binding of angiotensin II to angiotensin I
    b) May be as effective as ACE inhibitors without cough as a side effect
    c) May be less effective in African Americans
    d) Have been shown to decrease cardiovascular events
    e) Can help to prevent cardiac remodeling that results in left ventricular hypertrophy
    f) May delay progression of diabetic nephropathy and reduce albuminuria
    g) May be used with a beta-blocker in patients with systolic heart failure who cannot tolerate ACE inhibitors
    h) Possible hyperkalemia, especially in patients taking potassium supplements or potassium-sparing diuretics, or in those with reduced renal function
12. Beta-blockers
    a) Less effective in African Americans
    b) Decreased mortality in patients who have had an MI
    c) May mask hypoglycemia
    d) May increase or decrease blood glucose levels
    e) May increase serum triglycerides and decrease HDL
    f) May induce bronchospasm
    g) May exacerbate peripheral arterial insufficiency
    h) May decrease heart rate significantly
    i) Not all beta-blockers are equivalent; labetalol, carvedilol, and nebivolol have vasodilatory effects.
    j) In general, beta-blockers are less able to reduce left ventricular hypertrophy than other classes of drugs.
13. Mixed alpha- and beta-blocker: Labetalol, carvedilol
    a) Prompt decrease in blood pressure
    b) Orthostatic hypotension more frequent than with other blockers
    c) Does not alter serum lipids
14. Calcium channel blockers
    a) Verapamil and diltiazem prolong AV nodal conduction; therefore, they must be used with caution in patients who are taking beta-blockers.
    b) All calcium channel blockers except amlodipine and felodipine should be used cautiously in patients with CHF because these drugs have a negative inotropic effect on the heart.
    c) They have no effect on lipid concentrations.
15. Diuretics
    a) Low doses decrease mortality and cardiovascular events.
    b) Older adult patients can be effectively treated with smaller doses.
    c) Loop diuretics can be used to treat hypertension in patients with renal insufficiency (i.e., creatinine greater than 1.5 mg/dl).
    d) Thiazide-type diuretics increase the risk of new-onset diabetes mellitus.
16. Alpha-blockers
    a) Cause arterial and venous dilation
    b) Frequently cause postural hypotension, especially after first dose (increased incidence in older adults)
    c) Do not adversely affect blood lipids but may increase HDL
    d) Symptomatic relief of prostatism
E. Secondary hypertension: All patients with secondary hypertension will likely need a referral to an appropriate specialist.

1. Renal vascular disease: Most common of all secondary causes
   a) Potentially curable with renal artery angioplasty and stent placement
   b) Suspected if hypertension in patients younger than 30 years old, sudden worsening of hypertension after age 50 years, or treatment-resistant hypertension
2. Primary aldosteronism: Considered if patient has spontaneous hypokalemia, which can be accompanied by alkalosis
3. Pheochromocytoma
   a) Two to eight cases per million per year; can be familial
   b) Characterized by episodic hypertension with headache, diaphoresis, palpitations, pallor, abdominal pain, and weight loss
4. Obstructive sleep apnea (see Chapter 34)
   a) Prevalent and often associated with hypertension
   b) Treated with weight loss and continuous positive airway pressure, as appropriate
5. Cushing syndrome: 600 cases per million population, 50% of which are attributable to small cell lung cancer; treatment of surgery or medical management dependent on etiology
6. Coarctation of the aorta
   a) History of headaches, cold feet, claudication
   b) Treated with surgical correction
7. Polycystic renal disease: Familial; treated with supportive care

VII. Follow-up (Chobanian et al., 2004; Whelton et al., 2018)
   A. Encourage home monitoring; a recent finding indicated better control in patients who self-monitor their blood pressure.
   B. Once drug therapy is initiated, reevaluate monthly until goal is achieved and every three to six months thereafter.
   C. Follow up more often if comorbidities exist or the patient has stage II hypertension.

VIII. Referrals
   A. Cardiologist
      1. Hypertension at any stage with evidence of TOD
      2. Hypertension resistant to treatment
      3. Previously well-controlled blood pressure now resistant to treatment
      4. Hypertensive emergencies or urgencies
   B. Nephrologist: For patients with evidence of renal TOD
   C. Ophthalmologist: For patients with evidence of retinal TOD
   D. Neurologist: For patients with history of stroke and/or transient ischemic attack
   E. Endocrinologist: For patients with Cushing syndrome

The author would like to acknowledge Kathy Sharp, MSN, FNP-BC, AOCNP®, CCD, for her contribution to this chapter that remains unchanged from the previous edition of this book.

References

Asher, G.N., Corbett, A.H., & Hawke, R.L. (2017). Common herbal dietary supplement–drug interactions. *American Family Physician, 96*(2), 101–107. https://www.aafp.org/afp/2017/0715/p101.html

Bhagani, S., Kapil, V., & Lobo, M.D. (2018). Hypertension. *Medicine, 46*(9), 509–515. https://doi.org/10.1016/j.mpmcd.2018.06.009

Chobanian, A.V., Bakris, G.L., Black, H.R., Cushman, W.C., Green, L.A., Izzo, J.L., ... Wright, J.T., Jr. (2004, August). *The seventh report of the Joint National Committee on prevention, detection, evaluation, and treatment of high blood pressure* [NIH Publication No. 04-5320]. National Heart, Lung, and Blood Institute. http://www.nhlbi.nih.gov/guidelines/hypertension/jnc7full.htm

Cohen, J.B., Geara, A.S., Hogan, J.J., & Townsend, R.R. (2019). Hypertension in cancer patients and survivors: Epidemiology, diagnosis, and management. *JACC CardioOnoclogy, 1*(2), 238–251. https://doi.org/10.1016/j.jaccao.2019.11.009

Hong, K., Yu, E.S., & Chun, B.C. (2020). Risk factors of the progression to hypertension and characteristics of natural history during progression: A national cohort study. *PLOS ONE, 15*(3), e0230538. https://doi.org/10.1371/journal.pone.0230538

James, P.A., Oparil, S., Carter, B.L., Cushman, W.C., Dennison-Himmelfarb, C., Handler, J., ... Ortiz, E. (2014). 2014 evidence-based guideline for the management of high blood pressure in adults: Report from the panel members appointed to the Eighth Joint National Committee (JNC 8). *JAMA, 311*(5), 507–520. https://doi.org/10.1001/jama.2013.284427

Lewek, J., Bielecka-Dąbrowa, A., Maciejewski, M., & Banach, M. (2020). Pharmacological management of malignant hypertension. *Expert Opinion on Pharmacotherapy, 21*(10), 1189–1192. https://doi.org/10.1080/14656566.2020.1732923

Ohishi, M. (2018). Hypertension with diabetes mellitus: Physiology and pathology. *Hypertension Research, 41*(6), 389–393. https://doi.org/10.1038/s41440-018-0034-4

Poulter, N.R., Prabhakaran, D., & Caulfield, M. (2015). Hypertension. *Lancet, 386*(9995), 801–812. https://doi.org/10.1016/S0140-6736(14)61468-9

Smith, D.K., Lennon, R.P., & Carlsgaard, P.B. (2020). Managing hypertension using combination therapy. *American Family Physician, 101*(6), 341–349. https://www.aafp.org/afp/2020/0315/p341.html

Whelton, P.K., Carey, R.M., Aronow, W.S., Casey, D.E., Jr., Collins, K.J., Dennison Himmelfarb, C., ... Wright, J.T., Jr. (2018). ACC/AHA/AAPA/ABC/ACPM/AGS/APhA/ASH/ASPC/NMA/PCNA guideline for the prevention, detection, evaluation, and management of high blood pressure in adults: A report of the American College of Cardiology/American Heart Association Task Force on Clinical Practice Guidelines. *Circulation, 138*(17), e484–e594. https://doi.org/10.1161/CIR.0000000000000596

Wojtaszek, D., & Dang, D.K. (2014). MTM essentials for hypertension management. Part 2: Drug therapy considerations. *Drug Topics, 158*(5), 33–44. https://www.drugtopics.com/view/comprehensive-mtm-patients-cardiovascular-disease

CHAPTER 48

Hypotension

Rachael Fornwalt, MSN, AG–ACNP

I. Definition (Freeman et al., 2011; Freeman et al., 2018; Low & Tomalia, 2015; Tzur et al., 2019)
   A. An abnormally low blood pressure when compared to the patient's baseline pressure and associated systemic symptoms; in general, a systolic blood pressure less than 90 mm Hg and a diastolic pressure less than 60 mm Hg are considered to be abnormal.
   B. A decrease of 20 mm Hg or more in systolic blood pressure or a decrease of 10 mm Hg or more in diastolic pressure assuming the upright position or head-up tilt table testing; if heart rate is included, a rate increase of 15–30 bpm is significant upon standing.

II. Physiology/Pathophysiology (De Backer & Foulon, 2019; Freeman et al., 2011; Freeman et al., 2018; Lahrmann et al., 2006; Low & Tomalia, 2015)
   A. Normal
      1. Blood pressure is maintained as a result of the continuous regulation of cardiac output and systemic vascular resistance.
      2. The regulation takes place at the sites of the heart, pre- and postcapillary venule, and the kidneys.
      3. The autonomic nervous system and humoral influences stimulate or suppress the overall regulation of these sites.
      4. When standing, there is redistribution of blood volume with pooling of 300–800 ml of blood in the lower extremities. This causes decreased venous return to the heart and reduced cardiac filling pressure. The body responds to this diminished stroke volume and cardiac output by increasing sympathetic outflow to the heart and blood vessels and decreasing cardiac vagal nerve activity. By making these autonomic adjustments, vascular tone, heart rate, and cardiac contractility increase, thus stabilizing the arterial blood pressure.
      5. Likewise, contraction of skeletal muscle in the lower body prevents excessive pooling of blood, thus augmenting venous return to the heart.
   B. Pathophysiology
      1. Hypotension results from the disruption of cardiac output and systemic vascular resistance or the malfunction of the other regulatory systems; therefore, perfusion cannot meet the metabolic needs of the end organs.
      2. It can be classified as neurogenic (from autonomic system failure) or non-neurogenic (e.g., pump failure, venous pooling, medication induced).

III. Clinical features: Orthostatic hypotension is a common cardiovascular disease in older adult and frail individuals with multiple comorbidities. It is often the most disabling feature of autonomic dysfunction. Most cases of orthostatic hypotension are not neurologic in origin (Cheshire, 2019; Curigliano et al., 2016; Freeman et al., 2011; Lahrmann et al., 2006; Low & Tomalia, 2015; Magkas et al., 2019; Robinson & Kimpinski, 2019; Tzur et al., 2019).

A. Classified according to type
  1. Acute: Blood pressure has sudden drop with systolic less than 90 mm Hg or systolic drop of 40 mm Hg or more.
  2. Constitutional: Blood pressure is chronically lower than baseline.
  3. Orthostatic or postural: Blood pressure is normal but drops when the individual stands or changes positions.

B. Etiology
  1. Autonomic
    a) Parkinson disease
    b) Multiple system atrophy
    c) Lewy body syndrome
    d) Pure autonomic failure or Bradbury-Eggleston syndrome
    e) Neuropathies
      (1) Paraneoplastic autonomic neuropathy
      (2) Autoimmune autonomic neuropathy
      (3) Peripheral neuropathies
    f) Vascular and cardiac etiologies
  2. Distributive etiologies: Volume depletion, sepsis, drug induced
  3. Obstructive: Tension pneumothorax, emboli, stenosis
  4. Cardiac: Atrial arrhythmias, MI, heart failure, heart valve issues
  5. Postprandial hypotension: 15–20 minutes after meals, common in older adults
  6. Reflex syncope
  7. Cancer related: Autonomic, vascular, or immune related
    a) Brain tumors
    b) Small cell lung cancer
    c) Toxic neuropathies from chemotherapy: Vincristine, cisplatin, paclitaxel
    d) Paraneoplastic syndrome: Related to multiple types of cancer, particularly small cell lung cancer, myeloma, carcinoid tumor, thymoma (see Appendix M)
    e) Cetuximab and rituximab inducing hypotension
    f) Arrhythmias caused by microtubule inhibitors inducing hypotension
    g) Myocardial ischemia from 5-fluorouracil or capecitabine resulting in secondary hypotension
    h) Targeted therapies such as TKIs (e.g., alemtuzumab, trastuzumab, sunitinib, erlotinib, lapatinib, dasatinib) inducing heart failure or left ventricular failure, which may result in hypotension
    i) Biologics, especially IL-2 and denileukin diftitox
  8. Postural orthostatic hypotension syndrome
  9. Adrenal insufficiency
  10. Hypothyroidism (myxedema coma)
  11. Cardiac arrhythmias

C. History (Curigliano et al., 2016; Freeman et al., 2011; Freeman et al., 2018; Low & Tomalia, 2015)
  1. History of cancer and cancer treatment
  2. Current medications: Prescribed, over the counter
  3. History of presenting symptoms: Precipitating factors, onset, location, duration, associated symptoms (e.g., dizziness, light-headedness, syncope, chest discomfort, shortness of breath, vomiting, diarrhea, fever, chills, melena)
  4. Changes in ADLs

5. Past medical history: Recent infection, diabetes, hypothyroidism, neurodegenerative disease

6. Age older than 65 years

D. Signs and symptoms

1. Dizziness and light-headedness
2. Nausea and vomiting
3. Diarrhea
4. Fever and chills
5. Chest pain
6. Shortness of breath
7. Weakness
8. Fatigue
9. Cognitive impairment while in the upright position
10. Headache
11. Syncope

E. Physical examination

1. Vital signs

   a) Hypotension
   b) Fever indicating sepsis
   c) Recommended procedure

      (1) Have patient lie supine for 10 minutes, and obtain blood pressure and heart rate.
      (2) Take blood pressure and heart rate immediately after patient rises to a standing position, and ask about symptoms. Note whether the heart rate increases 10–15 bpm normally on rising.
      (3) Repeat blood pressure and heart rate after patient has been standing for three minutes.
      (4) Postural (orthostatic) hypotension diagnosis is made when, within two to five minutes of quiet standing (after a five-minute period of supine rest), one or both of the following is present.
         (a) At least a 20 mm Hg fall in systolic pressure
         (b) At least a 10 mm Hg fall in diastolic pressure

   d) A decreased blood pressure with increased heart rate may indicate non-neurogenic causes.
   e) A decreased blood pressure without increased heart rate may indicate neurogenic causes.

2. Integument

   a) Temperature: Hypothermia/hyperthermia
   b) Color: Pale, cold, clammy
   c) Poor skin turgor or dry mucous membranes indicating dehydration

3. Neurologic: Altered mental status

   a) Restlessness
   b) Agitation
   c) Confusion
   d) Lethargy
   e) Coma

4. Cardiac

   a) S_3 indicative of CHF
   b) S_4: May be present in MI
   c) Murmurs for valvular disease

      d) JVD in heart failure
   5. Pulmonary
      a) Rales: Pulmonary edema
      b) Rhonchi: Pneumonia
      c) Bilaterally equal breath sounds: Pneumothorax, hemothorax
   6. Extremities
      a) Weak or absent pulse
      b) Cool or mottled extremities
      c) Presence of edema
   7. Rectal: If bleeding is detected in stool guaiac test

IV. Diagnostic tests (Lahrmann et al., 2006)
   A. Laboratory
      1. CBC with differential to assess for anemia and leukocytosis in infection
      2. BUN and creatinine: Increased values potentially indicative of dehydration, metabolic acidosis, AKI, or sepsis
      3. Cultures, as indicated, to evaluate for sepsis of visible wounds, urine, and blood
      4. Thyroid function panel to evaluate for hypothyroidism
      5. Serum cortisol to evaluate for adrenal insufficiency
      6. Cardiac enzymes and BNP to evaluate for cardiac etiology of hypotension
   B. Radiology: Chest x-ray
      1. Heart size
      2. Evidence of CHF: Cardiomegaly
      3. Pulmonary edema
      4. Pneumonia: Infiltrates
      5. Pleural effusion
   C. Other
      1. ECG to assess for acute changes indicative of MI/ischemia, left ventricular hypertrophy, and dysrhythmia secondary to MI or electrolyte imbalances
      2. Echocardiogram to evaluate left ventricular function and valve status

V. Differential diagnosis (Ali et al., 2018; Magkas et al., 2019; Oommen et al., 2019; Robinson & Kimpinski, 2019)
   A. Cardiac and vascular
      1. Hypovolemia
      2. Pump failure
      3. Valvular dysfunction
   B. Distributive
      1. Septic shock (see Chapter 160)
      2. Anaphylactic shock (see Chapter 160)
      3. Drug induced
         a) ACE inhibitors
         b) Diuretics, especially potassium-sparing
         c) Nitrates
         d) Beta-blockers
         e) Central sympatholytics
         f) Alpha-blockers
         g) Tricyclic antidepressants
         h) Steroids from acute withdrawal
         i) Calcium antagonists

        j) Anxiolytics

        k) Sedatives/hypnotics

        l) Neuroleptics

        m) Antiparkinsonian drugs

        n) Antipsychotics of butyrophenone type

        o) Immunotherapy: IL-2, IFN, TNF

        p) Anaphylactic reactions (see Chapter 150)

    4. Neurogenic

    5. Acute adrenal insufficiency

  C. Obstructive

    1. Pneumothorax (see Chapter 31)

    2. Pericardial tamponade (see Chapter 50)

    3. Pulmonary emboli (see Chapter 33)

    4. PH (see Chapter 52)

    5. Aortic or mitral stenosis

  D. Neoplastic: Spinal lesions, space-occupying effusions in the chest

VI. Treatment for acute, sudden-onset hypotension

  A. Discontinue any causative IV medications or chemotherapy.

  B. Place patient in Trendelenburg or supine position with legs elevated.

  C. Use of oxygen

    1. Use is dependent on ABGs and patient's baseline pulmonary function, although it may be initiated immediately if patient is hypovolemic.

    2. Two liters by nasal cannula would be helpful and rarely affects carbon dioxide retention.

  D. Monitor urine output: Patient may be oliguric or nonoliguric.

    1. Use of a urinary catheter may be necessary.

    2. Urine output should be maintained at greater than or equal to 25–30 ml/hr.

  E. Volume replacement is determined by blood pressure, volume status, electrolyte status, and cardiovascular status.

  F. Vasoactive drugs are indicated in shock states (see Chapter 160).

  G. Diuretics are used only if CHF results in hypotension (see Chapter 42).

  H. Corticosteroids (e.g., hydrocortisone) are used to treat acute adrenal insufficiency (see Appendix K)

  I. Manage anaphylaxis, if suspected (see Chapter 150).

VII. Treatment for orthostatic hypotension (Ali et al., 2018; Cheshire, 2019; Freeman et al., 2011; Freeman et al., 2018; Isaacson et al., 2016; Magkas et al., 2019; Oommen et al., 2019)

  A. Midodrine, an alpha agonist, is the only approved therapy for postural hypotension. Administer 2.5–10 mg PO three times a day while awake.

  B. Fludrocortisone is the first-line treatment for orthostatic intolerance. It raises blood pressure via sodium retention. Initiate at 0.1 mg PO three times a week.

  C. Pyridostigmine has been used for treatment of orthostatic hypotension. Initiate at 60 mg PO three times a day.

  D. Droxidopa has demonstrated safety in treatment of neurogenic orthostatic hypotension in patients with primary autonomic failure. Initiate at 100 mg PO three times a day and titrate to response in increments of 100 mg three times a day every 24–48 hours. Do not exceed 600 mg three times a day.

  E. Caffeine alone may treat mild hypotension.

F. Desmopressin has been shown to be beneficial in patients with orthostatic hypotension who also have nocturnal polyuria. Low doses are recommended at bedtime. Initiate at 10–40 mcg as a nasal spray, or 0.1 to 0.2 mg PO daily as a tablet.

G. Considerations regarding hypotension

1. Hypotension from antihypertensives is relatively uncommon.
2. Pure vasodilating agents (e.g., dihydropyridine calcium channel blockers) are most likely to cause hypotension.
3. Patients not on a diuretic with serum sodium less than 135 mg/dl are more likely to have a marked drop in blood pressure with initiation of an ACE inhibitor or ARB.
4. Older adults typically have orthostatic hypotension secondary to decreased circulating volume and/or impaired peripheral vasoconstriction.
5. Most evidence supporting pharmacologic treatments was via trials on younger and middle-aged adults.
6. People with orthostatic hypotension have an approximately 50% higher risk of developing heart failure. In the future, orthostatic hypotension may be considered a marker of subclinical atherosclerosis.

H. Nonpharmacologic management (Ali et al., 2018; Magkas et al., 2019; Subbarayan et al., 2019)

1. Arise slowly in stages from supine to standing.
2. Avoid straining.
3. Use fall precautions.
4. Maintain hydration and avoid overheating.
5. Compression therapy may be beneficial.

VIII. Follow-up

A. Frequent to intermittent follow-up may be necessary depending on cause of hypotension and whether the condition becomes problematic.

B. A diastolic blood pressure that is less than 55–60 mm Hg may be associated with an increase in cardiovascular events and requires more frequent monitoring.

IX. Referrals

A. Cardiologist: If patient is not responding to treatment

B. Neurologist: For evaluation and treatment of autonomic system dysfunction

The author would like to acknowledge Kathy Sharp, MSN, FNP-BC, AOCNP®, CCD, for her contribution to this chapter that remains unchanged from the previous edition of this book.

References

Ali, A., Ali, N.S., Waqas, N., Bhan, C., Iftikhar, W., Sapna, F., … Ahmed, A. (2018). Management of orthostatic hypotension: A literature review. *Cureus, 10*(8), e3166. https://doi.org/10.7759/cureus.3166

Cheshire, W.P. (2019). Chemical pharmacotherapy for the treatment of orthostatic hypotension. *Expert Opinion on Pharmacotherapy, 20*(2), 187–199. https://doi.org/10.1080/14656566.2018.1543404

Curigliano, G., Cardinale, D., Dent, S., Criscitiello, C., Aseyev, O., Lenihan, D., & Cipolla, C.M., (2016). Cardiotoxicity of anticancer treatments: Epidemiology, detection, and management. *CA: A Cancer Journal for Clinicians, 66*(4), 309–325. https://doi.org/10.3322/caac.21341

De Backer, D., & Foulon, P. (2019). Minimizing catecholamines and optimizing perfusion. *Critical Care, 23*(Suppl. 1), 149. https://doi.org/10.1186/s13054-019-2433-6

Freeman, R., Wieling, W., Axelrod, F.B., Benditt, D.G., Benarroch, E., Biaggioni, I., … van Dijk, J.G. (2011). Consensus statement on the definition of orthostatic hypotension, neurally mediated syncope and the postural tachycardia syndrome. *Clinical Autonomic Research, 21*(2), 69–72. https://doi.org/10.1007/s10286-011-0119-5

Freeman, R., Abuzinadah, A.R., Gibbons, C., Jones, P., Miglis, M.G., & Sinn, D.I. (2018). Orthostatic hypotension: *JACC State-of-the-Art Review*. *Journal of the American College of Cardiology, 72*(11), 1294–1309. https://doi.org/10.1016/j.jacc.2018.05.079

Isaacson, S., Shill, H.A., Vernino, S., Ziemann, A., & Rowse, G.J. (2016). Safety and durability of effect with long-term, open-label droxidopa treatment in patients with symptomatic neurogenic orthostatic hypotension (NOH303). *Journal of Parkinson's Disease, 6*(4), 751–759. https://doi.org/10.3233/JPD-160860

Lahrmann, H., Cortelli, P., Hilz, M., Mathias, C.J., Struhal, W., & Tassinari, M. (2006). EFNS guidelines on the diagnosis and management of orthostatic hypotension. *European Journal of Neurology, 13*(9), 930–936. https://doi.org/10.1111/j.1468-1331.2006.01512.x

Low, P.A., & Tomalia, V.A. (2015). Orthostatic hypotension: Mechanisms, causes, management. *Journal of Clinical Neurology, 11*(3), 220–226. https://doi.org/10.3988/jcn.2015.11.3.220

Magkas, N., Tsioufis, C., Thomopoulos, C., Dilaveris, P., Georgiopoulos, G., Sanidas, E., ... Tousoulis, D. (2019). Orthostatic hypotension: From pathophysiology to clinical applications and therapeutic considerations. *Journal of Clinical Hypertension, 21*(5), 546–554. https://doi.org/10.1111/jch.13521

Oommen, J., Chen, J., Wang, S., Caraccio, T., & Hannah, A. (2019). Droxidopa for hypotension of different etiologies: Two case reports. *Pharmacy and Therapeutics, 44*(3), 125–144.

Robinson, L., & Kimpinski, K. (2019). Neurogenic orthostatic hypotension impairs information processing speed and attention. *Physiology and Behavior, 211,* 112682. https://doi.org/10.1016/j.physbeh.2019.112682

Subbarayan, S., Myint, P.K., Martin, K.R., Abraha, I., Devkota, S., O'Mahony, D., ... Soiza, R.L. (2019). Nonpharmacologic management of orthostatic hypotension in older people: A systematic review. The SENATOR ONTOP series. *Journal of the American Medical Directors Association, 20*(9), 1065–1073.e3. https://doi.org/10.1016/j.jamda.2019.03.032

Tzur, I., Izhakian, S., & Gorelik, O. (2019). Orthostatic hypotension: Definition, classification and evaluation. *Blood Pressure, 28*(3), 146–156. https://doi.org/10.1080/08037051.2019.1604067

Myocardial Infarction/ Acute Coronary Syndromes

Brenda K. Shelton, DNP, APRN-CNS, RN, CCRN, AOCN®

I. Definition: This cluster of disorders reflects varying degrees of symptomatic occlusion or narrowing of the coronary arteries, resulting in injury, ischemia, and necrosis of the myocardium. Two primary categories of disorders (ST-segment elevation and non–ST-segment elevation) are included in this constellation, indicating a spectrum of clinical manifestations (American Heart Association [AHA], 2016; Amsterdam et al., 2014; Bajaj et al., 2018; Bejik et al., 2019; Manolis et al., 2018).

   A. Non–ST-segment elevation acute coronary syndrome (NSTE-ACS) is a coronary artery occlusion that causes temporary or ongoing myocardial ischemia, with or without ECG changes or serum cardiac enzyme elevation. This category includes unstable angina and non–ST-segment elevation myocardial infarction (NSTEMI), as they are considered to be on the same continuum and may be difficult to differentiate in clinical presentation.

      1. Unstable angina: Defined as significant occlusion of coronary arteries leading to transient MI that may or may not reflect in ECG changes, without elevation of MI biomarkers

      2. NSTEMI: Coronary artery occlusion leading to release of specific cardiac biomarkers without ST-segment elevation (posterior wall infarction must be excluded)

   B. ST-segment elevation acute coronary syndrome (STE-ACS) is a coronary artery occlusion with two or more contiguous ST-segment elevations and an elevation of serum cardiac enzymes or new bundle branch block with ischemic repolarization patterns.

      1. Full-thickness muscle damage: A transmural wall infarction associated with development of a permanent conduction defect called a Q wave

      2. Partial wall thickness infarction: An "epidural" infarction not associated with a Q wave indicating a partial muscle infarction

      3. Subendocardial infarction: Subtle ECG changes that resolve but with cardiac enzyme release indicating some MI

   C. Any serum cardiac biomarker elevations indicate MI, whereas MI is identified as the presence of elevated biomarkers in addition to symptoms, ECG changes, or physical evidence of ischemia.

   D. Vasospastic angina, also known as *Prinzmetal angina*, may result in unstable angina or MI.

   E. *Reinfarction* is a term for an acute MI that occurs within 28 days of an incident or a recurrent MI. It is characterized by new ST-segment elevations or pathologic Q waves with increased biomarkers.

II. Physiology/Pathophysiology (AHA, 2016; Amsterdam et al., 2014; Filippo & Libby, 2017)
   A. Normal
      1. The heart is divided into four chambers. The top two chambers are the right and left atria, and the bottom two chambers are the right and left ventricles.
      2. Atria are small, thin-walled structures that act primarily as a reservoir for the blood returning to the heart from the veins throughout the body.
      3. The ventricles are large, thick-walled chambers that pump blood to the lungs (right ventricle) and throughout the body (left ventricle).
   B. Pathophysiology: Coronary syndromes are classified according to the area of the heart affecting specific coronary arteries or their major branches (see Table 49-1).
      1. Pathophysiology involves coronary artery occlusion or spasm, direct cardiac compromise, and sympathetic stimulation.
         a) Proposed mechanisms of occlusion
            (1) Plaque rupture with platelet adhesion causes an arterial occlusion.
            (2) Uppermost lipid layer of the plaque becomes unstable and may develop superficial erosion.
            (3) Clot enlargement occurs with clot-bound thrombin or microemboli causing occlusion.
         b) Hypercoagulability disorders cause independent clot formation without coronary artery plaques (e.g., acute promyelocytic leukemia).
         c) Coronary vasospasm narrows the artery, causing impaired flow. It may be a short-term vasospasm with increased cardiac demand or stimulant-induced arterial vasospasm (e.g., cocaine).
         d) Extreme vasoconstriction, such as that occurring with catecholamine release (e.g., pheochromocytoma), can occur.
      2. Initially after occlusion (first 24 hours), platelets and fibrin adhere to the rough edges of the occlusion, potentially extending the area of ischemia.
      3. Coronary artery occlusion leads to ischemia, injury, and necrosis if circulation is not restored.
         a) "Wave of injury" describes which of these three changes have occurred in the myocardium, as well as the depth of myocardial damage.
         b) Ischemia leads to the release of toxic metabolites (e.g., arachidonic acid, oxygen free radicals) that enlarge the area of ischemia and injury.
         c) Cardiac muscle or other structures (e.g., papillary muscle, conduction pathway, valves) deprived of oxygen lead to cell death and clinical manifestations typical of transmural MI (necrosis).
      4. Mechanisms of MI in patients with cancer are less likely to be atherosclerotic plaques and thromboses.
         a) Mediastinal radiation therapy at any dose causes microvascular changes that interfere with coronary blood flow.
         b) Demand ischemia from hypermetabolic processes or in conjunction with limited reserve (e.g., anemia) may be more common to induce MI.

III. Clinical features: Acute coronary syndromes typically occur when myocardial oxygen demand exceeds myocardial oxygen consumption. This imbalance is most often the result of coronary artery obstruction but may be caused by other cardiac and noncardiac physiologic processes that create excess demand of oxygen or limit oxygen delivery. Acute coronary syndrome is the most common cause of death worldwide. Its incidence is estimated to be more than 780,000 cases annually, with a male-to-female presentation ratio of 3:2 and a median presentation age of 68 years. Approximately 70% of presenting cases are NSTE-ACS, and these patients display

TABLE 49-1 **Electrocardiogram Diagnosis of Acute Coronary Syndromes: Correlation of Leads and Anatomic Structures**

Location	Associated Leads	Coronary Arteries Affected	Clinical Effects
Anterior wall	V_3–V_4	Left coronary artery (LCA)/left anterior descending artery (LAD) diagonal branch	Left ventricular failure with congestion Increased central venous pressure, congestion Dysrhythmias (e.g., tachycardia, heart block, ventricular dysrhythmias)
Anteroseptal	V_1–V_4	LCA/LAD diagonal and septal branches	Left ventricular failure with congestion Dysrhythmias (heart block)
Septum	V_1–V_2	LCA/LAD septal branch	Heart block and bundle branch block
Anterolateral	V_3–V_6, I, aVL	LAD diagonal and circumflex branches	Left ventricular failure with congestion Dysrhythmias (e.g., heart block, ventricular)
Lateral wall	V_5–V_6, I, aVL	LCA/left circumflex artery (LCF)	Left ventricular failure Heart block
Inferior wall (left ventricle)	II, III, aVF	Right coronary artery (RCA) posterior descending branch	Hypotension with sensitivity to nitrates Bradycardia usually without any heart blocks Papillary muscle rupture with murmur
Inferior wall (right ventricle)	II, III, aVF, right-sided V_4 (RV_4)	RCA proximal branch	Dysrhythmias (e.g., bradycardia, heart block, atrial dysrhythmias) Hypotension Increased jugular venous pressure Increased central venous pressure Volume dependence Clear lung fields Right-sided S_3 or S_4
Inferoposterior	II, III, aVF, with depression of precordial leads	RCA, proximal branches	Left ventricular failure Dysrhythmias
Posterior wall	V_1–V_4 (ST depression, not elevation)	LCA/LCF or RCA posterior descending branch	Left ventricular failure

Note. Based on information from American Heart Association, 2016; Amsterdam et al., 2014; Vogel et al., 2019.

more cardiac and noncardiac comorbidities than those presenting with STE-ACS (Abbott et al., 2019; AHA, 2016; Amsterdam et al., 2014; Aydin et al., 2019; Chang et al., 2018; DeVon et al., 2017; Diaz et al., 2019; D'souza, 2019; Long & Koyfman, 2018; Moore et al., 2019; Park et al., 2018; Suh et al., 2017; Tomaszewski et al., 2018; Vicent et al., 2017).

  A. Classification: Acute MIs are classified by the severity of left ventricular dysfunction (heart failure). Killip classification predicts prognosis based on degree of heart failure following an acute MI.

    1. Class I: Uncomplicated MI, no signs of pulmonary congestion or systemic hypoperfusion

    2. Class II: Mild heart failure, bilateral rales on lower lung auscultation, or presence of gallop heart sounds

      3. Class III: Pulmonary edema with or without intubation, bilateral rales in upper lung fields

      4. Class IV: Cardiogenic shock

B. Risk factors

      1. Modifiable risk factors include tobacco use, serum lipid levels, hypertension, diabetes mellitus, sedentary lifestyle, obesity, unhealthful diet, recreational drugs/medications, oral contraceptives, and vitamin D deficiency.

      2. Nonmodifiable risk factors include CKD, advancing age, gender, family/genetic history, and ethnicity/race.

      3. Chronic heart failure may lead to coronary artery incompetence and MI.

      4. Chronic renal disease induces small vessel disease and increased ventricular pressures, resulting in MI.

C. Etiology

      1. Hypercoagulability: Thrombocythemia

      2. Hyperviscosity: Hyperglycemia

      3. Malignancy

          a) Adenocarcinomas: Mucin-producing malignancies enhance clotting.

          b) Acute leukemia, especially high WBCs, high blast percentages, or progranulocytic variant

          c) Hyperviscosity disorders: Multiple myeloma, leukostasis in acute leukemia, sickle cell crisis

          d) Malignancy-associated Trousseau syndrome or DIC

          e) Cardiac tumors/heart infiltration with malignant cells: Tumors may infiltrate the myocardium or compress coronary arteries (most commonly lymphomas, sarcomas).

          f) Pheochromocytoma: Increased catecholamines and demand ischemia

          g) *JAK2* mutation–related diseases: Polycythemia vera, chronic leukemia

      4. Stimulant recreational drugs: Cocaine, speed balls, high-dose caffeine

      5. Anemia: Hematocrit less than 25% increases risk, particularly if preexisting CAD is present.

      6. Hypercalcemia

      7. HIV, especially when receiving antiretroviral agents

      8. Survivor of childhood cancer: Possible decreased growth hormone

      9. Radiation exposure to the heart: As little as 60 Gy has been associated with CAD; onset is 6–10 years after exposure.

     10. Medications: Cyclooxygenase-2 inhibitors, levodopa, dopamine, epinephrine, vitamin E (high consumption), nonselective beta-blockers, vitamin K (enhance hypercoagulability), corticosteroids, anesthetic agents

     11. Chemotherapy/immunotherapy/targeted therapy: Few agents alone cause cardiac disease but are specifically associated with coronary disease.

          a) Anthracyclines

          b) Antiangiogenic agents: Bevacizumab, ramucirumab

          c) Antimetabolites: Cytarabine, gemcitabine, fluoropyrimidines (e.g., 5-fluorouracil, capecitabine)

          d) Immunotherapy: IL-2, bortezomib, trastuzumab, cetuximab, G-CSF, rituximab

          e) Cisplatin, oxaliplatin

          f) Tamoxifen

          g) Taxanes

          h) TKIs: Imatinib, gefitinib, sorafenib, sunitinib

12. Noncardiovascular surgeries: Esophagectomy, head and neck resection, pneumo-nectomy; severing of the vagus nerve may contribute to risk.
13. Cardiovascular surgery: Coronary artery bypass

D. History
1. History of cancer and cancer treatments
2. Current medications: Prescribed, over the counter
3. History of presenting symptoms: Precipitating factors, onset, location, quality of pain, radiation, duration, associated symptoms
4. Changes in ADLs: Decreased activity tolerance
5. Past medical history: Cardiovascular disease, diabetes, hypercoagulability, DVT, glomerulonephritis, dysrhythmias, hyperlipidemia, sickle cell disease
6. Family history: Cardiovascular disease, hypercholesterolemia, first-degree relative younger than 50 years old with MI

E. Signs and symptoms: Figure 49-1 describes key clinical findings that identify high, inter-mediate, or low probability of an acute coronary syndrome.
1. Common symptoms: Chest pain, retrosternal pain, or chest pressure lasting more than 10 minutes; may radiate to one or both arms, the neck, or jaw; possible arm, neck, or jaw pain present without chest pain or pressure
2. Atypical symptoms: New or increased exertional dyspnea (most common), diapho-resis, nausea, vomiting, abdominal or epigastric pain, unexplained fatigue, palpita-tions, syncope, stabbing pleuritic pain
3. Common signs and symptoms of acute coronary syndrome in specific populations
   a) Women: Nausea, light-headedness or dizziness, syncope, extreme fatigue
   b) Chronic illness: Increased likelihood of atypical presentation
   c) Advanced age: Increased likelihood of absence of chest pain

---

FIGURE 49-1   **Chest Pain Suggestive of Myocardial Infarction**

High Probability of Ischemic Heart Disease
Clinical findings
- Chief symptom of chest or left arm pain plus current pain like prior documented angina or known coronary artery disease/myocardial injury
- Transient mitral regurgitation
- Hypotension
- Diaphoresis
- Pulmonary edema or crackles
Diagnostic test results
- New or presumably new tran-sient ST deviation (> 0.5 mm) or T-wave inversion (> 2 mm) with symptoms
- Elevated cardiac troponin I or troponin T
- Elevated creatine phosphoki-nase with muscle/brain sub-units (CPK-MB)

Intermediate Probability of Ischemic Heart Disease
None of the high likelihood find-ings and any of the following clinical findings
- Chief symptom of chest or left arm pain
- Age > 70 years
- Male
- Diabetes
- Extracardiac vascular disease
Diagnostic test results
- Fixed Q waves
- Abnormal ST segments or T waves that are not new
- Normal cardiac markers

Low Probability of Ischemic Heart Disease
Clinical findings
- Probable ischemic symptoms
- Recent cocaine use
- Chest pain reproduced by pal-pation
Diagnostic test results
- Normal electrocardiogram or T-wave flattening, or T-wave inversion in leads with domi-nant R waves
- Normal cardiac markers

Note. Based on information from American Heart Association, 2016; Amsterdam et al., 2014; Chang et al., 2018; D'souza, 2019; Tomaszewski et al., 2018.

F. Physical examination
   1. Vital signs
      a) Heart rate: Varies, as location of MI may cause bradycardia, tachycardia, or irregular rhythms
         (1) Persistent tachycardia is a particularly poor prognostic sign.
         (2) Right coronary artery occlusion causes bradycardia.
      b) Blood pressure: Normotensive when cardiac output is not severely compromised
         (1) In patients with acute infarction, blood pressure may be elevated.
         (2) Progressive hypotension, particularly with a narrow pulse pressure (less than 30 mm Hg), is a sign of severely compromised cardiac output with catecholamine-induced vasoconstriction.
         (3) Measure blood pressure in both arms to evaluate the possibility of aortic dissection or SVC syndrome.
      c) Tachypnea: Occurs as a result of reduced cardiac function and decreased cardiac output
      d) Low-grade fevers: Often present, representing an inflammatory response to tissue ischemia and injury
   2. Cardiac
      a) Auscultation of heart sounds: May be normal
         (1) Split S_1: Often normal, but split S_2 usually indicative of papillary muscle rupture
         (2) S_3 gallop: May be present in CHF
         (3) S_4 gallop: Often present, indicating an extensive anterior MI
      b) Irregular rhythm: May indicate ventricular ectopy
      c) Blowing systolic murmur: Indicative of mitral regurgitation and often present in an extensive anterior MI
      d) Holosystolic murmur: Often heard with inferior MI with papillary muscle rupture
      e) Pericardial friction rub: Heard as early as 24 hours after MI but usually 48–72 hours after MI; late onset (10–14 days after MI) usually indicative of Dressler syndrome (post-MI pericarditis)
      f) JVD: Considered positive at greater than 2 cm above the clavicle when patient is in 30° upright position, indicating right heart failure
      g) Pulses: Point of maximal impulse at heart apex but may be shifted laterally from left midclavicular line or below fifth intercostal space as a result of cardiomegaly dyskinesia
         (1) Peripheral pulses may be weaker. Weak, but bilaterally equal pulses indicate decreased cardiac output.
         (2) Pulsus alternans (alternating one strong, one weak) indicates high thoracic pressure or pericardial effusion.
         (3) Pulsus paradoxus (systolic decreases with inspiration) indicates high thoracic pressure, pericardial effusion, or tamponade (see Appendix D).
         (4) Weak, thready pulses indicate myocardial dysfunction with poor contractility.
      h) Lift or thrill may be palpable with severe murmurs. Large area of dyskinetic myocardium may cause systolic bulge along the left sternal border.
   3. Integumentary: Pallor or cyanosis, coolness, clamminess, or capillary refill less than three seconds indicative of inadequate peripheral tissue perfusion
   4. Pulmonary: May have shallow but equal respirations or labored respirations with nasal flaring and use of sternocleidomastoid muscles

     a) End-inspiratory fine crackles are characteristic of left ventricular dysfunction. Location of fine crackles correlates with the severity of the left ventricular dysfunction (e.g., further up in lung fields, more severe).

     b) Coarser crackles or wheezes may be present with pulmonary edema.

  5. Neurologic: Possible impaired mentation from poor perfusion

  6. Abdominal: Commonly manifests abnormalities, as blood shunts away from this system during acute MI and results in decreased bowel sounds

     a) Mesenteric ischemia-related abdominal pain is severe, diffuse, and not exacerbated by palpation.

     b) Rebound tenderness indicates bowel infarction.

     c) Right upper quadrant discomfort and hepatomegaly may be present and indicate congestive failure. It is prevalent after a severe hypotensive episode.

IV. Diagnostic tests (Alquézar-Arbé et al., 2018; AHA, 2016; Amsterdam et al., 2014; Aydin et al., 2019; Carey, 2016; Carr, 2019; Chang et al., 2018; Chen et al., 2019; Hof & von Eckardstein, 2019; Lippi & Sanchis-Gomar, 2018; Lyngbakken et al., 2019; Moore et al., 2019; Tomaszewski et al., 2018; Vaz et al., 2019; Vogel et al., 2019; Zelfani et al., 2019)

  A. Laboratory

    1. CBC to assess for anemia

    2. Cardiac markers (serum) (see Table 49-2)

    3. Creatine phosphokinase total greater than 115: Marks cardiac muscle death

TABLE 49–2 **Serum Cardiac Markers Indicative of Acute Coronary Syndromes**

Enzyme	Onset	Peak	Return to Normal	Normal or Significant Value[a]	Comments
Cardiac troponin I	3–6 hours	2–4 days	4–9 days	Significant > 300 mcg/ml	Most common, used routinely
Creatine phosphokinase (CPK)	4–6 hours	24 hours	2–3 days	Normal < 100 mcg/ml	–
Creatine phosphokinase myocardial band (CPK-MB)	4–6 hours	12–30 hours	2–3 days	Significant[b] > 10% of total	–
Highly sensitive cardiac troponin (HScTN)	30–90 mins	1–2 hours	2–3 days	Significant > 6 ng/L	False-positive results common and overestimate possibility of myocardial infarction
Lactate dehydrogenase (LDH)	8–12 hours	2–4 days	7–10 days	Normal 150–300 U/ml	–
LDH-1	6–24 hours	3–4 days	3–4 days	Significant > 30%–35% of total	–
Serum glutamic-oxaloacetic transaminase (SGOT)	8–12 hours	3–6 days	3–6 days	Normal 8–40 U/ml	–

[a] Laboratory units of measurement and normal values vary among institutions.
[b] Significant value for abnormal exists.

Note. Based on information from Alquézar-Arbé et al., 2018; American Heart Association, 2016; Amsterdam et al., 2014; Aydin et al., 2019; Chen et al., 2019; Lippi & Sanchis-Gomar, 2018; Lyngbakken et al., 2019.

4. Creatine phosphokinase with muscle/brain subunits (CPK-MB) (isoenzymes (greater than 5% of total CPK significant for MI): Specific for MI
5. Biomarkers that may be used to identify prognostic outcomes
   a) N-terminal prohormone BNP: Increased in ventricular overload or heart failure
   b) Homocysteine: Increased in cardiac disease
   c) CRP (inflammatory marker)
   d) Clinical conditions that may cause elevated biomarkers in the absence of MI: Atrial fibrillation, chronic renal failure, heart failure, hypovolemic stress
6. Chemistry to evaluate electrolytes and renal status
B. Radiology
   1. CT angiography of the heart: Used to verify noncardiogenic origin
   2. Nuclear and tomographic imaging
      a) Imaging may detect abnormal function when ECG is inconclusive and enzyme levels have returned to normal.
      b) Nuclear scans may be abnormal after any radiation to the heart region and may not be useful when symptoms of MI require evaluation.
   3. Cardiac MRI
      a) Imaging provides information to differentiate between reversible ischemia and permanent necrosis.
      b) It can identify left ventricular thrombus, which may occur with primary coronary intervention or in approximately 6% of large anterior MI.
C. Other
   1. ECG: See Table 49-3 for typical ischemia, injury, and prior infarct changes; see Table 49-1 for lead and location of infarct.
      a) More than one-half of patients with chest pain of probable coronary etiology do not have typical changes on ECG.
      b) Rhythm analysis in the frontal plane will show clear evidence of ST changes on the anterior heart but may miss lateral, inferior, or posterior injury. Sig-

TABLE 49-3	Electrocardiogram Changes of Ischemia, Injury, and Prior Injury	
Change	**Onset**	**Resolution**
Infarction		
T-wave elevation	Very early	Several hours
T-wave inversion	Within 1–2 hours	Several days to weeks (may be permanent)
ST-segment elevation and T wave	Within 1–2 hours	Several hours to days
Q wave	3 hours to several days	Permanent
Reversible Injury		
ST segment elevation	Within 1–2 hours	2–3 days (persistent elevation may indicate left ventricular aneurysm)
Reversible Ischemia		
T-wave inversion or flat, depressed T wave	With stress	Return to baseline with rest or medication (nitroglycerin)

Note. Based on information from American Heart Association, 2016; Amsterdam et al., 2014; Carey, 2016; Vogel et al., 2019.

nal-averaged cardiac monitoring helps to eliminate artifact and enhance accuracy of alarms.

 c) ECG changes that show ST elevations of 0.5 mm are considered potentially significant for ischemia or injury.

 d) Twelve-lead ECG shows ischemia and injury in a transmural MI of the left ventricle but may miss a significant right ventricular infarction. Right V_4 lead is most sensitive for right ventricular infarction.

 e) Continuous cardiac monitoring during diagnostic evaluation is routinely performed to assess for ischemic changes (ST segment monitoring) and dysrhythmias that occur with myocardial ischemia or injury.

2. Cardiac catheterization: It is the gold standard of diagnosis. If this technology is immediately available and the patient is stable, perform as an immediate diagnostic and therapeutic treatment modality.

 a) Catheterization permits immediate access to potentially reopen the vessel with angioplasty, coronary stent, or laser therapy.

 b) Suspicious symptoms based on patient presentation warrant proceeding with catheterization.

3. Echocardiogram

 a) Ejection fraction less than 40% after MI predicts for dysrhythmias and heart failure.

 b) It is not sensitive for stress- or exercise-induced cardiac ischemia and hypokinesis.

4. Exercise stress testing

 a) Testing is used for postinfarction follow-up to assess tolerance of exercise.

 b) It can differentiate high-risk angina from controlled or low-risk angina.

V. Differential diagnosis (Amsterdam et al., 2014; Bajaj et al., 2018; Diaz et al., 2019; Howard et al., 2019; Long & Koyfman, 2019; Uchida et al., 2018; Xiong et al., 2017; Zelfani et al., 2019)

A. Cardiac

1. Angina (see Chapter 40)
2. Aortic dissection/expanding aortic aneurysm
3. Cardiac contusion
4. Pericardial effusion/tamponade (see Chapter 50)
5. Dysrhythmia (see Chapter 45)
6. Endocarditis (see Chapter 46), pericarditis (see Chapter 50)
7. Myocarditis from infectious sources or immune therapies: Cytokines (e.g., IFN, IL), monoclonal antibodies (e.g., rituximab, cetuximab), antiangiogenic agents (e.g., bevacizumab), and checkpoint inhibitors (e.g., ipilimumab, nivolumab, pembrolizumab, avelumab, cemiplimab, durvalumab, atezolizumab)
8. SVC syndrome
9. Cardiac metastases of cancer
10. Hypercoagulability with subsequent coronary thrombus (see Chapter 122)
11. Cardiac valve disorder: Mitral valve prolapse, mitral regurgitation
12. Coronary spasm (Kounis syndrome): Antimicrobials (e.g., cefuroxime), antineoplastics (e.g., 5-fluorouracil)
13. Adrenergic surge: Pheochromocytoma

B. Pulmonary

1. Mediastinal diseases: Lung masses, carcinoid tumor, PE (see Chapter 33)
2. Pneumonia: Pleuritic chest pain (see Chapter 30)

C. GI

     1. Cholecystitis (see Chapter 68)
     2. Esophagitis
     3. Pancreatitis (see Chapter 77)
     4. Peptic ulcer disease (see Chapter 78)
     5. Gastroesophageal reflux/esophageal spasm (Chapter 71)
  D. Other
     1. Pectoral muscle injury or costochondritis
     2. Psychiatric disorders
     3. Sickle cell disease (see Chapter 119)
     4. HZV (see Chapter 22)

VI. Treatment (see Table 49-4; AHA, 2016; Amsterdam et al., 2014; Donisan et al., 2019; Dudzinski et al., 2018; Iliescu et al., 2018; Jneid et al., 2017; Larson et al., 2019; Singh et al., 2018; Skogestad & Aronsen, 2018; Tangvoraphonkchai & Davenport, 2018; Tavenier et al., 2018; Uchida et al., 2018; van der Weg et al., 2019; Vogel et al., 2019)

  A. Prevention: Recognition of risk factors and strategies directed to minimize risks
     1. Patients with more than two risk factors for CAD have their 10-year risk calculated. Patients with greater than 20% risk are screened every three to five years for the prevention of STEMI.
     2. Strategies to prevent risk of cardiovascular disease are implemented as appropriate (e.g., smoking cessation, weight loss).
     3. ASA 81 mg PO daily as prevention for MI has been common practice but has not been conclusively substantiated. Risks and benefits should be considered before implementing this strategy.
     4. Patients with cardiac disease should have a potassium threshold of 4 mEq/L and a magnesium threshold of 2 mEq/L.
     5. Identification of genes predisposing patients to cardiovascular disease permits exploration of high-risk families.
     6. Nutraceuticals have been used for reduction of CAD and risk for MI.

TABLE 49-4	Treatment of Acute Coronary Syndromes	
Treatment	**Rationale**	**Nursing Guidelines**
Interventional Cardiology		
Coronary artery bypass graft surgery	Host vessel or synthetic mesh grafts that replace occluded coronary arteries by circumventing occluded area	Concerns that bypass machine filters enhance hematogenous spread of cancer Requires postoperative anticoagulation
Coronary artery stent	Placement of small synthetic bypass links that permit rechanneling coronary blood flow past the site of small obstructions in easy-to-access areas of the coronary arteries	May be performed with minimally invasive surgery techniques Requires postoperative anticoagulation High reocclusion rate
Intracoronary thrombectomy	Extraction of the intracoronary clot through percutaneous intracoronary intervention	Immediate reversal of occlusive symptoms Can only be performed in large vessel disease

(Continued on next page)

TABLE 49-4	**Treatment of Acute Coronary Syndromes *(Continued)***	
Treatment	**Rationale**	**Nursing Guidelines**
Percutaneous transluminal coronary angioplasty	Opens occluded arteries with local pressure from an expanded balloon at the point of narrowing	Ideally performed immediately and prior to thrombolytic administration Reocclusion during hospitalization not uncommon Requires immediate availability of coronary artery bypass graft in case complications occur
Mechanical Circulatory Assist Devices		
Extracorporeal membrane oxygenation	Cardiac bypass that allows for complete heart rest; used in most severe cardiogenic shock and when short-term support is anticipated	Most effective emergent relief for cardiogenic shock or intractable dysrhythmias Requires expert intensive care unit team, perfusionist management Requires anticoagulation
Intra-aortic balloon pump	Balloon placed in the descending aorta that inflates with diastole, increasing coronary blood and reducing ischemia	Insertion of a large catheter in major artery possibly leads to vascular complications Requires intensive care unit care and expert monitoring of inflation times and effects on cardiac output
Ventricular assist devices	Short-term left or right ventricular assist devices that offer temporary support for the myocardial contraction until ischemia resolves and heart function improves; used when support is expected to exceed a few days or when long-term support or transplant is anticipated	Requires intensive care unit and expert monitoring of pump function Requires operative procedure and may not be performed quickly at the bedside May alter cardiac physiology and require long-term destination therapy or bridge to heart transplant Requires battery back-up and reliable electrical source Requires anticoagulation therapy
Medications		
Glyeoprotein IIb/IIIa platelet inhibitors (eptifibatide, abciximab, tirofiban)	Interferes with platelet membrane function by inhibiting fibrinogen binding, reducing platelet aggregation, and improving coronary stent survival	May inhibit other hematologic cell function (e.g., neutropenia)

Note. Based on information from American Heart Association, 2016; Amsterdam et al., 2014; Larson et al., 2019.

  a) Those with effects similar to calcium channel blockers include *Angelica*, garlic, ginger, *Ginkgo biloba*, grape seed, green tea, hawthorn, magnesium, and olive leaf.
  b) Those with effects similar to beta-blockers include grape seed, green tea, hawthorn, and magnesium.
  c) Coenzyme Q10 120 mg PO daily is thought to decrease the incidence of angina, dysrhythmias, and heart failure; however, its benefit is unproven.
 B. Patient education: Patient, family, and public education on early activation of emergency medical services includes the following.

1. Signs and symptoms of acute coronary syndromes
2. Use of ASA and nitroglycerin as immediate intervention for chest pain
3. Preventive health and lifestyle changes
4. Importance of taking medications as prescribed

C. Evaluation: Timeliness of screening and diagnostic workup is defined by national standards. The duration of ischemia is an independent predictor for postinfarction mortality.
   1. Professional evaluation is recommended within the first 10 minutes of presentation.
   2. Vital signs: Heart rate, respirations, blood pressure should be performed in both arms to rule out other causes.
   3. Oxygen saturation and administration of low-level oxygen for the first six hours after admission for possible MI has been routinely used but lacks definitive evidence for benefit. AHA recommends an oxygen saturation goal of 94%.
   4. IV access should be obtained.
   5. Twelve-lead ECG should be obtained. If not abnormal but symptoms are highly suspicious, it should be performed every 5–15 minutes.
   6. If inferior wall changes are present, right-sided ECG is performed.

D. From the time the patient enters emergency services to administration of reperfusion drug (if indicated) within 30 minutes, ASA, nitrates, platelet inhibitors, and fibrinolytics should be initiated.

E. When interventional cardiology is immediately available, medications may be delayed until cardiac catheterization or percutaneous transvenous coronary angioplasty can be performed (see Table 49-4).

F. Rest: Adequate rest decreases oxygen demand and consumption. Bronchodilator properties may enhance oxygenation.

G. Analgesics (see Appendix F): Reduced pain will decrease oxygen consumption, potentially preserving myocardium.
   1. Morphine sulfate often is used to enhance histamine release and decrease venous tone, causing venodilation and decreased preload, which decrease pulmonary artery pressure.
   2. Adverse effects such as hypotension, respiratory suppression, or reduced absorption of platelet inhibitors should be considered in selecting its use to manage chest pain.

H. Antiplatelet therapy: Indicated in unstable angina or evolving MI
   1. Two baby ASA (81 mg) PO or one adult ASA (325 mg chewable, non–enteric-coated tablet) PO should be administered immediately (even before confirmed diagnosis) to reduce platelet aggregation at occlusion site, preventing worsening ischemia and extension of MI. ASA *must* be chewed for immediate absorption.
   2. Other antiplatelet drugs include ticlopidine, clopidogrel, prasugrel, and ticagrelor, which act late in the clotting process and lessen the risk of reocclusion. Variability in clinical responses suggests that some genetic resistance to specific antiplatelet drugs may exist, so monitoring with stress testing or radiologic examination for reocclusion in the first month is recommended.

I. Thrombolytic therapy: Decreases infarct size, decreases mortality, preserves left ventricular function, and establishes reperfusion and coronary artery patency; used only when intervention reperfusion strategies are not possible
   1. Patient candidate criteria
      a) Chest pain less than six hours in duration; individual institutions may extend to 12 hours; benefit lasts up to 12 hours
      b) ST elevations greater than or equal to 1 mm on ECG in two consecutive leads
   2. Contraindications
      a) Active internal bleeding
      b) Intracranial/intraspinal surgery within prior two months

      c) Intracranial neoplasm or terminal illness

      d) Arteriovenous malformations or aneurysm

      e) Significant closed head/facial trauma within previous three months

      f) Pregnancy

      g) Comorbidities: Jaundice/hepatitis, renal failure, uncontrolled hypertension with systolic greater than 180 mm Hg, diastolic greater than 110 mm Hg, or systolic blood pressure variation between right and left arms greater than 15 mm Hg, severe blood dyscrasias, clotting disorders

      h) Relative contraindications: Surgery within prior 10 days, previous stroke, recent cardiopulmonary resuscitation for greater than 10 minutes, hemorrhagic retinopathy

  3. Intracoronary thrombolytics may be given through angiographic procedures when occluded vessel is visualized on catheterization.

      a) It is usually given via IV when immediate cardiac catheterization is not available, with successful reperfusion seen in 75%–80% of MIs.

      b) Symptoms/signs of myocardial reperfusion in thrombolytic therapy include rapid early rise and peak of enzymes, normalization of ST segment, and immediate relief of chest pain.

      c) Reperfusion dysrhythmias are seen during the first 10–20 minutes and up to two to four hours after administration. In particular, ventricular fibrillation or multifocal ventricular tachycardia is most observed.

J. Nitroglycerin: It is initially administered sublingually. The patient should have adequate salivation to dissolve tablet. It should be used with caution in patients who have received radiation to the head and neck area.

  1. Give 0.4 mcg sublingually every five minutes for three doses.

  2. Contraindications include systolic blood pressure less than 90 mm Hg or greater than 30 mm Hg below baseline, right ventricular infarction, bradycardia (less than 50 bpm), tachycardia (greater than 100 bpm), and phosphodiesterase inhibitor ingested for erectile dysfunction within past 24 hours (48 hours for tadalafil).

  3. Initiate IV nitroglycerin as soon as possible. Titrate to effect unless adverse effects are not tolerated.

      a) Prophylactic dose in patients with relieved chest pain is 10–50 mcg/min.

      b) Therapeutic dose routinely is 1 mcg/kg/min (50–150 mcg/min). No maximum dose exists.

      c) Advanced cardiovascular disease awaiting bypass surgery may require 300–600 mcg/min. It may decrease dose when hypotension occurs.

K. Weight-based heparin therapy: Bolus followed by continuous infusion

L. Beta-blocker: A beta-blocker can decrease myocardial oxygen consumption and decreases catecholamine effects on heart. Beta-1-selective agents are preferred (e.g., metoprolol). If the patient has clear ECG changes and is too hypotensive to tolerate nitrates and beta-blockers, greater benefit can be gained by administering beta-blockers.

  1. Loading dose is given until heart rate is 50–65 bpm. Blood pressure should be monitored. Metoprolol is usually given as a 5 mg IV every five minutes for three doses and then PO.

  2. Maintenance PO or IV bolus doses are given to sustain beta-blockade for four to seven days.

M. Primary coronary interventions are the preferred reperfusion strategy but may be limited in patients who will be unable to take antiplatelet therapy after the procedure.

  1. Interventions include percutaneous transcatheter arteriography with coronary stent balloon angioplasty or thrombectomy.

2. Left heart catheterization is required with intracoronary thrombolytic given concomitantly whenever possible followed by heparin infusion.
   a) It is indicated as immediate intervention if key clinical findings are present, such as heart rate greater than 100 bpm and systolic blood pressure less than 100 mm Hg or pulmonary edema (crackles) or signs of shock (cool and clammy).
   b) It usually requires long-term glycoprotein IIb/IIIa inhibitors, which increases risk of bleeding.
   c) Arterial line sheath usually is left in place for 8–34 hours in case repeat angiography is required.
   d) Interventions may include placement of coronary stents, balloon angioplasty, intracoronary thrombolytics, or thrombectomy.

N. Coronary artery bypass graft surgery: Indicated for refractory ischemia or when percutaneous transluminal coronary angioplasty has been unsuccessful

O. Unique treatment for right ventricular infarction
   1. Fluid loading: Up to 10 liters to achieve adequate preload volume
   2. Diuresis: May be required after the infarction is complete
   3. Atropine: 0.5 mg IV for symptomatic bradycardia
   4. Transcutaneous pacing: Early if atropine does not work

P. Long-term cardiovascular health to prevent recurrent MI
   1. Antiplatelet therapy
   2. Statins and niacin to enhance HDL cholesterol and lower LDL cholesterol
   3. Vitamin D to maintain high normal

Q. Management of complications of MI: Dysrhythmia, cardiogenic shock (high death rate), CHF, hypoxemia, bleeding secondary to antiplatelet/thrombolytic therapy, renal failure

R. Reperfusion dysrhythmias are common in first day after definitive coronary interventions.

S. Bleeding risks are associated with thrombocytopenia among patients with cancer, but evidence-based literature suggests no greater mortality or morbidity.

T. Long-term mechanical cardiovascular support may be achieved with left ventricular assist devices (LVADs), right ventricular assist devices (RVADs), and biventricular assist devices (BiVADs).
   1. Treated as bridge to transplant or destination therapy; heart transplant contraindicated
   2. Requires anticoagulation

VII. Follow-up (Amsterdam et al., 2014; Howard et al., 2019; Larson et al., 2019; Park et al., 2018)
   A. Frequent follow-up should be scheduled with a cardiologist in the first three months after MI to monitor for early postinfarction complications (e.g., dysrhythmias, pericarditis, heart failure, post-MI syndrome).
   B. Serial physical examination, 12-lead ECG, and exercise stress test should be performed annually.
   C. Therapeutic drug monitoring is required every three to four months after stabilization of dose for antidysrhythmics or anticoagulants.
      1. Anticoagulants: Coagulation profile usually every two to four weeks until stable, then every four to six months
      2. Antidysrhythmics: CBC every six months; rarely induces aplastic anemia
      3. Lipid-lowering drugs: LFTs at one month initially, then every six months
      4. Beta-blockers: Every 6–12 months to evaluate glucose intolerance
   D. Preventive health visits should be scheduled to assess adherence to lifestyle modifications.

VIII. Referrals (Chang et al., 2018; D'souza, 2019; Kirolos et al., 2019)
  A. Electrophysiologist: If refractory dysrhythmia is present
  B. Dietitian: To advise patients how to alter risk factors (e.g., obesity, hyperlipidemia)
  C. Mental health professional: To address difficulties with coping, depression, or behavior and lifestyle modification
  D. Genetic counselor: For families with high risk for cardiovascular disease
  E. Preventive cardiologist: May consult for risk factor analysis and modification; follow-up screening based on cancer treatment risk profile
  F. Cardiac rehabilitation: To ensure gradual return to ADLs while monitoring limitations from cardiovascular disease
    1. Effective recommendation (class I) from AHA and American College of Cardiology in treatment of patients with CAD
    2. Includes physical and psychological support and monitoring

References

Abbott, T.E.F., Pearse, R.M., Cuthbertson, B.H., Wijeysundera, D.N., & Ackland, G.L. (2019). Cardiac vagal dysfunction and myocardial injury after non-cardiac surgery: A planned secondary analysis of the measurement of exercise tolerance before surgery. *British Journal of Anaesthesia, 122*(2), 188–197. https://doi.org/10.1016/j.bja.2018.10.060

Alquézar-Arbé, A., Sanchís, J., Guillén, E., Bardají, A., Miró, Ò., & Ordóñez-Llanos, J. (2018). Cardiac troponin measurement and interpretation in the diagnosis of acute myocardial infarction in the emergency department: A consensus statement. *Emergencias, 30*(5), 336–349.

American Heart Association. (2016). *Advanced cardiovascular life support: Provider manual* (16th ed.). Author.

Amsterdam, E.A., Wenger, N.K., Brindis, R.G., Casey, D.E., Jr., Ganiats, T.G., Holmes, D.R., Jr., … Zieman, S.J. (2014). 2014 AHA/ACC guideline for the management of patients with non–ST-elevation acute coronary syndromes: A report of the American College of Cardiology/American Heart Association task force on practice guidelines. *Circulation, 130*(25), e344–e426. https://doi.org/10.1161/CIR.0000000000000134

Aydin, S., Ugur, K., Aydin, S., Sahin, İ., & Yardim, M. (2019). Biomarkers in acute myocardial infarction: Current perspectives. *Vascular Health and Risk Management, 15,* 1–10. https://doi.org/10.2147/VHRM.S166157

Bajaj, R., Jain, A.K., & Knight, C. (2018). Definitions of acute coronary syndromes. *Medicine, 46*(9), 528–532. https://doi.org/10.1016/j.mpmed.2018.06.006

Bejik, M.A., Vlastra, W.V., Delewi, R., van de Hoef, T.P., Boekholdt, S.M., Siauw, K.D., & Piek, J.J. (2019). Myocardial infarction with non-obstructive coronary arteries: A focus on vasospastic angina. *Netherlands Heart Journal, 27*(5), 237–245. https://doi.org/10.1007/s12471-019-1232-7

Carey, M.G. (2016). Acute coronary syndrome and ST segment monitoring. *Critical Care Nursing Clinics of North America, 28*(3), 347–355. https://doi.org/10.1016/j.cnc.2016.04.006

Carr, J.J. (2019). Calcium scoring for cardiovascular computed tomography: How, when and why? *Radiologic Clinics of North America, 57*(1), 1–12. https://doi.org/10.1016/j.rcl.2018.09.002

Chang, A.M., Fischman, D.L., & Hollander, J.E. (2018). Evaluation of chest pain and acute coronary syndromes. *Circulation, 36*(1), 1–12. https://doi.org/10.1016/j.ccl.2017.08.001

Chen, Y., Tao, Y., Zhang, L., Xu, W., & Zhou, X. (2019). Diagnostic and prognostic value of biomarkers in acute myocardial infarction. *Postgraduate Medical Journal, 95*(1122), 210–216. https://doi.org/10.1136/postgradmedj-2019-136409

DeVon, H.A., Vukovic, K., Ryan, C.J., Barnason, S., Zerwic, J.J., Pozehl, B., … Zimmerman, L. (2017). Systematic review of symptom clusters in cardiovascular disease. *Journal of Cardiovascular Nursing, 16*(1), 6–17. https://doi.org/10.1177/1474515116642594

Diaz, B., Elkbuli, A., Ehrhardt, J.D., Jr., McKenney, M., Boneva, D., & Hai, S. (2019). Pheochromocytoma-related cardiomyopathy presenting as broken heart syndrome: Case report and literature review. *International Journal of Surgery Case Reports, 55,* 7–10. https://doi.org/10.1016/j.ijscr.2018.12.003

Donisan, T., Balanescu, D.V., Palaskas, N., Lopez-Mattei, J., Karimzad, K., Kim, P., … Iliescu, C. (2019). Cardiac interventional procedures in cardio-oncology patients. *Cardiology Clinics, 37*(4), 469–486. https://doi.org/10.1016/j.ccl.2019.07.012

D'souza, E. (2019). An overview and awareness of acute coronary syndrome based on risk factors, early clinical assessment tools, and improving clinical outcomes. *Journal of Doctoral Nursing Practice, 12*(1), 125–130. https://doi.org/10.1891/2380-9418.12.1.125

Dudzinski, J.E., Gnall, E., & Kowey, P.R. (2018). A review of percutaneous mechanical support devices and strategies. *Reviews in Cardiovascular Medicine, 19*(1), 21–26. https://doi.org/10.31083/j.rcm.2018.01.904

Filippo, C., & Libby, P. (2017). Acute coronary syndromes: The way forward from mechanisms to precision treatment. *Circulation, 136*(12), 1155–1166. https://doi.org/10.1161/CIRCULATIONAHA.117.029870

Hof, D., & von Eckardstein, A. (2019). High-sensitivity troponin assays in clinical diagnostics of acute coronary syndrome. In C.W. Heizman (Ed.), *Methods of molecular biology: Vol. 1929. Calcium-binding proteins of the EF-hand superfamily: From basics to medical applications* (pp. 645–662). Springer. https://doi.org/10.1007/978-1-4939-9030-6_40

Howard, E., Steingart, M.R., Armstrong, G.T., Lyon, A.R., Armenian, S.H., Voso, M.T., ... Minotti, G. (2019). Cardiovascular events in cancer survivors. *Seminars in Oncology, 46*(6), 426–432. https://doi.org/10.1053/j.seminoncol.2019.01.007

Iliescu, C., Balanescu, D.V., Donisan, T., Giza, D.E., Muñoz Gonzalez, E.D., Cilingiroglu, M., ... Marmagkiolis, K. (2018). Safety of diagnostic and therapeutic cardiac catheterization in cancer patients with acute coronary syndrome and chronic thrombocytopenia. *American Journal of Cardiology, 122*(9), 1465–1470. https://doi.org/10.1016/j.amjcard.2018.07.033

Jneid, H., Addison, D., Bhatt, D.L., Fonarow, G.C., Godak, S., Grady, K.L., ... Pancholy, S. (2017). 2017 AHA/ACC clinical performance and quality measures for adults with ST-elevation and non–ST-elevation myocardial infarction. *Journal of the American College of Cardiology, 70*(16), 2048–2090. https://doi.org/10.1016/j.jacc.2017.06.032

Kirolos, I., Yakoub, D., Pendola, F., Picado, O., Kirolos, A., Levine, Y.C., ... Khouzam, R.N. (2019). Cardiac physiology in post myocardial infarction patients: The effect of cardiac rehabilitation programs—A systematic review and update meta-analysis. *Annals of Translational Medicine, 7*(17), 416. https://doi.org/10.21037/atm.2019.08.64

Larson, E.A., German, D.M., Shatzel, J., & DeLoughery, T.G. (2019). Anticoagulation in the cardiac patient: A concise review. *European Journal of Haematology, 102*(1), 3–19. https://doi.org/10.1111/ejh.13171

Lippi, G., & Sanchis-Gomar, F. (2018). "Ultra-sensitive" cardiac troponins: Requirements for effective implementation in clinical practice. *Biochemia Medica, 28*(3), 030501 https://doi.org/10.11613/BM.2018.030501

Long, B., & Koyfman, A. (2019). Infectious endocarditis: An update for emergency clinicians. *American Journal of Emergency Medicine, 36*(9), 1686–1692. https://doi.org/10.1016/j.ajem.2018.06.074

Lyngbakken, M.N., Myhre, P.L., Røsjø, H., & Omland, T. (2019). Novel biomarkers of cardiovascular disease: Applications in clinical practice. *Critical Reviews in Clinical Laboratory Sciences, 56*(1), 33–60. https://doi.org/10.1080/10408363.2018.1525335

Manolis, A.S., Manolis, A.A., Manolis, T.A., & Melita, H. (2018). Acute coronary syndromes in patients with angiographically normal or near normal (non-obstructive) coronary arteries. *Trends in Cardiovascular Medicine, 28*(8), 541–551. https://doi.org/10.1016/j.tcm.2018.05.006

Moore, A., Georne, H., Rajiah, P., Tanabe, Y., Saboo, S., & Abbara, S. (2019). Acute myocardial infarct. *Radiologic Clinics of North America, 57*(1), 45–55. https://doi.org/10.1016/j.rcl.2018.08.006

Park, J.Y., Guo, W., Al-Hijji, M., El Sabbagh, A., Begna, K.H., Haberman, T.M., ... Herrmann, J. (2018). Acute coronary syndromes in patients with active hematologic malignancies—Incidence, management, and outcomes. *International Journal of Cardiology, 275*, 6–12. https://doi.org/10.1016/j.ijcard.2018.10.008

Singh, R.B., Fedacko, J., Mojto, V., & Pella, D. (2018). Coenzyme Q10 modulates remodeling possibly by decreasing angiotensin-converting enzyme in patients with acute coronary syndrome. *Antioxidants, 7*(8), 99. https://doi.org/10.3390/antiox7080099

Skogestad, J., & Aronsen, J.M. (2018). Hypokalemia-induced arrhythmias and heart failure: new insights and implications for therapy. *Frontiers in Physiology, 9,* 1500. https://doi.org/10.3389/fphys.2018.01500

Suh, K.J., Lee, J.Y., Shin, D.-Y., Koh, Y., Bang, S.-M., Yoon, S.-S., ... Lee, J.-O. (2017). Analysis of adverse events associated with dasatinib and nilotinib treatments in chronic-phase chronic myeloid leukemia patients outside clinical trials. *International Journal of Hematology, 106*(2), 229–239. https://doi.org/10.1007/s12185-017-2225-1

Tangvoraphonkchai, K., & Davenport, A. (2018). Magnesium and cardiovascular disease. *Advances in Chronic Kidney Disease, 25*(3), 251–260. https://doi.org/10.1053/j.ackd.2018.02.010

Tavenier, A.H., Hermanides, R.S., Ottervanger, J.P., Ter Horst, P.G.J., Kedhi, E., & van 't Hof, A.W.J. (2018). Risks of opioids in ST-elevation myocardial infarction: A review. *Drug Safety, 41*(12), 1303–1308. https://doi.org/10.1007/s40264-018-0710-y

Tomaszewski, C.A., Nestler, D., Shah, K.H., Sudhir, A., & Brown, M.D. (2018). Clinical policy: Critical issues in the evaluation and management of emergency department patients with suspected non–ST-elevation acute coronary syndromes. *Annals of Emergency Medicine, 72*(5), e65–e106. https://doi.org/10.1016/j.annemergmed.2018.07.045

Uchida, K., Karube, N., Minami, T., Cho, T., Matsuki, Y., Nemoto, H., ... Masuda, M. (2018). Treatment of coronary malperfusion in type A acute aortic dissection. *General Thoracic and Cardiovascular Surgery, 66*(11), 621–625. https://doi.org/10.1007/s11748-018-1014-y

van der Weg, K., Prinzen, F.W., & Gorgels, A.P.M. (2019). Editor's choice—Reperfusion cardiac arrhythmias and their relation to reperfusion-induced cell death. *European Heart Journal: Acute Cardiovascular Care, 8*(2), 142–152. https://doi.org/10.1177/2048872618812148

Vaz, H.A., Guimaraes, R.B., & Dutra, O. (2019). Challenges in high-sensitive troponin assay interpretation for intensive therapy. *Revista Brasileira de Terapia Intensiva, 31*(1), 93–105. https://doi.org/10.5935/0103-507X.20190001

Vicent, L., Velásquez-Rodríguez, J., Valero-Masa, M.J., Díez-Delhovo, F., González-Saldívar, H., Bruña, V., ... Martínez-Sellés, M. (2017). Predictors of high Killip class after ST segment elevation myocardial infarction in the era of primary reperfusion. *International Journal of Cardiology, 248,* 46–50. https://doi.org/10.1016/j.ijcard.2017.07.038

Vogel, B., Claessen, B.E., Arnold, S.V., Chan, D., Cohen, D.J., Giannitsis, E., ... Mehran, R. (2019). ST-segment elevation myocardial infarction. *Nature Reviews Disease Primers, 5*(1), 39. https://doi.org/10.1038/s41572-019-0090-3

Xiong, N., Gao, W., Pan, J., Luo, X., Shi, H., & Li, J. (2017). Essential thrombocythemia presenting as acute coronary syndrome: Case reports and literature review. *Journal of Thrombosis and Thrombolysis, 44*(1), 57–62. https://doi.org/10.1007/s11239-017-1490-4

Zelfani, S., Manai, H., Laabidi, S., Wahabi, A., Akeri, S., & Daghfous, M. (2019). Pulmonary embolism mimicking acute myocardial infarction: A case report and review of literature. *Pan African Medical Journal, 33,* 275. https://doi.org/10.11604/pamj.2019.33.275.18517

Pericarditis/Pericardial Effusion/Pericardial Tamponade

Brenda K. Shelton, DNP, APRN–CNS, RN, CCRN, AOCN®

I. Definition: Three terms used to describe the clinical conditions of diminished pericardial stretch and increased pericardial pressure—pericarditis, pericardial effusion, and pericardial tamponade; may represent three separate entities or progression of a single pericardial disorder (Azarbal & LeWinter, 2017; Yusuf et al., 2016)

A. Pericarditis is inflammation of the lining surrounding the heart. It is termed *pericarditis* when inflammation is present but is termed *constrictive pericarditis* when fibrous bands restrict cardiac movement.

B. Pericardial effusion involves purulent, bloody, or malignant fluid accumulation within the pericardial sac.

C. Pericardial tamponade (cardiac tamponade) is fluid accumulation in the pericardial sac that is so great that normal filling and contraction or ejection capabilities fail.

D. Perimyocarditis is inflammation of the pericardial layer and myocardium characterized by elevations of cardiac troponins in addition to other symptoms.

II. Physiology/Pathophysiology (Azarbal & LeWinter, 2017; Honasoge & Dubbs, 2018; Murillo et al., 2016)

A. Normal

1. The intrapericardial pressure is subatmospheric (negative), which allows the return inflow of low-pressure venous blood into the right side of the heart.

2. The pericardium is a double-membrane fibrous sac that encloses the heart and the great blood vessels.

3. It is composed of an inner layer (epicardium) and outer fibrous layer (parietal pericardium).

4. The space between the two constitutes the pericardial cavity, which is filled with a small amount of serous fluid.

B. Pathophysiology: When the pericardium is constricted by fibrous bands or filled with fluid, the pressure in the pericardial sac is raised to a level that exceeds the normal filling pressure of the ventricle (see Table 50-1).

1. Initially, the primary pathophysiology is venous congestion caused by back pressure from compromised venous return of blood to the heart.

2. Later, when ventricular filling is more severely restricted, contraction capabilities fail. Then the disorder is characterized by symptoms of left ventricular failure.

TABLE 50-1	Etiologies of Pericardial Disease
Pathophysiologic Mechanism	**Examples of Etiologies**
Capillary permeability–induced fluid extravasation into the pericardium	Autoimmune disorders Hematologic malignancies Inflammatory cytokines given as anticancer therapy (e.g., interleukin-2, tumor necrosis factor) Medications causing endothelial damage (e.g., cytosine arabinoside), alkylating agents (e.g., busulfan, cyclophosphamide), retinoic acid syndrome Severe hypoalbuminemia White blood cell hematopoietic growth factors
Hemorrhage/fluid extravasation into the pericardium	Antiangiogenesis agents (e.g., bevacizumab) Chemotherapy-induced cardiomyopathy (e.g., cyclophosphamide) Displaced central venous catheter Post–cardiac surgery Post-viral syndrome: Epstein-Barr virus, human parvovirus, BK virus Renal failure (high incidence of progression to tamponade) Severe thrombocytopenia Traumatic injury (e.g., motor vehicle accident)
Malignant involvement	Breast cancer, especially infiltrating ductal carcinoma Endometrial/uterine cancer Head and neck cancer Hodgkin and non-Hodgkin lymphoma, especially primary effusion lymphoma (human herpes virus 6 or 8 related), HIV lymphoma, natural killer/T-cell or T-cell lymphoma subtypes Mesothelioma Multiple myeloma Non-small cell lung cancers, especially bronchogenic adenocarcinoma or anaplastic lymphoma kinase–positive tumors, and small cell lung cancer Ovarian cancer Pancreatic cancer Pheochromocytoma Prostate cancer Sarcomas (e.g., angiosarcoma, osteosarcoma) Thymic cancer
Pericardial inflammation with exudative fluid response	Immune antineoplastic therapies (e.g., cytokines, immune checkpoint inhibitors) Infectious disorders Myocardial injury Radiation exposure Renal failure (e.g., uric acid–related inflammation)
Severe chest venous congestion and obstruction of normal lymphatic fluid removal	Cardiomyopathy Esophageal cancer Lymphadenopathy disorders (e.g., HIV, hemophagocytic lymphohistiocytosis, chest lymphoma) Lymphangioleiomyomatosis Myocardial injury Myxedema/hypothyroidism Thoracic lymphatic duct obstruction from pulmonary infection or pulmonary tumor Thymic cancer

(Continued on next page)

TABLE 50-1	Etiologies of Pericardial Disease *(Continued)*
Pathophysiologic Mechanism	**Examples of Etiologies**
Unknown mechanism	Certain medications, including bortezomib, *BRC-ABL* inhibitors (e.g., imatinib), docetaxel/paclitaxel, multikinase inhibitors (e.g., sunitinib) Extramedullary hematopoiesis with leukemia or multiple myeloma Graft-versus-host disease

Note. Based on information from Azarbal & LeWinter, 2017; Colak et al., 2019; Niska et al., 2018; Raghunathan et al., 2017.

III. Clinical features: Approximately 10%–30% of patients with cancer experience some variation of this pericardial disorder during the course of illness, although the severity and reversibility vary. Small numbers of patients with pericardial effusion develop constrictive pericarditis. Incidence is overestimated in autopsy studies because evidence of effusion in late cancer may be common but not clinically significant, considering less than 1% with pericardial effusions at death had experienced clinical symptoms. Average survival after diagnosis of pericardial effusion, unless at the time of the initial cancer diagnosis, is four to six months (Azarbal & LeWinter, 2017; Carneiro et al., 2017; Colak et al., 2019; Imazio et al., 2015; Kalogeraki et al., 2016; Murillo et al., 2016; Niska et al., 2018; Oyakawa et al., 2018; Raghunathan et al., 2017; Yusuf et al., 2016).

A. Classifications of pericardial effusion
    1. Transudative effusions are the result of abnormal capillary permeability, LDH less than 200 U/L, protein less than 35 g/L, fluid-to-serum LDH ratio less than 0.6, and protein ratio less than 0.5. It is indicative of excessive fluid accumulation in nonmalignant conditions or lymphatic obstruction.
    2. Exudative effusions occur when an inflammatory stimulus is present and are characterized by LDH greater than 200 U/L, protein greater than 35 g/L, fluid-to-serum LDH ratio greater than 0.6, and fluid-to-protein ratio greater than 0.3. It is indicative of malignant or infectious process within the pericardium.

B. Risk factors (see Table 50-1)
    1. Malignancy involving the chest: It is the most common cause and occurs from spread to the pericardium and is associated with higher incidence of slow-developing tamponade.
    2. Thoracic lymphatic obstruction
    3. Radiation of 3,000–3,500 cGy to greater than 33%–42% of the heart region or fraction sizes greater than 300 cGy daily: Radiation pericarditis occurs in a small number of patients, and most develop a pericardial effusion.
    4. Chemotherapy (usually high dose) or immunotherapy agents that cause capillary permeability
    5. Infections that are prone to create large masses or lymphadenopathy, especially if occurring in the chest
    6. Medical conditions enhancing capillary permeability or fluid extravasation
    7. Catheter-infused fluid extravasation into the pericardial space: Rare but possible consequence from insertion of ventricular assist device, SVC stenting, or a displaced pleuropericardial shunt
    8. Acute vascular crises: Aortic dissection (related to trauma, aortic aneurysm), post–cardiac surgery bleeding, post–interventional cardiology procedures (e.g., insertion of pacemaker, flutter ablation)

C. Etiology (see Table 50-1)
    1. Most common causes of pericardial diseases in patients with cancer are drug- or treatment-induced capillary permeability and malignant cell invasion of the pericardium.

2. Exact etiology is often unknown, and in patients without cancer, infection is the most common cause. Fluid collection related to infection may be purulent and harbor infective organisms, or it may be serous and related to the inflammatory response of the pericardium.

D. History
1. History of cancer and cancer treatment that predispose to this complication
2. Current medications: Prescribed, over the counter (e.g., anticoagulants, hydralazine, penicillins, thrombolytics)
3. History of presenting symptoms: Precipitating factors, onset, location, duration
4. Changes in ADLs: Activity intolerance or profound fatigue
5. Past medical history: Infectious disease exposures, autoimmune or inflammatory disorders, idiopathic edema or fluid retention, chest injury (e.g., motor vehicular collision with steering wheel injury, blunt chest trauma)
6. Past surgical history: Aortic aneurysm repair, cardiac surgery

E. Signs and symptoms: Table 50-2 compares and contrasts key symptoms with each disorder.
1. The severity of signs and symptoms often reflects the chronicity of the problem.
   a) Rapidly developing effusions may present symptomatically with as little as 50–80 ml of fluid accumulation.
   b) In slowly developing effusions, the pericardium can stretch to accommodate the excess fluid, thus compensating for reduced cardiac output; symptoms may not present until greater than 1,000 ml of fluid has accumulated.
2. The common symptom reported by patients with malignancy-related pericardial disease is dyspnea.
3. For unexplained reasons, excessive yawning or hiccups have been associated with pericardial effusion.
4. Large pericardial effusions can compress the esophagus and cause dysphagia or hoarseness.

F. Physical examination: Table 50-3 compares and contrasts key findings with each disorder. Focus on cardiac examination.

TABLE 50-2 Symptoms of Pericarditis, Pericardial Effusion, and Pericardial Tamponade

Symptom	Pericarditis	Pericardial Effusion	Pericardial Tamponade
Chest pain	Severe, sharp, and localized Exacerbated by movement, deep breathing, or lying flat May be relieved, in part, by sitting up and leaning forward	Dull and diffuse Less positional	More often described as chest "heaviness" or absent
Cough	Not present	From congestive heart failure Characterized by pulmonary congestion	Severity depends on degree of left ventricular failure
Dyspnea	Mild to moderate From chest discomfort, alleviated partly by sitting up and leaning forward	Moderate to severe From congestive heart failure	Severe air hunger from low cardiac output and hypoxemia

Note. Based on information from Azarbal & LeWinter, 2017.

TABLE 50-3 **Physical Examination and Diagnostic Test Findings With Pericarditis, Pericardial Effusion, and Pericardial Tamponade**

Technique	Pericarditis	Pericardial Effusion	Pericardial Tamponade
Blood pressure	Narrow pulse pressure (rising diastolic rather than dropping systolic)	Hypotension: Diastolic blood pressure rises first; then the systolic pressure decreases (narrowing pulse pressure). The presence of a pulsus paradoxus > 10 mm Hg signifies resistance to the inflow of blood into the heart.	Systolic hypotension with narrow pulse pressure or large pulsus paradoxus Pulmonary artery pressures become almost equal because of equalization of the pressure within and around the heart.
Cardiac rhythm electrocardiogram findings	Normal sinus rhythm Low QRS voltage on electrocardiogram	Tachycardia is the earliest heart rate response to decreased cardiac output. Low QRS voltage is more prominent than with pericarditis. Bradycardia or heart block may occur with high thoracic pressure and poor coronary blood flow during inspiration.	High thoracic resistance leads to poor ventricular filling, particularly during inspiration. Bradycardia, heart block, or short periods of asystole may occur during inspiration. Electrical alternans (QRS alternating above and below isoelectric line) occurs in approximately 15% of patients.
Central venous pressure	Normal to slight elevation (10–12 cm of H_2O or 6–8 mm Hg)	Moderate elevation (15–18 cm of H_2O or 8–12 mm Hg)	Extremely high (18–26 cm of H_2O or 12–22 mm Hg), becoming close to ventricular or pulmonary artery pressures if a pulmonary artery catheter is in place
Heart sounds	Pericardial rub	Muffled heart sounds	Absent heart sounds
Hepatomegaly and splenomegaly	Rarely present When noted, usually mild size change but produces discomfort	Reflects degree of venous congestion Common finding in conjunction with slow-developing or chronic effusions	Reflects degree of congestion Common finding in conjunction with slow-developing or chronic effusions leading to tamponade
Jugular venous distention (JVD) and jugular venous pulsation (JVP)	Slight increase in JVD and JVP (2–4 cm above clavicle)	Bulging neck veins (JVD) and JVP near mandible, bilateral	Bulging neck veins (JVD) JVP producing a large continuous wave up the neck and to the chin (i.e., cannon waves)

(Continued on next page)

TABLE 50-3	Physical Examination and Diagnostic Test Findings With Pericarditis, Pericardial Effusion, and Pericardial Tamponade *(Continued)*		
Technique	Pericarditis	Pericardial Effusion	Pericardial Tamponade
Mental status	Normal	Awake, alert, oriented Anxious, restless	Alterations in mental status may be present if blood flow to the brain is impaired.
Peripheral edema	Trace-dependent edema initially noted Peripheral (especially lower extremities) and dependent edema will increase with progression of cardiac dysfunction.	Moderate 2+ to 3+ edema of the extremities (especially lower) with slow fluid accumulation Rapidly developing effusions produce minimal edema.	Severe upper and lower extremity edema may be present but actually reflects the severe effusion, not tamponade. Rapidly developing effusions produce minimal edema.
Point of maximal impulse	Normal	Shifted to the left (toward the axilla) or downward (toward sixth intercostal space)	Barely discernible but shifted laterally and downward if palpable
Strength and equality of pulses	Decreased peripheral pulses More diminished in lower extremities	Decreased peripheral pulses More diminished in lower extremities	Minimal carotid pulse Absent lower extremity pulses
Temperature	Fever	Normal	Normal
Urine output	Normal	Oliguria often is an early indicator of compromised cardiac output.	Anuria

Note. Based on information from Azarbal & LeWinter, 2017; Yusuf et al., 2016.

1. Findings vary according to the acuity of onset.
    a) In chronic, slowly developing effusions, evidence of progressive right heart failure reflecting obstruction to venous return may be the earliest clinical finding.
    b) Rapid onset of pericardial effusion reflects low cardiac output early in the disease process.
2. Findings differ between pericarditis, effusion, and tamponade based upon the level of inflammation or impaired pump function.
3. Findings that characteristically reflect poor tissue perfusion include low blood pressure, oliguria, cyanosis, diminished bowel sounds, and palpitations.
4. In acute-onset low cardiac output from pericardial disease, the first branch of the aortic arch provides the best tissue perfusion, resulting in perfusion to the brain or upper extremities even when the lower extremities are receiving little blood.

IV. Diagnostic tests: Refer to Table 50-3 for findings with pericarditis, pericardial effusion, and pericardial tamponade (Carneiro et al., 2017; Chalikias et al., 2017; Dadhich et al., 2016; Hamiel et al., 2015; Honasoge & Dubbs, 2018; Kligerman, 2019; Lekhakul et al., 2018; Saab et al., 2017; Sundling & Cibas, 2018; Yildirim et al., 2016).

A. Laboratory
   1. Laboratory markers of myocardial damage may indicate a combined pericardial disease and myocarditis and include elevated troponins, elevated ESR, increased LDH, and elevated N-terminal prohormone BNP levels.
   2. Some advocate obtaining serum values of LDH, protein, and glucose to compare with pericardial fluid.
   3. Pericardial fluid cytology via immunochemistry, flow cytometry, morphometry, or cytogenetics may be used to ascertain an etiology.
      a) Malignant effusions may be hemorrhagic, serosanguinous (majority), or serous.
      b) Confirmation of malignancy is present in 50%–88% of cases and only weakly associated with outcome.
      c) Targeted tumor markers may be evaluated, but their presence in fluid infiltrated with malignant cells is inconsistent (see Appendix O).
      d) Fluid cytology performs better than liquid biopsy.
   4. CBC is used to evaluate for increased WBCs with infection; low hematocrit/Hgb may be present.
   5. Renal profile is used to evaluate renal status and potential uremic etiology.
   6. Thyroid panel can be used to evaluate for hypothyroidism.
   7. Infectious evaluation is indicated with viral serologic testing and pericardial fluid viral culture.
B. Radiology
   1. Chest x-ray is used to evaluate the heart; lung fields are typically normal.
      a) Symmetric cardiac enlargement is more than one-half the diameter of the chest.
      b) Widened mediastinum or water-bottle silhouette of the heart and major vessels is seen as enhancement of a wider area centrally located in the chest near the major vessels.
   2. CT scan of chest is rarely performed but may be useful for needle-guided fluid removal when visualization with echocardiography is difficult.
C. Other
   1. Echocardiogram: Definitive diagnostic tool for confirmation of pericardial disease when technique includes bidimensional imaging with pulsed wave Doppler imaging
      a) When effusion or tamponade is present, fluid is visible within the pericardial sac. Fluid surrounding the heart presents an image of "swinging heart" where the heart appears to be floating within fluid.
         (1) Echocardiogram-diagnosed fluid thickness greater than 20 mm is associated with malignancy more than one-third of the time.
         (2) Fluid volume in pericardial sac does not reliably predict hemodynamic compromise.
      b) Restricted ventricular filling presents with impending cardiac tamponade, with right ventricular abnormalities occurring earlier in the disease process.
      c) Distorted or inadequate ventricular expansion is characteristic with all pericardial syndromes.
      d) Value is limited in evaluation of right heart, mediastinum, and paracardiac structures.
      e) Newer techniques using evaluation of tricuspid valve dynamics may be more helpful than analysis of fluid volume.
      f) Little added value exists in performing transesophageal echocardiogram rather than a three-dimensional Doppler study except when post–cardiac surgery pericardial effusion is suspected.

      g) Ejection fraction calculated from the echocardiogram provides a good estimation of the degree of compromise related to pericardial compression.

    2. Pericardial imaging: CT or cardiovascular MRI

      a) May be useful when echocardiogram results are indeterminate

      b) Helpful in determining if mediastinal masses include the pericardium

      c) More definitive in loculated effusions, constrictive pericarditis

    3. ECG (see Table 50-3)

      a) Pericarditis: Low-voltage QRS complexes, tachycardia, ST elevation with upright T waves and PR depression in all precordial leads

      b) Pericardial effusion: Low-voltage QRS complexes (especially limb leads), PR depression, precordial lead ST elevation tachycardia in approximately one-fourth of patients with early effusion

      c) Bradycardia/heart block in late effusion or impending tamponade

      d) Pericardial tamponade: Electrical alternans (alternating positive and negative deflected QRS complexes) occurs in a small number of patients but almost always signifies impending cardiac tamponade.

    4. Pericardial biopsy via pericardioscopy: Enhances diagnostic yield but should only be used when other diagnostic methods are ineffective and active treatment is intended

V. Differential diagnosis (Fardman et al., 2016; Saab et al., 2017; Schusler & Meyerson, 2018; Yildirim et al., 2016)

  A. Heart failure (see Chapter 42)

  B. SVC syndrome

  C. MI (see Chapter 49)

  D. Dissecting aortic aneurysm

  E. Tension pneumothorax (see Chapter 31)

  F. Cardiac metastasis

  G. Intrathoracic masses without pericardial effusions

  H. Pericardial infection

  I. TB (see Chapter 36)

  J. Pulmonary emboli (see Chapter 33)

  K. Advanced cirrhosis (see Chapter 69)

  L. Autoimmune disease

  M. Severe hypothyroidism (see Chapter 158)

  N. End-stage renal disease (see Chapter 86)

VI. Treatment: Definitive treatment of pericarditis is very different from treatment of pericardial effusion and tamponade (Azarbal & LeWinter, 2017; Colak et al., 2019; Fardman et al., 2016; Han et al., 2016; Imazio et al., 2015, 2017; Schusler & Meyerson, 2018; Yusuf et al., 2016).

  A. Proposed important variables to determine best treatment

    1. Size of effusion at end diastole

    2. Echocardiographic hemodynamic findings

    3. Etiology of pericardial effusion

  B. Pericarditis

    1. Observation alone may be indicated for mild symptoms.

    2. Pericarditis is an inflammatory process; anti-inflammatory agents are administered once hemorrhagic pericarditis is ruled out. Therapy usually is continued until symptoms subside or approximately two weeks (see Appendix E).

      a) Moderate-dose ASA: 650 mg PO every four hours

b) Moderate-dose NSAIDs: Ibuprofen 400–600 mg PO three times a day, for example

c) Colchicine: 2 mg PO daily; reported as helpful if uremia induced

d) Corticosteroids: May be used for symptomatic relief by patients with pericarditis refractory to NSAIDs or those who are terminally ill; rapid-acting agents (e.g., dexamethasone 4–10 mg PO or IV three times a day or hydrocortisone 125 mg IV four times a day) may be prescribed for a few weeks.

3. Concomitant gastroprotective therapy with omeprazole 20–40 mg PO daily or pantoprazole 40 mg PO or parenterally daily should be considered.

C. Pericardial effusion/pericardial tamponade

1. Treatment is based on cancer-related goals of care for the patient—palliation, control, or cure.

2. Observation alone may be the treatment of choice for mild or moderate pericardial effusion when the effusion is expected to resolve spontaneously.

3. In severe pericardial effusion and impending tamponade, maintaining spontaneous ventilation rather than inserting an invasive airway with positive pressure ventilation will enhance normal ventilation and induce negative thoracic pressures that will aid venous return.

4. Vigorous IV fluid administration (200–500 ml/hr): Despite clinical symptoms of heart failure, this has been the essential first intervention in impending tamponade to increase venous pressure above pericardial pressure, thus enhancing venous return. Immediate fluid challenge may be indicated but should be discontinued if hemodynamic parameters worsen.

5. Fluid removal: Severe pericardial effusion or tamponade with evidence of collapsed ventricles requires aspiration of pericardial fluid.

a) Fluid removal without definitive treatment of etiology has a 40% rate of recurrence.

b) Immediate fluid removal of large volume effusions can produce rebound fluid shifts with rapid fluid reaccumulation and signs of heart failure, termed *pericardial decompression syndrome.*

6. The method of fluid removal is based on the etiology and patient's hemodynamic status. See Table 50-4 for an overview of therapies.

7. Radiation: When malignant pericardial effusions are confirmed and slow-growing tumors amenable to radiation therapy are present, 100–200 cGy mediastinal radiation daily for three to four weeks may be administered. Intrapericardial injection phosphorus-32 (^{32}P) colloid with total radiation dose greater than 100 Gy has been used with some success.

8. Chemotherapy

a) When malignant pericardial effusions are confirmed and amenable to chemotherapy, specific systemic antitumor antineoplastic therapy is given.

b) Some advocate the administration of chemotherapy agents into the pericardial sac as a sclerosing agent, although this practice is uncommon.

(1) If performed, the physician usually administers at the time of fluid removal via pericardial catheter or pericardiocentesis.

(2) Common adverse effects include pain, fever, atrial fibrillation, and atrial flutter.

9. Fibrinolysis may be indicated in thick purulent, bloody, or chylous pericardial effusions. It is administered in a dose similar to that used for obstructed venous central catheters (e.g., tissue plasminogen activator 2 mg).

10. Diuretic therapy has not been clinically researched and is not supported by current pathophysiologic knowledge of effusions or cardiac tamponade.

TABLE 50-4	Methods for Removing Pericardial Fluid	
Treatment	**Technique**	**Nursing Implications**
Balloon pericardiotomy without continuous drainage	Catheter is inserted into pericardial sac and balloon inflated to open a hole in the pericardial sac; catheter is immediately removed, and pericardial fluid drains into the mediastinum.	It is indicated for short-term emergent removal of slowly or rapidly developing effusion. Preprocedural preparation is the same as pericardial catheter. Monitor for recurrent tamponade symptoms. Small studies suggest immediate results equivalent to pericardial catheter, but high incidence of procedural pain and reaccumulation exists. It may be appropriate only if unable to perform pericardial catheter drainage.
Pericardial catheter (may use to drain and remove or may leave in for several days)	Fluoroscopic-directed pericardial catheters have drainage and/or sclerosing. Many are "pigtail" with a corkscrew tail to hold in place.	It is indicated for short-term emergent removal of slow or rapidly developing effusion. It can be performed emergently with echocardiogram or fluoroscopic guidance. Preprocedural preparation: Administer minor sedation at bedside or in procedure room; semi-upright position may facilitate access to pericardial fluid; light meal permitted if clinical condition warrants. Maintain catheter patency and closed system. Account for drainage quantity, color, and consistency at each shift. Keep drainage bag below the level of the heart. Sudden cessation of drainage may indicate misplacement or clotting of the catheter; observe the patient for recurrent tamponade. Sudden increase in catheter drainage may indicate clotting abnormality. Report to the provider. Potential complications to observe include dysrhythmias, immediate pulmonary edema from fluid shifts with rapid fluid removal, infectious pericarditis, and post-procedure pericardial fibrosis. Complications may be reduced when catheter drainage is performed by ultrasound-guided technique. Flushing the catheter with approximately 3 ml of preservative-free normal saline may be performed every 4–8 hours as needed. If the drainage is extremely bloody, low-dose heparin may be used. Exit-site care: Catheter is not sutured in place but has a curled tip that should stay in the pericardial sac. Maintain a sterile dressing over exit site. Administer pain medication prior to sclerosing agent. Administer antipyretics if bleomycin is used. Clamp catheter for 2–4 hours after administration of sclerosing agent. Chemotherapy agents that have been administered via intrapericardial catheter include 5-fluorouracil, bevacizumab, bleomycin, cisplatin, and rituximab. Patients with a pigtail catheter that is not easy to remove should have an echocardiogram performed to ensure the catheter tip has not knotted.

(Continued on next page)

TABLE 50-4	Methods for Removing Pericardial Fluid *(Continued)*	
Treatment	**Technique**	**Nursing Implications**
Pericardial window	It is used for thoracotomy or subxiphoid thoracoscopy, or video-assisted thoracotomy surgery with resection of lower section of pericardial sac. A screen-like grid is placed to allow pericardial fluid drainage into mediastinum. Connecting window into pleura may be performed with equivalent results. Partial resection of pericardium may be performed if loculated effusions exist.	It is indicated for chronic severe effusions in a patient with otherwise good performance status. Newer techniques permit thoracoscopic approach without major surgery and general anesthesia. It is not indicated for diagnosis alone. Preoperative preparation is the same as with regular operative procedure with anesthetic. For postoperative thoracotomy, prevent pulmonary complications by encouraging coughing and deep breathing. For mediastinal chest tube care, monitor drainage (no bubbling from a mediastinal chest tube; tube is positioned in the epigastric region); perform usual chest tube exit-site care. Average duration of chest tube is 7 days. Inform patient/caregivers about symptoms of occlusion and reaccumulation.
Pericardiectomy	Pericardium is resected or stripped so there is no place for pericardial fluid to accumulate.	It is indicated for chronic, severe effusions in a patient with otherwise good performance status. Patient must be able to tolerate a thoracotomy procedure. It is used only after catheter or balloon fluid removal and pericardial window have failed. It is rarely performed because other therapeutic options are readily available. It is most commonly used with fibrous pericarditis, which occurs after radiation exposure to heart. Chronic congestive failure symptoms may be present after pericardiectomy.
Pericardioperitoneal shunt	Local anesthesia is used for percutaneous subxiphoid insertion of a Denver shunt that drains pericardial fluid into the abdomen.	It is indicated for palliative management of recurrent malignant effusions, particularly in patients with limited life expectancy. Preprocedural preparation is same as with pericardial catheter. Monitor for recurrent tamponade from occlusion of the shunt. It is rarely used given accessibility and ease of cardiac catheterization facilities.
Pericardiocentesis	It is the emergency bedside insertion of a needle into pericardial sac for removal of fluid; a long cardiac needle is attached to alligator clamp that is connected to V chest lead of the electrocardiogram machine. The needle is inserted subxiphoid and pointed toward the left shoulder; when injury curve occurs on electrocardiogram machine, needle is backed off and fluid aspirated.	It is indicated for life-threatening cardiac tamponade in presence of moderate to large pericardial effusion when open procedure cannot be performed promptly. Keep emergency equipment (e.g., crash cart, defibrillator) nearby during procedure. Use electrocardiogram machine and alligator clamp for evidence of position whenever possible (helps to avoid removal of intracardiac blood). Save aspirated fluid; pericardial fluid should not clot but will clot if it is withdrawn from the ventricle. Monitor return or strengthening of pulses during fluid removal. Monitor for pneumopericardium as complication of pericardiocentesis.

Note. Based on information from Azarbal & LeWinter, 2017; Colak et al., 2019; Fardman et al., 2016; Park & McGonigle, 2018; Schusler & Meyerson, 2018.

VII. Follow-up (Schusler & Meyerson, 2018; Yusuf et al., 2016)
   A. Pericarditis is followed clinically by physical examination and ECG. When the patient has repeated exposure to the triggering factor, frequent physical examinations (daily to weekly) and serial ECGs are monitored.
   B. Patients with pericardial effusion or a history of tamponade will have an echocardiogram one month after treatment and then at least every 6–12 months, depending upon the rate of accumulation during the first episode.

VIII. Referrals (Schusler & Meyerson, 2018)
   A. Radiation oncologist: May be indicated if the patient has a radiosensitive tumor that has not been maximally treated with radiation therapy
   B. Heart transplant program: May be indicated if the pericardial disease is related to a late or long-term effect of anticancer therapy and the patient is cured of cancer
   C. Home nurse visitation: Intermittent visits are required for many patients with effectively treated pericardial effusions for evaluation of symptoms signaling recurrence.
      1. Home oxygen therapy may be required.
      2. Home modifications to accommodate for limitations of ADLs may be necessary.
   D. Hospice: May be needed for patients in whom pericardial effusion is a manifestation of severe aggressive disease for symptomatic support
   E. Cardiologist, interventional radiologist, or thoracic surgeon: May be appropriate to assist with treatment, management, and drainage of the pericardium
   F. Mental health professional: May be helpful in assisting patients to cope with dyspnea through use of relaxation or distraction techniques

References

Azarbal, A., & LeWinter, M.M. (2017). Pericardial effusion. *Cardiology Clinics, 35*(4), 515–524. https://doi.org/10.1016/j.ccl.2017.07.005

Carneiro, F.P., Muniz-Junqueira, M.I., Pittella-Silva, F., de Vasconcelos Carneiro, M., Soares Takano, G.H., de Sousa Vianna, L.M., ... Barretto Motoyama, A. (2017). A panel of markers for identification of malignant and non-malignant cells in culture from effusions. *Oncology Reports, 38*(6), 3538–3544. https://doi.org/10.3892/or.2017.6022

Chalikias, G., Samaras, A., Ziakas, A., Kikas, P., Thomaidis, A., Drosos, I., ... & Tziakas, D. (2017). Novel echocardiographic prognostic markers for cardiac tamponade in patients with large malignant pericardial effusions: A paradigm shift from flow to tissue imaging. *Echocardiography, 34*(9), 1315–1323. https://doi.org/10.1111/echo.13620

Colak, A., Becit, N., Kaya, U., Ceviz, M., & Kocak, H. (2019). Treatment of pericardial effusion through subxiphoid tube pericardiostomy and computerized tomography- or echocardiography-guided percutaneous catheter drainage methods. *Brazilian Journal of Cardiovascular Surgery, 34*(2), 194–202. https://doi.org/10.21470/1678-9741-2018-0077

Dadhich, H., Toi, P.C., Siddaraju, N., & Sevvanthi, K. (2016). A comparative analysis of conventional cytopreparatory and liquid based cytological techniques (Sure Path) in evaluation of serous effusion fluids. *Diagnostic Cytopathology, 44*(11), 874–879. https://doi.org/10.1002/dc.23567

Fardman, A., Charron, P., Imazio, M., & Adler, Y. (2016). European guidelines on pericardial diseases: A focused review of novel aspects. *Current Cardiology Reports, 18*(5), 46. https://doi.org/10.1007/s11886-016-0721-1

Hamiel, U., Yeganeh, S., Carrasso, S., & Soboh, S. (2015). An alerting sign: Enlarged cardiac silhouette. *Cleveland Clinic Journal of Medicine, 82*(12), 801–803. https://doi.org/10.3949/ccjm.82a.14185

Han, A.J., Slomka, T., Mehrotra, A., Murillo, L.C., Alsafwah, S.F., & Khouzam, R.N. (2016). Paradoxical hemodynamic instability after pericardial window. *Echocardiography, 33*(8), 1251–1252. https://doi.org/10.1111/echo.13229

Honasoge, A.P., & Dubbs, S.B. (2018). Rapid fire: Pericardial effusion and tamponade. *Emergency Medicine Clinics of North America, 36*(3), 557–565. https://doi.org/10.1016/j.emc.2018.04.004

Imazio, M., Gaido, L., Battaglia, A., & Gaita, F. (2017). Contemporary management of pericardial effusion: Practical aspects for clinical practice. *Postgraduate Medicine, 129*(2), 178–186. https://doi.org/10.1080/00325481.2017.1285676

Imazio, M., Gaita, F., & LeWinter, M. (2015). Evaluation and treatment of pericarditis: A systematic review. *JAMA, 314*(14), 1498–1506. https://doi.org/10.1001/jama.2015.12763

Kalogeraki, A., Lazopoulos, G., Papadakis, G.Z., Tamiolakis, D., Karvela-Kalogeraki, I., Karvelas-Kalogerakis, M., ... Tzardi, M. (2016). Cytology of pericardial effusion due to malignancy. *Romanian Journal of Internal Medicine, 54*(3), 179–183. https://doi.org/10.1515/rjim-2016-0026

Kligerman, S. (2019). Imaging of pericardial disease. *Radiologic Clinics of North America, 57*(1), 179–199. https://doi.org/10.1016/j.rcl.2018.09.001

Lekhakul, A., Assawakawintip, C., Fenstad, E.R., Pislaru, S.V., Thaden, J.J., Sinak, L.J., & Kane, G.C. (2018). Safety and outcome of percutaneous drainage of pericardial effusions in patients with cancer. *American Journal of Cardiology, 122*(6), 1091–1094. https://doi.org/10.1016/j.amjcard.2018.06.002

Murillo, H., Santiago Restrepo, C., Marmol-Velez, J.A., Vargas, D., Ocazionez, D., Martinez-Jimenez, S., ... Baxi, A.J. (2016). Infectious diseases of the heart: Pathophysiology, clinical and imaging overview. *RadioGraphics, 36*(4), 963–983. https://doi.org/10.1148/rg.2016150225

Niska, J.R., Thorpe, C.S., Allen, S.M., Daniels, T.B., Rule, W.G., Schild, S.E., ... Mookadam, F. (2018). Radiation and the heart: Systematic review of dosimetery and cardiac endpoints. *Expert Review of Cardiovascular Therapy, 16*(12), 931–950. https://doi.org/10.1080/14779072.2018.1538785

Oyakawa, T., Muraoka, N., Iida, K., Kusuhara, M., Naito, T., & Omae, K. (2018). Characteristics of cellular composition in malignant pericardial effusion and its association with the clinical course of carcinomatous pericarditis. *Japanese Journal of Clinical Oncology, 48*(3), 291–294. https://doi.org/10.1093/jjco/hyx187

Park, C.Y., & McGonigle, N.C. (2018). Single-port thoracoscopic pericardial window under local anesthesia. *Innovations: Technology and Techniques in Cardiothoracic and Vascular Surgery, 13*(1), 62–64. https://doi.org/10.1097/IMI.0000000000000456

Raghunathan, D., Khilji, M.I., Hassan, S.A., & Yusuf, S.W. (2017). Radiation-induced cardiovascular disease. *Current Atherosclerosis Reports, 19*(5), 22. https://doi.org/10.1007/s11883-017-0658-x

Saab, J., Hoda, R.S., Narula, N., Hoda, S.A., Geraghty, B.E., Nasar, A., ... Giorgadze, T. (2017). Diagnostic yield of cytopathology in evaluating pericardial effusions: Clinicopathologic analysis of 419 specimens. *Cancer Cytopathology, 125*(2), 128–137. https://doi.org/10.1002/cncy.21790

Schusler, R., & Meyerson, S.L. (2018). Pericardial disease associated with malignancy. *Current Cardiology Reports, 20*(10), 92. https://doi.org/10.1007/s11886-018-1040-5

Sundling, K.E., & Cibas, E.S. (2018). Ancillary studies in pleural, pericardial, and peritoneal effusion cytology. *Cancer Cytopathology, 126*(Suppl. 8), 590–598. https://doi.org/10.1002/cncy.22021

Yildirim, M., Ustaalioglu, R., Erkan, M., Ustaalioglu, B.B.O., Demirbag, H., Yasaroglu, M., ... Okay, T. (2016). The diagnostic value of pericardial fluid and pericardial biopsy: Single center experiences. *Heart Surgery Forum, 19*(1), E23–E27. https://doi.org/10.1532/hsf.1328

Yusuf, S.W., Hassan, S.A., Mouhayar, E., Negi, S.I., Banchs, J., & O'Gara, P.T. (2016). Pericardial disease: A clinical review. *Expert Review of Cardiovascular Therapy, 14*(4), 525–539. https://doi.org/10.1586/14779072.2016.1134317

CHAPTER 51

Peripheral Vascular Disease

Deborah Kirk, DNP, FNP-BC, NP-C, AOCN®, FAANP

I. Definition (Gerhard-Herman et al., 2017; Krishna et al., 2015)
   A. Occlusive or inflammatory disease that develops within the peripheral arteries, veins, or lymphatics and alters blood flow
   B. Intermittent claudication: Muscular cramping/pain with exercise quickly relieved by rest; advanced pain signifies arteriosclerotic obstruction with pain occurring at rest.
   C. Peripheral artery disease: Type of peripheral vascular disease with problems only with blood flow through arteries

II. Physiology/Pathophysiology (Englund & Langham, 2020; Gerhard-Herman et al., 2017; Krishna et al., 2015)
   A. Normal
      1. Arteries are tough and less distensible vessels than veins that are subjected to more pressure where oxygenated blood flows through the body.
      2. Veins are less sturdy and more passive than arteries and carry unoxygenated blood back to the heart.
      3. Venous return is less forceful than blood flow through the arteries; veins contain valves to keep blood flowing in one direction.
      4. If blood volume increases significantly, the veins can expand and act as a repository for extra blood. This compensatory mechanism helps to diminish stress on the heart.
      5. The lymphatic system is made up of lymph fluid, the collecting ducts, and various tissues, including the lymph nodes, spleen, thymus, tonsils and adenoids, and Peyer patches.
   B. Pathophysiology
      1. Arterial embolism can cause obstruction by a thrombus or vegetation within the heart or aorta or from a venous thrombus.
      2. Vasospastic disorders are manifested with Raynaud phenomenon, in which cold exposure causes triphasic color response as a result of venous occlusion.
      3. Thromboangiitis obliterans is an inflammatory reaction that develops in veins and small arteries and leads to superficial thrombophlebitis and arterial obstruction with ulceration or gangrene of the digits in heavy smokers.
      4. Peripheral artery disease is the occlusion of lower-limb arteries most commonly caused by atherothrombosis.
      5. Atherothrombosis results in clinical ischemic events affecting the cerebral, coronary, and peripheral arterial circulation.
      6. Radiation damage to arteries causes intimal disruption and luminal stenosis, leading to occlusion.
      7. Pain occurs from imbalance between supply and demand of blood flow that fails to satisfy ongoing metabolic requirements.

III. Clinical features: The prevalence of peripheral artery disease in people aged 55 years and older is 10%–20%. This percentage increases with age. The majority of affected individuals are asymptomatic. Diagnosis of peripheral artery disease often is overlooked until the patient presents with life-threatening ischemia. Peripheral artery disease is a manifestation of the atherosclerotic process and is associated with an increased risk of cerebrovascular disease, cardiovascular disease, and death (Aboyans et al., 2018; Bauersachs et al., 2019; Criqui & Aboyans, 2015; Gerhard-Herman et al., 2017; Herrmann et al., 2016; Hossain et al., 2019; Tóth-Vajna et al., 2019).

A. Risk factors
1. Tobacco use
2. Dyslipidemia: High total cholesterol, low HDL
3. Age
4. Hyperhomocysteinemia
5. Physical inactivity
6. High-fat diet
7. Mediastinal irradiation
8. Hypertension
9. Diabetes mellitus
10. Chemotherapy: Cisplatin, nilotinib, ponatinib, IFN-α)

B. Etiology
1. Trauma
2. Hypertension
3. Diabetes mellitus: Prone to medial calcification of lower-limb arteries
4. Atherosclerosis: The major underlying disease contributing to peripheral vascular disease
   a) Arteriosclerotic plaques producing stenosis or occlusion of the arterial lumen often are segmentally distributed. Femoral and popliteal arteries are the most commonly affected.
   b) Other sites include the infrarenal abdominal aorta, aortic bifurcation, and iliac bifurcation artery.
   c) Pressure and blood flow are not significantly diminished until at least 75% of the vein is occluded.
5. Atherosclerosis obliterans is the most prevalent vascular disorder.
   a) Patients have an increased incidence of CAD because of shared risk factors associated with an increased incidence of MI.
   b) Femoral and popliteal arteries are most commonly affected.
6. Arteritis
7. Aneurysm
8. Embolism

C. History
1. History of cancer and cancer treatment
2. Current medications: Prescribed, over the counter
3. History of presenting symptoms: Precipitating factors, onset, location, duration, associated symptoms (e.g., leg pain at rest or with activity [dangling legs over side of bed relieves discomfort], hair loss on lower extremities, inability to have an erection)
4. Changes in ADLs: Activity intolerance
5. Past medical history: Atherosclerosis, diabetes, hypertension, hypercholesterolemia, renal problems
6. Family history: Atherosclerotic disease, hypercholesterolemia

   7. Social history: Tobacco use
  D. Signs and symptoms: Majority of patients are asymptomatic.
    1. True intermittent claudication
     a) Symptoms include cramping, tightness, tiredness, and aching.
     b) Pain is located in the buttock, hip, thigh, calf, or foot.
     c) It is exercise induced and not felt with standing.
     d) Distance walked before onset of pain is consistent.
     e) Pain is relieved when exercise or walking is discontinued.
    2. Pseudoclaudication
     a) Symptoms include cramping, tightness, tiredness, aching, tingling, weakness, and clumsiness.
     b) Pain is located in the buttock, hip, thigh, calf, or foot.
     c) Walking distance before pain onset is variable.
     d) Pain occurs with standing.
     e) Pain is relieved with sitting or position change.
    3. Numbness, weakness, or fatigue in the muscle groups of the lower extremities
    4. Impotence
    5. Hair loss, thickened nails, smooth and shiny skin
    6. Poorly healing wounds of the extremities
  E. Physical examination: Usually nonspecific
    1. Vital signs: Blood pressure in both arms; possible hypertension
    2. Integument
     a) Skin atrophy indicating loss of arterial perfusion
     b) Pallor or dependent rubor indicating poor venous return
     c) Cyanotic discoloration of digits, ulceration, necrosis, or gangrene indicating poor arterial flow
     d) Skin temperature: May be cool to touch
     e) Hair loss on lower extremities
     f) Poorly healing wounds
     g) Thickened nails
    3. Cardiac
     a) Palpate pulses: Decreased peripheral pulses at rest, which reduce with exercise
     b) Dependent rubor (redness)
     c) Aortic and groin regions auscultation for bruits
     d) Prolonged capillary refill
    4. Extremities: Limbs with severe insufficiency or obstruction will blanch when raised above the level of the heart while the patient is in a supine position.
     a) Pallor beyond 60 seconds is an ominous sign.
     b) A suddenly cold extremity is a sign of acute arterial occlusion.
     c) Inspect feet for color, temperature, and skin integrity.
     d) Assess muscle strength. Weakness indicates spinal stenosis.
     e) Assess for sensory loss indicating spinal stenosis.

 IV. Diagnostic tests (Aboyans et al., 2018; Criqui & Aboyans, 2015; Englund & Langham, 2020; Gerhard-Herman et al., 2017; Hossain et al., 2019; Tóth-Vajna et al., 2019)
  A. Laboratory
    1. Lipid profile to assess cholesterol, LDL, and HDL
    2. Homocysteine level elevated with cardiovascular disease
    3. Fasting blood sugar to detect diabetes
    4. BUN and creatinine to assess renal function

B. Radiology
1. CT angiography to view occlusion or stenosis
2. Magnetic resonance angiography to view occlusion or stenosis
3. Doppler ultrasound of blood flow measurements before and during exercise to localize stenosis
C. Other: Ankle-brachial index is a simple, noninvasive bedside tool for diagnosing peripheral artery disease that records the ratio of Doppler-recorded systolic pressures in the lower and upper extremities. A ratio less than 0.9 is diagnostic of peripheral artery disease.

V. Differential diagnosis (Aboyans et al., 2018; Bevan & White Solaru, 2020)
A. CAD
B. PE (see Chapter 33)
C. MI (see Chapter 49)
D. Pericarditis (see Chapter 50)
E. Endocarditis (see Chapter 46)
F. Raynaud phenomenon
G. Radiation-induced fibrosis
H. Antiphospholipid antibody syndrome
I. Dyslipidemia (see Chapter 44)
J. Peripheral neuropathy (see Chapter 143)
K. Neurogenic problems
1. Spinal stenosis
2. Disc disease
3. Tumor
4. Diabetes mellitus (see Chapter 151)
5. Alcohol use
L. Musculoskeletal problems
1. Popliteal entrapment
2. OA (see Chapter 105)
M. Lymphedema (see Chapter 112)
N. Superficial thrombophlebitis (see Chapter 164)
O. DVT (see Chapter 43)
P. SLE (see Chapter 110)

VI. Treatment (Aboyans et al., 2018; Bevan & White Solaru, 2020; Chionchio et al., 2019; Criqui & Aboyans, 2015; Gerhard-Herman et al., 2017; Hossain et al., 2019)
A. Nonpharmacologic
1. Lifestyle modifications: A daily supervised or structured exercise program is recommended in patients with claudication. The best exercise is daily walking to increase collateral circulation.
   a) Patients should walk to point of discomfort, stop briefly, and resume walking.
   b) Encourage 30–45 minutes daily (at least three days a week).
   c) Exercise bikes are an alternative to walking.
2. Careful foot care with regular inspection for signs of ulceration, skin necrosis, and infection
   a) Wash feet daily with mild soap and lukewarm water. Rinse thoroughly, and dry gently and completely, especially between toes.
   b) Apply moisturizing cream to feet but not between toes.
   c) Wear properly fitting shoes.
   d) Cut nails with extreme care straight across and even with the end of the toe.

3. Smoking cessation
   a) Nicotine patches: 21 mg daily for four to six weeks, then taper to lower dose (14 mg daily to 7 mg daily)
   b) Nicotine gum: 4 mg and 2 mg preparation with 12 pieces a day and taper to fewer pieces a day
   c) Bupropion: 300 mg PO daily
   d) Varenicline: 0.5 mg PO daily on days 1–3, then increased to 0.5 mg PO two times a day on day 4–7, then increased to 1 mg PO two times a day for 12 weeks; initiation of varenicline one week prior to quit date
   e) Hypnosis or acupuncture
   f) Development of a plan for quitting
   g) Referral to cessation program
4. Encourage weight reduction and reduced fat intake (e.g., Mediterranean diet).
5. Take aggressive measures to control major atherosclerotic risk factors, such as hypertension, dyslipidemia, diabetes mellitus, and smoking.

B. Pharmacologic
1. Treat dyslipidemia with a statin (see Chapter 44).
2. ASA: 81 mg PO daily; does not improve intermittent claudication but appears to delay progression and reduce the need for intervention; appropriate for patients with a history of transient ischemic attack or stroke, chronic stable angina, or peripheral artery disease
3. Clopidogrel: 75 mg PO daily for patients with transient ischemic attack or stroke, chronic stable angina, peripheral artery disease, or for those intolerant to ASA
4. Dipyridamole: 75–100 mg PO four times a day in combination with ASA for patients who experience a first episode of transient ischemic attack or stroke in the absence of clinically apparent CAD; also, for patients after revascularization surgery
5. ACE inhibitors (e.g., captopril): 25 mg PO two times a day or lisinopril 10 mg PO daily for management of hypertension
6. Cilostazol: 100 mg PO two times a day for claudication; a potent, reversible phosphodiesterase III inhibitor; allows for the increased availability of cyclic adenosine monophosphate, mediating many agonist-induced platelet inhibitory, vasodilatory, and vascular antiproliferative responses
7. Treat hypertension (see Chapter 47).
8. Treat diabetes mellitus (see Chapter 151).
9. Receive influenza vaccine yearly.

C. Surgery
1. Arterial revascularization surgery: For patients with severe claudication at rest or gangrene
2. Percutaneous angioplasty
   a) Incapacitating claudication interfering with work or lifestyle
   b) Limb salvage in people with limb-threatening ischemia
   c) Nonhealing ulcers and/or gangrene and vasculogenic impotence
3. Stent placement: Acute dissections and restenosis in native or bypassed grafts after angioplasty
4. Amputation: Performed if tissue loss has progressed beyond the point of salvage

VII. Follow-up (Bevan & White Solaru, 2020)
A. Perform follow-up monthly to evaluate patient's response to therapy.
B. Encourage patient to maintain lifestyle modifications.

    C. Revise follow-up PRN, including every six months for mild peripheral vascular disease (symptoms not interfering with lifestyle), every three months for moderate disease (symptoms begin to interfere with lifestyle), and monthly for severe disease (symptoms occur at rest).

VIII. Referrals
    A. Vascular surgeon: For surgical intervention
    B. Cardiologist: For patients with cardiac risk factors or symptoms of CAD, poorly controlled hypertension, and CHF
    C. Endocrinologist: For patients with diabetes mellitus

References

Aboyans, V., Ricco, J.-B., Bartelink, M.-L.E.L., Björck, M., Brodmann, M., Cohnert, T., ... Desormais, I. (2018). 2017 ESC guidelines of the diagnosis and treatment of peripheral arterial diseases, in collaboration with the European Society for Vascular Surgery (ESVS). *European Heart Journal, 39*(9), 763–821. https://doi.org/10.1093/eurheartj/ehx095

Bauersachs, R., Zeymer, U., Brière, J.-B., Marre, C., Bowrin, K., & Huelsebeck, M. (2019). Burden of coronary artery disease and peripheral artery disease: A literature review. *Cardiovascular Therapeutics, 2019,* 8295054. https://doi.org/10.1155/2019/8295054

Bevan, G.H., & White Solaru, K.T. (2020). Evidence-based medical management of peripheral artery disease. *Arteriosclerosis, Thrombosis, and Vascular Biology, 40*(3), 541–553. https://doi.org/10.1161/ATVBAHA.119.312142

Chionchio, A., Galmer, A., & Hirsh, B. (2019). Primary and novel lipid-lowering therapies to reduce risk in patients with peripheral arterial disease. *Current Treatment Options in Cardiovascular Medicine, 21*(12), 94. https://doi.org/10.1007/s11936-019-0791-7

Criqui, M.H., & Aboyans, V. (2015). Epidemiology of peripheral artery disease. *Circulation Research, 116*(9), 1509–1526. https://doi.org/10.1161/CIRCRESAHA.116.303849

Englund, E.K., & Langham, M.C. (2020). Quantitative and dynamic MRI measures of peripheral vascular function. *Frontiers in Physiology, 11,* 120. https://doi.org/10.3389/fphys.2020.00120

Gerhard-Herman, M.D., Gornik, H.L., Barrett, C., Barshes, N.R., Corriere, M.A., Drachman, D.E., ... Walsh, M.E. (2017). 2016 AHA/ACC guideline on the management of patients with lower extremity peripheral artery disease: A report of the American College of Cardiology/American Heart Association task force on clinical practice guidelines. *Journal of the American College of Cardiology, 69*(11), e71–e126. https://doi.org/10.1016/j.jacc.2016.11.007

Herrmann, J., Yang, E.H., Iliescu, C.A., Cilingirogu, M., Charitakis, K., Hakeem, A., ... Marmagkiolis, K. (2016). Vascular toxicities of cancer therapies: The old and the new—An evolving avenue. *Circulation, 133*(13), 1272–1289. https://doi.org/10.1161/CIRCULATIONAHA.115.018347

Hossain, P., Kokkinidis, D.G., & Armstrong, E.J. (2019). How to assess a claudication and when to intervene. *Current Cardiology Reports, 21*(12), 138. https://doi.org/10.1007/s11886-019-1227-4

Krishna, S.M., Moxon, J.V., & Golledge, J. (2015). A review of the pathophysiology and potential biomarkers for peripheral artery disease. *International Journal of Molecular Sciences, 16*(5), 11294–11322. https://doi.org/10.3390/ijms160511294

Tóth-Vajna, Z., Tóth-Vajna, G., Gombos, Z., Szilágyi, B., Járai, Z., Berczeli, M., & Sótonyi, P. (2019). Screening of peripheral arterial disease in primary health care. *Vascular Health and Risk Management, 15,* 355–363. https://doi.org/10.2147/VHRM.S208302

CHAPTER 52

Pulmonary Hypertension

Deborah Kirk, DNP, FNP-BC, NP-C, AOCN®, FAANP

I. Definition: Persistent elevation of the mean pulmonary artery pressure at rest (greater than 25 mm Hg) (Galiè et al., 2015; Simonneau et al., 2018)

II. Physiology/Pathophysiology (Gewillig & Brown, 2016; Guazzi & Naeije, 2017)
   A. Normal
      1. Normal blood flow through the pulmonary vasculature occurs without significant opposition to forward flow.
      2. The pulmonary vasculature is a high-capacitance and low-pressure system.
      3. Pulmonary vasculature size is balanced by vasodilator and vasoconstrictor mediators.
      4. The right ventricle is a smaller muscle mass than the left ventricle.
   B. Pathophysiology
      1. In pulmonary artery hypertension (PAH), vascular changes include vasoconstriction, smooth-muscle and endothelial cell proliferation, and thrombosis. Disturbances occur in the balance between vasoconstriction and vasodilators, prothrombotic and antithrombotic mediators, and growth factors.
      2. Chronic hypoxemia causes pulmonary vasoconstriction by a variety of actions on pulmonary artery endothelium and smooth muscle cells, including downregulation of endothelial nitric oxide synthetase.
      3. Arterioles usually have a small number of muscle fibers, which in PH become hypertrophied, leading to vasoconstriction and remodeling of the arteriole. An additional component of PH is the development of thrombosis because of stimulation of platelet aggregation by the vasoconstrictor thromboxane A2.
         a) Endothelium factors may contribute to the development of PH by releasing vasoconstrictors that cause prolonged vasoconstriction and resultant vascular remodeling.
         b) PH may develop as a result of an underlying disease state that causes hypoxia and hypoxic vasoconstriction in an effort to maintain a match between ventilation and perfusion. In chronic vasoconstriction, vascular remodeling and PH eventually will occur.
      4. Increased pulmonary artery pressures and pulmonary vascular resistance cause right ventricular hypertrophy and potential right ventricular failure. Right ventricular hypertrophy leads to tricuspid valve strain and eventual insufficiency.

III. Clinical features: PH is a complex, multifactorial disease that results in right heart failure and premature death. It is classified into five groups, with left heart disease the most common (Galiè et al., 2015; Herrmann et al., 2016; Hewes et al., 2020; Simonneau et al., 2018; Sonnweber et al., 2020; Thomas et al., 2019; Yaghi et al., 2020).

A. Classifications (see Table 52-1)
B. Etiology and risk factors (see Tables 52-1 and 52-2)
C. History
   1. History of cancer and cancer treatment (see Figure 52-1)
   2. Current medications: Prescribed, over the counter (see Table 52-2)
   3. History of presenting symptoms: Precipitating factors, onset, location, duration
   4. Changes in ADLs
   5. Past medical history: COPD, asthma, diabetes, CHF, HIV, renal/cardiac compromise or failure, congenital heart disease, thyroid disorder, sleep apnea
   6. Social history: Diet, smoking history (e.g., cigarettes, cigars, marijuana), alcohol use, illicit drug use

TABLE 52-1 Clinical Classifications and Etiology of Pulmonary Hypertension

Clinical Classification	Subcategories
Pulmonary arterial hypertension (group 1)	Idiopathic pulmonary arterial hypertension: Unknown cause Heritable: Linked to the *BMPR2* gene and subsequent changes in pulmonary vascular smooth muscle ALK1, endoglin (with or without hereditary hemorrhagic telangiectasia), SMAD9, CAV1, KCNK3 Associated with collagen vascular disease, congenital systemic-to-pulmonary shunts, portal hypertension, HIV infection, schistosomiasis, chronic hemolytic anemia, portal hypertension Associated with significant venous or capillary involvement (pulmonary veno-occlusive disease, pulmonary capillary hemangiomatosis) Persistent pulmonary hypertension of the newborn Drug and toxin induced
Pulmonary hypertension with left heart disease (group 2)	Systolic dysfunction Diastolic dysfunction Valvular disease Congenital/acquired left heart inflow/outflow obstruction and congenital cardiomyopathies
Pulmonary hypertension associated with lung diseases and/or hypoxemia (group 3)	Chronic obstructive pulmonary disease Interstitial lung disease Sleep disorder breathing Alveolar hypoventilation disorders Chronic exposure to high altitude Developmental abnormalities Other pulmonary diseases with mixed restrictive and obstructive pattern
Pulmonary hypertension because of chronic thrombotic and/or embolic disease (group 4)	Thromboembolic disease obstruction of proximal pulmonary arteries Thromboembolic disease obstruction of distal pulmonary arteries Nonthrombotic pulmonary embolism (e.g., tumor, parasites, foreign material)
Miscellaneous (group 5)	Hematologic disorders (e.g., myeloproliferative disorders) Systemic disorders (e.g., sarcoidosis, histiocytosis) Metabolic disorders (e.g., thyroid disorders, glycogen storage disease) Other (e.g., compression of pulmonary vessels from tumor, chronic renal failure, segmental pulmonary hypertension)

ALK1—activin receptor like kinase type 1; BMPR2—bone morphogenetic protein receptor type 2; HIV—human immunodeficiency virus

Note. Based on information from Simonneau et al., 2018.

TABLE 52-2	Updated Risk Factors and Associated Conditions Identified for Development of Pulmonary Arterial Hypertension

Strength of Evidence	Risk Factors
Definite	Aminorex, fenfluramine, dexfenfluramine, toxic rapeseed oil, benfluorex, methamphet-amines, dasatinib
Possible	Phenylpropanolamine, St. John's wort, cocaine, l-tryptophan, interferon-alpha, amphetamine-like drugs, alkylating agents, bosutinib, leflunomide, indirubin, direct-act-ing antiviral agents against hepatitis C virus

Note. From "Haemodynamic Definitions and Updated Clinical Classification of Pulmonary Hypertension," by F. Simonneau, D. Montani, D.S. Celermajer, C.P. Denton, M.A. Gatzoulis, M. Krowka, … R. Souza, 2018, *European Respiratory Journal, 53*(1), p. 7 (https://doi.org/10.1183/13993003.01913-2018). Copyright 2018 by European Respiratory Society. Adapted with permission.

D. Signs and symptoms
1. Shortness of breath
2. Dyspnea on exertion early, dyspnea at rest as disease progresses
3. Fatigue
4. Light-headedness or syncope (from decreased cardiac output)
5. Pedal edema and ascites (from right ventricular compromise or failure)
6. Angina
7. Abdominal distention (pain in right upper quadrant)
8. Dry cough
9. Hemoptysis
10. Hoarseness
11. Exercise-induced nausea and vomiting

E. Physical examination
1. Vital signs: Possible hypotension and tachycardia; weight gain with presence of edema
2. Pulmonary
   a) Respiratory rate and depth increased and shallow
   b) Auscultation
      (1) Clear auscultation if no underlying lung disease
      (2) Rales and symptoms of right ventricular failure as disease progresses
      (3) Wheeze and crackles usually absent
   c) Increased work of breathing
3. Cardiac
   a) Pulses, warmth of extremities, edema
   b) Heart sounds
      (1) Loud pulmonic sound

FIGURE 52-1	Examples of Cancer Treatments Associated With Pulmonary Hypertension

- Bleomycin
- Bortezomib
- Carfilzomib
- Cyclophosphamide
- Dasatinib
- Interferon alpha

Note. Based on information from Herrmann et al., 2016.

        (2) May have S_3 and/or S_4

        (3) May have systolic murmur from tricuspid regurgitation

     c) PAH specific

        (1) Cardiac: Left parasternal lift, accentuated component of S_2, pansystolic murmur of tricuspid regurgitation, diastolic murmur of pulmonary insufficiency

        (2) Neck: JVD

        (3) Abdominal: Hepatomegaly and ascites

        (4) Extremities: Peripheral edema, cool extremities

        (5) Skin: Telangiectasis

IV. Diagnostic tests (Galiè et al., 2015; Herrmann et al., 2016; Hewes et al., 2020; Simonneau et al., 2018; Yaghi et al., 2020)

  A. Laboratory: Not diagnostic for PH but helps to identify underlying problems

    1. CBC to evaluate for increased Hgb and hematocrit as a means of combating oxygen deficit; increased WBCs can be infection related, leading to pulmonary compromise.

    2. Chemistry panel to evaluate electrolytes and renal status, including LFTs; increased with cirrhosis or other liver disease

    3. ABGs to evaluate for hypoxia

    4. Autoantibody tests for SLE, scleroderma, and anticardiolipin antibodies to evaluate for rheumatoid factor as the underlying cause of PH with interstitial lung disease

    5. HIV serology to evaluate for HIV as the underlying cause of PH

    6. BNP: Elevated in ventricular overload; correlates with severity of right ventricular dysfunction and mortality in PAH

    7. Thyroid function test to evaluate for thyroid problems (common)

    8. Genetic testing: *BMPR2* gene mutation screening, *ACVRL1* and *ENG* genes

    9. Ferritin level and iron studies to evaluate for iron deficiency (common)

  B. Radiology

    1. Chest x-ray

     a) Posterior anterior and lateral are the preferred x-ray locations. Otherwise, anteroposterior should be used. Observe for enlarged heart, especially right ventricle. Note enlarged lung vessels suggestive of cardiac compromise.

     b) Pleural effusions may be associated with pulmonary venous hypertension related to left heart filling abnormality, pulmonary veno-occlusive disease, and pulmonary capillary hemangiomatosis.

     c) Hyperinflation may be associated with PH related to COPD.

     d) Marked asymmetry of enlarged central pulmonary arteries may be a symptom of chronic thromboembolic disease and related PH.

    2. CT imaging of the chest

     a) Abnormal lung vessels, blood clots

     b) Lung disease: Interstitial disease compressing blood vessels

    3. Cardiac MRI: Right ventricle size, function, blood flow

    4. Echocardiography: Initial study to evaluate right ventricular function, pulmonary systolic pressures and tricuspid valvular function, and bubble test for intracardiac or intrapulmonary shunts

    5. Ventilation/perfusion lung scan

     a) Chronic PE is usually one segmental size or larger perfusion defect.

     b) PH without ventilation/perfusion abnormality is more likely to be idiopathic PAH than chronic PE.

     c) Scans do not correlate well with severity of obstruction.

     d) Scan may mistakenly identify as clot when patient has sarcoma, large vessel pulmonary vasculitis, vascular compression, or pulmonary veno-occlusive disease.

   6. Pulmonary angiography: May be indicated if suspicion of chronic thromboembolic PH

C. Other

   1. Right heart catheterization: Gold standard diagnosis

     a) Establish or confirm diagnosis with central venous pressure, cardiac output, cardiac index, mixed venous oxygen saturations, pulmonary artery pressure, pulmonary vascular resistance, and pulmonary capillary wedge pressure readings. Measure blood pressure, heart rate, and response to acute vasodilator.

       (1) Mild PAH (mean pulmonary artery pressure of 25–35 mm Hg) is seen with emphysema and scleroderma-related interstitial lung disease.

       (2) Severe PAH (mean pulmonary artery pressure greater than 45 mm Hg) is uncommon in parenchymal lung disease and should exclude chronic pulmonary emboli and other etiologies of PH.

     b) Document pulmonary hemodynamics and cardiac output; identify intracardiac shunt—usually the result of uncorrected congenital heart disease. In a patient with a large ventricular–septal defect, high pulmonary pressure and flow states lead to right heart to left heart shunting of blood flow, leading to cyanosis. It is seen in patients who have or regenerate patent ductus arteriosus.

     c) Assess acute vasoreactivity to determine potential benefit of calcium channel blocker therapy in the setting of idiopathic PAH.

       (1) Decrease in mean pulmonary artery pressure of at least 10 mm Hg with mean pressure decreasing to 40 mm Hg or below with administration of short-acting vasodilator (IV prostacyclin, adenosine, or inhaled nitric oxide)

       (2) Accompanied by normal or increased cardiac output

       (3) Development of pulmonary edema during vasodilator therapy possibly indicative of development of pulmonary veno-occlusive disease or pulmonary capillary hemangioma, which is a contraindication to chronic vasodilator therapy

   2. ECG: Note signs consistent with increased heart size and change in rhythms/regularity. Right ventricular hypertrophy, strain, and right atrial dilation may be consistent with PAH.

   3. Overnight pulse oximetry to identify obstructive sleep apnea or hypopnea: Sleep studies may be appropriate to further evaluate for sleep apnea.

   4. Pulmonary function tests: Evaluate for restrictive or obstructive pattern and evaluate diffusing capacity of the lung; if less than 55%, this may be associated with future development of PAH.

   5. Exercise testing

     a) Six-minute walk test

       (1) Submaximal exercise test that is especially helpful in patients who cannot tolerate the maximal exercise test

       (2) Correlates inversely with functional class and survival in patients with idiopathic PAH

       (3) Does not necessarily correlate with pulmonary artery pressures

     b) Cardiopulmonary testing with gas exchange measurements

       (1) Reduced peak exercise oxygen consumption

(2) Reduced anaerobic threshold

(3) Findings indicating ventilation/perfusion mismatching, lactic acidosis at low work rate, arterial hypoxemia, and inability to sufficiently increase cardiac output and stroke volume

V. Differential diagnosis (Frost et al., 2018; Hussain et al., 2016; Sonnweber et al., 2020)

    A. COPD/COPD exacerbation (see Chapter 28)

    B. Asthma (see Chapter 28)

    C. Pulmonary edema (see Chapter 32)

    D. Pulmonary hemorrhage

    E. PE (see Chapter 33)

    F. Pleural effusion (see Chapter 29)

    G. Radiation- or chemotherapy-induced pulmonary disease

    H. Lung contusion

    I. CHF (see Chapter 42)

    J. Sleep apnea (see Chapter 34)

    K. Dilated cardiomyopathy (see Chapter 41)

    L. Connective tissue disorders

    M. Mitral stenosis

    N. Portal hypertension

    O. Pulmonic stenosis

    P. SLE (see Chapter 110)

    Q. Scleroderma

    R. Left-sided heart failure

    S. CAD

    T. Liver disease

    U. Sickle cell disease (see Chapter 119)

VI. Treatment (Galiè et al., 2015; Simonneau et al., 2018; Sommer et al., 2020; Sonnweber et al., 2020; Thomas et al., 2019; Yaghi et al., 2020)

    A. General

        1. Physical activity

            a) Maintain exercise regimen to prevent deconditioning, but watch for signs of increasing disease with development of dizziness, light-headedness, or severe dyspnea that may lead to syncopal episode.

            b) Suggest supervised rehabilitation within individual limits.

            c) Optimize QOL.

        2. Instruct patient and partner on contraceptive therapy to prevent pregnancy, which is contraindicated in patients with PH.

        3. Provide infection prevention education.

        4. Psychosocial support includes psychological, social, emotional, and spiritual options.

        5. Instruct on importance of medication adherence.

        6. Genetic counseling may be appropriate.

        7. Offer smoking cessation programs.

        8. Suggest participating in exercise and pulmonary rehabilitation for strength and training.

    B. Pharmacologic treatment

        1. Anticoagulants should be considered in certain types of PH.

            a) Careful use if patient has scleroderma, portopulmonary hypertension, or varices because of potential increased risk of bleeding *b)* Potential benefit in patients with right ventricular failure or venous stasis at increased risk of thromboembolism

2. Diuretics should be used to manage symptoms of fluid overload.
3. Maintain or increase oxygen delivery. Consider oxygen therapy to maintain saturation greater than 90% in patients with chronic hypoxemia.
4. Administer digitalis as indicated for control of atrial dysrhythmias (see Chapter 45) and right heart failure.
5. Iron replacement should be considered in those with iron deficiency (see Chapter 118).
6. Calcium channel blockers are recommended therapy for select patients; start with a low dose, and adjust according to heart rate (e.g., nifedipine 30 mg PO daily).
7. Endothelin receptor antagonists
   a) Endothelin-1 receptors are direct vasoconstrictors, stimulate the proliferation of vascular smooth muscle cells, induce fibrosis, and are proinflammatory mediators.
      (1) Endothelin A receptors cause sustained vasoconstriction and proliferation of vascular smooth muscle cells.
      (2) Endothelin B receptors mediate pulmonary endothelin clearance, induce production of nitric oxide and prostacyclin on endothelial cells, and stimulate vasoconstriction on vascular smooth muscle cells.
      (3) All may cause elevated LFTs.
   b) Drugs
      (1) Bosentan (initial dose): 62.5 mg PO two times a day
         (a) This endothelin A and B receptor antagonist works as a vasodilator, anti-inflammatory agent, and remodeling mediator.
         (b) Randomized controlled trials have shown improvement in exercise tolerance and time to worsening presentation.
         (c) Hepatotoxicity (increased aminotransferase levels) has been noted and was found to be dose dependent.
      (2) Ambrisentan (initial dose): 5 mg PO daily
         (a) It is a selective endothelin A blocker.
         (b) Randomized controlled trials have shown improved exercise tolerance and improvement in symptoms and hemodynamics.
         (c) Drug may cause significant acute hepatitis. Liver function monitoring is required.
      (3) Macitentan (initial dose): 10 mg PO daily
         (a) It is a dual endothelin antagonist.
         (b) Macitentan works to reduce morbidity and mortality and increase exercise capacity.
         (c) A reduction in Hgb occurs.
8. Phosphodiesterase inhibitors
   a) Phosphodiesterase inhibitors may facilitate the use of endogenous and exogenous nitric oxide to maintain pulmonary vasodilation.
   b) Drugs
      (1) Sildenafil
         (a) Phosphodiesterase type 5 inhibitor
         (b) 20 mg PO three times a day; doses lower than 20 mg three times a day are not recommended.
         (c) Side effects: Headache, flushing, dyspepsia, epistaxis
      (2) Tadalafil

        (a) Phosphodiesterase type 5 inhibitor

        (b) 2.5–40 mg PO daily

        (c) Side effects: Headache, flushing, dyspepsia, epistaxis

    (3) Vardenafil

        (a) Phosphodiesterase type 5 inhibitor

        (b) 5 mg PO two times a day

        (c) Side effects: Headache, flushing, dyspepsia, epistaxis

9. Prostacyclin therapy: Main product of arachidonic acid in the vascular endothelium

    a) Induces vascular smooth muscle relaxation, inhibits the growth of smooth muscle cells, and inhibits platelet aggregation

    b) In patients with moderately severe to severe PAH

    c) Drugs

        (1) Epoprostenol infusions have proved beneficial to increase functional status, decrease mean pulmonary artery pressure and mean pulmonary vascular resistance, and increase survival.

            (a) This survival advantage does not appear to be found in patients with scleroderma.

            (b) Interruption of the long-term infusion may be life threatening, and infusions require that patients and family members be able to manage catheters, infusion pumps, and intricacies of infusions (e.g., unstable at room temperature, must be reconstituted by the patient/caregiver, emergency planning for sudden cessation of infusion).

            (c) Infusions may serve as a bridge to lung transplantation.

        (2) Treprostinil is a prostacyclin analog that can be delivered via subcutaneous means, continuous IV, or inhalation. It is associated with pain and erythema at the infusion site. The half-life of the drug is approximately three hours, which makes interruptions less serious than with other IV agents.

        (3) Iloprost is a prostacyclin agent available as an IV, PO, or inhaled that has been tested and showed benefit in patients with New York Heart Association class III–IV symptomatology from idiopathic PAH, PAH from connective tissue disorders, and inoperable chronic thromboembolic PH. Frequent nebulized dosing (six to nine times daily) is required, as the half-life is approximately 20–25 minutes.

10. Transplantation

    a) Reserved for advanced PH that is not responsive to medical therapy

    b) May be single or bilateral lung transplantation or heart–lung transplantation

C. Subsets of PH

  1. Pulmonary venous hypertension

    a) Improve myocardial performance, including decreasing right ventricular preload with use of diuretic therapy.

    b) Relieve valvular defects with surgical intervention.

    c) Relieve direct compression of pulmonary veins with appropriate cancer treatment.

    d) Transplantation

        (1) Reserved for advanced PH that is not responsive to medical therapy

        (2) May require heart–lung transplantation for congenital heart defect

  2. PH associated with disorders of respiratory system or hypoxemia

    a) Oxygen therapy (16–24 hours a day) improves survival in patients with COPD.

    b) Altitude-based PH often resolves with relocation of patient to sea level.

    c) Treat underlying disease, such as COPD (see Chapter 28).
  3. PH caused by chronic thrombotic or embolic disease
    a) Dissolve or remove clots obstructing flow in major arteries.
    b) May require pulmonary endarterectomy; recommended selection criteria includes the following.
      (1) New York Heart Association functional class III or IV symptomatology
      (2) Preoperative pulmonary vascular resistance greater than 300 dyne/s/cm
      (3) Surgically accessible thrombus in the main, lobar, or segmental pulmonary arteries
      (4) No severe comorbidities
    c) Chronic vasodilator therapy may be beneficial for more peripheral lesions.
    d) Chronic anticoagulation therapy can be used with IVC filter insertion.
    e) Balloon pulmonary angioplasty is used for distal thromboembolism.
  4. PH caused by disorders directly affecting the pulmonary vasculature
    a) Relieve inflammatory disorders.
    b) Remove mechanical obstructions to restore flow through pulmonary vasculature.

VII. Follow-up (Galiè et al., 2015; Thomas et al., 2019)
  A. Perform frequent follow-up for serial measurements in monitoring disease progression.
    1. Functional status
    2. Exercise capacity
    3. Pulmonary hemodynamics
    4. Acute vasoreactivity
    5. Echocardiographic evaluation of right ventricular function/presence of pericardial effusion
    6. ECG for increased P-wave amplitude in lead II, an R pattern in lead V_1, and right ventricular hypertrophy
    7. Laboratory studies: BNP, endothelin-1, uric acid, troponin levels
  B. Follow-up appointments are dependent on severity of disease and should occur every 4–12 weeks.

VIII. Referrals (Yaghi et al., 2020)
  A. Cardiologist: For treatment options
  B. Thoracic surgeon or transplantation team: For possible transplantation
  C. Palliative care services
  D. Pulmonary rehabilitation: For exercise programs

References

Frost, A., Badesch, D., Gibbs, J.S.R., Gopalan, D., Khanna, D., Manes, A., … Torbicki, A. (2018). Diagnosis of pulmonary hypertension. *European Respiratory Journal, 55*(3), 1801904. https://doi.org/10.1183/13993003.01904-2018

Galiè, N., Humbert, M., Vachiery, J.-L., Gibbs, S., Lang, I., Torbicki, A., … Hoeper, M. (2015). 2015 ESC/ERS guidelines for the diagnosis and treatment of pulmonary hypertension. *European Respiratory Journal, 46*(4), 903–975. https://doi.org/10.1183/13993003.01032-2015

Gewillig, M., & Brown, S.C. (2016). The Fontan circulation after 45 years: Update in physiology. *Heart, 102*(14), 1081–1086. https://doi.org/10.1136/heartjnl-2015-307467

Guazzi, M., & Naeije, R. (2017). Pulmonary hypertension in heart failure: Pathophysiology, pathobiology, and emerging clinical perspectives. *Journal of the American College of Cardiology, 69*(13), 1718–1734. https://doi.org/10.1016/j.jacc.2017.01.051

Herrmann, J., Yang, E.H., Iliescu, C.A., Cilingirogu, M., Charitakis, K., Hakeem, A., … Marmagkiolis, K. (2016). Vascular toxicities of cancer therapies: The old and the new—An evolving avenue. *Circulation, 133*(13), 1272–1289. https://doi.org/10.1161/CIRCULATIONAHA.115.018347

Hewes, J.L., Lee, J.Y., Fagan, K.A., & Bauer, N.N. (2020). The changing face of pulmonary hypertension diagnosis: A historical perspective on the influence of diagnostics and biomarkers. *Pulmonary Circulation, 10*(1). https://doi.org/10.1177/2045894019892801

Hussain, N., Charalampopoulos, A., Ramjug, S., Condliffe, R., Elliot, C.A., O'Toole, L., ... Kiely, D.G. (2016). Pulmonary hypertension in patients with heart failure and preserved ejection fraction: differential diagnosis and management. *Pulmonary Circulation, 6*(1), 3–14. https://doi.org/10.1086/685021

Simonneau, G., Montani, D., Celermajer, D.S., Denton, C.P., Gatzoulis, M.A., Krowka, M., ... Souza, R., (2018). Haemodynamic definitions and updated clinical classification of pulmonary hypertension. *European Respiratory Journal, 53*(1), 1801913. https://doi.org/10.1183/13993003.01913-2018

Sommer, N., Ghofrani, H.A., Pak, O., Bonnet, S., Provencher, S., Sitbon, O., ... Kiely, D.G. (2020). Current and future treatments of pulmonary arterial hypertension. *British Journal of Pharmacology, 178*(1), 6–30. https://doi.org/10.1111/bph.15016

Sonnweber, T., Pizzini, A., Tancevski, I., Löffler-Ragg, J., & Weiss, G. (2020). Anaemia, iron homeostasis and pulmonary hypertension: A review. *Internal and Emergency Medicine, 15*(4), 573–585. https://doi.org/10.1007/s11739-020-02288-1

Thomas, C.A., Anderson, R.J., Condon, D.F., & de Jesus Perez, V.A. (2019). Diagnosis and management of pulmonary hypertension in the modern era: Insights from the 6th world symposium. *Pulmonary Therapy, 6*(1), 9–22. https://doi.org/10.1007/s41030-019-00105-5

Yaghi, S., Novikov, A., & Trandafirescu, T. (2020). Clinical update on pulmonary hypertension. *Journal of Investigative Medicine, 68*(4), 821–827. https://doi.org/10.1136/jim-2020-001291

Gastrointestinal

CHAPTER 53

Abdominal Pain

Jeannine M. Brant, PhD, APRN, AOCN®, FAAN

I. Definition: Pain originating from the abdomen and/or surrounding organs (American Pain Society, 2016)
  A. Acute: A sudden, severe experience of abdominal pain with unclear etiology that often requires immediate surgical or medical intervention; self-limiting
  B. Recurrent: Pain that recurs after apparent remission
  C. Chronic: Pain that persists over time, usually longer than three to six months

II. Physiology/Pathophysiology (Portenoy & Ahmed, 2018; Russo & Sundaramurthi, 2019)
  A. Normal: The abdominal cavity contains several visceral organs, including the liver, stomach, gallbladder, intestines, spleen, and kidneys. The peritoneum lines the cavity and forms a protective cover around abdominal structures.
  B. Pathophysiology: Pain arises from the viscera, body wall, or nerves and is attributed to ischemia, inflammation, muscle contraction, visceral spasm, distention, vascular disorders, metabolic disturbance, and neurologic disorders. Pain can also be referred from another source. Cross-communication between visceral afferents contributes to the diffuse perception of pain. Pathogenesis is dependent on origin of pain.
    1. Visceral pain: This diffuse, vague, poorly defined type of pain arises from autonomic nerve fibers in abdominal viscera. It is often perceived at the midline. Intestinal pain is often crampy.
    2. Somatic pain: This sharp, well-localized pain arises from somatic nerves in the parietal peritoneum and is often the result of the inflammatory processes. It often increases with movement.
    3. Referred pain: This pain is perceived at a distant site from the origin and is usually sharper and better localized than visceral pain. It is caused by the convergence of nerve pathways with the organ of origin or the linings of the viscera.

III. Clinical features: Numerous causes, ranging from acute, life-threatening emergencies to chronic functional disease and disorders of several organ systems, can generate abdominal pain. History is the critical diagnostic aspect of importance (Fink & Brant, 2018; Natesan et al., 2016; Park et al., 2016; Ruzga et al., 2019).
  A. Etiology: Location of the abdominal pain can assist in determining the etiology (see Figure 53-1).
  B. History
    1. History of cancer and cancer treatment: Intraperitoneal chemotherapy
    2. Current medications: Prescribed, over the counter
    3. History of presenting symptoms: Precipitating factors, onset, location, duration, pattern

FIGURE 53-1   Abdominal Pain Etiologies

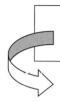

| **Generalized Pain** |
| Acute pancreatitis, appendicitis, bowel obstruction, diabetic ketoacidosis, gastroenteritis, mesenteric ischemia, peritonitis |

Epigastric
Aortic aneurysm; appendicitis (early); cancer of the colon, liver, esophagus, stomach, or pancreas; cholecystitis; colitis; gastroenteritis; herpes zoster; inflammatory bowel disease; lower lobe pneumonia; myocardial infarction or ischemia; pancreatitis

Right Upper Quadrant	**Left Upper Quadrant**
Biliary colic, cholecystitis, hepatitis, perforated duodenal ulcer	Colitis, gastritis, pancreatitis, peptic ulcer disease, pneumonia, pyelonephritis, splenomegaly, urinary tract infection

Umbilical
Aortic aneurysm, appendicitis, bowel obstruction, gastroenteritis, hernia, inflammatory bowel disease, mesenteric ischemia, pancreatitis

Right Lower Quadrant	**Left Lower Quadrant**
Appendicitis, cecal or Meckel diverticulitis	Sigmoid diverticulitis

Right or Left Lower Quadrants
Aortic aneurysm, bowel obstruction, cecal volvulus, colon or ovarian cancer, cystitis, diverticulitis, ectopic pregnancy, endometriosis, enteritis, hernia, inflammatory bowel disease, menstrual cramps, ovarian cyst/torsion, pelvic inflammatory disease, penetrating or perforating ulcer, prostatitis, psoas abscess, renal stones, salpingitis, testicular torsion

Note. Based on information from Avegno & Carlisle, 2016; Gans et al., 2015; Natesan et al., 2016; Ruzga et al., 2019.

    4. Changes in ADLs: Eating habits, elimination patterns
    5. For women
       a) History of menstrual cycle
       b) Abnormal vaginal bleeding or discharge, ectopic pregnancy
    6. Social history: Alcohol use, sexual history, adverse childhood events
  C. Signs and symptoms
    1. Upper GI tract: Nausea/vomiting, heartburn, dysphagia, halitosis, hematemesis, colic
    2. Lower GI tract: Abdominal distention, diarrhea or constipation, cramps, colic, dysuria (urgency or frequency), hematuria, melena, abnormal/missed menses (women), abnormal vaginal bleeding (women), bladder spasms, tenesmus suggesting perineal irritation
    3. Other: Syncope, jaundice, anorexia, fevers and chills
    4. Acute versus chronic
       a) Acute: Acute abdominal pain often involves autonomic factors (e.g., nausea and vomiting, profuse sweating, pallor, diarrhea, fear, anxiety). Other symp-

toms include bloating, anorexia, constipation, light-headedness, syncope, and weight loss. Blood vessel rupture, perforation, and abdominal sepsis should be considered for severe acute abdominal pain.

    b) Chronic: Symptoms include bloating, anorexia, constipation, light-headedness, syncope, and weight loss and can evolve from a variety of etiologic factors persisting longer than three to six months.

D. Physical examination

    1. Vital signs

      a) Blood pressure: Orthostatic, hypertension, hypotension

        (1) Postural changes secondary to obstruction, peritonitis, bowel infarction

        (2) Hypertension secondary to acute pain

        (3) Hypotension secondary to dehydration

      b) Pulse: Tachycardia (greater than 100 bpm) or bradycardia (less than 50 bpm)

      c) Respiration: Tachypnea (greater than 20 breaths per minute) with acute pain

      d) Temperature: Fever (greater than 38.3°C [101°F]) may indicate infection, but lack of fever does not rule out infectious etiology. Threshold for fever may change based on neutropenic status.

    2. General appearance

      a) Level of distress

      b) Positioning

        (1) Patient avoids movement: indicative of peritoneal irritation.

        (2) Patient is very restless: indicative of obstruction.

    3. Integument

      a) Jaundice and other stigmata of chronic liver disease

      b) Sclerae: Icterus suggestive of liver disease

      c) Rashes or lesions: Macules, papules, petechiae (pattern of distribution)

      d) Signs of trauma

      e) Poor skin turgor indicative of dehydration

      f) Ecchymotic areas indicative of DIC, liver disease

    4. Cardiovascular

      a) Murmurs/abnormal heart sounds: Ectopic beats with mesenteric ischemia

      b) Abdominal bruit: Abdominal aortic aneurysm

      c) JVD: Hepatomegaly associated with CHF

      d) Splinting indicative of inflammation

    5. Pulmonary: Breath sounds

      a) If diminished, could be suggestive of CHF or pneumonia

      b) Absent with consolidation

      c) Grating sound with pleural friction rub

    6. Abdominal

      a) Local tenderness, rebound tenderness, guarding tenderness located over affected digestive system in visceral pain

      b) Rigidity and rebound tenderness suggestive of peritoneal irritation and appendicitis

      c) Bowel sounds: High-pitched tinkling, bruits, or absent

      d) Distention: Obstruction, appendicitis, ascites

      e) Hepatosplenomegaly: Venous congestion associated with CHF, visible abdominal venous pattern indicative of portal hypertension

      f) Pulsatile/nonpulsatile masses: Aortic aneurysm

      g) Flank tenderness: Pyelonephritis

    7. Rectal: Includes prostate examination in men

       a) Masses

          (1) Heme-positive stools: Peptic ulcer disease or upper GI bleed

          (2) Prostate enlargement or with nodules suggestive of prostatitis

       b) Tenderness: Thrombosed hemorrhoids

       c) Gross rectal bleeding: Lower GI bleed (e.g., colon cancer)

   8. Pelvic examination to rule out pelvic inflammatory disease, STI, malignancy

       a) Vaginal or cervical discharge

       b) Cervical motion tenderness

       c) Adnexal masses or tenderness

   9. Male GU

       a) Testicular swelling, masses, or tenderness

       b) Scrotal masses or swelling

       c) Perineal edema

  10. Special tests (see Appendix D)

       a) Peritoneal irritation

          (1) Obturator sign: Have patient sit in supine position and flex knee to 90°; examiner immobilizes the ankle while performing internal/external rotation of the knee. Pain with rotation is positive.

          (2) Iliopsoas sign: Have patient sit in supine position and extend knee, attempting to flex thigh against resistance. Pain during maneuver is positive.

       b) Abdominal wall pain (Carnett test): With patient supine, palpate area of most intense tenderness. Palpate again with patient half sitting up. Pain that is intra-abdominal will not increase as tensed rectus muscles protect underlying viscus.

       c) Cholecystitis (e.g., Murphy sign): Have patient breathe in while palpating the edge of the liver. A positive sign is when patient stops breathing suddenly during inspiration because of pain.

  11. Surgical abdomen

       a) General overview: Extreme pallor, jaundice, restlessness, writhing with pain, rigidity, possible immobility

       b) Vital signs: High fever, tachypnea, irregular/thready pulse, orthostatic changes

       c) Abdominal: Absent or high-pitched bowel sounds, distended abdomen, severe localized tenderness, mass

IV. Diagnostic tests (Cartwright & Knudson, 2015; Gans et al., 2015; Ruzga et al., 2019)

  A. Laboratory studies

    1. CBC to evaluate for infection and anemia

       a) Elevated WBC count: Indicates inflammatory or infectious process

       b) Differential: Left shift indicates infection

       c) Low hematocrit and Hgb with bleeding

    2. BUN and creatinine, electrolytes, and glucose to evaluate for dehydration or imbalances

    3. Stool for occult or gross blood to evaluate for associated GI bleed

    4. Stool cultures to evaluate for infection

    5. Amylase/lipase: Elevated level potentially indicative of pancreatitis, perforation, or intestinal obstruction

    6. Urinalysis: Presence of hematuria or pyuria indicative of UTI/pyelonephritis

    7. Quantitative urine pregnancy test or beta human chorionic gonadotropin: For women of childbearing age to evaluate for ectopic pregnancy

    8. LFTs: May indicate hepatitis, cirrhosis, or hepatotoxicity with elevated values

         9. Peritoneal fluid cultures to evaluate for infection

    B. Radiology

         1. Plain and upright films of the abdomen to evaluate for obstructive processes, perforation (free air under diaphragm), ascites, and abnormal gas pattern

         2. Upper GI series to evaluate for ulcer, cancer, and small bowel obstruction

         3. CT scan to evaluate tumor status and rule out free intraperitoneal air and potential infectious complications

         4. Barium enema: If patient is bleeding; to evaluate for cancer and inflammatory bowel

         5. Abdominal ultrasound to evaluate for gallstones, biliary obstruction, ureteral obstruction, and uterine or ovarian mass and to visualize kidneys, liver, and pancreas for abnormalities

         6. IV pyelogram to evaluate for renal obstruction, mass, and stones

V. Differential diagnosis (Celli et al., 2018; Natesan et al., 2016; Portenoy & Ahmed, 2018; Ruzga et al., 2019)

    A. GI disorders

         1. Abdominal malignancies: Colon, gallbladder, gastric, GI stromal tumors, liver, pancreas, pelvic metastases

         2. Appendicitis

         3. Bowel obstruction and ileus (see Chapter 67)

         4. Cholecystitis/choledocholithiasis (see Chapter 68)

         5. Constipation (see Chapter 55)

         6. Crohn disease

         7. Diarrhea (see Chapter 56)

         8. Diverticulitis (see Chapter 70)

         9. Mucosal irritation/gastroenteritis/gastritis (see Chapter 72)

            a) *Clostridium difficile*

            b) Fungal infection: Candidiasis, aspergillosis, mucormycosis

            c) *Helicobacter pylori*

            d) Typhlitis

        10. Hepatomegaly (see Chapter 60)

        11. Hepatitis (see Chapter 74)

        12. Hernia

        13. Intestinal infarct or ischemia

        14. IBS (see Chapter 76)

        15. Pancreatitis (see Chapter 77)

        16. Peptic ulcer disease (see Chapter 78)

        17. Splenomegaly, splenic infarction (see Chapter 65)

        18. Ulcerative colitis

        19. Volvulus

        20. Malignant ascites

    B. GU disorders

         1. Women

            a) Ectopic pregnancy

            b) Endometriosis

            c) Menstrual cramps, premenstrual syndrome

            d) Ovarian complications: Cancer, cysts, adnexal torsion

            e) Pelvic inflammatory disease

            f) Salpingitis

            g) Uterine fibroids

    2. Men

       a) Prostate cancer

       b) Prostatitis (see Chapter 92)

       c) Seminal vesiculitis

       d) Testicular torsion/cancer

    3. Women and men

       a) Nephrolithiasis

       b) Pyelonephritis (see Chapter 94)

       c) Ureteral calculi or obstruction

       d) UTI (see Chapter 89)

C. Metabolic disorders

    1. Addison disease

    2. Diabetic ketoacidosis (see Chapter 151)

    3. Hypercalcemia (see Chapter 152)

    4. Hyperparathyroidism

    5. Porphyria

    6. Uremia

D. Cardiovascular disorders

    1. MI/ischemia/angina pectoris (see Chapter 49)

    2. Aortic aneurysm

    3. Sickle cell disease (see Chapter 119)

E. Pulmonary disorders

    1. PE (see Chapter 33)

    2. Pneumonia (see Chapter 30)

F. Neurogenic disorders: HZV (see Chapter 22)

G. Drug-induced disorders

    1. Chemotherapy and immunotherapy

       a) Vinca alkaloids: Ileus, constipation

       b) Antimetabolites, antitumor antibiotics: Diarrhea

       c) Anti–CTLA-4 therapy: Colitis, bowel perforation

       d) PD-1/PD-L1 inhibitors: Diarrhea, colitis

       e) PARP inhibitors: Abdominal pain

       f) Intraperitoneal chemotherapy

    2. Opioids: Ileus, constipation

    3. NSAIDs (see Appendix E): Peptic ulcer disease (see Chapter 78), esophagitis

    4. Alcohol: Cirrhosis, esophagitis, gastritis (see Chapters 69 and 72)

    5. SSRIs: Gastritis (see Chapter 72)

VI. Treatment (Brant et al., 2017; Eaton et al., 2017; Gans et al., 2015; Sundaramurthi et al., 2017)

A. Acute intervention

    1. Oxygen as indicated for hypoxia

    2. IV fluids for dehydrated status

    3. Dietary measures depending on the diagnosis: NPO, clear liquids, or low-fat/low-residue diet until the problem has resolved or has been diagnosed

    4. NG tube if nausea and vomiting are persistent or obstruction suspected

    5. Antibiotics with fever or suspected infection (see Appendix C)

B. Treatment of underlying cause

C. Comfort measures

    1. Opioids are a mainstay of abdominal pain management. Opioids increase pressure at the sphincter of Oddi, but benefits of opioid analgesics often outweigh risks (see Appendix F).

2. Coanalgesics
   a) Corticosteroids for visceral pain caused from abdominal distention
   b) Histamine receptor antagonists or PPIs for gastritis (see Chapter 72) or peptic ulcer disease (see Chapter 78)
   c) Antispasmodics, such as dicyclomine or hyoscyamine
   d) Local anesthetics for severe referred pain with hyperalgesia
D. Chronic abdominal pain interventions
   1. Intraspinal interventions can be used for chronic abdominal pain not relieved with other strategies (e.g., implantable intrathecal morphine pump).
   2. Nerve blocks may be beneficial.
      a) Celiac plexus block for pain related to pancreatic cancer
      b) Neurolytic superior hypogastric plexus block
E. Admission criteria for acute abdomen
   1. GI bleeding
   2. Signs of infection (impending sepsis)
   3. Significant intravascular volume depletion
   4. Bowel obstruction with nausea and vomiting
   5. Worsening of pain or tenderness during serial abdominal examination
   6. Biliary tree obstruction

VII. Follow-up (Natesan et al., 2016)
   A. Short term: Patients with nonacute abdomen; depending on the diagnosis, some disease states (e.g., reflux) require only dietary measures, whereas others (e.g., peptic ulcer disease) may require medical management.
   B. Long term: Patients requiring intensive measures (e.g., surgical intervention beginning with the postoperative or recovery period)
   C. Patients experiencing chronic symptoms (e.g., pancreatitis, reflux) need regular follow-up to monitor disease exacerbation and to determine if aggressive therapy should be initiated.

VIII. Referrals
   A. General surgeon/emergency department: For immediate referral of patients with acute abdomen or possible bowel obstruction
   B. Gynecologist: For immediate referral of women presenting with adnexal masses to a gynecologic oncologist or women who are pregnant
   C. Gastroenterologist: For patients with GI bleeding for guidance in evaluation or if the diagnosis is uncertain
   D. Urologist: For patients with severe UTI or with urolithiasis

References

American Pain Society. (2016). *Principles of analgesic use in the treatment of acute pain and cancer pain* (7th ed.). APS Press.

Avegno, J., & Carlisle, M. (2016). Evaluating the patient with right upper quadrant abdominal pain. *Emergency Medical Clinics of North America, 34*(2), 211–228. https://doi.org/10.1016/j.emc.2015.12.011

Brant, J.M., Eaton, L.H., & Irwin, M.M. (2017). Cancer-related pain: Assessment and management with Putting Evidence Into Practice interventions. *Clinical Journal of Oncology Nursing, 21*(Suppl. 3), 4–7. https://doi.org/10.1188/17.CJON.S3.4-7

Cartwright, S.L., & Knudson, M.P. (2015). Diagnostic imaging of acute abdominal pain in adults. *American Family Physician, 91*(7), 452–459. https://www.aafp.org/afp/2015/0401/p452.html

Celli, R., Kluger, H.M., & Zhang, X. (2018). Anti-PD-1 therapy-associated perforating colitis. *Case Reports in Gastrointestinal Medicine, 2018,* 3406437. https://doi.org/10.1155/2018/3406437

Eaton, L.H., Brant, J.M., McLeod, K., & Yeh, C.H. (2017). Nonpharmacologic pain interventions: A review of evidence-based practices for reducing chronic cancer pain. *Clinical Journal of Oncology Nursing, 21*(3), 54–79. https://doi.org/10.1188/17.CJON.S3.54-70

Fink, R.M., & Brant, J.M. (2018). Complex cancer pain assessment. *Hematology/Oncology Clinics of North America, 32*(3), 353–369. https://doi.org/10.1016/j.hoc.2018.01.001

Gans, S.L., Pols, M.A., Stoker, J., & Boermeester, M.A. (2015). Guideline for the diagnostic pathway in patients with acute abdominal pain. *Digestive Surgery, 32*(1), 23–31. https://doi.org/10.1159/000371583

Natesan, S., Lee, J., Volkamer, H., & Thoureen, T. (2016). Evidence-based medicine approach to abdominal pain. *Emergency Medical Clinics of North America, 34*(2), 165–190. https://doi.org/10.1016/j.emc.2015.12.008

Park, S.H., Videlock, E.J., Shih, W., Presson, A.P., Mayer, E.A., & Chang, L. (2016). Adverse childhood experiences are associated with irritable bowel syndrome and gastrointestinal symptom severity. *Neurogastroenterology Motility, 28*(8), 1252–1260. https://doi.org/10.1111/nmo.12826

Portenoy, R.K., & Ahmed, E. (2018). Cancer pain syndromes. *Hematology/Oncology Clinics of North America, 32*(3), 371–386. https://doi.org/10.1016/j.hoc.2018.01.002

Russo, M.M., & Sundaramurthi, T. (2019). An overview of cancer pain: Epidemiology and pathophysiology. *Seminars in Oncology Nursing, 35*(3), 223–228. https://doi.org/10.1016/j.soncn.2019.04.002

Ruzga, A., Jorgensen, B., & Thambi-Pillai, T. (2019). Evaluation of acute abdominal pain. *South Dakota Medicine, 72*(10), 478–484.

Sundaramurthi, T., Gallagher, N., & Sterling, B. (2017). Cancer-related acute pain: A systematic review of evidence-based interventions for Putting Evidence Into Practice. *Clinical Journal of Oncology Nursing, 21*(Suppl. 3), 13–30. https://doi.org/10.1188/17.CJON.S3.13-30

CHAPTER 54

Ascites

Kristina Mathey, MS, APRN–CNP, AOCNP®

I. Definition: Accumulation of more than 25 ml of fluid in the peritoneal cavity (Chen et al., 2018)

II. Physiology/Pathophysiology (Chen et al., 2018; Day et al., 2015; Kasztelan-Szczerbinska & Cichoz-Lach, 2019; Piano et al., 2018; Pose & Cardenas, 2017)
   A. Normal
      1. The peritoneal surface is a semipermeable membrane through which passive diffusion of water and solutes and exchanges between the abdominal cavity and the subperitoneal vascular and lymphatic channels occur.
      2. Fluid crosses the membrane at a rate of approximately 30–35 ml/hr.
   B. Pathophysiology
      1. Ascites is excessive fluid accumulation in the peritoneal cavity caused by increased renal sodium retention as a result of activation of the renin–angiotensin–aldosterone and sympathetic systems in response to marked vasodilation of the splanchnic circulation.
      2. Portal hypertension and sodium retention are hallmarks of ascites.

III. Clinical features: Malignant and nonmalignant ascites are associated with a poor prognosis. The most common cause is cirrhosis (Chen et al., 2018; Day et al., 2015; Kasztelan-Szczerbinska & Cichoz-Lach, 2019; Jayaraman et al., 2018; Piano et al., 2018; Pose & Cardenas, 2017; Venkat et al., 2019).
   A. Etiology
      1. Ascites occurs most frequently from decompensation of the following.
         a) Preexisting liver disease: Cirrhosis of which 60% will develop ascites within 10 years
         b) CHF
      2. Malignant ascites accounts for approximately 10% of all cases of ascites and is a manifestation of advanced disease. It may be presenting symptom at time of cancer diagnosis.
   B. History
      1. History of cancer and cancer treatment
      2. Current medications: Prescribed, over the counter, herbals
      3. History of presenting symptoms: Precipitating factors, onset, location, duration, associated symptoms (e.g., shortness of breath, weight gain, change in abdomen size, edema of ankles or legs, change in appetite)
      4. Changes in ADLs: Difficulty with dressing caused by increased abdominal girth and fatigue

     5. Past medical history: Liver disease, CHF, trauma, viral hepatitis, nonalcoholic fatty liver disease

     6. Social history: Alcohol use

C. Signs and symptoms

     1. Abdominal pain

     2. Abdominal fullness or pressure

     3. Abdominal distention: May be painless or associated with abdominal discomfort

     4. Shortness of breath

     5. Nausea

     6. Anorexia

     7. Early satiety

     8. Weight gain

     9. Flank pain

     10. Penile and scrotal edema

     11. Orthopnea

     12. Peripheral edema

     13. Altered bowel habits

     14. Increased abdominal girth

D. Physical examination: At least several hundred milliliters of fluid must be present to detect by physical examination. Flank dullness is noted on abdominal examination.

     1. Vital signs: Weight typically increased

     2. Pulmonary: Dullness and decreased or absent breath sound indicating pulmonary effusions, rales, or congestion

     3. Abdominal examination to confirm presence of fluid: Distention caused by the amount of fluid; deceptive because of bowel gas, stool from constipation, or bulky tumors

        a) Fluid wave on palpation, in the presence of ascites, will be positive.

        b) Assess for shifting dullness to ascertain ascites; dullness at the dependent side indicates ascites.

        c) Assess for the presence of a bulging flank.

        d) Increased venous distention occurs with abdominal distention.

        e) Monitoring abdominal girth is an unreliable gauge of fluid loss because of GI tract influences.

        f) Umbilicus may be flattened or slightly protuberant. A periumbilical nodule (Sister Mary Joseph's nodule) that is not bowel or omentum suggests an abdominal malignancy as a cause of ascites.

           (1) Grade 1 (mild): Detected only by ultrasound

           (2) Grade 2 (moderate): Symmetrical distention of the abdomen

           (3) Grade 3 (tense): Marked abdominal distention

     4. Edema: May be present in the extremities, sacrum, penis, scrotum, and other areas indicating ascites

     5. Integument: Palmar erythema and spider angiomata seen in cirrhosis

E. Assessment scale: Use NCI CTEP's Common Terminology Criteria for Adverse Events grading scale (NCI CTEP, 2017).

     1. Grade 1: Asymptomatic; clinical or diagnostic observation only; intervention not indicated

     2. Grade 2: Symptomatic; medical intervention needed

     3. Grade 3: Severe symptoms; invasive intervention needed

     4. Grade 4: Life-threatening consequences; urgent operative intervention indicated

     5. Grade 5: Death

IV. Diagnostic tests (Piano et al., 2018; Rudralingam et al., 2017; Venkat et al., 2019)
  A. Laboratory: Related to the underlying cause of ascites
    1. CBC
      a) Thrombocytopenia may be related to cirrhosis.
      b) Leukocytosis may be present with infection.
    2. Serum sodium: Hypervolemic hyponatremia with serum sodium concentration less than 135 mEq/L occurs in approximately one-half of patients with cirrhosis and ascites.
    3. Electrolytes to assess for azotemia and increased creatinine indicating renal failure: Electrolyte imbalance may be present.
    4. LFTs: Elevations may indicate liver damage or failure.
    5. PT, PTT: Prolongation suggests advanced liver disease.
    6. INR: It is elevated with cirrhosis.
    7. Amylase is elevated in pancreatic disorders.
    8. Diagnostic paracentesis
      a) It is central to determining cause of ascites and ruling out spontaneous bacterial peritonitis.
      b) Appearance is clear, bloody, cloudy, or milky.
      c) Test fluid for cell count and total protein, and determine the albumin gradient, culture and sensitivity, cytology, and amylase.
      d) Transudate fluid is clear or straw-colored with low protein content (less than 25 g/L), low specific gravity (less than 1.016), low cell count, and a high gradient difference in the albumin concentration between the serum and ascitic fluid.
      e) Exudate fluid has a low gradient difference in the albumin concentration and high protein (greater than 25 g/L).
      f) Serum-ascites albumin gradient or gap
        (1) This calculation helps to determine the cause of ascites. It is more useful than the traditional method of classifying ascites fluid as transudative or exudative.
        (2) The gradient is calculated by subtracting the albumin concentration of the ascitic fluid from the serum albumin concentration collected on the same day.
        (3) Patients with a high gradient (greater than 1.1 g/dl) are more likely to have cirrhosis, portal hypertension, alcoholic hepatitis, cardiac failure, hepatic failure, or portal vein thrombosis.
        (4) If gradient is greater than 1.1 g/dl, patients are more likely to respond to medical therapy such as diuretics.
        (5) Patients with a lower gradient (less than 1 g/dl) are more likely to have malignant ascites, peritoneal carcinomatosis, pancreatic or biliary ascites, peritoneal TB, nephrotic syndrome, bowel obstruction, or infarction. These patients and their condition do not respond well to diuretics.
      g) RBCs suggest hemorrhagic ascites, usually from malignancy, TB, or trauma.
      h) Amylase elevation suggests pancreatic disorders.
      i) Elevation of mononuclear cells (i.e., WBCs) suggests TB or fungal infection.
      j) Elevation of polymorphonuclear cells suggests bacterial infection.
      k) Nearly 100% of patients with peritoneal carcinomatosis will have positive cytology; however, approximately two-thirds of patients with malignancy-related ascites have peritoneal carcinomatosis.
      l) Culture fluid if infection is suspected.
      m) Bilirubin concentration may be indicative of bowel or biliary perforation.

n) White, milky fluid indicates chylous fluid; bloody fluid that clears during procedure may be related to trauma from the paracentesis.

9. Tumor markers may be indicated to detect malignancy-related ascites (see Appendix O).
10. Ammonia level: If encephalopathy is suspected, especially with altered mental status
11. Albumin: Decreased in malnutrition

B. Radiology
1. Abdominal ultrasound to confirm presence of ascites and rule out veno-occlusive disease
   a) Ascites becomes visible when volume approaches approximately 500 ml.
   b) Fluid etiology, amount, location, and ability to be drained can be assessed.
   c) Most abdominal ultrasounds focus on gallbladder and do not examine the spleen, necessitating the order of a complete abdominal ultrasound.
2. An abdominal CT scan or MRI may be indicated to identify source or disease progression.

V. Differential diagnosis (Kockerling et al., 2019; Piano et al., 2018; Venkat et al., 2019)
A. Alcohol-induced cirrhosis or hepatitis (see Chapters 69 and 74)
B. Cardiomyopathy (see Chapter 41)
C. Peritoneal disease
D. Portal hypertension
E. Hepatorenal syndrome
F. Acute tubular necrosis
G. Malignancy-related disorder
1. Adenocarcinoma of the peritoneum
2. Primary mesothelioma
3. Ovarian cancer
4. Chronic lymphocytic leukemia
5. Hepatocellular carcinoma
6. Peritoneal and abdominal metastasis
7. Liver metastasis
H. Liver disease
1. Acute liver disease: Drug toxicity (see Chapter 75), viral
2. Hepatic vein occlusion: Budd-Chiari syndrome
3. Bile ascites
4. Chronic liver disease: Substance abuse, toxicity, viral
5. Nonalcoholic steatohepatitis
I. Mesenteric inflammatory disease
J. Constrictive pericarditis (see Chapter 50)
K. Hemochromatosis (see Chapter 121)
L. Amyloidosis
M. TB peritonitis
N. IVC obstruction
O. Hypoalbuminemia
1. Nephrotic syndrome (see Chapter 91)
2. Protein-losing enteropathy
3. Malnutrition
P. Myxedema (see Chapter 158)
Q. Pancreatitis (see Chapter 77)
R. Chylous ascites
S. Ovarian overstimulation syndrome
T. Nephrogenic ascites

VI. Treatment: Under optimal conditions, the capacity to reabsorb ascitic fluid is no more than 700–900 ml daily; therefore, diuresis should proceed gradually (Caldwell et al., 2018; Chen et al., 2018; Jayaraman et al., 2018; Kasztelan-Szczerbinska & Cichoz-Lach, 2019; Piano et al., 2018; Pose & Cardenas, 2017; Rosenblatt et al., 2019; Venkat et al., 2019).

A. Monitor weight daily or every other day using the same scale.

B. Attempt dietary restriction of sodium to 2–4 g daily in patients with nonmalignant ascites (e.g., portal hypertension).

1. Noncompliance with dietary restriction sometimes is overlooked as a cause of refractory ascites.

2. In the absence of encephalopathy, protein intake of 50 g daily is recommended.

3. Free water fluid restriction is not necessary unless patients have hypervolemic hyponatremia with serum sodium less than 130 mEq/L, together with ascites and/or edema (see Chapter 155).

C. The goal of diuretic therapy should be a daily weight loss of 0.5–1 kg with edema and 0.25 kg without edema if diuresis has not occurred with dietary restriction of sodium.

1. Patients with grade 1 ascites do not require specific treatment but should avoid alcohol and foods with large amounts of salt.

2. Patients with grade 2 ascites are managed with sodium restriction and diuretics.

   a) Initiate spironolactone (50–100 mg PO daily) to reach weight loss goal. If needed, doses can be increased up to 400 mg PO daily.

   b) Furosemide can be added at 20–40 mg PO daily and increased up to 160 mg PO daily, if needed.

3. Diuretics can cause disturbances in fluid and electrolyte balance, including hyponatremia, dehydration, renal impairment, hyperkalemia, and hypokalemia; therefore, patients should be closely followed with serum and urine electrolyte measurements within the first two weeks of starting or modifying a dose.

D. Patients with grade 3 ascites are managed with large-volume paracentesis plus albumin, along with diuretics.

E. Therapeutic paracentesis is performed for symptomatic relief in patients with pain, shortness of breath, and cardiac dysfunction.

1. Paracentesis of up to 1 L daily may provide relief of acute respiratory symptoms; in portal hypertension, 3–4 L can be safely removed.

2. Care must be taken to preserve intravascular volume.

3. In larger-volume paracentesis (greater than 5 L), replacement of 25% albumin 6–8 g IV for each liter of ascitic fluid removed may prevent reduction in plasma volume. Of note, albumin does not reverse the underlying cause of ascites.

4. In larger-volume paracentesis, replacement of albumin 10 g IV for each liter of ascitic fluid removed may prevent reduction in plasma volume; however, this is rarely necessary.

5. Other volume expanders (e.g., dextran) may be used; however, their effect on morbidity and mortality is uncertain. Dextran may precipitate variceal hemorrhage in patients with portal hypertension.

6. Placement of a PleurX® subcutaneous tunneled catheter may reduce repeated paracentesis.

   a) Completion rate is similar to large volume paracentesis.

   b) When being used in the home setting, carefully instruct caregivers about the dangers of overdrainage, as well as the likelihood of reaccumulation.

F. Peritoneovenous shunts (e.g., LeVeen, Denver®) are used for patients who are refractory to all medical interventions and have disabling symptoms.

       1. Restrict use of shunts for patients with normal hepatic function.

       2. Shunts have poor outcomes and often fail early after placement; therefore, they usually are not indicated for malignant ascites.

   G. A TIPS is a nonsurgical technique to decompress the portal circulation by insertion of an intrahepatic stent between the hepatic vein and the portal vein using a transjugular approach. This prevents ascites by reducing portal pressure.

       1. Survival after TIPS insertion is related to the severity of liver function impairment.

       2. Occlusions and stenosis occur frequently and can lead to hepatic (i.e., portosystemic) encephalopathy in approximately 30% of patients.

   H. In patients with malignant ascites, systemic or intraperitoneal chemotherapy is aimed at the primary tumor. When the primary site is unknown, median survival rarely is affected by empiric therapy.

   I. Supportive measures to provide symptomatic relief (e.g., positioning, lower-extremity elevation, immersion in pool or whirlpool bath, use of pillows to support abdomen) may be beneficial and ultimately improve QOL for patients.

   J. Depending on the patient's condition, if the ascites is due to cirrhosis, a liver transplant may be an option.

VII. Follow-up: Dependent on disease state and cause

   A. Patients should schedule regular healthcare provider visits for physical examinations and to monitor laboratory values (e.g., BUN, creatinine, electrolytes, ammonia) and nutritional status.

   B. Shunt patency must be monitored with abdominal ultrasound at least every six months in patients who have undergone a TIPS insertion.

   C. Patients with peritoneovenous shunts need frequent monitoring of shunt function.

VIII. Referrals

   A. Dietitian: For dietary modification and counseling

   B. Gastroenterologist: If endoscopy is indicated for diagnostic purposes

   C. Surgeon: If biopsy is indicated or for shunt placement

   D. Internist: For newly diagnosed ascites, worsening encephalopathy, unexplained fever, increasing azotemia, and GI bleeding

   E. Home health: For in-home teaching, management of drainage and drainage devices

   F. Hospice: For palliative treatment to manage ascites, if appropriate

The author would like to acknowledge Miriam Rogers, EdD, APRN, AOCN®, CNS, for her contribution to this chapter that remains unchanged from the previous edition of this book.

References

Caldwell, J., Edriss, H., & Nugent, K. (2018). Chronic peritoneal indwelling catheters for the management of malignant and nonmalignant ascites. *Baylor University Medical Center Proceedings, 31*(3), 297–302. https://doi.org/10.1080/08998280.2018.1461525

Chen, B.S., Wong, S.H.C., Hawkins, S., & Huggins, L. (2018). Permanent peritoneal ports for the management of recurrent malignant ascites: A retrospective review of safety and efficacy. *Internal Medicine Journal, 48*(12), 1524–1528. https://doi.org/10.1111/imj.14137

Day, R., Hollywood, C., Durrant, D., & Perkins, P. (2015). Patient experience of non-malignant ascites and its treatment: A qualitative study. *International Journal of Palliative Nursing, 21*(8), 372–379. https://doi.org/10.12968/ijpn.2015.21.8.372

Jayaraman, S., Anand, J., & Hepsy, Y.S. (2018). Awareness, attitude and self-care activities related to management of ascites. *International Journal of Nursing Education, 10*(1), 132–138.

Kasztelan-Szczerbinska, B., & Cichoz-Lach, H. (2019). Refractory ascites—The contemporary view on pathogenesis and therapy. *PeerJ, 7,* e7855. https://doi.org/10.7717/peerj.7855

Kockerling, D., Nathwani, R., Forlano, R., Manousou, P., Mullish, B.H., & Dhar, A. (2019). Current and future pharmacological therapies for managing cirrhosis and its complications. *World Journal of Gastroenterology, 25*(8), 888–908. https://doi.org/10.3748/wjg.v25.i8.888

National Cancer Institute Cancer Therapy Evaluation Program. (2017). *Common terminology criteria for adverse events.* [v.5.0]. https://ctep.cancer.gov/protocoldevelopment/electronic_applications/docs/CTCAE_v5_Quick_Reference_8.5x11.pdf.

Piano, S., Tonon, M., & Angeli, P. (2018). Management of ascites and hepatorenal syndrome. *Hepatology International, 12*(1), 122–134. https://doi.org/10.1007/s12072-017-9815-0

Pose, E., & Cardenas, A. (2017). Translating our current understanding of ascites management into new therapies for patients with cirrhosis and fluid retention. *Digestive Diseases, 35*(4), 402–410. https://doi.org/10.1159/000456595

Rosenblatt, R., Tafesh, Z., Shen, N., Cohen-Mekelburg, S., Kumar, S., Lucero, C., ... Jesudian, A. (2019). Early paracentesis in high-risk hospitalized patients: Time for a new quality indicator. *American Journal of Gastroenterology, 114*(12), 1863–1869. https://doi.org/10.14309/ajg.0000000000000443

Rudralingam, V., Footitt, C., & Layton, B. (2017). Ascites matters. *Ultrasound, 25*(2), 69–79. https://doi.org/10.1177/1742271X16680653

Venkat, S., Maughan, K., III, Sandhu, J., Wempe, E.P., & Miller, Z.A. (2019). Malignant ascites: An overview of management with tunneled peritoneal drainage catheters. *Journal of Radiology Nursing, 38*(2), 106–109. https://doi.org/10.1016/j.jradnu.2019.01.009

CHAPTER 55

Constipation

Rebecca A. Hawkins, MSN, ARNP

I. Definition: Constipation differs from patient report versus a formal criteria (Gray, 2011; Hellström & Benno, 2019; Lacy, 2019; Simren et al., 2017).
   A. Patient report: A reduced frequency and ease of stool passage occurs from what is deemed as normal or expected from a usual pattern.
   B. Rome IV: At least two of the following criteria must be met for diagnosis of functional constipation.
      1. Straining during defecation
      2. Lumpy or hard stools
      3. Sensation of incomplete evacuation
      4. Sensation of anorectal obstruction/blockage
      5. Need for manual maneuvers to facilitate defecation
      6. Fewer than three defecations per week
   C. Chronic idiopathic constipation: This functional bowel disorder is characterized by difficult, infrequent, and/or incomplete defecation.

II. Physiology/Pathophysiology (Diaz et al., 2020; Müller-Lissner et al., 2017; Palit et al., 2012)
   A. Normal
      1. Elimination of fecal waste products requires coordination and function of the intestinal, muscular, and neural apparatuses.
         a) GI motility
         b) Mucosal transport
         c) Intact enteric nervous system
      2. The colon mixes and propels the contents through the bowel and absorbs water and electrolytes from stool.
      3. Propulsive movements, or peristalsis, move the contents forward in the colon and allow for absorption.
      4. Peristalsis occurs one to four times per day in response to strong mechanical stretching of the bowel and neural stimuli.
      5. Regular bowel function is dependent on the following.
         a) Absorption of water from intraluminal contents
         b) Normal peristalsis, propulsion of colonic contents at adequate rate
         c) Sensory awareness (via the cerebral cortex) of rectal filling
         d) Motor control of the anal sphincter with adequate rectal capacity
         e) Compliance with the urge to defecate by relaxation of the pelvic floor and anal sphincter

B. Pathophysiology: A decrease in colonic motility occurs as a result of metabolic and endocrine disturbances (Lalwani et al., 2019; Müller-Lissner et al., 2017; Rao et al., 2016; Sharma & Rao, 2017).

1. Peristalsis can become slow or sluggish, resulting in longer transit time and increased fluid absorption, which results in dry, hard stool.
2. Metabolic alterations decrease colonic contractions of smooth muscles, leading to slower motility.
3. Pelvic floor dysfunction is manifested by laxity of the pelvic floor muscles, impaired rectal sensation, and/or decreased anal canal and sphincter function.
4. Opioid-induced constipation causes delayed gastric emptying with constriction of the pyloric sphincter and impaired transit through the ileocecal sphincter and colon. This is caused by inhibition of the release of acetylcholine from the myenteric plexus, which leads to a relaxation of the longitudinal musculature of the colon and small intestine.

III. Clinical features: Normal frequency of bowel movements varies greatly, from two or three movements daily to one movement every three to five days. A change or decrease in the patient's normal frequency is significant. Most constipation is self-managed; subsequently, the prevalence of chronic constipation is hard to accurately determine. Constipation has been estimated to occur in 1.9%–27.2% of the U.S. population. Symptoms vary from patient to patient and impact all age groups. Constipation is a common complaint in older adults. Appropriate management requires an evaluation for secondary etiologies (e.g., systemic disorders, drug induced) (Bharucha & Wald, 2019; Diaz et al., 2020; Lacy, 2019; Palit et al., 2012; Pont et al., 2019; Rao et al., 2016; Schiller, 2019; Sharma & Rao, 2017).

A. Etiology: The etiology of constipation is varied, and multiple etiologies may exist at one time.

1. Medication induced
    a) Calcium supplements: Antacids
    b) Antiepileptics
    c) Antiemetics: 5-HT$_3$ antagonists
    d) Antihypertensives
    e) Antiparkinsonians
    f) Anticholinergics, antihistamines, first-generation antihistamines (see Appendix H)
    g) Antidepressants, antipsychotics
    h) Antitussives
    i) Antidiarrheal agents
    j) Vinca alkaloids
    k) Diuretics
    l) Iron supplementation
    m) Opioids
2. Metabolic causes: Dehydration, hypercalcemia, hypokalemia, uremia, hypothyroidism, diabetes
3. Neurologic causes: Cerebral tumors, SCC, sacral nerve infiltration, autonomic nervous system failure, Hirschsprung disease
4. Structural abnormalities: Pelvic tumor mass, radiation fibrosis, painful anorectal conditions, uncontrolled pain
5. Functional factors: Decreased food and fluids, lack of privacy or comfort when toileting, older age, decreased activity, confinement to bed, depression

B. History
1. History of cancer and cancer treatment
2. Current medications: Prescribed, over the counter (e.g., laxative use)
3. History of presenting symptoms: Precipitating factors, onset, location, duration
4. Changes in ADLs
5. Past medical history: Depression, diabetes, hypothyroidism, IBS, chronic laxative use
6. History of normal bowel habits
C. Signs and symptoms: Use a stool scale to obtain an accurate description, such as sausage shaped or pudding like.
1. Increased hardness of the stool or difficulty in moving bowels
2. Decreased frequency of defecation
3. Abdominal distention and bloating
4. Abdominal pain
5. Anal pain or tenderness
6. Nausea and vomiting
7. Tenesmus
8. Feeling of incomplete evacuation
9. Fecal impaction
D. Physical examination
1. Abdominal
   a) Normal, hypoactive, or no bowel sounds
   b) No hyperactive rushes or tinkles: Hyperactive rushes suggestive of obstruction
   c) No abdominal tenderness but possible distention
   d) Palpable stool in lower quadrants
2. Rectal
   a) Stool color and consistency; occult blood testing
   b) Masses, fissures, inflammation, and hard stool on inspection and palpation
   c) Sphincter control
   d) External or prolapsed hemorrhoids

IV. Diagnostic tests: Extensive testing usually is reserved for those with severe symptoms or a sudden change in number or consistency of bowel movements. Diagnostic workup is indicated for those with blood noted in the stool (Forootan et al., 2018; Gray, 2011; Hellström & Benno, 2019; Lalwani et al., 2019; Sharma & Rao, 2017; Simren et al., 2017).
A. Laboratory
1. Stool specimen for occult blood
2. Potassium level to evaluate for hypokalemia
3. TSH to evaluate for hypothyroidism after other causes have been eliminated
4. Calcium level to evaluate for hypercalcemia
5. BUN and creatinine levels to evaluate hydration status
6. Glucose or Hgb A1c, as indicated
B. Radiology
1. Abdominal flat plate x-ray to evaluate for obstruction
2. Colorectal transit study
   a) Used in chronic constipation
   b) Shows food transitioning through the colon
   c) Patient swallows capsules containing radioisotopes, which are followed through the colon by x-ray for three to seven days.
3. Anorectal function tests
   a) Diagnose constipation caused by abnormal functioning of the anus or rectum.

        b) Evaluate anal sphincter muscle function.

        c) Balloon expulsion test: A catheter or air-filled balloon is inserted into the anus and slowly pulled back through the sphincter muscle to measure tone and contractions.

        d) Defecography or magnetic resonance defecography: Defecography uses fluoroscopy and evaluates the anorectal area and the completeness of stool elimination and anorectal abnormalities. The magnetic resonance defecography eliminates radiation exposure.

    4. Colonic transit assessment test: Provides useful insights regarding overall colonic motor function, and can be performed using one of three methods

        a) Radio-opaque marker

        b) Wireless motility capsule

        c) Colonic and/or anorectal manometry

    5. Barium enema

        a) This views the rectum, colon, and lower part of the small intestine to locate abnormalities.

        b) Test will evaluate for obstruction, Hirschsprung disease, and decreased motility due to nerve damage.

        c) The colon is filled with barium, and an x-ray is taken to reveal abnormalities.

C. Other

    1. Sigmoidoscopy examination of the rectum and lower colon

    2. Colonoscopy examination of the rectum and entire colon

    3. Endoscopy when there are other warning signs, such as bleeding and new onset of constipation

D. Diagnostic criteria: Rome IV bowel disorders

    1. IBS

        a) IBS with predominant constipation (IBS-C)

        b) IBS with predominant diarrhea (IBS-D)

        c) IBS with mixed bowel habits (IBS-M)

        d) IBS unclassified (IBS-U)

    2. Functional constipation

    3. Functional diarrhea

    4. Functional abdominal bloating and distension

    5. Unspecified functional bowel disorder

    6. Opioid-induced constipation

V. Differential diagnosis (Bharucha & Wald, 2019; Hellström & Benno, 2019; Schiller, 2019)

A. Medication induced

    1. Opioids: Narcotic bowel syndrome (opioid-induced constipation)

    2. Anticholinergic agents

    3. Antidepressants

    4. 5-HT_3 receptor antagonist

    5. Chronic laxative use

    6. Vinca alkaloids and taxanes

    7. Iron preparations

    8. Calcium- or aluminum-containing antacids

    9. Diuretics

    10. Anticonvulsants

    11. Antispasmodics

    12. Antiparkinsonian drugs

B. Colonic tumors
C. Hypothyroidism (see Chapter 158)
D. IBS (see Chapter 76)
E. Diabetes mellitus (see Chapter 151)
F. Cushing syndrome
G. Diverticulitis (see Chapter 70)
H. Radiographic barium impaction
I. Dehydration
J. Immobility
K. Neurologic disorders
    1. SCC (see Chapter 145)
    2. Neuropathy
L. Electrolyte imbalances: Hypercalcemia and hypokalemia (see Chapters 152 and 153)
M. Emotional difficulties (see Chapters 161 and 162)

VI. Treatment (Bharucha & Wald, 2019; Diaz et al., 2020; Hayat et al., 2017; Lacy, 2019; Müller-Lissner et al., 2017; Pont et al., 2019; Sharma & Rao, 2017; Wang & Yin, 2015)
  A. Diet modification
    1. Encourage a high-fiber diet and increased fluid intake.
    2. Changing diet to treat constipation may not be sufficient or possible, especially in terminally ill patients.
    3. Diet will not affect constipation caused by opioids.
  B. Encourage activity and exercise, if appropriate.
  C. Set up a bowel regimen. It must be simple and used for prevention in patients receiving opioids (see Table 55-1).
    1. Chronic constipation, such as with the use of opioids, requires a stool softener and a laxative.

TABLE 55-1   **Pharmacologic Therapy for Constipation**

Therapy	Action	Onset	Examples	Comments
Bulk laxatives	Increase peristalsis by increasing size and weight of stool	12 hours to several days	Calcium polycarbophil, up to 1 tablespoon (2 g fiber) or 4 caplets (500 mg fiber/caplet), PO three times a day Methylcellulose 1 tablespoon (2 g) three times a day Psyllium 1 tablespoon (3.5 g fiber) PO once to three times a day	Laxatives work best with increased amounts of fluids and may not be feasible in patients with cancer.
Large bowel stimulants	Stimulate colonic motility	Several hours to days	Senna 1–6 tablets PO daily Bisacodyl 10–30 mg PO daily;10 mg suppository daily Phenolphthalein 1 or 2 tablets PO at bedtime Casanthranol plus docusate sodium 1 or 2 capsules PO once or three times a day	Stimulants can cause gastric irritation and are contraindicated in suspected intestinal obstruction or severe dehydration.

(Continued on next page)

TABLE 55-1	Pharmacologic Therapy for Constipation *(Continued)*			
Therapy	**Action**	**Onset**	**Examples**	**Comments**
Lubricants	Coat the stool and reduce friction	8 hours	Mineral oil 10–30 ml PO daily	Excessive doses can lead to seepage and malabsorption of fat-soluble vitamins.
Osmotic laxatives	Increase gastric, pancreatic, and small intestine secretion and increase motor activity of the small and large bowel	1–12 hours	Magnesium hydroxide (milk of magnesia) 30–60 ml PO Magnesium citrate 200 ml PO Sodium phosphate 30 ml PO or per enema	Avoid in patients with renal dysfunction. It may be problematic in patients with cardiac or renal disease.
	Nonabsorbable sugars that exert an osmotic effect in both the small and large intestines	30 minutes to several hours	Lactulose (5 grains/15 ml) 15–30 ml (up to 60 ml) PO daily Sorbitol 30–60 ml PO daily Glycerin suppository (2 or 3 g) per rectum for 15 minutes daily Polyethylene glycol 17 g PO in 8 oz water Polyethylene glycol 8.5–34 g PO daily in 240 ml (8 oz) liquid; not recommended for longer than 2 weeks Magnesium sulfate 5–10 gm in 240 ml water daily Magnesium citrate 200 ml PO daily	Watch for signs of dehydration, as it may cause nausea, bloating, and cramping.
Surfactants (softeners)	Reduce surface tension and allow penetration of water and fats into the stool	Several hours	Docusate sodium 50–500 mg PO daily Docusate calcium 240 mg PO daily	Softeners or surfactants are often used with other laxatives.
Other	Opioid binding at the mu-opioid receptor in periphery	Several hours	Methylnaltrexone 0.15 mg/kg subcutaneous every other day	Do not use with gastrointestinal obstruction or lesion of gastrointestinal tract.

Note. Based on information from Bharucha & Wald, 2019; Hayat et al., 2017; Müller-Lissner et al., 2017; Pont et al., 2019.

     2. If bowel program does not work within two days of initiating, change medications or classes of drugs.

D. Biofeedback is used for constipation caused by pelvic floor dysfunction and provides retraining of the pelvic floor muscles.

E. Acupuncture has been shown to improve chronic constipation.

F. Avoid suppositories or enemas in patients with thrombocytopenia or immunosuppression.

G. Probiotic supplements may be beneficial in relieving symptoms.

VII. Follow-up
  A. Short term: Patients should be called to see if bowel program is working within 24–48 hours of starting the medications.
  B. Long term: Patients with cancer, especially those on opioids, need constant follow-up regarding constipation and the effectiveness of their bowel program.

VIII. Referrals
  A. Dietitian: To make diet and hydration recommendations when appropriate
  B. Internist: If unable to relieve constipation effectively
  C. Oncologist: If patient needs to be admitted for narcotic bowel syndrome (opioid-induced constipation)
  D. Acupuncture: For those seeking complementary therapy for constipation

References

Bharucha, A.E., & Wald, A. (2019). Chronic constipation. *Mayo Clinic Proceedings, 94*(11), 2340–2357. https://doi.org/10.1016/j.mayocp.2019.01.031

Diaz, S., Bittar, K., & Mendez, M.D. (2020). Constipation. In *StatPearls*. https://www.ncbi.nlm.nih.gov/books/NBK513291

Forootan, M., Bagheri, N., & Darvishi, M. (2018). Chronic constipation: A review of literature. *Medicine, 97*(20), e10631. https://doi.org/10.1097/MD.0000000000010631

Gray, J.R. (2011). What is chronic constipation? Definition and diagnosis. *Canadian Journal of Gastroenterology, 25*(Suppl. B), 7B–10B.

Hayat, U., Dugum, M., & Garg, S. (2017). Chronic constipation: Update on management. *Cleveland Clinic Journal of Medicine, 84*(5), 397–408. https://doi.org/10.3949/ccjm.84a.15141

Hellström, P.M., & Benno, P. (2019). The Rome IV: Irritable bowel syndrome—A functional disorder. *Best Practice and Research: Clinical Gastroenterology, 40–41,* 101634. https://doi.org/10.1016/j.bpg.2019.101634

Lacy, B.E. (2019). Update on the management of chronic idiopathic constipation. *American Journal of Managed Care, 25*(Suppl. 4), S55–S62. https://www.ajmc.com/view/update-on-the-management-of-chronic-idiopathic-constipati

Lalwani, N., El Sayed, R.F., Kamath, A., Lewis, S., Arif, H., & Chernyak, V. (2019). Imaging and clinical assessment of functional defecatory disorders with emphasis on defecography. *Abdominal Radiology, 46*(4), 1323–1333. https://doi.org/10.1007/s00261-019-02142-9

Müller-Lissner, S., Bassotti, G., Coffin, B., Drewes, A.M., Breivik, H., Eisenberg, E., … Morlion, B. (2017). Opioid-induced constipation and bowel dysfunction: A clinical guideline. *Pain Medicine, 18*(10), 1837–1863. https://doi.org/10.1093/pm/pnw255

Palit, S., Lunniss, P.J., & Scott, S.M. (2012). The physiology of human defecation. *Digestive Diseases and Sciences, 57*(6), 1445–1464. https://doi.org/10.1007/s10620-012-2071-1

Pont, L.G., Fisher, M., & Williams, K. (2019). Appropriate use of laxatives in the older person. *Drugs and Aging, 36*(11), 999–1005. https://doi.org/10.1007/s40266-019-00701-9

Rao, S.S.C., Rattanakovit, K., & Patcharatrakul, T. (2016). Diagnosis and management of chronic constipation in adults. *Nature Reviews Gastroenterology and Hepatology, 13*(5), 295–305. https://doi.org/10.1038/nrgastro.2016.53

Schiller, L.R. (2019). Chronic constipation: New insights, better outcomes? *Lancet Gastroenterology and Hepatology, 4*(11), 873–882. https://doi.org/10.1016/S2468-1253(19)30199-2

Sharma, A., & Rao, S. (2017). Constipation: Pathophysiology and current therapeutic approaches. In B. Greenwood-Van Meerveld (Ed.), *Handbook of experimental pharmacology: Vol. 239. Gastrointestinal pharmacology* (pp. 59–74). Springer. https://doi.org/10.1007/164_2016_111

Simren, M., Palsson, O.S., & Whitehead, W.E. (2017). Update on Rome IV criteria for colorectal disorders: Implications for clinical practice. *Current Gastroenterology Reports, 19*(4), 15. https://doi.org/10.1007/s11894-017-0554-0

Wang, X., & Yin, J. (2015). Complementary and alternative therapies for chronic constipation. *Evidence-Based Complementary and Alternative Medicine, 2015,* 396396. https://doi.org/10.1155/2015/396396

CHAPTER 56

Diarrhea

Jeanne Held-Warmkessel, MSN, RN, AOCN®, ACNS-BC

I. Definition: Abnormal increase in frequency, volume, and/or liquid content of stool; more than three loose stools per 24-hour period; frequent loose stools with urgency (Reintam Blaser et al., 2015)

II. Physiology/Pathophysiology (Harb et al., 2014; Pezo et al., 2019; Prieux-Klotz et al., 2017; Raman, 2017; Reintam Blaser et al., 2015; Townsend et al., 2019)
   A. Normal
      1. Food is passed through the stomach to the bowel, where nutrients and water are absorbed.
      2. The majority of liquid is removed from the stool as it transits the bowel so that only 200 ml of water usually is present in a formed stool as it is evacuated.
      3. Peristaltic waves are responsible for the movement of stool through the bowel.
   B. Pathophysiology
      1. Osmotic diarrhea results from consumption of substances (food or drug) that create an increased amount of osmotic activity in the intestine. This increases the amount of water drawn into the colon and, thus, in the stool and usually is not associated with nocturnal stools.
      2. Secretory diarrhea is caused by a disruption in normal colonic epithelial cell transport of ions with increased intestinal mucosal secretion of fluid and electrolytes. It is associated with diurnal and nocturnal stools.
      3. Motility abnormalities occur when slow colon transit times allow bacterial overgrowth, which may cause diarrhea. Increased motility may cause reduced absorption.
      4. Exudative diarrhea results from alteration in the integrity of colonic mucosa from ulcers, inflammatory process, or radiation therapy.
      5. Malabsorptive diarrhea is caused by a combination of altered mucosal contiguity, altered bowel structure, or enzyme changes.
      6. Chemotherapy-induced diarrhea occurs due to a combination of intestinal inflammation, changes in villi, malabsorption, and secretory changes.
      7. Radiation-induced diarrhea/enteritis
         a) Acute: Radiation to intestines causes damage to crypt stem cells, resulting in apoptosis. Damage to the lining of the intestinal blood vessel may add to enteritis development.
         b) Chronic: Damage to blood vessels results in vasculature occlusion, leading to ischemia, fibrosis, telangiectasia, and additional changes resulting in malabsorption and altered intestinal motility.
      8. Inflammatory diarrhea occurs due to injury to mucosa and mucosal vasculature; checkpoint inhibitors induce inflammatory mucosal changes.

III. Clinical features: Diarrhea is classified as acute or chronic. Acute diarrhea lasts for no more than two weeks, and chronic diarrhea lasts for four weeks or longer. Diarrhea is subjective in its definition (Camilleri et al., 2017; Faiman, 2016; Harb et al., 2014; Mileto et al., 2019; Napolitano & Edmiston, 2017; Ong et al., 2017; Pezo et al., 2019; Raman, 2017; Reintam Blaser et al., 2015; Steffen et al., 2015).

A. Etiology (see Figure 56-1)

B. History

1. History of cancer and cancer treatment: Chemotherapy, immunotherapy
2. Current medications: Prescribed, over the counter; use of PPIs, H$_2$ blockers, laxatives, stool softeners, or antibiotics (e.g., beta-lactam agents, fluoroquinolones)
3. History of presenting symptoms: Patient's definition of diarrhea; precipitating factors, color, onset, consistency, duration, pattern, frequency, associated symptoms (e.g., abdominal pain, fever, weight loss, stool incontinence, cramps, vomiting, tenesmus, thirst, weakness, fecal impaction, GI bleeding [blood in or on stool], bloating, distention, nocturnal stools, rash)
4. Changes in ADLs and QOL
5. History of bowel habits
   a) Liquid versus formed stool, consistency
   b) Onset, volume, and frequency baseline versus current
   c) Color, odor, presence of undigested food or fat
   d) Presence of blood or mucus
6. Diet history: Food intolerance, aversions, lactase deficiency and milk product consumption, food allergies, consumption of wheat fiber, high fructose corn syrup, fatty foods, caffeine, sorbitol, mannitol, and xylitol
7. Past medical history: Inflammatory bowel disease, celiac disease, endocrine disorders, HIV infection, neurologic diseases, inflammatory arthritis, connective tissue disease, diabetes
8. Past surgical history: Bowel surgery, gastric bypass surgery, cholecystectomy

---

FIGURE 56-1 **Partial List of Etiologies for Acute and Chronic Diarrhea**

Acute
- Food/diet, sorbitol, lactose, ETOH (alcohol)
- Hyperosmolar foods, liquids
- Bacteria, virus, protozoal fungus, food poisoning
- Fecal impaction
- Radiation injury
- Partial bowel obstruction
- Premenstrual syndrome, dysmenorrhea
- Dihydropyrimidine dehydrogenase deficiency
- Medications, antimicrobials, laxatives
- Acute graft-versus-host disease
- Herbs/herbal supplements
- Bowel ischemia
- Traveler's diarrhea
- Colitis
- Neutropenic enterocolitis

Chronic
- Food/diet
- Medications
- HIV-induced diarrhea, chronic infections
- Fecal impaction, fecal incontinence
- Chronic radiation-induced enteritis
- Gastrointestinal tract surgical changes
- Colon cancer, hormone-producing malignancies
- Fistula
- Chronic graft-versus-host disease
- Inflammatory bowel diseases (e.g., ulcerative colitis, Crohn disease), diverticular disease, irritable bowel syndrome
- Malabsorption (bile acid)
- Motility disorders
- Alcoholism
- Collagen vascular diseases
- Endocrine disorders (e.g., diabetes), exocrine disorders, pancreatic enzyme deficiency
- Celiac disease

Note. Based on information from Camilleri et al., 2017; Raman, 2017; Reintam Blaser et al., 2015; Schiller et al., 201/.

9. Social history: Recent travel abroad or on a cruise; exposure to farm animals or animal feces; consumption of food or fluid contaminated with feces, well water, unpasteurized milk or its products, or raw seafood; similar illness in household; occupation (e.g., food handler, daycare worker)

C. Signs and symptoms
   1. Cramping, bloating, gas
   2. Abdominal pain
   3. Rectal urgency, tenesmus
   4. Fever combined with dizziness, bloody diarrhea, or abdominal pain suggestive of severe infection
   5. Dry mucous membranes
   6. Loose, watery, frequent stools
   7. Nocturnal diarrhea
   8. Thirst indicating dehydration
   9. Dizziness
   10. Nausea
   11. Blood in stool/rectal bleeding
   12. *Clostridium difficile* infection
       a) Mild to moderate severity: Cramps, abdominal pain, fever and malaise
       b) Colitis: Diarrhea, nausea, anorexia, mild to moderate abdominal pain with or without dehydration, fever, leukocytosis
       c) Fulminant colitis: Diarrhea or ileus, severe lower quadrant or diffuse abdominal pain, distention; may progress to toxic megacolon, renal failure, sepsis, septic shock, or acute surgical abdomen requiring ICU-level care

D. Physical examination
   1. Vital signs
      a) Blood pressure, pulse, and orthostatic vital signs to assess hydration status
      b) Weight loss
      c) Temperature to assess for signs of infection or inflammation
   2. Integument: Rash, poor skin turgor, and dry mucous membranes indicating dehydration
   3. Abdominal: Auscultation, percussion, and palpation of entire abdomen
      a) Tenderness or pain suggesting inflammation or infection
      b) Organomegaly or abdominal masses
      c) Distention indicating flatus
      d) Hyperactive or hypoactive bowel sounds
      e) Tympany indicating flatus
      f) Guarding indicating infection or peritoneal irritation
      g) Rebound tenderness indicating inflammation
      h) Stoma, scars
   4. Rectal
      a) Impaction, fissures, rectocele, mass, hemorrhoids
      b) Irritated perirectal or peristomal skin
      c) Stool testing for occult blood
      d) Sphincter tone, both at rest and when asked to constrict the sphincter
      e) Tenderness
      f) Stool color, odor, and appearance
   5. Lymph: Enlargement indicating infection or malignancy (see Appendix D)

IV. Diagnostic tests (Camilleri et al., 2017; Campbell et al., 2017; Cramer & Bresalier, 2017; Friedman et al., 2016; Harb et al., 2014; Mileto et al., 2019; Napolitano & Edmiston, 2017;

Ong et al., 2017; Pezo et al., 2019; Prieux-Klotz et al., 2017; Raman, 2017; Steffen et al., 2015; Townsend et al., 2019)

A. Laboratory

1. CBC: Increased WBC count present with infection
2. BUN–creatinine ratio: Increased ratio present with dehydration
3. Urine analysis to evaluate dehydration: Typically dark yellow or orange urine and concentrated
4. Serum electrolytes and ions: Decreased potassium and magnesium and increased or decreased sodium present with diarrhea
5. Testing for dihydropyrimidine dehydrogenase deficiency if patient is receiving 5-fluorouracil or capecitabine and diarrhea occurs with acute onset (i.e., 24–48 hours after initiating chemotherapy)
6. Testing for UGT1A1 polymorphism with early onset severe diarrhea with irinotecan therapy
7. Serum albumin: Low levels produce low oncotic pressure and result in intestinal edema and poor absorption of nutrients.
8. Blood cultures if patient is febrile
9. Thyroid hormone levels to assess for thyroid disorder
10. Blood glucose level to assess for diabetes
11. LFTs, enzymes, and bilirubin to assess for abnormalities suggesting liver etiology
12. Antitissue transglutaminase antibody and antiendomysial antibody if celiac disease suspected
13. Stool specimens
    a) *C. difficile* toxin stool specimen (combination testing for glutamate dehydrogenase and rapid enzyme immunoassay for toxin A and B) if patient has received a checkpoint inhibitor, has postantibiotic diarrhea, has been exposed to *C. difficile*, has had bowel surgery, has received immune suppression or chemotherapy, has been hospitalized, or has had febrile episodes: Stool consistency must be watery liquid and patient has had three or more liquid stools in 24 hours.
    b) Stool sample
       (1) Fecal leukocyte level, occult blood, fecal lactoferrin (inflammatory diarrhea)
       (2) Fecal calprotectin for inflammation; pH as indicated
       (3) Stool electrolytes to classify diarrhea type, especially secretory diarrhea
    c) Stool culture and sensitivity if travel-associated diarrhea or infection other than *C. difficile* is suspected
       (1) Use to isolate diarrhea of unknown cause. Often, it is not positive and is expensive. Culture should be sent if lactoferrin-positive or microscopy-positive for WBCs.
       (2) Use if patient is febrile or has bloody diarrhea, dehydration, abdominal pain, dizziness, or other systemic symptoms or diarrhea lasting two weeks or longer.
       (3) Test for ova, parasites, and protozoa in patients with HIV or those who have been traveling or exposed to contaminated water and had diarrhea lasting more than two weeks.
       (4) Special stains and antigen detection assays are available for pathogen detection.
    d) Stool for fecal fat: Use for chronic diarrhea. Presence of fat suggests malabsorption or pancreatic insufficiency. A 72-hour stool collection can be measured for fat content; patient must be on a diet including 100 g of fat daily for three days. Sudan stain identifies fatty diarrhea.

  e) For chronic diarrhea: A 24-hour stool collection for quantitative analysis and volume is used to evaluate for malabsorption or pancreatic insufficiency.

  f) Blood and mucus are visible in stool from exudative diarrhea.

14. Special studies

  a) Polymerase chain reaction testing for suspected *Campylobacter* infection in stool

  b) More than three stool samples to test for giardiasis

  c) Immunologic enzyme-linked immunosorbent assay (ELISA) of stool to identify giardia antigen

  d) Rapid ELISA tests for *Rotavirus*, cholera, *Cryptosporidium*, *Giardia*, and *Campylobacter*, if indicated

15. Antibody testing: For *Strongyloides* and schistosomiasis, most commonly seen in traveler's diarrhea

B. Radiology

  1. Plain abdominal film and obstruction series if partial bowel obstruction is suspected: Dilated bowel loops or U-shaped bowel loops will be demonstrated in the presence of obstruction. It may be used to assess for colitis, *C. difficile* colitis (polypoid mucosal thickening), or megacolon.

  2. CT scan: This preferred imaging modality is useful for identifying bowel wall thickening with neutropenic enterocolitis.

    a) *C. difficile*: Bowel wall thickening, mural thickening, accordion sign, double halo sign

    b) Checkpoint inhibitors: Bowel wall thickening or segmental colitis

  3. CT or magnetic resonance enterography: Methods are useful for radiation therapy enteritis evaluation of bowel and to reveal luminal changes, such as inflammation, bowel wall thickening, and stricture formation, along with other bowel wall and intraluminal changes.

  4. Small intestine contrast studies to evaluate for small bowel disease, obstruction, polyps, or cancer

  5. Ultrasound of abdomen: Bowel wall thickening, enlarged lymph nodes

  6. Contrast-enhanced ultrasound: Bowel tissue vascularization and perfusion, active inflammation

C. Other

  1. Sigmoidoscopy/colonoscopy

    a) If antibiotic-induced pseudomembranous colitis or bleeding is suspected

    b) Chronic diarrhea: To take biopsies and visualize intestinal lumen and lining

    c) Diarrhea induced by checkpoint inhibitors: For visualization and biopsies in presence of persistent grade 2 or higher diarrhea

  2. Upper endoscopy to take biopsies and cultures for chronic diarrhea

  3. Balloon-assisted enteroscopy to advance endoscope through small bowel to visualize bowel for abnormalities

  4. Patency capsule followed by video capsule endoscopy (if other tests negative)

V. Differential diagnosis (Campbell et al., 2017; Cramer & Bresalier, 2017; Faiman, 2016; Harb et al., 2014; Raman, 2017; Reintam Blaser et al., 2015; Schiller et al., 2017; Thiagarajah et al., 2015; Townsend et al., 2019)

  A. Diet induced

    1. High-osmolar foods and fluids, sugar substitute (e.g., sorbitol)

    2. Enteral tube feedings: Initiation or change in formula or rate of infusion, lack of fiber content in tube feeding formula in use, chronic enteral nutrition, high osmolar formula, bolus feedings

      3. Lactose intolerance

      4. Food allergy

      5. High-fiber diet, fatty diet

      6. Dietary deficiencies: Vitamin A, zinc

B. Infection

      1. Bacteria: *C. difficile*, food poisoning, toxicogenic *Escherichia coli, Yersinia, Salmonella, Shigella, Campylobacter*

      2. Protozoa: *Cryptosporidium, Giardia*

      3. Parasites

      4. Viruses: HIV/AIDS, viral gastroenteritis, CMV, norovirus, rotovirus

      5. Neutropenic enterocolitis: Necrotizing enterocolitis, typhlitis

C. Drug induced

      1. Antibiotics

      2. Systemic cancer therapy

         a) Chemotherapy

            (1) 5-Fluorouracil, capecitabine: May be life threatening in patients with dihydropyrimidine dehydrogenase deficiency

            (2) Irinotecan: Can be acute (within 24 hours after infusion [cholinergic response]) or delayed (6–14 days postinfusion); especially severe in patients with UGT1A1 polymorphism (*6 and *28)

            (3) Oxaliplatin, cisplatin

            (4) Taxanes

            (5) Cyclophosphamide

            (6) Cytarabine

            (7) Methotrexate

            (8) Topotecan

            (9) Doxorubicin, pegylated liposomal doxorubicin

            (10) Hyperthermic intraperitoneal chemotherapy (HIPEC)

         b) Immunotherapy: IL-2

         c) Targeted therapy (e.g., erlotinib, lapatinib, cetuximab, panitumumab) including checkpoint inhibitors (e.g., CTLA-4, PD-1, PD-L1): May cause colitis; incidence higher with combination therapy

         d) Proteosome inhibitors, immunomodulatory agents

      3. Laxatives

      4. Diuretics

      5. Antihypertensives

      6. Antiemetics and prokinetic agents: Metoclopramide, 5-HT$_3$ antagonists

      7. H$_2$ blockers, PPIs

      8. Sorbitol-based liquid medications

      9. EPO

     10. Antacids: Magnesium or calcium based

     11. NSAIDs: Ibuprofen (see Appendix E)

     12. Caffeine, alcohol

     13. Cholinergic medications

     14. Methylnaltrexone

     15. HIV therapeutics

D. Abdominal and pelvic radiation therapy, radiation proctitis, radiation enteritis

E. Surgery that interrupts or alters intestinal continuity or function

      1. Small or large bowel resection

      2. Ileostomy, colostomy, ileoanal anastomosis

   3. Billroth I or II, gastrectomy, gastric bypass surgery
   4. Pancreatectomy
   5. Biliary surgery
   6. Vagotomy
   7. Cholecystectomy
 F. Diseases of the bowel
   1. Malignancies that produce hormones: VIPomas (secrete vasoactive intestinal poly-peptide, known as VIP), carcinoid tumors, glucagonoma, neuroendocrine tumors, other solid tumors and lymphoma
   2. Inflammatory bowel diseases: Crohn disease, ulcerative colitis
   3. IBS (see Chapter 76)
   4. Partial bowel obstruction (see Chapter 67)
   5. Diverticulosis (see Chapter 70)
   6. Enterocolic fistula
   7. Villous adenoma
   8. Diabetes mellitus and other endocrine diseases (see Chapter 151)
   9. Collagen vascular diseases
   10. Malabsorption: Fatty acid, bile salt, carbohydrate, protein, short bowel, steatorrhea
   11. Sprue: Celiac disease
   12. Hyperthyroidism (see Chapter 157), hypoparathyroidism
   13. Bowel ischemia
   14. Small intestinal bacterial overgrowth
   15. Pancreatic enzyme insufficiency
   16. Neutropenic enterocolitis
 G. Psychiatric disorders: Anxiety, nervousness, opioid withdrawal in addiction (see Chapter 161)
 H. Fecal impaction with continuous oozing of liquid stool
 I. GVHD, organ rejection

VI. Treatment (Cramer & Bresalier, 2017; Enzler & Fojo, 2017; Faiman, 2016; Friedman et al., 2016; Harb et al., 2014; McDonald et al., 2018; Mileto et al., 2019; Napolitano & Edmiston, 2017; Ong et al., 2017; Prieux-Klotz et al., 2017; Puzanov et al., 2017; Steffen et al., 2015; Thiagarajah et al., 2015; Townsend et al., 2019)
 A. Diarrhea management of patients receiving chemotherapy is undergoing constant evolution. Consult with a medical oncologist for treatment of diarrhea lasting more than 24 hours or if the patient develops other symptoms.
 B. Severe, profuse, watery diarrhea is a life-threatening emergency requiring hospitalization for diarrhea management, parenteral hydration, and electrolyte replacement (see Chapters 152–156).
 C. Diet
   1. Maintain oral hydration, at least 64 oz of liquid daily; much of the fluid should contain electrolytes, such as sodium and potassium.
   2. Alterations in diet alone may sufficiently control cancer treatment–induced diarrhea.
   3. Eliminate offending food items; avoid lactose; reduce fiber; avoid greasy, fatty, and acidic foods; and avoid alcohol and high osmolar foods.
   4. Use fiber-based tube feeding formula. Reduce rate of infusion of tube feeding, reduce osmotic load of formula, or change concentration or type of formula.
   5. BRAT diet (bananas, rice, applesauce, white toast, decaffeinated tea) may be used for a short period of time. Add soft, easy-to-digest foods as diarrhea comes under control. Avoid lactose-containing products for a few weeks.

6. Recommend low-residue diet (e.g., small, frequent bland foods high in potassium, 3 L of fluid daily) that is high in protein.

7. Suggest isotonic oral diet supplements with added flavoring. Avoid hypertonic supplements and high-glucose foods, which increase diarrhea.

8. In patients receiving chemotherapy, use lactose-free dairy products during diarrhea period and for one week after diarrhea resolves.

9. Offer soups containing salt.

10. Provide low-fiber carbohydrates (e.g., rice, bread, potatoes without skin).

11. Encourage eating small meals and avoiding fatty, spicy foods.

D. Infection: Contact precautions

1. For positive *C. difficile* toxin, start appropriate antimicrobial therapy and stop causative agent, or replace with other antimicrobial if treatment is still required.

   a) Initial infection, nonsevere and severe: Give vancomycin 125 mg PO four times a day for 10 days or fidaxomicin 200 PO two times a day for 10 days. If these agents are not available and for nonsevere diarrhea only, give metronidazole 500 mg PO three times a day for 10–14 days.

   b) Initial infection, fulminant, complicated by hypotension, sepsis, ileus, or megacolon: Give vancomycin 500 mg PO four times a day or via NG tube with (if ileus present) metronidazole 500 mg IV every eight hours. In the presence of ileus, bowel obstruction or toxic megacolon, retention enema of vancomycin 500 mg/100 ml normal saline every 6, 8, or 12 hours may be added. Administer with caution to avoid additional mucosal injury from enema.

   c) Do not use antidiarrheal agents with *C. difficile* diarrhea.

2. Patients with fever and orthostatic symptoms, bloody stool, or severe abdominal pain: Begin antibiotic therapy with oral quinolone (e.g., ciprofloxacin).

3. Patients with an identified/suspected infection: Begin appropriate antibiotic therapy. Initiate antibiotics for patients with comorbidities, older adults, and patients with implants, prolonged symptoms, or relapsing diarrhea.

4. Traveler's diarrhea: This type is often bacterial and managed with antimicrobial therapy.

E. Secretory diarrhea

1. Somatostatin analog inhibits serotonin, vasoactive intestinal polypeptide, gastrin, and other hormones; onset is 30 minutes.

2. For example, give octreotide 100–200 mcg subcutaneous every eight hours. Titrate dose PRN to control diarrhea.

F. Antibiotics (oral fluoroquinolone such as levofloxacin 500 mg daily for seven days) should be instituted in patients receiving irinotecan when antidiarrheals administered for more than 24 hours are ineffective alone in managing diarrhea. If diarrhea persists beyond 48 hours with ongoing loperamide, admit patient to hospital, administer IV fluids and antibiotics, and change antidiarrheal medication to octreotide. Send stool to test for *C. difficile* and other pathogens as appropriate.

G. Antidiarrheals (antiperistalsis): Do not use antidiarrheal agents in patients with evidence of bowel obstruction, *C. difficile* infection, or inflammatory diarrhea.

1. Loperamide

   a) Chemotherapy-associated diarrhea: Standard dose is loperamide 4 mg PO (first dose), followed by 2 mg after each loose stool, up to 16 mg daily. It is also useful for radiation-associated diarrhea.

   b) Irinotecan-associated diarrhea: Aggressive high-dose therapy is required; give 4 mg at first evidence of diarrhea and then 2 mg every two hours (4 mg every four hours during night) until diarrhea-free for 12 hours.

    c) Persistent mild to moderate chemotherapy-associated diarrhea: If after 24 hours of persistent diarrhea, a more aggressive regimen as noted in "b" for irinotecan is recommended along with an antibiotic such as ciprofloxacin for seven days. If after 48 hours of high-dose loperamide (2 mg every two hours) the patient still has diarrhea, send stool for *C. difficile* testing; check CBC and comprehensive metabolic panel; administer parenteral fluids; replace electrolytes; and stop loperamide. Consider trying octreotide or tincture of opium.

    d) Complicated chemotherapy-associated diarrhea (e.g., nausea, vomiting, severe cramps, fever, sepsis, neutropenia, bleeding, dehydration): Admit to hospital, administer parenteral IV fluids, and replace electrolytes. Send stool to test for *C. difficile* and other pathogens. Administer octreotide 100–150 mcg subcutaneous every eight hours or 25–50 mcg/hr IV. Titrate dose up to 500 mcg subcutaneous every eight hours. Administer fluoroquinolone. If fluoropyrimidine-associated diarrhea continues and fluoropyrimidine toxicity is suspected, uridine triacetate is indicated.

    e) Mild diarrhea from checkpoint inhibitor: Use with caution, up to four doses a day of loperamide.

2. Diphenoxylate and atropine: It is not for use in patients with advanced liver disease because it can cause hepatic coma. Recommended dose is 5 mg PO four times a day. Titrate dose PRN. Stop if no response after two days.

3. Opium tincture: It is used to improve GI tract muscle tone and is given 0.3–1 ml PO four times a day, not to exceed 6 ml daily.

4. Paregoric: Give 5 ml PO diluted in water every three to four hours.

5. Psyllium: Give 1 teaspoon in 2 oz water PO. Titrate dose up to amount required to produce formed stool (chronic diarrhea only).

6. Atropine: Give 0.25–1 mg subcutaneous to treat or prevent irinotecan-induced acute diarrhea.

7. Bismuth salicylate: Use for traveler's diarrhea at eight tablets daily. Antibiotics are also effective (e.g., quinolone therapy).

8. Octreotide

    a) Give 100–150 mcg subcutaneous/IV every eight hours or 25–50 mcg/hr IV as a continuous infusion. Titrate dose to optimal effect. Octreotide may be useful for patients with opioid-resistant diarrhea. For carcinoid tumors and VIPomas, titrate octreotide to achieve best results and administer in two to four divided doses daily for two weeks and then give long-acting octreotide.

    b) Long-acting octreotide: Give 20 mg IM every 28 days.

    c) Lanreotide: Give 120 mg IM every four weeks for gastroenteropancreatic neuroendocrine tumors.

9. Uridine triacetate: Give 10 g PO every six hours for 20 doses. It is used as an antidote to fluoropyrimidines, for treatment of life-threatening diarrhea that develops within 96 hours after 5-fluorouracil or capecitabine treatment. Treatment is extremely expensive. Dihydropyrimidine dehydrogenase deficiency testing should be done prior to prescribing.

10. Oral steroids for grade 2 or higher diarrhea associated with immunotherapy and checkpoint inhibitor diarrhea and colitis: Give prednisone 0.5 mg/kg PO daily or higher (1 mg/kg). Doses up to 2 mg/kg PO daily are used for refractory or severe diarrhea or grade 2 diarrhea that does not improve after two to three days of a lower dose. Continue prednisone until diarrhea grade 1 or lower and follow with a steroid taper over four weeks. IV steroids are used if oral prednisone is not effective (e.g., methylprednisolone up to 2 mg/kg two times a day).

11. Infliximab: Give 5 mg/kg IV after two to three days, or up to five days dependent on patient and drug, of grade 3–4 diarrhea treated with higher dose systemic steroids and with no improvement or with clinical deterioration/worsening symptoms. It may be administered every two weeks, if needed.

12. Cholestyramine: Give to patients with bile salt malabsorption/overproduction to produce formed stool.

H. Rectal skin care

   1. Gently cleanse skin after each stool with a mild soap and water, rinse well, and pat dry or cleanse with an aloe-based baby wipe.
   2. Apply a soothing topical agent with skin barrier properties.
   3. Use sitz baths to soothe irritated tissues.

I. Patient education: All patients require hand hygiene and food safety education, when applicable.

   1. Balance fiber consumption with the amount of stool produced.
   2. Consume a minimum of 2–3 L of fluid daily. Fluid should contain glucose.
   3. Implement oral electrolyte replacement with sports drinks or oral replacement fluids containing glucose and electrolytes and cereal-based oral rehydration solutions.
   4. Eliminate diarrhea-producing foods (e.g., milk products, carbonated drinks, caffeinated drinks, gas-producing foods, spicy foods, alcohol).
   5. Add soluble fiber (e.g., oatmeal, apples, bananas) to diet to absorb fluid from bowel or use absorptive pharmacotherapy (e.g., cholestyramine 4 mg PO three times a day). Avoid insoluble fiber found in high-fiber foods (e.g., whole grains, prunes, popcorn, bran). Avoid sorbitol found in diet foods.
   6. Notify the nurse or provider if chemotherapy-associated diarrhea lasts longer than 24 hours or if the patient develops a fever.
   7. Instruct patient to keep a food diary.

J. Disimpact stool if impacted and start daily laxative regimen.

K. Radiation therapy–induced diarrhea is managed in the same manner as chemotherapy-associated diarrhea with loperamide.

VII. Follow-up: For patients treated for positive *C. difficile* toxin (McDonald et al., 2018; Mileto et al., 2019)

   A. If diarrhea recurs in patients treated initially with metronidazole, treat with vancomycin 125 mg PO four times a day for 10 days. For patients treated initially with vancomycin, treat with fidaxomicin 200 mg two PO times a day for 10 days. Refer patient to a gastroenterologist and an infectious disease specialist, especially if severely immunocompromised.

   B. Stop PPI use. Watch for signs and symptoms of toxic megacolon. If this occurs, surgery is urgently required to prevent mortality.

VIII. Referrals (Napolitano & Edmiston, 2017; Ong et al., 2017)

   A. Dietitian: For dietary education

   B. Gastroenterologist

      1. Consult gastroenterologist to perform sigmoidoscopy or colonoscopy or to assess and manage chronic diarrhea.
      2. Diarrhea lasting longer than four weeks is classified as chronic diarrhea and requires workup to determine the etiology so that effective treatment can be instituted.
      3. Post–radiation therapy bowel changes may occur two months or more after completion of radiation therapy.

   C. Enterostomal therapist: For patients with ostomies

D. Social worker: To assist patients with chronic diarrhea with coping and medication expenses

E. Internist: For hospitalization of patients with dehydration, electrolyte/acid-base imbalance, or fever, and high-risk patients, such as older adults, those who are immunosuppressed, or those with blood in stool

F. Infectious disease specialist: For recurrent *C. difficile* infection or immunocompromised patients

References

Camilleri, M., Sellin, J.H., & Barrett, K.E. (2017). Pathophysiology, evaluation, and management of chronic watery diarrhea. *Gastroenterology, 152*(3), 515–532.e2 https://doi.org/10.1053/j.gastro.2016.10.014

Campbell, J.M., Stephenson, M.D., Bateman, E., Peters, M.D.J., Keefe, D.M., & Bowen, J.M. (2017). Irinotecan-induced toxicity pharmacogenetics: An umbrella review of systematic reviews and meta-analyses. *Pharmacogenomics Journal, 17*(1), 21–28. https://doi.org/10.1038/tpj.2016.58.

Cramer, P., & Bresalier, R.S. (2017). Gastrointestinal and hepatic complications of immune checkpoint inhibitors. *Current Gastroenterology Report, 19*(1), 3. https://doi.org/10.1007/s11894-017-0540-6

Enzler, T., & Fojo, T. (2017). Long-acting somatostatin analogues in the treatment of unresectable/metastatic neuroendocrine tumors. *Seminars in Oncology, 44*(2), 141–156. https://doi.org/10.1053/j.seminoncol.2017.07.001

Faiman, B. (2016). Diarrhea in multiple myeloma. *Clinical Journal of Oncology Nursing, 20*(4), E100–E105. https://doi.org/10.1188/16.CJON.E100-E105

Friedman, C.F., Proverbs-Singh, T.A., & Postow, M.A. (2016). Treatment of the immune-related adverse events of immune checkpoint inhibitors: A review. *JAMA Oncology, 2*(10), 1346–1353. https://doi.org/10.1001/jamaoncol.2016.1051

Harb, A.H., Fadel, C.A., & Sharara, A.I. (2014). Radiation enteritis. *Current Gastrointestinal Reports, 16*(5), 383–391. https://doi.org/10.1007/s11894-014-0383-3

McDonald, L.C., Gerding, D.N., Johnson, S., Bakken, J.S., Carroll, K.C., Coffin, S.E., … Wilcox, M.H. (2018). Clinical practice guidelines for *Clostridium difficile* infection in adults and children: 2017 update by the Infectious Diseases Society of America (IDSA) and Society for Healthcare Epidemiology of America (SHEA). *Clinical Infectious Diseases, 66*(7), 987–994. https://doi.org/10.1093/cid/ciy149

Mileto, S., Das, A., & Lyras, D. (2019). Enterotoxic clostridia: *Clostridioides difficile* infections. *Microbiology Spectrum, 7*(3). https://doi.org/10.1128/microbiolspec.GPP3-0015-2018

Napolitano, L.M., & Edmiston, C.E., Jr. (2017). *Clostridium difficile* disease: Diagnosis, pathogenesis, and treatment update. *Surgery, 162*(2), 325–348. https://doi.org/10.1016/j.surg.2017.01.018.

Ong, G.K.B., Reidy, T.J., Huk, M.D., & Lane, F.R. (2017). Clostridium difficile colitis: A clinical review. *American Journal of Surgery, 213*(3), 565–571. https://doi.org/10.1016/j.amjsurg.2016.10.035

Pezo, R.C., Wong, M., & Martin, A. (2019). Impact of the gut microbiota on immune checkpoint inhibitor-associated toxicities. *Therapeutic Advances in Gastroenterology, 12.* https://doi.org/10.1177/1756284819870911

Prieux-Klotz, C., Dior, M., Damotte, D., Dreanic, J., Brieau, B., Brezault, C., … Coriat, R. (2017). Immune checkpoint inhibitor-induced colitis: Diagnosis and management. *Target Oncology, 12*(3), 301–308. https://doi.org/10.1007/s11523-017-0495-4

Puzanov, I., Diab, A., Abdallah, K., Bingham, C.O., Brogdon, C., Dadu, R., … Ernstoff, M.S. (2017). Managing toxicities associated with immune checkpoint inhibitors: Consensus recommendations from the Society for Immunotherapy of Cancer (SITC) toxicity management working group. *Journal for ImmunoTherapy of Cancer, 5*(1), 95. https://doi.org/10.1186/s40425-017-0300-z

Raman, M. (2017). Testing for chronic diarrhea. In G.S. Makowski (Ed.), *Advances in clinical chemistry: Vol. 79* (pp. 199–244). Elsevier. https://doi.org/10.1016/bs.acc.2016.09.004

Reintam Blaser, A., Deane, A.M., & Fruhwald, S. (2015). Diarrhoea in the critically ill. *Current Opinion in Critical Care, 21*(2), 142–153. https://doi.org/10.1097/MCC.0000000000000188

Schiller, L.R., Pardi, D.S., & Sellin, J.H. (2017). Chronic diarrhea: Diagnosis and management. *Clinical Gastroenterology and Hepatology, 15*(2), 182–193.e3. https://doi.org/10.1016/j.cgh.2016.07.028

Steffen, R., Hill, D.R., & DuPont, H.L. (2015). Traveler's diarrhea: A clinical review. *JAMA, 313*(1), 71–80. https://doi.org/10.1001/jama.2014.17006

Thiagarajah, J.R., Donowitz, M., & Verkman, A.S. (2015). Secretory diarrhoea: Mechanisms and emerging therapies. *Nature Reviews Gastroenterology and Hepatology, 12*(8), 446–457. https://doi.org/10.1038/nrgastro.2015.111

Townsend, T., Campbell, F., O'Toole, P., & Probert, C. (2019). Microscopic colitis: Diagnosis and management. *Frontline Gastroenterology, 10*(4), 388–393. https://doi.org/10.1136/flgastro-2018-101040

CHAPTER 57

Dysphagia

Kristina Mathey, MS, APRN-CNP, AOCNP®

I. Definitions (Abdel Jalil et al., 2015; Navaneethan & Eubanks, 2015; Schlottmann et al., 2018)
   A. Dysphagia: Sensation of abnormal swallowing or difficulty in swallowing
   B. Odynophagia: Pain with swallowing
   C. Achalasia: Absence of esophageal peristalsis and failure of the lower esophageal sphincter to relax in response to swallowing
   D. Globus: Intermittent or persistent nonpainful sensation of a lump in the throat with no structural lesion identified

II. Physiology/Pathophysiology (Ciucci et al., 2019; Khan et al., 2014; Kruger, 2014; Navaneethan & Eubanks, 2015)
   A. Normal
      1. The voluntary (oral) phase occurs when liquid or solid is ingested, masticated, and mixed with saliva. Food then navigates through the esophagus through a complex network of transfer and relaxation of the upper esophageal sphincter.
      2. As food enters the esophagus, the lower esophageal sphincter relaxes until peristaltic contraction has delivered the food bolus to the stomach.
   B. Pathophysiology
      1. Oropharyngeal dysphagia involves difficulty with the initiation of swallowing and commonly occurs with diseases of the nervous or musculoskeletal system. This presents as a component of a broader complex of neurologic deficits.
      2. Esophageal dysphagia involves difficulty after swallowing. Patients report food getting "stuck" in the throat or upper chest. This is caused by localized neuromuscular disorders or obstructive lesions.

III. Clinical features: History can provide a presumptive diagnosis in approximately 80% of patients. The type of food eliciting dysphagia (solid, liquid, or both), as well as its progression and timing, will provide important differential information. Intermittent dysphagia suggests a motility disorder, whereas persistent dysphagia is more likely related to an obstructive process. Stroke is the leading cause (Abdel Jalil et al., 2015; Chan & Balasubramanian, 2019; Kim & Kahrilas, 2019; Kruger, 2014; Navaneethan & Eubanks, 2015; Nawaz & Tulunay-Ugur, 2018).
   A. Etiology: Mechanical, dysmotility, or often times both
      1. Cranial nerve dysfunction affecting peristalsis: Stroke
      2. Radiation injury or reaction
      3. Failure of the lower esophageal sphincter to relax
      4. Diffuse esophageal spasm
      5. Esophageal stricture from cancer or benign reflux: Schatzki ring

      6. Extrinsic compression of the esophagus: Lung cancer, extrinsic lymph node compression

      7. Inflammatory processes related to infection: May or may not present with fever (e.g., Sjögren syndrome)

      8. Age-related changes: Loss of jaw strength, salivary production, or dentition; increased connective and fatty tissue in the tongue affecting the oral phase of swallowing; the esophageal phase can be delayed because of loss of upper esophageal elasticity.

  B. History: Key to etiology and workup

      1. History of cancer and cancer treatment

      2. Current medications: Prescribed, over the counter

      3. History of presenting symptoms: Precipitating factors, timing, onset, duration, solid versus liquid tolerance

      4. Changes in ADLs: Fatigue assessment

      5. Diet history: Change in appetite, avoidance of problematic foods, swallowing a corrosive substance

      6. Past medical history: GERD, stroke, esophageal infections, Barrett esophagus, immunosuppressive therapy, immunodeficiency

      7. Social history: Tobacco use, alcohol use

  C. Signs and symptoms

      1. Subjective sensation of difficulty swallowing

      2. Choking, cough, hiccups with eating

      3. Nausea and vomiting

      4. Substernal chest pain

      5. Eating food more slowly

      6. Pain with swallowing

      7. Sensation of heartburn or reflux

      8. Aspiration or regurgitation of fluid into the nose

      9. Halitosis or bad breath

    10. Sensation of a substernal lump

    11. Fatigue

    12. Weight loss: Intentional or unintentional

    13. Hoarseness: Late sign indicating laryngeal involvement with tumor

  D. Physical examination

      1. Vital signs: Changes related to fever, dehydration, or respiratory distress

      2. Integument: Hyperkeratosis on the palms and soles (a rare sign of esophageal carcinoma), collagen vascular diseases

      3. Neurologic: Mental status and cranial nerve function (e.g., gag reflex, palatal movement, tongue movement) (see Appendix A)

      4. HEENT

        a) Oral cavity and oropharynx for poor dentition, buccal lesions, tongue fasciculation, and asymmetric palate elevation

        b) Dentures for fit and any signs of irritation

      5. Neck

        a) Lymph node palpation for lymphadenopathy suggesting malignancy or inflammatory process (see Appendix D)

        b) Thyroid examination for masses or enlargement that may impinge on the esophagus

      6. Pulmonary: Decreased breath sounds, crackles, and consolidation suggestive of aspiration pneumonia

      7. Nutritional assessment: BMI for those with weight loss

IV. Diagnostic tests (Chan & Balasubramanian, 2019; Kim & Kahrilas, 2019)
  A. Laboratory: Guided by differential diagnosis
    1. CBC may reveal infectious, neoplastic, or inflammatory condition.
    2. Thyroid studies may reveal conditions causing compressive obstruction.
  B. Radiology: Barium swallow generally is the first step in the diagnostic process for motility disorders and provides a fluoroscopic record of swallowing difficulty and motor dysfunction.
    1. Barium swallow provides excellent sensitivity in determining the location and severity of an obstructing mass or lesion, allowing direct visualization of muscular strength and coordination.
    2. However, barium swallow procedure lacks sensitivity in identifying the nature of the lesion but is more sensitive in detection of esophageal strictures.
    3. Patients must be able to tolerate the supine position.
  C. Other
    1. Endoscopy: This procedure can identify esophageal anatomy. It is commonly the first step to evaluate solid food dysphagia, allowing more precise mucosal inspection and ability to biopsy.
      a) Upper GI endoscopy when a lesion is discovered and requires biopsy or if barium swallow is nondiagnostic
      b) Allows dilation to be performed with the diagnostic study if stricture is the problem
      c) Does not assess motor function
    2. High-resolution manometry
      a) Most sensitive technique to diagnose motility disorders (recent evidence)
      b) Uses up to 36 pressure transducers to provide panesophageal pressure tracing to evaluate peristaltic and sphincter function
    3. Swallowing study to evaluate the throat and esophagus

V. Differential diagnosis (Abdel Jalil et al., 2015; Aziz et al., 2016; Ciucci et al., 2019; Khan et al., 2014; Kruger, 2014; Nawaz & Tulunay-Ugur, 2018)
  A. Neuromuscular
    1. Pseudobulbar palsy
    2. Myasthenia gravis
    3. Multiple sclerosis
    4. Amyotrophic lateral sclerosis
    5. Huntington disease
    6. Parkinson disease
    7. Stroke (see Chapter 146)
  B. Structural
    1. Esophageal webs
    2. Esophageal or peptic strictures: Reflux strictures, Schatzki ring
    3. Esophageal cancer
    4. Head and neck cancer
    5. Zenker diverticulum: Weakness of the posterior hypopharyngeal wall
    6. Plummer-Vinson syndrome: Symptomatic hypopharyngeal webs occurring in women with iron deficiency
    7. Lymphadenopathy (see Chapter 111), mediastinal tumor
    8. Osteophytes, vascular compression, other extrinsic causes
    9. Aortic aneurysm
    10. Food impaction
    11. Goiter (see Chapter 158)

12. Postsurgical complications: Laryngectomy
13. Complications from chemotherapy and radiation
C. Functional
1. Inflammatory disorders: Erosive esophagitis
2. Eosinophilic esophagitis
3. Achalasia
4. Upper, lower, or distal esophageal sphincter dysfunction
5. Ineffective esophageal motility
6. Nutcracker esophagus
7. Scleroderma and other rheumatologic disorders
8. Decreased saliva production: Sjögren syndrome, radiation to the oral cavity
D. Medication induced: Doxycycline, tetracycline, potassium chloride, ferrous sulfate, NSAIDs, ASA

VI. Treatment (Chan & Balasubramanian, 2019; Ciucci et al., 2019; Iwakiri et al., 2016; Kroch & Madanick, 2017; Kruger, 2014; Kung et al., 2017)
A. Patients with reflux disease should be initially treated with maintenance therapy with a PPI and behavioral recommendation. If symptoms do not improve, consider increasing PPI to two times a day dosing and then change to another PPI or additional administration of a histamine H_2 receptor antagonist before sleep. PPIs have been shown to be inferior to H_2 blockers. Sodium alginate and antacids can be used for temporary improvement in conjunction with treatment.
   1. Acid-reducing medications
      a) PPIs: Omeprazole 20–40 mg PO, lansoprazole 15–30 mg PO, or pantoprazole 40 mg PO daily
      b) H_2 blockers: Cimetidine 200–400 mg PO or famotidine 20 mg PO two times a day
   2. Behavioral modifications
      a) Smoking cessation
      b) Limiting alcohol use
      c) Elevating head of bed during sleep at least eight inches
      d) Weight loss
      e) Avoiding food ingestion two hours prior to sleeping
      f) Decreasing acidic or reflexogenic foods (e.g., chocolate, mint, citrus, onion, peppermint, fatty foods) and beverages (e.g., coffee, caffeine, carbonation)
B. When possible, give medications in liquid form.
C. In patients with mild oropharyngeal dysphagia, behavioral modifications may be adequate.
   1. Advise patients to drink small quantities at a time, thoroughly chew all foods, and eat and swallow slowly.
   2. Patients should avoid cold foods if they worsen symptoms.
   3. The goal is to achieve adequate nutritional intake with minimal discomfort.
D. Antidepressants and cognitive behavioral therapy may be helpful for those with stress-related symptoms (see Appendix L).
E. Antifungal therapy is necessary in the treatment of patients with Candida esophagitis.
   1. Fluconazole 400 mg PO is used initially as loading dose, then 200–400 mg PO a day for 14–21 days. Voriconazole 200 mg PO two times a day is effective for patients unresponsive to fluconazole. The echinocandins (i.e., caspofungin, micafungin, and anidulafungin) are effective when fluconazole is ineffective; however, they are available in IV form and used mostly for hospitalized patients.
   2. Clotrimazole troches are administered by dissolving one 10 mg troche in the mouth (five times a day) for 7–14 days.

   3. Nystatin is administered at 100,000 U/ml or 5 ml PO by swish and swallowing four times a day for 7–14 days.
  F. Graded pneumatic dilation or laparoscopic surgical myotomy with partial fundoplication is indicated in patients with achalasia when conservative measures provide no relief.
  G. Botulinum toxin injection into the lower esophageal sphincter has also been shown to improve dysphagia in patients if other therapies are unsuccessful.
  H. Patients with esophageal carcinoma will require multimodal therapy.
    1. Endoscopic esophageal stent
    2. Radiation, chemotherapy, surgery, or combination depending on stage; may be curative
  I. Benign strictures usually are best managed with endoscopic dilation and/or stent placement.

VII. Follow-up (Kawamoto et al., 2018; Navaneethan & Eubanks, 2015; Nawaz & Tulunay-Ugar, 2018)
  A. Consistent follow-up with a dietitian to assess nutritional status
  B. Regular endoscopies if dilations are necessary
  C. Regular follow-up with an ear, nose, and throat medical and/or surgical oncologist for patients with head and neck or esophageal carcinoma or Barrett esophagus

VIII. Referrals (Ciucci et al., 2019)
  A. Dietitian: For dietary modifications and individual caloric recommendations; patients who aspirate during barium boluses may require a non-oral feeding program. Modifications in food textures can be suggested.
  B. Speech pathologist: For swallowing rehabilitation aiming to improve swallowing through exercises to improve impaired physiology; this is particularly used in those with oropharyngeal dysphagia and uses strategies such as postural adjustments, swallowing maneuvers, and dietary modifications. A speech pathologist can be beneficial to evaluate for aspiration.
  C. Gastroenterologist: For endoscopy, biopsy, and often for symptomatic management, dilation, and stenting in patients with an obstructive lesion
  D. Surgeon, medical oncologist, and/or radiation oncologist: For treatment planning collaboration following initial biopsy if malignant

The author would like to acknowledge Miriam Rogers, EdD, APRN, AOCN®, CNS, for her contribution to this chapter that remains unchanged from the previous edition of this book.

References

Abdel Jalil, A.A., Katzka, D.A., & Castell, D.O. (2015). Approach to the patient with dysphagia. *American Journal of Medicine, 128*(10), 1138.e17–1138.e23. https://doi.org/10.1016/j.amjmed.2015.04.026

Aziz, Q., Fass, R., Gyawali, C.P., Miwa, H., Pandolfino, J.E., & Zerbib, F. (2016). Esophageal disorders. *Gastroenterology, 150*(6), 1368–1379. https://doi.org/10.1053/j.gastro.2016.02.012.

Chan, M.Q., & Balasubramanian, G. (2019). Esophageal dysphagia in the elderly. *Current Treatment Options in Gastroenterology, 17*(4), 534–553. https://doi.org/10.1007/s11938-019-00264-z

Ciucci, M., Hoffmeister, J., & Wheeler-Hegland, K. (2019). Management of dysphagia in acquired and progressive neurologic conditions. *Seminars in Speech and Language, 40*(3), 203–212. https://doi.org/10.1055/s-0039-1688981

Iwakiri, K., Kinoshita, Y., Habu, Y., Oshima, T., Manabe, N., Fujiwara, Y., ... Shimosegawa, T. (2016). Evidence-based clinical practice guidelines for gastroesophageal reflux disease 2015. *Journal of Gastroenterology, 51*(8), 751–767. https://doi.org/10.1007/s00535-016-1227-8

Kawamoto, T., Nihei, K., Sasai, K., & Karasawa, K. (2018). Palliative radiotherapy and chemoradiotherapy in stage IVA/B esophageal cancer patients with dysphagia. *International Journal of Clinical Oncology, 23*(6), 1076–1083. https://doi .org/10.1007/s10147-018-1324-1

Khan, A., Carmona, R., & Traube, M. (2014). Dysphagia in the elderly. *Clinics in Geriatric Medicine,* 30(1), 43–53. https:// doi.org/10.1016/j.cger.2013.10.009.

Kim, J.P., & Kahrilas, P.J. (2019). How I approach dysphagia. *Current Gastroenterology Reports, 21*(10), 49. https://doi.org /10.1007/s11894-019-0718-1

Kroch, D.A., & Madanick, R.D. (2017). Medical treatment of gastroesophageal reflux disease. *World Journal of Surgery, 41*(7), 1678–1684. https://doi.org/10.1007/s00268-017-3954-2

Kruger, D. (2014). Assessing esophageal dysphagia. *Journal of the American Academy of Physician Assistants,* 27(5), 23–30. https://doi.org/10.1097/01.JAA.0000446227.85554.fb

Kung, Y.-M, Hsu, W.-H, Wu, M.-C, Wang, J.-W, Liu, C.-J, Su, Y.-C, ... Wang, Y.-K. (2017). Recent advances in the pharmacological management of gastroesophageal reflux disease. *Digestive Diseases and Sciences, 62*(12), 3298–3316. https:// doi.org/10.1007/s10620-017-4830-5.

Navaneethan, U., & Eubanks, S. (2015). Approach to patients with esophageal dysphagia. *Surgical Clinics of North America, 95*(3), 483–489. https://doi.org/10.1016/j.suc.2015.02.004

Nawaz, S., & Tulunay-Ugur, O.E. (2018). Dysphagia in the older patient. *Otolaryngologic Clinics of North America, 51*(4), 769–777. https://doi.org/10.1016/j.otc.2018.03.006

Schlottmann, F., Neto, R.M.L., Herbella, F.A.M., & Patti, M.G. (2018). Esophageal achalasia: Pathophysiology, clinical presentation, and diagnostic evaluation. *American Surgeon, 84*(4), 467–472.

CHAPTER 58

Heartburn/Indigestion/ Dyspepsia

Kristina Mathey, MS, APRN-CNP, AOCNP®

I. Definitions (Hachem & Shaheen, 2016; Moayyedi et al., 2017; Mounsey et al., 2020; Tomita et al., 2018; Vandenberghe et al., 2020)
   A. Heartburn: Retrosternal burning sensation
   B. Indigestion: Incomplete or imperfect digestion
   C. Dyspepsia: Predominant epigastric pain lasting at least one month that can be associated with other upper GI symptoms (e.g., epigastric fullness)
   D. Functional: Symptoms occurring for at least 12 weeks out of the past year in the setting of normal endoscopic findings with no underlying organic pathology to explain symptoms

II. Physiology/Pathophysiology (Iwakiri et al., 2016; Miwa et al., 2016; Tack & Carbone, 2017; Tomita et al., 2018)
   A. Normal
      1. The lower esophageal sphincter maintains a pressure barrier between the esophagus and the stomach.
      2. The hormone gastrin, alpha-adrenergic stimulation, and the vagus nerve promote relaxation of the smooth muscle of the lower esophageal sphincter.
      3. Primary peristalsis is essential for acid clearance from the esophagus.
   B. Pathophysiology
      1. Heartburn is the symptom produced by increased reflux at the esophagogastric junction and decreased clearance of stomach acid by gravity or esophageal peristalsis. This impairment leads to excessive esophageal acid exposure.
      2. Immunologic mechanisms mediated by cytokines, such as IL-8 and IL-1β, can potentially trigger inflammation, causing damage in esophageal sensitivity. This damage results in heartburn symptoms. Prostaglandin E2 (PGE2) and ATP, produced by esophageal epithelial cells, are likely candidates for mediators of heartburn symptoms.

III. Clinical features: Heartburn that persists despite PPI treatment is a frequent clinical problem with multiple potential causes. Functional dyspepsia is one of the most common GI disorders (Kroch & Madanick, 2017; Li et al., 2019; Mounsey et al., 2020; Schmulson, 2018; Spechler et al., 2019; Tack & Carbone, 2017; Vandenberghe et al., 2020).
   A. Etiology
      1. Pharmacologic agents that decrease lower esophageal sphincter tone
         a) Antibiotics

   b) NSAIDs
   c) Iron preparations
   d) Xanthines
   e) Beta-blockers
   f) Anticholinergics
   g) Calcium channel blockers
   h) Theophylline
   i) Digoxin
   j) Oral steroids
   k) Tricyclic antidepressants
   l) Opioids
   m) Estrogen replacement therapy
  2. Tobacco use
  3. Caffeine: Chocolate, coffee
  4. Ethanol
  5. High-fat or spicy foods
  6. Increased abdominal pressure from obesity, pregnancy, or ascites
  7. Delayed gastric emptying
  8. Alteration in esophageal mucosa
  9. Hiatal hernia, leading to progressive disruption of the diaphragmatic sphincter and resulting in increased susceptibility to reflux with abrupt increases of intra-abdominal pressure

B. History
  1. History of cancer and cancer treatment
  2. Current medications: Prescribed, over the counter, current measures to relieve discomfort, antacid use
  3. History of presenting symptoms: Precipitating factors, onset, location, duration, associated symptoms (e.g., dysphagia, nausea, vomiting, pain with swallowing, globus sensation, wheezing, hoarseness, early satiety, postprandial fullness and bloating)
  4. Changes in ADLs: Necessity to sleep on multiple pillows at night due to bothersome symptoms
  5. Past medical history: Hiatal hernia, ingestion of caustic materials, ulcers, IBS, gallstones, esophageal strictures, esophagitis, gastritis, trauma to the abdomen, throat, or esophagus
  6. Diet history: Food intolerances and time from ingestion of a meal until symptoms appear (as soon as 45 minutes); timing of last meal of the day in regard to bedtime
  7. Social history: Tobacco use, alcohol use

C. Signs and persistent symptoms
  1. Retrosternal burning that radiates upward
  2. Dull substernal discomfort or ache
  3. Feelings of abdominal distention
  4. Nausea and vomiting
  5. Sensation of reflux of gastric contents
  6. Worsening symptoms after meals with certain foods
  7. Worsening symptoms with food ingestion prior to sleep or when reclining after eating
  8. Dyspnea
  9. Pyrosis (sour or burning taste in mouth)
  10. Chronic, unexplained cough

D. Physical examination
  1. Vital signs: Unexplained weight loss indicative of possible malignancy or other condition

2. HEENT/oral cavity: Ulcers and thrush
3. Abdominal
   a) Epigastric tenderness on light or deep palpation indicating reflux
   b) Normal bowel sounds
   c) Masses and organomegaly indicating other conditions
   d) Murphy sign (if positive) indicative of gallbladder disease (see Appendix D)
   e) Abdominal distention indicating gas
   f) Abdominal ascites indicating other conditions
4. Lymph node: Cervical and supraclavicular lymph nodes for enlargement indicative of malignancy (see Appendix D)
5. Rectal: Stool testing for occult blood

IV. Diagnostic tests: A diagnosis can be made by careful clinical evaluation involving history taking with laboratory testing used in atypical, persistent, or severe cases. When history reveals uncomplicated heartburn with no evidence of underlying disease, proceed with treatment (Hachem & Shaheen, 2016; Iwakiri et al., 2016; Kroch & Madanick, 2017; Mounsey et al., 2020; Schmulson, 2018; Tack & Carbone, 2017).
   A. Laboratory
      1. CBC to evaluate for iron deficiency anemia
      2. *Helicobacter pylori* serology to evaluate for infection if a gastric or duodenal ulcer is present or suggested
      3. 24-hour esophageal pH monitoring in select cases when dietary and behavioral modifications, as well as medical therapy, have failed
   B. Radiology
      1. Testing for conditions other than uncomplicated dyspepsia, such as upper GI series
      2. Esophagram to evaluate for hiatal hernia and confirm gastroesophageal reflux
   C. Other: An endoscopy is performed when symptoms continue despite standard treatment to evaluate for esophagitis and hiatal hernia. It also allows direct visualization and biopsy when appropriate.

V. Differential diagnosis (Camilleri, 2016; Hachem & Shaheen, 2016; Kroch & Madanick, 2017; Schmulson, 2018; Spechler et al., 2019)
   A. Esophageal diseases
      1. Motility disorders: Achalasia, esophageal stricture scleroderma, diabetic neuropathy, amyloidosis, esophageal hypersensitivity
      2. GERD (see Chapter 71)
      3. Esophagitis
      4. Eosinophilic esophagitis
   B. Ulcers: Esophageal, gastric, or duodenal (see Chapter 78)
   C. Gastritis (see Chapter 72)
   D. Gastroparesis
   E. Cholelithiasis or biliary pathology (see Chapter 68)
   F. Pancreatitis (see Chapter 77)
   G. MI or other cardiac etiologies (see Chapter 49)
   H. Psychiatric disorders
      1. Anxiety disorders (see Chapter 161)
      2. Depression (see Chapter 162)
   I. Gastric or esophageal cancer: Dyspepsia is an uncommon but possible presentation.
   J. Rumination syndrome

VI. Treatment (Hachem & Shaheen, 2016; Kroch & Madanick, 2017; Kung et al., 2017; Li et al., 2019; Miwa et al., 2016; Mounsey et al., 2020; Spechler et al., 2019; Tack & Carbone, 2017; Tomita et al., 2018; Vandenberghe et al., 2020)

A. Lifestyle alterations

1. Discuss dietary modification. Eliminate foods that initiate or aggravate symptoms (e.g., chocolate, alcohol, oils, peppermint, garlic, onion, fatty foods).
2. Eliminate or decrease alcohol and caffeine intake.
3. Encourage smoking cessation.
4. Avoid eating for at least two hours before bedtime or reclining.
5. Drink fluids after eating to clear the esophagus.
6. Elevate the head of the bed six inches for sleeping or use a pillow wedge.
7. Eliminate or modify the dose of medications that reduce lower esophageal sphincter tone.
8. Eliminate medications that irritate esophageal mucosa.
9. Encourage weight loss, as indicated.
10. Promote salivation through oral lozenges or chewing gum to neutralize any reflux acid and increase the rate of esophageal acid clearance.
11. Routine use of complementary and alternative medicine therapies has not shown evidence of effectiveness and is not recommended.

B. Pharmacologic

1. Trial over-the-counter antacids after meals and at bedtime. Antacids could interfere with absorption of other medications and may result in alteration in bowel function (constipation or diarrhea). Equivalent store brands are available.
   a) Aluminum hydroxide, magnesium hydroxide, and simethicone 15–20 ml PO after meals and at bedtime
   b) Aluminum hydroxide plus magnesium hydroxide 15–30 ml PO after meals and at bedtime
   c) Calcium carbonate is widely available in oral form and may be taken two tablets PO every four hours PRN.

2. Trial H_2 blockers (H_2 receptor antagonists) to suppress acid secretion by competitively binding to H_2 receptors on the parietal cells, which reduces volume and acidity. Once-a-day dosing may be sufficient to control mild symptoms. Persistent use beyond a trial period is not recommended without an evaluation.
   a) Cimetidine: 200–400 mg two or three times a day or 800 mg PO at bedtime
   b) Famotidine: 20 mg two times a day or 40 mg PO at bedtime
   c) Nizatidine: 150 mg two times a day or 300 mg PO at bedtime

3. Trial PPIs for those with severe symptoms. PPIs strongly inhibit acid secretion. Persistent use of these agents is not recommended without an evaluation after the trial period to evaluate for more serious conditions such as GERD (see Chapter 71).
   a) PPIs have been found to be superior to H_2 receptor antagonists in resolving symptoms in four weeks and are often used as first-line drugs in treatment.
   b) At four weeks, resolution of symptoms is similar between agents and doses. Significant drug interaction occurs between clopidogrel and PPIs, potentially leading to an increased risk of cardiovascular events.
   c) Examples
      (1) Omeprazole over the counter: 20–40 mg PO daily
      (2) Lansoprazole over the counter: 15–30 mg PO daily
      (3) Esomeprazole: 20–40 mg PO daily
      (4) Pantoprazole: 40 mg PO daily

4. Trial promotility agents, which may cause diarrhea. Metoclopramide, 5–15 mg PO before meals and at bedtime, acts primarily on the lower esophageal sphincter and promotes peristalsis. Extrapyramidal reactions are a common side effect and should be monitored.

5. Institute *H. pylori* treatment if the patient is seropositive (see Chapter 78)

6. Treat infectious causes (e.g., candidal esophagitis, CMV, herpes simplex) as indicated.

C. Other procedures

1. Endoscopy with dilation: For patients with dysphagia and stricture

2. Antireflux surgery: Considered only if symptoms are incapacitating after gastroenterologist consultation

VII. Follow-up (Hachem & Shaheen, 2016; Kroch & Madanick, 2017; Moayyedi et al., 2017; Tack & Carbone, 2017)

A. Short term: Patients should be reevaluated within one month of instituting dietary modification and/or medications. Evaluation should include nutritional status, effect of modification on symptoms, and assessment of need for further diagnostic testing or intervention.

B. Long term: Patients with chronic or recurrent symptoms should be followed regularly.

1. These patients are at risk for development of GERD, severe esophagitis, strictures, and esophageal malignancy and should be referred for prolonged symptoms, workup, and management.

2. Patients with Barrett esophagus are at increased risk for development of esophageal adenocarcinoma. Some practitioners recommend periodic endoscopy for surveillance monitoring of patients with Barrett esophagus.

VIII. Referrals

A. Dietitian: For assistance with dietary modification, if appropriate

B. Gastroenterologist: For further evaluation if symptoms remain refractory after eight weeks of therapy or if endoscopy is indicated

C. Surgeon: If antireflux surgery is indicated

The author would like to acknowledge Miriam Rogers, EdD, APRN, AOCN®, CNS, for her contribution to this chapter that remains unchanged from the previous edition of this book.

References

Camilleri, M. (2016). Functional dyspepsia and gastroparesis. *Digestive Diseases, 34*(5), 491–499. https://doi.org/10.1159/000445226

Hachem, C., & Shaheen, N. (2016). Diagnosis and management of functional heartburn. *American Journal of Gastroenterology, 111*(1), 53–61. https://doi.org/10.1038/ajg.2015.376

Iwakiri, K., Kinoshita, Y., Habu, Y., Oshima, T., Manabe, N., Fujiwara, Y., … Shimosegawa, T. (2016). Evidence-based clinical practice guidelines for gastroesophageal reflux disease 2015. *Journal of Gastroenterology, 51*(8), 751–767. https://doi.org/10.1007/s00535-016-1227-8

Kroch, D.A., & Madanick, R.D. (2017). Medical treatment of gastroesophageal reflux disease. *World Journal of Surgery, 41*(7), 1678–1684. https://doi.org/10.1007/s00268-017-3954-2

Kung, Y.-M., Hsu, W.-H., Wu, M.-C., Wang, J.-W., Liu, C.-J., Su, Y.-C., … Wang, Y.-K. (2017). Recent advances in the pharmacological management of gastroesophageal reflux disease. *Digestive Diseases and Sciences, 62*(12), 3298–3316. https://doi.org/10.1007/s10620-017-4830-5

Li, J., Wang, F., Lv, L., Xu, L., Zeng, E., & Tang, X. (2019). Histamine H2 antagonists for functional dyspepsia: A protocol for a systematic review and meta-analysis. *Medicine, 98*(47), e18128. https://doi.org/10.1097/MD.0000000000018128

Miwa, H., Kondo, T., & Oshima, T. (2016). Gastroesophageal reflux disease–related and functional heartburn: Pathophysiology and treatment. *Current Opinion in Gastroenterology, 32*(4), 344–352. https://doi.org/10.1097/MOG.0000000000000282.

Moayyedi, P., Lacy, B.E., Andrews, C.N., Enns, R.A., Howden, C.W., & Vakil, N. (2017). ACG and CAG clinical guideline: Management of dyspepsia. *American Journal of Gastroenterology, 112*(7), 988–1013. https://doi.org/10.1038/ajg.2017.154

Mounsey, A., Barzin, A., & Rietz, A. (2020). Functional dyspepsia: Evaluation and management. *American Family Physician, 101*(2), 84–88. https://www.aafp.org/afp/2020/0115/p84.html

Schmulson, M. (2018). How to use Rome IV criteria in the evaluation of esophageal disorders. *Current Opinion in Gastroenterology, 34*(4), 258–265. https://doi.org/10.1097/MOG.0000000000000443.

Spechler, S.J., Hunter, J.G., Jones, K.M., Lee, R., Smith, B.R., Mashimo, H., ... Huang, G.D. (2019). Randomized trial of medical versus surgical treatment for refractory heartburn. *New England Journal of Medicine, 381*(16), 1513–1523. https://doi.org/10.1056/NEJMoa1811424

Tack, J., & Carbone, F. (2017). Functional dyspepsia and gastroparesis. *Current Opinion in Gastroenterology, 33*(6), 446–454. https://doi.org/10.1097/MOG.0000000000000393

Tomita, T., Oshima, T., & Miwa, H. (2018). New approaches to diagnosis and treatment of functional dyspepsia. *Current Gastroenterology Reports, 20*(12), 55. https://doi.org/10.1007/s11894-018-0663-4

Vandenberghe, A., Schol, J., Van den Houte, K., Masuy, I., Carbone, F., & Tack, J. (2020). Current and emerging therapeutic options for the management of functional dyspepsia. *Expert Opinion on Pharmacotherapy, 21*(3), 365–376. https://doi.org/10.1080/14656566.2019.1707805

CHAPTER 59

Hematemesis

Jeanne Held-Warmkessel, MSN, RN, AOCN®, ACNS-BC

I. Definition: Vomiting blood or coffee-ground emesis from esophagus, stomach, or duodenum (Farrar, 2018)

II. Physiology/Pathophysiology (Feinman & Haut, 2014)
   A. Normal: The GI tract has a robust blood supply, and the mucosal surface is composed of epithelial cells.
      1. The functions of the epithelial cells are transmembrane absorption and secretion.
      2. These functions facilitate the digestive tract in digestion and nutrient uptake.
      3. These cells act as a barrier against potentially harmful pathogens and mutagens in the lumen.
   B. Pathophysiology
      1. Bleeding from the GI mucosa occurs from tears, inflammation, irritation, ulceration, necrosis, or trauma, which results in stimulation of the GI pathways and initiates emesis.
      2. Bleeding source is mainly above the ligament of Treitz in the upper GI tract.
      3. Variceal and nonvariceal (majority) bleeds are typical sources.

III. Clinical features: Severity ranges from mild to overt bleeding that is potentially a life-threatening emergency. Bleeding may be described as coffee-ground emesis (signifying contact with gastric secretions) or as bright red. It may be categorized as variceal or nonvariceal. Occult blood in the emesis may not be readily apparent and can be identified only by testing. Bleeding may stop spontaneously (Farrar, 2018; Haddad et al., 2019; Kamboj et al., 2019; Nelms & Pelaez, 2018; Rahman & Saeian, 2016).
   A. Etiology
      1. Peptic ulcer disease: Most common cause of upper GI bleeding
      2. Portal varices, portal hypertension
      3. Gastritis
      4. Esophagitis
      5. Cancer
      6. Drug induced: Steroids, anticoagulants, NSAIDs
      7. Trauma
   B. History
      1. History of cancer and cancer treatment
      2. Current medications: Prescribed, over the counter, NSAIDs/ASA, steroids, anticoagulants, antiplatelet agents, direct oral anticoagulants, SSRIs
      3. History of presenting symptoms: Precipitating factors, onset, frequency, duration

    a) Ask patient to describe the color, volume, and consistency of blood vomited.

    b) Associated symptoms include change in bowel habits, blood per rectum, nose-bleeds, mouth bleeds, pain and its association with food, dizziness, weakness, shortness of breath, heartburn symptoms, and/or anorexia.

  4. Changes in ADLs

  5. Past medical history: Pancreatic disease, renal disease, peptic ulcer disease, chronic liver disease, cirrhosis, portal hypertension, prior GI bleeding, prior GI disease, prior surgery, esophageal varices, HIV, inflammatory bowel disease, heart disease, coagulation disorders, Peutz-Jeghers syndrome

  6. Past surgical history: Aortic aneurysm repair, any GI tract surgery

  7. Social history: Alcohol use, tobacco use

C. Signs and symptoms

  1. Retching and nausea

  2. Vomiting: Blood may or may not be visible. It may appear as coffee-ground emesis (old blood) or bright red (new blood).

  3. Pallor, jaundice

  4. Decreased level of consciousness

  5. Dizziness, light-headedness, weakness

  6. Abdominal pain: Epigastric (duodenal ulcer), relief with food (gastric ulcer)

  7. Anemia signs and symptoms: Chest pain, dyspnea, fatigue

D. Physical examination

  1. Vital signs and pulse oximetry (reassess frequently): Hypotension, orthostatic changes, resting tachycardia, and other signs of hypovolemia or shock; hemodynamic stability

    a) Loss of less than 500 ml blood: Few signs occur except in patients with preexisting anemia and in older adults.

    b) Loss of 1,000 ml blood (20% of blood volume): Tachycardia and/or orthostatic hypotension (decrease of 10 mm Hg) occurs alone or with light-headedness, nausea, thirst, and diaphoresis.

    c) Loss of 1,500 ml blood (30% of blood volume): Orthostatic hypotension develops, and previously listed signs and symptoms are present.

    d) Loss of 2,500 ml blood (40% of blood volume): Supine hypotension, pallor, and cool skin are present.

    e) Assess for weight loss.

  2. HEENT

    a) Oral cavity: Dry mucous membranes indicating poor hydration; bleeding source

    b) Tooth enamel: Acid damage caused by decalcification from gastric acid

    c) Nose: Bleeding

    d) Conjunctiva: Pallor

  3. Integument: Pallor, temperature, nailbed color and blanching, petechiae, ecchymosis, telangiectasias, jaundice, spider angioma, other signs indicating bleeding

  4. Lymph node: Regional lymph nodes for enlargement (e.g., left supraclavicular enlargement [Virchow node]) suggestive of intra-abdominal malignancy (see Appendix D)

  5. Abdominal: Liver size, ascites, pain, masses, tenderness, distention

    a) Hyperactive bowel sounds

    b) Rigidity and guarding indicating possibility of peritonitis from perforated gastroduodenal ulcer

  6. Rectal: Fissures, hemorrhoids, masses, stool color, stool testing for occult blood

  7. Mental status: Confusion

8. Cardiac examination, pulses, and capillary refill: Signs and symptoms associated with decreased circulating blood volume, which may affect cardiac function producing angina or myocardial ischemia
   a) Pulses: Increased rate, weak
   b) Capillary refill: Slow
   c) Tachycardia: Present at rest

IV. Diagnostic tests (Farrar, 2018; Kamboj et al., 2019; Nelms & Pelaez, 2018; Rahman & Saeian, 2016)
   A. Laboratory
      1. CBC with platelet count: Serial testing is required.
         a) Hgb and hematocrit: May not reflect extent of acute blood loss for 24–72 hours after bleeding begins
         b) Mean corpuscular volume: Low with chronic blood loss
         c) Ferritin: Low with chronic blood loss
         d) Low platelet count, thrombocytopenia: May contribute to bleeding
      2. Chemistry panel: Comprehensive metabolic panel
         a) Serial testing is required. BUN may be increased from hypovolemia and blood degradation from upper GI tract.
         b) Higher BUN–creatinine ratio often indicates an upper GI tract source.
      3. LFTs: Abnormal values present with liver disorders, which may promote upper GI bleeding (e.g., gastroesophageal varices, portal gastropathy).
      4. PT, PTT, and INR: Assess for bleeding disorders or prolonged clotting time. Results may not be accurate.
      5. Type and cross match: Note for transfusion.
      6. Cardiac enzymes: Assess in patients at risk for cardiac complications.
      7. Viscoelastic testing: Thromboelastography or rotation thromboelastomerty can occur.
   B. Radiology: CT angiography may be indicated with active bleeding when source has not been found during EGD.
   C. Other
      1. EGD: It is crucial to diagnose and treat bleeding source and to obtain biopsies of abnormal areas and for suspected malignancy. EGD is performed within 12–24 hours of onset of bleeding and must be done prior to discharge.
      2. NG tube: An NG tube is optional and may not provide useful information.
      3. Emesis: Visually inspect for blood, food, liquids, drugs, or other contents, and test for occult blood. Not everything red is blood. Some dyes used in foods and liquids are red.
      4. Selective celiac and selective mesenteric arteriography: Technique may be diagnostic or therapeutic.
      5. ECG: It should be performed in patients with cardiac history or symptomatology.
      6. If source is nose or mouth, consult ear, nose, and throat specialist and apply local pressure to control local bleeding.

V. Differential diagnosis (Feinman & Haut, 2014; Nelms & Pelaez, 2018; Rahman & Saeian, 2016)
   A. Esophageal
      1. Esophageal rupture, esophageal varices, esophageal tear
      2. GERD (see Chapter 71)
      3. Esophagitis, erosive esophagitis, aortoenteric fistula, esophageal ulcer from other causes (e.g., infection, radiation therapy, caustic ingestion, pill esophagitis)
      4. Infection: CMV, HSV, *Candida albicans*

B. Gastric
   1. Peptic ulcer disease (*Helicobacter pylori* infection): Most common cause of non-variceal bleeds (see Chapter 78)
   2. Mucosal erosion, stress ulcer, erosive gastritis (see Chapter 72)
   3. Gastric varices
   4. Hiatal hernia with erosions
   5. Dieulafoy lesion: Large artery in GI tract mucosa that erodes through mucosa and bleeds without associated ulceration
   6. Mallory-Weiss tear at gastroesophageal junction
   7. Gastric antral vascular ectasia
   8. Portal hypertensive gastropathy
   9. Radiation gastritis/arteriovenous malformations
C. Duodenal
   1. Erosive duodenitis
   2. Duodenal ulcers
   3. Crohn disease
D. Cancer
   1. Esophageal: Squamous or adenocarcinoma
   2. Gastric: Adenocarcinoma, lymphomas, GI stromal tumor
   3. GI tract metastases from other primary sites
   4. Duodenal cancer; pancreatic cancer invasion into duodenum
E. Connective tissue diseases that cause bleeding disorders: Pseudoxanthoma elasticum
F. Fistulas between large blood vessels and GI tract: Aortaenteric fistula
G. Arteriovenous malformations, angiodysplasia (e.g., dilated arteriole–venule–capillary network complex), vascular lesions
H. Bleeding secondary to lung etiology: Hemoptysis looking like hematemesis
I. Trauma or surgery of nose or mouth
J. Zollinger-Ellison syndrome
K. Hemobilia
L. Hemosuccus pancreaticus
M. Drug induced: NSAIDs/ASA (see Appendix E), antiplatelet agents, warfarin and other anticoagulants, steroids, alcohol, direct oral anticoagulants, unfractionated and LMWHs, oral and injectable factor Xa inhibitors, oral and injectable direct thrombin inhibitors, mitogen-activated protein kinase (MEK) inhibitors (e.g., trametinib, cobimetinib, binimetinib), caustic ingestion (e.g., lye)
N. Nose or oral bleeding
O. Left ventricular assist devices

VI. Treatment: Perform triage. Treatment may require emergency management depending on the patient's vital signs and hemodynamic stability. Transfer unstable or hemorrhaging patients to hospital/emergency department by ambulance, then to ICU if necessary. Some patients will require central venous monitoring. Other patients may have a slow bleed and are stable for outpatient workup (Baracat et al., 2016; Farrar, 2018; Feinman & Haut, 2014; Haddad et al., 2019; Hernández-Gea et al., 2018; Kamboj et al., 2019; Nelms & Pelaez, 2018; Rahman & Saeian, 2016; Stanley & Laine, 2019).
   A. Provide general support for hemodynamically unstable patients.
      1. Provide supplemental oxygen if pulse oximetry is less than 90%.
      2. Patient is NPO.
      3. Insert two large-gauge IV cannulas and rapidly replace lost fluid volume with isotonic (normal saline) fluids, but do not overhydrate.

4. Monitor intake and output.
5. Monitor central venous pressure and vital signs.
6. Transfuse packed RBCs and correct to Hgb of 7 mg/dl (higher with cardiac disease), particularly in presence of active bleeding or hypotension.
    a) Transfuse platelets and fresh frozen plasma dependent on patient situation.
    b) Administer platelets and fresh frozen plasma when three to four units or more of packed RBCs are rapidly infused or 1:1:1 with packed RBCs.
    c) For patients with acute hemorrhage, transfusion requirements are higher. Determine if massive transfusion protocol should be implemented.
B. Correct bleeding abnormalities.
    1. Initiate vitamin K 2.5–10 mg IV. It may be repeated to correct warfarin anticoagulation or vitamin K deficiency.
    2. Administer prothrombin complex concentrate with vitamin K.
    3. Reversal agents for direct oral anticoagulants are unclear.
        a) Dabigatran: Idarucizumab; may consider hemodialysis
        b) Rivaroxaban, apixaban: Andexanet alfa, prothrombin concentrate complex
        c) Edoxaban: Prothrombin concentrate complex
    4. Replace other clotting factors (e.g., factor VIII), as indicated.
C. Optional: Insert NG tube for assessment of gastric contents.
    1. Connect NG tube to low intermittent suction; lavage to assess for ongoing bleeding.
    2. Flush PRN to keep tube patent and assess blood loss.
D. Insert indwelling urinary catheter to monitor urine output, and watch patient for oliguria, which often is present with hypovolemia. Remove as soon as possible.
E. Bed rest: Elevate head of bed to 30°–45° to reduce risk of aspiration. With active bleeding, intubation may be needed to protect the airway during EGD.
F. Place airway and suction equipment at bedside in case of aspiration. Protect airway.
G. Upper endoscopy: Perform after initial stabilization to treat bleeding. Endoscopy can be performed thermally (e.g., bipolar electrocoagulation, heater probe). It can also be performed via injection of epinephrine or other vasoactive drugs, which should not be used alone but in combination with another endoscopic therapy. It can be used for peptic ulcer disease, combination therapy (recommended), or hemoclips or injection therapy with thermal coagulation (recommended). Thermal treatment and injection often are used in combination. Upper endoscopy can also be performed mechanically (e.g., bands, clips, loops). Biopsy all ulcers. Perform *H. pylori* testing.
    1. Therapy approaches are disease specific and should be performed within 12–24 hours of onset of bleeding.
    2. Patient assessment and hemodynamic stability should direct timing of endoscopy. Patients at high risk should be scoped sooner.
H. Medications
    1. Acid suppression with PPI for nonvariceal bleeding
        a) Start IV PPI to manage bleeding resulting from nonvariceal GI bleeding. Start prior to upper endoscopy.
            (1) Pantoprazole: 80 mg IV bolus followed by 8 mg/hr continuous IV infusion
            (2) Esomeprazole: 80 mg IV bolus followed by 8 mg/hr continuous IV infusion
            (3) Alternative: IV bolus PPI followed by intermittent high-dose PPI
        b) With bleeding from ulcers, IV bolus PPI followed by IV infusion of PPI is highly effective in reducing the risk of rebleeding. Continue IV infusion for 72 hours and then convert to two times a day PO dosing.
        c) Continue daily PO PPI after upper GI bleed caused by peptic ulcer disease for four to eight weeks.

2. Somatostatin analogs for variceal bleeding and cirrhosis
   a) Start IV octreotide 50 mcg IV bolus followed by 50 mcg/hr IV for five days in patients with acute variceal bleeding.
   b) PPIs and somatostatin analogs are not used together for variceal bleeding in patients with cirrhosis.
3. Antibiotics
   a) Reduce the risk of rebleeding and infection in patients with cirrhosis and gastroesophageal varices
   b) Recommended antibiotics for patients with cirrhosis
      (1) Short term (maximum seven days) antibiotic prophylaxis, such as norfloxacin 400 mg PO two times a day or ciprofloxacin 500 mg PO two times a day, should be administered to any patient with cirrhosis and GI hemorrhage.
      (2) In advanced cirrhosis, ceftriaxone 1 g IV daily is recommended.
4. Cardiac medications: Nonselective beta-blockers can be used to reduce hepatic venous pressure gradient if patient has cirrhosis and gastroesophageal varices (see Chapter 69) and evidence of portal hypertension; avoid use in active bleeding because it could interfere with cardiovascular responses.
5. Prokinetic agent: To empty stomach before endoscopy, give erythromycin 250 mg or 3 mg/kg infusion 30–120 minutes preprocedure.
6. Tranexamic acid: Evaluate if use is appropriate with severe bleeding.

I. Consult interventional radiology for arteriography with vasopressin infusion or embolization if EGD is unsuccessful in managing or locating source of bleeding. Minimal bleeding rate of 0.5–1 ml/minute is needed for visualization to occur.

J. Eliminate drug causes.

K. Administer oral iron supplements after patient is stable or PRN. This may cause dark stools, so carefully evaluate stool color and consistency prior to initiation of therapy (see Chapter 118).

L. If *H. pylori* is diagnosed, see Chapter 78 on peptic ulcer disease.

M. Portal hypertensive gastropathy: Pharmacologic (somatostatin and antibiotics) and endoscopy (with ligation therapy or other endoscopic therapy), or TIPS if more conservative approaches are unsuccessful

VII. Follow-up
   A. Monitor for further bleeding episodes and relapse of identified etiology.
   B. Most rebleeds occur within the first 72 hours after treatment.
   C. Patients requiring NSAID/ASA therapy must take ulcer prophylaxis.

VIII. Referrals (Farrar, 2018; Feinman & Haut, 2014; Nelms & Pelaez, 2018)
   A. Gastroenterologist: For immediate consultation to perform EGD, control bleeding, and perform follow-up endoscopy
   B. Medical internist or intensivist: For hospital admission, fluid and other resuscitation, and management of bleeding
   C. Surgeon: For crucial early consultation and ongoing evaluation, monitoring and prompt surgical interventions to correct bleeding etiology if other measures fail or are not appropriate, and for management of patients at risk of rebleeding
   D. Interventional radiologist: To perform angiogram and embolization of bleeding sites not controlled by endoscopic procedures or for patients too ill for surgery
   E. Cardiologist: As indicated for patients at risk or with cardiac history

References

Baracat, F., Moura, E., Bernardo, W., Pu, L.Z., Mendonça, E., Moura, D., … Ide, E. (2016). Endoscopic hemostasis for peptic ulcer bleeding: Systematic review and meta-analysis of randomized clinical trials. *Surgical Endoscopy, 30*(6), 2155–2168. https://doi.org/10.1007/s00464-015-4542-x

Farrar, F.C. (2018). Management of acute gastrointestinal bleed. *Critical Care Nursing Clinics of North America, 30*(1), 55–66. https://doi.org/10.1016/j.cnc.2017.10.005

Feinman, M., & Haut, E.R. (2014). Upper gastrointestinal bleeding. *Surgical Clinics of North America, 94*(1), 43–53. https://doi.org/10.1016/j.suc.2013.10.004

Haddad, F.G., El Imad, T., Nassani, N., Kwok, R., Al Moussawi, H., Polavarapu, A., … Deeb, L. (2019). In-hospital acute upper gastrointestinal bleeding: What is the scope of the problem? *World Journal of Gastrointestinal Endoscopy, 11*(12), 561–572. https://doi.org/10.4253/wjge.v11.i12.561

Hernández-Gea, V., Berbel, C., Baiges, A., & García-Pagán, J.C. (2018). Acute variceal bleeding: Risk stratification and management (including TIPS). *Hepatology International, 12*(Suppl. 1), S81–S90. https://doi.org/10.1007/s12072-017-9804-3

Kamboj, A.K., Hoversten, P., & Leggett, C.L. (2019). Upper gastrointestinal bleeding: Etiologies and management. *Mayo Clinic Proceedings, 94*(4), 697–703. https://doi.org/10.1016/j.mayocp.2019.01.022

Nelms, D.W., & Pelaez, C.A. (2018). The acute upper gastrointestinal bleed. *Surgical Clinics of North America, 98*(5), 1047–1057. https://doi.org/10.1016/j.suc.2018.05.004

Rahman, S.I.-U., & Saeian, K. (2016). Nonvariceal upper gastrointestinal bleeding. *Critical Care Clinics, 32*(2), 223–239. https://doi.org/10.1016/j.ccc.2015.12.002

Stanley, A.J., & Laine, L. (2019). Management of acute upper gastrointestinal bleeding. *BMJ, 364,* l536. https://doi.org/10.1136/bmj.l536

CHAPTER 60

Hepatomegaly

Richard Ornato, PA-C

I. Definition: Enlargement of the liver (Neal & Patel, 2017)

II. Physiology/Pathophysiology (Grus et al., 2017; Kowdley et al., 2019; Manne et al., 2018; Neal & Patel, 2017)
   A. Normal
      1. The liver span is approximately 6–12 cm and lies in the right upper quadrant of the abdomen, just below the diaphragm.
      2. Inferior surface lies close to the gallbladder, stomach, duodenum, and hepatic flexure of the colon.
      3. Each lobule is made up of liver cells (hepatocytes) radiating around a central vein from branches of the portal vein, hepatic artery, and bile duct.
      4. Bile is secreted by the hepatocytes into bile canaliculi and then to the hepatic ducts (left and right) that join with the cystic duct from the gallbladder to form the CBD. The CBD empties through the ampulla of Vater, which empties into the duodenum.
      5. The liver is a highly vascularized organ.
         a) The hepatic artery transports blood to the liver directly from the aorta, and the portal vein carries blood from the digestive tract and spleen to the liver.
         b) Three hepatic veins carry blood from the liver and empty into the IVC.
      6. Functions of the liver
         a) Metabolizes carbohydrates, fats, and proteins
         b) Converts glucose and stores it as glycogen; when stimulated, reconverts glycogen to glucose for secretion
         c) Uses cholesterol to form bile salts
         d) Metabolizes proteins to amino acids to albumin and converts their waste products to urea for excretion
         e) Stores several vitamins and iron
         f) Detoxifies potentially harmful substances
         g) Produces prothrombin, fibrinogen, and other substances for blood coagulation
         h) Conjugates and excretes steroid hormones
   B. Pathophysiology
      1. Hepatomegaly can result from destruction of the liver parenchyma, resulting in scarring and fat formation and indicating primary or secondary liver disease.
      2. In diabetes mellitus, hepatocellular glycogen accumulation can occur.
         a) During periods of hyperglycemia, glucose freely enters the hepatocytes, stimulating glycogen synthesis.

b) Accumulation of excessive amounts of glycogen in the hepatocytes is a function of intermittent episodes of hyperglycemia and hypoglycemia and the use of excessive insulin.

3. Nonalcoholic fatty liver disease is characterized by a fatty liver with infiltration of fat changing hepatocyte shape, resulting in swelling, cellular injury, and degeneration.

    a) This multifactorial process includes insulin resistance causing increased levels of fatty acids resulting in fatty infiltration of the liver.

    b) An increase in fatty acids eventually causes apoptosis of the hepatocytes.

4. Hemochromatosis is a genetic disorder more common in males of Northern European descent, causing hepatic iron deposits and enlargement of the liver. Clinically, the patient develops bronzing of the skin.

5. Hepatic venous obstruction can occur in the portal veins going to the liver or the hepatic veins going away from the liver (Budd-Chiari syndrome) to the IVC. This occlusive process causes increased hepatic sinusoidal pressure and portal hypertension.

III. Clinical features (Grus et al., 2017; Kowdley et al., 2019; Neal & Patel, 2017)

  A. Etiology

    1. Destruction of the liver by toxins, viruses (e.g., hepatitis A, B, C, and D), or bacteria

    2. Tumor involvement, primary or metastatic

    3. Alterations in hepatic venous outflow (e.g., from CHF, Budd-Chiari syndrome) or inflow causing hepatic ischemia (i.e., ischemic hepatitis)

    4. Extramedullary hematopoiesis

    5. Iron overload

    6. Obesity

    7. Autoimmune hepatitis

    8. Primary biliary cholangitis: Causes destruction of the bile ducts in the liver

    9. Primary sclerosis cholangitis: Causes destruction of intrahepatic and extrahepatic bile ducts

    10. Wilson disease: Genetic copper disorder

    11. Alpha-1 antitrypsin deficiency: Genetic disorder that affects liver and mainly the lungs

  B. History

    1. History of cancer and cancer treatment

    2. Current medications: Prescribed, over the counter (e.g., acetaminophen, oral contraceptives, androgenic steroids)

    3. History of presenting symptoms: Precipitating factors, onset, location, duration, associated symptoms (e.g., abdominal pain, fatigue, jaundice, color changes of stool or urine, somnolence)

    4. Changes in ADLs

    5. Social history: Alcohol use, illicit drug use, intranasal or IV drug use, tattoos, sexual activity

    6. Past medical history: Liver disease, hepatitis, cirrhosis, obesity, blood transfusion

    7. Family history: Liver disease

  C. Signs and symptoms

    1. Jaundice

    2. Confusion: End stage; from elevated serum ammonia level

    3. Right upper quadrant pain and fullness

    4. Nausea and vomiting

    5. Malaise

6. Fatigue, somnolence
7. Ascites
8. Light-colored stools
9. Dark urine
10. Anorexia
11. Weight loss
12. Pruritus

D. Physical examination
1. Integument
    a) Palmar surface inspection for erythema suggestive of chronic hepatitis
    b) Signs of excoriation
    c) Spider angioma: Seen on the head, neck, chest, arms, and upper abdomen almost exclusively in the drainage of the SVC, suggesting chronic hepatitis
    d) Acanthosis nigricans: Common finding from insulin resistance
    e) Jaundice
    f) Bronzing of the skin from excess iron deposition
2. HEENT/eye: Icteric sclerae and temporal wasting indicative of chronic disease
3. Cardiac: Heart murmurs, extra heart sounds, or rubs suggestive of CHF or tricuspid regurgitation
4. Abdominal
    a) Bruit, venous hum, or hepatic rub can occur.
        (1) Friction rubs are high-pitched and heard in association with respiration.
        (2) Venous hum is soft, low-pitched, and continuous, which occurs with increased collateral circulation between portal and systemic venous systems.
        (3) Scratch test is useful when the abdomen is distended (see Appendix D).
    b) Palpate the liver for contour and texture. Left lobe may be palpable in epigastrium.
        (1) Focal enlargement or rock-like consistency suggests tumor.
        (2) Tenderness suggests inflammation.
        (3) Rapid enlargement suggests right-sided heart failure.
        (4) Firmness and nodules suggest cirrhosis; nodules often are difficult to palpate.
        (5) Scarred cirrhotic liver may be small and not palpable.
    c) Percuss the liver margins to ascertain the size; normal vertical span is 6–12 cm, and normal midsternal span is 4–8 cm.
        (1) Normally, dullness is heard at the right costal margin or slightly below it.
        (2) Lower liver border that is more than 2–3 cm below the right costal margin suggests enlargement or downward displacement of the diaphragm secondary to pulmonary disease.
        (3) Upper liver border usually begins at the fifth to seventh intercostal space.
            (a) Upper border below the fifth to seventh intercostal space may indicate downward displacement or liver atrophy.
            (b) Dullness extending above the fifth to seventh intercostal space suggests upward displacement from ascites or masses.
    d) Assess fluid wave for ascites.
    e) Assessment of hepatojugular reflex is generally present and useful in differentiating hepatic congestion from primary intrahepatic liver disease or Budd-Chiari syndrome (see Appendix D).

IV. Diagnostic tests (Childs et al., 2016; Kowdley et al., 2019; Neal & Patel, 2017; Sweet et al., 2017)
   A. Laboratory
      1. LFTs: Enzymes may be elevated or normal.
         a) Serum glutamic–oxaloacetic transaminase or aspartate aminotransferase: Increased or normal
         b) Alkaline phosphatase: Increased or normal
      2. Serum albumin: Usually decreased
      3. Globulin levels: Often increased
      4. Bilirubin values: Usually elevated in obstructed diseases, acute and chronic hepatitis, end-stage liver disease, and drug toxicity
      5. Carcinoembryonic antigen value or alpha-fetoprotein levels: If hepatic metastasis or primary hepatic carcinoma is suspected (see Appendix O)
      6. Ferritin level: Increased in hemochromatosis
      7. PT: Usually increased in liver disease
      8. Glucose: Increased with diabetes
      9. Serum ammonia: May be elevated with hepatic encephalopathy
   B. Radiology
      1. Ultrasound: Best technique to assess liver size
      2. CT scan to evaluate the liver size, masses, and extrahepatic disease
   C. Other
      1. Biopsy of the liver, if necessary, to confirm diagnosis
      2. Diagnostic paracentesis to evaluate etiology (e.g., heart failure, cirrhosis)

V. Differential diagnosis (Kowdley et al., 2019; Long & Koyfman, 2018; Neal & Patel, 2017)
   A. Pulmonary etiology
      1. Lung hyperinflation
      2. COPD (see Chapter 28)
   B. Vascular congestion
      1. CHF (see Chapter 42)
      2. Tricuspid valve regurgitation
      3. Budd-Chiari syndrome
      4. Hepatic sinusoidal obstructive syndrome
      5. Hepatic infarction
      6. Constrictive pericarditis (see Chapter 50)
   C. Inflammatory disorders
      1. Hepatitis (see Chapter 74)
      2. Hepatotoxicity (see Chapter 75)
      3. Cirrhosis (see Chapter 69)
   D. Malignancy
      1. Hepatocellular carcinoma
      2. Metastatic cancer
   E. Infiltrative disorders
      1. Diabetes mellitus (see Chapter 151)
      2. Extramedullary hematopoiesis
      3. Amyloidosis
      4. Infection: TB (see Chapter 36), sarcoidosis, CMV
   F. Hematologic
      1. Hemolytic uremic syndrome
      2. Polycythemia vera (see Chapter 128)

      3. Thalassemia

      4. Hemochromatosis (see Chapter 121)

      5. Waldenström macroglobulinemia

      6. Hematologic malignancies

   G. Other

      1. Alcoholism

      2. Vitamin A toxicity

      3. HIV

      4. Cysts, adenomas

      5. Polycystic liver disease

      6. Drug induced: L-asparaginase, rituximab, anticholesterol agents, acetaminophen, anthracyclines, vinca alkaloids, erythromycin, cimetidine, halothane, isoniazid, tetracycline; all drugs metabolized by the liver have the potential to cause hepatotoxicity.

      7. Nonalcoholic fatty liver disease

      8. Nonalcoholic steatohepatitis

VI. Treatment: Dependent on underlying cause (Kowdley et al., 2019; Neal & Patel, 2017; Sweet et al., 2017)

   A. Avoid hepatotoxic medications.

   B. Place on a low-protein diet if in liver failure.

   C. Low-sodium diet may be needed if ascites is present.

   D. Administer regular phlebotomy treatments for hemochromatosis and polycythemia (see Chapters 121 and 128).

   E. Perform liver transplantation for severe hepatomegaly in polycystic liver disease.

   F. Control diabetes (see Chapter 151).

   G. Hepatic venous occlusion may require opening with balloon dilation and stenting or anticoagulation.

   H. Control obesity.

VII. Follow-up: Dependent on underlying cause

VIII. Referrals: Dependent on underlying cause

   A. Infectious disease specialist: To develop treatment plan for infections

   B. Oncologist: For evaluation and treatment of cancer

   C. Surgeon or interventional radiologist: For liver biopsy and transplantation

   D. Hematologist: For blood disorders

The author would like to acknowledge Dawn Camp-Sorrell, MSN, FNP, AOCN®, for her contribution to this chapter that remains unchanged from the previous edition of this book.

References

Childs, J.T., Esterman, A.J., Thoirs, K.A., & Turner, R.C. (2016). Ultrasound in the assessment of hepatomegaly: A simple technique to determine an enlarged liver using reliable and valid measurements. *Sonography, 3*(2), 47–52. https://doi.org/10.1002/sono.12051

Grus, T., Lambert, L., Grusová, G., Banerjee, R., & Burgetová, A. (2017). Budd-Chiari syndrome. *Prague Medical Report, 118*(2–3), 69–80. https://doi.org/10.14712/23362936.2017.6

Kowdley, K.V., Brown, K.E., Ahn, J., & Sundaram, V. (2019). ACG clinical guideline: Hereditary hemochromatosis. *American Journal of Gastroenterology, 114*(8), 1202–1218. https://doi.org/10.14309/ajg.0000000000000315

Long, B., & Koyfman, A. (2018). The emergency medicine evaluation and management of the patient with cirrhosis. *American Journal of Emergency Medicine, 36*(4), 689–698. https://doi.org/10.1016/j.ajem.2017.12.047

Manne, V., Handa, P., & Kowdley, K.V. (2018). Pathophysiology of nonalcoholic fatty liver disease/nonalcoholic steatohepatitis. *Clinical Liver Disease, 22*(1), 23–37. https://doi.org/10.1016/j.cld.2017.08.007.

Neal, K., & Patel, S. (2017). Hepatomegaly. *Cancer Therapy Advisor.* https://www.cancertherapyadvisor.com/home/decision-support-in-medicine/hospital-medicine/hepatomegaly-2

Sweet, P.H., Khoo, T., & Nguyen, S. (2017). Nonalcoholic fatty liver disease. *Primary Care: Clinics in Office Practice, 44*(4), 599–607. https://doi.org/10.1016/j.pop.2017.07.003.

CHAPTER 61

Jaundice

Richard Ornato, PA-C

I. Definition: Characteristic yellowing of the skin, sclera, and mucous membranes caused by the accumulation of bilirubin, a bile pigment, in the bloodstream (Abbas et al., 2016)

II. Physiology/Pathophysiology (Abbas et al., 2016; M. Chen et al., 2015; Dong et al., 2019; Fargo et al., 2017; Taylor & Wheatley, 2018)
   A. Normal: Healthy adults produce approximately 250 mg of bilirubin daily. Bilirubin is mainly the end product of Hgb degradation (70%–80%) from aged erythrocytes. An additional 20%–30% comes from the destruction of heme proteins (e.g., myoglobin, cytochrome P450 isoenzymes) by hepatocytes, and an insignificant portion is the result of ineffective erythropoiesis. This process of bilirubin production occurs during the prehepatic phase of bilirubin metabolism.
      1. The bilirubin initially produced through RBC destruction is referred to as unconjugated or indirect bilirubin.
         a) It is water insoluble and transported in the plasma bound to albumin.
         b) In healthy adults, approximately 90%–95% of circulating bilirubin is unconjugated.
      2. Once unconjugated bilirubin is transported to the liver, it is taken up by hepatocytes and converted to conjugated or direct bilirubin. This process happens during the intrahepatic phase.
      3. In the posthepatic phase, conjugated bilirubin is turned into bile and is stored in the gallbladder or travels into the duodenum, where it is eventually excreted in stool or turned into urobilinogen and reabsorbed or excreted in urine.
   B. Pathophysiology: Jaundice can be divided into three categories based on origin.
      1. Disorders of bilirubin metabolism
         a) Increased erythrocyte destruction: Hemolysis, ineffective erythropoiesis, transfusions, reabsorption of large hematomas
         b) Impaired uptake of bilirubin in hepatocytes: Secondary to drugs (e.g., rifampin)
         c) Impaired conjugation of bilirubin in the liver: Secondary to drugs (e.g., indinavir), Gilbert syndrome
      2. Liver disease
         a) Hepatocellular dysfunction occurs with direct effect on the hepatocytes.
         b) Hepatic disorders with cholestasis involve a compromised ability to transform bilirubin into bile as a result of diffuse hepatocellular injury or obstruction.
      3. Bile duct obstruction: Cholestatic jaundice is a result of impairment of bile flow between the hepatocytes and duodenum.

III. Clinical features: Jaundice may be evident when total serum bilirubin levels reach upward of 2.5–3 mg/dl. Clinically, however, it may take several days for visible signs (e.g., changes in skin color, sclera) to manifest. Jaundice can be classified as acute, subacute, or chronic and occurs in one of three phases of bilirubin metabolism: prehepatic, intrahepatic, or posthepatic. Clinical presentation ranges from asymptomatic to life threatening (see Table 61-1; Abbas et al., 2016; Björnsson, 2020; Fargo et al., 2017; Kovalic et al., 2019; Taylor & Wheatley, 2018; Wooton-Kee et al., 2015).

A. Risk factors

1. Cancer
2. Alcohol abuse
3. IV drug abuse, tattooing, unsafe sexual practices
4. Blood transfusions

TABLE 61-1   Clinical Features of Jaundice

Etiology	Onset	Signs/Symptoms	Laboratory	Physical Findings
Excess bilirubin production	Usually sudden	Pale yellow skin; dark stool	Normal aminotransferase levels Increased reticulocyte count Increased serum bilirubin (usually < 3.5 mg/dl) Decreased hemoglobin/hematocrit (hemolysis)	Splenomegaly, ecchymoses
Extrahepatic obstruction	Gradual	Jaundice; persistent pruritus; nausea, vomiting; mild to deep yellow-green skin; dark urine; clay-colored stool; fever; pain	Increased alkaline phosphatase, bilirubin, and transaminases Increased urine bilirubin Elevated serum amylase or lipase Possible leukocytosis If prothrombin time is increased, normalizes with vitamin K administration	Fever, abdominal tenderness, palpable abdominal mass
Impaired bilirubin conjugation	Neonatal type: First week of life, transient	Jaundice	Increased indirect bilirubin	Kernicterus
Impaired bilirubin uptake in the liver	Episodic, self-limiting	Mild jaundice	Increased indirect bilirubin	None
Intrahepatic cholestasis	Gradual	Anorexia, malaise, myalgias; mild to deep orange-yellow skin; dark urine; pale stool; pruritus	Increased alkaline phosphatase Increased direct/indirect bilirubin Increased urine bilirubin Increased prothrombin time Increased aspartate aminotransferase/serum glutamic-oxaloacetic transaminase	Ascites, abdominal veins, spider angioma, ecchymosis, hepatosplenomegaly, encephalopathy

Note. Based on information from Abbas et al., 2016; Fargo et al., 2017; Taylor & Wheatley, 2018; Wooton-Kee et al., 2015.

     5. Acute or chronic pancreatitis

     6. Gallstones

     7. Hepatitis: Acute or chronic

     8. Travel to underdeveloped countries

     9. Consumption of unsafe shellfish or other foods

    10. Certain medications: Acetaminophen, rifampin, statins

    11. Prior biliary tract surgery

    12. Certain autoimmune diseases: Primary sclerosing cholangitis

    13. Hereditary metabolic disease: Wilson disease

    14. Certain systemic diseases: Sarcoidosis, TB

B. Etiology

     1. Intrahepatic

        a) Infiltrative process: Malignancy; granulomatous diseases (e.g., sarcoidosis, mycobacterial infections)

        b) Inflammatory process: Primary biliary cirrhosis, GVHD

     2. Extrahepatic

        a) Intrahepatic or distal bile duct obstruction that leads to impaired hepatocytes

        b) Indirect damage to the liver, including pancreatitis; postoperative bile duct resection; neoplasms of the bile duct

     3. Hepatocellular injury due to viruses: Hepatitis B and C

     4. Hepatotoxins: Ethanol, acetaminophen, vitamin A

     5. Drugs: Isoniazid, phenytoin

     6. Metabolic disorders: Hemochromatosis, Wilson disease, nonalcoholic fatty liver disease

     7. Pregnancy induced: Preeclampsia, acute fatty liver

     8. Benign cholestasis

C. History

     1. History of cancer and cancer treatment

     2. Current medications: Prescribed, over the counter, herbal products

     3. History of presenting symptoms: Precipitating factors, onset, location, duration, associated symptoms (e.g., alteration in skin color, abdominal pain, fever, rigors, fatigue, myalgias, anorexia, weight loss, dyspepsia, nausea, vomiting, diarrhea, changes in stool color, pruritus)

     4. Changes in ADLs

     5. Past medical history: Blood or plasma transfusions, hepatitis, fat intolerance, biliary colic, surgical procedures, previous episodes of jaundice

     6. Family history: Liver disease or anemia

     7. Social history: Alcohol use, illicit drug use, occupation, exposure to toxins

     8. History of recent contact with a person with jaundice or viral hepatitis, recent foreign travel, recent consumption of raw shellfish or oysters

D. Signs and symptoms (see Table 61-1)

E. Physical examination

     1. Vital signs: Weight loss, fever

     2. General: Demeanor, energy level

     3. Integument: Discoloration of the skin (yellow)

        a) Jaundice

        b) Ecchymoses indicating clotting disorders, liver dysfunction, obstructive or hepatocellular disease

        c) Palmar erythema indicating acute or chronic liver failure

        d) Scratch marks indicating pruritus

        e) Hyperkeratosis indicating chronic cholestasis
        f) Pallor indicating anemia
        g) Gynecomastia: Sign of alcoholic liver disease

    4. Abdominal
        a) Tenderness indicating inflammation
        b) Hepatomegaly indicating liver disease
        c) Splenomegaly indicating cirrhosis
        d) Ascites or fluid wave indicating cirrhosis or malignancy
        e) Abdominal venous distention: Spider angiomas, portal hypertension as a result of acute or chronic liver damage
        f) Palpable abdominal mass indicating malignancy
        g) Palpable gallbladder: Known as Courvoisier sign; indication of CBD obstruction
        h) Charcot triad: Fever, jaundice, and right upper quadrant pain indicating gallstones
        i) Murphy sign: Hallmark of acute cholecystitis; tenderness on deep palpation under right costal margin (see Appendix D)

    5. Eye
        a) Sclera: Icterus
        b) Xanthoma of eyelids indicating chronic cholestasis
        c) Kayser-Fleischer rings around the iris: Present in Wilson disease

    6. Neurologic: Asterixis; flapping tremor of hands seen when encephalopathy present

IV. Diagnostic tests (Abbas et al., 2016; Fargo et al., 2017; Taylor & Wheatley, 2018)
    A. Laboratory (see Table 61-1)
        1. Initial testing
            a) CBC
                (1) Presence of schistocytes and increased reticulocytes are indicative of hemolysis.
                (2) Leukocytosis may be found with biliary tract obstructions or inflammation.
                (3) Thrombocytopenia is common in patients with cirrhosis or impaired splenic function due to portal hypertension.
            b) Serum total bilirubin and fractionated bilirubin: Normal total bilirubin levels range from 0.2–1 mg/dl; direct bilirubin 0.1–0.3 mg/dl; and indirect bilirubin 0.2–0.8 mg/dl.
                (1) Increased direct bilirubin indicates hepatocellular or cholestatic disease.
                (2) Increased indirect bilirubin indicates hemolysis.
                (3) Increased total and indirect bilirubin indicates disorders of bilirubin metabolism.
                (4) Increased direct bilirubin indicates bile duct obstruction.
            c) Transaminases (e.g., AST, ALT): Increases indicate hepatocellular injury due to ischemia, toxins, or viruses. This may not be useful in determining the etiology of jaundice in patients with chronic liver disease.
            d) Alkaline phosphatase, gamma-glutamyl transferase: Increased levels may indicate cholestasis. Levels three times the normal indicate obstruction (intrahepatic and extrahepatic) and prolonged cholestasis. It is more sensitive in liver injury than serum glutamic–oxaloacetic transaminase.
            e) Albumin: Low albumin indicates decreased liver function.
            f) Prealbumin: It is used to measure current nutritional status and decreased with poor nutritional status.

g) PT and INR: Prolonged PT and increased INR suggest cholestasis and obstruction; if not reversible with vitamin K administration, this suggests hepatocellular disease.

2. Secondary tests

a) Urine: Urinalysis provides a measure of bilirubin excretion. Increased values indicate cholestasis, obstruction, or hepatocellular injury.

b) Hepatitis A antibody, hepatitis B surface antigen, and hepatitis C antibody to assess for viral etiologies of jaundice

c) Amylase, lipase: Elevated with pancreatitis

d) Tumor markers, such as cancer antigen 19-9 (CA 19-9), carcinoembryonic antigen (CEA), or alpha fetoprotein, if suspected of or to confirm biliary or pancreatic carcinoma (CA 19-9), colorectal metastasis (CEA), or hepatocellular carcinoma (alpha fetoprotein)

e) IgM and IgG, antinuclear antibody, smooth muscle antibody, antimitochondrial antibody to evaluate for suspected autoimmune disorders

f) Ferritin, iron saturation to evaluate for secondary iron overload, or *HFE* gene for hemochromatosis and other anemias

g) Reticulocyte count: Increased with excess bilirubin production

B. Radiology

1. Abdominal ultrasound: Low-cost, noninvasive technique for evaluating obstructive jaundice

a) It is useful in determining the size of the hepatobiliary tree and revealing intra- or extrahepatic lesions and gallstones; it may not be useful in obese patients or patients with underlying bowel gas.

b) Ultrasound may not be able to accurately determine the exact location of the obstruction.

2. CT scan of the abdomen with contrast: Noninvasive, allows for accurate measurement of dilated bile ducts, and assesses size and location of hepatic masses, pancreatic lesions, and other space-occupying abdominal lesions

a) It is superior to ultrasound in obese patients.

b) Contrast may be contraindicated in some patients with renal insufficiency.

3. MRI of the abdomen

a) MRI is similar to CT but without the risk of radiation.

b) It is more sensitive than CT in differentiating metastasis, hemangiomas, hepatomas, and other liver lesions.

4. Magnetic resonance cholangiopancreatography: Noninvasive and provides function and anatomic information

a) It is more accurate than ultrasound or CT at detecting obstructions.

b) Standard MRI can be done simultaneously if there is suspicion for a hepatic or pancreatic mass.

5. Endoscopic retrograde cholangiopancreatography

a) This invasive procedure involves passing an endoscope into the duodenum, inserting a catheter into the ampulla of Vater, and injecting contrast into the bile duct.

b) It can identify obstructions in the biliary tree and allows for biopsies and brushings, as well as interventions including sphincterotomy, stone extraction, biliary stenting, and biliary stricture dilation.

6. Percutaneous transhepatic cholangiography

a) This invasive procedure involves passing a needle through the skin and hepatic parenchyma and into the biliary tract. It has been largely replaced by magnetic resonance cholangiopancreatography and endoscopic retrograde cholangiopancreatography.

   b) It may be useful when obstructions are proximal to the common hepatic duct or when ECRP cannot be completed.

   c) It allows for interventions including biopsies and stenting.

7. Endoscopic ultrasound

   a) This invasive procedure allows for visualization of the biliary tree and duodenum.

   b) It is useful in the detection of bile duct obstructions and allows for biopsies of suspected malignancies.

8. Cholescintigraphy (hepatobiliary iminodiacetic acid scan): It is limited in the presence of elevated bilirubin levels and not recommended for routine evaluation of jaundice.

C. Other

   1. Angiography: It is rarely used but helpful in patients with portal hypertension.

   2. Liver biopsy: Percutaneous liver biopsy can be done to obtain tissue from masses or lesions identified by other imaging methods.

V. Differential diagnosis (Abbas et al., 2016; Björnsson, 2020; Fargo et al., 2017; Kovalic et al., 2019; Taylor & Wheatley, 2018)

A. Prehepatic: Unconjugated hyperbilirubinemia

   1. Hemolysis: Hemolytic anemia (see Chapter 117), sickle cell disease (see Chapter 119), post–blood transfusion hemolysis

   2. Ineffective erythropoiesis: Thalassemia, iron (see Chapter 118) or folate deficiency (see Chapter 116)

   3. Reabsorption of large hematomas

B. Intrahepatic

   1. Unconjugated hyperbilirubinemia

      a) Hereditary disorders of bilirubin metabolism: Gilbert syndrome

      b) Drugs: Rifampin

   2. Conjugated hyperbilirubinemia: Drug induced (e.g., rifampin)

C. Liver disease

   1. Acute or chronic dysfunction

      a) Viral hepatitis (see Chapter 74)

      b) Wilson disease (rare), hemochromatosis (see Chapter 121), hepatotoxins (e.g., alcohol, medications, poison; see Chapter 75)

   2. Diffuse infiltrative disorders: Sarcoidosis, lymphoma, amyloidosis

   3. Inflammation of intrahepatic bile ducts and/or portal tracts

      a) GVHD

      b) Primary biliary cholangitis (see Chapter 69)

D. Obstruction of bile ducts

   1. Gallstones (see Chapter 68)

   2. Inflammation/infection: HIV/AIDS, hepatic arterial chemotherapy, postoperative strictures, primary sclerosing cholangitis

   3. Extrinsic compression of biliary tree: Pancreatitis (see Chapter 77), cancer

E. Common malignancies associated with jaundice

   1. Hepatocellular carcinoma

   2. Cholangiocarcinoma

   3. Gallbladder cancer

   4. Pancreatic cancer

   5. Ampullary cancer

   6. Duodenal cancer

   7. Metastatic cancer

   8. Lymphoma

VI. Treatment (Abbas et al., 2016; Björnsson, 2020; H.-L. Chen et al., 2018; Fargo et al., 2017; Taylor & Wheatley, 2018; Wooton-Kee et al., 2015)
   A. Obstructed bile ducts: Provide mechanical relief of obstruction.
      1. Removal of obstruction via surgery
      2. Palliative surgical bypass
      3. Stent placement
      4. Internal or external drain placement
      5. Sphincterotomy
      6. Balloon dilation of focal strictures
   B. Liver disease: Treat the underlying cause of the liver disease.
      1. Cessation of alcohol consumption
      2. Discontinuation of offending drug
      3. Antiviral therapy
   C. Management of pruritus (see Chapter 16)
      1. Antihistamines: Rarely provides significant relief
         a) Diphenhydramine: 25–50 mg PO four times a day
         b) Hydroxyzine: 25 mg PO three times a day
      2. Cholestyramine: 4–6 g PO 30 minutes before meals (absorbs bile acids); adverse effects: fat malabsorption, decreased absorption of other medications, constipation
      3. Emollients, mild fragrance-free soaps, less frequent bathing, lightweight clothing, short fingernails
   D. Management of cachexia (see Chapter 66)
      1. Nutritional supplements
      2. Dronabinol: 2.5–5 mg PO daily before lunch and dinner; started low and titrated slowly in older adult patients because of risk of CNS effects
      3. Megestrol: 400–800 mg PO daily

VII. Follow-up: Dependent on etiology and stage of disease

VIII. Referrals
   A. Gastroenterologist: For endoscopic retrograde cholangiopancreatography or endoscopic ultrasound
   B. Hepatologist: For evaluation and management of nonmalignant liver disease
   C. Hematologist: For patient with hemolytic anemia, thalassemia, or other blood disorders
   D. Surgeon: For gallstones and other surgically amenable conditions in curative or palliative cases
   E. Oncologist: For evaluation and treatment of malignant masses

The author would like to acknowledge Alison Ivey, RN, BSN, OCN®, CCRP, for her contribution to this chapter that remains unchanged from the previous edition of this book.

References

Abbas, M.W., Shamshad, T., Ashraf, M.A., & Javaid, R. (2016). Jaundice: A basic review. *International Journal of Research in Medical Sciences, 4*(5), 1313–1319. https://doi.org/10.18203/2320–6012.ijrms20161196

Björnsson, E.S. (2020). Epidemiology, predisposing factors, and outcomes of drug-induced liver injury. *Clinics in Liver Disease, 24*(1), 1–10. https://doi.org/10.1016/j.cld.2019.08.002

Chen, M., Suzuki, A., Borlak, J., Andrade, R.J., & Lucena, M.I. (2015). Drug-induced liver injury: Interactions between drug properties and host factors. *Journal of Hepatology, 63*(2), 503–514. https://doi.org/10.1016/j.jhep.2015.04.016.

Chen, H.-L., Wu, S.-H., Hsu, S.-H., Liou, B.-Y., Chen, H.-L., & Chang, M.-H. (2018). Jaundice revisited: Recent advances in the diagnosis and treatment of inherited cholestatic liver diseases. *Journal of Biomedical Science, 25,* 75. https://doi.org/10.1186/s12929-018-0475-8

Dong, V., Nanchal, R., & Karvellas, C.J. (2019). Pathophysiology of acute liver failure. *Nutrition in Clinical Practice, 35*(1), 24–29. https://doi.org/10.1002/ncp.10459

Fargo, M.V., Grogan, S.P., & Saguil, A. (2017). Evaluation of jaundice in adults. *American Family Physician, 95*(3), 164–168. https://www.aafp.org/afp/2017/0201/p164.html

Kovalic, A.J., Cholankeril, G., & Satapathy, S.K. (2019). Nonalcoholic fatty liver disease and alcoholic liver disease: Metabolic diseases with systemic manifestations. *Translational Gastroenterology and Hepatology, 4,* 65. https://doi.org/10.21037/tgh.2019.08.09

Taylor, T., & Wheatley, M. (2018). Jaundice in the emergency department: Meeting the challenges of diagnosis and treatment. *Emergency Medicine Practice, 20*(4), 1–24.

Wooton-Kee, C.R., Jain, A.K., Wagner, M., Grusak, M.A., Finegold, M.J., Lutsenko, S., & Moore, D.D. (2015). Elevated copper impairs hepatic nuclear receptor function in Wilson's disease. *Journal of Clinical Investigation, 125*(9), 3449–3460. https://doi.org/10.1172/JCI78991

CHAPTER 62

Melena

Jeanne Held-Warmkessel, MSN, RN, AOCN®, ACNS-BC

I. Definition: Foul-smelling, black, tarry stool associated with bleeding of an upper GI source, such as the esophagus, stomach, or duodenum, but may originate lower in the GI tract (Farrar, 2018)

II. Physiology/Pathophysiology (Jung & Moon, 2019; Stanley & Laine, 2019)
   A. Normal: The mucosal surface of the GI tract is composed of epithelial cells.
      1. The functions of the epithelial cells are transmembrane absorption and secretion.
      2. These functions facilitate the digestive tract in digestion and nutrient uptake.
      3. The epithelial cells act as a barrier against potentially harmful pathogens and mutagens in the lumen.
   B. Pathophysiology
      1. Blood is lost proximal to the ileocecal valve where Hgb is converted into hematin, which gives the stool a tarry appearance.
      2. Blood usually originates from the upper GI tract above the ligament of Treitz and is degraded as it passes through the small and large bowel.
      3. Right colonic bleeding or small bowel bleeding may cause melena when transit is slow.
      4. It indicates blood is in bowel for 14 hours or longer.
      5. Upper GI bleeding is categorized as either variceal or nonvariceal.
      6. The redder the blood, the faster the bleeding.

III. Clinical features: Melena may vary in severity from low, chronic blood loss to massive hemorrhage requiring intensive nursing care. Bleeding is overt (visible), obscure (recurrent bleeding in which source is not identified on upper endoscopy, colonoscopy, or small bowel radiography), or occult (not visible) (see Table 62-1; Farrar, 2018; Jung & Moon, 2019; Murphy et al., 2019; Nelms & Pelaez, 2018; Ohmiya et al., 2015; Rahman & Saeian, 2016; Stanley & Laine, 2019).
   A. Etiology
      1. Vascular: Varices, vascular lesions, angiodysplasia, small bowel bleeding, portal hypertension from liver disease
      2. Inflammatory
      3. Medications
      4. Tumors, cancer
      5. Diverticular disease
      6. Peptic ulcer disease
   B. History
      1. History of cancer and cancer treatment: Radiation therapy, abdominal surgery

TABLE 62-1	Clinical Features of Upper Gastrointestinal Bleed
Blood Loss	**Clinical Manifestation**
50–200 ml	Black, tarry stools; larger volumes may cause maroon stools.
< 500 ml	No associated hemodynamic instability
> 500 ml	Signs of hemodynamic instability
> 20% blood loss	Orthostatic blood pressure falls > 10 mm Hg or pulse rises > 10 beats per minute

Note. Based on information from Farrar, 2018; Nelms & Pelaez, 2018; Ohmiya et al., 2015.

2. Current medications: Prescribed, over the counter, NSAIDs/ASA, antiplatelet agents, anticoagulants, direct oral anticoagulants, SSRIs
3. History of presenting symptoms: Precipitating factors, onset, volume, frequency, duration, associated symptoms (e.g., dark red stool, black tarry stools, bleeding, dyspepsia, abdominal pain, back pain, anorexia, vomiting, vomiting blood, retching, dysphagia, indigestion, altered bowel habits, weight loss, fatigue)
4. Changes in ADLs
5. Past medical history: Ulcers, abdominal surgery, prior bleed or GI disorder, nosebleeds, mouth bleeding, liver disease, HIV, diverticular disease, recent GI procedures, pancreatitis, renal disease, heart failure, valvular heart disease, coagulation disorders, inflammatory bowel disease, Peutz-Jeghers syndrome, past surgical history
6. Social history: Alcohol use, tobacco use
7. Family history: Bowel disorders (e.g., Crohn disease, colitis, polyps, cancer, bleeding dyscrasia), coagulation disorders
8. Age: Older patients are at greater risk of bleeding from NSAID/ASA-related peptic ulcer disease.

C. Signs and symptoms
  1. Black, tarry stool
  2. Pallor
  3. Diaphoresis
  4. Dizziness and light-headedness
  5. Syncope
  6. Nausea and vomiting
  7. Thirst
  8. Bruising, hematuria, abnormal vaginal bleeding suggestive of coagulopathy
  9. Signs and symptoms of anemia: Fatigue, dyspnea, chest pain
  10. Abdominal pain
  11. Fatigue

D. Physical examination
  1. Vital signs and pulse oximetry: Hemodynamic instability
    a) Orthostatic hypotension, hypotension
    b) Tachycardia
    c) Possible lower GI bleed in patients who are hemodynamically stable
  2. Integument
    a) Rash, pallor, ecchymosis, petechiae, temperature, signs of liver or GI tract diseases (e.g., telangiectasias, angiomas, caput medusae)
    b) Nailbeds: Blanching; presence of rubor indicating inflammation from tissue injury
  3. HEENT: Nose and mouth for bleeding, oral telangiectasia, conjunctiva for pallor

4. Abdominal
   a) Distention
   b) Hyperactive bowel sounds: Upper GI source
   c) Tenderness, pain
   d) Masses
   e) Ascites
   f) Liver size
   g) Signs of peritonitis: Rebound tenderness, guarding
5. Rectal
   a) Stool testing for occult blood
   b) Rectal mass, tenderness, fecal impaction, passage of blood per rectum, hemorrhoids, fissures, stool color
6. Mental status: May be altered with decrease in blood volume
7. Cardiac, pulses, and capillary refill: May be decreased with loss of blood volume

IV. Diagnostic tests: Perform concurrently with treatment (Chopra et al., 2020; Farrar, 2018; Murphy et al., 2019; Nelms & Pelaez, 2018; Ohmiya et al., 2015; Rahman & Saeian, 2016; Stanley & Laine, 2019).
   A. Laboratory
      1. CBC with differential: Serial Hgb and hematocrit
         a) Indicating signs of anemia
            (1) Low mean corpuscular volume and low ferritin and iron to total iron-binding capacity ratio with chronic blood loss are signs of indicating anemia.
            (2) Fall in Hgb and hematocrit may not reflect volume of blood loss for 24–72 hours after bleeding begins.
            (3) Patients with melena often have a lower Hgb level than patients with hematemesis.
         b) Low platelet count indicating thrombocytopenia and increased risk of bleeding
      2. Coagulation studies: PT, PTT, and INR to assess for prolonged values, which facilitate bleeding
      3. LFTs to assess for abnormal values indicating liver disorders, total bilirubin
      4. CMP with BUN and creatinine: Increased BUN greater than or equal to 28 mg/dl; consider upper GI bleed; digested blood protein increases BUN.
      5. Type and crossmatch: If transfusion is needed and be prepared to transfuse
      6. Albumin: Low in liver dysfunction
      7. Electrolytes/chemistries to assess for imbalance from bleed
      8. Serum lactate level to assess for acidosis related to shock
      9. Cardiac enzymes in patients at risk for cardiac complications
      10. Test for *Helicobacter pylori*, as indicated
      11. Viscoelastic testing to assist with fluid resuscitation efforts
   B. Radiology
      1. Superselective celiac and mesenteric angiogram/arteriogram
         a) Perform after positive CT angiography or nuclear medicine scan.
         b) Use if endoscopic examination is negative.
         c) Use if massive bleeding precludes adequate endoscopic visualization.
         d) Perform if patient is unstable and cannot have adequate pre-endoscopic bowel preparation.
         e) Lesion must bleed at rate greater than or equal to 0.5 ml/min for angiography to be diagnostic.

        f) Perform to locate and control bleeding source prior to surgery.

        g) Use digital subtraction techniques for slow bleeding.

    2. CT scan of abdomen and pelvis to assess for tumors, masses, lymphadenopathy, liver disease, and hematoma formation

    3. Nuclear medicine: Radionuclide scanning

        a) Technetium-99m–labeled RBC scintigram is used.

        b) It is useful when colonoscopy or EGD is not diagnostic.

        c) Bleeding rate of more than 0.1 ml/min is needed for test to be useful.

        d) It should be performed before angiogram.

        e) Patient should be sent to angiography without a scan when massive bleeding is present.

    4. CT enterography/enteroclysis or magnetic resonance enterography/enteroclysis: For occult bleeding, small bowel bleeding source, or when endoscopy is nondiagnostic

    5. CT angiography: Useful in planning additional therapy such as surgery or angiography; no oral contrast required

  C. Other

    1. Upper endoscopy

        a) It is the preferred test to assess upper GI tract as potential source of bleeding.

        b) It should be performed as soon as possible; if patient is stabilized hemodynamically, it should be performed within 24 hours of onset of bleeding (12 hours with variceal bleeding or if patient not hemodynamically stable).

        c) Upper endoscopy should be used even if NG aspirate is negative for blood (bleeding source identified in 90% of cases).

        d) If ulcer or erosion is present, biopsy for *H. pylori.*

    2. Colonoscopy: Frequently the test of choice unless there is massive bleeding, bowel prep cannot be done, or patient is too unstable

        a) Colonoscopy can be done emergently to identify bleeding site and institute treatment; rapid purge bowel prep can be done for urgent colonoscopy.

        b) It should be performed within 24–48 hours of bleeding episode if upper GI evaluation is unrevealing.

    3. Anoscopy/proctosigmoidoscopy is not useful.

    4. Video capsule endoscopy is useful for difficult-to-find sources of GI bleeding; it can scan the entire small bowel.

    5. Double-balloon enteroscopy

        a) It can be performed via rectum or oral cavity.

        b) This technique may be used therapeutically to clip, biopsy, or remove polyps or other abnormalities.

    6. NG aspirate to assess for upper GI source: Not a reliable indicator of upper GI source in patients without hematemesis

    7. Pulse oximetry to assess oxygen saturation in massive GI bleed

    8. ECG to determine if myocardial ischemia or infarction related to blood loss in patients with or at risk for acute coronary syndrome is present

V. Differential diagnosis (Farrar, 2018; Feinman & Haut, 2014; Jung & Moon, 2019; Nelms & Pelaez, 2018; Ohmiya et al., 2015; Rahman & Saeian, 2016)

  A. Medications/drugs that promote GI bleeding

    1. NSAIDs/ASA: Most common etiology in older adults due to ulcer formation (see Appendix E)

    2. Corticosteroids

3. Anticoagulants, antiplatelet agents, direct oral anticoagulants

4. Alcohol induced, smoking induced

B. Peptic ulcer disease with or without associated *H. pylori* infection (see Chapter 78)

C. Gastritis (see Chapter 72)

D. Mallory-Weiss tear

E. Erosive gastritis, esophagitis, stress gastritis, esophageal ulcers

F. GERD (see Chapter 71)

G. Duodenal ulcer, duodenitis

H. Portal hypertensive gastropathy or colonopathy

I. Cancer

   1. Esophageal

   2. Gastric

   3. Small bowel

   4. Colorectal

   5. Metastasis

   6. Sarcomas

J. Gastric polyps, colon polyps, small bowel polyps, post-polypectomy bleeding

K. Esophageal varices/gastric varices, variceal hemorrhage

L. Infection: CMV enteritis, herpes simplex, *Candida albicans*, intestinal TB

M. Aortoenteric fistula: After repair of abdominal aortic aneurysm

N. Mesenteric vascular occlusion secondary to clot

O. GVHD

P. Pseudomelena: From iron, bismuth, licorice, beets, blueberries, charcoal

Q. Any cause of lower GI bleeding

   1. Crohn disease

   2. Infectious colitis

   3. Ulcerative colitis

R. Vascular ectasias/arteriovenous malformations, angiodysplasia

S. Hemobilia (fistula between splanchnic circulation and the biliary system)

T. Meckel diverticulum

U. Diverticular disease of colon or small bowel (see Chapter 70)

V. Dieulafoy lesion in GI tract, often stomach

W. Postsurgical anastomotic ulcerations

X. Hemosuccus pancreaticus

VI. Treatment: Administered concurrently with diagnosis because bleeding may range from minor to potentially life threatening and require intensive nursing level of care (Farrar, 2018; Feinman & Haut, 2014; Hernández-Gea et al., 2018; Nelms & Pelaez, 2018; Stanley & Laine, 2019)

A. General treatment and supportive measures

   1. Insert two large-gauge IV cannulas.

   2. Administer oxygen.

      a) If pulse oximetry is low or the patient has cardiopulmonary disease

      b) Oxygen saturation greater than 90% desirable

   3. Monitor vital signs continuously for hemodynamic instability.

   4. Monitor output; insert indwelling urinary catheter (consider short-term use to avoid infection).

   5. Monitor central venous pressure.

   6. Place on bed rest, to prevent syncope if hypotensive, and to conserve energy.

B. Fluid resuscitation: Infuse IV isotonic (normal saline) fluids. Avoid overhydration. Monitor fluid balance.

C. Blood transfusions
1. Administer packed RBCs PRN to maintain minimal Hgb of 7 g/dl (8 g/dl for patients with heart disease).
2. Correct bleeding abnormalities (e.g., prolonged PT) with transfusions of fresh frozen plasma; one unit often is administered after four units of packed RBCs, or use prothrombin complex concentrate. Avoid use in patients with cirrhosis and acute variceal bleeding.
3. Administer platelets to correct bleeding caused by thrombocytopenia.
4. Administer coagulation factors to correct identified deficiencies.
5. Massive transfusion protocol may be needed.
D. Medications
1. Administer vitamin K 2.5–10 mg IV to correct bleeding abnormalities from warfarin over anticoagulation or vitamin K deficiency, or use prothrombin complex with vitamin K. For severe bleeding, reversal agents may be used for direct oral anticoagulants.
2. Initiate IV PPI and administer for three days; convert to PO route when patient is stable and taking oral fluids, which is often administered for four to eight weeks. Do not use concurrently with octreotide.
3. Oral or IV iron supplements should be given after patient is stable (see Chapter 118).
4. Give octreotide 50 mcg IV bolus. Follow with IV infusion 50 mcg/hr up to five days for patients with acute variceal bleeding related to cirrhosis. These patients also need norfloxacin 400 mg PO two times a day or preferably IV ceftriaxone 1 g daily for seven days. This is not effective for lower GI bleeding.
5. Stop any causative agents, if possible. Consult cardiology PRN for patients who need ASA, direct oral anticoagulants, or antiplatelet agents.
6. Patients requiring NSAIDs must take ulcer prophylaxis.
7. Consider a prokinetic agent, such as erythromycin, to empty stomach prior to endoscopy.
8. If variceal bleeding, start vasoactive agent.
9. Propranolol for acute variceal bleeding reduces risk of rebleeding.
E. Procedures
1. Blood loss management
   a) Patient is placed on NPO.
   b) Insert NG tube to aspirate for blood. This is optional but may be used to remove blood clots prior to endoscopy.
   c) If aspirate is positive for blood, perform the following.
      (1) Leave NG tube in place to decompress stomach.
      (2) Approximate blood loss, and remove blood and lavage to prepare patient for endoscopy.
      (3) Flush PRN to keep tube patent.
2. Upper endoscopy is the preferred therapeutic approach. Perform within 24 hours of bleeding onset. Ulcers should be biopsied and *H. pylori* testing obtained. Colonoscopy should be performed if endoscopy is not diagnostic.
3. Consider selective arteriography with embolization.
4. TIPS should be placed for patients with portal hypertension and to reduce rebleeding risk.

VII. Follow-up: Monitor patients for further bleeding after discharge and relapse of identified etiology
A. Instruct patients to report blood in stool.

B. Perform repeat CBC and iron studies at next office visit and provide materials for home stool occult blood tests.

C. Perform repeat rectal examination and blood tests based on patient reports of blood in stool and at least annually if no further reports of bleeding (or more often based on assessment).

VIII. Referrals (Farrar, 2018; Feinman & Haut, 2014; Nelms & Pelaez, 2018; Stanley & Laine, 2019)

A. Gastroenterologist: For immediate consultation for diagnostic evaluation, including endoscopy, enteroscopy, and colonoscopy; management of rebleeding episodes; or when etiology not identified

B. Medical internist or hospitalist: For admission to hospital or ICU

C. Surgeon: For surgery if patient does not respond to endoscopic therapy or experiences rebleeding, if bleeding cannot be controlled, or for patients who fail other treatment options; early consultation recommended

D. Interventional radiologist: If bleeding is not controlled by endoscopy

E. Cardiologist: PRN for resumption of anticoagulants, antiplatelet agents, or ASA

References

Chopra, D., Rosenberg, M., Moayyedi, P., & Narula, N. (2020). Is blood urea concentration an independent predictor of positive endoscopic findings in presumed upper gastrointestinal bleeding? *Digestive Diseases, 38*(1), 77–84. https://doi.org/10.1159/000501549

Farrar, F.C. (2018). Management of acute gastrointestinal bleed. *Critical Care Nursing Clinics of North America, 30*(1), 55–66. https://doi.org/10.1016/j.cnc.2017.10.005

Feinman, M., & Haut, E.R. (2014). Upper gastrointestinal bleeding. *Surgical Clinics of North America, 94*(1), 43–53. https://doi.org/10.1016/j.suc.2013.10.004

Hernández-Gea, V., Berbel, C., Baiges, A., & García-Pagán, J.C. (2018). Acute variceal bleeding: Risk stratification and management (including TIPS). *Hepatology International, 12*(Suppl. 1), 81–90. https://doi.org/10.1007/s12072-017-9804-3

Jung, K., & Moon, W. (2019). Role of endoscopy in acute gastrointestinal bleeding in real clinical practice: An evidence-based review. *World Journal of Gastrointestinal Endoscopy, 11*(2), 68–83. https://doi.org/10.4253/wjge.v11.i2.68

Murphy, B., Winter, D.C., & Kavanagh, D.O. (2019). Small bowel gastrointestinal bleeding diagnosis and management—A narrative review. *Frontiers in Surgery, 6*, 25. https://doi.org/10.3389/fsurg.2019.00025

Nelms, D.W., & Pelaez, C.A. (2018). The acute upper gastrointestinal bleed. *Surgical Clinics of North America, 98*(5), 1047–1057. https://doi.org/10.1016/j.suc.2018.05.004

Ohmiya, N., Nakagawa, Y., Nagasaka, M., Tahara, T., Shibata, T., Nakamura, M., ... Hirata, I. (2015). Obscure gastrointestinal bleeding: Diagnosis and treatment. *Digestive Endoscopy, 27*(3), 285–294. https://doi.org/10.1111/den.12423

Rahman, S.I.-U., & Saeian, K. (2016). Nonvariceal upper gastrointestinal bleeding. *Critical Care Clinics, 32*(2), 223–239. https://doi.org/10.1016/j.ccc.2015.12.002

Stanley, A.J., & Laine, L. (2019). Management of acute upper gastrointestinal bleeding. *BMJ, 364*, l536. https://doi.org/10.1136/bmj.l536

CHAPTER 63

Nausea and Vomiting

Kristina Mathey, MS, APRN–CNP, AOCNP®

I. Definitions (Adel, 2017; Leach, 2019)
  A. Nausea: The subjective sensation or unpleasant feeling in the epigastrium and/or throat that leads to an unsettled stomach, which can be accompanied by the sensation of an impending need to vomit
  B. Vomiting: The physical, forceful expulsion of gastric contents via the mouth through stimulation of a multistep reflex pathway controlled by the brain
  C. Retching: The attempt to vomit without expulsion of gastric contents

II. Physiology/Pathophysiology (Adel, 2017; Bosnjak et al., 2016; Jordan et al., 2015; Leach, 2019; NCCN, 2020; Walsh et al., 2017)
  A. Normal
    1. A multistep reflex pathway controlled by the brain is responsible for vomiting.
      a) The vomiting center (VC) and the chemoreceptor trigger zone (CTZ) are two of the main brain stem centers that receive and integrate neurotransmitters responsible for nausea and vomiting.
      b) The VC is not a specific anatomical structure but a collection of nuclei in the medulla oblongata. The CTZ is located in the floor of the fourth ventricle and sits outside the blood–brain barrier, rendering it sensitive to CSF-borne stimuli, toxins, drugs, and other chemical derangements.
      c) The VC receives afferent impulses from the cerebral cortex, the vestibular system, the GI tract via vagal afferent fibers, pharynx, and cerebral cortex, as well as integrating input from the CTZ.
      d) Emetic transmitters (agonists), such as dopamine, serotonin, and substance P, are able to bind to their receptors found in the CNS and GI tract.
      e) Vomiting occurs when efferent impulses are sent from the VC to the salivation center, abdominal muscles, respiratory center, and cranial nerves.
    2. Nausea
      a) The stomach relaxes, and gastric acid secretion is inhibited.
      b) A single, retrograde, giant contraction of the small intestine causes the alkaline contents of the small bowel to be propelled into the stomach.
    3. Vomiting
      a) The abdominal muscles contract, and the periesophageal diaphragm relaxes.
      b) Compression of the stomach causes reflux of the contents through the esophagus and mouth.
  B. Pathophysiology
    1. Five principal neurotransmitter receptors mediate vomiting: M_1 (muscarinic), D_2 (dopamine), H_1 (histamine), 5-HT_3 (hydroxytryptamine), and NK_1 (neurokinin).

2. The efficacy of specific antiemetic agents is directly related to the affinity of an agent to a specific receptor.
3. Additional receptors involved in the emetogenic pathway include histamine, acetylcholine, endorphins, gamma-aminobutyric acid, and cannabinoids.
4. Metabolic chemicals resulting from paraneoplastic syndromes (see Appendix M), such as hypercalcemia, hyponatremia, and uremia, or metabolites from tumor proliferation or renal failure may stimulate the CTZ and VC, as well as the accumulation of drugs such as opioids and antibiotics.
   a) The accumulation of morphine metabolites can stimulate the vestibular apparatus, resulting in chronic nausea.
   b) The products of cellular breakdown after chemotherapy administration may contribute to nausea.
   c) Opioids directly stimulate the CTZ's serotonin and dopaminergic receptor sites.
5. Visceral alteration from gastric irritation, intestinal obstruction, or gastric, liver, or splenic distention may stimulate the vagus nerve. The vagal efferent fibers directly stimulate the VC by their release of histaminergic, serotoninergic, and cholinergic neurotransmitters. This can be related to obstruction of hollow viscus as well as stretched liver capsule.
6. Psychological factors (e.g., anxiety) stimulate the sympathetic nervous system, mediating the release of hormones from the pituitary and adrenal glands.
7. An increase in ICP in the CNS stimulates the histaminergic receptors in the VC.

III. Clinical features: Nausea and vomiting are common symptoms found in patients with cancer and are related to the primary cancer disease process, treatment of the underlying disease, and/or the coexisting disease and its treatment. The cause of these symptoms often is multifactorial. Nausea and vomiting are substantial and common (60%–80%) issues in patients with cancer. The prevalence of nausea and vomiting appears to increase as disease progresses (Leach, 2019; NCCN, 2020; Walsh et al., 2017).
   A. Etiology: Nausea and vomiting can be categorized according to underlying cause (e.g., chemical, impaired gastric emptying, visceral/serosal, cranial, vestibular, cortical).
      1. Approximately 62% of those with advanced cancer report nausea and vomiting.
      2. Effective treatment aims at treating the underlying cause.
         a) Constipation: Laxatives
         b) Hypercalcemia: Calcium-reduction agents and hydration
         c) Massive ascites: Paracentesis
         d) Opioids: Adjustment in dose of agent
      3. Most medications can produce nausea and vomiting.
      4. Regurgitation: Passive, retrograde flow of esophageal contents into oral cavity; occurs frequently with esophageal obstruction or gastroesophageal reflux
      5. Rumination: Eating disorder that can be confused with vomiting; occurs repetitively after meals but does not produce nausea or true vomiting
      6. Dyspepsia: Chronic or recurrent pain or discomfort in upper abdomen, usually caused by acid production or dysmotility etiologies
   B. History: Assessment and history are key to identify all etiology, as nausea and vomiting can lead to significant distress and impairment of QOL. It is important to focus on early assessment and intervention.
      1. History of cancer and cancer treatment
      2. Current medications: Prescribed, over the counter

3. History of presenting symptoms: Precipitating factors, onset, duration, associated symptoms (e.g., increased salivation, diaphoresis, tachycardia, diarrhea, retching, dysphagia, thirst)

   a) Inquire about character of vomitus (e.g., coffee-ground, feculent, bile).

   b) Inquire about volume and timing of emesis.

      (1) Opioid-induced nausea and vomiting usually occurs after initiation of opioids and is generally transient in nature, improving after one week of use.

      (2) Gastric stasis may present with feelings of early satiety, bloating, and nausea and vomiting soon after eating.

      (3) Malignant bowel obstruction is dependent ultimately on the level of obstruction.

         (a) In small bowel obstructions, nausea followed by large volume emesis is an early clinical feature often associated with central, colicky, and abdominal pain.

         (b) In large bowel obstructions, vomiting is often a later feature.

      (4) Nausea and vomiting from biochemical causes usually presents with constant symptoms and correlates with the initiation of a drug or development of a new relevant problem.

4. Changes in ADLs

5. Past medical history: Diabetes, liver disease, pancreatic disease, migraine headaches

C. Signs and symptoms: Dependent on etiology

   1. Decreased urine output secondary to dehydration

   2. Weight loss

   3. Constipation

   4. Pain: Abdominal, chest, head, ear

   5. Manifestations of hypokalemia: Malaise, fatigue, weakness, palpitations, paresthesia, cramps, restless legs syndrome

   6. Manifestations of metabolic alkalosis: Impaired mentation, hypotension, hypoventilation

   7. Viral symptoms: Malaise, myalgia, arthralgia, rhinorrhea, headache, stiff neck, vertigo, tinnitus, anorexia, chest pain, cough, fever (consider household members with similar symptoms)

   8. Neurologic symptoms: Headache, projectile vomiting, incoordination with altered vision, personality change, paralysis, convulsion, seizure

   9. Vestibular symptoms: Tinnitus, nausea worse with head motion or going from sitting to standing, decreased hearing, skull tenderness

   10. Impaired gastric emptying: Early satiety, postprandial fullness or abdominal bloating

D. Physical examination

   1. Vital signs

      a) Temperature: Decreased with dehydration, increased with infection

      b) Increased respirations in acidosis, respiratory abnormalities with increased ICP

      c) Orthostatic hypotension and tachycardia with dehydration, hypertension with bradycardia indicating increased ICP

      d) Weight loss with chronic nausea

   2. Neurologic

      a) Diagnostic signs of meningitis: Neck rigidity, Kernig and Brudzinski signs (see Appendix D), deconjugate ocular movements, pupillary abnormalities

      b) CNS involvement: Usually associated with some type of abnormal neurologic function, such as ataxia, abnormal coordination, or abnormal cranial nerve examination

    3. HEENT/oral cavity

        a) Dry mucous membranes indicating dehydration, *Candida* lesions or thrush (may exacerbate nausea)

        b) Teeth enamel erosion associated with chronic vomiting or bulimia

    4. Integument: Tenting skin turgor

    5. Cardiac: Regularity of rhythm to evaluate for dysrhythmia

    6. Abdominal: Hepatosplenomegaly, masses, ascites, rigidity, hyper-/hypoactive bowel sounds or tenderness

    7. Rectal: Fecal impaction

IV. Diagnostic tests: No gold standard diagnostic test exists for the etiology of nausea and vomiting. Many patients present with multifactorial symptoms. In most cases, the cause of nausea and vomiting can be determined from the history and physical examination.

  A. Laboratory

    1. CBC to evaluate WBC count for leukocytosis as sign of infection, as well as to evaluate Hgb for anemia

    2. Electrolytes: Potassium, magnesium, and chloride may be low in dehydration; sodium may be elevated or low; calcium may be elevated (hypercalcemia) and be a cause of nausea and vomiting. If albumin is low, calculate corrected calcium level for true calcium level evaluation.

    3. BUN and creatinine

        a) Ratio greater than 10:1 indicating fluid volume deficit

        b) Carbon dioxide: High in alkalosis

    4. Urinalysis: Specific gravity and osmolality increased in dehydration; chloride decreased in metabolic alkalosis

    5. LFTs: May be abnormal with liver metastases

    6. Elevated amylase in pancreatic disease

    7. Serum levels of drug toxicity: Digoxin, theophylline

    8. Serum beta-human chorionic gonadotropin if suspected pregnancy

  B. Radiology: Obtain only based on history and physical presentation if symptoms warrant.

    1. Abdominal flat plate and upright: Free intraperitoneal air if perforation or dilated loops of small bowel in mechanical small bowel obstruction

    2. Barium upper GI study: May show evidence of gastric outlet obstruction

    3. Abdominal ultrasound: May show blockage in the GI tract; a biliary obstruction can be noted but not bowel obstruction.

    4. Abdominal CT scan: May show bowel obstruction or a mass causing direct pressure on the bowel, as well as disease progression if history of abdominal malignancy or metastasis

    5. Brain CT scan or MRI: May show CNS involvement (e.g., brain metastasis)

  C. Other

    1. Upper endoscopy: May show evidence of gastric outlet obstruction, ulceration, tumor, gastritis, or esophagitis

    2. Saline load test: More than 400 ml residual 30 minutes after instillation of 750 ml of normal saline into the stomach indicating obstruction or gastroparesis

    3. ECG: Prominent U waves and QRS widening in hypokalemia; dysrhythmia

    4. Lumbar puncture to evaluate for increased ICP and meningitis

V. Differential diagnosis (Adel, 2017; Bosnjak et al., 2016; Leach, 2019; NCCN, 2020; Walsh et al., 2017)

  A. Treatment related

    1. Chemotherapy

    2. Radiation therapy to the abdomen, GI tract, or lumbosacral spine

    3. Surgery

    4. Drug induced

        a) Opioids (see Appendix F)

        b) Hormonal agents

        c) Antidepressants (see Appendix L)

        d) Antibiotics: beta-lactam agents, fluoroquinolones, tetracyclines

        e) NSAIDs (see Appendix E)

        f) Digoxin

        g) SSRIs

        h) Theophylline

        i) Anticonvulsants

        j) Iron

B. Malignancy related

    1. Hepatomegaly (see Chapter 60)

    2. Splenomegaly (see Chapter 65)

    3. CNS metastasis

    4. Vestibular neuroma

    5. Carcinoid tumor

    6. Paraneoplastic syndrome (see Appendix M)

    7. Abdominal carcinomatosis

C. GI

    1. Upper GI

        a) Gastroenteritis

        b) Peptic ulcer disease (see Chapter 78)

        c) Gastroparesis

        d) GERD (see Chapter 71)

    2. Lower GI

        a) Appendicitis

        b) Constipation (see Chapter 55)

        c) Diverticulosis (see Chapter 70)

    3. Hepatobiliary

        a) Biliary tract disease (cholecystitis; see Chapter 68)

        b) Hepatitis (see Chapter 74)

    4. Other

        a) Adhesions

        b) Bowel obstruction (see Chapter 67)

        c) Food poisoning

        d) Organ distention

        e) Pancreatitis (see Chapter 77)

        f) Peritonitis

        g) Superior mesenteric artery syndrome

        h) Zollinger-Ellison syndrome

        i) Sepsis

D. Endocrine

    1. Adrenal insufficiency caused by discontinuation of steroids

    2. Diabetic ketoacidosis

    3. Hyperparathyroidism

    4. Pregnancy

     5. Thyroid disease (see Chapters 157 and 158)

     6. Hypercalcemia (see Chapter 152)

   E. CNS

     1. Increased ICP

     2. Labyrinthitis

     3. Ménière disease

     4. Meningitis (see Chapter 141)

     5. Migraine headaches (see Chapter 137)

   F. Cardiac disease

     1. Glycoside treatment: Digoxin

     2. MI (see Chapter 49)

     3. CHF (see Chapter 42)

   G. Psychological

     1. Anxiety (see Chapter 161)

     2. Cyclical vomiting (conditioned response)

     3. Depression (see Chapter 162)

     4. Eating disorders

   H. Renal

     1. UTIs (see Chapter 89)

     2. Uremia

   I. Vestibular

     1. Primary vestibular disorder

     2. Acoustic neuroma

     3. Brain tumor or carcinomatous meningitis

   J. Pulmonary

     1. Secretions

     2. Cough (see Chapter 23)

   K. Substance abuse

     1. Drug withdrawal

     2. Binge drinking

   L. Pain

VI. Treatment: Direct treatment to the underlying disorder. Consider individual characteristics before initiation of a treatment plan (Adel, 2017; Leach, 2019; NCCN, 2020; Walsh et al., 2017).

   A. Clinical assessment will help to determine the most likely cause of symptoms.

     1. Identification of the pathway for the determined cause of nausea and vomiting will assist in treatment choice.

     2. Once the appropriate neurotransmitter receptor or receptors have been isolated, choose an antiemetic that antagonizes the identified receptor if possible.

     3. Administration of appropriate antiemetics (see Appendix P)

       a) Mechanistic approach: Generally used in clinical practice with the underlying principal to block the relevant emetogenic pathway by selecting an antiemetic that targets the pertinent receptors

       b) Empirical approach: Involves using drugs on the basis of generic tolerability and efficacy rather than specific receptor activity

   B. Identify and treat the consequences or complications of nausea and vomiting (e.g., dehydration, electrolyte imbalances; see Chapters 152–156).

   C. Nonpharmacologic treatment

     1. Muscle relaxation with guided imagery

  2. Hypnosis
  3. Music therapy
  4. Diversion or attention distraction
  5. Systematic desensitization
  6. Dietary modification: Small, frequent meals
  7. Acupuncture or acupressure: Point P6
  8. Control of odors from wounds or ulcers
D. NG tube placement or venting percutaneous endoscopic gastrostomy tube: Place for relief of symptoms and to alleviate bowel obstructions. Aspiration of more than 200 ml of fluid in a fasting patient may indicate obstruction or gastroparesis.

VII. Follow-up
A. Regularly assess the effectiveness of the treatment plan.
  1. If nausea or vomiting persists after 24 hours of antiemetic treatment, further evaluation is warranted.
  2. Monitor the patient for side effects; modify drugs and doses accordingly.
  3. Monitor electrolytes.
B. Self-care strategies and patient education should focus on the treatment plan, encouraging adherence, preventive measures, and appropriate follow-up medical/nursing consultation.

VIII. Referrals
A. Surgeon: For evidence of an acute dysfunction that may require surgical intervention
B. Oncologist or internist: For a progressive metastatic process or uncontrollable nausea and vomiting
C. Palliative care: For specialist care if symptoms persist

The author would like to acknowledge Pamela Hallquist Viale, RN, MS, AOCNP®, for her contribution to this chapter that remains unchanged from the previous edition of this book.

References

Adel, N. (2017). Overview of chemotherapy-induced nausea and vomiting and evidence-based therapies. *American Journal of Managed Care, 23*(14 Suppl.), S259–S265. https://www.ajmc.com/view/overview-of-chemotherapy-induced-nausea-and-vomiting-and-evidence-based-therapies-article

Bosnjak, S.M., Dimitrijevic, J., & Djordjevic, F. (2016). Cancer and chemotherapy-induced nausea and vomiting: A focus on olanzapine. *Current Opinion in Supportive and Palliative Care, 10*(2), 180–188. https://doi.org/10.1097/SPC.0000000000000206

Jordan, K., Jahn, F., & Aapro, M. (2015). Recent developments in the prevention of chemotherapy-induced nausea and vomiting (CINV): A comprehensive review. *Annals of Oncology, 26*(6), 1081–1090. https://doi.org/10.1093/annonc/mdv138

Leach, C. (2019). Nausea and vomiting in palliative care. *Clinical Medicine, 19*(4), 299–301. https://doi.org/10.7861/clinmedicine.19-4-299

National Comprehensive Cancer Network. (2020). *NCCN Clinical Practice Guidelines in Oncology (NCCN Guidelines®): Antiemesis* [v.1.2021]. https://www.nccn.org/professionals/physician_gls/pdf/antiemesis.pdf

Walsh, D., Davis, M., Ripamonti, C., Bruera, E., Davies, A. & Molassiotis, A. (2017). 2016 updated MASCC/ESMO consensus recommendations: Management of nausea and vomiting in advanced cancer. *Supportive Care in Cancer, 25*(1), 333–340. https://doi.org/10.1007/s00520-016-3371-3.

CHAPTER 64

Rectal Bleeding (Hematochezia)

Jeanne Held-Warmkessel, MSN, RN, AOCN®, ACNS-BC

I. Definition: Bright red to maroon blood excreted via the rectum, associated more often with lower GI tract bleeding from the jejunum, ileum, or colon and mixed with stool (Farrar, 2018)

II. Physiology/Pathophysiology (Aoki et al., 2019; Farrar, 2018)
   A. Normal: The mucosal surface of the GI tract is composed of epithelial cells.
      1. The functions of the epithelial cells are transmembrane absorption and secretion.
      2. The epithelial cells facilitate the digestive tract in digestion and nutrient uptake.
      3. These cells act as a barrier against potentially harmful pathogens and mutagens in the lumen.
   B. Pathophysiology
      1. Irritation, ulceration, or trauma of the GI mucosa will result in bleeding.
      2. Bleeding originates below the ligament of Treitz. Very brisk movement of blood from the right colon, small bowel, or stomach can lead to similar presentation and produce hemodynamic instability.

III. Clinical features: Bleeding is variable and may be pure or mixed with stool, clots, or diarrhea. Blood may be obvious or occult and may range from slow bleeding to a life-threatening hemorrhagic event to spontaneous cessation. It may be acute or chronic, or it may be continuous or intermittent. The colon will continue to eliminate blood even after active bleeding stops because of its storage capability. With an upper GI bleed, stool has bright red or dark red blood, and the patient is hemodynamically unstable (Aoki et al., 2019; Farrar, 2018; Jung & Moon, 2019; Oakland et al., 2019).
   A. Etiology: Up to 15% of lower GI bleeds have the bleeding origin in the upper GI tract.
      1. Anatomic: Diverticulosis—common cause, abrupt, may be massive
      2. Vascular
         a) Angiodysplasia, angioectasia, varices
         b) Ischemia
         c) Radiation induced
         d) Ectasias
         e) Dieulafoy lesion
      3. Inflammatory colitis
         a) Infectious
         b) Inflammatory bowel disease
      4. Neoplastic

         a) Polyp, postpolypectomy

         b) Carcinoma: Colon, anal, small bowel

         c) Pelvic irradiation: Anorectal

    5. Hemorrhoids

    6. Rectal ulcer

    7. Anal fissures: Minor bleeding with pain

    8. Rectal varices

    9. Other

         a) Trauma

         b) Aortoenteric fistula

         c) Drug induced

B. History

    1. History of cancer and cancer treatment, radiation therapy

    2. Current medications: Prescribed, over the counter, NSAIDs/ASA, steroids, antico-agulants, antiplatelet agents, direct oral anticoagulants

    3. History of presenting symptoms: Precipitating factors, onset, frequency, volume, duration, associated symptoms (e.g., bloating, urgency, weight loss, change in bowel habits, abdominal pain/cramping and its association with food, dyspepsia, nausea and vomiting, vomiting blood, diarrhea, constipation), color of blood, presence of clots, amount of blood passed per rectum

    4. Changes in ADLs

    5. Past medical history: Rectal or colon disease, hemorrhoids, anal fissure, prior episodes of bleeding, vascular disease, diverticular disease, upper GI tract disease or bleeding, HIV, human papillomavirus, liver disease, inflammatory bowel disease, cirrhosis, recent colonoscopy

    6. Social history: Alcohol use, smoking

    7. Family history: Polyps, hypercoagulable states, inflammatory bowel disease, cancer, bleeding dyscrasia

    8. Past surgical history: Abdominal aortic aneurysm repair, surgery of the bowel, prior biopsy of the rectum or colon

C. Signs and symptoms

    1. Visible blood at the rectum or passing of blood through rectum

    2. Vomiting, diarrhea, urgency, pain, tenesmus

    3. Light-headedness, dizziness, syncope

    4. Pallor

    5. Weakness

    6. Diaphoresis

    7. Pain: Tenderness, pain occurring with inflammation or ischemic colitis

    8. Palpitations

    9. Signs and symptoms of anemia: Fatigue, chest pain/angina

    10. Dyspnea/shortness of breath

D. Physical examination

    1. Vital signs and pulse oximetry: Assess for hemodynamic instability related to clinically significant blood loss. Upper GI blood loss produces a significantly lower blood pressure than a lower GI bleed. If the vital signs are stable, consider a lower GI bleed.

         a) Orthostatic hypotension

         b) Tachycardia

    2. Integument

         a) Lesions: Many GI disorders are associated with skin changes (e.g., telangiectasias).

         b) Pallor: Conjunctiva

     c) Temperature: Cold legs

     d) Petechiae, ecchymoses

  3. Abdominal

     a) Masses

     b) Ascites

     c) Tenderness (colitis), pain

     d) Distention

     e) Spider veins: Angioma

     f) Hyperactive bowel sounds

     g) Liver size

     h) Signs of peritonitis: Tenderness, guarding

     i) Bowel sounds: Typically normal

  4. Digital rectal: Hemorrhoids, fissures, masses, tenderness, stool impaction, stool color, blood, occult blood testing

  5. Cardiac

     a) Tachycardia

     b) Murmur with large blood loss

     c) Pulses and refill decreased with blood loss

  6. Pulmonary

     a) Dyspnea: Increased work of breathing

     b) Tachypnea

  7. Mental status altered with blood loss

IV. Diagnostic tests (Aoki et al., 2019; Farrar, 2018; Jung & Moon, 2019; Oakland et al., 2019; Speir et al., 2017)

  A. Laboratory tests

    1. CBC with differential

     a) Indicating signs of anemia

      (1) Low mean corpuscular volume and low ferritin, iron/total iron-binding capacity with chronic blood loss; no change with acute loss

      (2) Decrease in Hgb and hematocrit; may not reflect volume of blood loss for 24–72 hours after bleeding begins

     b) Platelets decreased indicating thrombocytopenia

    2. PT, PTT, and INR to assess for anticoagulation/coagulopathy, which increases the risk of bleeding

    3. LFTs and albumin: Abnormal values potentially indicative of liver dysfunction

    4. CMP with BUN and creatinine: Elevated BUN and creatinine indicating upper GI bleed; digested blood protein increases BUN value, as well as volume depletion.

    5. Type and crossmatch if transfusion is considered

    6. Electrolytes/chemistries to assess imbalance

    7. Serum lactate level to assess for acidosis related to shock

    8. Cardiac enzymes in patients at risk for cardiac complications

  B. Radiology

    1. Superselective angiography with embolization: Performed after CT angiography or scintigram (bleeding scan) when source of bleeding has been identified; used to control severe bleeding; useful if patient cannot tolerate a bowel prep; may be performed prior to planned surgical resection of bleeding source

     a) Perform if colonoscopy is not diagnostic, if patient is bleeding too much for a colonoscopy or is hemodynamically unstable for colonoscopy, or if surgery is planned.

      b) It is the procedure of choice if nuclear technetium-99m scan is positive or if CT angiography is positive.

      c) Lesion must be bleeding at the time of test to be useful in identifying bleeding site at greater than 0.5 ml/min. It can be performed quickly on patients who are hemodynamically unstable and should be initiated as soon as possible.

      d) Diverticular bleeding is the superselective embolization of intra-arterial vasopressin.

2. Contrast enema with flexible sigmoidoscopy: Not useful in active bleeding situations; useful to diagnose cancer and large polyps

3. Small bowel series: Used after other tests are unsuccessful in revealing source of chronic blood loss

4. Scintigraphy with technetium-99m–labeled RBCs: Tagged RBC scintigraphy not commonly used; may be useful if CT angiography, endoscopy, and colonoscopy are nondiagnostic in finding source of bleeding; useful with intermittent or slow rates of bleeding

      a) Labeled RBCs enter bowel at bleeding site.

      b) Lesion must be bleeding at time of technetium-99m colloid test to be useful in identifying bleeding site. Technetium-99m scans should be done over a period of 24 hours.

      c) It may be performed if NG aspirate, endoscopy, and colonoscopy do not reveal bleeding source.

      d) Angiography is used to control bleeding.

5. Plain abdominal x-ray: Should be performed prior to colonoscopy if perforation or obstruction is suspected

6. CT angiography: This sensitive and specific diagnostic tool is recommended for unstable patients with GI bleeding. It is useful in planning additional therapy such as colonoscopy, angiography, scintigraphy, or surgery. If the test is negative, also investigate an upper GI source. Hemodynamically unstable patients require a CT angiography followed by endoscopy or interventional radiology procedure to control bleeding if CT angiography is positive. The test is useful for patients who are hemodynamically unstable or unable to have a bowel prep and to plan therapy for unstable patients.

C. Other

1. Upper endoscopy: Should be performed to identify upper GI source if patient is hemodynamically unstable or if CT angiography does not reveal source of bleeding

2. NG aspirate to assess for upper GI source/upper endoscopy: Not usually performed; not a reliable test

3. Testing stool for occult blood, for possible infectious causes, and to help identify bleeding source

4. Proctosigmoidoscopy/anoscopy for bright red blood per rectum: May identify hemorrhoidal bleeding or anorectal disease/bleeding source

5. Colonoscopy: It is the preferred diagnostic procedure; oral bowel prep is recommended when lower GI bleed expected as etiology to improve diagnosis and treatment. Urgent colonoscopy can be done with rapid bowel prep. High-risk patients should have the procedure within 24 hours of presentation. Procedure is also used with hemodynamically stable patients and when CT angiography and anoscopy are negative.

6. Oxygen saturation with pulse oximetry

7. Enteroscopy of small bowel if colonoscopy and upper endoscopy are negative

8. Video capsule endoscopy: Wireless video cameras can take images of the small bowel to detect bleeding site when endoscopy and colonoscopy are negative. It is best performed within 48 hours of presentation of bleeding episode.

      9. ECG to assess for myocardial ischemia or infarction related to blood loss in patients with or at risk for acute coronary syndrome

V. Differential diagnosis (Aoki et al., 2019; Farrar, 2018; Oakland et al., 2019)
    A. Vascular abnormalities: Abnormal colon blood vessel structure with capillary dilation
        1. Vasculitis
        2. Vascular anomalies/angioectasia/arteriovenous malformation
        3. Mesenteric ischemia
        4. Colitis, ischemic colitis
        5. Varices
    B. Diverticular disease: Common etiology of lower GI bleed; often stops spontaneously (see Chapter 70)
    C. Cancer
        1. GI malignancies: Small bowel, colon, rectal, anal
        2. Metastases from other primary cancers
    D. Polyps
    E. Hemorrhoids: Internal; common cause (see Chapter 73)
    F. Rectal ulcer
    G. Small bowel or colorectal varices
    H. Lacerations, rectal trauma
    I. Fistula, rectovaginal, other malignancy-caused fistulas
    J. Anal fissure
    K. Drugs with anticoagulant activity, antithrombotic agents, direct oral anticoagulants
    L. Thrombocytopenia (see Chapter 129)
    M. Inflammatory bowel diseases
        1. Ulcerative colitis
        2. Crohn disease
        3. Ischemic colitis
        4. Infectious colitis
        5. Idiopathic
        6. Drug related
    N. Aortoenteric fistula (after abdominal aortic aneurysm repair)
    O. Radiation enteritis/colitis, proctitis: More than six months after radiation therapy
    P. Infection: HIV, *Clostridium difficile*, *Salmonella*, *Campylobacter*, other enteric pathogens causing hemorrhagic colitis
    Q. Brisk upper GI or small bowel bleed: More likely to cause hemodynamic instability
    R. Malabsorptive disorders, celiac disease
    S. Recent polypectomies
    T. Lymphoid nodular hyperplasia
    U. Anastomotic ulceration (after recent surgery)

VI. Treatment for lower GI bleed: Patients may require intensive level of care depending on severity of bleeding and hemodynamic instability. Patients are to be categorized as either stable or unstable. Stable patients are either major or minor (Aoki et al., 2019; Farrar, 2018; Oakland et al., 2019; Speir et al., 2017; Tabaja & Sidani, 2018).
    A. Insert two large-gauge IV cannulas and rapidly infuse isotonic (normal saline) fluids to achieve hemodynamic stability. Monitor central venous pressure.
    B. Monitor urine output, as oliguria may develop with hypovolemia.
    C. Check vital signs frequently for hemodynamic instability. Check pulse oximetry.

D. Transfuse with packed RBCs to minimal Hgb 7 g/dl. Patients with cardiovascular disease or patients with massive bleeding should receive more liberal RBC transfusion to Hgb 8 g/dl.
E. Provide supplemental oxygen PRN or if the patient has a history of cardiac disease.
F. Correct bleeding/coagulation problems.
   1. Administer vitamin K 2.5–10 mg IV if over anticoagulated from warfarin or from vitamin K deficiency.
   2. Administer platelets if platelet count is less than 50,000/mm^3.
   3. Use fresh frozen plasma to replace all clotting factors if coagulopathy is present.
   4. Administer prothrombin complex concentrate.
   5. Hold direct oral anticoagulants and antiplatelet agents and consider initiation of reversal agents for life-threatening bleeding. Consult cardiology immediately, especially for patients with stents or acute coronary syndrome.
G. Encourage bed rest to conserve energy and prevent syncope.
H. Perform colonoscopy for cautery, laser, polypectomy, or other methods to stop bleeding and for patients hemodynamically stable or with postpolypectomy bleeding.
I. Radiation proctitis: No standard therapy exists for management of this issue.
   1. Consult gastroenterologist.
   2. Consider oral sucralfate or sucralfate enemas. Consider adding oral metronidazole (dose 400 mg PO three times a day) to sucralfate enemas.
   3. Consider topical therapies (e.g., formalin, electrocautery, argon plasma coagulation, laser).
   4. Consider oral 5-aminosalicylic acid–containing medication, alone or with steroids or 5-aminosalicylic acid enemas.
   5. Short-chain fatty acid enemas may help treat acute radiation proctitis.
   6. Consider local hyperbaric oxygen when other therapy is not effective.
J. Iron supplements: When patient is stable, initiate ferrous sulfate 250–325 mg PO three times a day or iron salts (iron dextran, iron sucrose) IV PRN (see Chapter 118).
K. Consult interventional radiology for angiography with embolization after CT angiography when source of bleeding identified.
L. Consult surgery to resect bleeding source.
M. Stop agent identified as cause of bleeding.

VII. Follow-up: Monitor patient for further bleeding or for relapse from previously identified bleeding source. Patients with anorectal disease, angiodysplasia, and diverticular-induced bleeding are at a higher risk of rebleeding, as are patients taking anticoagulants or antiplatelet agents.

VIII. Referrals (Farrar, 2018)
A. Gastroenterologist: Immediate consult for endoscopy, colonoscopy/anoscopy, or proctosigmoidoscopy
B. Hospitalist, medical internist, or intensivist: For admission to hospital or ICU
C. Surgeon: For surgery when nonsurgical interventions are not successful, and the patient continues to bleed; for patients with aortoenteric fistula
D. Interventional radiologist: For angiography
E. Cardiology: For resumption of medications or replacement medications

References

Aoki, T., Hirata, Y., Yamada, A., & Koike, K. (2019). Initial management for acute lower gastrointestinal bleeding. *World Journal of Gastroenterology, 25*(1), 69–84. https://doi.org/10.3748/wjg.v25.i1.69.

Farrar, F.C. (2018). Management of acute gastrointestinal bleed. *Critical Care Nursing Clinics of North America, 30*(1), 55–66. https://doi.org/10.1016/j.cnc.2017.10.005

Jung, K., & Moon, W. (2019). Role of endoscopy in acute gastrointestinal bleeding in real clinical practice: An evidence-based review. *World Journal of Gastrointestinal Endoscopy, 11*(2), 68–83. https://doi.org/10.4253/wjge.v11.i2.68

Oakland, K., Chadwick, G., East, J.E., Guy, R., Humphries, A., Jairath, V., ... Hoare, J. (2019). Diagnosis and management of acute lower gastrointestinal bleeding: Guidelines from the British Society of Gastroenterology. *Gut, 68*(5), 776–789. https://doi.org/10.1136/gutjnl-2018-317807

Speir, E.J., Ermentrout, R.M., & Martin, J.G. (2017). Management of acute lower gastrointestinal bleeding. *Techniques in Vascular and Interventional Radiology, 20*(4), 258–262. https://doi.org/10.1053/j.tvir.2017.10.005

Tabaja, L., & Sidani, S.M. (2018). Management of radiation proctitis. *Digestive Diseases and Sciences, 63*(9), 2180–2188. https://doi.org/10.1007/s10620-018-5163-8.

CHAPTER 65

Splenomegaly

Kristina Mathey, MS, APRN-CNP, AOCNP®

I. Definition: Enlarged spleen by size or weight (Chow et al., 2016)

II. Physiology/Pathophysiology (McKenzie et al., 2018; Sjoberg et al., 2018)
   A. Normal: The major function of the spleen is continuous filtration of circulating blood.
      1. The normal spleen is located in the peritoneal cavity in the left upper quadrant adjacent to ribs 9–12.
      2. The normal-sized spleen abuts the stomach, colon, and left kidney, normally measuring up to 11 cm in craniocaudal length.
      3. The normal weight of an adult spleen is 70–200 g.
      4. The normal-sized spleen is usually not palpable in adults; however, it may be palpable during periods of altered body habitus and chest wall anatomy.
      5. The spleen is divided into two specific macroscopic compartments: red and white pulp.
         a) The white pulp is composed of lymphoid tissue and contains approximately one-fourth of the body's lymphocytes. Germinal centers exist where early B lymphocytes and plasma cells predominate. When foreign antigens are present in circulation, the spleen plays a role in immunologic response.
         b) The red pulp is composed of RBCs surrounding connective tissues, known as the cords of Billroth, and integrated with splenic sinusoids lined with macrophages. Its primary function is to filter blood of antigens, microorganisms, and defective RBCs.
      6. The normal spleen is the body's largest lymphoid organ and has many functions.
         a) Clearance of abnormal erythrocytes
         b) Removal of microorganisms and antigens
         c) Synthesis of IgG and the immune system peptides properdin and tuftsin
         d) Contains one-third of the body's circulating platelets
   B. Pathophysiology
      1. A spleen length of 11–20 cm indicates splenomegaly, and a length greater than 20 cm is indicative of massive splenomegaly. A spleen weighing 400–500 g indicates splenomegaly; greater than 1,000 g indicates massive splenomegaly.
      2. Pathologic splenomegaly results from any combination of three general pathophysiologic mechanisms.
         a) Hypertrophy or hyperplasia of normal splenic function results in exaggerated splenic function with enhanced filtration and phagocytosis of cellular components of blood, causing cytopenia.
         b) Infiltrative processes caused by focal lesions or diffuse infiltration, such as lymphomas, amyloidosis, and other malignant, benign, or metabolic conditions, can cause splenomegaly.

  c) Congestive processes resulting from blockage of the blood flow through splenic vasculature (e.g., portal hypertension), resulting in splenomegaly.

III. Clinical features (McKenzie et al., 2018; Rotbain et al., 2017; Sjoberg et al., 2018)
 A. Etiology: Splenic enlargement usually is secondary to other primary disorders. Splenomegaly varies and can be classified based on pathophysiologic mechanism.
  1. Hematologic: Lymphomas, leukemias, myeloproliferative disorders
  2. Infectious: An increase in immunologic activity and subsequent hyperplasia (e.g., endocarditis, infectious mononucleosis, HIV)
  3. Congestive: Pooled by blood (e.g., portal hypertension, splenic vein thrombosis, CHF)
  4. Inflammatory: Sarcoidosis, SLE, RA
  5. Infiltrative: Invasion by cells foreign to splenic environment (e.g., cancer metastasis, lipid storage diseases such as Gaucher disease, myeloid neoplasms); when the spleen is massively enlarged (greater than 8 cm below the left costal margin), non-Hodgkin lymphoma or myelofibrosis is likely the cause.
  6. Neoplastic: Physical infiltration by neoplastic cells (e.g., breast, colorectal, lung)
 B. History
  1. History of cancer and cancer treatment
  2. Current medications: Prescribed, over the counter
  3. History of presenting symptoms: Precipitating factors, onset, location, duration, associated symptoms (e.g., abdominal discomfort, bruising, bleeding)
  4. Changes in ADLs
  5. Past medical history: Abdominal injuries, immune disorders, blood disorders, recent infections or illnesses, abnormal bleeding, cardiac dysfunction
  6. Social history: Recent travel to tropical climates, alcohol use, IV drug use
 C. Signs and symptoms
  1. Petechiae, ecchymosis
  2. Fatigue
  3. Malaise
  4. Feeling of abdominal fullness or heaviness, especially in left upper quadrant
  5. Early satiety, anorexia
  6. Vague abdominal pain or localized pain in the left upper quadrant
  7. Referred pain to left shoulder
  8. Fever or night sweats
 D. Physical examination
  1. HEENT
   a) Petechiae indicating thrombocytopenia
   b) Exudates and erythema indicating infection
  2. Integument: Petechiae and ecchymosis indicating cytopenia
  3. Lymph node: Adenopathy upon palpation indicating signs of infection or malignancy (see Appendix D)
  4. Abdominal
   a) Physical examination techniques have a low sensitivity for detecting splenomegaly unless it is massive.
   b) When the spleen is enlarged, the lower edge moves down and to the right of the midclavicular line.
   c) Splenomegaly may present with upper quadrant fullness or bulging from beneath the left costal margin. During inspiration, the rounded edge of the spleen under the fingertips may be palpated.

       d) Percussion is used to identify the size and density of the spleen; dullness on full inspiration suggests spleen enlargement.

IV. Diagnostic tests (Gunes & Akturk, 2018; Nuffer et al., 2017; Parsi & Siripurapu, 2018; Rotbain et al., 2017; Sjoberg et al., 2018)
  A. Laboratory tests
    1. CBC with differential to evaluate for pancytopenia, which may be present with mild enlargement; thrombocytopenia common due to platelet sequestration
    2. Chemistry profile including LFTs to evaluate for liver failure
    3. Mononucleosis spot test, if indicated
    4. Rheumatologic panel to evaluate for RA, if indicated
    5. HIV testing if patient has known risk factors
    6. Bone marrow aspiration and biopsy, if indicated by CBC, to evaluate for hyperplastic marrow
    7. SPEP to evaluate for abnormal proteins
    8. Peripheral blood smear to evaluate the number, shape, size, and morphologic features of the blood cell, if indicated
  B. Radiology
    1. Ultrasound of the spleen has the highest validity to confirm splenomegaly and provide dimensions.
    2. Liver/spleen scan (with isotopes) can confirm splenomegaly and detect diffuse parenchymal disease in liver, which may be causing portal hypertension.
    3. CT or MRI scan of abdomen can delineate size and location of spleen, assess for presence of malignancy or ascites, and identify enlarged mesenteric or retroperitoneal lymph nodes. Both can identify lesions; however, MRI may be more useful to characterize a lesion that has already been identified.

V. Differential diagnosis (Huang et al., 2019; Kapoor et al., 2016; Mavilia et al., 2018; Sjoberg et al., 2018)
  A. Polycythemia vera (see Chapter 128)
  B. Waldenström macroglobulinemia
  C. Congenital syphilis
  D. HIV/AIDS
  E. Infection: Immune hyperplasia
    1. Mononucleosis: Epstein-Barr virus most common
    2. CMV
    3. Toxoplasmosis
    4. Chronic viral hepatitis
    5. Influenza
    6. Malaria
    7. Rickettsial infection: Rocky Mountain spotted fever
    8. Bacterial septicemia
    9. Fungal microabscesses: *Candida* most common
  F. Disordered immunoregulation: Inflammation
    1. Sarcoidosis
    2. RA (see Chapter 108)
    3. SLE (see Chapter 110)
    4. Felty syndrome
    5. Renal dialysis: Occurs in 10% of uremic patients

      6. Drug reactions

      7. Serum sickness

  G. Neoplasms: Infiltrative or myeloproliferative

      1. Leukemia: Acute and chronic

      2. Lymphomas

      3. Metastatic tumors: Rare

      4. Primary tumors: Rare

  H. Hemolytic disease: Phagocytic hyperplasia

      1. Spherocytosis

      2. Sickle cell disease (see Chapter 119)

      3. Thalassemia major

      4. Pyruvate kinase deficiency

      5. ITP (see Chapter 124)

  I. Infiltration

      1. Gaucher disease

      2. Niemann-Pick disease

      3. Amyloidosis

      4. Myelofibrosis

  J. Extramedullary hematopoiesis

  K. Splenic vein hypertension: Vascular congestion

      1. Cirrhosis (see Chapter 69)

      2. Splenic or portal vein thrombosis

      3. Chronic congestive hepatopathy (with or without CHF or cirrhosis)

  L. Endocrine

      1. Graves disease (see Chapter 157)

      2. Hashimoto thyroiditis (see Chapter 158)

  M. Hemophilia

  N. Chronic congestive splenomegaly: Banti syndrome

VI. Treatment: Directed at underlying cause of splenomegaly and generally restricted to either resolving the underlying condition, spleen reduction therapies, or radical splenectomy (Breccia et al., 2019; Kapoor et al., 2016; McKenzie et al., 2018; Parsi & Siripurapu, 2018; Sjoberg et al., 2018)

  A. Patients with polycythemia vera (see Chapter 128)

      1. Smoking cessation

      2. Phlebotomy (when hematocrit rises above approximately 50 g/dl): Avoid iron deficiency from excessive phlebotomy.

      3. Oxygen therapy

      4. Myelosuppressive therapy, only if unresponsive to conservative measures

  B. Patients with leukemia or lymphoma: Treatment is with chemotherapy or radiation therapy as indicated, depending on type and stage of disease.

  C. Patients with sarcoidosis: Treatment is aimed at relieving symptoms and active pulmonary disease, primarily with use of oral corticosteroids. This therapy is most effective if begun before pulmonary fibrosis occurs.

  D. Patients with congestive splenomegaly or secondary hypersplenism

      1. Splenectomy: Contraindicated in marrow failure; can be laparoscopic versus open depending on condition

      2. Irradiation: Reduces size, offers pain relief, and improves cytopenias

      3. TIPS

      4. Splenic embolization

E. Splenectomy considerations
1. It may be performed for symptom control in massive splenomegaly.
2. Immediate post-splenectomy leukocytosis and thrombocytosis may be noted.
3. Patients will be at significantly increased risk for infection from encapsulated organisms such as *Haemophilus influenzae*, *Streptococcus pneumoniae*, and *Neisseria meningitidis*. Pneumococcal, *H. influenzae*, and meningococcal vaccines should be given prior to surgery when possible or immediately afterward if splenectomy was done emergently.
4. The major operative risk for splenectomy is intraoperative and postoperative bleeding. Laparoscopic splenectomy may result in less postoperative morbidity.
5. Postoperatively, patients will be immunocompromised and will require careful monitoring for febrile illnesses.
F. Waldenström macroglobulinemia
1. A non-Hodgkin lymphoma characterized by the presence of cluster of differentiation 20 (CD20)-positive lymphoplasmacytic bone marrow infiltrate and elevated serum IgM monoclonal protein; both sporadic and familial forms exist.
2. Many patients are asymptomatic ("smoldering") and can be observed for months or years. No clear advantage exists for early therapy.
3. If hyperviscosity is present, plasmapheresis is used for initial management.
4. For patients who are symptomatic, initial treatment with rituximab-based regimens, with or without alkylating agents, is suggested.
5. Ibrutinib is reserved for patients who are unable to tolerate chemoimmunotherapy or have relapsed or refractory disease.
6. No standard therapy exists, and patients should be encouraged to participate in clinical trials. This lymphoma is incurable at present; goal of therapy is control.
G. Patient education
1. Instruct patients with splenomegaly to avoid activities that place them at risk for splenic injury or rupture (e.g., contact sports).
2. Post-splenectomy patients are at significantly increased risk for sepsis with encapsulated organisms (e.g., *S. pneumoniae*, *H. influenzae*, *N. meningitidis*).
   a) Signs and symptoms of infection, including fever, should be reported immediately.
   b) A viral infection may predispose patients to fulminant bacterial infection.
   c) Aggressive empiric therapy should be initiated in patients with sepsis of unknown origin.
   d) Prophylactic antibiotics are not recommended and may lead to the emergence of resistant infective organisms.

VII. Follow-up: Laboratory tests and healthcare provider visits will be dictated by the patient's underlying disease process.

VIII. Referrals
A. Internist: For patients who will require long-term follow-up
B. Infectious disease/AIDS specialist: For patients with newly diagnosed HIV infection or other major systemic infections; consultation for treatment planning
C. Pulmonologist: For patients with newly diagnosed sarcoidosis; referral based on stage and sites involved
D. Hematologist: For cytopenias or if hematologic malignancy is causative disease
E. Surgeon: If splenectomy is considered
F. Social worker: For patients with newly diagnosed malignancy or HIV infection

The author would like to acknowledge Miriam Rogers, EdD, APRN, AOCN®, CNS, for her contribution to this chapter that remains unchanged from the previous edition of this book.

References

Breccia, M., Luciano, L., Pugliese, N., Rossi, E., Tiribelli, M., Scalzulli, E., ... Palandri, F. (2019). Efficacy and safety of ruxolitinib and hydroxyurea combination in patients with hyperproliferative myelofibrosis. *Annals of Hematology, 98*(8), 1933–1936. https://doi.org/10.1007/s00277-019-03727-6

Chow, K.U., Luxembourg, B., Seifried, E., & Bonig, H. (2016). Spleen size is significantly influenced by body height and sex: Establishment of normal values for spleen size at US with a cohort of 1200 healthy individuals. *Radiology, 279*(1), 306–313. https://doi.org/10.1148/radiol.2015150887

Gunes, S.O., & Akturk, Y. (2018). Determination of splenomegaly by coronal oblique length on CT. *Japanese Journal of Radiology, 36*(2), 142–150. https://doi.org/10.1007/s11604-017-0704-1

Huang, M.-S, Chen, Y.-H., Wang, C.-W., Yao, M., & Kuo, S.-H. (2019). Low-dose splenic irradiation is an alternative therapy for symptomatic splenomegaly in patients with myelofibrosis. *Annals of Hematology, 98*(4), 1037–1040. https://doi.org/10.1007/s00277-018-3461-z

Kapoor, P., Paludo, J., & Ansell, S.M. (2016). Waldenstrom macroglobulinemia: Familial predisposition and the role of genomics in prognosis and treatment selection. *Current Treatment Options in Oncology, 17*(3), 16. https://doi.org/10.1007/s11864-016-0391-7

Mavilia, M., McAuliffe, A., Hafeez, S., & Vaziri, H. (2018). Hepatosplenic T cell lymphoma: A unifying entity in a patient with hemolytic anemia, massive splenomegaly, and liver dysfunction. *Clinical Journal of Gastroenterology, 11*(5), 364–370. https://doi.org/10.1007/s12328-018-0869-x

McKenzie, C.V., Colonne, C.K., Yeo, J.H., & Fraser, S.T. (2018). Splenomegaly: Pathophysiological bases and therapeutic options. *International Journal of Biochemistry and Cell Biology, 94,* 40–43. https://doi.org/10.1016/j.biocel.2017.11.011

Nuffer, Z., Marini, T., Rupasov, A., Kwak, S., & Bhatt, S. (2017). The best single measurement for assessing splenomegaly in patients with cirrhotic liver morphology. *Academic Radiology, 24*(12), 1510–1516. https://doi.org/10.1016/j.acra.2017.06.006

Parsi, S., & Siripurapu, V. (2018). Robotic-assisted splenectomy for massive splenomegaly secondary to sarcoidosis. *American Surgeon, 84*(6), 201–203. https://doi.org/10.1177/000313481808400608

Rotbain, E.C., Hansen, D.L., Schaffalitzky de Muckadell, O., Wibrand, F., Lund, A.M., & Frederiksen, H. (2017). Splenomegaly—Diagnostic validity, work-up, and underlying causes. *PLOS ONE, 12*(11), e0186674. https://doi.org/10.1371/journal.pone.0186674

Sjoberg, B.P., Menias, C.O., Lubner, M.G., Mellnick, V.M., & Pickhardt, P.J. (2018). Splenomegaly: A combined clinical and radiologic approach to the differential diagnosis. *Gastroenterology Clinics of North America, 47*(3), 643–666. https://doi.org/10.1016/j.gtc.2018.04.009

CHAPTER 66

Anorexia/Cachexia

Kristina Mathey, MS, APRN–CNP, AOCNP®

I. Definitions (Childs & Jatoi, 2019; Dev et al., 2017; Vagnildhaug et al., 2018; Zhang et al., 2018)
   A. Anorexia: Loss of appetite with or without weight loss
   B. Cachexia: A complex metabolic syndrome characterized by loss of muscle mass, with or without loss of fat mass, that cannot be fully reversed by conventional nutritional support and leads to progressive functional impairment; present when either weight loss exceeds 5% in six months or 2% in eight months, combined with BMI less than 20 kg/m^2 or sarcopenia
   C. Cachexia-anorexia syndrome: Progressive weight loss associated with malignancy characterized by loss of appetite (anorexia), skeletal muscle wasting, and reduced adipose tissue

II. Physiology/Pathophysiology (Aoyagi et al., 2015; Argilés et al., 2019; Dev et al., 2017; Ezeoke & Morley, 2015; Laviano et al., 2017)
   A. Normal
      1. Hunger is the physiologic need to eat.
      2. Appetite is the desire to eat that typically accompanies hunger.
      3. The hunger center is located in the hypothalamus.
      4. Thermostatic, glucostatic, normal digestive, and cerebral neurotransmitters influence appetite.
   B. Pathophysiology: When daily physiologic demands exceed the patient's dietary consumption, the body reserves are used to meet energy and protein needs.
      1. Cancer cachexia and anorexia mechanisms are complex, largely underestimated and untreated, and not fully understood.
         a) Cancer anorexia is believed to result from the impairment of the hypothalamic physiologic mechanism controlling eating behavior under normal conditions. The inflammatory response that occurs at the initiation of and throughout the cancer trajectory involves the brain areas that control the eating process. Neuroinflammation disrupts physiologic modulation of the activities of the hypothalamic satiety-mediating neurons and prophagic neurons.
         b) Insufficient oral intake is combined with complex metabolic abnormalities, leading to an increase in basal energy expenditure and resulting in a loss of lean body mass from skeletal muscle wasting.
         c) Cancer cachexia is characterized by an inflammatory response mediated by cytokines (e.g., IL-6, IL-2) and TNF-α, hypermetabolism and hormonal alterations with insulin resistance, and loss of skeletal muscle from protein breakdown and lipolysis.
         d) *Hypermetabolism* is defined as an elevated resting energy expenditure greater than 110% of predicted and can contribute to weight loss.

2. Secondary causes of cachexia and anorexia: Symptoms affecting appetite and overall nutrition (e.g., nausea, depression, pain, xerostomia, gastroparesis, constipation) contribute to a decrease in caloric intake and add a "starvation" component to the catabolic process.

III. Clinical features: Cancer anorexia occurs in one-half of all newly diagnosed patients with cancer. The overall prevalence of cancer cachexia has varied substantially in patients with advanced disease. Patients with cancer who have tumors that respond to treatment often regain weight; however, increased distress can cause treatment side effects, including continued weight loss. Cancer anorexia is of profound importance because of its implications for QOL, treatment responsiveness, and overall prognosis. Three stages of cancer cachexia exist: precachexia, cachexia, and refractory. Each stage is related to the amount and rate of weight loss (Dev et al., 2017; Ezeoke, & Morley, 2015; Zhang et al., 2018).

  A. Etiology
      1. More prevalent in patients with solid tumors, specifically lung and GI malignancies; less prevalent in hematologic malignancies and breast cancer
      2. Multifactorial (e.g., social, psychological, physiologic) rather than solely caused by poor dietary intake
          a) Inadequate intake
              (1) Changes in taste or smell of foods
              (2) Fear of provoking nausea, vomiting, abdominal cramping, and diarrhea
              (3) Disinterest in food
              (4) Tumors causing dysphagia or altered gut function
              (5) Alterations in the release of peripheral hormones that alter feeding: Ghrelin
          b) Associated symptoms of food aversion
              (1) Depression
              (2) Anxiety
              (3) Uncontrolled pain or nausea and vomiting
              (4) Xerostomia
              (5) Mucositis
          c) Malfunction of GI tract
              (1) Malabsorption
              (2) Substances released from or by the tumor: Proinflammatory cytokines, lactate
              (3) Tumors altering nutrients: Zinc deficiency
          d) Paraneoplastic syndrome (see Appendix M)
          e) Physiologic causes: Tumors causing hypoxia
  B. History: All patients with cancer should be screened for weight loss, muscle wasting, and nutritional status at diagnosis and throughout therapy (Dev et al., 2017; Laviano et al., 2017; Sadeghi et al., 2018).
      1. History of cancer and cancer treatment
      2. Current medications: Prescribed, over the counter
      3. History of presenting symptoms: Precipitating factors, onset, duration, associated symptoms (e.g., difficulty chewing and swallowing, sore throat, xerostomia, mucositis, dental caries, altered taste)
      4. Changes in ADLs: Evidence of interference of muscle wasting or edema (e.g., unable to bend over to put on pants due to ascites)
      5. Diet: History of typical 24-hour diet recall prior to cancer diagnosis and current 24-hour diet; use of nutritional supplements, vitamins, and minerals
      6. Family history: Reactions to food aversion, weight loss, and eating conflicts

    7. Screening tool

       a) The Patient-Generated Subjective Global Assessment tool is validated in patients with cancer but requires up to 15 minutes to perform and must be completed by a well-trained healthcare professional.

       b) The Malnutrition Universal Screening Tool is a validated, simple assessment tool that predicts mortality and incorporates BMI, weight loss, and acute disease score.

C. Signs and symptoms

    1. Significantly decreased weight over the past six months: BMI alone is limited in that it fails to identify proportion of bone, fat, and lean body mass. An international consensus group has proposed an alternative grading system.

       a) Grade 0: Weight-stable patients (loss ±2.4%) with BMI less than or equal to 25 kg/m^2 (median survival: 29 months)

       b) Grade 1: BMI 20–25 kg/m^2 and weight loss greater than or equal to 2.4%, or BMI less than or equal to 28 kg/m^2 and weight loss of 2.5%–6% (median survival: 14.6 months)

       c) Grade 2: BMI 20–28 kg/m^2 and weight loss of 2.5%–6%, or BMI less than or equal to 28 kg/m^2 and weight loss of 6%–11% (median survival: 10.8 months)

       d) Grade 3: BMI less than or equal to 20 kg/m^2 and weight loss of less than 6%, or BMI 20–28 kg/m^2 and weight loss of 6%–11%, or BMI 22–28 kg/m^2 and weight loss of 11%–15%, or BMI less than or equal to 28 kg/m^2 and weight loss greater than 15% (median survival: 7.6 months)

       e) Grade 4: BMI less than or equal to 20 kg/m^2 and weight stable or loss of less than 6%–11%, or BMI less than or equal to 22 kg/m^2 and weight loss of 11%–15%, or BMI less than or equal to 28 kg/m^2 and weight loss greater than 15% (median survival: 4.3 months)

    2. Emaciated appearance: Temporal wasting

    3. Loss of appetite

    4. Nausea and vomiting

    5. Fatigue/weakness

    6. Amenorrhea

    7. Polyuria

    8. Cold intolerance

D. Physical examination

    1. Vital signs

       a) Height and serial measurements of body weight

       b) BMI and anthropometric measurements: Typically decreased

       c) Blood pressure: Orthostatic hypotension

       d) Pulse: Tachycardia

       e) Respirations: Tachypnea

    2. Integument

       a) Dry skin with poor turgor

       b) Dry, brittle hair and nails

    3. HEENT: Poor dentition, mucositis, lesions, dry mucosal membranes, possible temporal wasting

    4. Cardiovascular: Irregular heart rate indicative of dysrhythmia, possible lower extremity edema

    5. Musculoskeletal: Loss of muscle mass, poor muscle tone, temporal wasting

    6. Abdominal: Protuberant distended abdomen in late stage from ascites

IV. Diagnostic tests (Del Fabbro, 2015; Dev et al., 2017; Sadeghi et al., 2018)
  A. Laboratory
    1. Hgb and hematocrit: May be decreased secondary to nutritional depletion
    2. Chemistry profile: Possible electrolyte alterations
       a) Sodium: May be decreased with weight loss, anorexia
       b) Potassium: May be decreased with weight loss, anorexia
    3. Serum albumin/serum protein: May be useful in measurement of nutrition status; will be low if malnourished; decreased prealbumin
    4. BUN–creatinine ratio: Helps to differentiate between dehydration and renal disease; will be increased with cachexia or volume depletion
    5. Cytokine mediators: Known to be abnormal (e.g., TNF, proteolysis-inducing factor, leptin); evaluation not recommended in routine clinical assessment
    6. CRP: Marker of inflammation and indication of catabolic drive; can be useful as prognostic value independent of tumor stage but has yet to be incorporated into screening or staging of cachexia
    7. Iron status
       a) Serum transferrin: Indicates visceral protein loss and may be depressed with extended periods of malnutrition
       b) Iron and iron saturation: Not specific in nutrition assessment
    8. Folate: Will be decreased in malnutrition
    9. TSH to evaluate for thyroid disorders
    10. HIV testing, as indicated
  B. Radiology
    1. Upper GI series or barium swallow to evaluate for obstructive process if symptoms warrant
    2. Other radiographic studies: CT, MRI, ultrasound, and chest x-ray to evaluate for progressive disease
    3. DEXA: Can distinguish lean body mass from fat-free mass and bone tissue as more accurate measure of weight; reserved mainly for the research setting

V. Differential diagnosis (Graul et al., 2016)
  A. Dementia
  B. CHF (see Chapter 42)
  C. COPD (see Chapter 28)
  D. Malignancy (primary or metastatic)
  E. Alcoholism
  F. Electrolyte imbalance (see Chapters 152–156)
  G. Multiple sclerosis
  H. RA (see Chapter 108)
  I. Hypoadrenalism
  J. Drug-induced disorders: Amphetamines, chemotherapy
  K. Depression (see Chapter 162)
  L. Anxiety (see Chapter 161)
  M. Fatigue (see Chapter 163)
  N. Pain
  O. Constipation (see Chapter 55)
  P. Impaired absorption
    1. Cholestasis
    2. Postgastrectomy
    3. Small bowel or pancreatic disease

      4. Parasitic infection: Giardiasis

      5. HIV/AIDS

      6. Mechanical obstruction

  Q. Increased nutrient loss

      1. Diabetes mellitus (see Chapter 151)

      2. Chronic diarrhea (see Chapter 56)

      3. Chronic nausea and vomiting (see Chapter 63)

      4. Hyperthyroidism (see Chapter 157)

VI. Treatment (Aoyagi et al., 2015; Argilés et al., 2019; Childs & Jatoi, 2019; Del Fabbro, 2015; Dev et al., 2017; Wang et al., 2019; Zhang et al., 2018)

  A. Treatment is centered on multifactorial etiologies and should be individualized, considering the patient's overall condition, mechanisms of weight loss, and goals of care. Currently, no standard guidelines exist for cachexia treatment with no cure; however, pharmacologic agents have been approved for support.

      1. Antineoplastic therapy to reduce tumor burden, pharmacologic anticachexia medications, nutritional counseling and support, physical activity to maintain muscle mass, and psychosocial support to patients and families must all be considered.

      2. Multidimensional treatment can be accomplished through an interprofessional approach.

  B. Patient education

      1. Discuss diet, and encourage frequent intake of high-calorie, high-protein foods throughout the day.

      2. Encourage activity as tolerated to stimulate appetite.

      3. Dietary counseling can help to increase caloric intake but may not affect QOL, overall nutritional status, or survival. It is imperative to educate patients and families that increasing caloric intake alone does not reverse the underlying anorexia/cachexia condition. The condition is unique from starvation and is a common sequela of dying with cancer.

  C. For associated symptoms, prescribe appropriate medications.

      1. Nausea and vomiting (see Chapter 63)

      2. Constipation (see Chapter 55)

      3. Diarrhea (see Chapter 56)

      4. Dysphagia (see Chapter 57)

  D. Anticipatory guidance: Continue to help patients to view their weight loss as a symptom with an expected pattern specific to their illness and treatment. Continue to offer encouragement, education, and hope through ongoing management.

  E. Consider the following medications for appetite stimulation and increased well-being.

      1. Megestrol acetate (600–800 mg PO daily; available in suspension) showed improved appetite and body weight compared to placebo in a minority of patients; however, no improvement in skeletal muscle mass and visceral proteins was found. Treatment should be weighed against potentially serious side effects. No overall evidence of improvement in QOL has been shown.

      2. The glucocorticoids dexamethasone (3–4 mg PO daily) or prednisone (20–40 mg PO daily) can improve appetite but not significantly improve body weight. Problematic side effects with long-term use include risk of adrenal insufficiency, insulin resistance, immunosuppression, and muscle myopathy.

      3. Dronabinol (2.5–5 mg PO daily) as a constituent of cannabis has been studied for appetite stimulation in patients with cancer; however, many placebo-controlled randomized trials have revealed no difference in appetite or QOL. Use with caution

and consider starting at lower doses in older adult patients because of the increased risk of CNS effects.

    F. Nonpharmacologic agents

        1. Nutrition: Dense protein and calorie supplementation may be of benefit, particularly with early intervention. Nutritional supplements can be recommended but should be consumed between meals and not be viewed as a meal replacement.

        2. Exercise: Physical activity has shown to increase insulin sensitivity, protein synthesis rate, and antioxidative enzyme activity and may lead to a suppression of the inflammatory response.

VII. Follow-up: Patients should be followed frequently to monitor weight with serial measurements and determine the effectiveness of interventions.

VIII. Referrals (Childs & Jatoi, 2019)

    A. Dietitian: For assessment of dietary intake and suggestions for nutritional supplements and elimination of mechanical barriers

    B. Psychological counseling: If depression or other emotional disturbances appear to be a contributing factor to weight loss; for suggestions on appropriate behavioral counseling, medication, and follow-up

    C. Medical, surgical, or radiation oncology: Depending on the underlying disease state and if treatment is an option

    D. Palliative care: To assist with symptom management

The author would like to acknowledge Margaret Quinn Rosenzweig, PhD, FNP-BC, AOCN®, for her contribution to this chapter that remains unchanged from the previous edition of this book.

References

Aoyagi, T., Terracina, K.P., Raza, A., Matsubara, H., & Takabe, K. (2015). Cancer cachexia, mechanism and treatment. *World Journal of Gastrointestinal Oncology, 7*(4), 17–29. https://doi.org/10.4251/wjgo.v7.i4.17

Argilés, J.M., Busquets, S., & López-Soriano, F.J. (2019). Cancer cachexia, a clinical challenge. *Current Opinion in Oncology, 31*(4), 286–290. https://doi.org/10.1097/CCO.0000000000000517

Childs, D.S., & Jatoi, A. (2019). A hunger for hunger: A review of palliative therapies for cancer-associated anorexia. *Annals of Palliative Medicine, 8*(1), 50–58. https://doi.org/10.21037/apm.2018.05.08

Del Fabbro, E. (2015). Current and future care of patients with the cancer anorexia-cachexia syndrome. *American Society of Clinical Oncology Educational Book, 35*, e229–e237. https://doi.org/10.14694/EdBook_AM.2015.35.e229

Dev, R., Wong, A., Hui, D., & Bruera, E. (2017). The evolving approach to management of cancer cachexia. *Oncology, 31*(1), 23–32. https://www.cancernetwork.com/view/evolving-approach-management-cancer-cachexia

Ezeoke, C.C., & Morley, J.E. (2015). Pathophysiology of anorexia in the cancer cachexia syndrome. *Journal of Cachexia, Sarcopenia and Muscle, 6*(4), 287–302. https://doi.org/10.1002/jcsm.12059

Graul, A.I., Stringer, M., & Sorbera, L. (2016). Cachexia. *Drugs of Today, 52*(9), 519–529. https://doi.org/10.1358/dot.2016.52.9.2545017

Laviano, A., Koverech, A., & Seelaender, M. (2017). Assessing pathophysiology of cancer anorexia. *Current Opinion in Clinical Nutrition and Metabolic Care, 20*(5), 340–435. https://doi.org/10.1097/MCO.0000000000000394

Sadeghi, M., Keshavarez-Fathi, M., Baracos, V., Arends, J., Mahmoudi, M., & Rezaei, N. (2018). Cancer cachexia: Diagnosis, assessment, and treatment. *Critical Reviews in Oncology/Hematology, 127*, 91–104. https://doi.org/10.1016/j.critrevonc.2018.05.006

Vagnildhaug, O.M., Balstad, T.R., Almberg, S.S., Brunelli, C., Knudsen, A.K., Kaasa, S., … Solhein, T.S. (2018). A cross-sectional study examining the prevalence of cachexia and areas of unmet need in patients with cancer. *Supportive Care in Cancer, 26*(6), 1871–1880. https://doi.org/10.1007/s00520 017-4022-z

Wang, J., Wang, Y., Tong, M., Pan, H., & Li, D. (2019). Medical cannabinoids for cancer cachexia: A systematic review and meta-analysis. *BioMed Research International, 2019*, 2864384. https://doi.org/10.1155/2019/2864384

Zhang, F., Shen, A., Jin, Y., & Qiang, W. (2018). The management strategies of cancer-associated anorexia: A critical appraisal of systematic reviews. *BMC Complementary and Alternative Medicine, 18,* 236. https://doi.org/10.1186/s12906-018-2304-8

CHAPTER 67

Bowel Obstruction/Ileus

Jeanne Held-Warmkessel, MSN, RN, AOCN®, ACNS-BC

I. Definition: Failure of intestinal materials to move forward in the normal manner (Katrancha & George, 2014)

II. Physiology/Pathophysiology (Flores-Funes et al., 2016; Hsu et al., 2019; Jaffe & Thompson, 2015; Katrancha & George, 2014; Reddy & Cappell, 2017; Venara et al., 2016)
   A. Normal: GI fluid secretion totals 7–8 L daily, which is mostly reabsorbed as it transits the length of the bowel.
   B. Pathophysiology
      1. Altered bowel motility
         a) Bowel becomes hyperactive above the obstruction, attempting to force bowel contents beyond the obstruction.
         b) Eventually, the bowel tires, stops its attempts to move the contents beyond the obstruction, and becomes dilated from swallowed air.
         c) Bowel below the obstruction continues to function and produce stool until the bowel is emptied below the obstruction.
         d) Swallowed air accounts for much of the trapped gas in bowel obstruction.
         e) Ileus is multifactorial and partly as a result of an altered sympathetic nervous system, causing altered smooth muscle contractions that normally produce intestinal propulsion. GI secretions then pool in the intestines.
         f) Tumor invasion into the nervous system that supplies bowel interferes with peristalsis.
      2. Loss of normal absorption capacity and the continued influx of fluids and electrolytes into the bowel cause bowel distention and deplete the intravascular volume.
         a) Distention causes mucosal edema and bowel ischemia.
         b) Fluid overload during the intraoperative period causes intestinal edema. This stimulates intracellular communication and results in smooth muscle relaxation and ileus.
         c) Vomiting causes hypovolemia and electrolyte loss.
      3. Bacterial overgrowth: Aerobic and anaerobic
         a) Overgrowth increases bowel gas, interferes with bowel absorption, and injures the bowel mucosa.
         b) Bacteria migrate through the bowel wall into the lymph nodes and bloodstream.
         c) Bacterial endotoxins enter the peritoneal cavity, allowing more bacteria to migrate through the bowel wall.
         d) Intraoperative bowel manipulation allows movement of particles out of the bowel through the bowel wall and also produces bowel lumen edema.

4. Damage to intestinal mucosa develops quickly when blood supply is impaired by increased intestinal intraluminal pressure from fluid accumulation. Fluids and electrolytes leak into the bowel, and the mucosa may slough and bleed. Sepsis may develop.

5. Inflammation

   a) Distant organ responses occur from the release of systemic inflammatory substances.

   b) Manipulation of bowel intraoperatively causes inflammation that results in postoperative ileus.

6. Pseudo-obstruction may be caused by adynamic ileus, Ogilvie syndrome, or toxic megacolon. Ogilvie syndrome is associated with autonomic nervous system dysfunction. The bowel functions as if obstructed, although no mechanical blockage is present.

III. Clinical features: Obstruction may be acute, chronic, intermittent, or recurrent. It can involve the small bowel (SBO), large bowel (LBO), or both and be complete or partial. Obstruction can also be strangulated or closed loop, and single or multiple areas may be affected. Ninety percent of bowel obstructions involve the small bowel. It should be determined if the patient is clinically stable or unstable, whether emergency surgical intervention is needed, and whether sepsis is present (Bower et al., 2018; Bragg et al., 2015; Hsu et al., 2019; Jaffe & Thompson, 2015; Katrancha & George, 2014; Paulson & Thompson, 2015; Reddy & Cappell, 2017).

A. Etiology

   1. Treatments

      a) Abdominal surgeries (e.g., GI, gynecologic, urology): Surgical complications may increase risk of ileus.

      b) Medications

      c) Radiation therapy–induced fibrosis

   2. Diseases

      a) Colon cancer, ovarian cancer

      b) Diverticulitis

      c) Inflammatory bowel disease, Crohn disease

      d) Hernia

   3. Other

      a) Adhesions

      b) Severe constipation

      c) Sepsis

      d) Volvulus, intussusception

B. History

   1. History of cancer and cancer treatment: Abdominal, ovarian, or colorectal cancer surgery, either open or laparoscopic; radiation therapy; prior bowel obstruction, including management and outcome

   2. Current medications: Prescribed, over the counter, opioid use

   3. History of presenting symptoms: Precipitating factors, onset, duration, associated symptoms (e.g., nausea, vomiting, bowel changes such as constipation, stool diameter or consistency [occasionally diarrhea may develop secondary to bacterial action on stool], abdominal pain, cramps or distention [patients describe that their pants or skirt feels tight], dizziness, flatus, time of vomiting in relation to food or fluid consumption, blood in stool, decreased urine output)

   4. Changes in ADLs

     5. Past medical history: Crohn disease, ulcerative colitis, other inflammatory bowel diseases, diverticulitis, abdominal, femoral, inguinal, incisional hernia

     6. Past surgical history: Abdominal or pelvic surgery, adhesions, hernia repair

C. Signs and symptoms: LBO symptoms occur slowly. Right colon obstructions produce symptoms later than left colon obstructions. SBOs occur quickly.

     1. Abdominal pain can be assessed using numeric pain rating scale, such as 0–10.

       a) Pain may be spasmodic, colicky, or crampy and located in the mid- to upper abdomen.

       b) Pain may be intermittent, diffuse, or localized.

       c) The more proximal the obstruction, the more frequent the episodes of pain.

       d) The longer the patient is obstructed, the weaker the bowel contractions.

       e) Constant severe or worsening pain suggests compromise of the bowel blood supply or perforation.

       f) LBO pain is located in periumbilical or hypogastric area.

     2. The more distal the obstruction, the worse the abdominal distention.

     3. Reduced amount, reduced caliber, or absence of stool can occur. As the distal bowel evacuates the remaining contents, stool will be eliminated, and constipation/obstipation occurs. No stool is produced with an ileus.

     4. Fever or chills can be suggestive of strangulation.

     5. Presence of peritonitis, perforation, sepsis, ischemia, strangulation, or severe abdominal pain is indicative of the need for urgent surgery after patient is stabilized.

     6. Retching, anorexia, nausea, and vomiting may be feculent with SBO. The more proximal the blockage, the worse the vomiting; the more distal the blockage, the longer it takes for vomiting to start.

     7. Flatus does not occur if the obstruction is complete or with an ileus.

     8. Dehydration can occur.

D. Physical examination

     1. Vital signs and pulse oximetry: Hypotension, orthostatic hypotension; tachycardia, tachypnea, and hypotension from hypovolemia; possible fever

     2. Neurologic: Changes in mental status from hypovolemia or electrolyte imbalances

     3. Integument: Radiation markings, abdominal mass or masses, scars for possible causes of obstruction (e.g., adhesions), skin and mucous membrane assessments for dehydration

     4. Pulmonary: Increased respiratory rate and decreased respiratory depth from pressure on the diaphragm secondary to obstruction

     5. Abdominal

       a) Tenderness: Direct on palpation, diffuse at site of blockage (variable); rebound tenderness, guarding, and rigidity indicative of bowel strangulation, ischemia, or perforation

       b) Distention: Baseline abdominal girth and size to assess response to treatment

       c) Bowel sounds: Usually hyperactive, high-pitched sounds above obstruction with periods of absence; as bowel tires, sounds stop; hypoactive with LBO; no bowel sounds with ileus

       d) Percussion: Tympany from air filled loops; dull with fluid filled loops

       e) Inguinal, femoral, or ventral hernia

       f) Masses that could be the cause of obstruction and ascites as a result of obstruction

       g) Enlarged liver

     6. Rectal examination: Impaction or masses; frank and occult blood testing

     7. Urine output: Reduced as a result of hypotension

IV. Diagnostic tests (Bower et al., 2018; Jaffe & Thompson, 2015; Paulson & Thompson, 2015; Reddy & Cappell, 2017)
  A. Laboratory
    1. Electrolytes
      a) Decreased potassium, chloride, and bicarbonate levels with bowel obstruction
      b) Increased phosphorus and potassium with bowel strangulation
      c) Loss of chlorides, sodium, and potassium with vomiting
    2. Comprehensive metabolic panel with BUN–creatinine: Increased ratio from intravascular volume depletion from vomiting and bowel sequestration of fluid; AKI
    3. CBC with differential: Increased WBC count with inflammation, ischemia, infection, or perforation
    4. LDH, amylase, and lipase: If strangulation is suspected, levels are increased, but the tests are not a reliable indicator. Increased amylase is associated with perforation.
    5. Blood pH, lactic acid
      a) Metabolic alkalosis: High intestinal obstruction
      b) Metabolic acidosis: Lower intestinal obstruction, ischemia, bowel infarction, bowel gangrene, intravascular volume depletion
      c) Lactic acid: With increase, associated with intestinal ischemia; contrast-enhanced CT scan of abdomen and pelvis recommended when associated with elevated amylase
    6. LFTs: Increased with gallstone ileus
    7. PT, PTT, and INR: Coagulation abnormality prior to surgery
    8. Blood cultures if sepsis suspected or with fever
    9. Intestinal fatty acid binding protein: New biomarker for intestinal injury; increased level of evidence of bowel ischemia
    10. Pregnancy test
    11. Laboratory tests repeated every six hours or per institution policy: CBC, basic metabolic panel, lactic acid to identify changes
  B. Radiology
    1. Serial plain abdominal radiographs: Flat (supine or prone) and upright, left (lateral or decubitus), chest x-ray, obstruction series
      a) In presence of complete SBO, x-rays show dilated bowel above obstruction, U-shaped bowel loops, minimal or no gas in large bowel, and air-fluid levels in multiple areas of bowel.
      b) With a partial or complete early SBO or ileus, gas is present in the large bowel. Upright radiographs may reveal free air in the abdomen, evidence of perforation.
      c) With a LBO, dilated large bowel present above obstruction and minimal or no gas is present below the obstruction. Air-fluid level is associated with acute obstruction.
      d) Water-soluble contrast material via NG tube followed by abdominal radiographs to monitor contrast passage may be considered.
      e) Portal venous gas, pneumoperitoneum, or pneumatosis may be seen.
    2. Multidetector CT scan/CT scan of abdomen and pelvis, with and without IV contrast, is the diagnostic test of choice for acute bowel obstruction.
      a) All patients with a diagnosis of suspected SBO require a CT scan.
      b) Scan is useful in determining if mechanical obstruction, ileus, or other pathology is causing the obstruction.
      c) Dilated bowel or bowel filled with air above obstruction, level or location of obstruction, etiology of obstruction (e.g., mass), complete versus partial obstruc-

tion, high-grade versus low-grade obstruction, metastases, inflammation, or ischemia can be noted.

    d) Test is useful if plain abdominal films are negative but patient has symptoms suggestive of bowel obstruction. Enteric contrast may be used with intermittent or low-grade obstruction.

  3. Contrast fluoroscopy (e.g., water-soluble contrast enema): Patient must be able to turn on the radiology table.

    a) Used for LBO to demonstrate area of blockage

    b) Small bowel follow-through contrast study

    c) Differentiates obstruction from pseudo-obstruction

    d) For low-grade or chronic-intermittent SBO

  4. Ultrasound if patient is unstable or pregnant: May be able to reveal cause of SBO and if complications are present

  5. Gastrografin® contrast administered by NG tube is both diagnostic and therapeutic.

    a) If 24 hours after NG tube instillation, SBO may resolve without surgery if contrast is seen in the colon. If the contrast is not seen, surgery will likely be needed.

    b) If administered by enema, it may be diagnostic and therapeutic.

C. Endoscopy

  1. Proctosigmoidoscopy to evaluate for LBO if a sigmoid mass or volvulus is suspected on CT: This method may be used to obtain biopsy. Therapeutic sigmoidoscopy may be able to untwist sigmoid volvulus. Carbon dioxide is preferred gas for insufflation.

  2. Colonoscopy to diagnose cancer or other obstructing lesions: It has limited utility because oral preparation cannot be taken in presence of bowel obstruction. It can be used to place colonic decompression tube or stent, or to decompress colon (enema prep may be used). Colonoscopy should not be performed in patients with complete obstruction or gangrenous bowel.

D. Paracentesis: If ascites is present, both therapeutic and diagnostic paracentesis and to assess for peritonitis

V. Differential diagnosis (Jaffe & Thompson, 2015; Paulson & Thompson, 2015; Reddy & Cappell, 2017)

  A. Mechanical

    1. Small bowel

      a) Adhesions: From prior abdominal surgery, intra-abdominal infection

      b) Hernia: Inguinal, ventral, femoral, or internal; hernias are more likely to cause strangulation of bowel.

      c) Malignancy, carcinomatosis

      d) Inflammatory edema or stenosis: Crohn disease, ischemia

      e) Abscess

      f) Gallstone ileus

      g) Foreign object, bezoars

      h) Intussusception, volvulus (bowel twisted on itself 180°)

    2. Large bowel: Sigmoid (most common)

      a) Malignancy originating intraluminally (e.g., colon cancer), extrinsically (e.g., ovarian cancer), or metastatically

      b) Diverticular disease, diverticulosis (see Chapter 70)

      c) Intussusceptions or volvulus

      d) Fecal impaction

      e) Strictures

    f) Cecal bascule

    g) External compression

    h) Hernia

    i) Gallstones, enteroliths, foreign bodies (see Chapter 68)

    j) Adhesions

    k) Inflammatory bowel disease

 B. Nonmechanical: Paralytic ileus secondary to the following

   1. Postoperative surgical complication, ileus

   2. Electrolyte imbalances: Hypokalemia, hyponatremia (see Chapters 152–156)

   3. Abdominal cavity inflammatory process: Infection, pancreatitis (see Chapter 77), peritonitis, inflammatory bowel disease

   4. Bowel blood vessel embolus or thrombus, acute mesenteric ischemia, ischemic colitis

   5. Fracture of spine, ribs, or pelvis: Possibly from reflex inhibition (see Chapter 102)

   6. MI: Impaired blood flow to bowel (see Chapter 49)

   7. Respiratory disorder: Pneumonia (see Chapter 30), PE (see Chapter 33)

   8. Retroperitoneal bleeding or inflammation: Ruptured abdominal aortic aneurysm, pyelonephritis (see Chapter 94)

   9. Drug-induced disorder

    a) Opioids

    b) Neurotoxicity from plant alkaloids: Vinblastine, vincristine

    c) Anticholinergics: Dicyclomine, hyoscyamine

    d) Diuretics causing hypokalemia

   10. Sepsis

   11. Paraneoplastic neuropathy (see Appendix M)

   12. Ogilvie syndrome

 C. Radiation therapy: Acute or late effects can occur months or years after treatment is completed.

   1. Early: Ulceration may cause contraction of the wall with resultant obstruction.

   2. Late: Scarring over a period of months to years may cause strictures.

 D. Strangulated (bowel dies quickly) versus nonstrangulated

 E. Perforation versus nonperforation

 F. Closed loop (two blockages) versus open loop (one blockage)

 G. Porphyria: A heme biosynthesis metabolic disorder causing an attack that can be confused with a bowel obstruction

VI. Treatment (Bower et al., 2018; Bragg et al., 2015; Flores-Funes et al., 2016; Hsu et al., 2019; Jaffe & Thompson, 2015; Katrancha & George, 2014; Lee et al., 2018; Olson et al., 2014; Paulson & Thompson, 2015; Reddy & Cappell, 2017)

 A. Complete bowel obstruction, strangulation, impaired or blocked blood supply, and perforation or other complications indicate the need for emergency surgery after stabilizing the patient. Patients with SBO who fail NG tube trial should have some type of intervention after three to five days.

 B. Partial bowel obstruction may be managed conservatively.

   1. Failure to improve indicates a need for surgical or invasive intervention.

   2. Medically managed patients require frequent assessment and monitoring so that surgery can be performed if bowel function is not restored.

   3. Presence of peritonitis, acidosis, high WBC count, or clinical instability are indicators for emergency surgery.

   4. LBO is managed similarly.

C. Relieve distention and vomiting by decompressing bowel.

    1. Insert NG tube and connect to low-intermittent suction or Salem Sump™ tube with antireflux valve to intermittent or continuous suction. Many patients have a trial of NG tube to suction and repeat abdominal radiographs and monitor response to decompression.

    2. Flush NG tube PRN to maintain patency.

    3. Patient is NPO.

    4. Monitor abdominal girth to assess response to bowel decompression. NG tube insertion and drainage should result in decreased abdominal girth and distention.

D. Replace fluids and electrolytes (see Chapters 152–156).

    1. Insert two large-gauge IV catheters. Start IV fluids; aggressive isotonic (normal saline or lactated ringers) fluid replacement may be needed. Avoid salt overload. Correct electrolyte imbalances.

    2. Insert indwelling urinary catheter to monitor urine output with hypovolemia or sepsis; oliguria often accompanies dehydration. Monitor intake and output closely. Balance fluid state between input and output. Remove bladder catheter as soon as possible to reduce infection risk.

    3. Correct metabolic acidosis with sodium bicarbonate in IV fluids (alkalosis occurs with proximal small bowel obstruction) to return pH to normal range.

    4. Monitor vital signs closely.

    5. Avoid overhydration resulting in fluid weight gain in patients with postoperative ileus and in patients being managed medically; excess IV fluids will increase bowel secretions resulting in more bowel edema and vomiting.

E. Relieve pain.

    1. Pain should decrease with NG tube decompression.

    2. Administer parenteral or topical opioids judiciously as they mask serious complications (see Appendix F).

    3. Reduce inflammation and provide symptom palliation with IV steroids.

F. Monitor frequently and regularly for signs and symptoms of ongoing complications and clinical deterioration (e.g., dry mouth, fever, nausea and vomiting, tachypnea, increased abdominal tenderness/pain, tachycardia, increasing WBC count, rigid abdomen, distention, hypoactive or absent bowel sounds, guarding, blood pressure changes, change in mental status, oliguria) indicating possible complications requiring surgery.

    1. Strangulation, bowel infarction, ischemia, necrosis

    2. Perforation

    3. Peritonitis

    4. Sepsis

    5. Respiratory compromise, aspiration

    6. Overhydration resulting in fluid weight gain in patients with postoperative ileus

G. Surgical intervention (e.g., laparotomy) may be required for patients with complete SBO or LBO, perforation, or ischemia to resect affected bowel or lyse adhesions or for patients who show no sign of clinical improvement.

    1. Consult surgery early in the admission.

    2. In selected patients, surgery offers a good outcome.

    3. For end-of-life patients, surgical interventions may relieve symptoms but frank discussion about goals of care is needed.

    4. For SBO due to adhesions, the majority of SBOs resolve if there is no evidence of peritonitis or complications. Surgery is needed if it does not resolve in three to five days.

H. Administer antibiotics, such as broad-spectrum agents with activity against gram-negative aerobes and anaerobes (see Appendix C).

I. Manage advanced or recurrent abdominal malignancy causing bowel obstruction.
  1. Percutaneous endoscopic gastrostomy/venting gastrostomy tube for continuous drainage in context of chronic obstruction
  2. Pain and symptom management
  3. Placement of self-expanding metallic stent for symptom palliation at end of life or when surgery is not an option; useful in open-loop obstruction, gastric outlet obstruction, and left-sided colon obstructions
  4. Tube decompression to prepare bowel for resection of malignant obstruction, symptom palliation at end of life

J. Provide parenteral nutrition if patient is NPO for five to seven days and improvement in QOL is expected with life expectancy of months to years. It is not recommended for patients at the end of life.

K. Ambulate with ileus to promote bowel function.

L. Manage emesis. Administer antiemetics; keep NG tube patent (see Appendix P).

M. Provide frequent oral care.

N. Manage secretions (e.g., palliative care, medically managed patients).
  1. Octreotide: 100 mcg subcutaneous three to four times a day, up to maximal dose of 1 mg daily; reduces volume of GI secretions; titrated dose; may be used postoperatively and administered intermittently; if no reduction in secretions, should be discontinued
  2. Dexamethasone: IV 6–16 mg daily with pantoprazole 40 mg daily

VII. Follow-up

A. Monitor for recurrence of obstruction after discharge.
  1. Patients with abdominal metastases may have recurrence of obstruction if not resected. If resected, reobstruction may still occur.
  2. Some patients may not be surgical candidates because of extensive carcinomatosis and are at risk for recurrence of obstruction.

B. Educate patients to call healthcare provider at first onset of symptoms so that prompt treatment can be instituted.

VIII. Referrals (Hsu et al., 2019; Jaffe & Thompson, 2015; Lee et al., 2018; Olson et al., 2014; Reddy & Cappell, 2017)

A. Surgeon: To evaluate and monitor patient for acute abdomen, perforation, ischemia or other complications and need for surgery; to evaluate patient for palliative surgery such as an ostomy

B. Gastroenterologist: For diagnostic evaluation and possible therapeutic endoscopy, stent placement, percutaneous endoscopic gastrostomy for straight drainage or feeding jejunal tube; for management of Ogilvie syndrome

C. Medical oncologist: If malignancy induced or if malignancy suspected

D. Interventional radiologist: For placement of percutaneous endoscopic gastrostomy for straight drainage or placement of feeding jejunal tube.

E. Radiologist: For diagnostic evaluation and monitoring of obstruction

F. Intensivist: For management of sepsis, hemodynamics, and metabolic derangements

G. Pain and palliative care team: To assist with pain, symptom management, and goals of care

H. Radiation oncologist: To determine if palliative radiation therapy may be helpful

References

Bower, K.L., Lollar, D.I., Williams, S.L., Adkins, F.C., Luyimbazi, D.T., & Bower, C.E. (2018). Small bowel obstruction. *Surgical Clinics of North America, 98*(5), 945–971. https://doi.org/10.1016/j.suc.2018.05.007

Bragg, D., El-Sharkawy, A.M., Psaltis, E., Maxwell-Armstrong, C.A., & Lobo, D.N. (2015). Postoperative ileus: Recent developments in pathophysiology and management. *Clinical Nutrition, 34*(3), 367–376. https://doi.org/10.1016/j.clnu.2015.01.016.

Flores-Funes, D., Campillo-Soto, Á., Pellicer-Franco, E., & Aguayo-Albasini, J.L. (2016). The use of coffee, chewing-gum and gastrograffin in the management of postoperative ileus: A review of current evidence. *Cirugía Española, 94*(9), 495–501. https://doi.org/10.1016/j.ciresp.2016.05.020

Hsu, K., Prommer, E., Murphy, M.C., & Lankarani-Fard, A. (2019). Pharmacologic management of malignant bowel obstruction: When surgery is not an option. *Journal of Hospital Medicine, 14*(6), 367–373. https://doi.org/10.12788/jhm.3187

Jaffe, T., & Thompson, W.M. (2015). Large-bowel obstruction in the adult: Classic radiographic and CT findings, etiology, and mimics. *Radiology, 275*(3), 651–663. https://doi.org/10.1148/radiol.2015140916.

Katrancha, E.D., & George, N.M. (2014). Postoperative ileus. *MedSurg Nursing, 23*(6), 387–390, 413.

Lee, Y.C., Jivraj, N., O'Brien, C., Chawla, T., Shlomovitz, E., Buchanan, S., … Lheureux, S. (2018). Malignant bowel obstruction in advanced gynecological cancers: An updated review from a multidisciplinary perspective. *Obstetrics and Gynecology International, 2018,* 1867238. https://doi.org/10.1155/2018/1867238

Olson, T.J.P., Pinkerton, C., Brasel, K.J., & Schwarze, M.L. (2014). Palliative surgery for malignant bowel obstruction from carcinomatosis: A systematic review. *JAMA Surgery, 149*(4), 383–392. https://doi.org/10.1001/jamasurg.2013.4059

Paulson, E.K., & Thompson, W.M. (2015). Review of small-bowel obstruction: The diagnosis and when to worry. *Radiology, 275*(2), 332–342. https://doi.org/10.1148/radiol.15131519

Reddy, S.R.R., & Cappell, M.S. (2017). A systematic review of the clinical presentation, diagnosis, and treatment of small bowel obstruction. *Current Gastroenterology Reports, 19*(6), 28. https://doi.org/10.1007/s11894-017-0566-9

Venara, A., Neunlist, M., Slim, K., Barbieux, J., Colas, P.A., Hamy, A., & Meurette, G. (2016). Postoperative ileus: Pathophysiology, incidence, and prevention. *Journal of Visceral Surgery, 153*(6), 439–446. https://doi.org/10.1016/j.jviscsurg.2016.08.010

CHAPTER 68

Cholecystitis

Richard Ornato, PA-C

I. Definition: Acute or chronic inflammation of the gallbladder, usually as a response to a cystic duct obstruction by a gallstone (Katabathina et al., 2015; Wilkins et al., 2017)

II. Physiology/Pathophysiology (European Association for the Study of the Liver, 2016; Wilkins et al., 2017)
   A. Normal: The gallbladder is a pear-shaped distensible organ approximately 4 × 8 cm in size with a normal capacity of 30–50 ml.
      1. The gallbladder lies in a fossa on the visceral surface of the liver, separating the right and left hepatic lobes.
      2. Posteriorly, it abuts the duodenum and the hepatic flexure of the colon, both hollow organs.
      3. The biliary tract starts at the hepatocyte canaliculi, which empties into the left and right hepatic ducts and then drains into the common hepatic duct.
      4. The cystic duct from the gallbladder joins the common hepatic duct, and together they form the CBD.
      5. Usually 8 cm long and 0.5–0.9 cm in diameter, the common hepatic duct empties into the duodenum at the ampulla of Vater. The pancreatic duct may join the CBD before it reaches the ampulla.
      6. Under normal circumstances, bile drains from the gallbladder into the duodenum via the CBD. The sphincter of Oddi prevents intestinal reflux into the CBD.
      7. The gallbladder stores bile, a yellow-colored fluid made in the liver from cholesterol, bile salts, and waste products.
         a) The major function of bile is to break down and metabolize fats.
         b) Bile also removes toxins from the liver, such as bacteria, viruses, drugs, or other foreign substances, and carries them to the intestines for removal.
         c) Normally, the liver produces approximately 1 L of bile daily.
         d) Bile contains water, cholesterol, phospholipids, bile salts, electrolytes, bilirubin, and other organic solutes.
   B. Pathophysiology
      1. Gallstones (cholelithiasis) are made by the precipitation of insoluble bile constituents including cholesterol, bilirubin, and calcium salts.
      2. Saturated bile may have impaired gallbladder motility, causing bile stasis and increasing the tendency for stone formation.
      3. Once inflammation of the gallbladder begins, additional inflammatory mediators are released. Prostaglandins, which are involved in gallbladder contraction and fluid absorption, probably play a central role in this process.

4. Infection of bile within the biliary system may have a role; however, not all patients with cholecystitis have infected bile.
5. Gallbladder outlet obstruction can lead to venous and lymphatic congestion and decreased blood supply. This, in turn, may cause gallbladder ischemia and necrosis.
6. Acalculous cholecystitis is inflammation of the gallbladder that may occur in the absence of gallstones. It occurs more often in immunosuppressed patients, patients with severe infections or severe systemic disease (e.g., CHF, diabetes), and postoperative patients.

III. Clinical features: Cholecystitis is considered the most common form of gallbladder disease and is an umbrella term that encompasses a variety of conditions concerned with the biliary system. Complications of acute cholecystitis include hepatic and intra-abdominal abscesses (Abraham et al., 2014; Alves de Oliveira et al., 2016; European Association for the Study of the Liver, 2016; Katabathina et al., 2015; Mou et al., 2019; Tazuma et al., 2017).
   A. Classification of gallstones
      1. Cholesterol stones
         a) Most prevalent in industrialized countries
         b) May be pure, large (greater than 2.5 cm), solitary, or mixed and multifaceted
      2. Pigmented stones
         a) Two types of pigmented stones are black and brown.
         b) The color of pigmented stones is determined by the amount of calcium bilirubinate in the stone.
         c) Black stones form exclusively in the gallbladder and are more common in older adults and patients with chronic hemolytic disorders, such as sickle cell disease or spherocytosis.
         d) Brown stones may form in the gallbladder or in the intra- or extrahepatic bile ducts and are commonly associated with infectious or parasitic processes.
   B. Risk factors
      1. Age older than 40 years
      2. Female
      3. Obesity
      4. Rapid weight loss
      5. Pregnancy
      6. Exogenous estrogens
      7. Diabetes
      8. Hemolysis
      9. Cirrhosis
      10. High-calorie and refined carbohydrate diet
      11. Total parenteral nutrition
      12. Ileal disease
      13. Certain cholesterol-reducing drugs
      14. Pancreatic insufficiency
      15. Cystic fibrosis
      16. Prior abdominal surgery
   C. Etiology
      1. Hereditary
      2. Dyslipidemia
      3. Calculous cholecystitis
      4. Infections
      5. Bile duct strictures
      6. Gallbladder ischemia

      7. Malignancy

      8. Acute acalculous cholecystitis

      9. Chronic cholecystitis: Repeated instances of mild gallbladder outlet obstruction

  D. History

      1. History of cancer and cancer treatments

      2. Current medications: Prescribed, over the counter, use of estrogen

      3. History of presenting symptoms: Precipitating factors, onset, duration, associated symptoms (e.g., abdominal pain, heartburn, indigestion)

      4. Changes in ADLs

      5. Past medical history: Diabetes, cystic fibrosis, pancreatic disease

      6. Diet recall: 24-hour intake

  E. Signs and symptoms: More than half (50%–90%) of people with gallstones are asymptomatic, whereas 2%–15% experience severe symptoms.

      1. Pain

         a) Pain from gallstones usually is felt in the upper right quadrant or epigastrium.

         b) It can be moderate and intermittent to severe and continuous.

         c) Pain may be localized to the right upper quadrant or diffuse to the right lower or other quadrants.

         d) Severe pain can be incapacitating, making it difficult or impossible for the patient to sit or stand.

         e) Pain in the right upper quadrant may radiate to the right side or back or right shoulder.

         f) Colicky-type pain lasting longer than 30 minutes usually follows a fatty meal.

      2. Nausea and vomiting

      3. Fever

      4. Dyspepsia

  F. Physical examination

      1. Vital signs

         a) Weight loss

         b) Possible elevated temperature

         c) Increased respiratory rate: Tachypnea (common)

      2. Integument: Jaundice present with obstruction

      3. Cardiac examination: Tachycardia (common)

      4. Abdominal (see Appendix D)

         a) Boas sign: Point tenderness in the region to the right of the 10th and 12th thoracic vertebrae, intrascapular region

         b) Murphy sign: A hallmark of acute cholecystitis—tenderness on deep palpation under the right costal margin

         c) Courvoisier sign: A palpable, dilated, nontender gallbladder in a patient with jaundice, usually suggesting cancer obstructing the CBD

         d) Guarding throughout the abdomen; no rigidity

         e) Tenderness present with an upper abdominal mass

         f) Palpable gallbladder

         g) Abdominal rigidity representing peritoneal inflammation

IV. Diagnostic tests (Abraham et al., 2014; Peterson et al., 2019; Schuster et al., 2019; Tazuma et al., 2017; Wilkins et al., 2017; Yokoe et al., 2018)

  A. Laboratory

      1. CBC: Many patients present with leukocytosis (greater than 10,000–20,000/mm³) with a left shift.

2. Chemistries
   a) Elevated alkaline phosphatase, transaminases, and bilirubin may be present.
   b) Jaundice may be evident when bilirubin levels are greater than 2.5 mg/dl.
   c) Choledocholithiasis should be considered in patients with a markedly elevated bilirubin level (greater than 3 mg/dl).
3. Potentially elevated serum amylase and lipase levels with pancreatitis
4. Gram stain, culture, and sensitivity of gallbladder fluid if infection suspected

B. Radiology
   1. Abdominal ultrasound is the current gold standard for evaluation of suspected cholecystitis. Ultrasound may be used to evaluate for the presence of biliary stones, sludge, and pericholecystic fluid.
      a) Can distinguish between acute cholecystitis, cholelithiasis, and choledocholithiasis
      b) Images the biliary tree and gallbladder (including gallbladder wall thickness)
      c) Less sensitive than CT for CBD stones
   2. Endoscopic ultrasound is very useful in evaluating choledocholithiasis.
      a) Highly accurate in assessing bile duct stones
      b) Allows for direct visualization of the bile ducts and general pancreatobiliary region
      c) Can detect tiny gallbladder and biliary stones less than 3 mm
      d) Not limited by obesity or bowel gas
   3. Oral cholecystography may be used in rare situations when the gallbladder is compressed, disallowing visualization of stones via ultrasound. The test takes up to 48 hours to complete and therefore is not useful in cases of acute cholecystitis.
   4. Cholescintigraphy (hepatobiliary iminodiacetic acid [HIDA] scan) involves nuclear imaging of the gallbladder and biliary tree. It is most often used in cases of acute cholecystitis.
      a) It can be performed in emergency situations, as it does not require fasting; results obtained in approximately 90 minutes
      b) It uses technetium-labeled HIDA or diisopropyl iminodiacetic acid (DISIDA). These compounds are injected and allow for visualization of the radioactivity in the gallbladder, biliary tree, and small intestine. In acute cholecystitis, the gallbladder is unable to be visualized. Conversely, one can diagnose a CBD obstruction when the bile ducts and gallbladder can be visualized but the radionuclide fails to enter the duodenum.
      c) False-positive results may happen in patients who are fasting or critically ill, as gallbladder motility is often impaired, leading to reduced clearance of the radionuclide.
   5. Endoscopic retrograde cholangiopancreatography is very useful in the detection of bile duct stones. The procedure involves passing an endoscope into the duodenum, inserting a catheter into the ampulla of Vater, and injecting contrast into the bile duct.
      a) An invasive procedure that should only be used when choledocholithiasis is highly suspected
      b) Advantages: Ability to perform therapeutic interventions during the procedure (e.g., sphincterotomy, stone extraction, biliary stenting, biopsies)
      c) Disadvantages: Postprocedure complications, including pancreatitis and bleeding
   6. CT is less sensitive than ultrasound for identifying gallstones but more sensitive in determining biliary dilation and CBD stones.
      a) Not limited by obesity or bowel gas

    b) Can identify portal hypertension, pseudocysts, peripancreatic fluid collections, pancreatic necrosis, and malignancies

    c) Indicated if suspected invasion of adjacent structures, abscess, inflammation, or obstruction

    d) Particularly sensitive to calcium stones; however, cholesterol stones are less easily visualized

    e) Disadvantages: Radiation exposure and administration of IV contrast, which may be limited in patients with renal disease

   7. Percutaneous transvenous coronary angioplasty (PTCA)

    a) Type of x-ray examination of the bile ducts inside and outside the liver; performed after a contrast medium is injected directly into a liver bile duct

    b) Used to determine obstruction in the CBD when a dilation of the hepatic biliary duct has been demonstrated on ultrasound; can reveal the location and nature of the obstruction

   8. Magnetic resonance cholangiopancreatography

    a) Noninvasive ultrafast magnetic resonance technique for imaging the pancreatobiliary tree

    b) Diagnostically accurate, not therapeutic

    c) Applications: Common duct stones, gallstones impacted in the neck or cystic duct not visible by ultrasound, intrahepatic or extrahepatic biliary dilation, cholangitis, pancreatic duct dilation

    d) Allows for simultaneous images of the abdomen (liver and pancreas) for detection of possible masses, fluid collections, abscesses, and pseudocysts, which is not possible with endoscopic retrograde cholangiopancreatography

    e) Can be used as initial diagnostic tool in patients who have contraindications to endoscopic retrograde cholangiopancreatography, older adult patients, and those with suspected stone in the bile duct

    f) Testing: If magnetic resonance cholangiopancreatography is negative, stop. If positive, perform stone extraction with endoscopic retrograde cholangiopancreatography or surgery.

   9. MRI

    a) Particularly helpful in assessing gallbladder perforation

    b) Shows soft tissue resolution and has high capability of finding small perforations that can be missed on ultrasound and CT

V. Differential diagnosis: Other causes of acute abdominal pain to consider include the following (Abraham et al., 2014; Peterson et al., 2019; Wilkins et al., 2017).

 A. Acute MI (see Chapter 49)

 B. Angina (see Chapter 40)

 C. Ruptured aortic aneurysm

 D. Appendicitis

 E. Acute pancreatitis (see Chapter 77)

 F. Intra-abdominal abscess

 G. Gastritis (see Chapter 72)

 H. Intestinal ischemia

 I. Intestinal obstruction (see Chapter 67)

 J. Peptic ulcer disease (see Chapter 78)

 K. Nephrolithiasis

 L. Renal colic

 M. Pleurisy

N. Pneumonia (see Chapter 30)

O. Pneumothorax (see Chapter 31)

P. Neoplasms

VI. Treatment: Management is dependent on clinical presentation and etiology. Patients with asymptomatic gallstones may not require intervention (Abraham et al., 2014; Higa & Irani, 2019; Mou et al., 2019; Rerknimitr & Pham, 2020; Schuster et al., 2019; Wilkins et al., 2017).

A. Supportive care

1. IV fluids, NPO, analgesics

2. The use of empiric antibiotics is controversial.

3. Antibiotics (see Appendix C): Indicated in patients with acalculous cholecystitis, emphysematous cholecystitis, or suspected gangrenous or perforated cholecystitis

a) Typically *Enterobacteriaceae* or *Enterococcus* species

b) Piperacillin/tazobactam: 3.375 g IV every six hours

c) Aztreonam: 2 g IV every eight hours

d) Ertapenem: 1 g IV every 24 hours

B. Surgery

1. Cholecystectomy

a) Indicated in symptomatic but otherwise stable patients

b) Should be performed within 72 hours of admission, unless the patient deteriorates clinically

c) Laparoscopic approach preferred over open cholecystectomy because of lower mortality rates and decreased recovery time

2. Emergent cholecystectomy

a) As a rule, emergency surgery should only be performed when a patient becomes progressively ill over 12 hours of medical treatment.

b) It should be performed when nonoperative decompression measures fail or are unavailable.

3. High-risk surgery patient characteristics

a) Previous cholecystitis

b) Choledocholithiasis

c) Diabetes

d) History of biliary tract intervention, sphincterotomy

e) Age older than 70 years

4. Interval cholecystectomy involves medical management of the acute phase of cholecystitis, followed by cholecystectomy 6–12 weeks later.

C. Nonsurgical patient management

1. Drainage via endoscopic or percutaneous cholecystostomy may be indicated in patients who are at high risk for surgical complications.

2. Therapeutic endoscopic retrograde cholangiopancreatography can be used in debilitated patients with CBD stones and intact gallbladders and when cholecystectomy and duct exploration are contraindicated.

3. Patients with gallstones who are not surgical candidates may benefit from oral bile salts. Bile salts, including ursodiol or chenodiol, are used in patients with a limited number of small (less than 15 mm) cholesterol stones.

a) Ursodiol: 8–10 mg/kg PO daily divided in two to three doses

b) Chenodiol: 250 mg PO two times a day initially for two weeks; increased by 250 mg daily each week until maximum tolerated dose is achieved; dose range usually 13–16 mg/kg daily in divided doses

    4. Lithotripsy uses high-pressure sound waves to break up gallstones. It is usually used in conjunction with bile salts.

  D. Decompression: Endoscopic route is initial choice for decompression of the biliary tree, especially if obstruction is below hepatic hilum or when intrahepatic ducts are dilated.

    1. PTCA is used to place a stent (particularly in debilitated patients in whom surgery is contraindicated) and can be used to relieve obstruction.

    2. It also is used to dissolve cholesterol stones by infusion of solvents via a percutaneous catheter placed above the stone.

    3. Stones can be dislodged and mobilized into the duodenum or withdrawn via a PTCA percutaneous catheter after the patient is treated with broad-spectrum antibiotics.

    4. Percutaneous cholecystectomy tube drainage is used for patients with cholangitis in the distal duct or if PTCA is unsuccessful.

VII. Follow-up

  A. Short term: 7–10 days after surgery or stone removal to assess pain, wound, and diarrhea

  B. Long term

    1. Postcholecystectomy pain

    2. Postoperative chronic diarrhea syndrome

VIII. Referrals

  A. Gastroenterologist: For cystic duct obstruction or choledocholithiasis

  B. Surgeon: For gallbladder removal or stone removal

The author would like to acknowledge Alison Ivey, RN, BSN, OCN®, CCRP, for her contribution to this chapter that remains unchanged from the previous edition of this book.

References

Abraham, S., Rivero, H.G., Erlikh, I.V., Griffith, L.F., & Kondamudi, V.K. (2014). Surgical and nonsurgical management of gallstones. *American Family Physician, 89*(10), 795–802. https://www.aafp.org/afp/2014/0515/p795.html

Alves de Oliveira, S.A., Jr., Véras Lemos, T.E., Costa de Medeiros, A., Jr., Dantas Freire, A., de Carvalho Garcia, C., de Sousa e Silva, R., … Araújo Filho, I. (2016). Acute acalculous cholecystitis in critically ill patients: Risk factors, diagnosis and treatment strategies. *Journal of the Pancreas, 17*(6), 580–586. http://pancreas.imedpub.com/acute-acalculous-cholecystitis-in-critically-ill-patients-risk-factors-diagnosis-and-treatment-strategies.php?aid=17273

European Association for the Study of the Liver. (2016). EASL clinical practice guidelines on the prevention, diagnosis, and treatment of gallstones. *Journal of Hepatology, 65*(1), 146–181. https://doi.org/10.1016/j.jhep.2016.03.005

Higa, J.T., & Irani, S.S. (2019). Endoscopic methods for gallbladder drainage. *Current Treatment Options in Gastroenterology, 17*(3), 357–366. https://doi.org/10.1007/s11938-019-00243-4

Katabathina, V.S., Zafar, A.M., & Suri, R. (2015). Clinical presentation, imaging, and management of acute cholecystitis. *Techniques in Vascular and Interventional Radiology, 18*(4), 256–265. https://doi.org/10.1053/j.tvir.2015.07.009

Mou, D., Tesfasilassie, T., Hirji, S., & Ashley, S.W. (2019). Advances in the management of acute cholecystitis. *Annals of Gastroenterology Surgery, 3*(3), 247–253. https://doi.org/10.1002/ags3.12240

Peterson, C.M., McNamara, M.M., Kamel, I.R., Al-Refaie, W.B., Arif-Tiwari, H., Cash, B.D., … Carucci, L.R. (2019). ACR Appropriateness Criteria® right upper quadrant pain. *Journal of the American College of Radiology, 16*(5 Suppl.), S235–S243. https://doi.org/10.1016/j.jacr.2019.02.013

Rerknimitr, R., & Pham, K.C. (2020). Practical approaches for high-risk surgical patients with acute cholecystitis: The percutaneous approach versus endoscopic alternatives. *Clinical Endoscopy, 53*(6), 678–685. https://doi.org/10.5946/ce.2019.186

Schuster, K.M., Holena, D.N., Salim, A., Savage, S., & Crandall, M. (2019). American Association for the Surgery of Trauma emergency general surgery guideline summaries 2018: Acute appendicitis, acute cholecystitis, acute diverticulitis, acute pancreatitis, and small bowel obstruction. *Trauma Surgery and Acute Care Open, 4*(1), e000281. https://doi.org/10.1136/tsaco-2018-000281

Tazuma, S., Unno, M., Igarashi, Y., Inui, K., Uchiyama, K., Kai, M., ... Shimosegawa, T. (2017). Evidence-based clinical practice guidelines for cholelithiasis 2016. *Journal of Gastroenterology, 52*(3), 276–300. https://doi.org/10.1007/s00535-016-1289-7

Wilkins, T., Agabin, E., Varghese, J., & Talukder, A. (2017). Gallbladder dysfunction: Cholecystitis, choledocholithiasis, cholangitis, and biliary dyskinesia. *Primary Care: Clinics in Office Practice, 44*(4), 575–597. https://doi.org/10.1016/j.pop.2017.07.002

Yokoe, M., Hata, J., Takada, T., Strasberg, S.M., Asbun, H.J., Wakabayashi, G., ... Yamamoto, M. (2018). Tokyo Guidelines 2018: Diagnostic criteria and severity grading of acute cholecystitis (with videos). *Journal of Hepato-Biliary-Pancreatic Sciences, 25*(1), 41–54. https://doi.org/10.1002/jhbp.515

CHAPTER 69

Cirrhosis

Deena Damsky Dell, MSN, APRN, AOCN®, LNC

I. Definition: Cirrhosis occurs through pathophysiologic changes in the liver due to hepatic injury, with extensive fibrosis and formation of regenerative nodules that result in architectural distortion of the liver caused by scar tissue slowly replacing normal functioning liver tissue. In the past, it was thought to be irreversible and require liver transplantation for cure; however, reversal potential exists when the cause is hepatitis B or C (with antiviral treatment), alcohol (with complete abstinence), or nonalcoholic fatty liver disease (with maintained weight loss) (Grgurevic et al., 2020; Nishikawa & Osaki, 2015).

II. Physiology/Pathophysiology (European Association for the Study of the Liver, 2018; Smith et al., 2019; Tsochatzis et al., 2014)
   A. Normal
      1. The liver lies in the right upper quadrant of the abdomen, below the diaphragm, and is composed of two predominant lobes (right and left). The right lobe has two additional minor segments.
      2. The liver is functionally divided into four sections by the portal blood flow.
      3. The liver plays an important role in the metabolism of carbohydrates, fats, proteins, vitamins, and iron; the detoxification of harmful substances; the production of antibodies; the conjugation and excretion of steroid hormones; and production of prothrombic fibrinogen and other substances for blood coagulation.
   B. Pathophysiology
      1. Hepatic lobules collapse from chronic exposure to toxins, bacteria, and viruses.
         a) Injury occurs, ranging from limited necrosis of liver cells to destruction of entire lobules with collapse of reticulin framework within the area.
         b) Repair process involves production of connective tissue (collagen) to bridge gaps within the liver structure and the regeneration of healthy hepatocytes, resulting in the formation of fibrous scars and nodules.
      2. Anatomic distortions caused by underlying collagen replacement change the liver's structure and increase intrahepatic resistance to blood flow. As a result, portal hypertension develops.

III. Clinical features: Liver failure appears when compensatory mechanisms fail because of decreased number of functioning hepatocytes or when resistance to portal venous flow results in symptomatic portal hypertension. Compensated cirrhosis occurs in up to 40% of patients (Carrion & Martin, 2019; Grgurevic et al., 2020; Lucier, 2019; National Institute for Health and Care Excellence, 2016; Tsochatzis et al., 2014).
   A. Etiology
      1. Primary

        a) Alcoholism

        b) Hepatitis B or C

        c) Nonalcoholic fatty liver diseases: Nonalcoholic steatohepatitis

    2. Secondary

        a) Autoimmune liver diseases

            (1) Autoimmune hepatitis

            (2) Primary or secondary biliary cirrhosis

            (3) Primary or secondary sclerosing cholangitis

        b) Inherited metabolic liver diseases

            (1) Hereditary hemochromatosis

            (2) Wilson disease

            (3) Alpha-1-antitrypsin deficiency

        c) Hepatotoxic drugs

        d) Chronic heart failure

        e) Hepatic sinusoidal obstruction syndrome: Veno-occlusive disease

        f) Cystic fibrosis

        g) Cryptogenic cirrhosis

B. History

    1. History of cancer and cancer treatment

    2. Current medications: Prescribed, over the counter

    3. History of presenting symptoms: Precipitating factors, onset, location, duration

    4. Changes in ADLs

    5. Past medical history: Viral hepatitis, alcohol use, diabetes, hereditary liver disorders, autoimmune diseases, blood transfusions

    6. Family history of liver disease

    7. Social history: Illicit drug use, travel

C. Signs and symptoms

    1. Compensated cirrhosis: Asymptomatic or mildly symptomatic

        a) Skin changes: Xanthomas, increased pigmentation, ecchymoses, spider angiomas, pruritus

        b) Vague abdominal pain, mild lower extremity edema

        c) Fatigue, sleep disturbances, decreased libido

        d) Anorexia, weight loss

    2. Uncompensated cirrhosis: Chronic liver failure

        a) Fatigue, weakness

        b) Anorexia/cachexia

        c) Heaviness and/or tenderness in right upper quadrant

        d) Abnormal endocrine function: Irregular menses, testicular atrophy, impaired sexual libido, impotence, gynecomastia (males)

        e) Jaundice: Tea-colored urine, sclera, mucous membranes

        f) Neurologic deficits: Confusion, asterixis

        g) Volume overload: Ascites, lower extremity edema

        h) Skin changes: Palmar erythema, spider angiomas, bruising, Muehrcke or Terry nails, caput medusa, pruritus

        i) Muscle cramps

    3. Alcoholic etiology

        a) Chylosis

        b) Night blindness

        c) Dupuytren contracture: Contracture of palmar fascia causing the ring and little fingers to bend into the palm

    4. Biliary cirrhosis

      a) Xanthelasma

      b) Pruritus, scratch marks

      c) Clubbing

    5. Portal hypertension

      a) Bleeding

      b) Ascites

      c) Abdominal wall venous distention

D. Physical examination

    1. Integument

      a) Jaundice

      b) Hyperpigmentation

      c) Purpura

      d) Vascular spiders, spider angiomas: Up to three on chest may be normal

      e) Palmar erythema

      f) Bruising

      g) Chylosis

      h) Xanthomas

    2. Thorax: Gynecomastia (males), loss of secondary hair

    3. HEENT

      a) Parotid enlargement

      b) Fetor hepaticus

    4. Abdominal

      a) Ascites

      b) Prominent abdominal wall veins

      c) Hepatosplenomegaly: Estimate liver span by percussion or scratch test (see Appendix D).

      d) Nodular liver with firm edge: Portal hypertension on palpation

      e) Presence of varicose veins radiating from the umbilicus (i.e., caput medusae)

      f) Scarred cirrhotic liver: May be small and not palpable

      g) Cruveilhier-Baumgarten murmur, an audible venous hum (heard best at the epigastrium), indicating portal hypertension

    5. Extremities

      a) Peripheral edema indicating chronic liver disease or failure

      b) Clubbing of fingers

      c) Hypertrophic osteoarthropathy

      d) Muscle cramps

    6. Neurologic: Findings indicating encephalopathy

      a) Mental status change

      b) Tremor

      c) Stupor

      d) Asterixis

    7. GU: Chronic liver failure

      a) Testicular atrophy

      b) Loss of pubic hair

    8. Rectal: Large hemorrhoids with portal hypertension

IV. Diagnostic tests (Fallatah, 2014; Grgurevic et al., 2020; Lucier, 2019; National Institute for Health and Care Excellence, 2016; Smith et al., 2019; Tsochatzis et al., 2014)

  A. Laboratory

1. Bilirubin
   a) Bilirubin may be normal if enough healthy cells remain to compensate for damaged cells and scar tissue.
   b) Total bilirubin is increased with significant hepatocellular damage.
   c) Increasing levels of direct bilirubin reflect worsening hepatic dysfunction in many cases. This does not distinguish between parenchymal injury with extensive hepatocellular necrosis and biliary obstruction.
2. Transaminases
   a) Aspartate aminotransferase: May be mildly elevated or normal
   b) Alanine transaminase: May be mildly elevated or normal
   c) If highly elevated, may indicate presence of additional acute processes such as drug toxicity, acute viral hepatitis, acute vascular compromise (hypotension or vascular thrombosis), acute biliary obstruction, or acute pancreatitis
3. Alkaline phosphatase: Usually increased
4. Albumin and Igs
   a) Albumin: Decreased; may be falsely elevated with dehydration
   b) IgA: May be elevated with alcoholic cirrhosis
   c) IgD: May be elevated with chronic hepatitis of cryptogenic cirrhosis
   d) Total globulin level: Usually increased
5. Gamma-glutamyl transferase: Elevated
6. PT and INR: Prolonged in advanced cirrhosis
7. Clotting factors: Decreased except for factor VIII
8. Blood ammonia: Increases with worsening of disease or in cases of infection or significant bleeding
9. Electrolytes: Hyponatremia and hypokalemia commonly present
10. Iron saturation and ferritin: Increased in hemochromatosis
11. Alpha fetoprotein: Usually increased with hepatocellular carcinoma or highly active inflammation
12. Viral hepatitis panel: May be positive
13. CBC: Leukopenia, anemia, and thrombocytopenia as a result of hypersplenism
14. Creatinine: Elevated in hepatorenal syndrome

B. Radiology
   1. Abdominal ultrasound: Identifies atrophy, surface nodularity, ascites, splenomegaly, biliary obstruction, gallstones, reversed portal flow, and portal vein thrombosis and screens for hepatocellular carcinoma
   2. CT scan of the abdomen: Used to confirm portal vein patency and to screen for the presence of hepatocellular carcinoma, especially with early arterial phase contrast
   3. MRI of the abdomen: Used to confirm the presence of hepatocellular carcinoma in dense cirrhotic liver, especially when used with IV contrast; test is expensive, and administration of MRI radiocontrast agents can be problematic in the presence of renal dysfunction; may identify severity of cirrhosis and reveal iron overload
   4. Magnetic resonance angiography: May confirm portal vein thrombosis
   5. Hepatobiliary iminodiacetic acid scan (nuclear medicine hepatobiliary imaging): Used to identify acute cholecystitis, high-grade biliary obstruction, and biliary leakage
   6. Guided diagnostic paracentesis to evaluate ascitic fluid

C. Other
   1. Doppler caput medusae: Assesses patency of hepatic and portal veins
   2. Endoscopic ultrasound: Used to visualize and biopsy masses in the liver and pancreas and associated lymph nodes

3. EGD: Identifies portal hypertensive gastropathy, gastroesophageal varices, and other possible sources of upper GI bleeding
4. Liver biopsy: Gold standard for cirrhosis diagnosis but usually not required unless transient elastography is not appropriate; determination of route based on presence of ascites, platelet count, and/or PT and INR
   a) Percutaneous: Normal INR, adequate platelets, and minimal ascites
   b) Transjugular: Highly abnormal INR, moderate thrombocytopenia, and/or moderate to large amount of ascites
   c) Laparoscopic core biopsy: Often provides adequate tissue for diagnosis; radiographically guided fine needle aspirate also available but provides less tissue
5. Transient elastography: Measures the degree of fibrosis in the liver; particularly helpful in patients with hepatitis C and/or patients with history of heavy alcohol intake
6. Acoustic radiation force imaging if transient elastography is not available to assess the underlying tissue structure and stiffness
7. Serum liver fibrosis test (e.g., FibroTest®/FibroSure®, FibroScan®): Uses a panel of serum markers to mathematically determine the probability of cirrhosis present in the patient

V. Differential diagnosis (Saad & Maria, 2017; Smith et al., 2019)
   A. Nephrotic syndrome (see Chapter 91)
   B. Right-sided heart failure (see Chapter 42)
   C. Myxedema (see Chapter 158)
   D. Malignant or benign biliary obstruction
   E. Celiac disease
   F. Thyroid dysfunction (see Chapters 157 and 158)
   G. Musculoskeletal disease
   H. Mononucleosis
   I. Alternative causes of encephalopathy
      1. Thiamine deficiency
      2. Uremia
      3. Drug-related delirium
   J. Alternative causes of upper GI bleeding
      1. Peptic ulcer disease (see Chapter 78)
      2. Mallory-Weiss syndrome
      3. Dieulafoy bleeding
   K. Alternative causes of portal hypertension
      1. Splenic vein thrombosis
      2. Schistosomiasis
      3. Cavernous transformation of the portal vein
   L. Cholangiocarcinoma
   M. Benign lesions
      1. Hepatic adenoma
      2. Hemangioma
      3. Focal fatty infiltration

VI. Treatment: Major goals are to slow or reverse disease, prevent and treat complications, prevent new insults to the liver, and determine if the patient is a candidate for liver transplantation (see Table 69-1; Bhattacharya et al., 2019; European Association for the Study of the Liver, 2018; Grgurevic et al., 2020; Kockerling et al., 2019; Mangray et al., 2015; National Institute for Health and Care Excellence, 2016; Smith et al., 2019; Tripathi et al., 2015; Tsochatzis et al., 2014).

TABLE 69-1	Pharmacologic Management of Cirrhosis		
Drug	**Indication**	**Dose**	**Comments**
Carvedilol (and other nonselective beta-blockers)	Lowering of portal venous pressure by decreasing cardiac output Esophageal varices	6.25–25 mg PO daily	Goal to decrease heart rate by 25% or to maintain heart rate at 50–60 beats per minute Primary prophylactic treatment of variceal bleeding More effective than selective beta-blockers
Cefotaxime	Spontaneous bacterial peritonitis	2 g IV every 8 hours for 5 days if creatinine < 1.5 mg/dl 1 g IV every 8 hours for 5 days if creatinine > 1.5 mg/dl	If low rate of bacterial resistance in the community, piperacillin/tazobactam; carbapenems are options in communities with high rates of bacterial resistance.
Ceftriaxone	Spontaneous bacterial peritonitis	2 g IV daily	If low rate of bacterial resistance in the community, piperacillin/tazobactam; carbapenems are options in communities with high rates of bacterial resistance.
Furosemide	Given with spironolactone for persistent edema/ascites	40–80 mg PO daily Maximum dose: 160 mg daily	Check weight, serum electrolytes, and renal function frequently. Administer in a ratio of 40:100 with spironolactone to counteract electrolyte imbalances.
Lactulose	Hepatic encephalopathy	30 ml PO every 2–4 hours Poor as enema: 300 ml lactulose solution in 700 ml saline or water	Adjust to produce 2–4 stools daily. May need aspiration precautions May need hydration
Metronidazole	Hepatic encephalopathy	500 mg PO three times a day	Reduces absorption of intestinal ammonia Can cause serious peripheral neuropathy
Neomycin sulfate	Hepatic encephalopathy	1 g PO two to four times a day	Reduces absorption of intestinal ammonia Prolonged use may result in hearing loss and renal failure. Synergistic side effects (ototoxicity and nephrotoxicity) with furosemide
Nitroglycerin (use with vasopressin)	Management of acute bleeding	50 mcg/min IV; may titrate up by 50 mcg every 15 minutes to keep systolic blood pressure at 100 mm Hg or greater Maximum infusion rate: 400 mcg/min	–

(Continued on next page)

TABLE 69-1   **Pharmacologic Management of Cirrhosis (Continued)**

Drug	Indication	Dose	Comments
Norfloxacin	Prophylaxis after an episode of spontaneous bacterial peritonitis	400 mg PO two times a day	Alternative is trimethoprim/sulfamethoxazole double strength 1 tablet PO daily
Octreotide (somatostatin analog)	Management of acute bleeding	50 mcg bolus followed by 25–50 mcg/hr by continuous infusion for 1–5 days	Direct splanchnic vasoconstrictor
Rifaximin	Hepatic encephalopathy	550 mg PO two times a day	Nonabsorbable broad-spectrum antibiotic Clinical trials show a trend toward better efficacy than neomycin or lactulose with better safety and tolerability.
Somatostatin	Management of acute bleeding	250 mcg bolus followed by 250–500 mcg/hr by continuous infusion for 1–5 days	Direct splanchnic vasoconstrictor
Spironolactone	Edema/ascites	100–200 mg PO daily as single dose or in divided doses Maximum dose: 400 mg PO daily	Inhibits hyperaldosteronism of portal hypertension Can cause tender gynecomastia and hyperkalemia
Torasemide	May be used if unresponsive to furosemide	5–10 mg PO daily Maximum dose: 40 mg PO daily	Check weight, serum electrolytes, and renal function frequently.
Vasopressin (use with nitroglycerin)	Management of acute bleeding if no somatostatin available Used with albumin to increase renal perfusion in hepatorenal syndrome	0.2 units/min IV, then increased by 0.2 units/min until bleeding is controlled Maximum tolerated dose: 2 units/min	Is a vesicant; administer by central line.
Vitamin K	Correction of clotting abnormalities	10 mg subcutaneous daily for three days	–

Note. Based on information from Bacon, 2018; Carrion & Martin, 2019; European Association for the Study of the Liver, 2018; Tripathi, 2015.

A. Lifestyle changes
  1. Eat a well-balanced diet. Nutritional supplementation may be needed to add calories and protein to diet.
     a) Zinc supplementation may correct zinc deficiency and help dysgeusia, anorexia, and muscle cramps.
     b) Restrict sodium to approximately 2 g daily in patients with edema and ascites. If edema is moderate and uncomplicated, a more liberal restriction of approximately 4–7 g daily may be allowed.

    c) Consider limiting protein load only in patients with active severe hepatic enceph-
alopathy.

2. Fluid restriction is not necessary except in the setting of severe hyponatremia (see
Chapter 155).

3. Take a multivitamin daily.

4. Cease alcohol use, and monitor for withdrawal.

5. Maintain appropriate weight.

6. Caution against the use of hepatotoxic drugs (e.g., acetaminophen [may use up to
2 g daily in divided doses], NSAIDs, certain herbs).

7. Vaccinate against hepatitis A and B, pneumonia, and flu.

8. Avoid opiates, as they can have prolonged hepatic clearance.

9. Low-dose benzodiazepine may be used if sedation is needed for alcohol withdrawal
and hepatic encephalopathy is not present.

10. Smoking cessation

    a) Smoking is associated with more severe fibrosis.

    b) Cannabis is associated with worsening fibrosis in chronic hepatitis C.

B. Pharmacologic treatment of cirrhosis

1. Aldosterone antagonists are the first choice of diuretics to manage moderate ascites
because they inhibit the hyperaldosteronism of portal hypertension.

    a) Spironolactone 100–200 mg PO daily is commonly used. Maximum is 400 mg
daily.

    b) If patient is unable to tolerate because of tender gynecomastia, amiloride
hydrochloride 5 mg PO daily is an alternative, although it is generally less
effective.

2. Loop diuretics will potentiate the effect of aldosterone antagonists.

    a) Coadminister with spironolactone in a ratio of furosemide (or equivalent loop
direct dose) 40 mg: spironolactone 100 mg PO, which may counteract electrolyte imbalances.

    b) Furosemide 40–80 mg PO daily is most commonly used; it may be increased
to 120–160 mg PO daily.

    c) Torasemide 5–10 mg PO daily may be considered if inadequate response to furo-
semide. Maximum daily dose is 40 mg.

3. Vasopressor midodrine hydrochloride 7.5 mg PO three times a day may be added
for recurrent/refractory ascites; transient beneficial effect has been seen.

C. Pharmacologic treatment of portal hypertension

1. Prevention of initial hemorrhage to lower portal venous pressure: Nonselective
beta-blockade to reduce venous pressure

    a) Carvedilol 6.25–25 mg PO

    b) Propranolol 20–180 mg PO two times a day

    c) Nadolol 40–160 mg PO daily

    d) Timolol 20–40 mg PO daily

2. Management of acute bleeding

    a) Administration of clotting factors, as indicated

    b) Packed RBCs to maintain Hgb 7–9 g/dl

    c) Platelet transfusion if actively bleeding or platelets less than 50,000/mm³

    d) Vasopressin: 20 units IV over 15–20 minutes, then 0.1–0.4 units/min, plus nitro-
glycerin 0.3 mg every hour sublingual or 0.2 mcg/min IV; used with caution in
patients with CHF or alcoholic cardiomyopathy

    e) Terlipressin, a synthetic analog of vasopressin: 2 mg IV every four to six hours
preferred over vasopressin; currently not available in the United States

D. Management of ascites: Most common complication of portal hypertension and cirrhosis (see Chapter 54)
   1. Therapeutic paracentesis: This procedure is used in refractory ascites, which is unresponsive to dietary sodium restriction and diuretics. It usually coincides with IV albumin to prevent renal failure.
   2. TIPS: This procedure may be necessary if ascites is refractory with prior measures. Prognosis is poor after TIPS; consideration is often given for liver transplantation.
   3. Surgical shunt: Peritoneovenous shunt (LeVeen shunt) has a high rate of complications, yet it may be useful in a few patients who are not candidates for transplantation or TIPS and are too obese or have too many abdominal surgical scars to permit safe, successful paracentesis.
E. Management of variceal hemorrhage
   1. Once varices have been identified, primary prevention is with nonselective beta-blockers or endoscopic intervention with endoscopic variceal band ligation.
   2. Octreotide, a direct splenic vasoconstrictor, 50 mcg IV bolus is given, followed by 50 mcg/hr for one to five days.
   3. If somatostatin or analog is not available, vasopressin is used.
   4. PPIs are not recommended except for treatment of peptic ulcers. Long-term use is associated with increased risk of spontaneous bacterial peritonitis, hepatic encephalopathy, and *Clostridium difficile* infection.
   5. Prophylactic antibiotics are used to prevent spontaneous bacterial pneumonitis in patients with advanced cirrhosis or renal insufficiency.
   6. TIPS placement is the percutaneous creation of a portacaval shunt in which a metal shunt is placed via angiographic guidance. It may be used in cases in which varices extend into proximal stomach and endoscopic and/or medical management fail to stop bleeding.
      a) May increase coagulopathy and hepatic encephalopathy
      b) Can occlude after placement and often is associated with poor prognosis
   7. Balloon tamponade allows short-term control (less than 24 hours) of variceal bleed. It is restricted to situations in which pharmacotherapy or endoscopic therapy is ineffective.
   8. Glue treatment of bleeding gastric varices can be used. Cyanoacrylate is effective in selected cases.
   9. Transfusion of RBCs or fresh frozen plasma can be considered, as indicated.
F. Management of spontaneous bacterial peritonitis: Infection of the ascitic fluid without an intra-abdominal source
   1. Hospitalized cirrhotic patients with ascites have a 30% chance of developing spontaneous bacterial peritonitis, which is associated with 25% in-hospital mortality. One-third of patients may be asymptomatic; therefore, all hospitalized patients with cirrhosis and ascites need diagnostic paracentesis.
   2. Diagnosis is made if ascitic fluid from peritoneal tap has an ANC greater than 250/mm^3, even if culture is negative.
   3. Prevalent organisms include *Escherichia coli, Streptococcus aureus, Klebsiella pneumoniae,* and *Enterococcus.*
   4. Appropriate antibiotics include third-generation cephalosporins, such as cefotaxime 2 g IV every eight hours or ceftriaxone 2 g IV daily, if there is a low rate of bacterial resistance in the community. Piperacillin/tazobactam or carbapenems are options in communities with high rates of bacterial resistance.
   5. Patients who have recovered from an episode will require spontaneous bacterial peritonitis prophylaxis, as 69% will have another episode within one year. Norflox-

acin 400 mg PO two times a day or trimethoprim/sulfamethoxazole double-strength 1 tablet PO daily are recommended.

    6. IV albumin (1.5 g/kg within six hours of diagnosis and followed by 1 g/kg on day 3) should be administered to patients with total serum bilirubin greater than 4 mg/dl, BUN greater than 30 mg/dl, or serum creatinine greater than 1 mg/d.

G. Management of hepatorenal syndrome: AKI can occur in a patient who has advanced liver disease due to cirrhosis. Minimal to no proteinuria is present.

    1. Discontinue any nephrotoxic agents and diuretics.

    2. Use albumin for volume expansion (1 g/kg up to 100 g/day)

    3. Vasoconstriction with octreotide plus midodrine, norepinephrine, or vasopressin may increase renal perfusion and mean arterial blood pressure.

    4. Prognosis is poor without a liver transplant.

H. Management of encephalopathy caused by gut-derived neurotoxins not being removed because of vascular shunting and decreased hepatic mass

    1. Hydrate and correct electrolytes (see Chapters 152–156).

    2. Monitor ammonia levels, which are typically elevated in venous sampling but have poor correlation with severity of disease.

    3. Initiate lactulose 30 ml PO every one to four hours; titrate to goal—production of two to three soft stools daily.

        a) Large amounts orally cause increased nausea and vomiting and potential aspiration.

        b) Diarrhea can lead to dehydration.

    4. Poorly absorbable or nonabsorbable antibiotics are used as adjuvant therapy if lactulose cannot be tolerated.

        a) Rifaximin 550 mg PO two times a day has fewer side effects than neomycin or metronidazole.

        b) If condition worsens, neomycin sulfate 250 mg PO three times a day, metronidazole 500 mg PO three times a day, or vancomycin 500 mg PO four times a day can be used. Neomycin and metronidazole can be alternated to reduce individual side effects.

I. Treat dyslipidemia (see Chapter 44) and diabetes (see Chapter 151) in case of nonalcoholic fatty liver disease and cirrhosis. Statins may be recommended for patients with hyperlipidemia nonalcoholic fatty liver disease or diabetes.

J. Use steroids or immunosuppressant agents to treat patients with autoimmune hepatitis (see Chapter 74).

VII. Follow-up: Dependent on etiology (Smith et al., 2019)

A. Yearly vaccinations for influenza

B. Screening for hepatocellular carcinoma with periodic serum alpha-fetoprotein and ultrasound every six months

C. Hepatitis A and B vaccinations, especially in patients with chronic hepatitis C

D. Pneumococcal vaccine

E. Prophylactic antibiotics for invasive procedures: Amoxicillin 2 g PO or clindamycin 600 mg PO

F. History of esophageal varices: Patient needs to be on nonselective beta-blocker or undergo variceal band ligation procedure.

G. If no esophageal varices, endoscopy every three years

VIII. Referrals

A. Hepatologist: For management of varices, periodic EGD, and liver cancer surveillance

B. Hematologist/oncologist: For treatment of anemia and coagulopathy or hepatocellular carcinoma
C. Alcohol/drug counselor: If appropriate
D. Dietitian: For assistance with protein–calorie malnutrition
E. Surgeon: For liver transplantation or resection or placement of portacaval shunts (infrequent)
F. Interventional radiologist: For placement of TIPS and biopsy of liver lesions

References

Bacon, B.R. (2018). Cirrhosis and its complications. In J.L. Jameson, A.S. Fauci, D.L. Kasper, S.L. Hauser, D.L. Longo, & J. Loscalzo (Eds.), *Harrison's principles of internal medicine* (20th ed., pp. 2405–2413). NY: McGraw-Hill.

Bhattacharya, C., Das-Mondal, M., Gupta, D., Sarkar, A.K., Kar-Purkayastha, S., & Konar, A. (2019). Infection in cirrhosis: A prospective study. *Annals of Hepatology, 18*(6), 862–868. https://doi.org/10.1016/j.aohep.2019.07.010

Carrion, A.F., & Martin, P. (2019). Renal dysfunction in cirrhotic patients. *American Journal of Gastroenterology, 114*(9), 1407–1410. https://doi.org/10.14309/ajg.0000000000000355

European Association for the Study of the Liver. (2018). EASL clinical guidelines for the management of patients with decompensated cirrhosis. *Journal of Hepatology, 69*(2), 406–460. https://doi.org/10.1016/j.jhep.2018.03.024

Fallatah, H.I. (2014). Noninvasive markers of liver fibrosis: An overview. *Advances in Hepatology, 2014,* 357287. https://doi.org/10.1155/2014/357287.

Grgurevic, I., Podrug, K., Mikolasevic, I., Kukla, M., Madir, A., & Tsochatzis, E.A. (2020). Natural history of nonalcoholic fatty liver disease: Implications for clinical practice and an individualized approach. *Canadian Journal of Gastroenterology and Hepatology, 2020,* 9181368. https://doi.org/10.1155/2020/9181368

Kockerling, D., Nathwani, R., Forlano, R., Manousou, P., Mullish, B.H., & Dhar, A. (2019). Current and future pharmacological therapies for managing cirrhosis and its complications. *World Journal of Gastroenterology, 25*(8), 888–908. https://doi.org/10.3748/wjg.v25.i8.888

Lucier, D. (2019). Cirrhosis. In F. Ferri (Ed.) *Ferri's clinical advisor 2019* (pp. 337–339). Elsevier.

Mangray, S., Zweit, J., & Puri, P. (2015). Zinc deficiency in cirrhosis: Micronutrient for thought? *Digestive Disease Science, 60*(10), 2868–2870. https://doi.org/10.1007/s10620-015-3854-y

National Institute for Health and Care Excellence. (2016). *Cirrhosis in over 16s: Assessment and management.* https://www.nice.org.uk/guidance/ng50

Nishikawa, H., & Osaki, Y. (2015). Liver cirrhosis: Evaluation, nutritional status, and prognosis. *Mediators of Inflammation, 2015,* 872152. https://doi.org/10.1155/2015/872152.

Saad, H., & Maria, R. (2017). Cirrhosis. *Cancer Therapy Advisor.* https://www.cancertherapyadvisor.com/home/decision-support-in-medicine/hospital-medicine/cirrhosis-2

Smith, A., Baumgartner, K., & Bositis, C. (2019). Cirrhosis: Diagnosis and management. *American Family Physician, 100*(12), 759–770. https://www.aafp.org/afp/2019/1215/p759.html

Tripathi, D., Stanley, A.J., Hayes, P.C., Patch, D., Milson, C., Mehrzad, H., … Christie, J.M. (2015) U.K. guidelines on management of variceal haemorrhage in cirrhotic patients. *Gut, 64*(11), 1680–1704. https://doi.org/10.1136/gutjnl-2015-309262

Tsochatzis, E.A., Bosch, J., & Burroughs, A.K. (2014). Liver cirrhosis. *Lancet, 383*(9930), 1749–1761. https://doi.org/10.1016/S0140-6736(14)60121-5

CHAPTER 70

Diverticulitis

R. Tim Davis, MSN, APRN

I. Definition (Munie & Nalamati, 2018)
   A. Diverticula are sac-like protrusions of mucosa through the muscular colon wall.
   B. Inflammation of a diverticulum leads to diverticulitis.

II. Physiology/Pathophysiology (Canadian Cancer Society, n.d.; Kupcinskas et al., 2019; Munie & Nalamati, 2018)
   A. Normal
      1. The colon is the longest part of the large intestine and receives almost completely digested food from the cecum.
      2. It absorbs water and nutrients and passes waste products (stool or feces) to the rectum.
      3. The colon is divided into four parts: the ascending, transverse, descending, and sigmoid colon.
   B. Pathophysiology
      1. Diverticula develop at points of weakness in the colonic wall corresponding to where the vasa recta penetrate the circular muscle layer to deliver blood to the colonic mucosa.
      2. Inflammation of the mucosal outpouching causes diverticulitis.
      3. The suspected mechanism of developing diverticulitis is bacterial overgrowth due to diverticular base obstruction by feces.
      4. When diverticulitis develops, there is increased intraluminal pressure during peristalsis within the segmented portion of colon where feces or partially digested food blocks the opening of the diverticula.
      5. Diverticular disease is complex with factors such as chronic low-grade inflammation, alteration of intestinal microflora, and alteration in colon motility.

III. Clinical features: Diverticular disease is one of the most common causes of lower GI hemorrhage and is the leading differential diagnosis for patients presenting with brisk rectal bleeding. Diverticulitis is the third most common GI illness that leads to hospitalization and is the leading cause for elective colon resection. It can present as an acute or chronic process or as uncomplicated or complicated disease. Complicated disease includes episodes associated with perforation, abscess, fistula, obstruction, or stricture. Left-sided diverticula is predominant in the United States, and right-sided (cecal) diverticula is predominant in Asia (Böhm, 2015; Copeland & St. Clair Jones, 2019; Feuerstein & Falchuk, 2016; Kupcinskas et al., 2019; Lembcke, 2015; Munie & Nalamati, 2018; Rezapour et al., 2018; Violi et al., 2018).
   A. Etiology: Exact etiology is unknown.
      1. Aging: Incidence increases with age.
      2. Obesity

      3. Tobacco use

      4. Low-fiber diet in combination with high fat or red meat intake

      5. Sedentary lifestyle or lack of exercise

      6. Medications: Opioids, NSAIDs, steroids

      7. Comorbidities: Hypertension, diabetes mellitus, polycystic kidney disease

      8. Genetic syndromes: Marfan syndrome, Ehlers-Danlos syndrome, Williams syndrome, Coffin-Lowry syndrome

      9. HIV infection

    10. Immunocompromised

B. History

      1. History of cancer and cancer treatment

      2. Current medications: Prescribed, over the counter

      3. History of presenting symptoms: Precipitating factors, onset, location, duration

      4. Changes in ADLs

      5. Past medical history: IBS, hypertension, diabetes

      6. Past surgical history: Surgical resection for diverticula

      7. Social history: Sedentary lifestyle, tobacco use, alcohol use

      8. Family history: Monozygotic twin or same-gender dizygotic twins with diverticular disease, genetic disorders

      9. Diet history: High fat or red meat intake, fiber intake

C. Signs and symptoms: Can be asymptomatic; symptoms dependent on the underlying inflammatory process

      1. Abdominal pain: Most common symptom

         a) Usually, pain is located in the left lower quadrant because of sigmoid colon involvement.

         b) Patients may experience right lower quadrant pain.

      2. Nausea and vomiting: Noted in approximately 50% of patients due to possible bowel obstruction or an ileus from peritoneal irritation

      3. Low-grade fever

      4. Changes in bowel habits

         a) Constipation: Approximately 50%

         b) Diarrhea: Approximately 30%

         c) Hematochezia: Rare

      5. Urinary urgency, frequency, or dysuria due to irritation to the bladder from colon inflammation

      6. Associated with perforation or peritonitis: Hypotension, oliguria, changes in mentation, cool/clammy skin

      7. Rectal tenderness in the presence of distal abscess or disease

D. Physical examination

      1. Vital signs: Fever, tachycardia, or hypotension

      2. Abdominal

         a) Tenderness: Most common

         b) Guarding

         c) Rebound tenderness

         d) Presence of a palpable mass

         e) Bowel sounds

            (1) Hyperactive or increased with obstruction

            (2) Typically hypoactive or decreased

            (3) Normal in some cases

      3. Rectal: Mass

IV. Diagnostic tests (Bugiantella et al., 2015; Lembcke, 2015; Štimac et al., 2019; Strate & Morris, 2019)
- A. Laboratory
    1. CBC: May reveal mild leukocytosis (normal in up to 45% of patients), decreased hematocrit and Hgb in presence of bleeding
    2. CMP: Baseline assessment of electrolytes, renal function, and liver function
    3. Serum amylase and lipase: Normal to mildly elevated
    4. Urinalysis: May reveal sterile pyuria due to adjacent inflammation
    5. Pregnancy test, if indicated
    6. Stool studies
        - *a)* Infectious etiology if diarrhea present
        - *b)* Hemoccult for blood
    7. CRP: Possible elevation; used as an inflammatory marker
- B. Radiology
    1. CT scan of abdomen and pelvis with oral and IV contrast: Imaging of choice with 94%–99% sensitivity and specificity
        - *a)* Presence of localized bowel wall thickening greater than 4 mm
        - *b)* Increased soft tissue density in pericolonic fat secondary to fat stranding and acute inflammation
        - *c)* Diverticula and segmental narrowing
        - *d)* Pericolonic edema and exudates
        - *e)* Ascites
        - *f)* Abscess
    2. Abdominal ultrasound: Less expensive and easily accessible
        - *a)* Hypoechoic peridiverticular inflammation
        - *b)* Peridiverticular abscess formation (with and without gas bubbles)
        - *c)* Thickening of the bowel wall greater than 4 mm
        - *d)* Presence of diverticula
    3. MRI of abdomen and pelvis with similar findings compared to CT scan without the risk of radiation
    4. Abdominal plain film to evaluate for ileus or obstruction
        - *a)* Air-fluid levels within the small and large intestine (secondary to possible ileus or obstruction)
        - *b)* Soft tissue densities secondary to abscess
- C. Other: Colonoscopy to evaluate for diverticular disease and bleeding or to differentiate inflammatory bowel disease

V. Differential diagnosis (Lembcke, 2015; Štimac et al., 2019)
- A. IBS (see Chapter 76)
- B. Colorectal cancer
- C. Acute appendicitis
- D. Inflammatory bowel disease
- E. Ischemic colitis
- F. Infectious colitis
- G. Ovarian cyst or torsion
- H. Ectopic pregnancy
- I. Cystitis (see Chapter 89)
- J. Nephrolithiasis
- K. Constipation (see Chapter 55)
- L. Hernia
- M. Renal colic

VI. Treatment: Therapy is aimed at decreasing acute inflammation, preventing recurrence, and managing acute and chronic symptoms (Brandimarte et al., 2019; Bugiantella et al., 2015; Feingold et al., 2014; Regenbogen et al., 2014; Sallinen et al., 2015; Stollman et al., 2015; Strate & Morris, 2019; You et al., 2019).

A. Outpatient treatment is recommended in afebrile, clinically stable patients with uncomplicated diverticulitis.

B. Criteria for inpatient treatment

1. Complicated diverticulitis with perforation, abscess, obstruction, and/or fistula: Hinchey classification has been used to distinguish four stages of complicated diverticulitis due to colonic perforation.

a) Stage I: Localized abscess

b) Stage II: Pelvic abscess

c) Stage III: Purulent peritonitis

d) Stage IV: Feculent peritonitis

2. Uncomplicated diverticulitis with sepsis, microperforations, fever greater than 102.5°F (39.2°C), significant leukocytosis, immunosuppressed, severe abdominal pain, diffuse peritonitis, inability to tolerate oral intake, age older than 70 years, and/or failed outpatient treatment

C. Nonpharmacologic measures

1. Outpatient: No evidence exists for dietary restrictions in acute uncomplicated diverticulitis. Prescribe clear liquid diet with progression (soft to regular) as symptoms improve.

2. Inpatient: Typically, complete bowel rest or clear liquids with progression (soft to regular) as symptoms improve.

a) NG tube placement, as indicated

b) IV fluids

D. Pharmacologic measures

1. Outpatient treatment: Oral antibiotics, typically 7–10 days

a) Ciprofloxacin (500 mg every 12 hours) plus metronidazole (500 mg every eight hours)

b) Levofloxacin (750 mg daily) plus metronidazole (500 mg every eight hours)

c) Trimethoprim/sulfamethoxazole one double-strength tablet (trimethoprim 160 mg; sulfamethoxazole 800 mg) every 12 hours plus metronidazole (500 mg) every eight hours

d) Moxifloxacin (400 mg daily) used with patients who are intolerant of both metronidazole and beta lactams

e) Amoxicillin/clavulanate one tablet (amoxicillin 875 mg; clavulanate 125 mg) every eight hours or Augmentin® XR two tablets (amoxicillin 1 g; clavulanate 62.5 mg) every 12 hours

2. Inpatient treatment is based on whether the patient has complicated or uncomplicated disease. Repeat imaging is recommended with no clinical improvement within two to three days of receiving IV antibiotics.

a) Low-risk regimens

(1) Ertapenem 1 g IV daily

(2) Piperacillin/tazobactam 3.375 g IV every six hours

(3) Cefazolin 1–2 g IV every eight hours; metronidazole 500 mg IV every eight hours

(4) Ceftriaxone 2 g IV daily; metronidazole 500 mg IV every eight hours

(5) Cefotaxime 2 g IV every eight hours; metronidazole 500 mg IV every eight hours

   (6) Ciprofloxacin 400 mg IV every 12 hours; metronidazole 500 mg IV every eight hours

   (7) Levofloxacin 750 mg IV daily; metronidazole 500 mg IV every eight hours

  b) High-risk regimens

   (1) Imipenem/cilastatin 500 mg IV every six hours

   (2) Meropenem 1 g IV every eight hours

   (3) Doripenem 500 mg IV every eight hours

   (4) Piperacillin/tazobactam 4.5 g IV every six hours

   (5) Cefepime 2 g IV every eight hours; metronidazole 500 mg IV every eight hours

   (6) Ceftazidime 2 g IV every eight hours; metronidazole 500 mg IV every eight hours

 3. Opioids (see Appendix F)

E. Surgical management

 1. Intervention is necessary for abscess, peritonitis, obstruction, fistula, or failure to improve after several days of medical management or recurrence after successful medical management.

 2. Approximately one-quarter of patients with acute diverticulitis will require surgical intervention during the course of their disease.

VII. Follow-up (Feingold et al., 2014; Vennix et al., 2014; You et al., 2019)

A. Reassess in two to three days after initiation of antibiotic therapy and then weekly until resolution of symptoms.

B. Reassess in six to eight weeks (after successful inpatient or outpatient treatment).

 1. Consider chronic smoldering disease for persistent symptoms.

 2. Monitor for complications (e.g., abscess, bowel obstruction, perforation, fistula).

 3. Monitor for recurrence. Up to 42% of patients have one or more recurrent attacks after nonoperative management.

C. Colonoscopy is recommended six to eight weeks after resolution of diverticulitis unless performed in the past year.

VIII. Referrals

A. Gastroenterologist: For colonoscopy

B. Surgeon: For surgical intervention

C. Nutritionist: For dietary counseling for high-fiber, lean, healthy diet

References

Böhm, S.K. (2015). Risk factors for diverticulosis, diverticulitis, diverticular perforation, and bleeding: A plea for more subtle history taking. *Viszeralmedizin, 31*(2), 84–94. https://doi.org/10.1159/000381867

Brandimarte, G., Bafutto, M., Kruis, W., Scarpignato, C., Mearin, F., Barbara, G., ... Malfertheiner, P. (2019). Hot topics in medical treatment of diverticular disease: Evidence pro and cons. *Journal of Gastrointestinal and Liver Diseases, 28*(Suppl. 4), 23–29. https://doi.org/10.15403/jgld-554

Bugiantella, W., Rondelli, F., Longaronia, M., Mariania, E., Sanguinetti, A., & Avenia, N. (2015). Left colon acute diverticulitis: An update on diagnosis, treatment and prevention. *International Journal of Surgery, 13*, 157–164. https://doi.org/10.1016/j.ijsu.2014.12.012

Canadian Cancer Society. (n.d.). The colon and rectum. https://www.cancer.ca/en/cancer-information/cancer-type/colorectal/colorectal-cancer/the-colon-and-rectum

Copeland, E., & St. Clair Jones, A. (2019). Diverticular disease and diverticulitis: Causes, symptoms and treatment. *Pharmaceutical Journal.* https://doi.org/10.1211/PJ.2019.20206352

Feingold, D., Steele, S.R., Lee, S., Kaiser, A., Boushey, R., Buie, W.D., & Rafferty, J. (2014). Practice parameters for the treatment of sigmoid diverticulitis. *Diseases of the Colon and Rectum, 57*(3), 284–294. https://doi.org/10.1097/DCR.0000000000000075

Feuerstein, J.D., & Falchuk, K.R. (2016). Diverticulosis and diverticulitis. *Mayo Clinic Proceedings, 91*(8), 1094–104. https://doi.org/10.1016/j.mayocp.2016.03.012.

Kupcinskas, J., Strate, L.L., Bassotti, G., Torti, G., Herszènyi, L., Malfertheiner, P., ... Tursi, A. (2019). Pathogenesis of diverticulosis and diverticular disease. *Journal of Gastrointestinal and Liver Diseases, 28*(Suppl. 4), 7–10. https://doi.org/10.15403/jgld-551

Lembcke, B. (2015). Diagnosis, differential diagnoses, and classification of diverticular disease. *Viszeralmedizin, 31*(2), 95–102. https://doi.org/10.1159/000380833

Munie, S.T., & Nalamati, S.P.M. (2018). Epidemiology and pathophysiology of diverticular disease. *Clinics in Colon and Rectal Surgery, 31*(4), 209–213. https://doi.org/10.1055/s-0037-1607464

Regenbogen, S.E., Hardiman, K.M., Hendersen, S., & Morris, A.M. (2014). Surgery for diverticulitis in the 21st century: A systematic review. *JAMA Surgery, 149*(3), 292–303. https://doi.org/10.1001/jamasurg.2013.5477

Rezapour, M., Ali, S., & Stollman, N. (2018). Diverticular disease: An update on pathogenesis and management. *Gut and Liver, 12*(2), 125–132. https://doi.org/10.5009/gnl16552

Sallinen, V., Mali, J., Leppäniemi, A., & Mentula, P. (2015). Assessment of risk for recurrent diverticulitis: A proposal of risk score for complicated recurrence. *Medicine, 94*(8), e557. https://doi.org/10.1097/MD.0000000000000557

Štimac, D., Nardone, G., Mazzari, A., Crucitti, A., Maconi, G., Elisel, W., ... DiMario, F. (2019). What's new in diagnosing diverticular disease. *Journal of Gastrointestinal and Liver Diseases, 28*(Suppl. 4), 17–22. https://doi.org/10.15403/jgld-553

Stollman, N., Smalley, W., & Hirano, I. (2015). American Gastroenterology Association Institution guidelines on the management of acute diverticulitis. *Gastroenterology, 149*(7), 1944–1949. https://doi.org/10.1053/j.gastro.2015.10.003

Strate, L.L., & Morris, A.M. (2019). Epidemiology, pathophysiology, and treatment of diverticulitis. *Gastroenterology, 156*(5), 1282–1298.e1. https://doi.org/10.1053/j.gastro.2018.12.033

Vennix, S., Morton, D.G., Hahnloser, D., Lange, J.F., & Bemelman, W.A. (2014). Systematic review of evidence and consensus on diverticulitis: An analysis of national and international guidelines. *Colorectal Disease, 16*(11), 866–878. https://doi.org/10.1111/codi.12659

Violi, A., Cambiè, G., Miraglia, C., Barchi, A., Nouvenne, A., Capasso, M., ... Di Mario, F. (2018). Epidemiology and risk factors for diverticular disease. *Acta Biomedica, 89*(Suppl. 9), 107–112. https://doi.org/10.23750/abm.v89i9-S.7924

You, H., Sweeny, A., Cooper, M.L., Von Papen, M., & Innes, J. (2019). The management of diverticulitis: A review of the guidelines. *Medical Journal of Australia, 211*(9), 421–427. https://doi.org/10.5694/mja2.50276

CHAPTER 71

Gastroesophageal Reflux Disease

Diane G. Cope, PhD, APRN, BC, AOCNP®

I. Definition: Regurgitation of GI contents into the esophagus with or without manifestations of esophageal, laryngeal, or pulmonary injury (Kellerman & Kintanar, 2017)

II. Physiology/Pathophysiology (Chen & Brady, 2019; Clarrett & Hachem, 2018; Pandit et al., 2018; Savarino et al., 2017)
    A. Normal
        1. The lower esophageal sphincter maintains a pressure barrier between the esophagus and the stomach.
        2. The hormone gastrin, alpha-adrenergic stimulation, and the vagus nerve promote relaxation of the smooth muscle of the lower esophageal sphincter.
    B. Pathophysiology
        1. Absence of the high-pressure barrier between the stomach and the esophagus increases reflux.
        2. Intermittent relaxation of the lower esophageal sphincter as a result of inhibitory reflexes triggered by gastric distention increases reflux.
        3. Inflammation of the esophageal mucosa delays peristalsis, increasing the time that gastric reflux remains in the esophagus; salivation and neutralization of gastric secretions are decreased.
        4. Reduced gastric storage capacity and increased postprandial intragastric pressure from conditions such as partial gastric resection can increase reflux.

III. Clinical features: Heartburn typically described as a burning sensation in the sternal area during the postprandial period; symptoms occurring two or more days a week (mild) or more than one day a week (moderate to severe) can be troublesome (Chen & Brady, 2019; Pandit et al., 2018; Richter & Rubenstein, 2018).
    A. Etiology
        1. Abnormalities of the lower esophageal sphincter
            a) Incompetent lower esophageal sphincter
                (1) Drug induced: Hormones, anticholinergics, calcium antagonists, theophylline, meperidine
                (2) Nicotine
                (3) Alcohol
                (4) Caffeine
                (5) Foods: High-fat, acidic, spicy, chocolate, or mints

        b) Decreased lower esophageal sphincter tone: Gastric distention from obesity or ascites

  2. Impaired esophageal peristalsis

      a) Sleeping, which ceases swallowing

      b) Lying in a horizontal position, which increases time of gastric reflux contact with the esophageal mucosa

  3. Gastric emptying abnormalities

B. History

  1. History of cancer and cancer treatment

  2. Current medications: Prescribed, over the counter

  3. History of presenting symptoms: Precipitating factors, onset, duration, associated symptoms (e.g., voice changes, respiratory problems)

  4. Changes in ADLs

  5. History of dietary contributing factors: Spicy foods, acidic foods

  6. Social history: Tobacco use, alcohol use

C. Signs and symptoms

  1. Acid regurgitation and heartburn: Most common symptom

      a) Presents as substernal burning

      b) Usually occurs after meals

      c) Aggravated by position change

  2. If reflux becomes severe, esophageal, laryngeal, or pulmonary injury may occur, exhibiting the following symptoms.

      a) Chest pain

      b) Sore throat

      c) Dyspepsia

      d) Vomiting

      e) Belching

      f) Chronic cough

      g) Hoarseness

      h) Wheezing

      i) Sensation of lump in throat

  3. Dental erosions

  4. Hematemesis

  5. Weight loss

  6. Dysphagia

  7. Nausea: Infrequent

D. Physical examination

  1. Vital signs: Unexplained weight loss indicative of malignancy

  2. Integument: Signs of compromised nutritional status (e.g., poor skin turgor, loss of subcutaneous fat)

  3. HEENT: Erythematous oropharynx, halitosis, acid erosion of teeth

  4. Abdominal

      a) Abdominal appearance usually is normal, but slight distention may be present.

      b) Mild pain may be elicited upon palpation of the epigastric area.

      c) Listen for bowel sounds, typically normal.

  5. Rectal: Occult blood, bright red blood, melena

IV. Diagnostic tests: Can be based on clinical symptoms alone in patients with classical symptoms (Gyawali & Fass, 2018; Kandulski et al., 2018; Pandit et al., 2018; Sandhu & Fass, 2017; Savarino et al., 2017; Vaezi et al., 2017)

    A. Laboratory: 24-hour pH monitoring (sensitivity and specificity of 70%–96%)

    B. Radiology: Barium upper GI radiographic examination to detect sequelae of GERD (e.g., ulceration, obstruction, stricture)

    C. Other: Upper endoscopy to detect sequelae of GERD (e.g., esophagitis, ulceration, stricture, Barrett esophagus)

V. Differential diagnosis

    A. Cardiac disease

    B. Lower respiratory infections

    C. Gastric or duodenal ulcer disease (see Chapter 78)

    D. Cholelithiasis (see Chapter 68)

    E. Esophageal infections: *Candida*

    F. Barrett esophagus

    G. Gastritis (see Chapter 72)

    H. Pill-induced esophagitis

VI. Treatment (McFarlane, 2018; Pandit et al., 2018; Sandhu & Fass, 2017)

    A. Postural measures

        1. Place head of bed on six- to eight-inch blocks.

        2. Avoid recumbent position for at least two hours after eating.

    B. Dietary measures

        1. Reduce meal size and avoid late or large evening meals.

        2. Selective elimination of fatty diet, spices, sweets, acidic foods, caffeine, alcohol, peppermint, spearmint, chewing gum, carbonated beverages, and chocolate could be considered if patients note correlation with GERD symptoms and improvement with elimination.

    C. Lifestyle modifications

        1. Smoking cessation

        2. Weight reduction

        3. Avoidance of tight-fitting garments

    D. Pharmacologic interventions

        1. Modify or discontinue medications that decrease lower esophageal sphincter pressure (e.g., theophylline, anticholinergics, calcium antagonists, hormones).

        2. Antisecretory drugs: For erosive esophagitis, PPI are more effective than H_2 blockers.

            a) H_2 blockers

                (1) Cimetidine: 400 mg PO two times a day or 800 mg at bedtime

                (2) Famotidine: 20 mg PO two times a day or 40 mg at bedtime

                (3) Nizatidine: 150 mg PO two times a day

            b) PPIs: Take 30 minutes prior to breakfast.

                (1) Esomeprazole: 20–40 mg PO daily

                (2) Dexlansoprazole: 30–60 mg delayed-release capsule PO daily

                (3) Omeprazole: 20–40 mg PO daily

                (4) Omeprazole/sodium bicarbonate: 20–40 mg PO daily

                (5) Lansoprazole: 15–30 mg PO daily

                (6) Pantoprazole: 40 mg PO daily

                (7) Rabeprazole: 20 mg PO daily

        3. Gastrokinetic drugs: Increases lower esophageal sphincter pressure and enhances gastric emptying

            a) Metoclopramide: 5–15 mg PO before meals and at bedtime

            b) Bethanechol (Urecholine®): 25 mg PO four times a day

    4. Mucosal protectant: Sucralfate 1 g PO four times a day before meals and at bedtime

    5. Antacids

        a) Sodium bicarbonate: Two tablets dissolved in six ounces of water every four hours PO PRN, not to exceed eight a day

        b) Calcium carbonate: Two tablets PO every four hours PRN

        c) Magnesium and aluminum hydroxides: 10–20 ml PO one hour after meals and at bedtime

        d) Magnesium and aluminum hydroxides and simethicone: 10–20 ml PO one hour after meals and at bedtime

    6. Treat appropriately for *Helicobacter pylori* (see Chapter 78).

VII. Follow-up

    A. Short term: Symptoms should improve in four weeks with H_2 receptor antagonist, antacids, and lifestyle modifications. Patients may also be treated with a PPI for a maximum of eight weeks of therapy. If no improvement after eight weeks, refer to gastroenterologist.

    B. Long term

        1. Encourage continued lifestyle modifications.

        2. Consider maintenance therapy after response with H_2 receptor antagonists.

VIII. Referrals

    A. Dietitian: To assist with dietary modifications

    B. Cardiologist: If chest pain is suspected to have cardiac origin

    C. Gastroenterologist: For further evaluation if symptoms are refractory after eight weeks of therapy

References

Chen, J., & Brady, P. (2019). Gastroesophageal reflux disease: Pathophysiology, diagnosis, and treatment. *Gastroenterology Nursing, 42*(1), 20–28. https://doi.org/10.1097/SGA.0000000000000359

Clarrett, D.M., & Hachem, C. (2018). Gastroesophageal reflux disease (GERD). *Missouri Medicine, 115*(3), 214–218.

Gyawali, C.P., & Fass, R. (2018). Management of gastroesophageal reflux disease. *Gastroenterology, 154*(2), 302–318. https://doi.org/10.1053/j.gastro.2017.07.049

Kandulski, A., Moleda, L., & Müller-Schilling, M. (2018). Diagnostic investigations of gastroesophageal reflux disease: Who and when to refer and for what test? *Visceral Medicine, 34*(2), 97–100. https://doi.org/10.1159/000488184

Kellerman, R., & Kintanar, T. (2017). Gastroesophageal reflux disease. *Primary Care: Clinics in Office Practice, 44*(4), 561–573. https://doi.org/10.1016/j.pop.2017.07.001

McFarlane, B. (2018). Management of gastroesophageal reflux disease in adults: A pharmacist's perspective. *Integrated Pharmacy Research and Practice, 7*, 41–52. https://doi.org/10.2147/IPRP.S142932

Pandit, S., Boktor, M., Alexander, J.S., Becker, F., & Morris, J. (2018). Gastroesophageal reflux disease: A clinical overview for primary care physicians. *Pathophysiology, 25*(1), 1–11. https://doi.org/10.1016/j.pathophys.2017.09.001

Richter, J.E., & Rubenstein, J.H. (2018). Presentation and epidemiology of gastroesophageal reflux disease. *Gastroenterology, 154*(2), 267–276. https://doi.org/10.1053/j.gastro.2017.07.045

Sandhu, D.S., & Fass, R. (2017). Current trends in the management of gastroesophageal reflux disease. *Gut and Liver, 12*(1), 7–16. https://doi.org/10.5009/gnl16615

Savarino, E., Bredenoord, A.J., Fox, M., Pandolfino, J.E., Roman, S., & Gyawali, C.P. (2017). Expert consensus document: Advances in the physiological assessment and diagnosis of GERD. *Nature Reviews Gastroenterology and Hepatology, 14*(11), 665–676. https://doi.org/10.1038/nrgastro.2017.130

Vaezi, M.F., Pandolfino, J.E., Vela, M.R., & Shaheen, N.J. (2017). White paper AGA: Optimal strategies to define and diagnose gastroesophageal reflux disease. *Clinical Gastroenterology and Hepatology, 15*(8), 1162–1172. https://doi.org/10.1016/j.cgh.2017.03.021

CHAPTER 72

Gastritis

Kristina Mathey, MS, APRN–CNP, AOCNP®

I. Definition: Inflammation of the gastric mucosa (Minalyan et al., 2017; Sipponen & Maaroos, 2015)
   A. Metaplastic atrophic gastritis or gastric atrophy: A chronic form of gastritis associated with inflammation in the mucous membrane, mucosal thinning, loss of specialized cells in the gastric glands, and changes in epithelial cell types; includes two main subtypes: autoimmune and environmental (caused by *Helicobacter pylori*)
   B. Autoimmune atrophic gastritis: A chronic form of gastritis in which the body mistakenly attacks healthy stomach cells, including cells that produce intrinsic factor, which is responsible for vitamin B_{12} absorption

II. Physiology/Pathophysiology (Huang et al., 2017; Joo, 2017; Sipponen & Maaroos, 2015; Soma, 2016)
   A. Normal
      1. The stomach has three sections that lie transversely in the upper abdominal cavity below the diaphragm.
         a) Upper portion referred to as the fundus
         b) Middle section referred to as the body
         c) Distal portal referred to as the pylorus
      2. Hydrochloric acid and digestive enzymes are secreted in the stomach to break down fats and proteins.
      3. Pepsin is secreted to digest proteins, amylase breaks down carbohydrates, and gastric lipase acts on emulsified fats.
   B. Pathophysiology
      1. Chronic gastritis is a multistep, lifelong, progressive inflammation. As gastritis occurs, there is a failure of secretion of hydrochloric acid and intrinsic factor from oxyntic glands, leading to corpus atrophy and failure in synthesis and secretion of gastrin-17 from antral G cells in antral atrophy.
      2. Erosive gastritis is most commonly caused by *H. pylori* and can develop through the use of NSAIDs or from immune-mediated causes.
         a) *H. pylori* is a gram-negative rod that resides under the gastric mucosal layer next to epithelial cells. It causes hypochlorhydria, resulting in an excess of nitrites and N-nitroso compounds, a theoretical link to atrophy and metaplasia. Initial infection causes acute gastritis followed by chronic inflammation. If left untreated, this can lead to atrophic gastritis.
         b) *H. pylori* infection is the major cause of chronic gastritis, gastric mucosa–associated lymphoid tissue lymphoma, and gastric adenocarcinoma.
         c) *H. pylori* is thought to be transmitted by a GI–oral route.

(1) *H. pylori* can be cured through eradication of the bacterium resulting in normalization of the gastric mucosa.

(2) Carcinogenic risk is modified by strain-specific bacterial components, host responses, and/or specific host–microbe interactions.

(3) A synergistic relationship between NSAID use and *H. pylori* exists, leading to increased risk of gastritis when both are present.

(4) Endoscopic findings in gastritis include erythema, mucosal erosions, absence of rugal folds, and presence of visible vessels.

(5) Histologic findings of gastritis can vary over a wide spectrum, ranging from epithelial hyperplasia with minimal inflammation to extensive epithelial cell damage with infiltration by inflammatory cells.

d) NSAIDs inhibit cyclooxygenase, the enzyme that controls prostaglandin synthesis, weakening the mucosa and increasing sensitivity to acid and pepsin.

III. Clinical features: Gastritis may be asymptomatic to symptomatic with symptoms poorly correlated with endoscopic changes. It is characterized as acute or chronic. *H. pylori* infects more than 50% of the global population. A primary prevention strategy is through the eradication of *H. pylori* in regions with a high incidence of gastric adenocarcinoma (Best et al., 2018; Massironi et al., 2019; Minalyan et al., 2017; Sipponen & Maaroos, 2015).

A. Risk factors

1. NSAIDs: Especially high-dose, non–cyclooxygenase-2 inhibitor, and long-acting NSAIDs used longer than three months (see Appendix E)

2. Other medications: Corticosteroids, acarbose, bisphosphonates, iron, metformin, orlistat, potassium chloride, oral antibiotics, herbs (e.g., garlic, ginkgo, saw palmetto, feverfew, chaste tree berry, white willow)

3. Demographics

a) Age older than 60 years

b) Female gender

c) Residence in a developing country: Prevalence of *H. pylori* in Asian Americans, African Americans, and Hispanics is similar to that in people in developing countries.

d) Poor socioeconomic conditions and poor hygiene

e) Family overcrowding

f) Possible ethnic or genetic predisposition: Chronic gastritis of the autoimmune type has shown to be a recessive multigenic disease of possible Northern European heritage.

B. Etiology

1. Erosive gastritis

a) NSAIDs

b) *H. pylori*

c) Other causes: Alcohol use, ASA use, stress during severe illness, portal hypertension

d) In immunocompromised patients: Erosive gastritis may be caused by bacterial infection, CMV, or fungal infections of the stomach lining.

2. Nonerosive gastritis, called nonulcer dyspepsia/gastropathy

a) Pernicious anemia results from an autoimmune gastritis of the fundic gland from vitamin B_{12} deficiency. It causes mucosal atrophy (atrophic gastritis) and achlorhydria. It is a relatively uncommon cause but is a risk factor for gastric carcinoid tumors and adenocarcinoma of the stomach.

b) A postinfectious or postinflammatory origin has been proposed for nonerosive gastritis.

c) H. pylori infection is present in 30%–50% of the population; most are asymptomatic, and only a minority develop erosive gastritis or peptic ulcer disease. The reasons are unclear but may be the virulence of the strain of *H. pylori* and differences in host defense mechanisms. The more cytotoxic the strain, the more active and aggressive, leading to chronic gastritis.

d) People with nonerosive gastritis are more likely to experience anxiety or depression or have multiple somatic complaints.

e) Chemotherapy agents can cause mucosal injury, particularly mitomycin C and 5-fluorouracil.

f) Monoclonal antibodies have been associated with severe enteritis.

g) Radiation therapy to the upper abdomen and total body irradiation for HSCT have been associated with gastric mucosal injury.

C. History
1. History of cancer and cancer treatment
2. Current medications: Prescribed, over the counter
3. History of presenting symptoms: Precipitating factors, onset, duration, associated symptoms (e.g., weight loss, fatigue, nausea, vomiting, bloody stools, bloody vomitus)
4. Changes in ADLs
5. Past medical history: Peptic ulcer disease
6. Social history: Tobacco, alcohol, and caffeine use; stress
7. Family history: Gastric cancer
8. Travel history

D. Signs and symptoms
1. Alarm symptoms for risk of gastric cancer or peptic ulcer disease prompting further evaluation
   a) Age older than 45 years
   b) Rectal bleeding or melena
   c) Weight loss greater than 10%
   d) Anemia
   e) Dysphagia
   f) Abdominal mass
   g) Jaundice
   h) Anorexia/early satiety
   i) Dyspepsia
   j) Protracted vomiting
2. Erosive gastritis
   a) Often asymptomatic
   b) Upper GI bleed: Most common clinical manifestation
      (1) Coffee-ground emesis
      (2) Blood in NG aspirate
      (3) Melena
3. Nonerosive gastritis/nonulcer dyspepsia/gastropathy
   a) May have a transient clinical illness with acute infection characterized by nausea and abdominal pain for several days
   b) Dysmotility-like dyspepsia: Indigestion with bloating, belching, and fullness
   c) Nausea and/or vomiting, often postprandial
   d) Anorexia
   e) Gnawing or burning sensation in the epigastric region that is relieved by food, antacids, or antisecretory drugs

      4. Autoimmune atrophic gastritis with symptoms of B_{12} deficiency
- *a)* Chest pain
- *b)* Generalized fatigue
- *c)* Tinnitus
- *d)* Dizziness or light-headedness
- *e)* Heart palpitations
- *f)* Confusion
- *g)* Tinging or numbness in arms or legs
- *h)* Unsteady gait

E. Physical examination
  1. Abdominal
- *a)* May have epigastric tenderness to deep palpation
- *b)* Normal bowel sounds
- *c)* No masses palpable
- *d)* No organomegaly

  2. Rectal
- *a)* No rectal masses
- *b)* Stool testing for occult blood

IV. Diagnostic tests (El-Zimaity et al., 2018; Sipponen & Maaroos, 2015)
A. Laboratory
1. CBC to evaluate for anemia
2. Ferritin and iron level if anemic: *H. pylori* has been shown to impair iron uptake.
3. Chemistry profile to evaluate liver abnormalities
4. *H. pylori* enzyme-linked immunosorbent assay (ELISA): Consensus to "test and treat" using laboratory-based serologic testing for IgG antibodies
   - *a)* Presence of antibodies suggests active infection in symptomatic patients not previously treated and has a strong negative predictive value.
   - *b)* This is the most commonly used test because of convenience, but it is less accurate than the urea breath test or stool antigen test.
5. Rapid, office-based whole blood tests for IgG antibodies: Available but not as accurate
6. Urea breath: Reliable test for cure and more reliable than serology in identifying active infection
   - *a)* It is usually hospital based and is more expensive than serology.
   - *b)* PPI use must be held two weeks prior to testing and antibiotics held for four weeks for accuracy of testing.
7. Stool antigen test to measure *H. pylori* antigens and for cure
   - *a)* It is less expensive and less invasive than the urea breath test.
   - *b)* Fresh stool is required for testing.
8. Low pepsinogen I and II: Useful test in screening patients at high risk for gastric cancer; has limitations; can only be used to diagnose atrophic corpus gastritis
9. GastroPanel®: Complete test, including an assay of the plasma levels of gastrin-17, assays of pepsinogen I and pepsinogen II, and the *H. pylori* serology
10. Vitamin B_{12} level to evaluate for deficiency

B. Radiology: Upper GI series; least sensitive test for gastritis and will not allow biopsy
C. Other
  1. Endoscopy with biopsy should be reserved for patients with alarm symptoms or who have failed treatment.

2. Biopsy is required to differentiate among acute, chronic active, and chronic gastritis and gastropathy. The Sydney system and its updated guidelines are used for interpretation of the microscopic appearancc in biopsy specimens.
3. Biopsy will reveal the typical spiral-shaped bacilli, but prior treatment may change the appearance of the bacteria.
4. Multiple biopsies are needed to confirm diagnosis.
5. Lymphoid follicles may be present on biopsy, representing an immune response to the bacteria, and are involved in the pathogenesis of primary gastric lymphoma.

V. Differential diagnosis (El-Zimaity et al., 2018)
  A. Peptic ulcer disease (see Chapter 78)
  B. GERD (see Chapter 71)
  C. Gastric carcinoma and gastric lymphoma
  D. Biliary tract disease
  E. Food poisoning
  F. Viral gastroenteritis
  G. Nonulcer dyspepsia
  H. Sarcoidosis
  I. Isolated granulomatosis gastritis
  J. Patients with severe pain at presentation
    1. Perforating or penetrating ulcer
    2. Pancreatic disease (see Chapter 77)
    3. Esophageal rupture
    4. Ruptured aortic aneurysm
    5. Ureteral colic
    6. MI (see Chapter 49)
  K. Patients with GI bleeding at presentation
    1. Esophageal varices or severe esophagitis
    2. Mallory-Weiss tear
    3. Arteriovenous malformation
    4. Crohn disease

VI. Treatment (Chang & Hu, 2015; Hu et al., 2017; Huang et al., 2017; Massironi et al., 2019; Minalyan et al., 2017)
  A. Treatment is based on underlying cause.
    1. Erosive gastritis
      a) Eliminate the cause, if possible.
      b) Discontinue the use of all NSAIDs (see Appendix E).
      c) Encourage smoking cessation.
      d) Encourage decreased alcohol and caffeine intake.
      e) Dietary modification plays no specific role.
    2. If NSAID use is necessary
      a) Use lowest effective dose.
      b) Switch to nonacetylated salicylate 500–3,000 mg PO daily in divided doses or a nonacidic NSAID, meloxicam 7.5–15 mg daily PO, or a cyclooxygenase-2 NSAID, celecoxib 200 mg PO daily.
      c) Coadminister a PPI, H_2 blocker, or mucosal protectant with the NSAID.
        (1) Naproxen sodium plus esomeprazole: 375 mg/20 mg PO or 500 mg/20 mg PO two times a day

        (2) Ibuprofen plus famotidine: 800 mg/26.6 mg PO three times a day

        (3) Diclofenac plus misoprostol: 50 mg/200 mcg or 75 mg/200 mcg PO two times a day

     d) Coadminister a mucosal protective agent misoprostol 100 mcg PO two times a day, and titrate weekly up to 200 mcg PO two times a day.

   3. Treatment options for erosive gastritis

     a) Antacids: Administered one and three hours after meals

     b) H_2 receptor blockers: Generally given for six to eight weeks

        (1) Cimetidine: 400 mg PO two times a day or 800 mg at bedtime

        (2) Famotidine: 20 mg PO two times a day or 40 mg at bedtime

        (3) Nizatidine: 150 mg PO two times a day or 300 mg PO at bedtime

     c) PPIs: Generally given for four to eight weeks

        (1) Esomeprazole: 20–40 mg PO daily

        (2) Omeprazole: 20–40 mg PO daily

        (3) Lansoprazole: 15–30 mg PO daily

        (4) Pantoprazole: 40 mg PO daily

        (5) Rabeprazole: 20 mg PO daily

        (6) Dexlansoprazole: 60 mg PO daily

        (7) Long-term use of PPIs

          (a) Associated with decreased absorption of certain medications, including ketoconazole, itraconazole, iron, and clopidogrel; pantoprazole has not been shown to interact with clopidogrel.

          (b) Possible development of gastric polyps, vitamin B_{12} deficiency, and bone fractures

     d) Mucosal protective agents

        (1) Sucralfate: 1 g PO four times a day for six to eight weeks

        (2) Misoprostol: 100 mcg PO two times a day; titrated weekly up to 200 mcg four times a day

B. Treatment options for *H. pylori* gastritis: Successful eradication of *H. pylori* is a major component in treating gastritis; however, the rate of eradication after traditional triple therapy is decreasing with standard amoxicillin plus clarithromycin-based therapy as the result of antibiotic resistance, poor compliance, and rapid metabolism of PPIs. It is essential to know the antibiotic resistance data in the population treated to avoid this triple therapy unless it has been proven to achieve success rates locally. Several strategies, including bismuth quadruple therapy, have been proposed to increase eradication rate. Treatment should last for 10–14 days.

   1. First-line treatment: Triple therapy and PPI oral drugs

     a) PPI: Omeprazole 20 mg two times a day, lansoprazole 30 mg two times a day, rabeprazole 20 mg two times a day, or pantoprazole 40 mg two times a day

     b) Plus antibiotic therapy: Clarithromycin 500 mg two times a day and amoxicillin 1 g two times a day

     c) Prevpac® triple therapy of amoxicillin, clarithromycin, and lansoprazole available prepackaged

     d) If patient is allergic to penicillin, substitute metronidazole 500 mg PO two times a day for amoxicillin.

   2. Second-line treatment: Bismuth quadruple oral therapy

     a) PPI two times a day

     b) Antibiotics: Metronidazole 250 mg four times a day plus tetracycline 500 mg four times a day

     c) Bismuth subsalicylate: 120 mg four times a day

      d) Helidac®, metronidazole, tetracycline, and Pepto-Bismol® available prepackaged
   C. Pernicious anemia resulting from autoimmune atrophic gastritis: Lifelong replacement with cobalamin (vitamin B_{12}) 1,000 mcg IM daily or every other day for a week, followed by a weekly administration for one to two months, and then monthly lifelong

VII. Follow-up
   A. Short term
      1. Patients should be seen two to four weeks after initiating therapy for symptom evaluation and to confirm compliance with medication.
      2. Stool antigen test or urea breath test is useful to determine eradication of *H. pylori* after treatment, especially if symptoms have not resolved entirely.
   B. Long term: One-third of patients with bleeding ulcers rebleed in one to two years; these patients require close follow-up every two to three months.

VIII. Referrals
   A. Gastroenterologist: For endoscopy, acute GI bleed, evaluation of severe pain, and acute symptomatology
   B. Surgeon: For evaluation in acute GI bleed, severe pain, and acute symptomatology

The author would like to acknowledge Kristine Turner Story, RN, MSN, APRN, BC, for her contribution to this chapter that remains unchanged from the previous edition of this book.

References

Best, L.M.J., Takwoingi, Y., Siddique, S., Selladurai, A., Gandhi, A., Low, B., … Gurusamy, K.S. (2018). Non-invasive diagnostic tests for *Helicobacter pylori* infection. *Cochrane Database of Systematic Reviews, 2018*(3). https://doi.org/10.1002/14651858.CD012080.pub2

Chang, S.-S., & Hu, H.-Y. (2015). *Helicobacter pylori*: Effect of coexisting diseases and update on treatment regimens. *World Journal of Gastrointestinal Pharmacology and Therapeutics, 6*(4), 127–136. https://doi.org/10.4292/wjgpt.v6.i4.127

El-Zimaity, H., Choi, W.-T., Lauwers, G.Y., & Riddell, R. (2018). The differential diagnosis of *Helicobacter pylori* negative gastritis. *Virchows Archiv, 473*(5), 533–550. https://doi.org/10.1007/s00428-018-2454-6

Hu, Y., Zhu, Y., & Lu, N.-H. (2017). Novel and effective therapeutic regimens for *Helicobacter pylori* in an era of increasing antibiotic resistance. *Frontiers in Cellular and Infection Microbiology, 7,* 168. https://doi.org/10.3389/fcimb.2017.00168

Huang, C.-C., Tsai, K.-W., Tsai, T.-J., & Hsu, P.-I. (2017). Update on the first-line treatment for *Helicobacter pylori* infection—A continuing challenge from an old enemy. *Biomarker Research, 5,* 23. https://doi.org/10.1186/s40364-017-0103-x

Joo, M. (2017). Rare gastric lesions associated with *Helicobacter pylori* infection: A histopathological review. *Journal of Pathology and Translational Medicine, 51*(4), 341–351. https://doi.org/10.4132/jptm.2017.04.03

Massironi, S., Zilli, A., Elvevi, A., & Invernizzi, P. (2019). The changing face of chronic autoimmune atrophic gastritis: An updated comprehensive perspective. *Autoimmunity Reviews, 18*(3), 215–222. https://doi.org/10.1016/j.autrev.2018.08.011

Minalyan, A., Benhammou, J.N., Artashesyan, A., Lewis, M.S., & Pisegna, J.R. (2017). Autoimmune atrophic gastritis: Current perspectives. *Clinical and Experimental Gastroenterology, 10,* 19–27. https://doi.org/10.2147/CEG.S109123

Sipponen, P., & Maaroos, H.-I. (2015). Chronic gastritis. *Scandinavian Journal of Gastroenterology, 50*(6), 657–667. https://doi.org/10.3109/00365521.2015.1019918

Soma, N. (2016). Diagnosis of *Helicobacter pylori*–related chronic gastritis, gastric adenoma and early gastric cancer by magnifying endoscopy. *Journal of Digestive Diseases, 17*(10), 641–651. https://doi.org/10.1111/1751-2980.12404

CHAPTER 73

Hemorrhoids

Karen A. Roesser, MSN, RN, AOCNS®

I. Definition: Swollen and inflamed veins in the lower rectum; may be internal or external (Gardner et al., 2020; Margetis, 2019)

II. Physiology/Pathophysiology (Davis et al., 2018; Gardner et al., 2020; Kline, 2015; Lohsiriwat, 2015; Margetis, 2019)
   A. Normal: Hemorrhoids are normal vascular structures in the anal canal. They are mucosal vascular cushions present in all individuals.
      1. The anal canal is approximately 2.5–4 cm in length and opens onto the perineum.
      2. The rectum and anus form the terminal portions of the GI tract.
      3. Internal and external hemorrhoids communicate with one another and drain into the internal pudendal veins and ultimately into the IVC.
      4. Hemorrhoids aid in the closure of the anal canal at rest and help to prevent incontinence secondary to stool and flatus. They account for approximately 20% of resting anal pressure.
      5. The dentate line is a landmark separating anal (squamous) and colonic (columnar) mucosa in the anal canal.
         a) This border area is a zone of transition between the rectum and anal canal mucosa.
         b) The dentate line is important in differentiating between external and internal hemorrhoids.
   B. Pathophysiology
      1. Hemorrhoids arise from a plexus of dilated arteriovenous channels and connective tissue with the veins arising from the superior and inferior hemorrhoidal veins. Plentiful anastomoses exist between these two veins and the middle rectal vein, thus connecting to the portal and systemic circulations.
      2. These veins are located in the submucosal layer in the lower rectum. They are classified by their anatomic origin within the anal canal and by their position relative to the dentate line.
      3. Internal hemorrhoids arise from the superior hemorrhoidal plexus and are located above or proximal to the dentate line. At the dentate line, they are anchored to the underlying muscle by the mucosal suspensory ligament.
         a) Hemorrhoids are derived from embryonic endoderm and lined with the columnar epithelium of the anal mucosa.
         b) Hemorrhoids are innervated by visceral pain receptors.
         c) This cushion of tissue located above the dentate line is associated with a diminished pain sensation.

4. External hemorrhoids arise from the inferior hemorrhoidal plexus and are located below or distal to the dentate line.
   - *a)* These hemorrhoids develop from ectoderm and are covered by squamous epithelium.
   - *b)* Numerous somatic pain receptors, including the pudendal nerve and the sacral plexus, are contained within this epithelium, making this anoderm area sensitive.
5. Both types of hemorrhoids often coexist, resulting in mixed hemorrhoids (external and internal) across the dentate line.

III. Clinical features: External hemorrhoids are more likely to cause pain or burning sensation. Internal hemorrhoids do typically cause pain but may become symptomatic when prolapse and excessive engorgement occurs. This leads to stretching of the suspensory muscles and eventual prolapse of rectal tissue through the anal canal. It may be difficult to establish whether symptoms are caused by internal or external hemorrhoids, particularly when patients present with mixed disease (Cohee et al., 2020; Davis et al., 2018; Gardner et al., 2020; Kline, 2015; Margetis, 2019; Sandler & Peery, 2019).

A. Etiology: Cause may be different in individual patients.
   1. Inadequate fiber intake
   2. Heredity
   3. Carcinomas: Especially pelvic tumors
   4. Constipation
   5. Increased straining with stools accompanied by Valsalva maneuver
   6. Sitting for defecation, as opposed to squatting
   7. Diarrhea: Contributes to hemorrhoidal development secondary to irritation; associated with comorbid diseases (e.g., colitis, malabsorption, intestinal bypass, chronic pancreatitis)
   8. Result of pregnancy/vaginal delivery
   9. Loss of muscle tone: Old age, surgery, episiotomy, anal intercourse
   10. Hepatic disease
   11. Obesity
   12. Spinal cord injury

B. History
   1. History of cancer and cancer treatment
   2. Current medications: Prescribed, over the counter
   3. History of presenting symptoms: Precipitating factors, onset, duration, associated symptoms (e.g., pain, itching, or burning during or after a bowel movement; blood in stool or on the toilet paper; fecal soiling)
   4. Changes in ADLs
   5. Past medical history: Pregnancy, liver disease, chronic constipation, bowel habits
   6. Past surgical history: Episiotomy
   7. Family history: Hemorrhoids
   8. Social history: Diet recall, occupation, prolonged sitting, heavy lifting

C. Signs and symptoms
   1. Anal itching/pruritus ani
   2. Anal pain during defecation or between bowel movements due to thrombosis
   3. Bleeding: Most commonly seen after defecation and visible on surface of stool or toilet paper
   4. Constipation/diarrhea
   5. External burning sensation

      6. Difficulty sitting for prolonged periods

      7. Feeling of incomplete defecation

      8. Fecal soiling

      9. Prolapse

  D. Physical examination

      1. Vital signs: Unexplained weight loss indicative of malignancy

      2. Abdominal: Normal bowel sounds and no abdominal tenderness

      3. Perirectal and anal

          a) External: Examination performed in the prone, knee–chest, or lateral decubitus position; visible, palpable masses on inspection; protuberant purplish nodules covered by mucosa (prolapsed internal hemorrhoids); examination at rest and with straining

          b) Digital rectal: Usually no palpable masses unless external, in which case a firm mass on the anal surface may be palpated

              (1) Not tender unless thrombosed: A rope-like mass is felt.

              (2) Rectal vault usually smooth: Internal hemorrhoid usually cannot be palpated unless thrombosed.

              (3) Rectal mass as a source of bleeding

              (4) Mucoid discharge suggesting infection or lesion

          c) Internal: Best visualized with a slotted anoscope but can be seen on retroflexion with an endoscope (proctosigmoidoscopy)

IV. Diagnostic tests (Cengiz & Gorgun, 2019; Cohee et al., 2020; Davis et al., 2018; Gardner et al., 2020; Pillant-Le Moult et al., 2015)

  A. Laboratory: Not typically required for diagnostic purposes

      1. Hemoccult stool testing

          a) Will be positive if any blood is present

          b) Not reliable as first-line diagnosis

      2. CBC only if suspected infection or anemia

  B. Radiology: Not indicated

  C. Other: Endoscopy

      1. Colonoscopy

          a) For rectal bleeding not typical of hemorrhoids: Significant risk factors for colonic malignancy or rectal bleeding with negative anorectal examination

          b) Patients older than age 50 years: Colonoscopy before focusing on internal hemorrhoids

          c) Strong family history of colorectal cancer or history of advanced adenoma

          d) Positive fecal immunochemical testing

          e) If bleeding does not completely resolve: Should be performed despite the age of the patient

      2. Anoscopy and flexible sigmoidoscopy: To verify diagnosis and assess hemorrhoids

          a) Internal hemorrhoids are graded on a scale of I–IV (see Table 73-1). Grading is helpful for treatment guidance.

          b) No widely used classification system exists for external hemorrhoids.

V. Differential diagnosis (Cohee et al., 2020; Davis et al., 2018; Lohsiriwat, 2015; Mott et al., 2018)

  A. Anorectal conditions causing acute or chronic symptoms or bleeding can be divided into those with or without anorectal pain (see Figure 73-1).

TABLE 73-1	Internal Hemorrhoid Grading and Treatment	
Grade	**Descriptions**	**Treatment**
I	Hemorrhoids visible only on anoscopy; often bleed and may bulge into lumen but do not prolapse below the dentate line	Respond to medical therapy Do not require anoscopic or surgical therapy
II	Hemorrhoids prolapsed below the dentate line and out of the anal canal with defecation or straining, but spontaneously reduce	Some patients will respond to medical therapy. If recurrent or chronic symptoms, often require anoscopic therapies
III	Hemorrhoids prolapsed below the dentate line and out of the anal canal with defecation or straining; require manual reduction into their normal position	Usually do not respond to medical therapies alone Respond well to banding or other surgical therapies
IV	Hemorrhoids prolapsed and stay below the dentate line; are irreducible and may strangulate	Some patients may respond to banding or other anoscopic therapies to control bleeding. Most patients respond best to surgical interventions.

Note. Based on information from Banov et al., 1985; Davis et al., 2018; Gardner et al., 2020; Lohsiriwat, 2015.

    B. Uncomplicated or untreated internal hemorrhoids are not usually associated with pain. Significant anal pain suggests the presence of a nonhemorrhoidal anorectal condition (e.g., anal fissure, anorectal abscess).

  VI. Treatment (Cengiz & Gorgun, 2019; Cohee et al., 2020; Gardner et al., 2020; Garg, 2016; Lohsiriwat, 2015; Perera et al., 2012; Sheikh, 2019)
    A. Conservative measures
       1. Avoidance of direct pressure, especially with thrombosed external hemorrhoids
       2. Changes in bathroom habits that lead to straining and downward pressure (e.g., spending 3–5 minutes on the commode, avoiding reading while on it)
       3. Limiting frequency of defecation to once daily
       4. Sitz baths two to three times a day using warm water (40°C [104°F]) to relieve tissue edema and sphincter spasm; may be used with Epsom salts (1 cup salt/2 quarts water)
       5. High-fiber diet with increased water intake (5–6 teaspoons of fiber with 500–600 ml of water); a detailed listing of the fiber content of various foods should be provided to patients.
       6. Use of phlebotonics consisting of plant extracts, such as flavonoids, or synthetic compounds, such as calcium dobesilate
          a) Phlebotonics can decrease venous inflammation associated with venous disorders including hemorrhoids, increase vascular tone, reduce venous capacity, decrease capillary permeability, and facilitate lymphatic drainage.
          b) A Cochrane Review demonstrated a statistically significant benefit in outcomes for symptoms of pruritus bleeding, discharge and leakage, and overall symptom improvement.
    B. Pharmacology
       1. Stool softeners/stimulant laxatives: Titrate upward PRN.
          a) Docusate sodium: 100 mg PO two a day to start, then every day; maximum dose: 360 mg PO daily; 283 mg daily per rectum

        b) Docusate and senna: 1–2 tablets PO (50 mg docusate sodium and 8.6 mg sennosides per tablet) to start at bedtime; maximum dose: 200 mg PO daily for docusate sodium and 34.4 mg sennosides PO daily

    2. Bulk laxatives (e.g., psyllium, methylcellulose, calcium polycarbophil): Patients must be able to increase fluid intake.

        a) Patients should take 1 teaspoon PO mixed in water or one or two tablets as directed at bedtime. Treatment should aim for dose of 20–30 g daily of fiber.

        b) Fiber supplementation is recommended as the best means to consistently modify stool texture.

    3. Topical preparations: These preparations can alleviate the pain and itching associated with hemorrhoids. Treatments should not be used for longer than one week, as they may lead to side effects such as contact dermatitis with analgesic creams or mucosal atrophy with steroid creams.

        a) Hydrocortisone acetate 25 mg: Apply cream or ointment rectally two times a day.

        b) Pramoxine 1%/hydrocortisone acetate 1%: Apply cream rectally two times a day.

        c) Witch hazel: Apply rectally after each bowel movement.

    4. Analgesic topical rectal preparations: To help alleviate pain

        a) Nupercainal® anesthetic: Use three to four times daily.

        b) Hydrocortisone, topical anesthetic, emollient, and protectant: Use three to four times daily.

        c) Calmoseptine® topical ointment: Use three to four times daily.

        d) Lidocaine 2.5% cream: Use two times a day.

    5. Systemic analgesics: Used in treating pain associated with thrombosed hemorrhoids or in postsurgical thrombectomy (see Appendices E and F)

        a) Acetaminophen: 650 mg PO every four to six hours PRN

        b) NSAIDs: May be used rather than opioids to avoid side effect of constipation; should be avoided if there is bleeding

    6. Suppositories are painful to insert and are generally ineffective because they may end up in the rectum rather than the anal canal, where internal hemorrhoids are located.

  C. Surgery (Albuquerque, 2016; Lohsiriwat, 2015; Sandler & Peery, 2019)

    1. Indications for surgical interventions

FIGURE 73-1   **Differential Diagnosis of Anorectal Conditions Causing Pain or Bleeding**

Painless
- Internal hemorrhoids
- Anal fistula
- Polyps (anal or rectal)
- Early cancer (1° or 2°)[a]
- Radiation telangiectasia
- Kaposi sarcoma
- Rectal varices
- Postsurgical anastomotic ulcer
- Postpolypectomy ulcer
- Skin tags

Painful
- Thrombosed external hemorrhoids
- Mixed hemorrhoids
- Anal fissure
- Anal trauma (e.g., anal sex)
- Advanced cancer
- Rectal abscess with or without fistula
- Anal warts
- Fecal impaction
- Foreign body
- Rectal prolapse
- Proctitis ani
- Proctitis or colitis
- Inflammatory bowel disease

---

[a] 1° refers to cancers originating in the anorectum; 2° cancers are metastatic to the anorectum.

Note. Based on information from Cohee et al., 2020; Mott et al., 2018; Ohning et al., 2009.

a) Surgery may be proposed after failure of medical and nonoperative therapy.

b) Symptomatic grades III–IV or mixed internal and external hemorrhoids could be another indication for surgery.

c) Surgery would be offered for symptomatic hemorrhoids in the presence of a concomitant anorectal condition (e.g., anal fissure, condyloma) that requires surgery.

d) Patient preference after discussion of the treatment options could result in the decision to undergo surgery.

2. Closed excisional hemorrhoidectomy used for grades III–IV

a) This is the most common procedure performed for external hemorrhoids.

b) Elliptical incision is made to remove the redundant anoderm and hemorrhoidal tissue, which is closed with an absorbable suture.

c) This is superior to open excisional hemorrhoidectomy for long-term patient satisfaction and continence.

3. Open excisional hemorrhoidectomy: Used for grades III–IV

a) This option is the same as closed procedure, except excision and ligation without mucosal closure.

b) Some physicians prefer this approach because of decreased risk of infection.

4. Stapled hemorrhoidectomy (stapled hemorrhoidopexy): Used for grades II–IV

a) Intraluminal circular stapling device is used as an alternative to conventional surgical hemorrhoidectomy.

b) This is not appropriate for treatment of external hemorrhoids.

c) It is used more commonly for patients with bleeding or prolapsed internal hemorrhoids who have failed rubber band ligation.

5. Doppler-guided hemorrhoidectomy

a) A Doppler-guided/assisted hemorrhoid artery ligation through use of an anoscope can identify each hemorrhoid artery for ligation.

b) Potential benefits are lack of tissue excision and possibly less pain.

D. Office-based procedures for treatment of internal hemorrhoids

1. Rubber band ligation: Commonly used for grades I–II and select patients with grade III

a) Procedure is performed without local anesthesia and without preparation of the bowel with an enema.

b) Placement of the rubber band causes strangulation of the blood supply to the mucosa with resulting tissue necrosis and sloughing in one to two weeks.

c) Only one hemorrhoid should be banded on the first visit to determine the patient's tolerance to the procedure.

d) This procedure is shown to be superior to sclerotherapy and infrared coagulation.

2. Sclerotherapy: Used for grades I–II

a) Sclerosing agents, such as quinine and urea hydrochloride or 5% phenol in oil, are injected into the submucosa at the base of the hemorrhoid. This leads to fibrosis and scarring.

b) Sclerotherapy can be safely used in patients on anticoagulation as it does not involve sloughing.

c) Only two sites should be sclerosed to decrease the risk of complications.

3. Bipolar electrocautery: Used for grades I–II

a) Method of electrocautery is applied in one-second pulses of 20 W at the base of the hemorrhoid until underlying tissue is coagulated.

b) Three or four applications of energy are needed for each hemorrhoidal complex. Several hemorrhoids can be treated during each session.

4. Infrared coagulation: Used for grades I–II

    a) Infrared radiation is generated by a tungsten–halogen lamp and applied onto the hemorrhoid tissue via a probe tip.

    b) Tip of probe is placed superior to hemorrhoid cushion and delivers pulses of energy (heat).

    c) Three or four applications of energy are needed for each hemorrhoidal complex. Several hemorrhoids can be treated during each session.

VII. Follow-up

    A. Conservative therapy requires no follow-up if symptoms have spontaneously resolved using a nonsurgical treatment, especially for nonthrombosed external hemorrhoids or for grades I–II internal hemorrhoids.

    B. Higher-grade hemorrhoids usually require closer follow-up after a procedure is performed; follow-up generally occurs one to two weeks after the procedure.

    C. Monitor for the following complications: Thrombosis, bleeding, secondary infection, ulceration, incontinence, and anemia (rare) after surgical intervention.

VIII. Referrals

    A. Gastroenterologist/surgeon: For patients who do not respond to conservative measures for further evaluation

    B. Surgeon: Immediate referral for patients with thrombosed hemorrhoids that cause severe pain and bleeding, resulting in strangulation and ulceration

References

Albuquerque, A. (2016). Rubber band ligation of hemorrhoids: A guide for complications. *World Journal of Gastrointestinal Surgery, 27*(9), 614–620. https://doi.org/10.4240/wjgs.v8.i9.614

Banov, L., Knoepp, L.F., Jr., Erdman, L.H., & Alia, R.T. (1985). Management of hemorrhoidal disease. *Journal of the South Carolina Medical Association, 81*(7), 398–401.

Cengiz, T.B., & Gorgun, E. (2019). Hemorrhoids: A range of treatments. *Cleveland Clinic Journal of Medicine, 86*(9), 612–620. https://doi.org/10.3949/ccjm.86a.18079

Cohee, M.W., Hurff, A., & Gazewood, J.D. (2020). Benign anorectal conditions: Evaluation and management. *American Family Physician, 101*(1), 24–33. https://www.aafp.org/afp/2020/0101/p24.html

Davis, B.R., Lee-Kong, S.A., Migaly, J., Feingold, D.L., & Steele, S.R. (2018). The American Society of Colon and Rectal Surgeons clinical practice guidelines for the management of hemorrhoids. *Diseases of the Colon and Rectum, 61*(3), 284–292. https://doi.org/10.1097/DCR.0000000000001030

Gardner, I.H., Siddharthan, R.V., & Tsikitis, V.L. (2020). Benign anorectal disease: Hemorrhoids, fissures, and fistulas. *Annals of Gastroenterology, 33*(1), 9–18. https://doi.org/10.20524/aog.2019.0438

Garg, P. (2016). Why should a good proportion of hemorrhoids not be operated on?—Let's TONE up. *Diseases of the Colon and Rectum, 59*(6), 583–585. https://doi.org/10.1097/DCR.0000000000000560

Kline, R.P. (2015). Operative management of internal hemorrhoids. *Journal of the American Academy of Physician Assistants, 28*(2), 27–31. https://doi.org/10.1097/01.JAA.0000459809.87889.85

Lohsiriwat, V. (2015). Treatment of hemorrhoids: A coloproctologist's view. *World Journal of Gastroenterology, 21*(31), 9245–9252. https://doi.org/10.3748/wjg.v21.i31.9245

Margetis, N. (2019). Pathophysiology of internal hemorrhoids. *Annals of Gastroenterology, 32*(3), 264–272. https://doi.org/10.20524/aog.2019.0355

Mott, T., Latimer, K., & Edwards, C. (2018). Hemorrhoids: Diagnosis and treatment options. *American Family Physician, 97*(3), 172–179. https://www.aafp.org/afp/2018/0201/p172.html

Ohning, G.V., Machicado, G.A., & Jensen, D.M. (2009). Definitive therapy for internal hemorrhoids—New opportunities and options. *Reviews in Gastroenterological Disorders, 9*(1), 16–26.

Perera, N., Liolitsa, D., Iype, S., Croxford, A., Yassin, M., Lang, P., ... van Issum, C. (2012). Phlebotonics for haemorrhoids. *Cochrane Database of Systematic Reviews, 2012*(8). https://doi.org/10.1002/14651858.CD004322.pub3

Pillant-Le Moult, H., Aubert, M., & De Parades, V. (2015). Classical treatment of hemorrhoids. *Journal of Visceral Surgery, 152*(2 Suppl.), S3–S9. https://doi.org/10.1016/j.jviscsurg.2014.09.012

Sandler, R.S., & Peery, A.F. (2019). Rethinking what we know about hemorrhoids. *Clinical Gastroenterology and Hepatology, 17*(1), 8–15. https://doi.org/10.1016/j.cgh.2018.03.020

Sheikh, P. (2019). Management of hemorrhoidal disease: Medical management. *Medicographia, 41*(2), 64–70.

CHAPTER 74

Hepatitis

Karen L. Pitman, RN, MSN, ARNP, NP-C

I. Definition (Mohsen & Levy, 2017)
   A. Hepatitis is an inflammation of the liver and a group of viral infections (most commonly A, B, and C) that affect the liver.
   B. Autoimmune hepatitis is a generally progressive, chronic liver disease associated with chronic hepatic inflammation.

II. Physiology/Pathophysiology (CDC, 2020; Mohsen & Levy, 2017; Soi et al., 2019)
   A. Normal
      1. The liver lies in the right upper quadrant of the abdomen just below the diaphragm and is functionally divided into the right and left lobes. The right and left lobe each contain a smaller lobe. The caudate lobe extends from the posterior side of the right lobe and wraps around the IVC. The quadrate lobe, which is inferior to the caudate lobe, extends from the posterior side of the right lobe and wraps around the gallbladder.
      2. The liver plays an important role in the metabolism of carbohydrates, fats, and protein into biologically useful materials and is responsible for the production of the majority of proteins circulating in the plasma.
      3. The liver performs many other critical functions, including synthesis of clotting factors; storage of glycogen, minerals, and vitamins; and synthesis of blood proteins such as albumin.
   B. Pathophysiology
      1. The hepatic inflammatory process or immune response of the liver is produced by the actions of immune cells, such as monocytes, neutrophils, and dendritic cells, which initiate and maintain hepatic inflammation through the production of cytokines and chemokines.
      2. The inflammatory response may also include lymphocytes, other nonmononuclear cells, as well as cell necrosis.
         a) Microscopic findings include hepatocellular necrosis, inflammatory infiltrates, and liver cell regeneration.
         b) The histologic pattern in the variety of hepatitis diseases cannot be clearly recognized nor used as a predictor of illness severity. Variability in the lesions may account for the differences in liver damage.
      3. Typical morphologic changes include the portal, periportal, and lobular areas or may involve the entire liver.
      4. Types of viruses
         a) Hepatitis A (HAV): This RNA enteric virus is a member of the *Picornaviridae* family. Its replication appears limited to the liver, and it is transmitted primar-

ily person-to-person through the fecal–oral route or the consumption of contaminated food or water.

b) Hepatitis B (HBV): This DNA virus is a member of the *Hepadnaviridae* family, with at least eight main genotypes (A–H). Replication is largely confined to the liver; however, extrahepatic replication at several sites has been shown. Transmission is generally via the percutaneous or permucosal route, through infected blood or body fluids, sexual contact, contaminated needles, or childbirth.

c) Hepatitis C (HCV): This RNA-enveloped virus is a member of the *Flaviviridae* family and has six genotypes and more than 100 subtypes. HCV may be transmitted via direct contact with infected body fluids and is a blood-borne virus. Although sexual transmission of the C virus can occur, it is primarily transmitted via the parenteral route.

d) Hepatitis D (HDV): It is a virus-like particle with a hepatitis B surface antigen (HBsAg) coating and an internal or delta antigen. Three genotypes are known. HDV requires coinfection with HBV. It is transmitted through direct contact with blood.

e) Hepatitis E (HEV): This nonenveloped, single-stranded RNA enteric virus is a member of the *Hepeviridae* family and has at least five genotypes. It is transmitted primarily via contaminated water or food typically found in areas of poor sanitation and contamination. HEV is a self-limited disease and does not result in chronic infection.

III. Clinical features: Hepatitis may present without symptoms, as a subclinical illness, or as fulminant hepatic failure. A different type of virus is responsible for each type of transmitted viral hepatitis. Hepatitis can occur as a result of medications, illicit drug use, toxins, and alcohol use. Four clinical stages are identified: incubation period, preicteric phase, icteric phase, and convalescent phase. Not all individuals experience each phase. Viral hepatitis is the leading cause of liver cancer and the most common reason for liver transplantation. An estimated 4.4 million Americans are living with chronic hepatitis, mainly HBV and HCV, and most do not know they are infected. Approximately 80,000 new infections occur each year (CDC, 2020; Mohsen & Levy, 2017; Shin & Jeong, 2018; Terrault et al., 2018)

A. Etiology (see Table 74-1).

B. Classification of viral hepatitis (see Table 74-1)
   1. Hepatitis A virus (HAV)
   2. Hepatitis B virus (HBV)
   3. Hepatitis C virus (HCV; formerly identified as non-A, non-B)
   4. Hepatitis D virus (HDV)
   5. Hepatitis E virus (HEV)
   6. Hepatitis F virus (isolated in human stool)
   7. Hepatitis G virus (seen in liver transplant recipients and caused by chronic liver disease)

C. History
   1. History of cancer and cancer treatment
   2. Current medications: Prescribed, over the counter
   3. History of presenting symptoms: Precipitating factors, onset, location, duration
   4. Changes in ADLs
   5. Past medical history: Exposure to blood or body fluids, blood transfusions
   6. Social history: Recent foreign travel, alcohol use, illicit drug use, tattoos, sexual orientation, similar illness in household contacts

D. Signs and symptoms: Some individuals (especially children) may be asymptomatic (see Table 74-1). General symptoms may include fever, malaise, fatigue, anorexia, and jaundice. Generally, hepatitis lasting less than six months is acute, and hepatitis with symptoms persisting beyond six months is chronic.

1. The incubation or preclinical period occurs from the time of exposure to the development of symptoms. Transmission of disease is of concern.

2. The preicteric or prodromal phase occurs from appearance of symptoms to development of jaundice. Symptoms may include fever, malaise, anorexia, aversion to smoking, nausea, vomiting, and abdominal pain.

3. Icteric phase symptoms include jaundice, abdominal tenderness, dark urine, gray-colored stools, fever, and pruritus. Rarely, high fever, marked abdominal pain, jaundice, and the development of hepatic encephalopathy associated with coma and seizures may occur, leading to death in 70%–90% of patients.

4. The convalescent phase includes slow resolution of symptoms. General fatigue and malaise may continue.

E. Physical examination

1. Integument

   a) Jaundice: Yellowing of eyes or skin; mucous membranes
   b) Skin excoriation from severe pruritus
   c) Rash: Common in HBV; maculopapular, hives, erythema

2. Abdominal

   a) Hepatomegaly (enlarged and/or tender liver) with smooth, regular border indicative of acute hepatitis
   b) Enlarged, firm, nodular liver indicative of potential chronic hepatitis
   c) Splenomegaly
   d) Inguinal lymphadenopathy
   e) Ascites

3. Neurologic: Late-stage or chronic fulminant hepatitis (when the liver is unable to detoxify harmful substances and produces additional proteins), causing peripheral edema and bleeding; lethargy; confusion; somnolence; forgetfulness; stupor; and coma

4. Extremities: Peripheral edema, which is present in late-stage hepatitis

IV. Diagnostic tests (Mohsen & Levy, 2017; Wilkins et al., 2019)

A. Laboratory

1. Specific serologic assays to confirm hepatitis (see Table 74-1)

   a) Hepatitis A IgM (HAV-IgM) is a marker of acute infection and may remain positive for four to six months. It indicates past infection or immunization as well as lifelong protection.
   b) Hepatitis B surface antigen (HBsAg) reflects current or chronic hepatitis B infection. A person with persistent HBsAg should be considered infectious.
   c) Hepatitis B surface antibody (anti-HBs) reflects past infection or successful immunization.
   d) Hepatitis B core antibody (anti-HBc) indicates immunity due to current or past infection.
   e) Hepatitis B e antigen (HBeAg) is positive in the early course of infection and may persist in chronic disease. It indicates a high level of infectiousness or carrier state.
   f) Hepatitis B e antibody (anti-HBe) is a later marker indicating conversion from HBeAg. It signifies an inactive carrier.
   g) Hepatitis C antibody (anti-HCV or HCVAb) reflects current or past infection.

TABLE 74-1	Characteristics of Hepatitis A Through Hepatitis E				
Characteristics	**HAV**	**HBV**	**HCV**	**HDV**	**HEV**
Epidemiology	Worldwide, sporadic, and epidemic Foodborne outbreaks Daycare-related exposures Household and sexual contacts Most common among school-aged children and young adults	Worldwide Higher prevalence: Africa, Asia, and South America; seen in infancy and childhood	Worldwide 2%–3% of world's population with chronic HCV Major cause of nonepidemic hepatitis 1.5%–4.4% of general population with positive HCV antibodies Leading reason for liver transplantation	Worldwide Associated with HBV as coinfection or superinfection Self-limited or chronic progression	Not endemic to United States Epidemic in Asia, North and West Africa Waterborne outbreaks Common in young adults Uncommon in children and older adults
Incubation period	2–6 weeks; average 3–4 weeks	2–6 months; average 2–3 months	2–24 weeks; average 6–9 weeks	1–24 weeks; average 2–8 weeks	2–9 weeks; average 4–6 weeks
Transmission	Fecal–oral route; person to person Contaminated water and food not cooked or handled after cooking; mollusks from contaminated water; produce such as lettuce and strawberries; poor sanitation Rarely: Blood transfusions, sexual contact Greatest infectivity 2 weeks before onset of symptoms	Illicit drug use Percutaneous and per-mucosal exposure: blood, saliva, semen, vaginal fluids Sexual contact Perinatal Needlestick, accidental Tattooing and acupuncture Community razors, toothbrushes	Illicit drug use Percutaneous blood exposure Transfusion Perinatal Needlestick, accidental (rate approximately 3%–10% after needlestick) Tattooing, piercing Less frequently: sexual contact	Illicit drug use Blood and serous body fluids Parenteral exposure (common in drug-injecting population and hemophiliacs) Sexual contact Coinfection with HBV	Fecal–oral route; person to person (uncommon) Contaminated water and food supply

(Continued on next page)

TABLE 74-1   Characteristics of Hepatitis A Through Hepatitis E *(Continued)*

Characteristics	HAV	HBV	HCV	HDV	HEV
Clinical signs and symptoms	Can be asymptomatic Malaise, anorexia, nausea, vomiting, fever, abdominal pain, jaundice, dark urine, hepatomegaly, lymphadenopathy	Can be asymptomatic Malaise, abdominal pain, diarrhea, anorexia, nausea, vomiting, fever, muscle and joint pain, jaundice, rash	Commonly asymptomatic Malaise, anorexia, nausea, vomiting, abdominal pain, jaundice	Resembles those of HBV; always associated with coexistent HBV infection; superinfection with HBV more severe than coinfection	Similar to HAV
Onset	Abrupt; severity related to age	Insidious	Insidious	Abrupt	Abrupt
Specific tests	Anti-HAV Anti-HAV IgM Liver function tests	Anti-HBs HBsAg HBcAg Anti-HBc HBeAg Liver function tests	Anti-HCV (if negative during acute phase, repeat in six months) RIBA (additional test to confirm presence of antibodies) HCV RNA Liver function tests	Anti-HDV (anti-delta)	Anti-HEV (not commercially available; test available at CDC) Exclusion of other hepatitis Liver function tests
Vaccine	Combination HAV and HBV vaccines (tetra- and pentavalent vaccines)	HBIg, in combination Combination HAV and HBV vaccines (tetra- and pentavalent vaccines)	None	HBV vaccine prevents HDV infection.	None
Treatment	No specific treatment	No specific treatment IFN-α, lamivudine, adefovir, and others may help chronic carriers.	No specific treatment Combination therapy: pegylated IFN with ribavirin	No specific treatment	None

anti-HAV—antibodies to HAV; anti-HAV IgM—immunoglobulin M antibodies to hepatitis A virus; anti-HBc—hepatitis B core antibody; anti-HBs—antibody to hepatitis B surface antigen; anti-HCV—hepatitis C antibody; anti-HDV—antibodies to HDV; anti-HEV—antibodies to HEV; CDC—Centers for Disease Control and Prevention; HAV—hepatitis A; HBcAg—hepatitis B core antigen; HBeAg—hepatitis B e antigen; HBIg—hepatitis B immunoglobulin; HBsAg—hepatitis B surface antigen; HBV—hepatitis B virus; HCV—hepatitis C virus; HDV—hepatitis D virus; HEV—hepatitis E virus; IFN-α—interferon-alpha; RIBA—recombinant immunoblot assay

Note. Based on information from Centers for Disease Control and Prevention, 2020; Doshani et al., 2019; Mohsen & Levy, 2017.

        (1) To confirm positive anti-HCV, additional testing is required (e.g., recombinant immunoblot assay [RIBA], polymerase chain reaction, RNA).

        (2) HCV genotyping should also be performed to aid in selection of an appropriate treatment regimen.

   h) Hepatitis D (HBsAg and HDV antibody) reflects acute infection or disease.

        (1) IgM anti-HBc positive indicates coinfection.

        (2) IgG anti-HBc positive indicates superinfection.

   i) Hepatitis E

        (1) IgM HEV antibody levels generally increase approximately four weeks after infection and remain detectable for two to six months after the onset of illness. These levels are used to detect acute or recent infection.

        (2) HEV RNA can be detected just prior to symptom onset but becomes undetectable after approximately three weeks.

        (3) The virus will continue to shed in the stool for approximately two weeks. Negative HEV RNA does not preclude recent infection.

        (4) HEV IgG elevated reactivity indicates the presence of acute HEV.

  2. LFTs

   a) AST is an enzyme that processes proteins and is released into the bloodstream if the liver is damaged. AST may be noted to rise 1.5–15 times normal levels during acute HEV.

        (1) Elevated AST is characteristic of hepatitis.

        (2) AST generally will be elevated in the early prodromal period, will peak before jaundice is maximal, and its levels will fall slowly during the convalescent phase.

   b) ALT is a metabolism enzyme that is released into the bloodstream if the liver is damaged. ALT may be noted to rise to 1.5–15 times normal levels during acute infection. ALT is generally higher than AST with the exception of alcohol-induced hepatitis, where the reverse is generally seen.

   c) In chronic HCV, an increase in ALT and AST ranges from 1–20 times the upper limits.

  3. Bilirubin: A byproduct of the normal breakdown of RBCs in the liver

   a) If the liver is damaged, bilirubin levels rise in the bloodstream and may cause jaundice.

   b) Total bilirubin is all the bilirubin in the blood, whereas direct bilirubin measures only the bilirubin that has been processed by the liver and attached to other chemicals.

  4. Prothrombin: Protein made by the liver that contributes to blood clotting; typically normal in acute hepatitis and prolonged with more severe liver necrosis and fulminant hepatic failure

  5. SPEP: Hypergammaglobulinemia with autoimmune hepatitis

B. Radiology: To identify fatty infiltration of the liver, imaging (e.g., ultrasound, MRI, CT) may be useful to evaluate for obstructions but does not identify inflammation of the liver.

C. Other: Liver biopsy generally is not necessary in acute hepatitis but is indicated in the following situations.

  1. When the patient has severe or fulminant hepatitis to assess extent of disease and whether transplantation is urgently needed

  2. When diagnosis is not clear despite clinical and serologic data

  3. If more than one explanation of acute hepatitis is considered, particularly in patients with a significant history of alcohol use

V. Differential diagnosis: Includes infectious as well as noninfectious hepatitis (Kwong et al., 2019)

   A. Bacterial infections: Pneumococcal pneumonia

   B. Viral infections

      1. Hepatitis A–G

      2. CMV

      3. Epstein-Barr virus

      4. HSV

      5. VZV

      6. Rubella

      7. Rubeola (measles)

      8. Coxsackievirus

      9. Adenovirus

      10. Yellow fever

   C. Drug or toxin induced

      1. Acetaminophen

      2. Over-the-counter pain and fever medications: NSAIDs, ASA

      3. Chlorpromazine

      4. Halothane

      5. Methotrexate

      6. Isoniazid

      7. Phenytoin

      8. Methyldopa

      9. Inhaled anesthetics

      10. Phenothiazine

      11. Immune checkpoint inhibitors: CTLA-4, PD-1, PD-L1, monoclonal antibodies

   D. Autoimmune hepatitis

   E. Cancer of the liver or metastasis

   F. Radiation hepatitis with doses greater than 2,500 cGy to the liver

   G. Reactivation of hepatitis from cancer therapy: Rituximab

   H. Alcoholic hepatitis

VI. Prevention (Abara et al., 2017; Angelidakis et al., 2018; CDC, 2020; Doshani et al., 2019; Ezeanolue et al., 2017; Hwang et al., 2015; Schillie et al., 2018)

   A. Vaccine recommendations

      1. Hepatitis A vaccine: 1 ml IM

         a) Typically administered in two doses, six months apart

         b) Effective four weeks after receiving vaccine

         c) Booster given a minimum of six months later

         d) Individuals to immunize

            (1) All people who wish to achieve immunity from HAV

            (2) Travelers or workers traveling to countries where HAV is common

            (3) People who have chronic liver disease; use IV or non-IV drugs; or are homosexuals

            (4) People who receive clotting-factor concentrates; work with HAV in experimental laboratory settings; or food handlers when health authorities or private employers determine vaccination to be appropriate

            (5) People who anticipate close personal contact with an international adoptee from a country of high or intermediate endemicity during the first 60 days following the adoptee's arrival in the United States

(6) Adults aged 40 years or younger with recent (within two weeks) exposure to HAV; for adults older than 40 years with recent exposure to HAV (within two weeks), Ig is preferred over HAV vaccine.

2. Hepatitis B vaccine: 1 ml IM
   a) Typically given in three doses: Initially, one month later, and six months later
   b) Given IM into the arm
   c) Individuals to immunize
      (1) All people who wish to achieve immunity from HBV
      (2) All infants and adolescents not yet vaccinated
      (3) Household and sexual partners of people who are HBsAg–positive
      (4) IV drug users; sexually active people with multiple sexual partners
      (5) Homosexuals
      (6) People with HIV
      (7) People seeking STI evaluation or treatment
      (8) Hemodialysis patients and those with renal disease that may result in dialysis
      (9) Healthcare personnel and public safety workers who may be exposed to blood
      (10) Clients and staff of institutions for the developmentally disabled
      (11) Inmates of long-term prisons
      (12) International travelers to certain regions (e.g., Africa, Asia, South America)
      (13) People with chronic liver disease

3. All patients should be screened for HBsAg by a sensitive method before the start of immunosuppressive therapy.
   a) HBcAg and anti-HBs testing should be performed in patients who are HBsAg–negative and will receive intensive immunosuppressive therapy.
   b) Prophylaxis with a nucleoside analog, such as lamivudine 100 mg PO daily, is essential for prevention of HBV reactivation in patients who are HBsAg–positive.

B. Management of close contacts of people with HAV
   1. HAV vaccine 1 ml IM (Havrix® or Vaqta®) should be given for postexposure prophylaxis and administered concurrently with Ig at a separate anatomic injection site.
   2. Ig given 0.02 mg/kg of body weight IM is recommended as soon as possible after exposure. Use of Ig after more than two weeks after exposure is not indicated.

C. Management of individuals exposed to HBV (see Table 74-2)
   1. For immediate management, wash with soap and water, apply disinfectant to puncture wounds and cutaneous injuries, and flush exposed mucous membrane with copious amounts of water/saline.
   2. Draw blood to determine HBV antibody status, if unknown. It is not necessary to do further testing on individuals who have had a known positive antibody response following a series of three doses of vaccine.
   3. Hepatitis B Ig (HBIg) should be given for prophylactic treatment to exposed susceptible individuals.
      a) Give 0.06 ml/kg IM as a single dose for adults as soon as possible within 24 hours of a high-risk exposure. It can be given in conjunction with HBV but at different anatomical sites.
      b) Initiate HBV vaccine series.
   4. HBV vaccine is typically administered IM in three doses (initially, one month later, and six months later) into the deltoid muscle.

TABLE 74-2	Recommended Postexposure Prophylaxis for Hepatitis B Virus		
Vaccination and Antibody Response Status of Exposed Person[a]	**Treatment**		
	Source HBsAg[b] Positive	**Source HBsAg[b] Negative**	**Source Unknown or Not Available for Testing**
Unvaccinated	HBIG[c] × 1 and initiate HB vaccine series[d]	Initiate HB vaccine series	Initiate HB vaccine series
Previously vaccinated			
• Known responder[e]	No treatment	No treatment	No treatment
• Known nonresponder[f]	HBIG × 1 and initiate revaccination or HBIG × 2[g]	No treatment	If known high risk source, treat as if source were HBsAg positive
• Antibody response unknown	Test exposed person for anti-HBs[h] 1. If adequate,[e] no treatment is necessary 2. If inadequate,[f] HBIG × 1 and HB vaccine booster	No treatment	Test exposed person for anti-HBs 1. If adequate,[d] no treatment is necessary 2. If inadequate,[d] administer vaccine booster and recheck titer in 1–2 months

[a]Persons who have previously been infected with HBV are immune to reinfection and do not require postexposure prophylaxis.

[b]Hepatitis B surface antigen.

[c]Hepatitis B immune globulin; dose is 0.06 mL/kg intramuscularly.

[d]Hepatitis B vaccine.

[e]A responder is a person with adequate levels of serum antibody to HBsAg (i.e., anti-HBs >10 mIU/mL).

[f]A nonresponder is a person with inadequate response to vaccination (i.e., serum anti-HBs < 10 mIU/mL).

[g]The option of giving one dose of HBIG and reinitiating the vaccine series is preferred for nonresponders who have not completed a second 3-dose vaccine series. For persons who previously completed a second vaccine series but failed to respond, two doses of HBIG are preferred.

[h]Antibody to HBsAg.

HB—hepatitis B; HBIG—hepatitis B immunoglobulin; HBsAg—hepatitis B surface antigen

Note. From "Updated U.S. Public Health Service Guidelines for the Management of Occupational Exposures to HBV, HCV, and HIV and Recommendations for Postexposure Prophylaxis," by Centers for Disease Control and Prevention, 2014, *MMWR Recommendations and Reports, 50*(RR-11), p. 22. https://npin.cdc.gov/publication/mmwr-updated-us-public -health-service-guidelines-management-occupational-exposures-hbv.

VII. Treatment: Current guidelines, diagnostic workup, and management of HBV continue to evolve, and clinicians are urged to refer to the most current recommendations from CDC (www.cdc.gov/hepatitis/index.htm) (Mohsen & Levy, 2017; Pozza et al., 2017; Terrault et al., 2018; Thuener, 2017; Wahid, 2020; Yurdaydin, 2017).

    A. All individuals on chemotherapy and immunosuppressive therapy should be evaluated for HBV, and a determination should be made for treatment or prophylaxis, especially if they are at high risk of HBV reactivation.

        1. Testing should include HBsAg, anti-HBs, and anti-HBc.

        2. Dose modifications must be calculated for hepatic and renal impairment. Ongoing evaluation of the patient's current medications is required, and limit those metabolized in the liver.

    B. Seven FDA-approved drugs are now available to treat patients living with HBV. Five are administered orally. Almost 90% of patients with HBV treated with one of the new oral medications achieve viral suppression.

1. IFN-α: Subcutaneous several times a week for six months to a year
2. Pegylated IFN: 180 mcg once a week via subcutaneous injection for six months to a year
3. Lamivudine: 100 mg PO daily for one year or longer
4. Adefovir dipivoxil: 10 mg PO daily for one year or longer
5. Entecavir: 0.5 mg PO daily for at least one year
6. Telbivudine: 600 mg PO daily for at least one year
7. Tenofovir: 300 mg PO daily for at least one year
8. Tenofovir alafenamide: 25 mg PO daily with food for at least one year
9. Antidepressants: Should be initiated with the use of IFN because depression is a major side effect (see Appendix L)

C. For patients with HCV, the standard of care since 2015 is a combination of direct-acting antiviral drugs. Sofosbuvir, daclatasvir, and sofosbuvir/ledipasvir combination are part of preferred regimens. This new regimen may reduce the required length of treatment, improve response rates, and allow for IFN-free regimens for some HCV genotypes.

   1. Previous treatment regimens consist of a long-acting IFN injection combined with oral doses of ribavirin. With this regimen, almost one-half of patients achieve eradication of the infection.

   2. The use of HCV antiviral regimens should be managed ideally in consultation with a specialist. For each HCV genotype, multiple approved regimens are available.

     a) Patient adherence is critical to successful treatment of HCV.

     b) Drug resistance may develop over time.

     c) Pegasys® IFN monotherapy: 180 mcg subcutaneous once weekly for 48 weeks; IFN as monotherapy: 9 mcg subcutaneous three times a week for 24 weeks

     d) Ribavirin (often given with IFN): 800–1,200 mg PO, based on body weight, in two divided doses taken with food

D. No specific treatment exists for HAV. The body typically clears the virus on its own. In most cases, the liver heals completely in a month or two without damage. Supportive care is prescribed to control symptoms of fatigue, nausea, and loss of appetite.

E. Pegylated IFN-α remains the only drug currently used for the treatment of HDV infection and has not been shown to be highly effective. Only patients with compensated HDV-associated liver disease should be considered for treatment with IFN-α. HDV treatment is focused on dealing with symptoms or complications of the virus.

   1. Most people recover completely within a few months. Chronic HDV can develop, leading to liver damage or liver cancer.

   2. Although no specific regimens or drugs are approved to treat chronic HDV, liver transplantation is the only therapeutic choice for individuals with decompensation liver disease or advanced liver disease.

   3. HDV only occurs as a coinfection with HBV, so HBV immunization will prevent HDV.

F. Management of HEV is focused on prevention, relying on clean drinking water, good sanitation, and proper personal hygiene. The virus is generally self-limiting and resolves within two to six weeks.

   1. Travelers to endemic areas should avoid drinking water or other beverages that may be contaminated and should avoid eating uncooked shellfish.

   2. Care should be taken in the preparation of uncooked fruits or vegetables.

   3. No specific treatment exists for HEV.

G. For more than three decades, corticosteroids, either alone or in combination with azathioprine (75–100 mg PO daily), have been the mainstay drug therapy for patients with autoimmune hepatitis.

H. In most patients with alcoholic hepatitis, the illness is mild. No specific treatment is required except alcohol abstinence. Ensure good nutrition and supplemental vitamins, including folate and thiamine. For severe damage, see Chapter 69 on cirrhosis.

I. Immune checkpoint inhibitor–induced hepatitis is treated with corticosteroid therapy. Mycophenolate mofetil can be used for steroid-refractory cases.

VIII. Follow-up
  A. Short term
    1. Monitor LFTs during the acute phase regularly and specifically for three to six months.
    2. Monitor ALT, AST, alkaline phosphatase, bilirubin levels, and PT one or two times weekly and every one to two weeks until normal.
    3. Provide education for prevention of transmission and good health maintenance.
      a) Refrain from donating blood, organs, tissues, or semen.
      b) Practice safe sex.
      c) Refrain from sharing razors and toothbrushes.
    4. Monitor CBC and ALT monthly while on IFN or ribavirin.
    5. Monitor for depression two to four weeks after beginning IFN therapy.
  B. Long term
    1. HAV is typically a self-limiting disease. Monitor older adult patients for acute liver failure.
    2. HBV
      a) If HBsAg is positive, repeat every one to two months until it is undetectable.
      b) HBeAg is requested when HBsAg is positive. This indicates a high likelihood of infectivity.
      c) The presence of HBsAg and HBeAg four to six months after acute disease indicates chronic carrier state.
    3. HCV
      a) When serology for HCV is negative initially, recheck antibodies in six months. If positive, conduct further follow-up to rule out chronic HCV.
      b) To confirm a positive anti-HCV, conduct a follow-up HCV RNA.
      c) HAV and HBV vaccination is recommended for all HCV-positive patients.
    4. Monitor for chronic liver damage and the development of liver carcinoma.

IX. Referrals: Upon positive serology or persistent abnormal LFTs
  A. Infectious disease specialist: To develop treatment plan
  B. Gastroenterologist/hepatologist: To perform liver biopsy and to consider liver transplantation
  C. Public health departments: For reportable disease
  D. CDC Advisory Committee on Immunization Practices

The author would like to acknowledge Gayle K. Gilmore, RN, MA, MIS, for her contribution to this chapter that remains unchanged from the previous edition of this book.

References

Abara, W.E., Qaseem, A., Schillie, S., McMahon, B.J., & Harris, A.M. (2017). Hepatitis B vaccination, screening, and linkage to care: Best practice advice from the American College of Physicians and the Centers for Disease Control and Prevention. *Annals of Internal Medicine, 167*(11), 794–804. https://doi.org/10.7326/M17-1106

Angelidakis, G., Hwang, J.P., Dandachi, D., Economides, M.P., Hosry, J., Granwehr, B.P., & Torres, H.A. (2018). Universal screening for hepatitis C: A needed approach in patients with haematologic malignancies. *Journal of Viral Hepatitis, 25*(9), 1102–1104. https://doi.org/10.1111/jvh.12913

Centers for Disease Control and Prevention. (2020). The ABCs of hepatitis—For health professionals. http://www.cdc.gov/hepatitis/Resources/Professionals/PDFs/ABCTable.pdf

Doshani, M., Weng, M., Moore, K.L., Romero, J.R., & Nelson, N.P. (2019). Recommendations of the Advisory Committee on Immunization Practices for use of hepatitis A vaccine for persons experiencing homelessness. *Morbidity and Mortality Weekly Report, 68*(6), 153–156. https://doi.org/10.15585/mmwr.mm6806a6

Ezeanolue, E., Harriman, K., Hunter, P., Kroger, A.T., & Pellegrini, C. (2017). *General best practice guidelines for immunization: Best practices guidance of the Advisory Committee on Immunization Practices (ACIP).* https://www.cdc.gov/vaccines/hcp/acip-recs/general-recs/index.html

Hwang, J.P., Somerfield, M.R., Alston-Johnson, D.E., Cryer, D.R., Feld, J.J., Kramer, B.S., ... Artz, A.S. (2015). Hepatitis B virus screening for patients with cancer before therapy: American Society of Clinical Oncology provisional clinical opinion update. *Journal of Clinical Oncology, 33*(19), 2212–2220. https://doi.org/10.1200/JCO.2015.61.3745.

Kwong, S., Meyerson, C., Zheng, W., Kassardjian, W.A., Stanzione, N., Zhang, K., & Wang, H.L. (2019). Acute hepatitis and acute liver failure: Pathologic diagnosis and differential diagnosis. *Seminars in Diagnostic Pathology, 36*(6), 404–414. https://doi.org/10.1053/j.semdp.2019.07.005

Mohsen, W., & Levy, M.T. (2017). Hepatitis A to E: What's new? *Internal Medicine Journal, 47*(4), 380–389. https://doi.org/10.1111/imj.13386

Pozza, R., Hill, C., Hefner, A.M., Vawter, B., & Hassanein, T. (2017). Hepatitis C infection: Updates on treatment guidelines. *Nurse Practitioner, 42*(5), 14–23. https://doi.org/10.1097/01.npr.0000515423.38284.28

Schillie, S., Vellozzi, C., Reingold, A., Harris, A., Haber, P., Ward, J.W., & Nelson, N.P. (2018). Prevention of hepatitis B virus infection in the United States: Recommendations of the Advisory Committee on Immunization Practices. *MMWR Recommendations and Reports, 67*(1), 1–31. https://doi.org/10.15585/mmwr.rr6701a1

Shin, E.-C., & Jeong, S.-H. (2018). Natural history, clinical manifestations, and pathogenesis of hepatitis A. *Cold Spring Harbor Perspectives in Medicine, 8*(9), a031708 https://doi.org/10.1101/cshperspect.a031708

Soi, V., Daifi, C., Yee, J., & Adams, E. (2019). Pathophysiology and treatment of hepatitis B and C infections in patients with end-stage renal disease. *Advances in Chronic Kidney Disease, 26*(1), 41–50. https://doi.org/10.1053/j.ackd.2018.10.004

Terrault, N.A., Lok, A.S.F., McMahon, B.J., Chang, K.-M., Hwang, J.P., Jonas, M.M., ... Wong, J.B. (2018). Update on prevention, diagnosis, and treatment of chronic hepatitis B: AASLD 2018 hepatitis B guidance. *Hepatology, 67*(4), 1560–1599. https://doi.org/10.1002/hep.29800

Thuener, J. (2017). Hepatitis A and B infections. *Primary Care: Clinics in Office Practice, 44*(4), 621–629. https://doi.org/10.1016/j.pop.2017.07.005

Wahid, B. (2020). Successful treatment of HBV, HCV, & HEV with 12-week long use of tenofovir, sofosbuvir, daclatasvir, and ribavirin: A case report. *Journal of Infection and Public Health, 13*(1), 149–150. https://doi.org/10.1016/j.jiph.2019.06.004

Wilkins, T., Sams, R., & Carpenter, M. (2019). Hepatitis B: Screening, prevention, diagnosis, and treatment. *American Family Physician, 99*(5), 314–323. https://www.aafp.org/afp/2019/0301/p314.html

Yurdaydin, C. (2017). Recent advances in managing hepatitis D. *F1000Research, 6,* 1596. https://doi.org/10.12688/f1000research.11796.1

CHAPTER 75

Hepatotoxicity

Karen A. Roesser, MSN, RN, AOCNS®

I. Definition: Injury to the liver following inhalation, ingestion, or parenteral administration of pharmacologic or chemical agents, including herbal or dietary supplements; results in distortion of normal liver architecture that may affect liver function (Shehu et al., 2017)

II. Physiology/Pathophysiology (O'Brien et al., 2015; Ramadori et al., 2008; Su et al., 2019)
   A. Normal
      1. Metabolic functions of the liver
         a) Carbohydrate metabolism: Maintains blood glucose levels, provides energy for cells, stores excess carbohydrates as glycogen and fat
         b) Fat metabolism: Synthesizes and degrades fats to fatty acids; synthesizes and degrades triglycerides, cholesterol, phospholipids, and lipoproteins; forms bile salts through metabolism of cholesterol
         c) Protein metabolism: Synthesizes and releases plasma proteins and enzymes, oxidizes amino acids, converts ammonia to urea, synthesizes blood clotting factors (e.g., I, II, V, VII, IX, X)
         d) Transforms drugs into active metabolites or harmless substances for excretion
         e) Synthesizes hormones and cytokines (e.g., IL-8, IL-6) and plays a role in endocrine function and sex hormone metabolism (e.g., insulin-like growth factor 1, thrombopoietin, EPO)
         f) Plays significant role in the breakdown of heme; receives unconjugated bilirubin bound to albumin, which undergoes conjugation to become hydrophilic
      2. Normal filtration functions: Kupffer cells are specialized macrophages of the liver and remove bacteria, antigens, by-products of coagulation, and other harmful substances from the blood.
      3. Normal storage functions
         a) Sinusoids hold blood for shunting into general circulation.
         b) The liver stores and/or metabolizes the fat-soluble vitamins (e.g., A, D, E) and the water-soluble vitamin B_{12}. Although vitamin K is not stored or metabolized in the liver, it is essential for coagulation factors II, VII, IX, and X and proteins C and S.
         c) The liver stores copper and iron minerals.
      4. Normal excretion of bilirubin
         a) After formation in reticuloendothelial cells, bilirubin is bound to albumin and transported to the liver, conjugated, and excreted into the bile.
         b) Bilirubin is then excreted via the biliary tree into the small intestine.
         c) Intestinal bacteria reduce conjugated bilirubin into urobilinogen, which is excreted in stool or urine or reabsorbed into portal blood.

B. Pathophysiology
  1. Pathologic changes of the liver are broadly categorized as neoplastic, inflammatory, fibrotic, or necrotic.
     a) Cirrhosis represents an advanced stage of fibrosis resulting in liver failure and portal hypertension often requiring liver transplantation.
     b) Hepatotoxicity may lead to acute or chronic liver diseases.
  2. Damage to hepatocytes
     a) Leads to impaired metabolism and elimination of bilirubin
     b) Depresses synthesis of factors I, II, V, VII, IX, and X
     c) Diminishes glucose synthesis
     d) Decreases lactate uptake or increases intracellular lactate generation
     e) Triggers hepatocellular injury from direct toxin effects or as an idiosyncratic reaction

III. Clinical features: Clinical presentation varies widely and can mimic other forms of acute and chronic liver disease (Ahmad & Odin, 2017; Fisher et al., 2015; García-Cortés et al., 2016; Shehu et al., 2017).
  A. Risk factors
     1. Alcohol use
     2. Drugs known to cause hepatotoxicity
     3. Age older than 55 years
     4. Obesity
     5. Hepatitis, especially C
     6. Genetic polymorphism of cytochrome P450 isoenzyme resulting in cytochrome P450 enzyme induction or inhibition
     7. More common in women
     8. History of HIV/AIDS
     9. Malnourishment
     10. African Americans and Hispanics more susceptible to isoniazid toxicity
     11. Long-acting drugs
  B. Etiology
     1. Drug-induced liver injury
        a) Intrinsic-predictable: Dose-dependent manner
        b) Idiosyncratic drug-induced liver injury: Unpredictable, non-dose-dependent manner
     2. Herbal and dietary supplements
        a) Illicit anabolic steroids for bodybuilding
        b) Green tea extracts
        c) Vitamin A
        d) Linoleic acid
        e) Products sold for weight loss: Herbalife®, Hydroxycut®, ma huang extract, garcinia cambogia
     3. Cirrhosis: Result of prolonged liver injury
     4. Mechanisms causing elevated bilirubin
        a) Overproduction of bilirubin
        b) Reduction in hepatic uptake or conjugation; impairment of cytochrome P450 activity
        c) Decreased biliary excretion
           (1) By cell mechanisms: Intrahepatic cholestasis
           (2) By duct obstruction: Extrahepatic cholestasis

C. History
1. History of cancer and cancer treatment
2. Current medications: Prescribed, over the counter, with particular attention to drugs associated with hepatotoxicity (e.g., herbal and other dietary supplements)
3. History of presenting symptoms: Precipitating factors, onset (including with new medications), location, duration
4. Changes in ADLs
5. Past medical history: Organ transplantation, hepatitis, exposure to hepatitis-infected individuals, recent episodes of hypotension
6. Social history: Alcohol use, illicit (recreational) drug use, recent foreign travel
7. Family history: Hereditary liver diseases

D. Signs and symptoms
1. Varying degrees of jaundice
2. Varying color changes in urine and stool
3. Pruritus
4. Edema
5. Ecchymosis
6. Malaise: Anorexia, fatigue, headache, muscle and joint aches, and low-grade fever suggesting hepatitis

E. Physical examination
1. Vital signs: Fever suggestive of hepatitis
2. Integument
   a) Jaundice
   b) Ecchymosis, petechiae
   c) Skin rash: Stevens-Johnson syndrome or Lyell syndrome suggestive of drug hypersensitivity
3. HEENT: Icteric sclera
4. Neurologic: Altered behavior, level of orientation, mental status, asterixis
5. Cardiac and pulmonary: Signs of CHF (e.g., peripheral edema, extra heart sounds, rales, jugular venous distention—may suggest hepatic congestion)
6. Abdominal
   a) Tenderness: Represents inflammation, especially right upper quadrant pain; severe right upper quadrant tenderness with respiratory arrest on inspiration (Murphy sign) suggestive of cholecystitis or occasionally ascending cholangitis (see Appendix D)
   b) Decreased bowel sounds suggestive of obstruction, ileus
   c) Hepatomegaly suggestive of liver disease
   d) Splenomegaly: Palpated in cirrhosis
   e) Ascites: Cirrhosis or malignancy with peritoneal spread
   f) Abdominal venous distention: Spider angiomas and portal hypertension
   g) Palpable gallbladder: Known as Courvoisier sign; indicates CBD obstruction
   h) Charcot triad: Fever, jaundice, and right upper quadrant pain indicating gallstones

IV. Diagnostic tests (Goodman, 2017; Kullak-Ublick et al., 2017; Zimmerman, 1968)
   A. Laboratory: No single gold standard test is available for drug-induced hepatotoxicity; however, proposed thresholds have been established (see Table 75-1).
      1. Serum aminotransferase: Elevated levels indicate liver injury from either cell necrosis or increased cell permeability.

TABLE 75-1	Thresholds for Diagnosis of Drug-Induced Liver Injury
Laboratory Test	**Laboratory Value**
ALT	≥ 5 × ULN
Alkaline phosphatase	≥ 2 × ULN
ALT + total bilirubin	ALT ≥ 3 × ULN + total bilirubin ≥ 2 × ULN[a]

[a]Referred to as Hy's Law, which anticipates a 10% risk of mortality/liver transplantation

ALT— alanine aminotransferase; ULN—upper limit of normal

Note. Based on information from Kullak-Ublick et al., 2017; Zimmerman, 1968.

a) ALT: It is a specific indicator of liver damage, primarily localized to the liver, with lower enzymatic activities found in skeletal muscle and heart tissue.

b) AST: It is generally sensitive for liver disease. Elevation of AST is often greater than ALT in alcohol-related liver disease. AST is localized in the heart, brain, skeletal muscle, and liver tissue and released from damaged myocytes, as well as hepatocytes. The ratio of serum AST to ALT can be used to differentiate liver damage from other organ damage.

2. Alkaline phosphatase: It is released by disorders affecting the bile duct; markedly elevated levels reflect hepatotoxicity, cholestasis (especially drug-induced cholestasis), and extrahepatic and intrahepatic obstruction. If elevated, alkaline phosphatase isoenzymes may be ordered to determine the etiology of the elevation (e.g., bone, liver, intestine).

3. Gamma-glutamyl transferase: It is marker of hepatobiliary injury, especially cholestasis and biliary effects, but lacks specificity. Gamma-glutamyl transferase may be used in conjunction with alkaline phosphatase to distinguish liver origin from bone.

4. Serum bilirubin

   a) Total bilirubin is a composite of indirect (nonhepatic) and direct (hepatic) bilirubin and is a product of Hgb degradation and a marker of hepatobiliary injury, especially cholestasis and biliary effects. In acute hepatic injury, total bilirubin can be a better indicator of disease.

   b) Elevated indirect (unconjugated) bilirubin indicates liver damage and is seen in hemolytic anemia, congenital enzyme deficiencies, and severe chronic hepatic damage. Unconjugated hyperbilirubinemia (greater than 80% of the total bilirubin is indirect) suggests hemolysis or Gilbert syndrome.

   c) Elevated direct (conjugated) bilirubin reflects excess amounts excreted into serum from obstruction of bile ducts as seen in viral hepatitis, cirrhosis, obstruction to bile flow (e.g., gallstones, cancer of the head of the pancreas or ampulla of Vater), and drug-induced hepatotoxicity. Conjugated hyperbilirubinemia (greater than 50% of the total bilirubin is direct) suggests hepatocellular dysfunction or cholestasis.

5. PT: A PT greater than 1.5 indicates either vitamin K deficiency caused by prolonged jaundice and malabsorption of vitamin K or significant hepatocellular dysfunction. Failure to correct with parenteral administration of vitamin K indicates severe hepatocellular injury.

6. Albumin: Low level suggests a chronic process, such as cirrhosis or cancer; normal level suggests an acute process, such as viral hepatitis or choledocholithiasis.

   7. Viral hepatitis screening, as indicated
   8. CBC: Assessment for peripheral eosinophilia (with fever and rash, suggests drug allergy), granulocytopenia, thrombocytopenia, or hemolytic anemia
B. Radiology
   1. Abdominal ultrasound: Determines the size of the hepatobiliary tree and any evidence of mechanical biliary obstruction and reveals intra- or extrahepatic lesions and gallstones; may not be useful in obese patients or those with underlying bowel gas
   2. CT scan of the abdomen: Shows dilated bile ducts and assesses soft abdominal masses, pancreatic lesions, and other space-occupying lesions
   3. MRI of the abdomen: More sensitive than CT in differentiating metastasis, hemangiomas, hepatomas, and other liver lesions
   4. Percutaneous transvenous coronary angioplasty: Visualizes the biliary tree; indicated to evaluate obstruction when ultrasound and CT scan are positive
   5. Endoscopic retrograde cholangiopancreatography: Best to visualize the biliary tree in patients with obstruction
   6. Hepatobiliary iminodiacetic acid scan: Evaluates gallbladder disease by means of nuclear imaging
   7. Angiography: Rarely used but helpful in patients with portal hypertension
C. Other
   1. Liver biopsy is useful in identifying the cause of hepatic injury, as well as the pathology of masses or lesions identified by other imaging methods.
   2. A clinical scale such as the Roussel Uclaf Causality Assessment Method (RUCAM) scale and/or the Maria and Victorino criteria may be used to establish a causal relationship between the suspected offending drug and liver damage if suspected drug-induced or herb-induced liver injury (see Table 75-2).

V. Differential diagnosis (Kleiner, 2017; Kullak-Ublick et al., 2017)
A. Portal and hepatic circulation disturbances
   1. Portal hypertension
   2. Budd-Chiari syndrome: Thrombosis of hepatic vein
   3. CHF (see Chapter 42)
   4. Veno-occlusive disease
B. Hepatobiliary tract disorders
   1. Primary biliary cirrhosis (see Chapter 69)
   2. Primary sclerosing cholangitis
   3. Wilson disease: Inherited disorder of metabolism creating copper overload
   4. Malignancy
   5. Cholecystitis (see Chapter 68)
C. Hepatocellular disturbances
   1. Hepatitis (see Chapter 74)
   2. Cirrhosis (see Chapter 69)
   3. Alpha-1-antitrypsin deficiency
   4. Hemochromatosis (see Chapter 121)
   5. Hepatic failure
   6. Reye syndrome
   7. Diabetes mellitus (see Chapter 151)
   8. Coagulation disorders (see Chapter 122)
   9. Pregnancy-related conditions of liver
   10. Shock liver: Hepatic ischemia

| TABLE 75-2 | Roussel Uclaf Causality Assessment Method Scale |

	Type of Liver Injury				
Criteria	Hepatocellular		Points	Cholestatic/Mixed		Points
Time of onset of the event	First exposure	Rechallenge	–	First exposure	Rechallenge	–
Time from drug intake until reaction onset	5–90 days	1–15 days	+2	5–90 days	1–90 days	+2
	< 5 or > 90 days	> 15 days	+1	< 5 or > 90 days	> 90 days	+1
Time from drug withdrawal until reaction onset	≤ 15 days	≤ 15 days	+1	≤ 30 days	≤ 30 days	+1
Risk factors	Alcohol use (> 2 days in women; > 3 days in men)		+1	Alcohol use or pregnancy		+1
	Age ≥ 55 years		+1	Age ≥ 55 years		+1
Course of the reaction Percentage difference between alanine transaminase peak and upper limit of normal	≥ 50% improvement in 8 days		+3	–		
	≥ 50% improvement in 30 days		+2	≥ 50% improvement in 180 days		+2
	Lack of information or no improvement Decreased ≥ 50% after 30 days +0		+0	Lack of information or no improvement		+0
	Decreased < 50% after 30th day or Recurrent increase		-2	Decreased < 50% in 180 days		+1

Score Analysis
≤ 0: Relationship with the drug excluded
1–2: Unlikely
3–5: Possible
6–7: Probable
≥ 8: Highly likely

Note. Based on information from Danan & Teschke, 2016; Kullak-Ublick et al., 2017.

D. Drug induced: Any hepatotoxic drugs are included. Prescribed drugs account for greater than 50% of cases of acute liver failure.
   1. Acetaminophen: Represents the majority of drug-induced acute liver failure
   2. Anesthetics: Halothane
   3. Anti-TB drugs: Isoniazid, rifampin
   4. Antidiabetic agents: Oral sulfonylureas
   5. Anticonvulsants: Phenytoin, valproic acid
   6. Antibiotics: Amoxicillin/clavulanate, ciprofloxacin, erythromycin, sulfonamides
   7. Antipsychotics: Chlorpromazine
   8. Antivirals: Ritonavir, indinavir
   9. Antidepressants

        a) Serotonin-norepinephrine reuptake inhibitors: Duloxetine

        b) Tricyclics

10. Hormonal agents: Estrogens, antiestrogens
11. Cholesterol-lowering agents: Niacin, statins
12. Chemotherapy: Vinca alkaloids, taxanes, regorafenib
13. Cardiovascular agents: Methyldopa, amiodarone
14. Immunotherapy: IFN-β1a
15. Antifungals: Fluconazole, ketoconazole, itraconazole, posaconazole, voriconazole
16. NSAIDs (see Appendix E)
17. Herbal agents: Hepatotoxicity is one of the most frequently reported side effects of complementary and alternative medicine products, such as green teas, valerian root, ma huang ephedra alkaloid (a weight loss agent), mistletoe, and kava products.

VI. Treatment (Andrade et al., 2019; Fisher et al., 2015)
   A. If drug induced, discontinue offending agent.
   B. Treatment is based on specific irritant to the liver and is largely supportive based on symptomatology.
   C. Observe presenting symptoms and correlate to the degree of toxicity.
   D. Reevaluate medications PRN and exchange for a different class that has either less or no potential for hepatotoxicity.
   E. Consider liver transplantation in select situations, typically with idiosyncratic drug reaction that causes acute liver failure.

VII. Follow-up
   A. Monitor laboratory values at periodic intervals until they begin to normalize or have normalized.
   B. Manage symptoms until complete resolution of toxicity.
   C. Mild symptoms may resolve if offending agent is removed. Persistent symptoms and abnormal laboratory values indicate need for further workup.

VIII. Referrals
   A. Gastroenterologist: For initial consult
   B. Hepatologist: For more clinical complex scenarios requiring expertise

References

Ahmad, J., & Odin, J.A. (2017). Epidemiology and genetic risk factors of drug hepatotoxicity. *Clinics in Liver Disease, 21*(1), 55–72. https://doi.org/10.1016/j.cld.2016.08.004

Andrade, R.J., Chalasani, N., Björnsson, E.S., Suzuki, A., Kullak-Ublick, G.A., Watkins, P.B., ... Aithal, G.P. (2019). Drug-induced liver injury. *Nature Reviews Disease Primers, 5*(1), 58. https://doi.org/10.1038/s41572-019-0105-0

Danan, G., & Teschke, R. (2016). RUCAM in drug and herb induced liver injury: The update. *International Journal of Molecular Sciences, 17*(1), 14. https://doi.org/10.3390/ijms17010014

Fisher, K., Vuppalanchi, R., & Saxena, R. (2015). Drug-induced liver injury. *Archives of Pathology and Laboratory Medicine, 139*(7), 876–887. https://doi.org/10.5858/arpa.2014-0214-RA

García-Cortés, M., Robles-Díaz, M., Ortega-Alonso, A., Medina-Caliz, I., & Andrade, R.J. (2016). Hepatotoxicity by dietary supplements: A tabular listing and clinical characteristics. *International Journal of Molecular Sciences, 17*(4), 537. https://doi.org/10.3390/ijms17040537

Goodman, Z.D. (2017). Phenotypes and pathology of drug-induced liver disease. *Clinics in Liver Disease, 21*(1), 89–101. https://doi.org/10.1016/j.cld.2016.08.006

Kleiner, D.E. (2017). Drug-induced liver injury: The hepatic pathologist's approach. *Gastroenterology Clinics of North America, 46*(2), 273–296. https://doi.org/10.1016/j.gtc.2017.01.004

Kullak-Ublick, G.A., Andrade, R.J., Merz, M., End, P., Benesic, A., Gerbes, A.L., & Aithal, G.P. (2017). Drug-induced liver injury: Recent advances in diagnosis and risk assessment. *Gut, 66*(6), 1154–1164. https://doi.org/10.1136/gutjnl-2016-313369

O'Brien, L., Hosick, P.A., John, K., Stec, D.E., & Hinds, T.D., Jr. (2015). Biliverdin reductase isozymes in metabolism. *Trends in Endocrinology and Metabolism, 26*(4), 212–220. https://doi.org/10.1016/j.tem.2015.02.001

Ramadori, G., Moriconi, F., Malik, I., & Dudas, J. (2008). Physiology and pathophysiology of liver inflammation, damage and repair. *Journal of Physiology and Pharmacology, 59*(Suppl. 1), 107–117.

Shehu, A.I., Ma, X., & Venkataramanan, R. (2017). Mechanisms of drug-induced hepatotoxicity. *Clinics in Liver Disease, 21*(1), 35–54. https://doi.org/10.1016/j.cld.2016.08.002

Su, W., Mao, Z., Liu, Y., Zhang, X., Zhang, W., Gustafsson, J.-A., & Guan, Y. (2019). Role of HSD17B13 in the liver physiology and pathophysiology. *Molecular and Cellular Endocrinology, 489,* 119–125. https://doi.org/10.1016/j.mce.2018.10.014

Zimmerman, H.J. (1968). The spectrum of hepatotoxicity. *Perspectives in Biology and Medicine, 12*(1), 135–161. https://doi.org/10.1353/pbm.1968.0004

CHAPTER 76

Irritable Bowel Syndrome

Kristina Mathey, MS, APRN–CNP, AOCNP®

I. Definition: A functional bowel disorder in which recurring abdominal pain is associated with a change in stool frequency or form (Ford et al., 2017; Nelkowska, 2020; Ooi et al., 2019)

II. Physiology/Pathophysiology (Defrees & Bailey, 2017; Ford et al., 2017; Harris & Baffy, 2017; Kim & Kim, 2018; Nelkowska, 2020)
   A. Normal
      1. Small intestines begin at the pyloric orifice, joining the large intestine at the ileocecal valve.
      2. The CBD and pancreatic duct open into the first section of the small intestine, referred to as the duodenum.
      3. The second section is the jejunum, and the third section is the ileum.
      4. The ileocecal valve between the ileum and large intestine prevents backflow of fecal material.
      5. Digestion is completed with pancreatic enzymes, bile, and the small intestine, where nutrients are absorbed through small intestine walls.
   B. Pathophysiology: A diverse disorder with many factors implicated in pathogenesis, which is still not clearly understood
      1. Immune-mediated factors alter gut function, such as infection of normal gut microbiota leading to postinfectious IBS.
      2. Alterations in the diversity of the normal gut microbiota, known as dysbiosis, specifically a decrease in *Lactobacillus* and *Bifidobacterium* species, can lead to activation of the immune system, leading to low-grade inflammation of the gut, which disrupts the gut–brain axis interaction.

III. Clinical features: IBS occurs more commonly in women than men; however, men may be underdiagnosed. Diagnosis is based on symptoms; no precise biomarker or diagnostic test exists. IBS often manifests in childhood, though peak prevalence is in early adulthood. Symptoms may arise or become aggravated by stress and anxiety (Basnayake, 2018; Defrees & Bailey, 2017; Ford et al., 2017; Harris & Baffy, 2017; Hellström & Benno, 2019; Lacy & Patel, 2017).
   A. Etiology: Studies have identified a combination of factors that contribute to the syndrome.
      1. Genetic, gut–brain dysregulation, hormonal influences, diet, and GI factors have been proposed as potential causes.
      2. IBS is common as a result of various interactions between genetic and environmental factors.
      3. Changes in the gut microbe and release of inflammatory mediators (cytokines or chemokines) may be responsible for CNS disorders that arise after development of IBS symptoms.

B. History
   1. History of cancer and cancer treatment
   2. Current medications: Prescribed, over the counter
   3. History of presenting symptoms: Precipitating factors, onset, duration, associated symptoms (e.g., abdominal pain [must be present for diagnosis], weight loss, fever, night sweats, nausea, vomiting)
   4. Changes in ADLs
   5. History of altered bowel habits: History of stool consistency, relief with defecation
   6. Social history: Dietary intake recall, current stress level
C. Signs and symptoms: Diagnosis is based on symptoms.
   1. Hallmark of IBS is abdominal pain relieved by defecation or change in stool consistency. The Bristol Stool Form Scale is a useful tool to help differentiate stool types (see www.ibscounsel.com/Diagnosis/BristolStool).
   2. According to the Rome IV criteria, IBS is defined as greater than or equal to three months of persistent symptoms with symptom onset at least six months before diagnosis occurring greater than or equal to one day per week and associated with two or more criteria.
      a) Related to defecation
      b) Associated with change in stool frequency
      c) Associated with change in stool appearance
   3. If patients meet Rome IV criteria with no alarm features, a positive diagnosis of IBS can be made without resorting to a battery of tests.
   4. Four IBS subtypes include diarrhea predominant (IBS-D), constipation predominant (IBS-C), mixed (IBS-M), or unspecified (IBS-U).
   5. Abdominal pain
      a) Poorly localized but often occurs in the lower abdomen
      b) May be initiated by or worsen with meals
      c) May be initiated or exacerbated by stress or anxiety
      d) May include bloating
      e) Does not awaken the patient from sleep
      f) May worsen with menses
   6. Other GI symptoms
      a) Indigestion
      b) Nausea
      c) Early satiety
      d) Intermittent dyspepsia
   7. Red flag symptoms (see Figure 76-1)
D. Physical examination
   1. Abdominal
      a) Normal bowel sounds
      b) Soft, nondistended abdomen
      c) Normal to slightly tympanic to percussion
      d) No tenderness or mild left lower quadrant tenderness on palpation
      e) No abdominal masses; tender, cord-like sigmoid present in the left lower quadrant
   2. Rectal: May have increased sensitivity to rectal examination, no rectal masses

IV. Diagnostic tests: No current biomarkers are available. Routine diagnostic testing is not recommended in patients with typical IBS symptoms and no red flag features (see Figure 76-1). Initial testing should be minimally invasive. In the case of red flag symptoms or

---

FIGURE 76-1   **Red Flags in Evaluating for Irritable Bowel Syndrome**

- Anemia
- Family history of colon cancer, inflammatory bowel disease, or celiac disease
- Fever
- Hemoccult-positive stools
- New or recent onset in people aged > 50 years
- Nighttime symptoms
- Palpable abdominal or rectal mass
- Persistent diarrhea or severe constipation
- Recent antibiotic use
- Rectal bleeding
- Travel to areas with parasitic diseases
- Weight loss

Note. Based on information from Ford et al., 2018; Lacy & Patel, 2017.

worsening symptoms, the following tests may be appropriate to assess for other etiologies (Barros et al., 2019; Basnayake, 2018; Bellini et al., 2020; Lacy et al., 2016; Lacy & Patel, 2017; Ooi et al., 2019).
   A. Laboratory
      1. CBC to evaluate for microcytic anemia
      2. Serologic testing to evaluate for celiac disease (e.g., tissue transglutaminase antibodies [tTG-IgA])
      3. CRP and faecal calprotectin level to evaluate for inflammation, elevation suggestive of inflammatory bowel disease
      4. Electrolytes to evaluate metabolic complications of diarrhea; hypokalemia can cause decreased bowel contractility and produce an ileus.
      5. Stool studies as indicated with diarrhea for culture and sensitivity, ova and parasites if recent travel, *Clostridium difficile* if recently on antibiotics
      6. Stool testing for occult blood
   B. Radiology: Abdominal film to evaluate for obstruction in IBS-C
   C. Other
      1. Sigmoidoscopy or colonoscopy: If patient age is older than 50 years with no previous colonoscopy; mass or lesion is suspected; fecal occult stool is positive; or for persistent diarrhea or constipation to evaluate for cancer, inflammatory bowel disease, or colitis
      2. Low fermentable, oligosaccharides, disaccharides, monosaccharides, and polyols (FODMAP) diet
      3. Psychological assessment if anxiety or depression is suspected as a cause of symptoms

V. Differential diagnosis (Barros et al., 2019; Defrees & Bailey, 2017)
   A. Malabsorption
      1. Food intolerance
      2. Lactose intolerance
      3. Bile acid malabsorption
      4. Exocrine pancreatic insufficiency
      5. Carbohydrate intolerance
   B. Functional disorders: Nonulcer dyspepsia (see Chapter 58)
   C. Organic disorders
      1. GERD (see Chapter 71)

    2. Peptic ulcer disease (see Chapter 78)

    3. Malignant lesions

    4. Inflammatory bowel disease

    5. Gallstones and biliary spasm

    6. Infectious diarrhea (See Chapter 56)

    7. Diverticulosis (see Chapter 70)

    8. Bowel obstruction (see Chapter 67)

    9. Diabetic autonomic neuropathy (see Chapter 151)

    10. Peripheral neuropathy (see Chapter 143)

    11. Celiac disease

    12. Microscopic colitis

    13. GI cancers

  D. Psychiatric disorders

    1. Anxiety (see Chapter 161)

    2. Depression (see Chapter 162)

    3. Somatization disorders

VI. Treatment: Treatment is primarily supportive with a large placebo effect. Establishing a trusting, therapeutic relationship with the patient is essential (Barros et al., 2019; Basnayake, 2018; Bellini et al., 2020; Defrees & Bailey, 2017; Ford et al., 2017; Ford et al., 2018; Kim & Kim, 2018; Nelkowska, 2020; Staudacher, 2017).

  A. Provide education and reassurance as to the benign nature of the disease and the overall lack of progression to a more serious condition.

  B. Use a 14-day diary to accurately characterize and categorize symptoms.

  C. Increase exercise and reduce daily stress.

  D. Dietary modifications

    1. Eat smaller, frequent meals.

    2. Avoid offending agents such as lactose, alcohol, caffeine, and foods that increase flatulence (e.g., beans, onions, celery, carrots, raisins, bananas, apricots, prunes, brussels sprouts, wheat germ, pretzels, bagels).

    3. Insoluble fibers are more likely to worsen abdominal pain and bloating; however, soluble fibers (e.g., psyllium) improve symptoms, especially in patients with constipation subtype.

    4. Low-FODMAP diet

      a) FODMAP foods contain short-chain carbohydrates and are poorly absorbed by the small intestine, leading to an osmotic effect in the colon with excess gas production, pain, and diarrhea. High-FODMAP diets are associated with dysbiosis, inflammation, barrier dysfunction, and visceral hypersensitivity.

      b) Patients with IBS-D should consider this diet, which eliminates many staple foods.

        (1) Carbohydrates and sugar alcohols occur in some foods naturally or as an additive.

        (2) Foods include fructose (e.g., fruits, vegetables), fructan (e.g., fructose found in some grains and vegetables), lactose (e.g., diary), galectins (e.g., legumes), and polyols (e.g., artificial sweetener).

      c) Dietary intervention involves FODMAP intake restriction for three to four weeks to test for symptom response. When symptom reduction is achieved, some FODMAP carbohydrates can be reintroduced individually to test for tolerance with the goal of long-term symptom control and a nutritionally adequate diet.

    d) This diet is guided by a qualified clinician or nutritionist.

E. Use of soluble fiber may relieve symptoms; however, data are limited.

    1. Psyllium: 1 teaspoon to 1 tablespoon PO three times a day

    2. Methylcellulose: 0.5–1 tablespoon PO three times a day

    3. Calcium polycarbophil: 1–2 tablets PO three times a day

F. Management of pain

    1. Antispasmodic agents have shown short-term benefit.

        a) Dicyclomine: 20–40 mg PO four times a day

        b) Hyoscyamine sulfate: 0.125–0.25 mg PO every four hours PRN

    2. Antidepressants may be beneficial because of the potential role of the brain–gut axis and abnormal central pain processing. Antidepressants manipulate visceral hypersensitivity and abnormal pain sensitization (see Appendix L).

        a) Tricyclic antidepressants: Most benefit for patients with IBS-D with known side effect of constipation

            (1) Amitriptyline: 10–50 mg PO at bedtime

            (2) Desipramine: 25–100 mg PO at bedtime

        b) SSRIs: Most benefit in patients with IBS-C with known side effect of diarrhea

            (1) Paroxetine: 10–40 mg PO daily

            (2) Sertraline: 25–100 mg PO daily

            (3) Citalopram: 10–40 mg PO daily

            (4) Escitalopram: 10–20 mg PO daily

            (5) Fluoxetine: 20–40 mg PO daily

G. Management of diarrhea (see Chapter 56)

    1. Loperamide: 4 mg PO initially, then 2 mg after each loose stool; maximum 16 mg; beneficial to take preprandial to decrease overall number of stools

    2. Bile salt sequestrants

        a) Cholestyramine: 9 g PO two or three times a day

        b) Colestipol: 2 g PO one or two times a day

    3. Eluxadoline: 100 mg PO two times a day

    4. 5-HT$_3$ antagonists: Alosetron 0.5–1 mg PO two times a day; only for women with severe IBS-D who have failed other treatments and meet conditions of an FDA-mandated physician–patient agreement; referral to a gastroenterologist and registry required

H. Management of constipation: Osmotic agents (see Chapter 55)

    1. Lactulose: 15–30 ml PO daily

    2. Sorbitol: 15–30 ml PO daily

    3. Polyethylene glycol: 17 g PO daily

    4. Lubiprostone: 8 mcg PO two times a day in women older than 18 years

    5. Linaclotide: 290 mcg PO daily

    6. Tenapanor: 50 mg PO two times a day

I. Antibiotics: Rifaximin is a minimally absorbed agent beneficial in those with IBS-D; however, relapse is usual, and mode of action is unclear given evidence the microbiome is not altered.

J. Probiotics: Treatment of discomfort and bloating may be accomplished by alteration of disrupted bowel flora. Probiotics are attenuated bacteria that can be beneficial to the host and reduce symptoms; however, it is unclear on the most beneficial strain or dose. Small studies have shown superiority of *Lactiplantibacillus plantarum.*

K. Prebiotics: This special form of dietary fiber enhances normal gut flora (e.g., garlic, onion); however, they have no evidence of clinical benefit.

L. Complementary therapies (Defrees & Bailey, 2017; Ford et al., 2017)

1. Peppermint oil: This oil has antispasmodic properties caused by smooth muscle relaxation through the blockade of calcium channels. It has shown to be more effective than placebo but may exacerbate heartburn.
2. Apple cider vinegar: Its antimicrobial, antifungal, and antiviral properties, as well as probiotics and prebiotics, may repair the GI system.
3. Acupuncture: Several studies have shown benefit for pain versus placebo, but no improvement in overall symptoms has been found.
4. Reassurance, relaxation, hypnotherapy (guided hypnosis), and other cognitive behavioral therapies: These techniques may provide symptom relief; however, no randomized controlled trials have proved efficacy.

VII. Follow-up
    A. Short term: It is important to establish a trusting therapeutic relationship. See patients frequently at the time of diagnosis, and less often as control is achieved.
    B. Long term
        1. For new symptoms PRN
        2. Annually for routine follow-up

VIII. Referrals
    A. Dietitian: For dietary interventions and modification
    B. Gastroenterologist: For refractory or disabling symptoms
    C. Behavioral health specialist: For behavior modification techniques

The author would like to acknowledge Kristine Turner Story, RN, MSN, APRN, BC, for her contribution to this chapter that remains unchanged from the previous edition of this book.

References

Barros, L.L., Farias, A.Q., & Rezaie, A. (2019). Gastrointestinal motility and absorptive disorders in patients with inflammatory bowel diseases: Prevalence, diagnosis and treatment. *World Journal of Gastroenterology, 25*(31), 4414–4426. https://doi.org/10.3748/wjg.v25.i31.4414.

Basnayake, C. (2018). Treatment of irritable bowel syndrome. *Australian Prescriber, 41*(5), 145–149. https://doi.org/10.18773/austprescr.2018.044

Bellini, M., Tonarelli, S., Nagy, A.G., Pancetti, A., Costa, F., Ricchiuti, A., ... Rossi, A. (2020). Low FODMAP diet: Evidence, doubts, and hopes. *Nutrients, 12*(1), 148. https://doi.org/10.3390/nu12010148

Defrees, D.N., & Bailey, J. (2017). Irritable bowel syndrome: Epidemiology, pathophysiology, diagnosis, and treatment. *Primary Care: Clinics in Office Practice, 44*(4), 655–671. https://doi.org/10.1016/j.pop.2017.07.009

Ford, A.C., Lacy, B.E., & Talley, N.J. (2017). Irritable bowel syndrome. *New England Journal of Medicine, 376*(26), 2566–2578. https://doi.org/10.1056/NEJMra1607547.

Ford, A.C., Moayyedi, P., Chey, W.D., Harris, L.A., Lacy, B., Saito, Y.A., & Quigley, E.M.M. (2018). American College of Gastroenterology monograph on management of irritable bowel syndrome. *American Journal of Gastroenterology, 113*(Suppl. 2), 1–18. https://doi.org/10.1038/s41395-018-0084-x

Harris, L.A., & Baffy, N. (2017). Modulation of the gut microbiota: A focus on treatments for irritable bowel syndrome. *Postgraduate Medicine, 129*(8), 872–888. https://doi.org/10.1080/00325481.2017.1383819.

Hellström, P.M., & Benno, P. (2019). The Rome IV: Irritable bowel syndrome—A functional disorder. *Best Practice and Research: Clinical Gastroenterology, 40–41*, 101634. https://doi.org/10.1016/j.bpg.2019.101634

Kim, Y.S., & Kim, N. (2018). Sex-gender differences in irritable bowel syndrome. *Journal of Neurogastroenterology and Motility, 24*(4), 544–558. https://doi.org/10.5056/jnm18082

Lacy, B.E., Mearin, F., Chang, L., Chey, W.D., Lembo, A.J., Simren, M., & Spiller, R. (2016). Bowel disorders. *Gastroenterology, 150*(6), 1393–1407. https://doi.org/10.1053/j.gastro.2016.02.031

Lacy, B.E., & Patel, N.K. (2017). Rome criteria and a diagnostic approach to irritable bowel syndrome. *Journal of Clinical Medicine, 6*(11), 99. https://doi.org/10.3390/jcm6110099

Nelkowska, D.D. (2020). Treating irritable bowel syndrome through an interdisciplinary approach. *Annals of Gastroenterology, 33*(1), 1–8. https://doi.org/10.20524/aog.2019.0441

Ooi, S.L., Correa, D., & Pak, C. (2019). Probiotics, prebiotics and low FODMAP diet for irritable bowel syndrome—What is the current evidence? *Complementary Therapies in Medicine, 43,* 73–80. https://doi.org/10.1016/j.ctim.2019.01.010

Staudacher, H.M. (2017). Nutritional, microbiological and psychosocial implications of the low FODMAP diet. *Journal of Gastroenterology and Hepatology, 32*(Suppl. 1), 16–19. https://doi.org/10.1111/jgh.13688

CHAPTER 77

Pancreatitis

R. Tim Davis, MSN, APRN

I. Definition: Inflammation of the pancreas usually associated with sudden onset upper abdominal pain or epigastric pain with elevation in serum pancreatic enzymes (Gardner et al., 2020; Shah et al., 2018)

II. Physiology/Pathophysiology (Barry, 2018; Derrick et al., 2019; Gardner et al., 2020; Ince & Baysal, 2014; Pham & Forsmark, 2018; Quinlan, 2014)
  A. Normal
    1. Large gland that lies behind the stomach and beside the duodenum or upper part of the small intestine
    2. Facilitates digestion of carbohydrates, proteins, and fat by secreting digestive enzymes into the small intestine, functioning as an exocrine gland
    3. Releases insulin and glucagon into the bloodstream
  B. Pathophysiology
    1. Acute: Gradual or sudden onset initiated by an acute injury; consists of three phases
      a) Premature activation of trypsin occurs within pancreatic acinar cells, which leads to activation and release of injurious pancreatic digestive enzymes.
      b) Intrapancreatic inflammation occurs through a variety of mechanisms and pathways.
      c) Extrapancreatic inflammation results in widespread toxicity and damage to specific organs (e.g., acute respiratory syndrome).
      d) Acute pancreatitis diffusely involves a large portion of the entire pancreas with a predominantly neutrophilic inflammatory response.
    2. Chronic: Pathophysiology of chronic pancreatitis remains unclear.
      a) Generally, it is the result of long-standing damage to the pancreas from chronic alcohol consumption resulting in tissue damage and scarring.
      b) Other causes can produce chronic pancreatitis, resulting in a progressive destruction of exocrine tissue and fibrosis and possibly loss of endocrine tissue.
      c) It is a patchy focal disease characterized by a mononuclear infiltration and fibrosis process.

III. Clinical features: Chronic pancreatitis has a variable course, ranging from mild to severe and life threatening, depending on degree of pancreatic damage. The severity of disease can be determined using a multifactor scoring system (e.g., 2012 revision of the Atlanta classification, Ranson criteria, APACHE II and III) and imaging studies. Chronic pancreatitis is more common in men than women and typically presents with unrelenting pain of varying duration (Banks et al., 2013; Chatila et al., 2019; Crockett et al., 2018; Gardner et al., 2020; Mao, 2019; Quinlan, 2014).

A. Etiology
1. Alcoholism
2. Gallstones
3. Hyperlipidemia
4. Hereditary chronic pancreatitis
5. Drug induced
6. Post–endoscopic retrograde cholangiopancreatography
7. Pancreatic duct injury
8. Biliary sludge/microlithiasis
9. Biliary obstruction
10. Infections
11. Anatomic or physiologic pancreatic anomalies
12. Idiopathic

B. History
1. History of cancer and cancer treatment
2. Current medications: Prescribed, over the counter
3. Presenting symptoms: Precipitating factors, onset, location, duration, associated symptoms (e.g., weight loss, abdominal pain)
4. Changes in ADLs
5. Past medical history: Recent abdominal surgery or trauma, biliary disease or gallstones, cholecystectomy or pancreatic surgery, pancreatitis, acute or chronic pancreatitis, pancreatic cancer, diabetes
6. Social history: Alcohol use, illicit drug use
7. Family history: Pancreatitis
8. Autoimmune disease suggestive of autoimmune pancreatitis

C. Signs and symptoms: Similar in both acute and chronic pancreatitis, but pain may be more severe in chronic pancreatitis
1. Upper abdominal/epigastric pain: Radiates to the back, mimics MI in chronic states, or can initially be painless
2. Initial pain: Worsens after eating or drinking, especially fatty foods; typically, becomes constant over time
3. Indigestion, abdominal fullness, distension
4. Clay-colored stools
5. Decreased urine output
6. Frequent hiccups
7. Nausea and vomiting
8. Fever
9. Jaundice/scleral icterus
10. Weight loss: Chronic pancreatitis

D. Physical examination
1. Vital signs
   a) Tachycardia in acute pancreatitis
   b) Blood pressure: Normal or slightly increased
   c) Respirations: Shallow from pain or tachypnea with severe pancreatitis
   d) Fever: Low grade with acute disease
   e) Hypotension in severe acute pancreatitis
2. HEENT: Xanthoma and lipemia retinalis secondary to hyperlipidemia
3. Pulmonary
   a) Presence of basilar consolidation with decreased breath sounds suggestive of severe pancreatitis

        b) Absent sounds indicating effusion

   4. Abdominal

        a) Spider angioma and thickening of palmar sheaths present with alcohol-induced pancreatitis

        b) Rebound tenderness with guarding

        c) Hypoactive/absent bowel sounds indicating ileus

        d) Flank or periumbilical ecchymosis suggestive of severe pancreatitis

        e) Distention

        f) Cullen sign (ecchymosis and edema in the subcutaneous tissue around the umbilicus) in acute pancreatitis suggestive of intraperitoneal hemorrhage (see Appendix D)

        g) Grey Turner sign (ecchymosis of the flank) present in acute pancreatitis suggestive of retroperitoneal bleeding (see Appendix D)

IV. Diagnostic tests (Esteban-Zubero, 2018; Gardner et al., 2020; Quinlan, 2014; Türkvatan et al., 2015)

   A. Laboratory

      1. Acute

        a) Increased amylase and serum lipase greater than or equal to three times ULN: Serum lipase is preferred for sensitivity and specificity. It is not necessary to measure both at the same time.

        b) Increased ALT/AST in alcoholic hepatitis or choledocholithiasis

        c) Hyperbilirubinemia in alcoholic or biliary obstruction

        d) Hyperglycemia if endocrine function is compromised

        e) Hypocalcemia suggestive of cardiovascular involvement

        f) Leukocytosis with destructive pancreatic process

        g) Increased Hgb secondary to hemodilution

        h) Increased coagulation panel

      2. Chronic

        a) Possible normal amylase/lipase

        b) Hyperglycemia from endocrine compromise

        c) Stool for chymotrypsin, elastase, and fat typically positive because of an alteration in lipid metabolism

        d) Hyperbilirubinemia suggestive of biliary obstruction or hepatic involvement

   B. Radiology

      1. Acute

        a) Contrast-enhanced CT: Standard imaging; shows pancreatic enlargement, ill-defined border, heterogeneous attenuation, segmental-focal involvement, fluid collections, pseudocysts, venous thrombosis of the splenic vein, and necrosis (nonenhancement of greater than 3 cm or 30% of pancreatic volume on CT, considered CT sign of necrosis)

        b) Noncontrast CT: Cannot evaluate for pancreatic necrosis and vascular complications

        c) Ultrasound (transabdominal or endoscopic): Excellent for detecting pancreatobiliary disease such as bile duct calculi or sludge

        d) Endoscopic retrograde cholangiopancreatography in combination with sphincterotomy for gallstone removal and drainage of infected bile in severe pancreatitis (not used as a diagnostic modality): Magnetic resonance cholangiopancreatography or endoscopic ultrasound used to determine if an endoscopic retrograde cholangiopancreatography required

      e) MRI
         (1) Similar to contrast-enhanced CT but with better tissue characterization of pancreatic parenchyma
         (2) Distinguishes fluid from liquefied necrotic tissue and detection of calculi and pancreas divisum
         (3) Characterizes an abnormal or disconnected pancreatic duct and fluid collection
      f) Abdominal angiography: Excellent for detection of vascular abnormalities
   2. Chronic
      a) Abdominal ultrasound to assess for pseudocyst formation and calcification
      b) Magnetic resonance cholangiopancreatography: Identifies ductal deformity, retained CBD stones, pancreatic stones, and strictures

V. Differential diagnosis (Gardner et al., 2020; Quinlan, 2014)
  A. Mesenteric ischemia or infarction
  B. Biliary colic
  C. Dissecting aortic aneurysm
  D. Inferior wall MI (see Chapter 49)
  E. Intestinal obstruction (see Chapter 67)
  F. Acute cholelithiasis (see Chapter 68)
  G. Trauma
  H. Cancer of pancreas
  I. SLE (see Chapter 110)
  J. Peptic ulcer disease (see Chapter 78)
  K. Cholecystitis (see Chapter 68)
  L. Hepatitis (see Chapter 74)
  M. Autoimmune pancreatitis

VI. Treatment: Primarily supportive, with pain medicine and hyperhydration (to maintain hemodynamic stability); ICU care if patient has sustained major organ failure or surgery for infected pancreatic necrosis; should identify precipitating factors (Crockett et al., 2018; Derrick et al., 2019; Esteban-Zubero et al., 2018; Forsmark et al., 2016; Gardner et al., 2020; Krenzer, 2016; Mao, 2019; Pham & Forsmark, 2018; Quinlan, 2014)
  A. Pain management (see Appendix F)
    1. Morphine or equivalent dose of fentanyl or hydromorphone
      a) A patient-controlled analgesia pump is preferred at 1 mg/hr with a demand dose of 0.5–2.5 mg every 5–10 minutes in opioid-naïve patients.
      b) Doses may need to be increased in patients with prior exposure.
      c) Use oral formulations (e.g., morphine, hydromorphone, oxycodone) if patient is not on bowel rest.
    2. Ketorolac: 15–30 mg PO or IV every six hours
      a) Maximum daily dose is 120 mg.
      b) Reduce dose by 50% for those older than 65 years and with renal impairment.
      c) Maximum duration is five days.
  B. Hydration: Vigorous to counteract hypovolemia related to third-space volume loss, vomiting, and diaphoresis
    1. Hypovolemia is associated with the development of necrotizing pancreatitis.
    2. Intravascular volume depletion leads to hemoconcentration (hematocrit greater than or equal to 44%), tachycardia, hypotension, reduced urine output, prerenal azotemia, and BUN–creatinine ratio greater than 20.

C. Oxygen: To prevent or minimize pancreatic necrosis and improve survival
D. Nutrition: Patient should be NPO. Introduce food as soon as pain subsides and patient can tolerate. Enteral (preferred) or parenteral nutrition should be initiated as appropriate if patient is NPO for more than five days.
E. PPIs: In partial or total pancreatic necrosis; omeprazole 20 mg PO daily
F. Pancreatic enzymes: In severe necrotizing pancreatitis (no role in interstitial pancreatitis) (e.g., lipase 500–2,500 units/kg PO meal)
G. Antibiotics: Controversial; carbapenems (e.g., imipenem) in infected necrotizing pancreatitis; limited to two weeks (see Appendix C); prophylactic antibiotics not recommended in acute pancreatitis
H. NSAIDs and acetaminophen: Useful in chronic pancreatitis (see Appendix E)
I. Endoscopic ultrasound–guided celiac plexus block: Used in chronic pancreatitis
J. Octreotide: Controversial; used in chronic pancreatitis; inhibits pancreatic secretion; 0.5 mg IM three times a day used in clinical trials
K. Cessation of alcohol use and smoking
L. Low-fat diet in chronic pancreatitis because complex foods cannot be digested because loss of exocrine function, resulting in significant protein and fat deficiencies; approximately 20 g daily recommended

VII. Follow-up (Quinlan, 2014)
A. Encouragement of alcohol abstinence
B. Management of underlying states: Hyperglyceridemia, cholelithiasis
C. Laboratory evaluation: Pseudocyst should be suspected if enzymes remain elevated weeks after an acute episode.
D. Periodic monitoring in chronic pancreatitis for diabetes and vitamin D deficiency

VIII. Referrals (Esteban-Zubero et al., 2018; Gardner et al., 2020)
A. Surgery: For cholecystectomy and/or endoscopic sphincterotomy for patients with gallstones
B. Counseling services for alcohol and smoking cessation programs (as appropriate): For patients with alcoholic pancreatitis

The author would like to acknowledge Faith A. Mutale, MSN, CRNP, for her contribution to this chapter that remains unchanged from the previous edition of this book.

References

Banks, P.A., Bollen, T.L., Dervenis, C., Gooszen, H.G., Johnson, C.D., Sarr, M.G., … Vege, S.S. (2013). Classification of acute pancreatitis—2012: Revision of the Atlanta classification and definitions by international consensus. *Gut, 62*(1), 102–111. https://doi.org/10.1136/gutjnl-2012-302779

Barry, K. (2018). Chronic pancreatitis: Diagnosis and treatment. *American Family Physician, 97*(6), 385–393. https://www.aafp.org/afp/2018/0315/p385.html

Chatila, A.T., Bilal, M., & Guturu, P. (2019). Evaluation and management of acute pancreatitis. *World Journal of Clinical Cases, 7*(9), 1006–1020. https://doi.org/10.12998/wjcc.v7.i9.1006

Crockett, S.D., Wani, S., Gardner, T.B., Falck-Ytter, Y., & Barkun, A.N. (2018). American Gastroenterological Association Institute guideline on initial management of acute pancreatitis. *Gastroenterology, 154*(4), 1096–1101. https://doi.org/10.1053/j.gastro.2018.01.032

Derrick, D., Frandy, F., & Wirawan, A.D. (2019). Acute pancreatitis: Etiology, pathogenesis, pathophysiology and the current trend in its management and prevention. *Indonesian Journal of Gastroenterology, Hepatology, and Digestive Endoscopy, 20*(1), 27–37. http://www.ina-jghe.com/index.php/jghe/article/view/691

Esteban-Zubero, E., Cabrera-Falcón, E., Ribagorda-Tejedor, S., Alatorre-Jiménez, M.A., López-García, C.A., Marín-Medina, A., ... Gomez-Ramos, J.J. (2018). Current trends in management of acute pancreatitis: A review. *Annals of Gastroenterology and the Digestive System, 2,* 1006. https://doi.org/10.33582/2637-4501/1006

Forsmark, C.E., Vege, S.S., & Wilcox, C.M. (2016). Acute pancreatitis. *New England Journal of Medicine, 375*(20), 1972–1981. https://doi.org/10.1056/NEJMra1505202

Gardner, T.B., Adler, D.G., Forsmark, C.E., Sauer, B.G., Taylor, J.R., & Whitcomb, D.C. (2020). ACG clinical guideline: Pancreatitis. *American Journal of Gastroenterology, 115*(3), 322–339. https://doi.org/10.14309/ajg.0000000000000535

Ince, A.T., & Baysal, B. (2014). Pathophysiology, classification and available guidelines of acute pancreatitis. *Turkish Journal of Gastroenterology, 25*(4), 351–357. https://doi.org/10.5152/tjg.2014.13005

Krenzer, M.E. (2016). Understanding acute pancreatitis. *Nursing, 46*(8), 34–40. https://doi.org/10.1097/01.NURSE.0000484959.78110.98

Mao, E. (2019). Intensive management of severe acute pancreatitis. *Annals of Translational Medicine, 7*(22), 687. https://doi.org/10.21037/atm.2019.10.58

Pham, A., & Forsmark, C. (2018). Chronic pancreatitis: review and update of etiology, risk factors, and management. *F1000Research, 17*(7), 607. https://doi.org/10.12688/f1000research.12852.1

Quinlan, J.D. (2014). Acute pancreatitis. *American Family Physician, 90*(9), 632–639. https://www.aafp.org/afp/2014/1101/p632.html

Shah, A.P., Mourad, M.M., & Bramhall, S.R. (2018). Acute pancreatitis: Current perspectives on diagnosis and management. *Journal of Inflammation Research, 11,* 77–85. https://doi.org/10.2147/JIR.S135751

Türkvatan, A., Erden, A., Türkoğlu, A., Seçil, M., & Yener, Ö. (2015). Imaging of acute pancreatitis and its complications. Part 1: Acute pancreatitis. *Diagnostic and Interventional Imaging, 96*(2), 151–160. https://doi.org/10.1016/j.diii.2013.12.017

CHAPTER 78

Peptic Ulcer Disease

Jeanne Held-Warmkessel, MSN, RN, AOCN®, ACNS-BC

I. Definition: Cavity-shaped disruption of integrity of the gastric or duodenal mucosal layer (muscularis mucosa) resulting from gastric acid secretions with extension into submucosa or muscularis propria (Boltin et al., 2019; Malfertheiner & Schulz, 2020)

II. Physiology/Pathophysiology (Boltin et al., 2019; Chey et al., 2017; Kamboj et al., 2017; Kempenich & Sirinek, 2018; Lanas & Chan, 2017; Melcarne et al., 2016; Sheldon & Eckert, 2017)
   A. Normal: The epithelial cells of the stomach are protected from pepsin and hydrochloric acid, the major components of gastric secretions that digest food through the following methods.
      1. Rapidly reproducing mucosal lining
      2. Secretion of bicarbonate to neutralize acid
      3. Mucus production promoted by blood supply and prostaglandin release
   B. Pathophysiology
      1. *Helicobacter pylori*–associated ulcer
         a) Bacteria secrete an enzyme, urease, which protects the bacteria as a result of stomach acid.
         b) Bacteria produce an inflammatory response, causing mucosal tissue damage in the stomach and duodenum.
         c) *H. pylori* infection affects the neural pathways and alters acid production, either hypo- or hypersecretion.
         d) Excess acid results in duodenitis and duodenal ulcer.
         e) *H. pylori* causes pangastritis with hyposecretion. Gastric ulcers form as a result of mucosal atrophy.
         f) Not all people with *H. pylori* develop ulcers. Other mechanisms, such as genetics, are present that allow for ulcer formation.
      2. ASA and NSAIDs cause gastric ulcers by interfering with the protective effect of prostaglandins in the stomach. *H. pylori* infection increases the risk of ulcer formation and bleeding in patients taking ASA and NSAIDs.
      3. Duodenal ulcers may develop from elevated levels of acid secretion and enhanced gastric emptying, even in the absence of *H. pylori* or ASA and NSAIDs (e.g., Zollinger-Ellison syndrome).
      4. Nicotine/tobacco, alcohol, chemotherapy, and drug abuse (e.g., cocaine, amphetamine) can cause ulcers by promoting ulcerogenic factors and reducing protective factors.
      5. Stress ulcers may form in the presence of life-threatening (i.e., ICU level of care) trauma or illness (e.g., hypoperfusion of gastric mucosa secondary to use of vasopressors) or large-scale disasters (e.g., earthquakes).

III. Clinical features: Peptic ulcer disease continues to be a source of significant morbidity and mortality worldwide. Approximately two-thirds of patients found to have peptic ulcer disease are asymptomatic. Most cases are associated with *H. pylori* infection, the use of NSAIDs, or both (Boltin et al., 2019; Farrar, 2018; Kavitt et al., 2019; Kempenich & Sirinek, 2018; Lanas & Chan, 2017; Malfertheiner & Schulz, 2020; Melcarne et al., 2016).

A. Risk factors
1. *H. pylori* infection
2. NSAID/ASA use: Low-dose ASA, antiplatelet agents
3. Stress
4. Chronic renal insufficiency
5. Alcohol abuse, cocaine or methamphetamine use
6. High caffeine use, fasting
7. COPD
8. Radiation to the stomach causing mucosal damage
9. Heart disease
10. CMV infection
11. Crohn disease
12. Advanced liver disease: Portal gastropathy, cirrhosis
13. Chemotherapy, antiangiogenesis agents
14. Tobacco use

B. Etiology
1. Bacterial
   a) *H. pylori*: Bacteria are present in the majority of patients with duodenal ulcers and approximately 70% of patients with gastric ulcers. Presence of *H. pylori* increases NSAID-associated risk for complications.
   b) *Mycobacterium avium* complex
   c) *Treponema pallidum* (syphilis)
   d) HIV/AIDS and phlegmonous gastritis (alpha- or beta-hemolytic streptococci)
2. Viral: Rarely causes ulcers
   a) HSV-1
   b) CMV
3. Drug induced
   a) ASA/NSAIDs, cyclooxygenase-2 inhibitors (see Appendix E)
   b) Chemotherapy: Hepatic artery floxuridine infusion
   c) Cocaine
   d) Steroids
   e) Digitalis
   f) Oral potassium chloride
   g) Oral bisphosphonates

C. History
1. History of cancer and cancer treatment: Chemotherapy, radiation therapy
2. Current medications: Prescribed; over the counter; PPI, H$_2$ antagonist, and antacid use; past antimicrobial use
3. History of presenting symptoms: Precipitating factors, onset, location, duration, association with food, nighttime epigastric pain, nocturnal awakening with pain
4. Changes in ADLs
5. Social history: Tobacco use, drug use, alcohol use, caffeine consumption
6. Past medical history: COPD, cirrhosis, chronic kidney insufficiency, metabolic disorders, diabetes, alpha-2-antitrypsin deficiency, heart disease, CMV infection, prior ulcer, infection with *H. pylori*, Zollinger-Ellison syndrome

  7. Past surgical history: Gastric surgery, bariatric surgery

D. Signs and symptoms

  1. Gnawing or burning epigastric pain: Pain occurs two to three (up to five) hours after meals and at night. It may occur in the right or left upper quadrants or radiate to the back. Food consumption, PPIs or H_2 blockers, or antacids reduce pain. In some patients, food increases pain. Duodenal ulcers are associated with pain when the stomach is empty and during the night. Relief occurs with food or antacid. Patients complain of feeling hungry.

  2. Ulcers: When taking ASA/NSAIDs or in older adults, ulcers may perforate or bleed before symptoms develop.

  3. Anorexia, nausea, vomiting, hyperphagia

  4. Weight loss/gain

  5. Heartburn, indigestion, reflux, referred back pain, or left shoulder pain

  6. Dyspepsia, fullness, belching, bloating, distention, fatty food intolerance

  7. If ulcer bleeds, hematemesis or melena may occur along with abdominal pain.

  8. Signs and symptoms of anemia, such as fatigue, shortness of breath, headache, or dizziness

  9. Signs and symptoms of gastric outlet obstruction (rare), such as nausea or vomiting, pain, early satiety, bloating, dehydration

  10. Penetration of bowel wall: Penetration results in severe pain.

  11. Fistula formation: Fever, tenderness, abdominal pain

  12. Perforation: Sudden acute epigastric abdominal pain

E. Physical examination: Nonspecific

  1. Abdominal

   a) Pain elicited on palpation

   b) Masses and organomegaly

   c) Acute epigastric abdominal tenderness suggestive of perforation

   d) Guarding (voluntary and involuntary) with rigidity suggestive of ulcer perforation

  2. Rectal: Stool testing for occult blood

  3. Vital signs: Hemodynamic status for tachycardia with or without hypotension associated with peritonitis

IV. Diagnostic tests (Boltin et al., 2019; Chey et al., 2017; Farrar, 2018; Kamboj et al., 2017; Kavitt et al., 2019; Kempenich & Sirinek, 2018; Lanas & Chan, 2017; Nelms & Pelaez, 2018)

A. Laboratory: CBC (Hgb/hematocrit if bleeding is suspected), comprehensive metabolic panel, LFTs, pancreatic enzymes for baseline and to evaluate for abnormalities

B. Radiology

  1. Acute abdomen series to evaluate for obstruction

  2. Upper GI series to assess if an ulcer has limited usefulness; endoscopy preferred diagnostic test

C. Other

  1. *H. pylori* testing required for all patients diagnosed with a peptic ulcer, mucosa-associated lymphoid tissue lymphoma, or dyspepsia who are younger than age 60 years

   a) Test choices

    (1) Enzyme-linked immunosorbent assay (ELISA)

    (2) Serum *H. pylori* antibody test: Serology for IgG blood levels of antibodies induced by bacterial infection with *H. pylori*; not affected by medications; unable to differentiate between active disease and past exposure; remains positive after successful treatment

(3) Carbon-13 or carbon-14 urea breath test: Six-hour pretest fasting required; accurate and noninvasive
    (a) The patient drinks a labeled urea solution, which the bacteria metabolize.
    (b) Twenty to thirty minutes later, a series of breath samples are taken and sent for analysis for the presence of labeled carbon dioxide, which is released only from bacterial metabolism of urea.
    (c) Human cells do not have the enzyme urease necessary to metabolize urea in the solution.
    (d) Test is useful for determining outcome of therapy.
(4) Fecal antigen test is used for *H. pylori*.
(5) Biopsy urease test or histology test (biopsy and culture) is performed during endoscopy.
    b) Antiulcer drugs (e.g., bismuth compounds) and antibiotics taken up to four weeks and PPIs taken two weeks before tests for *H. pylori* (except serology) will cause false-negative results.
    c) Other drugs (e.g., misoprostol, sucralfate) taken one week prior to the breath test will interfere with test accuracy.
    d) Cimetidine taken two weeks prior to the breath test interferes with test accuracy.
2. Upper endoscopy: Test is performed for ulcer diagnosis and for treatment and management of bleeding. For biopsy to rule out gastric malignancy or infection, specimens for *H. pylori* testing/culture should be taken from two to three areas of the stomach, and the biopsies tested for urease activity. This is the diagnostic test of choice.
    a) It should be done within 24 hours of hospital admission for bleeding ulcer.
    b) It is required for patients with new dyspepsia (age 50 years or older), trouble swallowing, weight loss, upper GI cancer history in family, GI bleeding, left supraclavicular lymphadenopathy, abdominal mass, or vomiting.
3. Gastric analysis should be performed to quantitatively assess acid secretions (uncommonly used).

V. Differential diagnosis (Boltin et al., 2019; Farrar, 2018; Lanas & Chan, 2017)
  A. Infection with *H. pylori*, CMV, *Helicobacter heilmannii*
  B. Medication/drug induced: Drug abuse such as cocaine
  C. GI disorders
    1. Inflammatory disease (e.g., Crohn disease), celiac disease
    2. Zollinger-Ellison syndrome, gastrinoma
    3. Gastritis, gastroduodenitis (see Chapter 72)
    4. Pancreatitis (see Chapter 77)
    5. Cholecystitis (see Chapter 68)
    6. Gastric or duodenal cancer, pancreatic cancer, lymphoma, gastric mucosa-associated lymphoid tissue lymphoma
    7. Idiopathic ulcer: *H. pylori*-negative, NSAID-negative ulcer
    8. Radiation therapy–induced gastritis
    9. Systemic mastocytosis
    10. Behçet disease
    11. Cirrhosis with portal hypertension (see Chapter 69)
    12. Vasculitis

VI. Treatment: If patient relapses after initial treatment, reevaluate and retreat. Treatment is an ongoing, continuous evolution. Consult the most recent literature and experts in the field of *H. pylori* management. Antimicrobial resistance is developing to clarithromycin (Chey et al., 2017; Chiu, 2019; Freedberg et al., 2017; Kavitt et al., 2019; Kempenich, & Sirinek, 2018; Lanas & Chan, 2017; Malfertheiner & Schulz, 2020; Melcarne et al., 2016).

A. Antibiotics

    1. For patients with peptic ulcer disease who are positive for *H. pylori*, treat with combination therapy with a PPI and two antibiotics or bismuth with a PPI and two antibiotics. **Do not** use monotherapy.

    2. Treatment options: Antimicrobial choice is dependent on local antimicrobial resistance to *H. pylori*. If local clarithromycin resistance rate is greater than 15%, do not use clarithromycin. Treatment choice is based on prior antimicrobial exposure and microbial allergies. Patients with any prior macrolide therapy should not receive clarithromycin.

        a) Administer therapy.

            (1) Bismuth quadruple therapy: Bismuth subcitrate 120–300 mg PO four times a day or 300 mg bismuth subsalicylate PO four times a day, tetracycline 500 mg PO four times a day, and metronidazole 250 mg PO four times a day (500 mg three to four times a day) and standard dose PPI for 10–14 days; useful for patients previously treated with clarithromycin or in areas with clarithromycin resistance

            (2) Clarithromycin triple therapy: PPI two times a day plus clarithromycin 500 mg PO two times a day and amoxicillin 1,000 mg PO two times a day (Prevpac®); contains lansoprazole 30 mg PO as the PPI; can replace the amoxicillin with metronidazole 500 mg PO three times a day

            (3) Concomitant therapy standard dose: PPI two times a day, amoxicillin 1,000 mg PO, clarithromycin 500 mg PO two times a day, plus nitroimidazole 500 mg PO for 10–14 days

            (4) Sequential therapy: PPI two times a day, amoxicillin 1,000 mg PO two times a day for five to seven days, followed by five to seven days of PPI two times a day, clarithromycin 500 mg PO two times a day, and nitroimidazole 500 mg PO two times a day

        b) Caution is advised with the use of metronidazole and alcohol, as it may cause an Antabuse® (disulfiram) effect.

B. Non–*H. pylori* peptic ulcer

    1. In patients taking NSAIDs, stop agents if possible. Continued use will interfere with ulcer healing. Patients requiring NSAIDs need peptic ulcer disease prophylaxis and ongoing therapy after ulcer healing. A PPI (regular dose strength) with naproxen (low cardiovascular risk) or celecoxib is recommended for patients requiring NSAID therapy. Patients requiring long-term, low-dose ASA therapy or long-term NSAID therapy need to be tested for *H. pylori* and, if positive, treated to eradicate the organism to reduce their risk of peptic ulcer disease. Use the lowest dose of NSAID for the shortest period of time possible. Evaluate the patient's response after NSAID dose reductions.

    2. PPIs are the preferred agent for NSAID–associated ulcers. Treat for more than eight weeks; for recurrent symptoms, add four to eight weeks of therapy. No evidence exists that high-dose PPI is better than standard dose PPI.

        a) Omeprazole: 20–40 mg PO

        b) Esomeprazole: 20–40 mg PO

        c) Lansoprazole: 15–30 mg PO

        d) Pantoprazole: 40–80 mg PO

        e) Rabeprazole: 20–40 mg PO

        f) Agents are most effective when taken immediately before eating a meal.

    g) Agents interfere with ketoconazole absorption and increase absorption of digoxin and may inhibit clopidogrel activity.

    h) Drugs are metabolized in the liver by cytochrome P450 isoenzyme CYP2C19. Drug–drug interactions may occur.

    i) PPIs may increase the risk of osteoporosis and hip fractures with long-term use, especially in older adults. They interfere with calcium absorption from hypochlorhydria and by interfering with osteoclast activity.

    j) PPIs may increase the risk of *Clostridium difficile* colitis by producing hypochlorhydria.

  3. Antacids are not used as first-line therapy but are contraindicated in patients with renal insufficiency.

  4. Bismuth is a colloid that coats ulcers and has direct antibacterial activity. Long-term use may cause neurotoxicity.

C. Patient education

  1. Avoid smoking because cigarette smoke blocks bicarbonate release in the stomach and interferes with drug efficacy.

  2. Diet

    a) Avoid foods and fluids that cause pain or increase symptoms, such as pepper, alcohol, and caffeine-containing foods and liquids. Avoid acidic foods and fatty foods. A bland diet may be more tolerable.

    b) Reduce weight if obese.

  3. Medications to avoid include over-the-counter and nonprescribed medications containing NSAIDs and ASA (see Appendix E).

  4. Stress causes increased acid secretion; implement relaxation and quiet diversion.

D. Endoscopy: Used to diagnose infection and malignancy and to treat active bleeding associated with complicated peptic ulcer disease

E. Interventional radiology: If endoscopy is unsuccessful in controlling bleeding

F. Surgery: If endoscopy and interventional radiology are not effective in stopping bleeding

VII. Follow-up (Chey et al., 2017; Kamboj et al., 2017; Lanas & Chan, 2017; Nelms & Pelaez, 2018)

A. Improvement should be noted after several weeks of treatment. Healing should occur within six to eight weeks of treatment, depending on ulcer size. If healing does not occur as expected, assess for therapy adherence and ongoing NSAID use. Gastric ulcer will need a second-look endoscopy to ensure complete healing.

B. Repeat urea breath test no earlier than four weeks after treatment to avoid false-negative results. Repeat breath test is recommended for all patients. Repeat breath test in patients with ongoing symptoms after treatment and for patients with bleeding or complicated ulcers, mucosa-associated lymphoid tissue lymphoma, or gastric cancer, if *H. pylori* was diagnosed. Discontinue use of PPI two weeks prior to test. Fecal antigen test may also be used.

C. Development of fatigue, tachycardia, pallor, coffee-ground emesis, hematemesis, or black stools indicates bleeding or hemorrhage, and prompt medical or surgical intervention is required.

D. Perforation requires prompt emergency surgical intervention. Peritonitis develops quickly over the next 6–12 hours.

E. Serology will remain positive after successful treatment. *H. pylori* IgG blood levels decrease slowly after *H. pylori* treatment.

F. Educate patients to maintain smoking cessation.

G. Bleeding peptic ulcer disease: Approximately 15%–20% of patients will experience rebleeding. Repeat endoscopy after eight weeks of treatment may be done, especially in patients with recurrent symptoms. High-risk patients may benefit from a second-look endoscopy, including patients at risk for gastric cancer and those with appropriately treated nonhealing ulcers.

VIII. Referrals (Farrar, 2018; Nelms & Pelaez, 2018)
   A. Gastroenterologist: For EGD (initial and second look), treatment of active and recurrent bleeding and refractory ulcers, and recurrent *H. pylori* infection, failed frontline therapy and patients requiring low-dose ASA therapy
   B. Interventional radiologist: For angiography with embolization for bleeding if endoscopic intervention is unsuccessful
   C. Surgeon: For recommended surgical consultation for bleeding ulcers
      1. If bleeding is not controlled by endoscopic or radiologic interventions or if perforation or other complications, such as hypotension and rebleeding or hemorrhage, are present
      2. Older patients who tolerate ongoing bleeding poorly
      3. Hemodynamic instability after three units of packed RBCs
      4. For large ulcers, stomach and posterior duodenal ulcers that may benefit from early surgery
   D. Smoking cessation programs

References

Boltin, D., Niv, Y., Schütte, K., & Schulz, C. (2019). Review: *Helicobacter pylori* and non-malignant upper gastrointestinal diseases. *Helicobacter, 24*(Suppl. 1), e12637. https://doi.org/10.1111/hel.12637

Chey, W.D., Leontiadis, G.I., Howden, C.W., & Moss, S.F. (2017). ACG clinical guideline: Treatment of *Helicobacter pylori* infection. *American Journal of Gastroenterology, 112*(2), 212–238. https://doi.org/10.1038/ajg.2016.563

Chiu, P.W.Y. (2019). Endoscopic management of peptic ulcer bleeding: Recent advances. *Clinical Endoscopy, 52*(5), 416–418. https://doi.org/10.5946/ce.2018.182

Farrar, F.C. (2018). Management of acute gastrointestinal bleed. *Critical Care Nursing Clinics of North America, 30*(1), 55–66. https://doi.org/10.1016/j.cnc.2017.10.005

Freedberg, D.E., Kim, L.S., & Yang, Y.-X. (2017). The risks and benefits of long-term use of proton pump inhibitors: Expert review and best practice advice from the American Gastroenterological Association. *Gastroenterology, 152*(4), 706–715. https://doi.org/10.1053/j.gastro.2017.01.031

Kamboj, A.K., Cotter, T.G., & Oxentenko, A.S. (2017). *Helicobacter pylori*: The past, present, and future in management. *Mayo Clinic Proceedings, 92*(4), 599–604. https://doi.org/10.1016/j.mayocp.2016.11.017

Kavitt, R.T., Lipowska, A.M., Anyane-Yeboa, A., & Gralnek, I.M. (2019). Diagnosis and treatment of peptic ulcer disease. *American Journal of Medicine, 132*(4), 447–456. https://doi.org/10.1016/j.amjmed.2018.12.009

Kempenich, J.W., & Sirinek, K.R. (2018). Acid peptic disease. *Surgical Clinics of North America, 98*(5), 933–944. https://doi.org/10.1016/j.suc.2018.06.003

Lanas, A., & Chan, F.K.L. (2017). Peptic ulcer disease. *Lancet, 390*(10094), 613–624. https://doi.org/10.1016/S0140-6736(16)32404-7

Malfertheiner, P., & Schulz, C. (2020). Peptic ulcer: Chapter closed? *Digestive Diseases, 38*(2), 112–116. https://doi.org/10.1159/000505367

Melcarne, L., García-Iglesias, P., & Calvet, X. (2016). Management of NSAID-associated peptic ulcer disease. *Expert Review of Gastroenterology and Hepatology, 10*(6), 723–733. https://doi.org/10.1586/17474124.2016.1142872

Nelms, D.W., & Pelaez, C.A. (2018). The acute upper gastrointestinal bleed. *Surgical Clinics of North America, 98*(5), 1047–1057. https://doi.org/10.1016/j.suc.2018.05.004

Sheldon, R., & Eckert, M. (2017). Surgical critical care: Gastrointestinal complications. *Surgical Clinics of North America, 97*(6), 1425–1447. https://doi.org/10.1016/j.suc.2017.08.002

Genitourinary

CHAPTER 79

Abnormal Vaginal Bleeding (Menorrhagia)

Lindsay Tedder, MSN, APRN, WHNP-BC

I. Definition (Jordahl-Iafrato et al., 2019; Munro, 2014; Munro et al., 2018)
   A. In premenopausal women
      1. Chronic: Bleeding from the uterus with abnormal volume, regularity, and/or timing and present for a majority of the past six months
      2. Acute: Episode of heavy bleeding requiring immediate intervention to prevent further blood loss
   B. In postmenopausal women: Spontaneous uterine bleeding occurring more than 12 months from date of last menstrual cycle

II. Physiology/Pathophysiology (Jordahl-Iafrato et al., 2019; Levy-Zauberman et al., 2017; Munro et al., 2018; Whitaker & Critchley, 2016)
   A. Normal
      1. Women of reproductive age experience cyclic menstrual bleeding in three phases: follicular, ovulatory, and luteal.
      2. Normal blood loss is 5–8 ml, with regularity of menses ±2–20 days.
   B. Pathophysiology
      1. A menstrual cycle less than 24 days or more than 38 days, or a menstrual flow less than 4.5 days or more than 8 days, is considered abnormal.
      2. Abnormal vaginal bleeding is caused by hormonal changes, bleeding disorders, or ovulatory dysfunction.

III. Clinical features: Abnormal uterine bleeding is a common condition that leads to increased healthcare costs and decreased QOL. Menorrhagia is an excessive blood loss that impairs a woman's life physically, emotionally, and socially (Bradley & Gueye, 2016; Jordahl-Iafrato et al., 2019; Marnach & Laughlin-Tommaso, 2019; Munro et al., 2018; Whitaker & Critchley, 2016).
   A. Classification
      1. Structural (PALM)
         a) **P**olyp: Focal epithelial proliferation developed from endometrium
         b) **A**denomyosis
         c) **L**eiomyoma
         d) **M**alignancy/hyperplasia: Cervical and endometrial carcinomas, uterine sarcomas
      2. Nonstructural (COEIN)

    a) **C**oagulopathy: Constitutional coagulation disorders, anticoagulation and anti-platelet treatment

    b) **O**vulatory dysfunction: Anovulatory cycles from physiologic puberty, perimenopause, polycystic ovary syndrome (PCOS), treatments altering dopaminergic metabolism

    c) **E**ndometrial disorders: Atrophic, eutrophic, hypertrophic

    d) **I**atrogenic: Bleeding related to hormonal treatments

    e) **N**ot otherwise classified: Special entities, vascular anomalies, chronic endometritis

3. Special cases not in PALM/COEIN: Isthmocele, cesarean scar defect, retained products of conception

B. Etiology
1. Inherited or acquired coagulopathy
2. Eating disorders, stress, excess exercise
3. Genital tract pathology
4. Dysfunctional uterine bleeding
5. Medication induced: Anticoagulants, hormones, intrauterine devices

C. History
1. History of cancer and cancer treatment
2. Current medications: Prescribed, over the counter (e.g., hormonal, contraceptives, anticoagulants, SSRIs, antipsychotics, tamoxifen, herbals)
3. History of presenting symptoms: Precipitating factors, onset, location, and duration, associated symptoms (e.g., fevers, chills, increasing abdominal girth, pelvic pressure or pain, bowel or bladder dysfunction, vaginal discharge or odor)
4. Changes in ADLs
5. Past medical history: Menopausal status, PCOS, hypothyroidism, hyperprolactinemia, hypothalamic or adrenal disorder
6. Bleeding pattern: Quantity, frequency of changing pads/tampons, presence of clots, timing during menstrual cycle, impact on QOL
7. Sexual/reproductive history: Contraceptives, STIs, cervical screening, possibility of pregnancy, desire for future fertility, known infertility
8. Family history: Coagulation or thromboembolic disorders, hormone-sensitive cancers

D. Physical examination
1. Vital signs: Fever indicating infection; weight and BMI obesity present with PCOS
2. Neck: Enlarged thyroid or nodules indicating thyroid dysfunction
3. Abdominal: Striae noted with PCOS, palpable mass, tenderness indicating endometritis or pelvic inflammatory disease
4. Integument: Bruising and petechiae indicating bleeding disorder, hirsutism, male hair pattern, acanthosis nigricans indicating PCOS or hyperandrogenism
5. Genitalia: Vulva, vagina, and anus for drainage; irritation, erythema, hemorrhoids, lesions, or open areas indicating trauma, infection, or other source for bleeding
6. Bimanual pelvic
    a) Presence of active bleeding and its volume
    b) Uterine enlargement suggestive of presence of fibroid, adenomyosis, or infection
    c) Adnexa palpitation to evaluate for pelvic tenderness or pelvic mass indicating pelvic inflammatory disease or uterine or adnexal pathology
    d) Source of bleeding: Vulva, vagina, cervical surface, cervical os, urethra, anus
    e) Clitoromegaly suggesting PCOS
7. Rectal: Mass, internal hemorrhoids, bleeding from rectum

IV. Diagnostic tests (Bradley & Gueye, 2016; Jordahl-Iafrato et al., 2019; Levy-Zauberman et al., 2017; Marnach & Laughlin-Tommaso, 2019; Munro, 2014; van Hanegem et al., 2016)
   A. Laboratory
      1. Pregnancy test, beta-human chorionic gonadotropin, if indicated
      2. CBC with platelets to evaluate for anemia, elevated WBC indicating infection or leukemia, low platelets
      3. Ferritin to evaluate for iron deficiency
      4. Thyroid panel to evaluate for hypothyroidism or hyperthyroidism
      5. Coagulation tests: PT, PTT, fibrinogen, thrombin time, or von Willebrand diagnostic panel to evaluate for coagulopathy if indicated from family history or chronic bleeding
      6. FSH, luteinizing hormone, and estradiol levels to assess for premature ovarian insufficiency
      7. Serum androgens to evaluate for excess indicating hirsutism or hypothalamic dysfunction with poor nutrition or excessive exercise
      8. Prolactin and testosterone levels to evaluate for ovulatory dysfunction
      9. Vaginal cultures if suspected to evaluate for genital tract infection (e.g., *Chlamydia trachomatis, Neisseria gonorrhoeae*)
      10. Pap smear to evaluate for cervical cancer
   B. Radiology
      1. Transvaginal ultrasound measurement of endometrial thickness to evaluate for endometrial neoplasia; alternative to endometrial sampling in postmenopausal women
      2. Pelvic ultrasound to evaluate for uterus or adnexa pathology
   C. Other
      1. Hysteroscopy can be used to evaluate for endometrial polyps, endometrial thickening, and submucosal leiomyoma.
      2. Postmenopausal women with spontaneous bleeding with an endometrial lining greater than 4 mm should undergo endometrial sampling.

V. Differential diagnosis (Jordahl-Iafrato et al., 2019; Munro et al., 2016, 2018; van Hanegem et al., 2016)
   A. Hormonal imbalances
      1. Medication induced: Oral contraceptive pills, hormone replacement therapies
      2. PCOS
      3. Adrenal hyperplasia
      4. Cushing disease
      5. Hypothyroid or hyperthyroid disease (see Chapters 157 and 158)
   B. Anatomic changes
      1. Adenomas
      2. Leiomyomas
      3. Polyps of cervix or endometrium
      4. Cervical dysplasia
      5. Endometrial hyperplasia
   C. Malignancy: Cervical, uterine, ovarian
   D. Underlying disease
      1. Coagulopathies (see Chapter 122)
      2. Blood dyscrasias
      3. Celiac disease
   E. Complications of pregnancy

F. Excessive dieting, exercise, stress

G. Injury from trauma: Foreign body, intrauterine devices, sexual abuse, assault

H. Inflammation of genital tract

I. Medication induced: Anticoagulants, hormone therapy, tamoxifen

VI. Treatment (Bofill Rodriguez et al., 2019; Bradley & Gueye, 2016; Heikinheimo & Fraser, 2017; Jordahl-Iafrato et al., 2019; Lethaby et al., 2019; Levy-Zauberman et al., 2017; Marnach & Laughlin-Tommaso, 2019; Whitaker & Critchley, 2016)

A. Underlying medical conditions should be treated, such as thyroid disorder (see Chapters 157 and 158) or coagulation disorder (see Chapter 122).

B. Surgical management

1. Polyp or fibroids: Resection of abnormal growth

2. Adenomyosis: Hysterectomy or adenomyomectomy

3. Malignancy: Surgery with or without adjuvant treatment, high-dose progestogens, palliation (includes radiation)

4. Uterine curettage for abnormal bleeding without pathologic cause

5. Endometrial ablation

   a) Ovulatory dysfunction: Lifestyle modification of monitoring stress, excessive exercise, weight management

   b) Antibiotics for endometritis or pelvic inflammatory disease: Ceftriaxone 250 mg IM daily, plus doxycycline 100 mg PO two times a day for 14 days, plus metronidazole 400 mg PO two times a day for 14 days

C. Hormonal treatment

1. Combined contraceptives: Used in cases without anatomical focal lesions; action based on inhibition of hypothalamic–pituitary axis and endometrial atrophy

   a) Acute: Monophasic 35 mcg estradiol PO three times a day for seven days, then daily dosing for three weeks

   b) Heavy menstrual bleeding: Cyclic monophasic or triphasic oral pill, extended or continuous monophasic oral pill, transdermal patch, vaginal ring

2. Conjugated equine estrogen: For acute bleeding, 25 mg IV every four to six hours for 24 hours

3. Oral progestins: Action based on endometrial atrophy; limited to patients with endometrial hypertrophy who wish to preserve fertility

   a) Acute: Medroxyprogesterone acetate 20 mg PO three times a day for seven days

   b) Heavy menstrual bleeding: Oral medroxyprogesterone acetate 2.5–10 mg PO, norethindrone 2.5–5 mg PO, megestrol acetate 40–320 mg PO, or micronized progesterone 200–400 mg PO; without ovulatory dysfunction, one tablet daily starting day five for 21 days; with ovulatory dysfunction, one tablet daily for two weeks every four weeks

4. Progesterone injection: Medroxyprogesterone acetate 150 mg IM injection every 12 weeks

5. Levonorgestrel-releasing intrauterine system: Placement every five years; releases 20 mcg daily; used without anatomical focal lesion

6. Gonadotropin-releasing hormone agonists: Based on inhibition of the gonadal axis, responsible for hypogonadism with endometrial atrophy and secondary amenorrhea (e.g., leuprolide 7.5 mg IM every month, goserelin 3.6 mg pellet subcutaneous every 28 days)

D. Nonhormonal

1. NSAIDs (see Appendix E)

2. Ibuprofen: 600–800 mg PO every six to eight hours, respectively
3. Tranexamic acid: 1.3 g PO every eight hours for five days

VII. Follow-up
  A. Short term
    1. Bleeding and response to treatment
    2. Reevaluated if treating infection
  B. Long term: Specific to condition

VIII. Referrals
  A. Gynecologist: For prolonged or repeated bleeding
  B. Other specialists: Dependent on underlying chronic condition

The author would like to acknowledge Joanne Lester, PhD, CNP, AOCN®, for her contribution to this chapter that remains unchanged from the previous edition of this book.

References

Bofill Rodriguez, M., Lethaby, A., & Farquhar, C. (2019). Nonsteroidal anti-inflammatory drugs for heavy menstrual bleeding. *Cochrane Database of Systematic Reviews, 2019*(9). https://doi.org/10.1002/14651858.CD000400.pub4

Bradley, L.D., & Gueye, N.-A. (2016). The medical management of abnormal uterine bleeding in reproductive-aged women. *American Journal of Obstetrics and Gynecology, 214*(1), 31–44. https://doi.org/10.1016/j.ajog.2015.07.044

Heikinheimo, O., & Fraser, I. (2017). The current status of hormonal therapies for heavy menstrual bleeding. *Best Practice and Research: Clinical Obstetrics and Gynaecology, 40,* 111–120. https://doi.org/10.1016/j.bpobgyn.2017.01.001

Jordahl-Iafrato, M.A., Reed, H., Hadley, S.K., & Kolman, K.B. (2019). A systematic approach to chronic abnormal uterine bleeding. *Journal of Family Practice, 68*(2), 82–92. https://www.mdedge.com/familymedicine/article/195849/womens-health/systematic-approach-chronic-abnormal-uterine-bleeding

Lethaby, A., Wise, M.R., Weterings, M.A.J., Bofill Rodriguez, M., & Brown, J. (2019). Combined hormonal contraceptives for heavy menstrual bleeding. *Cochrane Database of Systematic Reviews, 2019*(2). https://doi.org/10.1002/14651858.CD000154.pub3

Levy-Zauberman, Y., Pourcelot, A.-G., Capmas, P., & Fernandez, H. (2017). Update on the management of abnormal uterine bleeding. *Journal of Gynecology Obstetrics and Human Reproduction, 46*(8), 613–622. https://doi.org/10.1016/j.jogoh.2017.07.005

Marnach, M.L., & Laughlin-Tommaso, S.K. (2019). Evaluation and management of abnormal uterine bleeding. *Mayo Clinic Proceedings, 94*(2), 326–335. https://doi.org/10.1016/j.mayocp.2018.12.012

Munro, M.G. (2014). Investigation of women with postmenopausal uterine bleeding: Clinical practice recommendations. *Permanente Journal, 18*(1), 55–70. https://doi.org/10.7812/TPP/13-072

Munro, M.G., Critchley, H.O.D., & Fraser, I.S. (2016). Research and clinical management for women with abnormal uterine bleeding in the reproductive years: More than PALM-COEIN. *BJOG, 124*(2), 185–189. https://doi.org/10.1111/1471-0528.14431

Munro, M.G., Critchley, H.O.D., & Fraser, I.S. (2018). The two FIGO systems for normal and abnormal uterine bleeding symptoms and classification of causes of abnormal uterine bleeding in the reproductive years: 2018 revisions. *International Journal of Gynecology and Obstetrics, 143*(3), 393–408. https://doi.org/10.1002/ijgo.12666

van Hanegem, N., Breijer, M., Slockers, S.A., Zafarmand, M.H., Geomini, P.M.A.J., Catshoek, R., ... Timmermans, A. (2016). Diagnostic workup for postmenopausal bleeding: A randomised controlled trial. *BJOG, 124*(2), 231–240. https://doi.org/10.1111/1471-0528.14126

Whitaker, L., & Critchley, H.O.D. (2016). Abnormal uterine bleeding. *Best Practice and Research: Clinical Obstetrics and Gynaecology, 34,* 54–65. https://doi.org/10.1016/j.bpobgyn.2015.11.012

CHAPTER 80

Amenorrhea

Stephanie Jackson, DNP, MSN, RN, AOCNS®, BMTCN®

I. Definition: The absence of menstrual bleeding, a normal feature in woman who are prepubertal, pregnant, and postmenstrual (Fourman & Fazeli, 2015; Pereira & Brown, 2017; Yoon & Cheon, 2019)

A. Primary: Lack of menses by age 16 years in the presence of normal growth and secondary sexual characteristics

B. Secondary: Lack of menses after the onset of menarche; oligomenorrhea, or the absence of menses after more than 35 days

II. Physiology/Pathophysiology (Marsh & Grimstad, 2014; Pereira & Brown, 2017; Yoon & Cheon, 2019)

A. A normal menstrual cycle is the progression of hormonal events that produce a developed follicle to release an egg for implantation. The target organs include the hypothalamus, pituitary gland, ovaries, and uterus.

1. Physiologically, the hypothalamus releases pulses of gonadotropin-releasing hormone to stimulate the anterior pituitary to release FSH and luteinizing hormone (LH).

2. Puberty development extends over a three-year period.

3. These two hormones stimulate the ovary to produce estrogen (estradiol), androgens (testosterone), and progesterone, resulting in the release of an egg.

4. The number of oocytes present at birth is close to one million. By puberty, the number is reduced to 300,000. This dramatic loss is a complex process of apoptosis, development, and ovulation, which leaves close to 1,000 oocytes by natural menopause around age 50 years.

5. FSH, LH, progesterone, and estradiol cycle are necessary components for menstruation and reproductive functions.

6. Estrogen stimulates the endometrium, which results in proliferation for egg implantation. After ovulation, if the egg is not fertilized, the uterus sheds its lining.

7. Menstrual flow passes through the cervix and down through the vagina.

B. Pathophysiology: Amenorrhea occurs when part of the functional hypothalamus, pituitary gland, ovaries, uterus, cervix, or vaginal canal malfunctions.

1. Anovulatory amenorrhea involves the disruption of the hypothalamic–pituitary–ovarian axis.

2. Hypothalamic dysfunction typically represents a functional disorder of gonadotropin-releasing hormone, leading to a loss of LH and failure to ovulate.

3. Pituitary dysfunction results from an inhibited gonadotropin-releasing hormone and impaired gonadotropin production.

4. Ovarian dysfunction can cause a hypergonadotropic response, leading to marked serum elevations in LH and FSH and low levels of estrogen and progesterone.

5. Chemotherapy accelerates the natural ovarian aging process by causing damage in steroid-producing cells (granulose and theca cells) and apoptotic death of a fraction of primordial follicles.

   a) The extent of damage is dependent on the patient's age, the type of chemotherapy, and the dose given. Cumulative dose adds more risk than dose rate.

   b) Ovarian dysfunction can occur at any point during the planned chemotherapy protocol.

   c) Menses may become irregular or stop and may resume in some patients many years after chemotherapy has ended.

   d) Alkylating agents (particularly non–cell cycle specific) and hormone therapy present the greatest risk.

   e) Natural menopause prior to the start of chemotherapy increases the rate of permanent ovarian failure.

6. Total abdominal irradiation, pelvic irradiation, or a lumbar spinal radiation field increases the risk for ovarian failure when radiation scatters to sites outside the abdomen and pelvis, affecting the gonadal system.

   a) Median dose is less than 2 Gy for permanent oocyte loss, and permanent ovarian failure can be seen with approximately 4–5 Gy of total pelvic nodal irradiation (e.g., treatment for cervical cancer, Hodgkin lymphoma).

   b) Ovarian function may resume when eggs in small radioresistant follicles mature and resume functioning.

   c) Lead shielding of the ovary or transposition of the ovaries (surgical procedure) out of the treatment field may reduce ovarian damage.

   d) Total body irradiation performed as part of HSCT conditioning delivers approximately 8–12 Gy, which destroys ovarian function within three months in most women.

7. Ovulatory amenorrhea occurs as the result of chromosomal abnormalities or other congenital anatomic genital abnormalities that obstruct menstrual flow.

III. Clinical features (Klein et al., 2019; Pereira & Brown, 2017; Yoon & Cheon, 2019)
   A. Etiology
      1. Delayed puberty
      2. Virilization
      3. Pregnancy
      4. Cancer treatment induced
      5. Drug induced
      6. Brain or pituitary tumor
      7. Hyperprolactinemia
      8. Anorexia
      9. Extreme weight loss
      10. Emotional or physical stress
      11. Polycystic ovary syndrome
      12. Functional hypothalamic anovulation
      13. Hypo- or hyperthyroidism
      14. Genital abnormality: Turner syndrome
      15. Congenital abnormality
      16. Pelvic tumor
      17. Adrenal tumor
      18. Cushing syndrome

B. History
   1. History of cancer and cancer treatment
   2. Current medications: Abuse of cocaine and opioids, antiepileptics, oral contraceptives, drugs that affect dopamine or sex hormones
   3. History of presenting symptoms: Precipitating factors, onset, duration, associated symptoms (e.g., recent weight changes over past four to six months, exercise patterns, stress)
   4. Changes in ADLs
   5. History of menstrual cycle: Age at menarche (if occurred); regularity, duration, and flow of menses; date of last menstrual period
   6. History of puberty: Age at breast development, growth spurt, presence of axillary and pubic hair
   7. Past medical history: Gynecologic procedures, hypothalamic disorders, pituitary disorders, hypothyroidism, ovarian disorders, endometriosis, pelvic inflammatory disease, infertility, STIs, chronic illness (e.g., Crohn disease, cystic fibrosis, sickle cell disease)
   8. Family history: Menstrual problems, infertility, endocrine diseases, autoimmune diseases, congenital anomalies
C. Signs and symptoms
   1. Pituitary disorders: Galactorrhea, headaches, visual field defects
   2. Hypothyroidism: Fatigue, weight gain, cold intolerance
   3. Hyperthyroidism: Palpitations, nervousness, tremor, heat intolerance
   4. Androgen excess: Acne, hirsutism, voice changes
   5. Estrogen deficiency: Hot flashes, night sweats, sleep disturbances, vaginal dryness, decreased libido
   6. Emotional lability: Anxiety, depression, irritability, decreased cognition
   7. Urinary symptoms: Dysuria, frequency, urge, incontinence
   8. Vaginal pruritus and/or dyspareunia
D. Physical examination
   1. Body composition: Height and weight for substantial increase or decrease
   2. HEENT
      a) Hair distribution for signs of androgen deficiency: Male pattern baldness
      b) Eye: Signs of increased ICP suggestive of intracranial tumor
      c) Skin: Presence of acne, hirsutism, hair loss suggestive of increased androgen
      d) Facial hair: Excess hair distribution suggestive of increased androgen
      e) Thyroid: Presence of enlarged thyroid or palpable nodules
   3. Neurologic: Evidence of cranial nerve deficits suggestive of intracranial tumor (see Appendix A)
   4. Breast
      a) Presence of galactorrhea indicative of inappropriate prolactin release
      b) Masses, edema, abnormal dimpling, skin changes, nipple discharge
      c) Excess axillary hair quantity indicative of increased androgen
   5. Abdominal
      a) Abdominal striae in nulliparous women indicative of hypercortisolism
      b) Obesity with fat concentration in the trunk suggestive of high androgen levels
      c) Abdominal mass or organomegaly
   6. Gynecologic
      a) Presence of ambiguous genitalia, fused labia, or other abnormalities
      b) Hair distribution on the external genitalia and pubis
      c) External genitalia and vagina for evidence of low estrogen levels

      (1) Dry, pale, atrophic mucosa with alkaline pH

      (2) Minimal cervical mucus

         (*a*) Clitoris for enlargement indicative of elevated androgen levels

         (*b*) Vaginal canal for reddened or thin mucosa, imperforate hymen, vaginal septum defect preventing menstrual flow, or vaginal stenosis

         (*c*) Cervical assessment for signs of stricture or blockage preventing menstrual flow; patency of cervix

         (*d*) Uterus and ovaries for enlargement or mass

  7. Extremities: Excess hair distribution or increased muscle mass indicative of increased androgen levels

  8. Dysmorphic features indicative of Turner syndrome: Webbed neck, short stature, low hairline

IV. Diagnostic tests: Dependent on suspected cause of primary or secondary amenorrhea (Klein et al., 2017; Klein et al., 2019; Yoon & Cheon, 2019)

  A. Laboratory

    1. CBC and metabolic panel to rule out chronic diseases

    2. Qualitative beta-human chorionic gonadotropin (βHCG): Must be completed first to evaluate for pregnancy; results reported as positive or negative (secondary amenorrhea)

      a) Urine βHCG: Modern day tests can detect levels as low as 20 mIU/ml.

      b) Normal intrauterine pregnancy βHCG levels will double every 48 hours.

    3. TSH level to evaluate for hypothyroidism or hyperthyroidism: Normal is less than 5 mU/L.

    4. Serum prolactin level to evaluate for hyperprolactinemia: Normal is 10–25 ng/ml.

    5. Free and total testosterone to evaluate for hyperandrogenism, ovarian or adrenal tumor, and Cushing syndrome

    6. Serum FSH, LH, and estradiol to evaluate for hypothalamic, pituitary dysfunction, perimenopausal, or menopausal state

      a) Normal levels: FSH 5–30 IU/L (mid-cycle levels will be twice the baseline level); LH 5–20 IU/L (mid-cycle levels will be three times the baseline level)

      b) Hypothalamic amenorrhea, polycystic ovary syndrome: If FSH and LH levels are repeatedly low or normal; estradiol levels normal to low

      c) Ovarian failure/postmenopausal: If FSH and LH levels are repeatedly high; estradiol less than 50 pg/ml

         (1) If exhibiting signs of hirsutism: Serum dehydroepiandrosterone sulfate, 17-hydroxyprogesterone level, free testosterone levels to evaluate for androgen excess

         (2) If elevated FSH and workup suggestive of possible autoimmune etiology: CBC, ESR, antinuclear antibody, rheumatoid factor, total protein, albumin/globulin ratio, morning cortisol level, phosphorus, and calcium to evaluate for autoimmune disorder

         (3) Chromosome karyotype studies: If FSH greater than 20 IU/L and prolactin and TSH normal

  B. Radiology

    1. Pelvic ultrasound when polycystic ovary syndrome or suspicion of ovarian mass: Congenital abnormalities of the uterus, cervix, and vagina may also be identified.

    2. Abdominal CT scan when androgen-secreting adrenal tumors suspected

    3. MRI of sella turcica anterior pituitary: If galactorrhea or prolactin level greater than 100 ng/ml or patient has symptoms of increased ICP to evaluate for prolactinoma

or CNS abnormality; MRI for clinical manifestations of associated headaches, profound estrogen deficiency, hyperprolactinemia, and elevated gonadotropins

4. Uterine ultrasound in presence of ambiguous βHCG: Increase less than 60% in 48 hours, rapid elevation, or suspected hydatidiform mole

5. Hysterosalpingography or hysteroscopy to evaluate for evidence of tubal blockage or uterine scarring, fibroid, or polyp

6. DEXA scan to evaluate for bone loss if estrogen levels low

V. Differential diagnosis (Klein et al., 2017; Klein et al., 2019; Yoon & Cheon, 2019)
   A. Anovulatory amenorrhea
      1. Hypothalamic dysfunction, structural
      2. Genetic disorders: Prader-Willi syndrome
      3. Infiltrative disorders of the hypothalamus: Sarcoidosis
      4. Irradiation of the hypothalamus
      5. Traumatic brain injury
      6. Tumors of the hypothalamus
   B. Hypothalamic dysfunction, functional
      1. Cachexia (see Chapter 66)
      2. Chronic disorders: GI, respiratory, hematologic, renal, hepatic
      3. Dieting
      4. Malabsorption syndromes: Celiac disease
      5. Drug abuse: Alcohol, illicit drugs
      6. Eating disorders: Anorexia nervosa, bulimia
      7. Excessive physical exercise
      8. HIV infection and immunodeficiency
      9. Psychiatric disorders: Stress, depression, schizophrenia, obsessive–compulsive disorder
      10. Psychoactive drugs
   C. Pituitary dysfunction
      1. Hyperprolactinemia
      2. Disorders of the pituitary: Hemochromatosis (see Chapter 121), TB (see Chapter 36)
      3. Kallmann syndrome
      4. Sheehan syndrome
      5. Traumatic brain injury
      6. Brain tumor: Meningioma, craniopharyngioma, glioma
      7. Tumors of the pituitary
   D. Ovarian dysfunction
      1. Autoimmune disorders that result in autoimmune oophoritis: Myasthenia gravis, thyroiditis, vitiligo
      2. Chemotherapy induced
      3. Pelvic irradiation
      4. Genetic abnormalities including chromosomal abnormalities: Turner syndrome, fragile X syndrome
      5. Gonadal dysgenesis
      6. Metabolic disease: Addison disease, diabetes (see Chapter 151), galactosemia
      7. Viral infections: Mumps
   E. Other endocrine dysfunctions
      1. Androgen insensitivity syndrome
      2. Congenital adrenal virilism
      3. Cushing syndrome

    4. Drug-induced virilization: Androgens, antidepressants, danazol
    5. Hyperthyroidism (see Chapter 157)
    6. Hypothyroidism (see Chapter 158)
    7. Obesity
    8. Polycystic ovary syndrome
    9. True hermaphroditism
    10. Ovarian or adrenal tumors producing androgens
    11. Tumors producing estrogen or human chorionic gonadotropin
 F. Congenital genital abnormalities
    1. Cervical stenosis
    2. Imperforate hymen
    3. Pseudohermaphroditism
    4. Transverse vaginal septum
    5. Vaginal or uterine aplasia
 G. Acquired uterine abnormalities
    1. Asherman syndrome
    2. Endometrial TB
    3. Obstructive fibroids and polyps

VI. Treatment: Directed at the underlying disorder (Klein et al., 2017; Klein et al., 2019; Pereira & Brown, 2017; Yoon & Cheon, 2019)
  A. Treat symptoms and long-term effects of estrogen deficiency (see Chapter 90). A combination approach works best of education, nutritional support, lifestyle modification, counseling, physical activity, and several pharmacologic agents.
  B. Treat symptoms of estrogen excess.
  C. Minimize hirsutism and long-term effects of androgen excess.
  D. Depression: Manage with antidepressant medications and counseling (see Chapter 162).
  E. Osteoporosis: Manage patients based on age and risk factors for vitamin D deficiency (see Chapter 106).
  F. Cardiovascular disease: Risk may be decreased and managed by a daily exercise regimen and lifestyle changes (e.g., proper diet, limiting alcoholic intake, avoidance of smoking, hypertension control, lipid control).

VII. Follow-up
  A. Short term: Patients treated with estrogen or progesterone therapy should be followed after starting therapy to assess for response or side effects.
  B. Long term: Patients should be seen in one year, then followed periodically to determine if amenorrhea is resolving or is occurring because of premature menopause.

VIII. Referrals
  A. Reproductive endocrinologist: For recommendations for treatment of delayed puberty, virilization, ovarian failure, and other hormone-based abnormalities
  B. Surgeon: For surgical options for anatomic genital tract abnormalities
  C. Fertility specialist: For counseling, options, and treatment
  D. Internal medicine specialist: To manage chronic disease (e.g., hypertension, immunodeficiency, sarcoidosis, TB)
  E. Rheumatologist: To recommend management of autoimmune disorders
  F. Clinical psychologist or psychiatrist: To recommend or manage treatment for depression, anxiety, drug abuse, suspected eating disorders, and psychiatric disorders
  G. Medical oncologist: For evaluation and management of malignancies

The author would like to acknowledge Dana L. Viviano, RN, BSN, for her contribution to this chapter that remains unchanged from the previous edition of this book.

References

Fourman, L.T., & Fazeli, P.K. (2015). Neuroendocrine causes of amenorrhea—An update. *Journal of Clinical Endocrinology and Metabolism, 100*(3), 812–824. https://doi.org/10.1210/jc.2014-3344

Klein, D.A., Emerick, J.E., Sylvester, J.E., & Vogt, K.S. (2017). Disorders of puberty: An approach to diagnosis and management. *American Family Physician, 96*(9), 590–599. https://www.aafp.org/afp/2017/1101/p590.html

Klein, D.A., Paradise, S.L., & Reeder, R.M. (2019). Amenorrhea: A systematic approach to diagnosis and management. *American Family Physician, 100*(1), 39–48. https://www.aafp.org/afp/2019/0701/p39.html

Marsh, C.A., & Grimstad, F.W. (2014). Primary amenorrhea: Diagnosis and management. *Obstetrics and Gynecological Surgery, 69*(10), 603–612. https://doi.org/10.1097/OGX.0000000000000111

Pereira, K., & Brown, A.J. (2017). Secondary amenorrhea: Diagnostic approach and treatment considerations. *Nurse Practitioner, 42*(9), 34–41. https://doi.org/10.1097/01.NPR.0000520832.14406.76.

Yoon, J.Y., & Cheon, C.K. (2019). Evaluation and management of amenorrhea related to congenital sex hormonal disorders. *Annals of Pediatric Endocrinology and Metabolism, 24*(3), 149–157. https://doi.org/10.6065/apem.2019.24.3.149

CHAPTER 81

Dysuria

Faith A. Mutale, MSN, CRNP, and Cecile B. Miller, MSN, CRNP

I. Definition: Burning, tingling, or stinging of the urethra and meatus associated with voiding (Alpay et al., 2018; Michels & Sands, 2015)

II. Physiology/Pathophysiology (Michels & Sands, 2015)
   A. Normal: The bladder is a muscular, membranous reservoir for urine storage and expulsion. Urine is discharged from the bladder through the urethra. Bladder capacity is approximately 400–600 ml of urine in a healthy adult.
   B. Pathophysiology: Dysuria results from chemical irritation, inflammatory/infectious conditions, bladder irritation, or stricture, causing difficulty initiating urination and usually associated with burning or pain.

III. Clinical features: Approximately 50% of women experience dysuria at some time in their lives. Dysuria is less common among men (Chu & Lowder, 2018; Geerlings, 2016; Gupta et al., 2017; Michels & Sands, 2015; Tan & Chlebicky, 2016).
   A. Risk factors
      1. In women, a short urethra increases risk for infection.
         a) Atrophic vaginitis, candidiasis, bacterial vaginosis
         b) Urinary catheterization
         c) Pelvic surgery or previous urologic procedure
         d) Dermatologic conditions: Irritant or contact dermatitis, lichen sclerosus, lichen planus, psoriasis, Stevens-Johnson syndrome, Behçet disease
         e) Anxiety and depression
      2. In men, a short urethra may enlarge the prostate or cause infection.
      3. Age older than 40 years
   B. Etiology
      1. Bacterial UTI: Urethritis, schistosomiasis
      2. Obstruction due to prostate enlargement strictures, diverticula; stent in bladder or urethra; pelvic mass
      3. Drug induced: Cyclophosphamide, ifosfamide
      4. Allopurinol and intravesical therapy: Bacillus Calmette-Guérin
      5. Personal hygiene irritants: Sprays, gels, powders, soaps
      6. Contraceptive devices
      7. STIs
      8. Neoplasms: Bladder, prostate, or penile cancers; vaginal/vulvar and renal cell tumor
   C. History
      1. History of cancer and cancer treatment
      2. Current medications: Prescribed, over the counter

3. History of presenting symptoms: Precipitating factors, onset, location, duration, associated symptoms (e.g., flank tenderness; back pain; hematuria; urinary urgency, frequency, and hesitancy)
4. Changes in ADLs
5. Past medical history: UTIs, stress incontinence, and known abnormalities; STIs, unprotected sex, number of partners, method of contraception, and pregnancy; urethral or vaginal discharge; diabetes mellitus; vaginal atrophy; traumatic vaginal or pelvic injury and/or surgery; exposure to chemicals, dyes, and solvents; recent hospitalization and instrumentation

D. Signs and symptoms
1. Burning suggestive of urethral inflammation
2. Urgency
3. Frequency
4. Urethral or vaginal discharge, malodorous urine
5. Hematuria

E. Physical examination
1. Vital signs: Fever with kidney infection (often absent in older adults)
2. Abdominal: Suprapubic tenderness or guarding suggestive of cystitis (not always present), palpable bladder indicating retention or bladder mass
3. Posterior thorax: Tender costovertebral angle on palpation; consistent with renal inflammation; not always present
4. Male GU
   a) Possible urethral discharge and erythema with STIs or penile cancer
   b) Tender prostate suggestive of prostatitis
   c) Increased bacterial count in prostatic secretions or void suggestive of infection
   d) Scrotal: Consistent with epididymitis when pain is unilateral
5. Gynecologic
   a) External genitalia examination for discharge, odor, labial irritation, or herpes simplex lesions suggestive of STIs; prolapsed bladder; evidence of trauma
   b) Cervical motion tenderness to evaluate for pelvic inflammatory disease

IV. Diagnostic tests (Alpay et al., 2018; Chu & Lowder, 2018; Gupta et al., 2017; Huttner et al., 2015; Michels & Sands, 2015; Nik-Ahd et al., 2018; Tan & Chlebicky, 2016)
A. Laboratory
1. Urinalysis
   a) Color usually dark yellow (concentrated) or amber (hematuria)
   b) Pyuria indicative of UTI
      (1) Absence of pyuria indicating a vaginal cause for dysuria
      (2) Sterile pyuria suggestive of renal TB
      (3) WBC casts suggestive of renal parenchymal infection
      (4) RBCs indicating serious underlying pathology, including malignancy
   c) Presence of one organism on high-power field suggesting clinically significant bacteria in urine
2. Urine culture
   a) A colony count greater than 100,000 organisms/ml provides high specificity but poor sensitivity.
   b) *Escherichia coli* is the most common organism causing UTI.
      (1) Gram-positive organism (e.g., *Enterococcus, Staphylococcus aureus*, group B streptococci) are also common in UTI.

(2) *Staphylococcus epidermis* or diphtheroids are skin flora and are considered contaminants.

(3) *Candida* seldom is correlated with symptoms of UTI and most likely is related to vaginal secretions in the urine sample.

3. Urine cytology, as appropriate, in patients at high risk for malignancy
4. Pregnancy test, as appropriate, in women of childbearing age
5. Culture drainage
   a) Urethral or cervical discharge suggestive of STI
   b) Vaginal cultures to assess for bacterial vaginitis or *Candida* infections

B. Radiology
   1. Renal ultrasound to assess for obstruction or masses
   2. Bladder ultrasound to assess for obstruction
   3. Kidney, ureter, and bladder x-ray if renal tract stones suspected

C. Other: Cystoscopy, if indicated, for persistent symptoms

V. Differential diagnosis (Alpay et al., 2018; Michels & Sands, 2015; Nik-Ahd et al., 2018)
   A. UTI: Cystitis (see Chapter 89)
   B. Urethritis: Reiter syndrome
   C. Other infections in the urinary tract: STIs, pyelonephritis, acute bacterial prostatitis (see Chapters 92 and 94)
   D. Urethral stricture: Urinary obstruction (e.g., calculus)
   E. Benign prostatic hypertrophy, chronic bacterial prostatitis, nonbacterial prostatitis (see Chapters 87 and 92)
   F. Tumor: Prostate, bladder, cervix, kidney, ureter, urethra
   G. Gynecologic disorders: Postmenopausal atrophic vaginitis (see Chapter 85), prolapse of uterus, cystocele, rectocele, dysmenorrhea
   H. Pelvic peritonitis and abscess: STIs, vulvovaginitis (see Chapter 85)
   I. Psychological abnormalities
   J. Mechanical or chemical irritation: Sexual abuse, incidental trauma
   K. Interstitial cystitis (see Chapter 89)
   L. Polycystic kidneys
   M. Renal cysts
   N. Sickle cell disease (see Chapter 119)
   O. Overactive bladder

VI. Treatment: Determining treatment is dependent on the cause of the pain. Painful urination can be caused by infection, inflammation, pathology of the bladder, prostate, or malignancy (Alpay et al., 2018; Chu & Lowder, 2018; Geerlings, 2016; Gupta et al., 2017; Gupta et al., 2011; Michels & Sands, 2015; Nik-Ahd et al., 2018).
   A. Symptomatic treatment for dysuria: Phenazopyridine HCL 200 mg PO three times a day for one to two days; provides symptomatic relief within hours of the first dose; will turn urine red-orange
   B. Symptomatic treatment for bladder spasms
      1. Oxybutynin: 5 mg PO two to three times a day, titrated up to 20 mg PO daily in divided doses; or extended release 5 or 10 mg PO daily, titrated up to 30 mg PO daily
      2. Tolterodine tartrate: 1–2 mg PO two times a day; or extended-release 2–4 mg PO daily
   C. Treatment of dysuria with pyuria is dependent on organism. Antibiotic alternatives include the following (see Appendix C).
      1. Uncomplicated cystitis

      a) Trimethoprim/sulfamethoxazole: One double-strength (160 mg/800 mg) tablet PO two times a day for three days

      b) Nitrofurantoin macrocrystals: 100 mg PO two times a day for five to seven days; should not be prescribed to men

  2. Pyelonephritis and complicated cystitis

      a) Give ciprofloxacin 500 mg PO two times a day, Cipro® XR 500 mg once daily, or trimethoprim/sulfamethoxazole double strength (160 mg/800 mg).

      b) Minimum duration of therapy is generally 7–14 days for pyelonephritis and complicated cystitis; agent should be narrowed based on antimicrobial susceptibilities.

VII. Follow-up: In asymptomatic patients PRN

VIII. Referral: Care of a specialist is paramount in some conditions.

  A. If the cause is not apparent

  B. Urologist/oncologist: If neoplasm is suspected; for management and long-term follow-up of sequelae from cancer treatment

  C. For symptoms persisting despite thorough assessment, advice, and treatment in primary care

References

Alpay, Y., Aykın, N., Korkmaz, P., Güldüren, H.M., & Çağlan, F.C. (2018). Urinary tract infections in the geriatric patients. *Pakistan Journal of Medical Sciences, 34*(1), 67–72. https://doi.org/10.12669/pjms.341.14013

Chu, C.M., & Lowder, J.L. (2018). Diagnosis and treatment of urinary tract infections across age groups. *American Journal of Obstetrics and Gynecology, 219*(1), 40–51. https://doi.org/10.1016/j.ajog.2017.12.231

Geerlings, S.E. (2016). Clinical presentations and epidemiology of urinary tract infections. *Microbiology Spectrum, 4*(5). https://doi.org/10.1128/microbiolspec.UTI-0002-2012

Gupta, K., Grigoryan, L., & Trautner, B. (2017). Urinary tract infection. *Annals of Internal Medicine, 167*(7), ITC49–ITC64. https://doi.org/10.7326/AITC201710030

Gupta, K., Hooton, T.M., Naber, K.G., Wullt, B., Colgan, R., Miller, L.G., ... Soper, D.E. (2011). International clinical practice guidelines for the treatment of acute uncomplicated cystitis and pyelonephritis in women: A 2010 update by the Infectious Diseases Society of America and the European Society for Microbiology and Infectious Diseases. *Clinical Infectious Diseases, 52*(5), e103–e120. https://doi.org/10.1093/cid/ciq257

Huttner, A., Verhaegh, E.M., Harbarth, S., Muller, A.E., Theuretzbacher, U., & Mouton, J.W. (2015). Nitrofurantoin revisited: A systematic review and meta-analysis of controlled trials. *Journal of Antimicrobial Chemotherapy, 70*(9), 2456–2464. https://doi.org/10.1093/jac/dkv147

Michels, T.C., & Sands, J.E. (2015). Dysuria: Evaluation and differential diagnosis in adults. *American Family Physician, 92*(9), 778–788. https://www.aafp.org/afp/2015/1101/p778.html

Nik-Ahd, F., Ackerman, A.L., & Anger, J. (2018). Recurrent urinary tract infections in females and the overlap with overactive bladder. *Current Urology Reports, 19*(11), 94. https://doi.org/10.1007/s11934-018-0839-3

Tan, C.W., & Chlebicky, M.P. (2016). Urinary tract infections in adults. *Singapore Medical Journal, 57*(9) 485–490. https://doi.org/10.11622/smedj.2016153

CHAPTER 82

Hematuria

Faith A. Mutale, MSN, CRNP, and Cecile B. Miller, MSN, CRNP

I. Definition: Abnormal presence of RBCs in urine; microscopic or gross/macroscopic (Bolenz et al., 2018; Moloney et al., 2014)

II. Physiology/Pathophysiology (Bolenz et al., 2018; Moloney et al., 2014; Niemi & Cohen, 2015)
   A. Normal
      1. Fewer than 100 RBCs are excreted into the urine per minute.
      2. Normal urine contains a small number of cells and other formed elements shed from the urinary system.
   B. Pathophysiology: Any process that results in infection, inflammation, or injury to GU structures can result in hematuria.
      1. Increased excretion to 3,000–5,000 RBCs per minute (three or more RBCs/high-power field), or an Addis count greater than 500,000 RBCs per 12 hours, results in microscopic hematuria.
      2. Excretion of greater than 1 million RBCs per minute results in gross hematuria.
      3. Presence of eight RBCs/high-power field may suggest a serious underlying problem, including malignancy.
      4. Irritation or damage to the urothelium and urethra (cystitis and urethritis) can result in hematuria.
      5. An increased risk of malignancy exists in patients presenting with microscopic hematuria.

III. Clinical features: The degree of hematuria does not correlate with severity of underlying cause. Asymptomatic microscopic hematuria can range from minor findings that do not require treatment to highly significant life-threatening symptoms. Asymptomatic hematuria occurs at a rate of 0.2%–21% and can be intermittent, even in patients subsequently diagnosed with a GU malignancy. Macroscopic hematuria carries an approximate risk of 10%–34.5% of malignancy and requires complete evaluation (Bolenz et al., 2018; Moloney et al., 2014).
   A. Risk factors
      1. Exposure to chemicals or dyes: Cyclophosphamide, benzenes, aromatic amines
      2. Age older than 35 years
      3. Male gender
      4. Analgesia abuse: NSAIDs
      5. Prior urologic malignancy and pelvic irradiation, prior chemotherapy with cyclophosphamide
      6. Smoking
      7. Irritative voiding symptoms: Urgency dysuria, frequency, nocturia
      8. Exposure to aristolochic acid

      9. Chronic UTIs

     10. Indwelling Foley catheter

B. Etiology: RBCs in urine can originate from anywhere in the urinary tract, which is divided into glomerular and nonglomerular.

    1. Glomerular causes

      a) Hereditary nephritis: Alport syndrome

      b) Thin glomerular basement membrane disease

      c) IgA nephropathy: Berger disease; most common in men aged 10–29 years following acute illness

      d) Postinfectious glomerulonephritis

    2. Nonglomerular causes

      a) Infections and inflammatory conditions: Pyelonephritis, cystitis

      b) Urolithiasis/renal stones

      c) Neoplasms: Renal cell carcinoma, bladder

      d) Benign prostatic hypertrophy

      e) Chemotherapy agents: Cyclophosphamide, ifosfamide

      f) Medications: NSAIDs, oral anticoagulants

      g) Systemic factors: Hemophilia, leukemia, renal vein thrombosis, embolic renal infarction, sickle cell disease, endometriosis

      h) Strenuous activity such as jogging (runner's hematuria) or sexual activity

      i) Menstruation

      j) Postprocedure

      k) Arteriovenous malformation/angiomyolipoma

C. History: Important to direct care management

    1. History of cancer and cancer treatment

    2. Current medications: Prescribed, over the counter, phenazopyridine, hydroxychloroquine

    3. History of presenting symptoms: Precipitating factors, onset, location, duration, associated symptoms (e.g., joint pain, swelling, diarrhea, rash, gross hematuria, transient or persistent UTIs/urinary symptoms)

    4. Changes in ADLs

    5. Past medical history: Recent urologic procedures or instrumentation, sexual activity, STIs, edema, and arrhythmias suggestive of nephrotic syndrome

    6. Recent trauma or injury to the pelvis or flank regions; diet and strenuous exercise history

    7. Family history: Nephritis, polycystic kidney disease, sickle cell disease

D. Signs and symptoms

    1. Urine may be blood-tinged, grossly bloody, or smoky brown or cola in color. Color identifies when blood appears in urine.

      a) Initial hematuria includes bright red blood at onset of urination suggesting a urethral origin.

      b) Terminal hematuria includes blood at the end of urination suggesting a site near the bladder neck or prostate.

      c) Total hematuria includes bleeding throughout voiding suggesting a bleeding site above bladder neck.

      d) Long-standing blood in the urinary tract deteriorates and gives urine a smoky, brownish color suggesting a bleeding site above the bladder neck.

      e) Clots in urine are almost always indicative of glomerular origin.

    2. Urinary frequency

    3. Dysuria characterized as sharp and burning

    4. Urinary urgency

    5. Suprapubic or flank pain or tenderness

    6. Fever and/or chills

    7. Nocturia

    8. Foul-smelling urine

    9. Proteinuria greater than 500 mg daily suggestive of glomerular source

  E. Physical examination

    1. Vital signs

      a) Fever associated with flank pain suggestive of pyelonephritis

      b) Possible hypertension noted in glomerulonephritis

    2. Integument: Petechiae or mottling suggestive of possible coagulopathy process

    3. Abdominal: Lower abdominal and pelvic tenderness, masses, and bruits; positive abdominal bruit suggestive of vascular process such as aneurysm or arteriovenous malformation; costovertebral angle tenderness indicating possible mass

    4. Lymph nodes: Inguinal masses or adenopathy (see Appendix D)

    5. Posterior thorax: Costovertebral angle tenderness indicating ureteral obstruction or kidney infection

    6. GU

      a) Urethral orifice and external genitalia assessment for drainage, ulceration, and stenosis for evidence of STIs

      b) Prostate enlargement, nodules, or pain

    7. GU: Lacerations suggestive of possible trauma

    8. HEENT: Periorbital edema indicative of possible nephrotic syndrome

IV. Diagnostic tests (Bauer et al., 2019; Bolenz et al., 2018; Moloney et al., 2014; Niemi & Cohen, 2015; Ziegelman et al., 2017)

  A. Laboratory

    1. Urine

      a) Dipstick: This quick, inexpensive test is nondiagnostic (affected by food, drugs, alkaline urine pH, contamination with oxidizing agents, and myoglobinuria associated with spurious hematuria) and must be done in combination with microscopic examination of urine.

      b) Urinalysis: It is the gold standard. Urinalysis is helpful in distinguishing between glomerular from nonglomerular causes of hematuria.

        (1) WBC casts suggestive of pyelonephritis or interstitial nephritis

        (2) RBCs in specimen indicative of urinary tract disease including possible malignancy

        (3) Cellular casts, dysmorphic RBCs suggestive of a glomerular cause; glomerulonephritis

        (4) Positive cytology indicative of a urothelial malignancy and warrants referral to oncology

        (5) Proteinuria or an elevated creatinine suggestive of a glomerular cause

        (6) Presence of proteinuria, cellular casts, and dysmorphic (abnormally shaped) RBCs warranting nephrology workup

      c) Urine culture

        (1) Isolation of infectious organism

        (2) WBC count of more than 100,000/mm³ indicative of infection

    2. CBC: WBC count elevated with infection

    3. PT and PTT: Prolonged in coagulopathies

    4. Prostate-specific antigen: For prostate lesions, benign prostatic hypertrophy, or prostatitis

     5. Urine cytology: Detection of urothelial malignancy

  B. Radiology

     1. Multidetector CT urography: Increased sensitivity and specificity for detection of calculi and malignancy in upper urinary tract

     2. CT: Most sensitive and gold standard for detection of intrarenal and extrarenal masses, calculi, upper tract urothelial masses, and extrinsic lesions; secondary role; to rule out calculi or other types of obstruction in GU tract

     3. Magnetic resonance urography: Evolving technology with increasing role in detection of malignancy independent of excretory function; inferior to multidetector CT urography and not adequate for detection of calculi

     4. Renal and bladder ultrasound: Avoids exposure to ionizing radiation; useful for detection and characterization of renal masses, cysts, obstruction, hydronephrosis, or abdominal aortic aneurysm

     5. IV urography (IVU; same as IV pyelogram): For evaluation of structural and urological abnormalities in the upper urinary tract; blood flow, obstructive lesions (major disadvantage is inability to distinguish cysts from malignant masses)

     6. Retrograde pyelography with fluoroscopy: Performed in combination with cystoscopy for better visualization and characterization of ureters; performed under sedation or general anesthesia

     7. CT urography: Preferred in patients with renal insufficiency or allergy to dye; visualizes upper urinary tract, including renal parenchyma and urothelium

     8. Conventional radiography (kidney, ureter, and bladder [KUB] radiograph): Limited utility and not a routinely recommended diagnostic tool

  C. Other

     1. Cystoscopy

       a) Recommended in all patients with gross hematuria for direct visualization of the bladder, as well for biopsy in patients at risk for cancer

       b) Recommended in patients presenting with microscopic hematuria and in those who are aged 35 years or older

     2. Kidney angiography: Useful for vascular malformation assessment

V. Differential diagnosis (Bolenz et al., 2018; Casto, 2016; Niemi & Cohen, 2015)

  A. Diseases

     1. Urothelial cancers: Bladder, kidney, prostate

     2. Systemic conditions: Malignant hypertension, sickle cell disease, diabetes

     3. UTI (see Chapters 89 and 92)

     4. BPH (see Chapter 87)

     5. Intrinsic kidney disease

     6. Coagulopathy (see Chapter 122)

     7. Renal stones

  B. Medications

     1. Oral anticoagulants

     2. Chemotherapy agents

  C. Radiation therapy

     1. External beam: Pelvic field total dose is 650–780 cGy.

     2. Brachytherapy: Seed implants to the prostate; symptoms usually resolve within 12 months after treatment but may persist for years.

  D. Hemorrhagic cystitis (see Chapter 88)

  E. Rhabdomyolysis (see Chapter 159)

  F. Trauma

VI. Treatment: Dependent on underlying cause, such as infection, calculi, or malignancy (Bauer et al., 2019; Bolenz et al., 2018; Carocci et al., 2018; Linder et al., 2014; Matz & Hsieh, 2017; Moloney et al., 2014; Niemi & Cohen., 2015; Pitto & García-Perdomo, 2017; Ziegelman et al., 2017; Zwaans et al., 2016)

  A. Infection: Antibiotic regimen is dependent on the organism isolated.

    1. Trimethoprim/sulfamethoxazole: One double-strength (160 mg/800 mg) tablet PO two times a day for three days for uncomplicated infection

    2. Ciprofloxacin: 250 mg PO two times a day for three days; Cipro® XR: 500 mg PO daily for three days; ofloxacin: 200 mg PO two times a day for three days

    3. Nitrofurantoin macrocrystals: 100 mg PO two times a day for five days; not recommended for men

  B. Drug-induced hemorrhagic cystitis

    1. Administer hyperhydration before and during high-dose cyclophosphamide and ifosfamide therapy. Encourage oral fluids.

    2. Use mesna (a uroprotectant) prior to cyclophosphamide and ifosfamide infusions and then repeat two and six hours or three and six hours after or administer as a continuous infusion, which is practice or protocol dependent.

  C. Active bleeding

    1. Continuous bladder irrigation with normal saline

    2. Intravesical instillation of alum, silver nitrate, aminocaproic acid, or formalin (reserved for refractory bleeding in patients with good renal function who have failed initial treatment)

    3. Cystoscopy with fulguration of bleeding sources

    4. Cystectomy with urinary diversion, as appropriate

  D. Tumor: Appropriate management of underlying process

VII. Follow-up

  A. Short term: Assess resolution of symptoms and efficacy of interventions within a few days to a week. Urinalysis is warranted after six weeks in patients with infection.

  B. Long term: Monitor HSCT recipients treated with high-dose cyclophosphamide for potential long-term bladder sequelae.

  C. Perform initial and periodic cytology in patients at high risk for malignancy at 6, 12, 24, and 36 months. For persistent or recurrent asymptomatic microscopic hematuria after initial evaluation, consider follow-up risk assessment within three to five years.

VIII. Referrals (Bolenz et al., 2018)

  A. If findings suggest a glomerular source of bleeding, referral to nephrologist is necessary for further evaluation and management for the following.

    1. All patients on anticoagulation therapy

    2. Acutely elevated creatinine

    3. Dysmorphic RBCs, RBC casts, and WBC casts

  B. Refer to urology for evaluation in patients at increased risk for malignancy.

  C. Refer to urology for asymptomatic hematuria for evaluation. This requires urinalysis annually for two years after negative urinalysis.

References

Bauer, S.R., Carroll, P.R., & Grady, D. (2019). Hematuria practice guidelines that explicitly consider harms and costs. *JAMA Internal Medicine, 179*(10), 1362–1364. https://doi.org/10.1001/jamainternmed.2019.2269

Bolenz, C., Schröppel, B., Eisenhardt, A., Schmitz-Dräger, B.J., & Grimm, M.-O. (2018). The investigation of hematuria. *Deutsches Ärzteblat International, 115*(48), 801–807. https://doi.org/10.3238/arztebl.2018.0801

Carocci, K.F., Levy, J., Hanna, D., Edwards, D., Nordsiek, M., Brian, M., ... Belkoff, L. (2018). A case of formalin instillation secondary to refractory gross hematuria in a patient with radiation cystitis. *Clinical Research in Urology, 1*(1), 1–4. https://asclepiusopen.com/clinical-research-in-urology/volume-1-issue-1/8.php

Casto, J. (2016). What is causing this patient's hematuria. *Journal of the American Academy of Physician Assistants, 29*(9), 54–56. https://doi.org/10.1097/01.JAA.0000490950.02814.6a

Linder, B.J., Tarrell, R.F., & Boorjian, S.A. (2014). Cystectomy for refractory hemorrhagic cystitis: Contemporary etiology, presentation and outcomes. *Journal of Urology, 192*(6), 1687–1692. https://doi.org/10.1016/j.juro.2014.06.030

Matz, E.L., & Hsieh, M.H. (2017). Review of advances in uroprotective agents for cyclophosphamide- and ifosfamide-induced hemorrhagic cystitis. *Urology, 100,* 16–19. https://doi.org/10.1016/j.urology.2016.07.030

Moloney, F., Murphy, P.K., Twomey, M., O'Connor, O.J., & Maher, M.M. (2014). Hematuria: An imaging guide. *Advances in Urology, 2014,* 414125. https://doi.org/10.1155/2014/414125

Niemi, M.A., & Cohen, R.A. (2015). Evaluation of microscopic hematuria: A critical review and proposed algorithm. *Advances in Chronic Kidney Disease, 22*(4), 289–296. https://doi.org/10.1053/j.ackd.2015.04.006

Pitto, C.M., & García-Perdomo, H.A. (2017). Interventions to treat hemorrhagic cystitis: A systematic review and meta-analysis. *Supportive Care in Cancer, 25*(7), 2043–2046. https://doi.org/10.1007/s00520-017-3731-7

Ziegelman, M.J., Boorijian, S.A., Joyce, D.D., Montgomery, B.D., & Linder, B.J. (2017). Intravesical formalin for hemorrhagic cystitis. A contemporary cohort. *Canadian Urological Association Journal, 11*(3–4), E79–E82. https://doi.org/10.5489/cuaj.4047

Zwaans, B.M.M., Chancellor, B.M., & Lamb, L.E. (2016). Modeling and treatment of radiation cystitis. *Urology, 88,* 14–21. https://doi.org/10.1016/j.urology.2015.11.001

CHAPTER 83

Oliguria/Anuria/Azotemia

Gary Shelton, DNP, MSN, NP, ANP-BC, AOCNP®, ACHPN

I. Definitions (Kellum et al., 2016; Perner et al., 2017; Schetz & Hoste, 2017; Schortgen & Schetz, 2017; van der Zee et al., 2017)

    A. Oliguria relates to a reduction in urinary volume (less than 0.5 ml/kg/hr for children and adults or 400–500 ml in 24 hours) or an output of urine below which end-products of metabolism cannot be excreted (e.g., urea, potassium, creatinine, medications).

    B. Anuria, literally, is without urine or a urinary output less than 100 ml daily.

    C. Azotemia is the retention of nitrogenous waste products normally cleared by the kidney, with greater than 50% reduction in GFR, thus affecting fluid and electrolyte balance.

II. Physiology/Pathophysiology (Kellum et al., 2016; Pham et al., 2017; Schetz & Hoste, 2017; Schortgen & Schetz, 2017; Yang et al., 2016)

    A. Normal: Urine is fluid secreted from the blood by the kidneys, stored in the bladder, and usually discharged voluntarily through the urethra.

        1. Urine is noncloudy, clear to amber in color, slightly acidic, and with deposits of phosphate.

        2. Urine mostly consists of water and other solids, such as urea, uric acid, creatinine, ammonia, chlorides, calcium, magnesium, and phosphorus. It should be negative of protein or blood.

    B. Pathophysiology: Oliguria, anuria, and azotemia can result from prerenal mechanisms (inadequate renal perfusion), acute causes (intrarenal hemodynamic causes/intrinsic renal damage), or postrenal processes (generally obstructive/outside of kidney).

III. Clinical features (Kellum et al., 2016; Klein et al., 2018; Perner et al., 2017; Pham et al., 2017; Schetz & Hoste, 2017; Schortgen & Schetz, 2017; Yang et al., 2016)

    A. Etiology

        1. Obstruction in the urinary tract

        2. Renal parenchymal disease

        3. Renal arterial occlusion, atheroembolism

        4. Cortical necrosis

        5. Glomerulonephritis, interstitial nephritis

        6. Acute tubular necrosis, acute cortical necrosis

        7. Hypovolemia: Diarrhea, diuresis, poor intake, dehydration

        8. "Third space" losses: Peritonitis, sepsis

        9. Nephrotoxic medication

        10. Preexisting renal disease: Diabetes, atherosclerosis

    B. History

      1. History of cancer and cancer treatment: Platinum-based therapies, other nephrotoxic therapies
      2. Current medications: Prescribed, over the counter
      3. History of presenting symptoms: Precipitating factors, onset, location, duration, what worsens or relieves symptoms
      4. Changes in ADLs
      5. Past medical history: Stomach or intestinal bleeding, CHF, cirrhosis, nephrotic syndrome, peritonitis, bowel obstruction, diabetes mellitus, hypertension
      6. Recent history of receiving contrast dyes

  C. Signs and symptoms
      1. Hypovolemia and prerenal azotemia
          a) Poor tissue turgor
          b) Thirst
          c) Dizziness, light-headedness, orthostatic dizziness
          d) Weight loss
          e) Dry mucous membranes
          f) Tachycardia
      2. CHF or cirrhosis of the liver
          a) Edema
          b) Shortness of breath
      3. Postrenal failure
          a) Edema
          b) Confusion
          c) Nausea and vomiting
          d) Flank pain

  D. Physical examination
      1. Vital signs
          a) Orthostatic hypotension indicative of hypovolemia
          b) Tachycardia indicative of hypovolemia
          c) Weight loss or gain: May be present depending on etiology
      2. Abdominal
          a) Hepatomegaly indicative of cirrhosis or CHF
          b) Hepatojugular reflux in supine or semirecumbent position indicative of cirrhosis (see Appendix D)
          c) Distended bladder and flank pain indicative of postrenal obstructive AKI
      3. Integument: Poor skin turgor, dry skin, xerostomia indicating hypovolemia
      4. Lower extremities: Pitting edema indicative of cirrhosis, CHF, or obstruction
      5. Pulmonary
          a) Rales indicative of CHF
          b) Inability to lie flat without shortness of breath indicative of CHF
      6. Cardiac
          a) Sinus tachycardia indicating hypovolemia
          b) S_3 gallop sound indicating CHF
          c) Collapsed neck veins indicating hypovolemia
          d) JVD indicating CHF or cirrhosis of the liver
      7. Rectal: Enlarged prostate indicative of postrenal failure
      8. GU: If Foley catheter is present, obstruction indicative of postrenal failure

IV. Diagnostic tests (Amathieu et al., 2017; Kellum et al., 2016; Klein et al., 2018; Perner et al., 2017; Schetz & Hoste, 2017; Schortgen & Schetz, 2017)

   A. Laboratory
      1. Urinalysis: Urine amount decreased
         a) Prerenal: Normal or may have slight protein or RBCs
         b) AKI: Casts, presence of RBCs, WBCs, protein
         c) Postrenal: Crystals, WBCs, RBCs, bacteria
      2. Urinary sodium
         a) Prerenal: Less than 20 mEq/L
         b) AKI: Greater than 40 mEq/L
         c) Postrenal: Variable
      3. Urinary osmolality
         a) Prerenal: Greater than 600 mOsm/kg
         b) AKI: Less than 350 mOsm/kg
         c) Postrenal: Variable
      4. A 24-hour urine collection, including creatinine and protein, may be a better reflection of urinary volume and may indicate renal failure.
      5. Chemistries
         a) BUN–creatinine ratio: 10–14:1 in renal parenchymal disease
         b) BUN–creatinine ratio: 20:1 in prerenal disease
         c) Hyperchloremic acidosis: Suggests tubular dysfunction and interstitial disease
   B. Radiology
      1. Technetium scanning to distinguish vascular occlusion from obstructive uropathy and renal parenchymal disease
      2. Ultrasound to evaluate for renal obstruction; avoid dye
      3. Retrograde pyelography if questions of obstruction remain after the previously mentioned procedures are completed

V. Differential diagnosis (Kellum et al., 2016; Perner et al., 2017; Schetz & Hoste, 2017; Schortgen & Schetz, 2017)
   A. Volume depletion
      1. Shock (see Chapter 160)
      2. Dehydration
      3. GI fluid volume loss, diarrhea, vomiting (see Chapters 56 and 63)
      4. Cutaneous loss, burns
      5. Third-space loss
   B. CHF (see Chapter 42)
   C. Cirrhosis (see Chapter 69)
   D. Nephrotic syndrome (see Chapter 91)
   E. Peritonitis
   F. Obstructive uropathy
      1. Urethral obstruction/stricture
      2. Bilateral ureteral obstruction
      3. Neurogenic bladder
      4. Prostatic enlargement (see Chapter 87)
   G. Vascular disease
      1. Acute renal arterial obstruction
      2. Renal vein obstruction
      3. Dissecting arterial aneurysm
      4. Hemorrhage
   H. Renal parenchymal disease
      1. Diffuse acute glomerular disease

    a) Acute glomerulonephritis
    b) Acute vasculitis
    c) IgA nephropathy
    d) Diabetes mellitus (see Chapter 151)
    e) Diabetes insipidus
2. Acute tubular necrosis
    a) Prolonged prerenal failure
    b) Nephrotoxic agents
    c) Sepsis
    d) Myoglobinuria
3. Acute interstitial nephritis
    a) Hypersensitivity to methicillin, ampicillin, NSAIDs, cephalosporins, sulfonamides (see Appendices C and E)
    b) Uric acid nephropathy
    c) Obstructive uropathy
4. Postcontrast media in preexisting renal failure
    a) Multiple myeloma (myelomatosis)
    b) Diabetes mellitus (see Chapter 151)

VI. Treatment (Klein et al., 2018; Perner et al., 2017; Schetz & Hoste, 2017; Schortgen & Schetz, 2017; van der Zee et al., 2017)
  A. Diagnosis to guide treatment
    1. Perform catheter placement to monitor output.
    2. Attempt to establish a urine output with volume challenge or diuretics and administration of fluids (contraindicated in CHF).
    3. Relieve vascular obstruction.
    4. Relieve obstruction with surgical intervention or stent placement.
  B. Correct electrolyte imbalances (see Chapters 152–156).
  C. Measure strict intake and output and daily weights.
  D. Discontinue all nephrotoxic medications and avoid radiographic studies with IV contrast.
  E. If oliguria and hypotension persist in a well-hydrated patient, consider vasopressors.
  F. Consider renal nutritionist if restrictions in protein intake are warranted or for dietary replacement needs.

VII. Follow-up: Follow-up is dependent on underlying etiology. Serial observations are necessary to measure serum creatinine.

VIII. Referral: Nephrologist to collaborate for evaluation and initial management

References

Amathieu, R., Al-Khafaji, A., Sileanu, F.E., Foldes, E., DeSensi, R., Hilmi, I., & Kellum, J.A. (2017). Significance of oliguria in critically ill patients with chronic liver disease. *Hepatology, 66*(5), 1592–1600. https://doi.org/10.1002/hep.29303

Kellum, J.A., Bellomo, R., & Ronco, C. (2016). Does this patient have acute kidney injury? An AKI checklist. *Intensive Care Medicine, 42*(1), 96–99. https://doi.org/10.1007/s00134-015-4026-4

Klein, S.J., Lehner, G.F., Forni, L.G., & Joannidis, M. (2018). Oliguria in critically ill patients: A narrative review. *Journal of Nephrology, 31*(6), 855–862. https://doi.org/10.1007/s40620-018-0539-6

Perner, A., Prowle, J., Joannidis, M., Young, P., Hjortrup, P.B., & Pettilä, V. (2017). Fluid management in acute kidney injury. *Intensive Care Medicine, 43*(6), 807–815. https://doi.org/10.1007/s00134-017-4817-x.

Pham, P.-C., Reddy, P., Qaqish, S., Kamath, A., Rodriguez, J., Bolos, D., ... Pham, P.-T. (2017). Cisplatin-induced renal salt wasting requiring over 12 liters of 3% saline replacement. *Case Reports in Nephrology, 2017,* 8137078. https://doi.org/10.1155/2017/8137078

Schetz, M., & Hoste, E. (2017). Understanding oliguria in the critically ill. *Intensive Care Medicine, 43*(6), 914–916. https://doi.org/10.1007/s00134-016-4537-7.

Schortgen, F., & Schetz, M. (2017). Does this critically ill patient with oliguria need more fluids, a vasopressor, or neither? *Intensive Care Medicine, 43*(6), 907–910. https://doi.org/10.1007/s00134-017-4744-x

van der Zee, E.N., Egal, M., Gommers, D., & Groeneveld, A.B.J. (2017). Targeting urine output and 30-day mortality in goal-directed therapy: A systematic review with meta-analysis and meta-regression. *BMC Anesthesiology, 17,* 22. https://doi.org/10.1186/s12871-017-0316-4

Yang, Y., Li, H.-Y., Zhou, Q., Peng, Z.-W., An, X., Li, W., ... Mao, H.-P. (2016). Renal function and all-cause mortality risk among cancer patients. *Medicine, 95*(20), e3728. https://doi.org/10.1097/MD.0000000000003728

CHAPTER 84

Urinary Incontinence

Wendy H. Vogel, MSN, FNP, AOCNP®

I. Definition: An involuntary, uncontrolled loss of urine producing a social and hygienic problem, as perceived by the patient, family, or caregivers, as well as the potential for physical and psychological problems; several types of urinary incontinence exist (Wilson & Waghel, 2016; see Table 84-1).

II. Physiology/Pathophysiology (Juszczak et al., 2019; Potts & Payne, 2018; Sharma & Chakrabarti, 2018; Smith, 2018; Weledji et al., 2019)
   A. Normal
      1. The bladder is a hollow muscular organ lined by mucosa. The detrusor muscle of the bladder normally is under simultaneous sympathetic and parasympathetic con-

TABLE 84-1	Types of Incontinence
Type	**Description**
Functional	Associated with chronic impairments of physical and/or cognitive function, such as dementia or poor performance status; a diagnosis of exclusion
Mixed	Associated with both stress and other characteristics
Overflow	Associated with overdistention of the bladder and resulting overflow of urine; may be caused by adverse drug effects, fecal impaction, obstruction, or neurologic conditions
Sensory urgency	Associated with decreased bladder elasticity and increased bladder pressure; severe urgency and bladder hypersensitivity without detrusor overactivity; may be caused by cystitis secondary to radiation, interstitial disease, or radical pelvic surgery
Sphincteric	Associated with urethral hypermotility and/or intrinsic sphincter deficiency; may be caused by surgery, lumbosacral disorder, aging, or hyperestrogenism
Stress	Associated with physical activity that increases abdominal pressure, such as running, jumping, sneezing, or coughing
Transient	Associated with an acute medical problem, such as infection, and usually resolves with correction of underlying problem
Urgency	Associated with strong, sudden desire to void, usually due to involuntary detrusor contractions

Note. Based on information from Nambiar et al., 2018; Panesar, 2014; Wilson & Waghel, 2016.

trol. The bladder stores urine produced by the kidneys with a normal capacity of approximately 300–400 ml.

    a) During the filling phase, sympathetic tone predominates, whereas parasympathetic tone is inhibited.

    b) During voluntary emptying, parasympathetic stimulation produces detrusor contraction, and sympathetic tone decreases. The external sphincter muscles of the pelvic floor relax, and abdominal muscles tighten. The urethra facilitates continence.

    c) A reflex arc between the detrusor muscle and the brain stem initiates and amplifies bladder contraction by parasympathetic stimulation. The reflex arc is under cortical inhibition.

  2. Continence is dependent on four factors.

    a) Detrusor stability

    b) Sphincter or pelvic competence

    c) Central autonomic nervous system function

    d) Pelvic floor muscles

B. Pathophysiology

  1. Excessive and inappropriate bladder detrusor muscle contraction reduces bladder volume capacity, causing frequent incomplete voiding. The mechanism involves decreased or loss of cortical inhibition of detrusor contraction.

  2. Detrusor overactivity may occur from bladder irritation or detrusor hyperreflexia.

  3. Sphincter or pelvic incompetence occurs from pelvic floor laxity that develops from partial denervation, which reduces sphincter tone.

  4. Interference with sensation and coordination of the detrusor and sphincter activity above the sacral area of the spinal cord leads to detrusor spasticity and outlet obstruction.

  5. Detrusor hypotonia results from long-standing outlet obstruction, detrusor insufficiency (usually from lower motor neuron damage), overextension, or impaired sensation.

  6. Frontal lobe dysfunction caused by cortical compromise results in the inability to void independently, despite having an intact urinary system.

III. Clinical features: Urinary incontinence is one of the most prevalent health problems in the United States, occurring in more than 20 million women and 6 million men (Irwin, 2019). It occurs in up to 40% of adult women and 14% of adult men. Incontinence remains underreported, underdiagnosed, and undertreated and may occur following cancer or cancer treatment. Incontinence is not a normal sign of aging (Handler & Rosenman, 2019; Juszczak et al., 2019; Kołodyńska et al., 2019; Nambiar et al., 2018; Potts & Payne, 2018; Smith, 2018).

A. Risk factors

  1. Gender: Twice as common in women than in men

  2. Pregnancy

  3. Childbirth

  4. Menopause

  5. Structure of the female GU tract

  6. Age older than 60 years

  7. Obesity

  8. Diet that contributes to bladder urgency or diuresis: Caffeine, carbonated beverages

  9. Environment not conducive to voiding comfort: Lack of access, privacy, cleanliness, or safety

  10. Low estrogen levels

11. Comorbidities: Hypertension, stroke, constipation, prostate disease
12. Tobacco use
13. Race/ethnicity: Less common in African American women
14. Certain medications: Sympathomimetics, tricyclic antidepressants, alpha-blockers, ACE inhibitors
15. High-impact activities: Jumping, running

B. Etiology: Manifestations of underlying disease
   1. Detrusor impairment
      a) Bladder infection or chronic cystitis
      b) Dementia
      c) Pelvic irradiation
      d) Detrusor hyperreflexia or hypertrophy
   2. Stress incontinence
      a) Occurs during coughing, sneezing, laughing, or other physical activity
      b) Most commonly caused by bladder neck/urethral hypermobility and intrinsic sphincteric deficiency
      c) Develops with aging, hormonal changes, deliveries (vaginal), and following urologic surgery
      d) Perineal injury, neurogenic disorders
   3. Urge incontinence/overactive bladder: Associated with frequent, small voids
      a) Enlarged prostate: Outlet obstruction
      b) Infection: Acute
      c) Cystocele
      d) Multiple sclerosis, Parkinson disease, stroke, disc problems
      e) Irritable bladder disorders: Postinterstitial bladder chemotherapy
      f) Primary urothelial tumors, bladder tumor
      g) Medications: Psychotropic
   4. Overflow incontinence: Associated with outlet obstruction with an intermittent or slow stream, hesitancy, and sensation of incomplete void
      a) Diabetes mellitus
      b) Medications with anticholinergic effects, opioids
      c) Sacral cord lesion
      d) Bladder outlet obstruction
      e) Increased alcohol use
   5. Functional incontinence
      a) Psychiatric disease
      b) Functional impairment
   6. Transient (reversible) incontinence
      a) Medications
      b) UTI
      c) Mental impairment
      d) Decreased mobility

C. History: History-taking is enhanced by acknowledging embarrassment about symptoms and demonstrating sensitivity.
   1. History of cancer and cancer treatment
   2. Current medications: Prescribed, over the counter
   3. History of presenting symptoms: Precipitating factors, onset, location, duration, associated symptoms (e.g., polydipsia, fever, weight gain/loss, dysuria, pain/discomfort, changes in bowel habits or sexual function)
   4. Changes in ADLs

     5. Past medical history: Diabetes, stroke, hypertension, heart failure, chronic constipation, dementia, prostate problems, Parkinson disease, changes in sexual functioning

     6. Past surgical history: Surgery of the prostate, colon, or bladder; gynecologic surgery

     7. Family history: Urge incontinence

     8. Voiding diary

  D. Signs and symptoms: May characterize a simple mechanical disorder of the urinary system or may be the direct or indirect result of a serious underlying illness

     1. Nocturia

     2. Dysuria

     3. Hesitancy

     4. Straining

     5. Interrupted stream

     6. Hematuria

     7. Pain

     8. Frequency

     9. Urgency

    10. Increased leakage, dribbling, or weak stream

    11. Changes in bowel habits or sexual function

  E. Physical examination

     1. Abdominal

       a) Masses and areas of fullness or tenderness on palpation

       b) Bladder palpation after patient voids for masses and distention

     2. Genital (men)

       a) Abnormalities of foreskin, glans penis, and perineal skin

       b) Prostate palpation for enlargement

     3. Pelvic (women)

       a) Vaginal atrophy, bladder prolapse, perineal skin abnormality, tenderness, cystocele, rectocele, enterocele, muscle tone

       b) Contact dermatitis and skin breakdown from chronic exposure to urine-soaked pads

       c) Asking patient to cough or performing Valsalva maneuver; absence of urine if continence is intact

     4. Rectal: Rectal sensation, tone, fecal impaction, sphincter tone, masses

     5. Neurologic: Nerve roots S2–S4 (see Appendix B) to determine deficits above, within, or distal to the autonomic reflex arc

       a) Bulbocavernosus reflex assessment by squeezing the clitoris or glans penis, which normally will cause the anal sphincter to contract

       b) Anal tone similar to bladder sphincter tone; if the patient can contract anal sphincter voluntarily, the autonomic reflex arc is intact.

       c) Cognitive functioning and altered mental status

IV. Diagnostic tests (Bettez et al., 2012; de Vries & Heesakkers, 2018; Nambiar et al., 2018)

  A. Laboratory

     1. Urinalysis to evaluate for hematuria, glycosuria, and proteinuria

     2. Urine culture to evaluate for bacteriuria or pyuria

     3. Urine cytology to screen for bladder cancer, if appropriate

     4. Renal panel to evaluate renal status

     5. Elevated prostate-specific antigen suggestive of benign prostatic hypertrophy or cancer

     6. Vaginal swabs to culture for *Ureaplasma urealyticum* and chlamydia

B. Radiology
   1. IV pyelogram to assess upper urinary tract
   2. Ultrasound to evaluate upper urinary tract and kidneys
   3. Voiding cystourethrogram to evaluate lower urinary tract integrity
   4. Plain x-rays to evaluate kidneys, ureters, and bladder
C. Urodynamics
   1. Cystometrogram tests for urinary stress incontinence, bladder compliance, urine flow rate, and bladder and intra-abdominal pressures
   2. Video urodynamics: Combines fluoroscopy and urodynamics to assess anatomy and function of the bladder
   3. Electromyography: Measures the electrical activity of the external urethral sphincter or anal sphincter to document innervation of pelvic floor muscle
   4. Postvoid residual (bladder scan) to determine residual urine
   5. Cystoscopy to evaluate presence of bladder lesions or urinary obstructive process

V. Differential diagnosis (Kołodyńska et al., 2019; Nambiar et al., 2018; Smith, 2018)
   A. Infection (see Chapters 89, 92, and 94)
   B. Overactive bladder
   C. Renal stones
   D. Spinal cord injury (see Chapter 145)
   E. Malignancy
   F. BPH (see Chapter 87), prostatitis (see Chapter 92)
   G. Drug induced (see Table 84-2)
   H. Multiple sclerosis
   I. Uterine prolapse

VI. Treatment: Begin with the least invasive approach. Treatment is dependent on type of urinary incontinence and patient status (American Urological Association, 2019; Bettez et al., 2012; de Vries & Heesakkers, 2018; Handler & Rosenman, 2019; Irwin, 2019; Kołodyńska et al., 2019; Nambiar et al., 2018; Potts & Payne, 2018; Syan & Brucker, 2016).
   A. Behavioral: To improve bladder control
      1. Bladder training for urge and stress incontinence, timed voiding
      2. Habit training for urge incontinence
      3. Prompted toileting in frail or cognitively impaired patients; use of an absorbent pad and frequent changes to prevent skin irritation; use of bedside commodes and mobility aids
      4. Pelvic muscle exercises (e.g., Kegel exercises) for urge and stress incontinence
      5. Restriction of fluid, including coffee, tea, and alcohol; timing of fluid intake
      6. Avoidance of diuretics before periods of recumbency
      7. Maintenance of healthy weight, control of obesity
      8. Avoiding dairy products to assess total and incremental voided volumes, frequency, diurnal distribution, and other factors
      9. Hygiene self-care measures for chronic pad users to prevent contact dermatitis
   B. Pharmacologic
      1. Elimination or decrease in doses of offending pharmacologic agents (see Table 84-2)
      2. Drugs for stress and urge incontinence
         a) Anticholinergic agents
            (1) Oxybutynin
               (a) Immediate release: 2.5 mg PO two to three times a day, may titrate up to 20 mg daily in divided doses

TABLE 84-2	Characteristics of Drugs That Affect Continence	
Medication	**Potential Effects**	**Comments**
Alcohol	Urinary frequency	Can cloud sensorium, impair mobility, and induce diuresis, resulting in incontinence
Alpha-blockers	Stress incontinence (women), urinary retention (men)	Relax urinary sphincter
Anticholinergics	Urinary retention	Side effects of drugs with anticholinergic properties include urinary retention with associated urinary frequency and overflow incontinence. Many over-the-counter medications, such as those commonly taken for insomnia, coryza, pruritus, and vertigo, have anticholinergic effects.
Antidepressants	Urinary retention	Have anticholinergic properties
Antihypertensives	Bladder outlet relaxation	Sphincter tone in the proximal urethra can be decreased by alpha-2 agonists, causing urinary retention.
Antipsychotics	Urinary retention, sphincter relaxation	Have anticholinergic properties
Calcium channel blockers	Urinary retention, frequency	Reduce smooth muscle contractility in the bladder and occasionally can cause urinary retention and overflow incontinence
Cytotoxic agents (e.g., cyclophosphamide, ifosfamide)	Urinary frequency, urgency, dysuria	Irritates the lining of the bladder causing chemical cystitis
Diuretics	Urinary frequency, urgency	A brisk diuresis induced by loop diuretics (e.g., furosemide, ethacrynic acid, bumetanide) can overwhelm bladder capacity and lead to polyuria, frequency, and urgency, thereby precipitating incontinence in a frail older person.
Opioids	Urinary retention	Have anticholinergic properties
Sedatives/hypnotics	Urinary sphincter relaxation	Benzodiazepines, especially long-acting agents (e.g., flurazepam, diazepam), may accumulate in older adults and cause confusion and secondary incontinence.

Note. Based on information from Nambiar et al., 2018; Panesar, 2014.

        (b) Extended release: 5 mg PO daily, may titrate up to 30 mg PO daily
        (c) Transdermal patch: Equivalent to 3.9 mg PO daily; twice a week to the abdomen, hip, or buttock
        (d) Topical 10% gel: 1 g (approximately 1 ml) daily to the thigh, abdomen, upper arm, or shoulder
    (2) Tolterodine
        (a) Immediate release: 1–2 mg PO two times a day
        (b) Extended release: 2–4 mg PO daily
    (3) Trospium
        (a) Immediate release: 20 mg PO two times a day

    (b) Extended release: 60 mg PO daily
   (4) Solifenacin 5–10 mg PO daily; darifenacin 7.5–15 mg PO daily; fesotero-
    dine 4–8 mg PO daily; mirabegron 25–50 mg PO daily
    (a) Indicated for overactive bladder with urge incontinence
    (b) Increases bladder capacity, decreases involuntary contractions
    (c) Adverse reactions: Dry eyes and mouth, constipation, blurred vision,
     orthostatic hypotension
  b) Antispasmodics: Use with caution or avoid in patients with heart disease, renal
   or hepatic impairment, history of QT prolongation, or glaucoma. Antispasmodic
   drugs depress smooth muscle activity.
   (1) Oxybutynin: Doses noted previously
   (2) Flavoxate: 100–200 mg PO three to four times a day
  c) Estrogen
   (1) Increases the density of alpha-receptors in the urethra and increases the
    vascularity of the urethral mucosa
   (2) Topical estrogen cream 0.5 g two times weekly or estradiol table 10 mcg
    two times weekly
   (3) Limited clinical data are available on therapeutic effects; however, it might
    be most useful in postmenopausal women with atrophic vaginitis or intrin-
    sic sphincter deficiency.
  d) Botulinum toxin: Approved for urinary incontinence in patients with neurologic
   conditions, such as spinal cord injury or multiple sclerosis, who have overactive
   bladder; given by intradetrusor injections via cystoscopy
 C. Surgical
  1. Management of stress incontinence
   a) Retropubic or laparoscopic suspension
   b) Sling (primarily female): Suburethral synthetic polypropylene mesh sling place-
    ment is the most common surgery currently performed for stress incontinence.
   c) Artificial sphincter, cystocele repair
   d) Urethral bulking: Periurethral/transurethral injection
   e) Surgically implanted devices that activate or inhibit muscle action
  2. Management of urge incontinence
   a) Augmentation cystoplasty: Open, laparoscopic
   b) Removal of inflammatory or obstructive lesion
  3. Management of overflow incontinence: Surgical interventions to relieve obstruction
 D. Supportive
  1. Required after or in conjunction with initial attempts to control incontinent episode by collecting incontinent urine
  2. External catheters (e.g., condom, Texas catheter with leg bag), indwelling urinary
   catheters, intermittent self-catheterization, external pads, diapers

VII. Follow-up (de Vries & Heesakkers, 2018; Handler & Rosenman, 2019; Nambiar et al., 2018;
 Potts & Payne, 2018)
 A. Short term
  1. Dependent on the nature and etiology of incontinence
  2. Ongoing need for education and reinforcement of self-care techniques
 B. Long term
  1. Long-term adaptation to urinary incontinence
  2. Adverse effects of long-term urinary incontinence: Skin alterations, depression,
   impaired sexual functioning, reduced work productivity, loss of self-esteem

VIII. Referrals (Nambiar et al., 2018; Potts & Payne, 2018)
  A. Urologist
    1. Uncertain diagnosis or inability to develop a reasonable management plan based on the diagnostic evaluation; failure to respond to medication trial
    2. Incontinence associated with recurrent symptomatic UTI
    3. Hematuria without infection
    4. Presence of known or suspected prostate nodule, primary bladder tumor, pelvic mass, or lymph node enlargement causing bladder outlet obstruction
  B. Enterostomal therapist: If self-care skills concerning urinary care are required
  C. Neurology: For suspected spinal cord injury

References

American Urological Association. (2019). AUA position statement on the use of vaginal mesh for the surgical treatment of stress urinary incontinence (SUI). https://www.auanet.org/guidelines/use-of-vaginal-mesh-for-the-surgical-treatment-of-stress-urinary-incontinence

Bettez, M., Tu, L., Carlson, K., Corcos, J., Gajewski, J., Jolivet, M., & Bailly, G. (2012). 2012 update: Guidelines for adult urinary incontinence collaborative consensus document for the Canadian Urological Association. *Canadian Urological Association Journal, 6*(5), 354–363. https://doi.org/10.5489/cuaj.12248

de Vries, A.M., & Heesakkers, J.P.F.A. (2018). Contemporary diagnostics and treatment options for female stress urinary incontinence. *Asian Journal of Urology, 5*(3), 141–148. https://doi.org/10.1016/j.ajur.2017.09.001

Handler, S.J., & Rosenman, A.E. (2019). Urinary incontinence: Evaluation and management. *Clinical Obstetrics and Gynecology, 62*(4), 700–711. https://doi.org/10.1097/GRF.0000000000000488

Irwin, G.M. (2019) Urinary incontinence. *Primary Care, 46*(2), 233–242. https://doi.org/10.1016/j.pop.2019.02.004

Juszczak, K., Ostrowski, A., Bryczkowski, M., Adamczyk, P., & Drewa, T. (2019). A hypothesis for the mechanism of urine incontinence in patients after radical prostatectomy due to urinary bladder hypertrophy. *Advances in Clinical and Experimental Medicine, 28*(3), 391–395. https://doi.org/10.17219/acem/79935

Kołodyńska, G., Zalewski, M., & Rożek-Piechura, K. (2019). Urinary incontinence in post-menopausal women—Causes, symptoms, treatment. *Menopause Review, 18*(1), 46–50. https://doi.org/10.5114/pm.2019.84157

Nambiar, A.K., Bosch, R., Cruz, F., Lemack, G.E., Thiruchelvam, N., Tubaro, A., ... Burkhand, F.C. (2018). EAU guidelines on assessment and nonsurgical management of urinary incontinence. *European Urology, 73*(4), 596–609. https://doi.org/10.1016/j.eururo.2017.12.031

Panesar, K. (2014). Drug-induced urinary incontinence. *U.S. Pharmacist, 39*(8), 24–29. https://www.uspharmacist.com/article/druginduced-urinary-incontinence

Potts, J.M., & Payne, C.K. (2018). Urinary urgency in the elderly. *Gerontology, 64*(6), 541–550. https://doi.org/10.1159/000492330

Sharma, N., & Chakrabarti, S. (2018). Clinical evaluation of urinary incontinence. *Journal of Midlife Health, 9*(2), 55–64. https://doi.org/10.4103/jmh.JMH_122_17

Smith, A. (2018). Understanding overactive bladder and urgency incontinence: What does the brain have to do with it? *F1000Research, 7,* 1869. https://doi.org/10.12688/f1000research.16418.1

Syan, R., & Brucker, B. (2016). Guideline of guidelines: Urinary incontinence. *BJU International, 117*(1), 20–33. https://doi.org/10.1111/bju.13187

Weledji, E.P., Eyongeta, D., & Ngounou, E. (2019). The anatomy of urination: What every physician should know. *Clinical Anatomy, 32*(1), 60–67. https://doi.org/10.1002/ca.23296

Wilson, J.A., & Waghel, R.C. (2016). The management of urinary incontinence. *U.S. Pharmacist, 41*(9), 22–26. https://www.uspharmacist.com/article/the-management-of-urinary-incontinence

CHAPTER 85

Vaginitis

Karen A. Roesser, MSN, RN, AOCNS®

I. Definitions (Gaydos et al., 2017; Paavonen & Brunham, 2018)
   A. Vulvovaginitis: An inflammation of the vulvovaginal mucosa that may be infectious or noninfectious
   B. Bacterial vaginosis (BV): An overgrowth of anaerobic bacteria in the vagina that lacks inflammation
   C. Desquamative inflammatory vaginosis (DIV): Aerobic bacteria in the vagina associated with inflammation; also referred to as aerobic vaginitis
   D. Vulvovaginal candidiasis (VVC): An overgrowth of *Candida*

II. Physiology/Pathophysiology (CDC, 2021; Faught & Reyes, 2019; Mills, 2017; Neal et al., 2020; Paavonen & Brunham, 2018; Yano et al., 2019)
   A. Normal
      1. The vagina is a musculomembranous tube that forms the passageway between the cervix and the vulva. The vulva is the female external genitalia lying posterior to the mons veneris, which consists of the labia majora, labia minora, clitoris, vestibule of the vagina, and vaginal opening.
      2. In most women, the vaginal canal is normally colonized by many bacteria, including the hydrogen peroxide–producing *Lactobacillus* species. *Lactobacillus crispatus* and *Lactobacillus jensenii* are common lactobacilli in the vagina of healthy women and account for 70%–90% of the total microbiome in a healthy vagina.
         a) Lactobacilli react with glycogen to produce lactic acid.
         b) The lactic acid helps to maintain an acidic environment, normally with a pH of 3.8–4.2.
         c) The acidic secretions allow the vagina to be naturally resistant to bacterial infection.
      3. The vaginal canal flora also may contain organisms from the *Candida* genus; 10%–20% of healthy asymptomatic women under conditions of normal pH will have *Candida* in their lower genital tract.
   B. Pathophysiology
      1. Any condition in which the balance of bacteria and yeast is altered results in overgrowth and causes symptoms.
         a) The precise conditions required for pathogenesis are not known.
         b) Absence or a decrease in peroxidase-producing lactobacilli appears to be important in the development of anaerobic bacterial infections.
         c) The presence of a gene polymorphism associated with a diminished production of mannose-binding lectin is important in women with recurrent vulvovaginal yeast infections.

2. Some chemotherapy agents (e.g., pegylated liposomal doxorubicin) or radiation therapy can cause a vaginal mucositis/vulvovaginitis similar to that seen in the oral cavity as a result of an inflammatory reaction.

3. BV can occur when the normal vaginal flora becomes altered.
   a) The term *bacterial vaginosis* reflects a number of species of bacteria that naturally live in the vaginal area and may grow to excess.
   b) The abundance of anaerobes leads to a greater presence of proteolytic carboxylase enzymes.
      (1) These enzymes in an alkaline environment result in a chain reaction, leading to squamous epithelial cell exfoliation, subsequent discharge, and the creation of a characteristic fishy odor.
      (2) These anaerobic bacteria, which include *Atopobium vaginae, Gardnerella vaginalis, Mobiluncus mulieris, Prevotella*, BV-associated bacterium 2, and *Megasphaera*, have an enhanced ability to stick to the sloughed epithelial cells, covering cell borders, and are referred to as *clue cells*. They occur in the absence of rods, which indicates an absence of lactobacilli.
   c) Persistence after antimicrobial therapy may occur because of the formation of a biofilm protecting the BV-causing bacteria.

4. DIV can occur when there is a microbial imbalance in the normal vaginal microbiome associated with inflammation.
   a) DIV is less understood than BV.
   b) Bacteria associated with this typically consist of *Escherichia coli, Staphylococcus aureus*, group B streptococci, or *Enterococcus faecali*.

5. VVC occurs when the normal vaginal flora becomes altered.
   a) A change in the vaginal environment is necessary before the yeast exerts a pathologic action.
   b) *Candida* organisms probably access the vagina via migration across the perianal area from the rectum.
   c) Acute inflammation of the vulva and vaginal mucosa is induced by overgrowth of *Candida* organisms.

III. Clinical features: Vaginitis is one of the most common causes of patient visits to gynecologists, primary care providers, and urgent care centers. The most common infectious causes of vaginitis are BV (22%–50%), DIV (7%–12%), VVC (17%–39%), and trichomoniasis (4%–35%). They may be infectious or noninfectious in origin (Coudray & Madhivanan, 2020; Donders et al., 2017; Gaydos et al., 2017; Javed et al., 2019; Mills, 2017; Neal et al., 2020; Paavonen & Brunham, 2018; Reiter & Kellogg Spadt, 2019; Yano et al., 2019).
   A. Risk factors
      1. Vaginitis
         a) Chemotherapy
         b) Radiation to vulva area
         c) Sexually active
         d) Pregnancy
         e) Menopause-induced atrophy
      2. BV
         a) Use of antibiotics causing a reduction in the lactobacilli development of the alkaline environment
         b) Douching
         c) Use of higher doses of spermicide nonoxynol-9
         d) Smoking

      e) Use of an intrauterine contraceptive device

      f) New or multiple sexual partners

      g) Unprotected sexual intercourse

      h) Homosexual relationships: Lesbian patients whose female partners have BV; oral–genital sex

      i) Foreign bodies: Tampons

      j) Pregnancy

      k) Phase of menstrual cycle: The pH of vagina is least acidic on days just prior to and during menstruation, leading to increased risk of infections during this time.

      l) Decreased estrogen level: After menopause

      m) Sociodemographic factors: Younger age, African American or Mexican American, having less than a high school education, living at or near the federal poverty level

3. DIV

      a) Etiology unknown

      b) Perimenopausal Caucasian women

      c) Genetic predisposition for abnormal immune insult to vaginal mucosa

4. Candidiasis

      a) Vaginal or systemic antibiotic use

      b) Diet high in refined sugars

      c) Uncontrolled diabetes mellitus, especially non–*albicans Candida* species

      d) Increased estrogen levels: The use of oral contraceptives (especially when estrogen dose is high), pregnancy, estrogen therapy

      e) Immunosuppression: Use of corticosteroids

      f) HIV infection

      g) Genetic susceptibility

      h) Contraceptive devices: Vaginal sponges, diaphragms, and intrauterine devices are all associated but not consistently. Spermicides are not associated with *Candida* infection.

      i) New sexual partner: Does not appear to be related to lifetime number of sexual partners or frequency of coitus

      j) Unprotected sexual intercourse

      k) Homosexual relationships

      l) No evidence linking VVC with hygienic habits or wearing tight or synthetic clothing

B. Etiology

  1. Vaginitis

      a) BV

      b) Trichomoniasis

      c) VVC

      d) Estrogen deficiency resulting in atrophic vaginitis

      e) Erosive lichen planus

      f) Allergens resulting in irritant or allergic contact dermatitis

  2. BV: Most common vaginal infection in premenopausal women

      a) Not classified as an STI, yet BV considered sexually associated

      b) Associated with replacement of *Lactobacillus* species with high concentrations of *Prevotella* species, *Mobiluncus* species, *G. vaginalis*, *Ureaplasma urealyticum*, and *Mycoplasma* species

  3. DIV

      a) Existence not universally accepted by clinicians

      b) Etiology uncertain

4. Candidiasis: Second most common cause; *Candida albicans* accounts for the majority of infections.

    a) VVC is not traditionally considered to be an STI.

    b) Candidiasis is classified as uncomplicated or complicated disease.

    c) Infection is caused by *Candida albicans* or non-*Candida albicans* species, such as *Candida tropicalis, Candida glabrata, Candida krusei, Candida kefyr, Candida guilliermondii, Candida parapsilosis,* or *Saccharomyces cerevisiae. Candida albicans* is responsible for approximately 65%–90% of the vaginal *Candida* species infections, and non-*albicans Candida* species are responsible for up to 30%.

C. History

  1. History of cancer and cancer treatment

  2. Current medications: Prescribed, over the counter, suppositories or topical agents used in the vulvovaginal area, antibiotics, hormonal agents, estrogen, steroids

  3. History of presenting symptoms: Precipitating factors, onset, location, duration, frequency, severity

  4. Changes in ADLs

  5. Past medical history

    a) Allergies, especially to peripads, scented tampons, contraceptives, condoms, spermicides, and vulvovaginal or environmental products used in the vaginal area

    b) Menstrual and obstetric history

      (1) Last menstrual period: Menstruation altering the natural vaginal pH

      (2) Pregnancy history: Preterm deliveries

      (3) Contraceptive history: Use of oral contraceptives, intrauterine devices, diaphragm with spermicide for contraception

      (4) Menopause/perimenopause: History of atrophic vaginitis

      (5) Methods used to alleviate vaginal symptoms

      (6) Tampons, douches, pads, vaginal deodorants

    c) Comorbidities: Diabetes, HIV/AIDS, infections requiring antibiotic use, immunosuppressive disorders such as SLE, previous vaginal infections, history of pelvic inflammatory disease

    d) Sexual history

      (1) Number of sexual partners

      (2) Frequency of sexual intercourse

      (3) History of STIs

      (4) Use of sexual devices

      (5) Partner history of *Candida* infections

D. Signs and symptoms

  1. Vaginitis: Pruritus

  2. BV: Approximately one-half of patients are asymptomatic.

    a) Symptoms are often inconclusive. Malodorous "fishy smelling" discharge is more noticeable after coitus and during menses; discharge is clear, off-white or gray, thin, and homogenous.

    b) Pruritus, pain, and vaginal inflammation (erythema, edema) are typically absent; neutrophils are absent.

    c) Dysuria and dyspareunia rarely occur.

  3. DIV

    a) Purulent vaginal discharge that is homogeneous and yellowish with no fishy smell

    b) Strong inflammatory reaction

        c) Vulvar irritation

        d) Severe dyspareunia

        e) Pruritus

        f) Vaginal mucosal erythema with ecchymotic lesions or erosions present in severe cases

    4. VVC: Often inconclusive and unspecific

        a) Frequent pruritus

        b) Vulvar burning/pain

        c) Dysuria

        d) Dyspareunia

        e) Symptoms: Frequently emerge one week before menses and disappear with the onset of menstruation

        f) Vaginal discharge: May or may not be present; white, thick, and without pronounced odor

        g) Vulvar symptoms: Erythema, edema, and swelling, particularly near the introitus

E. Physical examination

    1. Vital signs: Fever potentially indicative of infection

    2. Abdominal: Generalized lower abdominal tenderness, guarding, or rebound indicative of pelvic inflammatory disease

    3. External genitalia: Odor, signs of erythema, discharge, edema, rashes/lesions, atrophy of vagina; malodor indicative of BV

    4. Pelvic

        a) Insert the speculum and assess vaginal vault for atrophy (loss of rugae), erythema, edema, inflammation, lesions, odor, or presence of discharge.

           (1) BV: Increased thin, milky white, or gray discharge adherent to the vaginal walls with fishy odor

           (2) DIV: Purulent yellow to green vaginal discharge with deep red erythema of the vagina and erosions with well-defined borders

           (3) *Candida*: Cottage cheese–like odorless vaginal discharge

           (4) Atrophic vaginitis: Yellow or greenish odorless vaginal discharge

           (5) Discharge: Minimal if vaginitis is related to contact irritation or allergens

        b) Assess cervix for erythema, discharge, or lesions.

        c) Perform bimanual examination with attention to cervical motion tenderness to rule out mucopurulent cervicitis or pelvic infection.

    5. Lymph node: Inguinal node palpitation to evaluate for adenopathy associated with pelvic infections (see Appendix D)

IV. Diagnostic tests (CDC, 2021; Gaydos et al., 2017; Mills, 2017; Neal et al., 2020; Paavonen & Brunham, 2018; Paladine & Desai, 2018; Reiter & Kellogg Spadt, 2019; Yano et al., 2019)

  A. Laboratory

    1. Check pH of vaginal secretions. Apply pH paper directly to pooled vaginal fluid or to a vaginal fluid sample on a cotton swab. Smear the fluid from the swab on the pH paper. Observe immediately for color changes and compare to the color chart on the dispenser.

        a) Less than 4.7: Normal

        b) Greater than 4.7: VVC

        c) Greater than or equal to 4.7: BV

        d) Greater than or equal to 4.7: DIV

        e) pH varies: Trichomoniasis

    2. Fresh wet-mount microscopy: Apply 0.9% saline to slide with vaginal secretions.

    a) BV will reveal greater than 20% clue cells, few WBCs, and decreased lactobacilli.

    b) DIV will reveal neutrophils, immature parabasal cells, absence of clue cells, and abundance of polymorphic cocci and bacilli. This is the preferred method of diagnosing desquamative inflammatory vaginitis, as Gram staining does not discriminate between BV and DIV.

    c) Candidiasis will reveal yeast or hyphal cells.

3. Vaginal Gram stain: This test assesses the vaginal cells using the Nugent score.

    a) Some consider it to be the gold standard because of a higher sensitivity in diagnosing BV by reviewing types of rods identified. No gram-positive rods is 4 points; many gram-negative or variable rods is 4 points; many curved gram-variable rods is 2 points.

    b) Scores greater than or equal to 7 are considered consistent with BV.

    c) Compared with Nugent scoring by vaginal Gram stain, Amsel criteria have a sensitivity of 92%.

    d) Evidence reveals that the Gram stain procedure harms part of the lactobacillary flora and favors the nonlactobacillary flora, leading to a false overemphasis of abnormal flora in Gram stains when compared with wet mounts.

    e) BV is diagnosed by finding three of four Amsel criteria.

      (1) Thin, homogenous discharge

      (2) Vaginal pH greater than 4.5

      (3) More than 20% of the epithelial cells are clue cells on fresh wet mount.

      (4) Fishy odor after addition of 10% potassium hydroxide in water

4. Apply drop of 10% potassium hydroxide to slide with vaginal secretions to assess for fishy odor of BV (whiff test) or inspect for *Candida*.

5. Culture of cervix is only indicated to evaluate for gonorrhea or chlamydia. It has no role in diagnosing BV or DIV.

6. Rapid diagnostic test may confirm infection if microscopy cannot be performed.

    a) This rapid test can confirm BV (e.g., FemExam card test, QuickVue®, Pip Activity TestCard™).

    b) A rapid yeast detection test (SavvyCheck™ Vaginal Yeast Test) can be performed by the patient and costs less than yeast culture.

7. For recurrently symptomatic women with negative wet mounts and normal pH, consider a vaginal culture for *Candida*.

8. If patient is HIV positive, obtain cluster of differentiation 4 lymphocyte count.

9. Glucose: Hyperglycemia contributes to candidiasis.

B. Radiology: Not indicated

V. Differential diagnosis (Coudray & Madhivanan, 2020; Javed et al., 2019; Mills, 2017; Neal et al., 2020; Paavonen & Brunham, 2018; Paladine & Desai, 2018)

A. BV

B. VVC

C. Atrophic vaginitis

  1. With secondary bacterial infection

  2. Postpartum or breastfeeding

  3. Menopause (see Chapter 90)

D. Trichomonal vaginitis

E. Infectious vaginitis

  1. Group A streptococcal vaginitis

  2. Ulcerative vaginitis from *S. aureus*/toxic shock syndrome

  3. Idiopathic vaginal ulceration in patients who are HIV positive

    F. DIV
        1. Noninfectious because of chemotherapy
        2. Infectious
        3. Radiation-induced inflammation
    G. Irritant contact dermatitis resulting in chemical vaginitis
    H. Allergic contact dermatitis (see Chapter 20)
     I. Collagen vascular disease, pemphigus syndromes, Behçet syndrome
     J. Erosive lichen planus
    K. Idiopathic vaginitis
    L. Genital herpes
    M. Mechanical irritation with decreased vaginal lubrication in menopause and perimenopause
    N. Cervicitis
    O. Pediculosis
    P. Lichen sclerosus
    Q. Vulvar carcinoma
    R. Physiologic leukorrhea

VI. Treatment (CDC, 2021; Faught & Reyes, 2019; Han et al., 2015; Javed et al., 2019; Mills, 2017; Neal et al., 2020; Paavonen & Brunham, 2018; Reiter & Kellogg Spadt, 2019)
    A. Noninfectious vaginitis: No specific treatment exists. Keep area clean and dry and monitor for infection.
    B. BV
        1. It may resolve spontaneously.
        2. Treatment is indicated if symptomatic, to prevent postoperative infection in those with asymptomatic infection prior to abortion or hysterectomy, or to reduce the risk of acquiring an STI, including HIV.
        3. Studies show intravaginal and oral antibiotic preparations to be equally effective. Oral regimens have longer treatment duration and a higher incidence of systemic side effects than vaginal administration.
           a) Of those treated, approximately 50%–60% will have a recurrence within 12 months of treatment.
           b) Metronidazole may not be an ideal empirical agent, as *A. vaginae* is resistant and thus predictive of a high risk of recurrence of infection.
        4. Pharmacology: Initial recommended treatments
           a) Metronidazole: 500 mg PO two times a day for seven days
           b) Metronidazole gel: 0.75% one full applicator (5 g) applied intravaginally once daily at bedtime for five days
           c) Clindamycin 2%: 5 g applied intravaginally once daily at bedtime for seven days
           d) Avoid intercourse until infection or vaginitis is improved, usually 48–72 hours with BV and three to five days after chemotherapy treatment.
        5. Complementary and alternative medicine: Because of the impact on QOL with recurrent BV/vaginitis, many women are using complementary and alternative therapies independently. The use of recolonization with 30 days of the oral probiotic *Lactobacillus,* in addition to seven days of metronidazole therapy, has been suggested but is not recommended because of a lack of efficacy.
        6. Patient counseling regarding adherence to prescribed treatments, hygienic practices, and treatment of symptomatic same-sex partner is important to prevent recurrence.
    C. DIV
        1. May be chronic or recurrent

2. Treatment options not tested in randomized controlled trials
3. Pharmacologic: Initial recommended treatment
   a) Clindamycin 2% cream: Intravaginally daily at bedtime for one to two weeks; maintenance therapy considered one or two times a week for two to six months
   b) Hydrocortisone: 12.5 mg intravaginal suppository two times a day for two months, then daily for two months, then one to three times per week as maintenance therapy; higher doses of hydrocortisone in a 10% cream potentially superior
   c) Official treatment guidelines not developed

D. Candidiasis
   1. Uncomplicated VVC
      a) Characteristics
         (1) Sporadic, infrequent
         (2) Mild to moderate signs/symptoms
         (3) Probable infection with *C. albicans*
         (4) Healthy, nonpregnant woman
      b) Current research
         (1) Current research has found that oral and intravaginal routes for treatment are equally effective.
         (2) RCTs have found that although no significant difference exists in side effects between the two routes, intravaginal medications often are less likely to cause nausea, abdominal pain, or headache while increasing vulvar irritation and vaginal discharge.
         (3) Women may be given the choice of route based on cost, medical history, and patient preferences.
      c) Pharmacology
         (1) Over-the-counter treatment for uncomplicated VVC: Intravaginal antifungal suppositories/ointments for one to seven days
            (a) Clotrimazole 2%: 5 g intravaginally once daily at bedtime for three days; clotrimazole 1% (Gyne-Lotrimin® 7) 5 g intravaginally once daily at bedtime for 7–14 days
            (b) Miconazole 2%: 5 g intravaginally once daily at bedtime for seven days, or 100 mg vaginal suppository once daily at bedtime for seven days
            (c) Tioconazole 6.5%: 5 g intravaginally in a single dose at bedtime
         (2) Prescription for uncomplicated VVC: Fluconazole 150 mg PO for one dose
   2. Complicated VVC
      a) Characteristics
         (1) Poorly controlled diabetes, immunosuppression, debilitation
         (2) Severe signs and symptoms
         (3) *Candida* species other than *C. albicans*, particularly *C. glabrata* (non-albicans)
         (4) History of recurrent VVC: Four or more infections per year
      b) Pharmacology
         (1) Prescription intravaginal suppositories/ointments for complicated VVC
            (a) Second dose of fluconazole given three days after the first dose
            (b) Any azole: Intravaginally daily for 7–14 days
            (c) Boric acid: 600 mg gelatin capsule intravaginally once daily at bedtime for 14 days; indicated for non-albicans candidiasis
         (2) Oral agents: Fluconazole 150 mg PO every 72 hours for three doses
   3. Recurrent VVC: Fluconazole for 7–14 days

        a) Fluconazole: 150 mg PO every three days for three doses

        b) Fluconazole: 150 mg PO every week for six months

        c) Clotrimazole: 200 mg cream intravaginally two times weekly for six months

        d) Use of any of the topical azoles previously noted at bedtime

   4. Lifestyle modifications to reduce recurrence of candidal infections

        a) Behavioral changes may rarely be beneficial for some women (e.g., avoiding panty liners and pantyhose, drinking cranberry juice).

        b) Treatment should also be directed at the sexual dysfunction (e.g., vaginal dryness or dyspareunia) and marital discord that frequently accompany chronic vaginitis.

VII. Follow-up

   A. Follow-up is necessary if symptoms do not improve with treatment.

   B. Annual Pap smear and pelvic examination are recommended.

VIII. Referrals

   A. Gynecologist: If patient symptoms are unresolved or if recurrent infection

   B. Infectious disease specialist: If patient is HIV-positive

References

Centers for Disease Control and Prevention. (2021). Sexually transmitted infections treatment guidelines, 2021. https://www.cdc.gov/std/treatment-guidelines/default.htm

Coudray, M.S., & Madhivanan, P. (2020) Bacterial vaginosis—A brief synopsis of the literature. *European Journal of Obstetrics, Gynecology, and Reproductive Biology, 245,* 143–148. https://doi.org/10.1016/j.ejogrb.2019.12.035

Donders, G.G.G., Bellen, G., Grinceviciene, S., Ruban, K., & Viera-Baptista, P. (2017). Aerobic vaginitis: No longer a stranger. *Research in Microbiology, 168*(9–10), 845–858. https://doi.org/10.1016/j.resmic.2017.04.004

Faught, B.M., & Reyes, S. (2019). Characterization and treatment of recurrent bacterial vaginosis. *Journal of Women's Health, 28*(9), 1218–1226. https://doi.org/10.1089/jwh.2018.7383

Gaydos, C.A., Beqaj, S., Schwebke, J.R., Lebed, J., Smith, B., Davis, T.E., ... Cooper, C.K. (2017). Clinical validation of a test for the diagnosis of vaginitis. *Obstetrics and Gynecology, 130*(1), 181–189. https://doi.org/10.1097/AOG.0000000000002090.

Han, C., Wu, W., Fan, A., Wang, Y., Zhang, H., Chu, Z., ... Xue, F. (2015). Diagnostic and therapeutic advancements for aerobic vaginitis. *Archives of Gynecology and Obstetrics, 291*(2), 251–257. https://doi.org/10.1007/s00404-014-3525-9

Javed, A., Parvaiz, F., & Manzoor, S. (2019). Bacterial vaginosis: An insight into the prevalence, alternative treatments regimen and its associated resistance patterns. *Microbial Pathogenesis, 127,* 21–30. https://doi.org/10.1016/j.micpath.2018.11.046

Mills, B.B. (2017). Vaginitis: Beyond the basics. *Obstetrics and Gynecology Clinics of North America, 44*(2), 159–177. https://doi.org/10.1016/j.ogc.2017.02.010

Neal, C.M., Kus, L.H., Eckert, L.O., & Peipert, J.F. (2020). Noncandidal vaginitis: A comprehensive approach to diagnosis and management. *American Journal of Obstetrics and Gynecology, 222*(2), 114–122. https://doi.org/10.1016/j.ajog.2019.09.001

Paavonen, J., & Brunham, R.C. (2018). Bacterial vaginosis and desquamative inflammatory vaginitis. *New England Journal of Medicine, 379*(23), 2246–2254. https://doi.org/10.1056/NEJMra1808418

Paladine, H.L., & Desai, U.A. (2018). Vaginitis: Diagnosis and treatment. *American Family Physician, 97*(5), 321–329. https://www.aafp.org/afp/2018/0301/p321.html

Reiter, S., & Kellogg Spadt, S. (2019). Bacterial vaginosis: A primer for clinicians. *Postgraduate Medicine, 131*(1), 8–18. https://doi.org/10.1080/00325481.2019.1546534

Yano, J., Sobel, J.D., Nyirjesy, P., Sobel, R., Williams, V.L., Yu, Q., ... Fidel, P.L. (2019). Current patient perspectives of vulvovaginal candidiasis: Incidence, symptoms, management and post-treatment outcomes. *BMC Women's Health, 19,* 48. https://doi.org/10.1186/s12905-019-0748-8

CHAPTER 86

Acute Kidney Injury

Mary W. Dunn, MSN, RN, OCN®, NP-C

I. Definition (Gameiro et al., 2018; Makris & Spanou, 2016; Thomas et al., 2015)

    A. Acute kidney injury (AKI) is an abrupt (usually reversible) deterioration of GFR. GFR gives a rough measure of functioning nephrons.

    B. AKI occurs with a rise in serum creatinine (sCr) greater than or equal to 0.3 mg/dl over a 48-hour period, sCr greater than or equal to 1.5 times baseline value within seven days prior, or urine volume less than or equal to 0.5 ml/kg/hr for six hours.

    C. AKI is formally referred to as *acute renal failure*.

II. Physiology/Pathophysiology (Makris & Spanou, 2016; Osterman & Liu, 2017)

    A. Normal

        1. The kidneys are two organs located in the posterior retroperitoneal space.

        2. Kidney functions include removing metabolic waste products, regulating fluid and electrolytes, and maintaining acid-base balance through filtration of blood.

        3. The nephron is the functional unit of the kidney. Each kidney contains approximately 1.25 million nephrons.

        4. Renal blood flow normally drains 20% of the cardiac output (1,000 ml/min).

        5. Renal perfusion begins at the afferent arterioles. The afferent loop becomes the glomerulus, a web of capillaries responsible for filtration. The efferent loop extends from the glomerulus.

        6. Renal perfusion is maintained by cardiac output, renal perfusion pressure, and glomerular hemodynamic factors.

        7. Mechanisms of control in renal function include the cardiovascular, nervous, endocrine, and compensatory systems.

            a) Cardiovascular system: Responsible for provision of adequate plasma at a constant rate to promote regulation of water and electrolytes, maintenance of blood pressure and hydrostatic pressure, and preservation of vascular resistance required for filtration

            b) Nervous system: Influences fluid balance by regulating thirst mechanism and by controlling essential receptors

                (1) Chemoreceptors: Located in carotid and aortic bodies; send messages to vasomotor center to increase blood flow

                (2) Baroreceptors: Sense change in blood pressure and activate the hypothalamus to produce ADH

                (3) Osmoreceptors: Sense changes in osmolality and activate the hypothalamus to alter ADH production

            c) Endocrine system: Triggered by the nervous system

          (1) ADH: Produced by hypothalamus and secreted by posterior pituitary; increases permeability of the nephron membrane to water, allowing for increased fluid absorption

          (2) Aldosterone: Produced by adrenal cortex in response to fluid deficits; alters absorption and water excretion

       d) Compensatory system

          (1) Renin–angiotensin system: Kidney secretion of renin as response to a decline in blood pressure; combines with angiotensin 1 to cause vasoconstriction, leading to increased hydrostatic pressure, to improve filtration at the glomerulus

          (2) Autoregulation: Maintains renal blood flow by regulating resistance of blood flow in circulation

B. Pathophysiology

  1. Prerenal: Renal hypoperfusion; leads to decreased GFR as a response to various extrarenal insults

  2. Intrinsic: Classified according to site of injury (e.g., tubules, glomeruli, interstitium, intrarenal vessels); represents true kidney disease

  3. Postrenal: Results from obstruction of urine outflow, which increases intratubular pressure and decreases GFR

  4. Stages of AKI

    a) Onset: From time of the precipitating event until tubular injury occurs

    b) Oliguric or anuric: Decrease in urine output or nonoliguric; usually lasts 10–14 days; retention of endogenous metabolites and fluid

    c) Diuretic: Days to weeks after oliguria indicating nephrons have recovered enough to produce urine; occurs before full correction and electrolyte imbalances

    d) Baseline GFR: Recovers to 70%–80% in one to two years

III. Clinical features (Gallieni et al., 2018; Hertzberg et al., 2017; Makris & Spanou, 2016; Moore et al., 2018)

A. Risk factors

  1. CKD

  2. Impaired left ventricular systolic function

  3. Advanced age

  4. Diabetes

  5. Dehydration

  6. Nephrotoxic drugs

  7. Patients with cancer: Antineoplastic agents, sepsis, metabolic disturbances, primary thrombotic microangiopathies, direct involvement of the kidney by cancer

B. Etiology

  1. Prerenal

    a) Hypovolemia

      (1) GI loss: Emesis, diarrhea

      (2) Blood loss: Trauma, surgery

      (3) Renal loss: Diuretics, mineralocorticoid deficiency, postobstructive diuresis

      (4) Skin loss: Burns

    b) Decreased cardiac output

    c) Decreased effective circulating volume

      (1) CHF

      (2) Liver failure

     d) Impaired renal autoregulation
        (1) NSAIDs
        (2) ACE inhibitors: ARBs
        (3) Cyclosporins
2. Intrinsic
  a) Small vessels
     (1) Acute glomerulonephritis
     (2) Vasculitis
     (3) Thrombotic thrombocytopenia purpura/hemolytic uremic syndrome
     (4) DIC
     (5) Atheroembolism
     (6) Malignant hypertension
     (7) Calcineurin inhibitors
     (8) Sepsis
     (9) Infections with secondary glomerulonephritis: Hepatitis B or C, HIV
  b) Tubular
     (1) Toxic acute tubular necrosis
        (a) Endogenous: Rhabdomyolysis, hemolysis
        (b) Exogenous
           i. Iodinated contrast
           ii. Platinum-based chemotherapy
           iii. Aminoglycosides
           iv. Heavy metals
           v. NSAIDs
           vi. Zoledronic acid
     (2) Ischemic acute tubular necrosis
     (3) Sepsis
  c) Intratubular
     (1) Endogenous
        (a) Myeloma proteins
        (b) Uric acid: Tumor lysis syndrome
        (c) Cellular debris
     (2) Exogenous: Acyclovir, methotrexate
  d) Interstitium
     (1) Allergic reaction
        (a) Penicillin
        (b) PPIs
        (c) NSAIDs
        (d) Rifampin
     (2) Infection
        (a) Severe pyelonephritis
        (b) Sepsis
        (c) *Legionella*
     (3) Infiltration: Lymphoma, leukemia
     (4) Inflammatory
        (a) Sepsis
        (b) Sjögren syndrome
        (c) Tubulointerstitial nephritis uveitis
  e) Large vessels
     (1) Renal artery embolus, dissection, vasculitis

        (2) Renal vein thrombosis

        (3) Abdominal compartment syndrome

  3. Postrenal

    a) Bladder outlet obstruction/lower urinary tract obstruction

      (1) BPH

      (2) Prostate cancer

      (3) Neurogenic bladder

      (4) Anticholinergic drugs

      (5) Obstructed urethral catheters

      (6) Calculi

      (7) Urethral strictures

    b) Pelviureteric obstruction

      (1) Intraluminal obstruction

        (a) Calculi

        (b) Blood clots

        (c) Sloughed renal papillae

      (2) Infiltration of ureteric wall: Malignancy

      (3) External compression

        (a) Retroperitoneal fibrosis

        (b) Malignancy

        (c) Abscess

        (d) Intraoperative damage

C. History

  1. History of cancer and cancer treatment

  2. Current medications: Prescribed, over the counter

  3. History of presenting symptoms: Precipitating factors, onset

  4. Changes in ADLs

  5. Past medical history: CKD, diabetes mellitus, cardiac disease, BPH, urolithiasis

  6. Social history: Poor nutritional intake or fluid loss

  7. Recent surgery, trauma, diagnostic tests, or procedures using nephrotoxic contrast

D. Signs and symptoms: Dependent on cause, rate, and severity of kidney function decline

  1. Lower extremity edema

  2. Decreased urine output

  3. Fatigue

  4. Difficulty concentrating

  5. Anorexia, weight loss

  6. Nausea

  7. Shortness of breath

  8. Flank pain

  9. Suprapubic pressure and tenderness

  10. Fever

  11. Myalgias

  12. Seizures

E. Physical examination

  1. Vitals signs

    a) Weight increase: CHF, renal injury

    b) Hypertension: Fluid overload

    c) Hypotension: Hypovolemia

2. General: Weakness, fatigue
3. HEENT: Xerostomia, low jugular venous pressure
4. Pulmonary: Basilar crackles indicative of fluid overload or cardiac disease
5. Cardiac: Irregular rhythm with electrolyte imbalance
6. Abdominal
   a) Ascites indicative of portal hypertension or chronic liver disease
   b) Splenomegaly indicative of portal hypertension or chronic liver disease
   c) Pain on palpation: As urea increases and decomposes in the GI tract, ammonia is produced, leading to capillary fragility and ulcer formation.
7. Neurologic
   a) Asterixis: Tremulousness, loss of reflexes, uremic buildup
   b) Confusion, drowsiness, coma
      (1) Encephalopathy: Uremic buildup
      (2) Cerebral edema: Fluid buildup
8. Integument
   a) Pruritic rash: Nephritis, drug reaction
   b) Poor turgor: Dehydration
   c) Palmar erythema indicative of vascular instability
9. Rectal: Enlarged prostate; possible BPH as cause of bladder outlet obstruction

IV. Diagnostic tests (Gameiro et al., 2018; Kellum, 2016; Mehta et al., 2007; Osterman & Liu, 2017)
   A. Laboratory
      1. CBC
         a) RBCs: Anemia possibly indicative of acute blood loss, hemolysis, or chronic loss of EPO
         b) Eosinophilia potentially indicative of nephritis
      2. BUN (end point of metabolism): Varies daily with intake; poor indicator of renal damage; increased with high protein diet and decreased with anorexia
      3. Creatinine (end product of muscle metabolism): Minimal variability daily; best marker for GFR; changes greater than 50% indicative of renal damage
      4. BUN–creatinine ratio: Normal considered 20:1
         a) Prerenal: Greater than or equal to 20:1
         b) Intrinsic: 10–20:1
         c) Postrenal: Normal or elevated
      5. Electrolytes: Hyponatremia, hyperkalemia, hyperphosphatemia, hyperuricemia (e.g., tumor lysis syndrome), hypocalcemia, metabolic acidosis
      6. SPEP: If high, risk for multiple myeloma
      7. GFR: Calculated by using sCr and creatinine clearance; important to identify stability
      8. Other: Antinuclear antibody, hepatitis serologies, blood cultures
      9. Urinalysis
         a) RBC casts: Proliferative glomerulonephritis
         b) WBC casts: Interstitial inflammation (e.g., acute tubular necrosis, acute interstitial nephritis)
         c) Protein: Glomerulonephritis
         d) Occult blood: Rhabdomyolysis, hemolysis
         e) Specific gravity: Increased with dehydration, decreased with diuresis
         f) Bacteria: Pyelonephritis
         g) Osmolality: Loss of concentrating ability is an early finding in AKI.
            (1) Less than 350 mOsm/kg: Tubular damage

          (2) Greater than 500 mOsm/kg: Prerenal origin; reflects hypovolemic stimulus to the secretion of ADH and the maintenance of normal tubular function

      h) Fractional excretion of sodium (FENa): Helpful in patients with oliguria

         (1) Calculation

           (a) (Urinary sodium × sCr) / (serum sodium × urinary creatinine) × 100 = FENa

           (b) FENa less than 1%: Prerenal

           (c) FENa greater than 2%: Intrinsic

      i) Urine protein electrophoresis: If concern for multiple myeloma

   B. Radiology

     1. Ultrasound

      a) Small echogenic indicative of CKD

      b) Hydronephrosis indicative of postrenal obstructions

     2. CT scan: Identifies mass or hemorrhage

   C. Other

     1. Bladder scan: Postvoid residual

     2. Renal biopsy: If noninvasive evaluation unable to establish a diagnosis

     3. ECG: Possible dysrhythmias that develop secondary to electrolyte imbalances

   D. Classification and staging: Different criteria have been published, including Risk, Injury, Failure, Loss of Kidney Function, End-Stage Kidney Disease (RIFLE) in 2004; Acute Kidney Injury Network (AKIN) classification in 2007; and the Kidney Disease Improving Global Outcomes (KDIGO) classification, which merged the RIFLE and AKIN data (see Table 86-1).

TABLE 86-1   **Classification and Staging of Acute Kidney Injury**

AKI Stage	Urine Output	RIFLE	AKIN	KDIGO
1	< 0.5 ml/kg/hr for 6–12 hrs	**R**isk: sCr > 1.5 × increase within 7 days, sustained for > 24 hrs	sCr 1.5–2 × baseline, or > 0.3 mg/dl absolute sCr increase within 48 hrs	sCr 1.5–1.9 x baseline over 7 days or > 0.3 mg/dl absolute increase over 48 hrs
2	< 0.5 ml/kg/hr for > 12 hrs	**I**njury: sCr > 2 × increase	sCr > 2–3 × baseline	sCr 2–2.9 × baseline
3	< 0.3 ml/kg/hr for > 24 hrs or anuria for > 12 hrs	**F**ailure: sCr > 3 × increase, or sCr increase > 4 mg/dl (with increase of 0.5 mg/dl), or initiation of RRT	sCr > 3 × baseline, or sCr increase to > 4 mg/dl (with increase of 0.5 mg/dl), or initiation of RRT	sCr > 3 × baseline, or sCr increase to > 4 mg/dl, or initiation of RRT
–	–	**L**oss: Complete loss of kidney function for > 4 weeks	–	–
–	–	**E**nd-stage kidney disease for > 3 months	–	–

AKI—acute kidney injury; AKIN—Acute Kidney Injury Network; hr—hour; KDIGO—Kidney Disease Improving Global Outcomes; RIFLE—Risk, Injury, Failure, Loss of Kidney Function, End-Stage Kidney Disease; RRT—renal replacement therapy; sCr—serum creatinine

Note. Based on information from Bellomo et al., 2004; Kellum et al., 2012; Mehta et al., 2007.

V. Differential diagnosis (Makris & Spanou, 2016; Osterman & Liu, 2017)
   A. Chronic renal failure
   B. CHF (see Chapter 42)
   C. Chronic hypertension (see Chapter 47)
   D. Dehydration
   E. Infection
   F. BPH (see Chapter 87)
   G. Glomerulonephritis
   H. Nephrotoxicity
   I. Pyelonephritis (see Chapter 94)
   J. Hemolytic uremic syndrome
   K. Nephrotic syndrome (see Chapter 91)

VI. Treatment (Cerdá et al., 2016; Hertzberg et al., 2017; Kellum et al., 2012; Mohsenin, 2017; Moore et al., 2018; Sykes et al., 2018)
   A. Prevention
      1. Early assessment of at-risk patients
      2. Reduction in the use of multiple nephrotoxic medications (e.g., prescription, over the counter)
      3. Use of cytoprotectants with nephrotoxic chemotherapy
      4. Hydration and urine alkalization in patients at risk for tumor lysis syndrome
      5. Prevention of contrast-induced nephropathy: Ensure adequate hydration and coordinate diagnostic tests to limit repeat testing until clearance of contrast.
      6. Prior to administration of radiocontrast dye: Use low-osmolar contrast agents and hold metformin for 48 hours after contrast and assess sCr prior to restart.
   B. Correction of underlying causes
      1. Prerenal volume loss: Replacement should target type of fluid lost (e.g., crystalloid, blood, plasma). Perform fluid resuscitation with small boluses to monitor effect and prevent fluid shifts.
      2. Intrinsic renal injury
         a) Treatment of contributing comorbidities
         b) Treatment of infection
         c) Removal of nephrotoxic drugs
      3. Postrenal causes: Prompt relief of obstruction; transurethral or suprapubic bladder catheterization; percutaneous nephrostomy tube or ureteral stent may be required for ureteral obstructions.
   C. Medical management of AKI
      1. Elimination of nephrotoxic agents
      2. Volume management
         a) Hypovolemia: Volume expansion and vasopressors
            (1) Dopamine: Low-dose infusion is used to minimize kidney injury by dilating afferent and efferent arterioles.
            (2) Other vasopressors used in the ICU setting include norepinephrine and vasopressin.
         b) Hypervolemia
            (1) Fluid and sodium restriction
            (2) Diuretics: Used in the past with fluid bolus; now controversial
      3. Treatment of metabolic acidosis or metabolic alkalosis
      4. Correction of electrolyte imbalances
         a) Hyponatremia: Fluid restriction (see Chapter 155)

      b) Hyperkalemia: Potassium-restricted diet (see Chapter 153)

      c) Hypocalcemia (see Chapter 152)

      d) Hyperuricemia: In tumor lysis syndrome (e.g., allopurinol, rasburicase)

      e) Hyperphosphatemia (see Chapter 156)

      f) Hypomagnesemia (see Chapter 154)

    5. Correction of malnutrition: AKI is a hypercatabolic state leading to alteration in protein, amino acid, carbohydrate, and lipid metabolism.

  D. Renal replacement therapy: Therapy is indicated if refractory to medical management. Data are conflicting as to when dialysis should be initiated.

    1. Peritoneal dialysis: Temporary intraperitoneal catheter is placed. Dialysate solution is instilled into the peritoneal cavity to promote clearance of wastes through peritoneal membranes and ultrafiltration of water.

    2. Hemodialysis: Vascular access is through the femoral, internal jugular, or subclavian vein. This process intermittently removes solutes and volume for three to four hours a day for several days a week.

    3. Continuous renal replacement therapy for patients who are not hemodynamically stable occurs 24 hours a day, seven days a week.

VII. Follow-up (Silver & Siew, 2017)

  A. Frequent monitoring of renal function and other laboratory tests

  B. Determined by underlying cause of AKI

VIII. Referrals (Silver & Siew, 2017)

  A. Nephrologist: For management of chronic renal disease and if dialysis indicated; if initial interventions fail to improve the AKI; if AKI occurs as a complication of an unrelated condition and further treatment is dependent on nephrology input (e.g., AKI secondary to chemotherapy)

  B. Endocrinologist: For management of abnormal metabolic function

  C. Urologist: For management of obstruction

  D. Cardiologist: For management of CHF and arrhythmias

The author would like to acknowledge Marianne Davies, RN, MSN, CNS-BC, AOCNP®, for her contribution to this chapter that remains unchanged from the previous edition of this book.

References

Bellomo, R., Ronco, C., Kellum, J.A., Mehta, R.L., & Palevsky, P. (2004). Acute renal failure—Definition, outcome measures, animal models, fluid therapy and information technology needs: The Second International Consensus Conference of the Acute Dialysis Quality Initiative (ADQI) group. *Critical Care, 8,* R204. https://doi.org/10.1186/cc2872

Cerdá, J., Baldwin, I., Honore, P.M., Villa, G., Kellum, J.A., & Ronco, C. (2016). Role of technology for the management of AKI in critically ill patients: From adoptive technology to precision continuous renal replacement therapy. *Blood Purification, 42*(3), 248–265. https://doi.org/10.1159/000448527

Gallieni, M., Cosmai, L., & Porta, C. (2018). Acute kidney injury in cancer patients. In X. Ding, M.H. Rosner, & C. Ronco (Eds.), *Contributions to nephrology: Vol. 193. Acute kidney injury—Basic research and clinical practice* (pp. 137–148). Karger. https://doi.org/10.1159/000484970

Gameiro, J., Fonseca, J.A., Jorge, S., & Lopes, J.A. (2018). Acute kidney injury definition and diagnosis: A narrative review. *Journal of Clinical Medicine, 7*(10), 307. https://doi.org/10.3390/jcm7100307

Hertzberg, D., Rydén, L., Pickering, J.W., Sartipy, U., & Holzmann, M.J. (2017). Acute kidney injury—An overview of diagnostic methods and clinical management. *Clinical Kidney Journal, 10*(3), 323–331. https://doi.org/10.1093/ckj/sfx003

Kellum, J.A. (2016). Diagnostic criteria for acute kidney injury: Present and future. *Critical Care Clinics, 31*(4), 621–632. https://doi.org/10.1016/j.ccc.2015.06.001

Kellum, J.A., Lameire, N., Aspelin, P., Barsoum, R.S., Burdmann, E.A., Goldstein, S.L., … Uchino, S. (2012). KDIGO clinical practice guideline for acute kidney injury. *Kidney International Supplements, 2*(1), 1–138. https://doi.org/10.1038/kisup.2012.1

Makris, K., & Spanou, L. (2016). Acute kidney injury: Definition, pathophysiology, and clinical phenotypes. *Clinical Biochemist Reviews, 37*(2), 85–98.

Mehta, R.L., Kellum, J.A., Shah, S.V., Molitoris, B.A., Ronco, C., Warnock, D.G., & Levin, A. (2007). Acute Kidney Injury Network: Report of an initiative to improve outcomes in acute kidney injury. *Critical Care, 11,* R31. https://doi.org/10.1186/cc5713

Mohsenin, V. (2017). Practical approach to detection and management of acute kidney injury in critically ill patient. *Journal of Intensive Care, 5,* 57. https://doi.org/10.1186/s40560-017-0251-y

Moore, P.K., Hsu, R.K., & Liu, K.D. (2018). Management of acute kidney injury: Core curriculum 2018. *American Journal of Kidney Diseases, 72*(1), 136–148. https://doi.org/10.1053/j.ajkd.2017.11.021

Osterman, M., & Liu, K. (2017). Pathophysiology of AKI. *Best Practice and Research Clinical Anaesthesiology, 31*(3), 305–314. https://doi.org/10.1016/j.bpa.2017.09.001

Silver, S.A., & Siew, E.D. (2017). Follow-up care in acute kidney injury: Lost in transition. *Advances in Chronic Kidney Disease, 24*(4), 246–252. https://doi.org/10.1053/j.ackd.2017.05.008

Sykes, L., Nipah, R., Kalra, P., & Green, D. (2018). A narrative review of the impact of interventions in acute kidney injury. *Journal of Nephrology, 31*(4), 523–535. https://doi.org/10.1007/s40620-017-0454-2

Thomas, M.E., Blaine, C., Dawnay, A., Devonald, M.A.J., Ftouh, S., Laing, C., … Ostermann, M. (2015). The definition of acute kidney injury and its use in practice. *Kidney International, 87*(1), 62–73. https://doi.org/10.1038/ki.2014.328

CHAPTER 87

Benign Prostatic Hyperplasia

Myriam J. Cadet, PhD, APRN, MSN, FNP-C

I. Definition: Nonmalignant enlargement of the prostate gland and bladder dysfunction (Madersbacher et al., 2019)

II. Physiology/Pathophysiology (Foo, 2017; Skinder et al., 2016)
   A. Normal: The prostate gland is an organ that surrounds the urethra at the bladder neck in men.
      1. It is a slow-growing organ until puberty, at which it doubles in size. It begins to grow again by age 25 years.
      2. Dihydrotestosterone (DHT) is necessary for prostate growth.
   B. Pathophysiology: The exact pathophysiology is not clear, but it is thought to involve hormonal changes.
      1. Men produce both testosterone and estrogen. As men age, testosterone levels drop disproportionately to estrogen, resulting in increased cellular activity.
      2. Accumulation of DHT in older men results in prostate enlargement, causing the gland to press against the urethra.
      3. If untreated, irreversible damage may occur. Myohypertrophy and collagenosis may lead to storage dysfunction and reduction of contractile tissue.
      4. BPH may lead to obstructive neuropathy, bladder decompensation, acute urinary retention, infection, or bladder calculi.

III. Clinical features (Barry et al., 1992; Patel & Parsons, 2014; Pearson & Williams, 2014; Skinder et al., 2016; Vasanwala et al., 2017)
   A. Risk factors
      1. Age: Occurs in 50% of men older than 60 years and greater than 80% of men older than 90 years
      2. Family history of BPH
      3. Sedentary lifestyle
      4. Obesity
      5. African American ethnicity
      6. Diet high in starches and meat
      7. Excessive alcohol use
   B. Etiology
      1. Age
      2. Endocrine: Increased DHT and estrogen
      3. Inadequate opening of the bladder neck sphincter resulting from stimulation of the alpha-adrenergic nerve endings
      4. Drugs: Anticholinergics and sympathomimetics cause contractile and increased outflow resistance of the bladder, respectively.

C. History
  1. History of cancer and cancer therapy
  2. Current medications: Prescribed, over the counter
  3. History of presenting symptoms: Precipitating factors, onset, location, duration
  4. Changes in ADLs
  5. Past medical history: Hypertension, prior surgical procedures of the urinary tract, diabetes mellitus, neurologic disease, recurrent UTIs
  6. Family history of BPH, prostate cancer
  7. Voiding diary for two weeks
D. Signs and symptoms: The signs and symptoms are consistent with either obstruction or irritation. Severity of symptoms is assessed using the International Prostate Symptom Score or the American Urological Association Symptom Index (AUA-SI). Both are validated, short, self-administered questionnaires measuring a patient's own experience of symptoms. The higher the score, the more severe the condition, with a cutoff score of 8.
  1. Voiding (obstructive) symptoms
    a) Hesitancy, weak stream
    b) Decreased force and caliber of stream
    c) Straining to urinate
    d) Double urinating
    e) Sensation of incomplete bladder emptying
    f) Postvoid dribbling
  2. Storage (irritative) symptoms
    a) Urgency
    b) Frequency
    c) Nocturia
E. Physical examination
  1. Abdominal
    a) Bladder distention, urinary retention
    b) Bladder distention, tenderness, mass, pain on palpitation
  2. Digital rectal: To determine the size of the prostate
    a) Normal prostate size is 2.5–3 cm in diameter.
    b) Normal prostate is smooth with the median sulcus palpated.
    c) A prostate height-to-width ratio greater than or equal to 0.8 cm and a prostate volume greater than 30 ml suggest a bladder outlet obstruction.
    d) Irregularly shaped or nodular prostate may be indicative of a prostate lesion.
    e) Only the posterior and lateral aspects of the prostate can be palpated, and 40% of cancerous lesions occur interiorly.
    f) Prostate lesions are palpable when greater than or equal to 1.5 cm.
    g) Sphincter tone should be assessed.
  3. Musculoskeletal: Ambulatory and neuromuscular function of lower extremity function to evaluate for neurologic causes of urinary problems

IV. Diagnostic tests (Foster et al., 2018; Vasanwala et al., 2017)
  A. Laboratory
    1. Urinalysis to evaluate for infection or hematuria; hematuria potentially indicative of a serious GU issue, such as malignancy or calculi; pyuria suggestive of complicated UTI
    2. Routine measurement of serum creatinine to assess for renal function and obstruction not recommended in the initial evaluation of lower urinary tract symptoms secondary to BPH

3. Prostate-specific antigen (PSA) test in patients older than 50 years of age or with a family history of prostate cancer: Increased PSA greater than age guideline suggestive of prostatitis or prostate cancer

4. AUA-SI score: Defines severity of symptoms with mild (0–7), moderate (8–19), and severe score (20–35)

B. Radiology

1. Transabdominal ultrasound and transrectal ultrasonography: Transrectal preferred to assess bladder and ureters for obstruction; prostate size and shape assessment

2. IV pyelogram to assess urinary tract

3. MRI more accurate but is costly to assess urinary tract

4. CT scan of abdomen/pelvis: Recurrent UTIs, urolithiasis, renal insufficiency, hematuria, history of urinary tract surgery; preferred test for smaller cysts or masses

C. Other

1. Peak urinary flow rate (Qmax): A measure of how quickly urine is flowing; reduced rate possibly indicative of obstruction with a Qmax less than 10 ml/s

2. Post-void residual urine volume greater than or equal to 50 ml indicative of potential bladder dysfunction as a result of medication failure and need for surgery

3. Cystoscopy to determine the size of the prostate for direct visualization or intervention

4. Tissue biopsy for diagnosis

V. Differential diagnosis (Pearson & Williams, 2014)

A. Prostate cancer

B. Urethral stricture

C. Neurogenic bladder

D. UTI (see Chapter 89)

E. Bacterial or nonbacterial prostatitis (see Chapter 92)

VI. Treatment: Symptom dependent (Barry et al., 1992; Foster et al., 2018; Lokeshwar et al., 2019; Vasanwala et al., 2017)

A. Mild to moderate symptoms (AUA-SI score 0–7) and not bothersome: Watchful waiting; no antibiotic use, behavioral management program (e.g., limit fluid, treat constipation, bladder training, complete voiding)

B. Moderate to severe symptoms (AUA-SI score greater than or equal to 8): Drug therapy or surgery

1. Medication: Reduction of prostate size or prostatic smooth muscle tone is observed. Single-agent therapy is the mainstay of treatment; however, combination therapy may be required for patients who have a larger baseline prostate gland (30 g) and elevated PSA levels (greater than 1.6 ng/ml).

a) Alpha-blockers: Nonselective and selective; cause smooth muscle relaxation; doxazosin 4 mg PO daily; terazosin 1–10 mg PO daily, maximum dose 20 mg PO daily; alfuzosin 10 mg PO daily; tamsulosin 0.4–0.8 mg PO daily or silodosin 8 mg PO daily with meals

(1) Improvement of symptoms and flow rate occurs via relaxation of smooth muscle tone in the prostate and bladder neck. Tamsulosin is the most cost-effective but causes ejaculatory dysfunction.

(2) Blockers may lower blood pressure (nonselective) by decreasing peripheral vascular resistance; dose should be administered in the evening initially to minimize hypotension. Use with caution in patients on an antihypertensive. The phosphodiesterase type 5 inhibitors sildenafil and var-

denafil may potentiate the hypotensive effects of terazosin and doxazosin. Risks with tadalafil are less clear. Titrate terazosin and doxazosin to prevent hypotension.

    (3) Side effects include syncope, headache, postural hypotension, palpitations, impotence, falls, head trauma, and weight gain.

    (4) Avoid selective alpha-1A blockers in patients undergoing cataract surgery, as they may cause intraoperative floppy iris syndrome; assess patient prior to initiating cataract therapy.

  b) 5-Alpha-reductase inhibitors: Choice in proven prostate enlargement; finasteride 5 mg daily or dutasteride 0.5 mg PO daily; prostate therapy started greater than 30 g; clinical improvement in three to six weeks

    (1) Decrease prostate volume by suppressing 5-alpha-reductase enzyme conversion of testosterone to DHT.

    (2) Decrease symptoms, prostate size, risk of urinary retention, and likelihood of surgery.

    (3) Full effects may take several months before relief.

    (4) Side effects include decreased libido, impotence, and ejaculatory dysfunction; these symptoms tend to decrease with longer treatment duration. Sexual dysfunction, such as gynecomastia, can occur.

    (5) These inhibitors may cause a significant reduction in PSA levels, which is important information when screening for prostate cancer.

  c) Combination therapy with alpha-blockers and 5-alpha-reductase inhibitors: Effective in patients with refractory symptoms, a grossly enlarged prostate, or elevated PSA levels (e.g., doxazosin, finasteride); decreases clinical progression and long-term risk of acute urinary retention and surgery; more efficacious in men with larger prostate glands, not in men with only moderate BPH

  d) Other: Anticholinergic agents; oxybutynin 5 mg PO two to three times a day, started low at 2.5 mg PO in older adults; tolterodine 1–2 mg PO two times a day; caution with post-void residual urine greater than 250–300 ml

2. Minimally invasive procedures

  a) Transurethral needle ablation uses radiofrequency energy to remove prostate overgrowth. It is effective in improving voiding symptoms and has a lower risk of adverse events than with transurethral resection of the prostate, which is a treatment option for men with lower urinary tract symptoms attributed to BPH.

  b) Transurethral microwave thermotherapy has higher rates of retreatment over transurethral resection of the prostate.

  c) Transurethral ethanol injection (endoscopic procedure) is currently under investigation.

3. Surgery: A surgical procedure might be indicated in patients with refractory retention, recurrent gross hematuria, recurrent UTIs, and renal insufficiency due to BPH, bladder calculi, or symptoms refractory to medical management. No recommendation to perform surgery exists solely for asymptomatic bladder diverticulum.

  a) Transurethral resection of the prostate is the mainstay for BPH surgical treatment for men with lower urinary tract symptoms attributed to BPH. Complications of prostate resection through the bladder include the following.

    (1) Retrograde ejaculation

    (2) Erectile dysfunction

    (3) Transurethral resection syndrome: Hyponatremia, hypervolemia

    (4) Bleeding, potential transfusion

(5) Bladder neck contracture or urethral stricture

(6) Prostate perforation with extravasation

b) Transurethral incision of the prostate includes resection of the prostate through an incision in the bladder. This does not cause ejaculatory or fertility dysfunction. Treat prostates less than 30 g for lower urinary tract symptoms attributed to BPH.

c) Laser vaporization prostatectomy is a procedure that uses regional anesthesia. It causes tissue coagulation. Treatment is particularly useful for patients with severe cardiac or pulmonary comorbidities. It has the best cost-effectiveness ratio of all interventional therapies. Complications are reoperation, incontinence, and blood transfusion.

d) Transurethral laser coagulation (e.g., visual laser ablation) is another option.

e) Open prostatectomy is the option of choice for severely enlarged and obstructive prostate; large prostates are greater than 60 g.

VII. Follow-up

A. In two to four weeks, assess for persistent symptoms (e.g., hematuria, dysuria, irritation). Patient prescribed alpha blockade should be assessed within one or two weeks.

B. Assess for symptoms of retrograde ejaculation (occurs less frequently with laser vaporization). Teach medication side effects, including gynecomastia, dizziness, or impotence.

C. Follow-up annually or as symptoms occur. Annual screening is recommended for prostate cancer with digital rectal examination and PSA.

VIII. Referral: Urologist for long-term management

The author would like to acknowledge Faith A. Mutale, MSN, CRNP, for her contribution to this chapter that remains unchanged from the previous edition of this book.

References

Barry, M.J., Fowler, F.J., Jr., O'Leary, M.P., Bruskewitz, R.C., Holtgrewe, H.L., Mebust, W.K., & Cockett, A.T. (1992). The American Urological Association symptom index for benign prostatic hyperplasia. *Journal of Urology, 148*(5), 1549–1557. https://doi.org/10.1016/s0022-5347(17)36966-5

Foo, K.T. (2017). Pathophysiology of clinical benign prostatic hyperplasia. *Asian Journal of Urology, 4*(3), 152–157. https://doi.org/10.1016/j.ajur.2017.06.003

Foster, H.E., Barry, M.J., Dahm, P., Gandhi, M.C., Kaplan, S.A., Kohler, T.S., ... McVary, K.T. (2018). Surgical management of lower urinary tract symptoms attributed to benign prostatic hyperplasia: AUA guideline. *Journal of Urology, 200*(3), 612–619. https://doi.org/10.1016/j.juro.2018.05.048

Lokeshwar, S.D., Harper, B.T., Webb, E., Jordan, A., Dykes, T.A., Neal, D.E., Jr., ... Klaasen, Z. (2019). Epidemiology and treatment modalities for the management of benign prostatic hyperplasia. *Translational Andrology and Urology, 8*(5), 529–539. https://doi.org/10.21037/tau.2019.10.01

Madersbacher, S., Sampson, N., & Culig, Z. (2019). Pathophysiology of benign prostatic hyperplasia and benign prostatic enlargement: A mini-review. *Gerontology, 65*(5), 458–464. https://doi.org/10.1159/000496289

Patel, N.D., & Parsons, J.K. (2014). Epidemiology and etiology of benign prostatic hyperplasia and bladder outlet obstruction. *Indian Journal of Urology, 30*(2), 170–176. https://doi.org/10.4103/0970-1591.126900

Pearson, R., & Williams, P.M. (2014). Common questions about the diagnosis and management of benign prostatic hyperplasia. *American Family Physician, 90*(11), 769–774. https://www.aafp.org/afp/2014/1201/p769.html

Skinder, D., Zacharia, I., Studin, J., & Covino, J. (2016). Benign prostatic hyperplasia: A clinical review. *Journal of the American Academy of Physician Assistants, 29*(8), 19–23. https://doi.org/10.1097/01.JAA.0000488689.58176.0a

Vasanwala, F.F., Wong, M.Y.C., Ho, H.S.S., & Foo, K.T. (2017). Benign prostatic hyperplasia and male lower urinary symptoms: A guide for family physicians. *Asian Journal of Urology, 4*(3), 181–184. https://doi.org/10.1016/j.ajur.2017.05.003

CHAPTER 88

Hemorrhagic Cystitis

Faith A. Mutale, MSN, CRNP

I. Definition: Diffuse inflammatory bladder condition that leads to mucosal bleeding (Linder et al., 2014; Zwaans et al., 2016)

II. Physiology/Pathophysiology (Linder et al., 2014; Zwaans et al., 2016)
  A. Normal: The bladder is a muscular, membranous reservoir for urine storage and expulsion. Urine is discharged from the bladder through the urethra. Capacity is approximately 400–600 ml of urine.
  B. Pathophysiology: Results from mucosal damage to the bladder's transitional epithelium and blood vessels by toxins, bacteria, viruses, chemotherapy drugs, radiation, or other disease processes
    1. Injury to urothelium of the bladder occurs from metabolites of oxazaphosphorine alkylating agents, such as fludarabine, cabazitaxel, cyclophosphamide, ifosfamide, busulfan, doxorubicin, and dacarbazine.
      a) Excreted acrolein (a toxin liver metabolite) binds to the bladder mucosa and causes erythema, inflammation, ulceration, necrosis, and hemorrhage. Acrolein urotoxicity is related to increased exposure of the urothelium to the acrolein.
      b) Disruption of bladder mucosa integrity by lesions leads to microscopic or frank hemorrhage.
    2. Mucosal damage from pelvic radiation therapy leads to microscopic progressive obliterative endarteritis that causes mucosal ischemia and reperfusion injury, ulceration, and bleeding.
    3. Herpes simplex or adenovirus can alter bladder mucosa, resulting in hemorrhagic cystitis.
    4. Acute urethral syndrome can cause submucosal hemorrhage or interstitial cystitis that can be caused by chlamydia infection.

III. Clinical features: Hemorrhagic cystitis may occur as an emergent event or may precede a history of microscopic hematuria (Linder et al., 2014; Zwaans et al., 2016).
  A. Etiology: Infectious and noninfectious
    1. Infectious: Due to either the direct effects or activation of dormant viruses in the kidney, ureter, or bladder
      a) Adenoviruses
      b) Polyomavirus
    2. Noninfectious
      a) Chemotherapy, mainly with alkylating oxazaphosphorine (e.g., cyclophosphamide, ifosfamide): Occurs in 6%–40% of patients without uroprotection; dose related; occurs in less than 5% of patients receiving uroprotection with mesna
      b) Carcinoma of bladder

      c) Pelvic irradiation: Occurs in 25% of patients; at a median of 35 months after radiation therapy

         (1) Common in patients receiving conventional pelvic radiation therapy

         (2) Dose dependent; occurs in 6%–9% of patients receiving full dose

         (3) Severe in less than 5% of patients receiving full dose

         (4) Common in patients receiving radiation to a large area (volume)

      d) HSCT

         (1) Occurs in approximately 10%–20% of recipients

         (2) More common in matched unrelated donors and unrelated cord blood transplants

         (3) Median duration of hemorrhagic cystitis of 27–73 days

         (4) Higher risk in autologous recipients after myeloablative therapy

   3. Drug induced: Rare

      a) Penicillins with extended use: Symptoms may take up to two weeks after initiation.

      b) Danazol in patients with hereditary angioedema

   4. Chemically induced: Related to exposure to urotoxic agents such as derivatives of aniline, a compound found in dyes, marking pens, and shoe polish, and toluidine, which is found in shoe polish and pesticides

 B. History: Important to guide care management

   1. History of cancer and cancer treatment

   2. Current medications: Prescribed, over the counter

   3. History of presenting symptoms: Precipitating factors, onset, duration

   4. Changes in ADLs

   5. Social history: Occupational and chemical exposure

 C. Signs and symptoms

   1. Hematuria: Variable degrees, ranging from slightly blood-tinged urine to gross hematuria with clots and hemorrhage

   2. Dysuria

   3. Frequency

   4. Urgency

   5. Abdominal discomfort

   6. Suprapubic pain

   7. Bladder spasms; in men, can cause severe penile pain

   8. Flank pain

 D. Physical examination

   1. Vital signs

      a) Fever indicative of possible infection

      b) Blood pressure and pulse for signs of extreme blood loss

   2. Abdominal

      a) Suprapubic fullness, bladder distension, discomfort, or pain indicating bladder irritation upon palpitation

      b) Costovertebral angle tenderness suggestive of kidney infection

   3. Posterior thorax: Costovertebral angle tenderness suggestive of ureteral obstruction or kidney infection

   4. Pelvic (women): Vaginitis, urethral mass

   5. GU (men): Testes, penis, digital rectal examination (prostate)

IV. Diagnostic tests (Linder et al., 2014)

 A. Laboratory

   1. Urinalysis: Distinguish infectious from noninfectious causes.

2. CBC: Hgb and hematocrit are decreased with blood loss, particularly in patients with chronic hemorrhagic cystitis. WBCs may be elevated in infection.

3. Basic metabolic panel and coagulation studies: Tests may reflect sequelae of primary condition. Assess renal function.

4. Urine studies for viruses, as appropriate: Perform viral culture and enzyme-linked immunosorbent assay (ELISA) test.

B. Radiology

1. Renal ultrasonography with kidney, ureter, and bladder to assess for stones

2. CT: Urography to assess for stones

3. IV pyelography to evaluate urinary tract

C. Other

1. Cystoscopy: In patients with severe symptoms; delayed in active bleeding to visualize source of bleeding

2. Voiding cystourethrography to assess abnormalities in urethra and bladder and whether urine flow is normal as bladder empties

V. Differential diagnosis (Linder et al., 2014; Ziegelman et al., 2017)

A. Cystitis (see Chapter 89)

B. BPH, chronic prostatitis (see Chapters 87 and 92)

C. Carcinoma of bladder, prostate, uterus, cervix, or rectum

D. Renal cell carcinoma: Late sign suggesting invasion of vascular or collecting system

E. Calculus disease (urolithiasis): Presents as renal colic and hematuria

F. Trauma

G. Glomerular disease

H. Sickle cell disease (see Chapter 119)

I. Viral infection: CMV, BK polyomavirus, adenovirus type 11

J. Systemic coagulopathies

K. Anticoagulation therapy (see Chapter 122)

VI. Treatment: Treat underlying etiology or disease following American Urology Association guidelines (Alesawi et al., 2014; Gowda et al., 2019; Linder et al., 2014; Pitto & García-Perdomo, 2017; Ziegelman et al., 2017; Zwaans et al., 2016).

A. Cystoscopy with clot evacuation and fulguration: Surgical approach is used.

B. Bladder irrigation: The irrigation process is manual or continuous and uses a three-way catheter following the American Urology Association algorithm. Intravesical instillation with alum is initial treatment for patients with good renal function and for those who do not respond to continuous bladder irrigation. Irrigation induces vasoconstriction and decreases capillary permeability, resulting in hemostasis (aminocaproic acid).

C. Alum is associated with encephalopathy in patients with renal insufficiency. It may cause bladder wall necrosis and perforation.

D. Bladder embolization: Surgical approach is used.

E. Prevention of chemotherapy-induced hemorrhagic cystitis: American Society of Clinical Oncology guidelines recommend administration of mesna with saline diuresis or saline diuresis alone in patients undergoing high-dose cyclophosphamide for HSCT. Guidelines should be referred to for complete dosing recommendations and administration.

1. Mesna dose is dependent on chemotherapy dose. It is administered prior to chemotherapy and repeated four and eight hours after chemotherapy or as a continuous infusion (practice dependent).

2. Discontinue chemotherapy if hemorrhagic cystitis develops.

    3. Administer hydration with 0.5 normal saline to maintain urine output greater than 150 ml/hr.

  F. Hyperbaric oxygen for radiation-induced hemorrhagic cystitis induces capillary angiogenesis.

    1. Average of 20–30 sessions required for approximately 60 minutes for each treatment

    2. Not a good option for acutely ill patients

  G. Embolization of the iliac artery or superior vesical arteries is used in severe cases.

  H. Antibiotic or antiviral therapy is used as appropriate with infection (see Appendix C).

  I. Chondroitin sulfate and sodium hyaluronate are used for prevention of radiation-induced hemorrhagic cystitis.

  J. Oxybutynin chloride: Give 5 mg PO two to three times a day for bladder spasms.

  K. Aminocaproic acid: Administer 200 mg mixed in a liter of saline solution given via IV until bleeding resolves or PO 100–150 mg/kg in divided doses. Assess patient for thromboembolic events. Upper GU bleeding must be ruled out prior to oral administration.

  L. Intravesical instillation of silver nitrate causes chemical cauterization of the urothelium.

  M. Formalin instillation is in refractory settings and performed in operating room.

  N. Nephrostomy diversion is an option.

  O. Cystectomy is used as a last resort.

  P. Blood transfusion should be given PRN for blood loss.

  Q. Intravesical instillation of tacrolimus is under investigation in patients with radiation-induced hemorrhagic cystitis.

VII. Follow-up (Ziegelman et al., 2017; Zwaans et al., 2016)

  A. Assess for refractory symptoms frequently.

  B. Long-term follow-up includes bladder ultrasonography in patients with previous exposure to alkylating chemotherapy agents, pelvic irradiation, and formalin.

VIII. Referrals (Ziegelman et al., 2017; Zwaans et al., 2016)

  A. Urologist: For management of patients with radiation- or chemotherapy-induced fibrosis

  B. Hyperbaric specialist: For hyperbaric oxygen therapy, as appropriate, in patients with prior pelvic radiation exposure

References

Alesawi, A.M., El-Hakim, A., Zorn, K.C., & Saad, F. (2014). Radiation-induced hemorrhagic cystitis. *Current Opinion in Supportive and Palliative Care, 8*(3), 235–240. https://doi.org/10.1097/SPC.0000000000000073

Gowda, G.G., Vijaykumar, R., & Tigga, M.P. (2019). Endovascular management of radiation-induced hemorrhagic cystitis. *Indian Journal of Palliative Care, 25*(3), 471–473. https://doi.org/10.4103/IJPC.IJPC_6_19

Linder, B.J., Tarrell, R.F., & Boorjian, S.A. (2014). Cystectomy for refractory hemorrhagic cystitis: Contemporary etiology, presentation and outcomes. *Journal of Urology, 192*(6), 1687–1692. https://doi.org/10.1016/j.juro.2014.06.030.

Pitto, C.M., & García-Perdomo, H.A. (2017). Interventions to treat hemorrhagic cystitis: A systematic review and meta-analysis. *Supportive Care in Cancer, 25*(7), 2043–2046. https://doi.org/10.1007/s00520-017-3731-7

Ziegelman, M.J., Boorijian, S.A., Joyce, D.D., Montgomery, B.D., & Linder, B.J. (2017). Intravesical formalin for hemorrhagic cystitis. A contemporary cohort. *Canadian Urological Association Journal, 11*(3–4), E79–E82. https://doi.org/10.5489/cuaj.4047

Zwaans, B.M.M., Chancellor, M.B., & Lamb, L.E. (2016). Modeling and treatment of radiation cystitis. *Urology, 88,* 14–21. https://doi.org/10.1016/j.urology.2015.11.001.

CHAPTER 89

Lower Urinary Tract Infection (Cystitis)

Mary W. Dunn, MSN, RN, OCN®, NP-C

I. Definition: Infection of the bladder (Bonkat et al., 2018; Dubbs & Sommerkamp, 2019; Tan, & Chlebicki, 2016)
   A. Acute simple cystitis is an infection confined to the bladder.
   B. Other types of lower UTIs include urethritis, acute prostatitis, chronic prostatitis, and complicated UTI (i.e., special populations).

II. Physiology/Pathophysiology (Hickling et al., 2015; McLellan & Hunstad, 2016)
   A. Normal
      1. The urinary tract is composed of epithelial tissue that extends from the kidneys to the urethral meatus.
      2. The urinary tract contains a continuous stream of sterile urine.
   B. Pathophysiology
      1. Bacteria can enter the urinary tract through three pathways.
        a) Ascension from the urethra into the bladder, then up the ureters to the kidneys
        b) Lymphatic channels from GI or pelvic origin: Rare
        c) Hematogenous route to the kidneys: Rare in healthy individuals
      2. Most of the causative microorganisms originate in the GI tract.
      3. Standard threshold for bacteriuria is greater than or equal to 100,000 colony-forming units (CFU)/ml. Women with symptomatic pyuria may have lower midstream urine counts (e.g., less than 100,000 CFU/ml but greater than 100 CFU/ml).
      4. The most common infecting organism is *Escherichia coli.*

III. Clinical features: UTIs, including cystitis, are common bacterial infections that primary care providers encounter. When cystitis is suspected, it is crucial to determine its classification: asymptomatic bacteriuria, uncomplicated cystitis, pyelonephritis, prostatitis, or complicated UTI (Bonkat et al., 2018; Chu & Lowder, 2018; Dubbs & Sommerkamp, 2019; Foxman, 2014; Kolman, 2019; McLellan & Hunstad, 2016).
   A. Risk factors
      1. Female gender: Shorter distance from anus to urethra
      2. Sexual activity
      3. Intercourse with use of a spermicide-containing contraceptive
      4. Anatomic abnormalities: Neurogenic bladder, bladder/urethral obstruction
      5. Diabetes mellitus
      6. BPH

      7. Urinary retention

      8. Obesity

      9. Prior UTI

     10. Trauma/manipulation: Insertion of urinary catheter

     11. Advanced age

     12. Pregnancy

     13. Chronic renal failure

     14. Chronic catherization

B. Etiology

      1. Enteric, usually gram-negative bacteria

        a) *E. coli* (greater than 80%)

        b) *Klebsiella, Proteus mirabilis, Pseudomonas aeruginosa*

      2. Gram-positive bacteria: Less frequent; *Staphylococcus saprophyticus, Enterococcus faecalis, Streptococcus agalactiae*

C. History

      1. History of cancer and cancer treatment

      2. Current medications: Prescribed, over the counter

      3. History of presenting symptoms: Precipitating factors, onset, duration

      4. Changes in ADLs

      5. Past medical history: STIs, UTIs, urolithiasis, prostatitis, diabetes, immunocompromised state

      6. Social history: Sexual practices, birth control method

D. Signs and symptoms

      1. Dysuria

      2. Urinary frequency

      3. Urinary urgency

      4. Suprapubic pain

      5. Hematuria

      6. Urinary incontinence

      7. Malodorous and cloudy urine

      8. Older adult or debilitated patients: Historically, generalized signs or symptoms, such as falls, altered mental status, decline in functional status, and fatigue, have prompted evaluation for UTI. Newer data suggest no association between these changes and bacteriuria, so further evaluation should be individualized.

      9. Fever, chills, pelvic/perineal/flank pain suggestive of complicated UTI or pyelonephritis

E. Physical examination

      1. Vital signs: Fevers; uncommon in simple cystitis

      2. Abdominal: Bladder distention, suprapubic tenderness

      3. Posterior thorax: Flank or costovertebral tenderness indicative of upper tract pathology (e.g., pyelonephritis)

      4. Pelvic (women)

        a) Vaginitis

        b) Urethral mass

        c) Lesions, drainage, or irritation suggestive of STI

      5. GU (men)

        a) Lesion of scrotum and penis indicating STI or malignancy

        b) Testes and scrotum masses and tenderness indicative of prostatitis

        c) Digital rectal examination to assess prostate for enlargement or tenderness suggestive of prostatitis or BPH

IV. Diagnosis and testing (Bonkat et al., 2018; Chu & Lowder, 2018; Dubbs & Sommerkamp, 2019; Kolman, 2019; Tonolini & Ippolito, 2016)
   A. Laboratory
      1. Men
         a) Urinalysis: Pyuria typically present
         b) Urine culture: Midstream urine culture with greater than or equal to 1,000 CFU/ml of a predominant species
      2. Women
         a) Most women with symptoms of acute simple cystitis do not warrant additional testing and can be diagnosed clinically.
         b) Urinalysis can be useful in women who have clinical features that are suggestive but not clearly diagnostic of cystitis.
      3. Urinalysis: Possible abnormalities with cystitis
         a) Color: Dark yellow, cloudy, amber, or red
         b) Pyuria: Greater than 2–5 WBCs per high-power field
         c) Leukocyte esterase: Enzyme released into the urine by WBCs indicating infection
         d) Nitrite: Forms when bacteria reduce the nitrate present in normal urine
         e) RBCs: Increased tissue destruction
      4. Urine culture: Collected to determine specific organism
         a) All men presenting with symptoms of cystitis should have a urine culture.
         b) Women
            (1) If symptoms persist after treatment
            (2) Recurrent infection after adequate treatment
      5. Pregnancy test, if indicated
   B. Radiology
      1. Not indicated for acute simple cystitis
      2. Indications for IV pyelogram
         a) Women with recurrent UTIs to evaluate for renal abnormalities
         b) Complicated UTIs
         c) Persistent microhematuria (greater than or equal to 3 RBCs/high-power field) in the absence of obvious cause: Symptomatic UTI, instrumentation
   C. Other: Routine cystoscopy is unwarranted but may be useful in certain scenarios, including if symptoms persist with negative urine culture, in gross hematuria with negative urine culture, and with abnormal imaging.

V. Differential diagnosis (Michels & Sands, 2015)
   A. Acute abdominal disorder
   B. Acute pyelonephritis (see Chapter 94)
   C. Bladder obstruction
   D. Cervicitis
   E. Chemotherapy-induced cystitis
   F. Diabetes mellitus (see Chapter 151)
   G. GU cancer
   H. Prostatitis (see Chapter 92)
   I. Radiation-induced cystitis
   J. Salpingitis
   K. Urethritis
   L. Urolithiasis
   M. Vaginitis (see Chapter 85)
   N. Overactive bladder

VI. Treatment (Anger et al., 2019; Bonkat et al., 2018; Chu & Lowder, 2018; Dubbs & Sommer-kamp, 2019; Flores-Mireles et al., 2015; Gupta et al., 2011; Kolman, 2019; Naber & Wagenlehner, 2019; Nicolle et al., 2019)
   A. First-line pharmacologic therapy: Dependent on the source (see Appendix C)
      1. Nitrofurantoin: 100 mg PO two times a day for five days
      2. Trimethoprim/sulfamethoxazole: 160 mg/800 mg PO two times a day for three days
      3. Fosfomycin: 3 g PO for one dose
      4. Alternative antimicrobials: Dependent on patient allergies, concern for resistance
      5. Urinary analgesic: Phenazopyridine 200 mg PO three times a day for two days
   B. Unresolved cystitis: Positive urine culture after completion of antibiotic therapy; treated with 7–14-day course of appropriate antibiotic if persistent positive urine culture within 7–14 days after initial treatment
   C. Recurrent cystitis: Greater than or equal to two infections in six months or greater than or equal to three infections in one year; continuous (three months then reassess) or post-coital antibiotic prophylaxis
   D. Prevention
      1. Behavioral changes: Liberal fluid intake, modify contraception, postcoital voiding, wiping from front to back to avoid perineal contamination
      2. Topical estrogen for postmenopausal women (see Chapter 90)
      3. Options with unclear benefit: Cranberry products, probiotics, antiseptics, D-mannose
   E. Asymptomatic bacteriuria: In healthy premenopausal and postmenopausal women, recommendation is no screening or treatment.

VII. Follow-up (Bonkat et al., 2018)
   A. Short term: Symptomatic relief occurs within hours to three days after starting antibiotics; follow-up urine culture is not needed in patients with acute simple cystitis whose symptoms resolve with antibiotics.
   B. Long term: Follow-up includes urine culture after three months on prophylactic antibiotics.

VIII. Referrals (Tan & Chlebicki, 2016)
   A. Urologist: For recurrent cystitis, urolithiasis, anatomic abnormalities, hematuria with negative urine culture, persistent urinary symptoms with negative urine culture, and cystitis in young men
   B. Gynecologist: For vaginitis, STIs, pelvic organ prolapse

The author would like to acknowledge Diane G. Cope, PhD, ARNP-BC, AOCNP®, for her contribution to this chapter that remains unchanged from the previous edition of this book.

References

Anger, J., Lee, U., Ackerman, A.L., Chou, R., Chughtai, B., Clemens, J.Q., ... Chai, T.C. (2019). Recurrent uncomplicated urinary tract infections in women: AUA/CUA/SUFU guideline. *Journal of Urology, 202*(2), 282–289. https://doi.org/10.1097/JU.0000000000000296

Bonkat, G., Pickard, R., Bartoletti, R., Cai, T., Bruyère, F., Geerlings, S.E., ... Wagenlehner, F. (2018). *EAU guidelines on urologic infections.* European Association of Urology. https://uroweb.org/wp-content/uploads/EAU-Guidelines-on-Urological-Infections-2018-large text.pdf

Chu, C.M., & Lowder, J.L. (2018). Diagnosis and treatment of urinary tract infections across age groups. *American Journal of Obstetrics and Gynecology, 219*(1), 40–51. https://doi.org/10.1016/j.ajog.2017.12.231.

Dubbs, S.B., & Sommerkamp, S.K. (2019). Evaluation and management of urinary tract infection in the emergency department. *Emergency Medicine Clinics of North America, 37*(4), 707–723. https://doi.org/10.1016/j.emc.2019.07.007

Flores-Mireles, A.L., Walker, J.N, Caparon, M., & Hultgren, S.J. (2015). Urinary tract infections: Epidemiology, mechanisms of infection, and treatment options. *Nature Reviews Microbiology, 13*(5), 269–284. https://doi.org/10.1038/nrmicro3432.

Foxman, B. (2014). Urinary tract infection syndromes: Occurrence, recurrence, bacteriology, risk factors, and disease burden. *Infectious Disease Clinics of North America, 28*(1), 1–13. https://doi.org/10.1016/j.idc.2013.09.003

Gupta, K., Hooton, T.M, Naber, K.G., Wullt, B., Colgan, R., Miller, L.G., ... Soper, D.E. (2011). International clinical practice guidelines for treatment of acute uncomplicated cystitis and pyelonephritis in women: A 2010 update by the Infectious Diseases Society of America and the European Society for Microbiology and Infectious Diseases. *Clinical Infectious Disease, 52*(5), e103–e120. https://doi.org/10.1093/cid/ciq257

Hickling, D.R., Sun, T.-T., & Wu, X.-R. (2015). Anatomy and physiology of the urinary tract: Relation to host defense and microbial infection. *Microbiology Spectrum, 3*(4). https://doi.org/10.1128/microbiolspec.UTI-0016-2012

Kolman, K.B. (2019). Cystitis and pyelonephritis: Diagnosis, treatment, and prevention. *Primary Care: Clinics in Office Practice, 46*(2), 191–202. https://doi.org/10.1016/j.pop.2019.01.001

McLellan, L.K., & Hunstad, D.A. (2016). Urinary tract infection: Pathogenesis and outlook. *Trends in Molecular Medicine, 22*(11), 946–957. https://doi.org/10.1016/j.molmed.2016.09.003

Michels, T.C., & Sands, J.E. (2015). Dysuria: Evaluation and differential diagnosis in adults. *American Family Physician, 92*(9), 778–788. https://www.aafp.org/afp/2015/1101/p778.html

Naber, K.G., & Wagenlehner, F.M.E. (2019). Novel antibiotics in the treatment of urinary tract infections. *European Urology Focus, 5*(1), 10–12. https://doi.org/10.1016/j.euf.2018.11.012

Nicolle, L.E., Gupta, K., Bradley, S.F., Colgan, R., DeMuri, G.P., Drekonja, D., ... Siemieniuk, R. (2019). Clinical practice guideline for the management of asymptomatic bacteriuria: 2019 update by the Infectious Diseases Society of America. *Clinical Infectious Diseases, 68*(10), 1611–1615. https://doi.org/10.1093/cid/ciz021

Tan, C.W., & Chlebicki, M.P. (2016). Urinary tract infections in adults. *Singapore Medical Journal, 57*(9), 485–490. https://doi.org/10.11622/smedj.2016153

Tonolini, M., & Ippolito, S. (2016). Cross-sectional imaging of complicated urinary infections affecting the lower tract and male genital organs. *Insights Into Imaging, 7*(5), 689–711. https://doi.org/10.1007/s13244-016-0503-8

CHAPTER 90

Menopausal Symptoms and Menopause

Stephanie Jackson, DNP, MSN, RN, AOCNS®, BMTCN®

I. Definition (Roberts & Hickey, 2016)
   A. Natural menopause is the transition from the time of the onset of menstrual cycle changes until one year after the final menstrual period. The transition occurs at a median age of 47 years and lasts for five to eight years.
   B. Primary ovarian insufficiency is defined as menopause before age 40 years and is considered abnormal.
   C. Induced menopause is an abrupt cessation of menses related to chemical or surgical intervention.

II. Physiology/Pathophysiology (Palacios et al., 2019; Santoro et al., 2015)
   A. Normal
      1. The hypothalamus releases gonadotropin-releasing hormone to stimulate the anterior pituitary to release FSH and luteinizing hormone (LH).
      2. At premenopause, the ovary is composed of eggs surrounded by granulosa cells in a sac or follicle.
      3. The follicle responds to FSH and LH by developing and producing estrogen, and ovulation occurs.
      4. At menopause, the ovary contains no follicles and does not respond to FSH or LH.
      5. The follicular granulosa cells also produce diminishing levels of inhibin, a hormone that inhibits the synthesis and release of FSH, which allows the anterior pituitary to release more FSH.
      6. The ovaries and adrenal glands synthesize androstenedione (an androgen), which is converted to estrone (a weak estrogen) in peripheral tissue, liver, fat, and hypothalamic nuclei.
   B. Pathophysiology
      1. Menopause is a normal process of aging in women as a result of a diminished number of ovarian and primary follicles.
      2. There is a decreased production of LH and ovulation no longer takes place, resulting in a decrease in estrogen and in the ability to conceive.

III. Clinical features: Typically, women start to experience perimenopausal symptoms in their mid-40s and go through menopause at an average age of 51 years; however, women undergoing cancer treatment may develop premature menopause at any age. Menopause is a natural physiologic process and is described as a normal stage of life (Palacios et al., 2019; Santoro et al., 2015).

A. Risk factors for early menopause
1. Chemotherapy agents
    a) Degree of occurrence is based on age, drug dose, and duration of treatment.
    b) Women older than age 40 years are at greater risk.
2. Hormonal agents: Tamoxifen, aromatase inhibitors
3. Chromosome defects: Turner syndrome
4. Autoimmune disease: RA
5. Epilepsy
6. Smoking
7. Thyroid disease
8. Pelvic irradiation
9. Oophorectomy or hysterectomy

B. Etiology
1. Medication induced
2. Cancer treatment
3. Surgical procedures: Hysterectomy with bilateral oophorectomy
4. Aging process
5. Primary ovarian insufficiency

C. History
1. History of cancer and cancer treatment
2. Current medications: Prescribed, over the counter, herbal products
3. History of presenting symptoms: Precipitating factors, onset, frequency, severity, duration, associated symptoms (e.g., hot flashes, night sweats, insomnia)
4. Changes in ADLs
5. Current or past use of complementary and alternative methods to manage menopausal symptoms: Stress management techniques, massage, acupuncture, chiropractic, dietary soy, naturopathic, homeopathic
6. Menstrual and obstetric history
    a) Menarche
    b) Time between periods: Flow, length, changes in menses
    c) Character of menses
    d) History of pregnancies, miscarriages, abortions, stillbirths, premature births, complications
    e) Use of hormone therapy, including birth control pills, or gynecologic and obstetric procedures
7. Past medical history: Heart disease, overweight, hypertension, congenital or acquired hyperlipidemia, diabetes mellitus, osteoporosis, depression, hysterectomy
8. Family history: Osteoporosis, heart disease, cancer, early menopause

D. Signs and symptoms
1. Hot flashes
2. Night sweats
3. Insomnia
4. Fatigue
5. Anxiety/tension
6. Depression
7. Irritability
8. Migraines
9. Joint pains

10. Stomach upset
11. Loss of concentration
12. Loss of self-esteem/confidence
13. Forgetfulness
14. Dysuria, urinary frequency, stress incontinence
15. Vaginal dryness, pruritus, dyspareunia
16. Urethral atrophy
17. Stress incontinence, frequency, urgency, dysuria
18. Decreased libido

E. Physical examination
    1. Vital signs and height: Hypertension and decreased height, which may be present with estrogen deficiency
    2. Neck: Hypothyroidism or hyperthyroidism on palpitation; symptoms similar to menopausal symptoms
    3. Breast: Atrophy present with long-term estrogen deficiency
    4. Musculoskeletal: Weakness or discomfort to evaluate for osteoporosis
    5. Pelvic: Prolapse of the vagina, bladder, or rectum; vaginal atrophy with dyspareunia and/or mucosal dryness with prolonged low estrogen levels

IV. Diagnostic studies: Studies usually are not necessary to diagnose menopause. Symptoms and clinical manifestations direct diagnosis (American College of Obstetricians and Gynecologists, 2018; Fourman & Fazeli, 2015; Klein et al., 2019; Pereira & Brown, 2017).

A. Laboratory
    1. FSH and estradiol levels to confirm diagnosis of menopause
        a) FSH greater than 50 mIU/ml
        b) Estradiol less than 50 pg/ml
    2. To evaluate for other medical causes of symptoms
        a) CBC to assess for anemia
        b) Electrolytes to evaluate for hypokalemia
        c) Serum glucose to assess for diabetes mellitus
        d) LFTs to assess for liver disease
        e) Thyroid function tests to evaluate for thyroid disease
        f) Beta human chorionic gonadotropin to assess for pregnancy in selected patients
    3. Lipid profile: Important screening tools at the start of menopause
        a) LDL rises: LDL less than 130 mg/dl is within normal limits.
        b) Total HDL to LDL cholesterol ratio rises: Total HDL:LDL cholesterol ratio less than 7.5 is within normal limits.
        c) HDL becomes lower: HDL greater than 70 mg/dl is within normal limits.
        d) Total cholesterol less than 200 mg/dl and triglycerides 50–250 are within normal limits.

B. Radiology
    1. Mammogram to assess for breast lesions or abnormalities, especially if hormone therapy will be initiated
    2. DEXA to measure bone density with decreased estrogen and increased risk for bone loss
        a) DEXA can be used to measure whole-body bone mass. Typically, it measures the bone density in the radius, hip, and spine.
        b) Bone mineral density is reported in grams per centimeters squared (g/cm^2); bone mineral content is reported in grams. Results are determined in comparison with those of age-, sex-, and race-matched controls.

        c) Reports indicate whether bone mineral density is normal or above or below levels of the comparison group. Results help to predict risk of fracture by estimating the standard deviation from the matched controls.

           (1) Results greater than –2.5 indicate osteoporosis and require treatment.

           (2) Patients with results of –1.5 to –2.5 may be treated or be observed at regular intervals.

    3. Transvaginal ultrasound, as indicated

        a) Used to exclude ovarian pathology in patients with an abnormal adnexal mass or suspicious clinical features (e.g., GI distress, abdominal pain, abnormal vaginal bleeding); consideration to obtain cancer antigen 125, if indicated

        b) Used to exclude endometrial pathology in patients taking tamoxifen

        c) To evaluate an enlarged or irregular uterus

  C. Other: Endometrial biopsy to assess for malignancy, as indicated

V. Differential diagnosis (Fourman & Fazeli, 2015; Klein et al., 2019)

  A. Estrogen excess or deficiency, perimenopausal condition

  B. Metabolic

    1. Hyperthyroidism or hypothyroidism (see Chapters 157 and 158)

    2. Polycystic ovary syndrome

    3. Pheochromocytoma

    4. Carcinoid syndrome

    5. Anorexia (see Chapter 66)

  C. Pregnancy

  D. Panic attacks (see Chapter 161)

  E. Drug induced

    1. Endocrine drug therapy: Levothyroxine sodium, liothyronine sodium, corticotropin, cosyntropin, desmopressin acetate, calcitonin

    2. Sympathomimetic drugs: Mephentermine sulfate, metaraminol, norepinephrine bitartrate

    3. Tamoxifen

    4. Aromatase inhibitors

    5. Oral contraceptives

    6. Nicotinic acid

    7. Niacin and nitrates

    8. Chemotherapy, especially alkylating agents

    9. Antipsychotic drugs: Risperidone, olanzapine

    10. Phenothiazines

    11. Dopamine-affecting drugs: Reserpine, verapamil, cimetidine, opioids, tricyclic antidepressants

  F. Lymphoma

  G. Metastatic disease

  H. Retroperitoneal irradiation

  I. Hysterectomy

VI. Treatment (Cobin & Goodman, 2017; Kaplan & Mahon, 2014; Kaunitz & Manson, 2015; Klein et al., 2019; Minkin, 2019; North American Menopause Society, 2018; Palacios et al., 2019; Pinkerton et al., 2019; Roberts & Hickey, 2016; Santoro et al., 2015)

  A. Guidance should be provided about symptoms and treatment options. Patient medical history, risk assessment for cardiovascular disease, osteoporosis, and cancer (especially estrogen-dependent tumors), frequency and intensity of symptoms, and benefits and risks of treatment should be considered. Most patients will need nonhormone-based symptom management.

B. Treatment for those at risk for cardiovascular disease, diabetes, cancer, or osteoporosis
   1. Primary prevention
      a) Avoid tobacco use.
      b) Adhere to a balanced, nutrient-dense diet; maintain BMI of 18.5–24.9 kg/m².
      c) Exercise 20–30 minutes for four to seven days per week using a combination of aerobic exercise, weight-bearing exercise, strength training with weights, and stretching.
      d) Manage dyslipidemia with lipid-lowering medications (see Chapter 44).
      e) Manage hypertension with antihypertensive medications (see Chapter 47).
      f) Preventive measures of osteoporosis include calcium intake 1,000 mg PO daily (in divided doses) for those on hormone therapy or 1,500 mg PO daily in divided doses plus vitamin D₃ (cholecalciferol) 400–800 IU PO daily plus use of bisphosphonates (see Chapter 106).
   2. Secondary prevention of cardiovascular disease
      a) Antiembolism prophylaxis for those with documented PE or DVT (see Chapters 33 and 43)
      b) Beta-blockers and ACE inhibitors for those with documented cardiovascular disease
   3. Secondary prevention for those with documented osteoporosis (see Chapter 106)
C. Symptom management without hormone therapy
   1. Hot flashes
      a) Mild to moderate and does not interfere with typical functioning
         (1) Stress management techniques: Meditation, yoga, visualization, hypnosis, cognitive behavioral therapy, biofeedback
         (2) Dressing in layers using loose, cotton clothing
         (3) Drinking an adequate amount of cold water
         (4) Creating an environment that provides movement of air, such as a fan or open window with breezes
         (5) Avoiding tobacco and alcohol use
         (6) Avoiding hot, humid weather and confining spaces
         (7) Avoiding stress, caffeine, alcohol, hot drinks, and spicy foods
         (8) Vitamin E: 400–1,200 IU PO daily
         (9) Regular exercise: Specifics of exercise to reduce hot flashes are unknown.
         (10) Weight loss
      b) Moderate to severe and interferes with typical functioning
         (1) SSRIs
            (a) Paroxetine: 10 mg PO daily for seven days, then 20 mg daily or paroxetine controlled release 12.5 mg or 25 mg PO daily; 62%–65% decrease in hot flashes; should be avoided in patients on tamoxifen; possible drug interactions that decrease efficacy of tamoxifen
            (b) Venlafaxine extended release: 37.5 mg PO daily for seven days, then may increase to maximum of 75 mg PO daily; or venlafaxine 37.5 mg PO one or two times a day
            (c) Citalopram: 20 mg PO daily
            (d) Fluoxetine: 20 mg PO daily; 50% decrease in hot flashes
         (2) SSRIs and norepinephrine reuptake inhibitors: Desvenlafaxine 50 mg PO daily
         (3) Psychotropic medications: Gabapentin 300 mg PO three times a day
         (4) If previous agents are not effective or contraindicated
            (a) Clonidine: Initially 0.1 mg PO daily or 0.1 mg PO two times a day

      (b) Clonidine: 0.1 mg daily transdermal therapeutic system every seven days; applied to nonhairy skin on upper outer arm or chest; has been shown to reduce hot flashes by 20%

      (c) Megestrol acetate: 40 mg PO daily or 20 mg two times a day, which can be tapered to 20 mg every other day after one month; has been shown to reduce hot flashes by 20%

      (d) Medroxyprogesterone: 400 mg IM single dose; has shown efficacy

      (e) Mirtazapine: 7.5 mg PO every night for two weeks, then 15 mg PO every night for one week, then may increase to 30 mg PO every night

2. Vaginal dryness and dyspareunia: Mild to moderate

    a) Use strategies that promote the flexibility of the vagina (e.g., regular intercourse, vaginal dilator), improve muscle tone and circulation, decrease the chance of atrophy, and maintain the acidic pH of the vagina to reduce the risk of vaginal and bladder infections.

    b) Avoid products that may increase symptoms of dryness (e.g., perfumes, antihistamines, soaps, deodorants, powders, spermicides, panty liners, synthetic fabrics, tight clothing).

    c) Use vaginal moisturizers and lubrication products.

    d) Use estrogen vaginal ring/tablets (see Table 90-1) and/or creams (see Table 90-2).

3. Decreased libido/altered sexuality

    a) Mild to moderate symptoms

      (1) Provide anticipatory guidance to assist patients with altered self-concept, body image, perceptions of sexuality, potential changes, and interventional strategies.

      (2) Encourage use of stress management techniques (e.g., meditation, yoga, visualization, biofeedback).

TABLE 90-1	Estrogen Vaginal Ring/Tablets
Drug	**Dose/Comments**
Estradiol	Administer 7.5 mcg daily. Insert into the upper third of the vagina once every 3 months. It is not necessary to use progestins when using this vaginal ring. It may be offered to patients with breast cancer for genitourinary symptoms.
Estradiol acetate	Administer 0.05–0.1 mg daily. Insert into the upper third of the vagina once every 3 months.

Note. Based on information from North American Menopause Society, 2018; Palacios et al., 2019; Pinkerton et al., 2019; Roberts & Hickey, 2016; Santoro et al., 2015.

TABLE 90-2	Estrogen Vaginal Creams
Drug	**Dose/Comments**
Conjugated estrogen 0.625 mg/g	Use a 42.5 g tube and 0.5–2 g applicator. Administer every day, 3 weeks on, 1 week off.
Estradiol (0.01%) 0.1 mg/g	Use a 42.5 g tube and 1–4 g applicator. Administer every day for 1–2 weeks, then 1–3 times a week thereafter.

Note. Based on information from North American Menopause Society, 2018; Palacios et al., 2019; Pinkerton et al., 2019; Roberts & Hickey, 2016; Santoro et al., 2015.

      (3) Recommend a nutrient-rich diet to optimize BMI.

      (4) Suggest regular exercise.

      (5) Encourage communication and expression of needs.

      (6) Encourage behavioral techniques such as mutual massage of the patient with partner.

      (7) Emphasize symptom management of fatigue, weight gain, depression, anxiety, and poor sleep.

    b) Moderate to severe symptoms: Estrogen with methyltestosterone (see Table 90-3); used for women who experience sexual dysfunction or lack of libido after menopause, except for women with hormone-based cancers

      (1) These drugs are to be administered cyclically on a short-term basis.

      (2) Side effects of testosterone can cause deepening of the voice, weight gain, an increase in body hair, balding of scalp hair, and acne.

      (3) Estrogen with methyltestosterone may increase the effects of oral anticoagulant and insulin therapy.

      (4) Drug should be discontinued if jaundice, hypertension, hypercalcemia, or edema occurs.

4. Poor sleep

  a) Recommend regular aerobic exercise.

  b) Use stress management techniques (e.g., meditation, yoga, visualization) that have been shown through research to improve sleep.

  c) Avoid alcohol use.

  d) Avoid or decrease intake of caffeine, especially late in the day.

  e) Eat a light dinner.

5. Encourage strategies to assist with the feelings of fatigue (see Chapter 163).

6. Encourage strategies to assist with urinary incontinence (see Chapter 84).

7. Skin dryness

  a) Protect skin from the sun through use of sunscreen, hats, and clothing.

  b) Avoid cigarette smoke, including secondhand smoke.

  c) Drink 8–10 glasses of water daily.

  d) Apply skin moisturizers daily, especially after bathing while the skin is still moist.

  e) Avoid deodorant soaps.

8. Decreased cognitive function

  a) Avoid smoking or secondhand smoke.

  b) Maintain normotensive blood pressure.

  c) For those with diabetes, maintain good diabetic control to prevent vascular complications.

TABLE 90-3	Estrogen With Methyltestosterone
Drug	**Dose/Comments**
Esterified estrogen with methyltestosterone	Administer esterified estrogen 0.625 mg PO and methyltestosterone 1.25 mg PO. Take 3 weeks on, 1 week off.
Esterified estrogen with methyltestosterone	Give esterified estrogen 1.125 mg PO and methyltestosterone 2.5 mg PO. Administer cyclically.

Note. Based on information from North American Menopause Society, 2018; Palacios et al., 2019; Pinkerton et al., 2019; Roberts & Hickey, 2016; Santoro et al., 2015.

    d) Perform regular mental exercises, such as crossword puzzles, mathematics, reading, and learning a new subject.

D. Symptom management with hormone therapy for select patients after full discussion of risks and benefits: The risks associated with hormone therapy change with age and should be considered when prescribing to treat symptoms. Hormone therapy may be natural, conjugated equine, or synthetic and may be taken in pill, cream, or patch form. Use of hormone therapy in breast or endometrial cancer survivors is contraindicated for most women. Hormone therapy may be considered in some women with severe symptoms after full discussion of options, risks, and benefits. Tables 90-1 to 90-8 describe current hormone therapy drugs.

    1. Estrogen only

      a) Titrate to keep serum estradiol level at 50–150 pg/ml to treat symptoms and minimize side effects.

      b) Unopposed estrogen regimens only may be prescribed for women without a uterus and may be taken on a continuous basis.

      c) Women with a uterus require estrogen plus progesterone (generally given three weeks on, one week off) to avoid a 20% increase in the risk of endometrial cancer.

      d) If hormone therapy is discontinued, taper over a three-month period.

      e) Estrogen pills or tablet formulation (see Table 90-4)

        (1) Estrogens that are non-naturally occurring in humans (e.g., conjugated equine estrogen, ethinyl estradiol) have elevated potency in the liver relative to their estrogen potential.

        (2) Side effects may include nausea, breast tenderness, weight gain, fluid retention, dizziness, headaches, breakthrough bleeding, gallbladder disease, and yeast infections.

        (3) Fewer side effects are experienced with vaginal creams and rings.

        (4) Estrogen pills or tablets are contraindicated in women with undiagnosed vaginal bleeding, active liver disease, or active thromboembolic disorders.

TABLE 90-4	Estrogen Pills
Drug	**Dose/Comments**
Conjugated equine estrogen	0.3 mg daily; available as 0.45, 0.625, 0.9, and 1.25 mg
Conjugated estrogen, from soybean	0.625–1.25 mg daily; available as 0.3, 0.45, and 0.9 mg
Esterified estrogen	1.25 mg daily; available as 0.3, 0.625, 1.25, and 2.5 mg
Estradiol acetate	0.45 mg daily; available as 0.45 and 0.9 mg
Estrone sodium sulfate (as estropipate)	0.75–6 mg daily; available as 0.75, 1.5, and 3 mg (equivalent to 0.625, 1.25, and 2.5 mg tablets)
Estropipate	0.625 (0.75 mg)–1.25 (1.5 mg); may give 0.75–6 mg of estropipate daily
Micronized estradiol	1–2 mg daily; available as 0.5, 1, and 2 mg
Synthetic conjugated estrogen	0.3 mg daily; available as 0.3, 0.45, 0.625, 0.9, and 1.25 mg

Note. Based on information from North American Menopause Society, 2018; Palacios et al., 2019; Pinkerton et al., 2019; Roberts & Hickey, 2016; Santoro et al., 2015.

TABLE 90-5	Estrogen and Estrogen/Progesterone Patches
Drug	**Dose/Comments**
Estradiol	Take 0.014 mg daily. Apply single patch weekly.
	Take 0.025–0.05 mg daily. Apply two patches weekly. Drug is available as 0.025, 0.05, 0.075, and 0.1 mg daily patches. Take 3 weeks on, 1 week off with uterus or continuous if no uterus.
	Take 0.025–0.1 mg daily. Apply single patch weekly. Drug is available as 0.025, 0.0375, 0.05, 0.06, 0.075, and 0.1 mg daily patches. Take 3 weeks on, 1 week off.
	Take 0.05–0.1 mg daily. Apply two patches weekly. Take 3 weeks on, 1 week off with uterus or continuous if no uterus. Drug is also available as Vivelle-Dot® in strengths of 0.025, 0.0375, and 0.075 mg daily.
Estradiol with levo-norgestrel	Take estradiol 0.045 mg daily with levonorgestrel 0.015 mg daily. Apply single patch weekly.
Estradiol with nore-thindrone acetate	Take estradiol 0.05 mg with norethindrone acetate 0.14 mg. Apply patch twice weekly for 28-day cycle. Drug is also available as estradiol 0.05 mg and norethindrone acetate 0.25 mg.

Note. Based on information from North American Menopause Society, 2018; Palacios et al., 2019; Pinkerton et al., 2019; Roberts & Hickey, 2016; Santoro et al., 2015.

(5) They are also usually contraindicated in women with a history of breast, endometrial, or hormone-based cancer.

f) Estrogen patches (see Table 90-5)

(1) Patches are applied to a clean, dry area of the trunk (e.g., lower abdomen, upper buttocks).

(2) Patches should not be applied to the breasts, waistline, or an area that receives direct sunlight. Rotate sites of application. Patients can shower, bathe, and swim with the patch.

(3) Patients with a uterus should have cyclic administration of the patch (i.e., three weeks on, one week off).

(4) In some patients, patches cause skin irritation and rashes; a different patch should be tried if this occurs.

g) Estrogen vaginal ring/tablets (see Table 90-1)

(1) Rings or tablets are used to treat the GU symptoms of vaginal dryness, pruritus, dyspareunia, urgency, and dysuria.

(2) Progesterone use is not necessary when using the vaginal ring.

(3) A ring is inserted into the upper third of the vagina once every three months.

(4) The ring does not interfere with sexual intercourse.

(5) If the ring should fall out within a three-month time period, it can be washed with lukewarm water and reinserted.

(6) Fewer side effects occur than with oral or patch estrogens.

h) Estrogen vaginal creams (see Table 90-2)

(1) These creams are used to relieve moderate or severe painful intercourse caused by menopausal changes.

(2) Estrogen is absorbed in systemic circulation for about one month until the vaginal mucosa becomes cornified; then, systemic absorption is minimal.

(3) Women with a uterus must take progesterone when using vaginal cream, as it causes a buildup of the endometrial lining.

(4) The woman's partner can absorb estrogen during intercourse; men can develop breast tissue if a sufficient amount enters their bloodstream on a regular basis.

(5) Creams have fewer side effects than oral or patch estrogens.

2. Estrogen with cyclic progesterone (see Table 90-6)

   a) Estrogen is taken on days 1–25 and progesterone on days 16–25 of each month.

   b) Estrogen is taken daily and progesterone on days 1–10 or 16–25 of each month.

   c) Patients may experience side effects of estrogen/progesterone use, such as vaginal discharge, uterine bleeding, breast tenderness, genital irritation/itching, uterine cramping, nervousness, fatigue, and lower tolerance to glucose.

3. Estrogen plus progesterone (see Table 90-6)

   a) The disadvantage of these combinations is irregular and unpredictable menses in the first year of treatment.

   b) Once the regimen is established, menses usually will disappear.

   c) Side effects are the same as estrogen with cyclic progesterone.

4. Estrogen with methyltestosterone (see Table 90-3)

   a) This combination is used for women who experience a lack of libido after menopause.

   b) Drugs are to be administered cyclically on a short-term basis.

   c) Side effects of testosterone can cause deepening of the voice, weight gain, an increase in body hair, balding of scalp hair, and acne.

5. Progestin (see Table 90-7)

   a) Progestin is used in conjunction with estrogen for the prevention of endometrial hyperplasia.

TABLE 90-6	Estrogen/Progesterone Combination Pills
Drug	**Dose/Comments**

Conjugated estrogen with medroxyprogesterone acetate	• 0.625 mg Premarin® maroon tablet on days 1–14
	• Light-blue tablet containing 0.625 mg of conjugated estrogen with 5 mg of medroxyprogesterone acetate on days 15–28
	  – 0.3 mg/1.5 mg tablet PO daily
	  – Also available as 0.45 mg/1.5 mg; 0.625 mg/2.5 mg; or 0.625 mg/5 mg tablets

Estradiol	• 0.5 mg with norethindrone 0.1 mg tablet PO daily • 1 mg with norethindrone 0.5 mg tablet PO daily • 0.5 mg with drospirenone 0.25 mg tablet PO daily • 1 mg with drospirenone 0.5 mg tablet PO daily
Estradiol/norgestimate	• Estradiol 1 mg with norgestimate 0.09 mg • Peach-colored estradiol tablet daily for 3 days followed by white estradiol/norgestimate tablet for 3 days • Regimen repeated continuously without interruption
Ethinyl estradiol	• 2.5 mcg with norethindrone 0.5 mg, 1 tablet PO daily • 5 mcg with norethindrone 1 mg, 1 tablet PO daily

Note. Based on information from North American Menopause Society, 2018; Palacios et al., 2019; Pinkerton et al., 2019; Roberts & Hickey, 2016; Santoro et al., 2015.

TABLE 90-7	Progestins
Drug	**Dose/Comments**
Medroxyprogesterone acetate	Take 5–10 mg on days 1–10 or 16–25 of each month. Drug is available in 2.5, 5, and 10 mg (scored) tablets.
Natural micronized progesterone	Take 200–400 mg every night for 10–12 days/month. Drug is available as 100, 200, and 300 mg capsules.
Norethindrone acetate (synthetic progesterone)	Take 2.5–10 mg on days 16–25 of each month. Drug is available as 5 mg (scored) tablets.

Note. Based on information from North American Menopause Society, 2018; Palacios et al., 2019; Pinkerton et al., 2019; Roberts & Hickey, 2016; Santoro et al., 2015.

> b) Side effects of progestin may include fluid retention, weight gain, uterine cramps, bloating, breast tenderness, depression, headache, nervousness, dizziness, weakness, and lower tolerance to glucose.
>
> c) Progestin is contraindicated in those with undiagnosed vaginal bleeding, hormone-based cancers, thromboembolic disorders, or liver dysfunction or disease.
>
> d) Natural micronized progesterone has been found to have fewer side effects (e.g., fluid retention, weight gain, depression, breast tenderness) than those associated with synthetic progestin.
>
> 6. Progesterone vaginal cream: Micronized natural progesterone
> 7. Other preparations (see Table 90-8)

VII. Follow-up
    A. Short term: Reevaluate in one to three months for effectiveness of treatment, adequate hormonal serum levels, or any side effects.
    B. Long term: Perform annual follow-up, including periodic Pap smear and lipid panel, as indicated.

TABLE 90-8	Other Preparations
Drug	**Dose/Comments**
Estradiol 0.06% gel	Apply one pump (0.87 g) daily to clean, dry, unbroken skin of upper arm. Reevaluate periodically.
Estradiol gel	Take one packet daily applied to 5 × 7 inch area of dry skin on upper thigh. Alternate thighs daily. Drug is available as 0.25, 0.5, 0.75, and 1 mg.
Estradiol hemihydrate	Take 2.5 mg/g topical emulsion, 3.48 g daily. Rub contents of two pouches onto thigh daily over 3 minutes (a pouch per leg); rub excess on hands onto buttocks.
Estradiol spray	Take 1.53 mg/spray transdermal spray daily; initially spray once daily to the skin on the inside of the forearm between elbow and wrist. Increase to 2–3 sprays if needed. Do not spray in the same area.
Estradiol valerate 10, 20, and 40 mg/ml	Take 5–10 mg daily by deep intramuscular injection in gluteal muscle; take 10–20 mg every 4 weeks.

Note. Based on information from North American Menopause Society, 2018; Palacios et al., 2019; Pinkerton et al., 2019; Roberts & Hickey, 2016; Santoro et al., 2015.

VIII. Referrals (Pereira & Brown, 2017)
A. Gynecologist or reproductive endocrinologist: For women who do not respond to initial treatment, have severe symptoms, have abnormal bleeding, require a dilation and curettage, or endometrial biopsy
B. Internist or endocrinologist: For evaluation of medical conditions inducing menopause
C. Urologist: For those with GU symptoms unrelieved by treatment strategies
D. Psychiatric nurse, psychiatrist, or psycho-oncologist: To assist with adjustment to situational stress or to distinguish between mood disturbance, clinical depression, and psychiatric illness
E. Sex therapist: For assessment and management of sexual dysfunction

The author would like to acknowledge Giselle J. Moore-Higgs, ARNP, PhD, AOCN®, for her contribution to this chapter that remains unchanged from the previous edition of this book.

References

American College of Obstetricians and Gynecologists. (2018). ACOG committee opinion No. 734: The role of transvaginal ultrasonography in evaluating the endometrium of women with postmenopausal bleeding. *Obstetrics and Gynecology, 131*(5), e124–e129. https://doi.org/10.1097/AOG.0000000000002631

Cobin, R.H., & Goodman, N.F. (2017). American Association of Clinical Endocrinologists and American College of Endocrinology position statement on menopause—2017 update. *Endocrine Practice, 23*(7), 869–880. https://doi.org/10.4158/EP171828.PS

Fourman, L.T., & Fazeli, P.K. (2015). Neuroendocrine causes of amenorrhea—An update. *Journal of Clinical Endocrinology and Metabolism, 100*(3), 812–824. https://doi.org/10.1210/jc.2014-3344

Kaplan, M., & Mahon, S. (2014). Hot flash management: Update of the evidence for patients with cancer. *Clinical Journal of Oncology Nursing, 18*(Suppl. 6), 59–67. https://doi.org/10.1188/14.CJON.S3.59-67

Kaunitz, A.M., & Manson, J.E. (2015). Management of menopausal symptoms. *Obstetrics and Gynecology, 126*(4), 859–876. https://doi.org/10.1097/AOG.0000000000001058

Klein, D.A., Paradise, S.L., & Reeder, R.M. (2019). Amenorrhea: A systematic approach to diagnosis and management. *American Family Physician, 100*(1), 39–48. https://www.aafp.org/afp/2019/0701/p39.html

Minkin, M.J. (2019). Menopause: Hormones, lifestyle, and optimizing aging. *Obstetrics and Gynecology Clinics of North America, 46*(3), 501–514. https://doi.org/10.1016/j.ogc.2019.04.008

North American Menopause Society. (2018). The 2017 hormone therapy position statement of the North American Menopause Society. *Menopause, 25*(11), 1362–1387. https://doi.org/10.1097/GME.0000000000001241

Palacios, S., Stevenson, J.C., Schaudig, K., Lukasiewicz, M., & Graziottin, A. (2019). Hormone therapy for first-line management of menopausal symptoms: Practical recommendations. *Women's Health, 15*. https://doi.org/10.1177/1745506519864009

Pereira, K., & Brown, A.J. (2017). Secondary amenorrhea: Diagnostic approach and treatment considerations. *Nurse Practitioner, 42*(9), 34–41. https://doi.org/10.1097/01.NPR.0000520832.14406.76

Pinkerton, J.V., Conner, E.A., & Kaunitz, A.M. (2019). Management of menopause and the role for hormone therapy. *Clinical Obstetrics and Gynecology, 62*(4), 677–686. https://doi.org/10.1097/GRF.0000000000000487

Roberts, H., & Hickey, M. (2016). Managing the menopause: An update. *Maturitas, 86,* 53–58. https://doi.org/10.1016/j.maturitas.2016.01.007

Santoro, N., Epperson, C.N., & Mathews, S.B. (2015). Menopausal symptoms and their management. *Endocrinology and Metabolism Clinics of North America, 44*(3), 497–515. https://doi.org/10.1016/j.ecl.2015.05.001

CHAPTER 91

Nephrotic Syndrome

Gary Shelton, DNP, MSN, NP, ANP-BC, AOCNP®, ACHPN

I. Definition: A constellation of features, both clinical and laboratory, that confirms heavy proteinuria and hypoalbuminemia and affects the glomeruli (Candelier & Lorenzo, 2020; Kodner, 2016)

II. Physiology/Pathophysiology (Candelier & Lorenzo, 2020; Hogan et al., 2016; Kodner, 2016; Königshausen & Sellin, 2017; McCloskey & Maxwell, 2017)
   A. Normal
      1. Barriers in the glomerular basement membrane restrict passage of ionic plasma proteins.
         a) One barrier is charge specific, allowing only ions carrying specific charges to pass through the membrane.
         b) The other barrier normally prevents larger molecules, including protein, from passing through the membrane.
      2. The glomerular barrier within the kidneys is a complex sieve allowing for high filtration rates of water and small- to medium-sized molecules, restricting albumin and larger proteins. The glomerular filtration barrier consists of endothelial cells, basement membrane, and podocytes.
      3. Normal average protein excretion is 40–50 mg daily.
   B. Pathophysiology
      1. Damage to glomerulus from primary disease results in severe proteinuria.
      2. Hypoalbuminemia occurs from proteinuria. Symptoms of nephrotic syndrome worsen as serum albumin falls below 2.5 g/dl.
      3. An increase in circulating plasma factor causes an increase in albumin exertion secondary to increased permeability of glomeruli. Postulated examples are T-cell–derived humoral factor, vascular permeability factor, and hemopexin.
      4. Salt retention and decreased oncotic pressure result in edema.
      5. Increased hepatic synthesis produces hyperlipidemia, particularly hypercholesterolemia and hypertriglyceridemia, thought to be a result of low oncotic pressure and urinary loss of regulatory proteins.
      6. Increased risk of clotting (hypercoagulability state) results from antithrombin III loss in urine.
      7. Loss of charge selectivity in basement membrane produces minimal change glomerulopathy, occurring mainly in children and related to immunochemical response.
      8. Loss of size selectivity in basement membrane produces membranous glomerulonephritis, thought to be caused by collection of immunochemicals in the subepithelial membrane of the glomerular capillaries.

9. Minimal change disease is thought to be caused by an imbalance in the T-lymphocyte population.

III. Clinical features: Nephrotic syndrome can be of idiopathic (primary) or systemic disease (secondary) origin. Nephrotic syndrome in adults commonly signals serious underlying disease. It generally presents with marked edema, proteinuria, hypoalbuminemia, and hyperlipidemia. The idiopathic form is probably the most harmful and comprises two entities, referred to as *minimal change disease* and *focal segmental glomerulosclerosis* (Candelier & Lorenzo, 2020; Gupta et al., 2019; Kodner, 2016; Mahalingasivam et al., 2018; McCloskey & Maxwell, 2017).

A. Etiology
1. Primary glomerulonephropathy: Primary renal disease
   a) Minimal change glomerulopathy: Primary cause of nephrotic syndrome in children
   b) Idiopathic membranous glomerulonephritis
   c) Focal segmental glomerulonephritis
   d) Membranoproliferative glomerulonephritis
   e) IgA nephropathy
   f) Congenital nephrotic syndrome
2. Secondary glomerulonephropathy
   a) Diabetes mellitus: Most common cause of nephrotic syndrome in adults
   b) Collagen vascular disorders: SLE nephritis
   c) Amyloidosis
   d) Dysproteinemias: Multiple myeloma, light chain deposition disease, heavy chain deposition disease, immunotactoid/fibrillary glomerulonephritis
   e) Infectious diseases: HIV, hepatitis B, hepatitis C, syphilis, malaria, schistosomiasis, TB, leprosy
   f) Malignant neoplasms: Solid adenocarcinomas, such as lung, breast, and colon; Hodgkin lymphoma; multiple myeloma; others
   g) Drugs or toxins: NSAIDs, gold, penicillamine, probenecid, mercury, captopril, heroin
   h) Other: Preeclampsia, chronic allograft rejection, bee sting, mercury, venoms, poison ivy

B. History
1. History of cancer and cancer treatment
2. Current medications: Prescribed, over the counter, supplements
3. History of presenting symptoms: Precipitating factors, onset, location, associated symptoms (e.g., edema, worsening edema, altered urinary pattern, dizziness, tachycardia, abdominal pain, diarrhea)
4. Changes in ADLs
5. Past medical history: SLE, diabetes mellitus, hypertension, amyloidosis, renal disorders, current or past infection
6. Family history: Diabetes mellitus, renal disorders
7. Social history: Recent travel

C. Signs and symptoms
1. Periorbital and pedal edema
2. Dyspnea/orthopnea
3. Changes in urinary pattern, usually an increase in urinary frequency
4. Hematuria: May or may not be present
5. Anorexia
6. Malaise

D. Physical examination: Typically nonspecific depending on etiology; edema most common

    1. Vital signs

        a) Orthostatic hypotension or hypertension and tachycardia

        b) Increase in weight with edema

    2. Integument: Color, turgor (especially of extremities), pallor accentuated by edema

    3. Cardiac

        a) S_3 or S_4 if CHF is present

        b) JVD indicating heart failure

        c) Potential tachycardia present with anemia or SLE

        d) Peripheral edema often seen with nephrotic syndrome

    4. Pulmonary

        a) Rales present in heart failure

        b) Absent breath sounds, increased vocal fremitus, pleural friction rub, egophony present over effusion

    5. Abdominal

        a) Hepatomegaly indicating accumulation of protein

        b) Hepatojugular reflex indicating heart failure (see Appendix D)

        c) Ascites

    6. HEENT: Periorbital edema

    7. Scrotal: Edema

IV. Diagnostic tests (Kodner, 2016; Mahalingasivam et al., 2018; McCloskey & Maxwell, 2017)

  A. Laboratory

    1. Random urine dipstick for semiquantitative measure of proteinuria: Quantitation of urinary protein is indicated when a random urine sample indicates greater than a trace of protein (generally 3+ to 4+ in nephrotic syndrome).

    2. 24-hour urine for quantitation of protein excretion: Normal is less than 150 mg daily; patients excreting greater than 3 g daily have nephrotic-range proteinuria.

    3. Albumin: Hypoalbuminemia less than 30 g/L accompanied by edema is characteristic of nephrotic syndrome and with protein malnutrition.

    4. Vitamin D level: Deficiency is common with nephrotic syndrome.

    5. Electrolytes: Imbalances can be present with nephrotic syndrome.

    6. Serologic studies to consider for systemic causes

        a) Antinuclear antibodies indicative of SLE

        b) Complement, serum, or urine protein electrophoresis for amyloid, light chain disease, or multiple myeloma

        c) Syphilis serology, HIV, hepatitis B, and hepatitis C for infectious etiology

        d) Atrial natriuretic peptide often elevated in nephrotic syndrome

        e) Cryoglobulins for diagnosis of mixed cryoglobulinemia caused by hepatitis C

        f) Lipid panel to evaluate for dyslipidemia, which is common in nephrotic syndrome

        g) Glucose and Hgb A1c to evaluate for diabetes

        h) Serum drug levels if toxicity indicated as etiology

    7. Hypercoagulable evaluation with high incidence of thrombus (see Chapter 43)

  B. Radiology: If indicated, ultrasound, chest x-ray, CT, and endoscopy to evaluate for renal abnormality or other etiology

  C. Renal biopsy: Required to establish a diagnosis to distinguish primary glomerular disease from secondary glomerular diseases, such as amyloidosis or diabetes mellitus, and to determine severity of disease

D. Diagnostic criteria
  1. Persistent nephrotic-range proteinuria (urinary protein level exceeding 3–3.5 g daily): Heavy proteinuria (100 mg/dl or greater) is associated with a spectrum of clinical issues, including sodium retention, hyperlipoproteinemia, and thrombo-embolic and infectious complications.
  2. Hypoalbuminemia: Persistent protein leaking into the urine causes hypoalbumin-emia (serum level less than 2.5 g/dl) and hypercholesterolemia.
  3. Edema: It is progressive and generally in the lower extremity. Periorbital edema, genital edema, ascites, and effusions can occur.
  4. Weight gain
  5. Hyperlipidemia, lipiduria
  6. Fatigue

V. Differential diagnosis: Nephrotic syndrome results from a primary renal or secondary systemic disease (Gupta et al., 2019; Kodner, 2016; Mahalingasivam et al., 2018).
  A. Amyloidosis
  B. Preeclampsia
  C. Edema-forming conditions
    1. CHF (see Chapter 42)
    2. Malnutrition
    3. Cirrhosis (see Chapter 69)
    4. Protein-losing enteropathy
  D. Infectious diseases
    1. Endocarditis (see Chapter 46)
    2. Syphilis
    3. Hepatitis B or C (see Chapter 74)
    4. HIV
    5. Malaria
  E. Malignant neoplasms or multiple myeloma
  F. SLE (see Chapter 110)
  G. Immune reactions
  H. Drug reactions
    1. Gold
    2. Penicillamine
    3. NSAIDs (see Appendix E)
    4. Captopril
    5. IFN-α
    6. Heroin
  I. Environmental antigens
    1. Poison ivy
    2. Inhaled antigens
    3. Bee sting
  J. Diabetes mellitus (see Chapter 151)

VI. Treatment (Gupta et al., 2019; Kodner, 2016; Königshausen & Sellin, 2017; Mahalingasivam et al., 2018; McCloskey & Maxwell, 2017; Siligato et al., 2018)
  A. Treat underlying condition (e.g., edema, dyslipidemia, hypertension).
  B. Reduction of proteinuria
    1. ACE inhibitors and/or ARB to reduce proteinuria: Enalapril 2.5–20 mg PO daily may reduce proteinuria regardless of blood pressure.

    2. Low-protein diet: Evidence for use of this intervention is unclear; however, it may play a role in reducing proteinuria.

  C. Immunologic interventions

    1. IFN-α for hepatitis-associated nephrotic syndrome: Standard therapy is 5 million units subcutaneous daily for 16 weeks for hepatitis B and 3 million units three times weekly for 16 weeks for hepatitis C (see Chapter 74).

    2. Colchicine at standard doses may prevent progression of renal disease.

  D. Steroid therapy is the standard treatment when the underlying cause is not known. Oral prednisone 2 mg/kg daily is the usual dose.

  E. Sodium restriction: Less than 1 g daily

  F. Loop diuretics, often at increased doses, to increase sodium excretion: Furosemide 80–120 mg IV daily

  G. Treat dyslipidemia (see Chapter 44) and hypertension (see Chapter 47) if present.

  H. Immunosuppressive drugs (e.g., cyclophosphamide, chlorambucil, cyclosporine) other than steroids may be useful, though choice is controversial.

  I. Prophylactic anticoagulation is not recommended.

  J. Monitor for skin breakdown from edema.

VII. Follow-up: Dependent on etiology

VIII. Referral (Kodner, 2016)

  A. Nephrologist: If further evaluation is warranted, autoimmune process is suspected, etiology is unknown, or renal biopsy is necessary

  B. Medical oncologist/hematologist depending on findings: For hypercoagulable state or neoplasm

  C. Endocrinologist: For management of diabetes

References

Candelier, J.-J., & Lorenzo, H.-K. (2020). Idiopathic nephrotic syndrome and serum permeability factors: A molecular jigsaw puzzle. *Cell and Tissue Research, 379*(2), 231–243. https://doi.org/10.1007/s00441-019-03147-y

Gupta, S., Pepper, R.J., Ashman, N., & Walsh, S.B. (2019). Nephrotic syndrome: Oedema formation and its treatment with diuretics. *Frontiers in Physiology, 9,* 1868. https://doi.org/10.3389/fphy.2018.01868

Hogan, M.C., Reich, H.N., Nelson, P.J., Adler, S.G., Cattran, D.C., Appel, G.B., ... Lieske, J.C. (2016). The relatively poor correlation between random and 24-hour urine protein excretion in patients with biopsy-proven glomerular diseases. *Kidney International, 90*(5), 1080–1089. https://doi.org/10.1016/j.kint.2016.06.020.

Kodner, C. (2016). Diagnosis and management of nephrotic syndrome in adults. *American Family Physician, 93*(6), 479–485. https://www.aafp.org/afp/2016/0315/p479.html

Königshausen, E., & Sellin, L. (2017). Recent treatment advances and new trials in adult nephrotic syndrome. *BioMed Research International, 2017,* 7689254. https://doi.org/10.1155/2017/7689254

Mahalingasivam, V., Booth, J., Sheaff, M., & Yaqoob, M. (2018). Nephrotic syndrome in adults. *Acute Medicine, 17*(1), 36–43. https://acutemedjournal.co.uk/journal/volume-17/volume-17-issue-1-pages-1-56-2018/nephrotic-syndrome-adults

McCloskey, O., & Maxwell, A.P. (2017). Diagnosis and management of nephrotic syndrome. *Practitioner, 261*(1801), 11–15. https://www.thepractitioner.co.uk//Symposium/Renal-Medicine/9859-/Diagnosis-and-management-of-nephrotic-syndrome

Siligato, R., Cernaro, V., Nardi, C., De Gregorio, F., Gembillo, G., Costantino, G., ... Santoro, D. (2018). Emerging therapeutic strategies for minimal change disease and focal and segmental glomerulosclerosis. *Expert Opinion on Investigational Drugs, 27*(11), 839–879. https://doi.org/10.1080/13543784.2018.1540587

Prostatitis/Lower Urinary Tract Symptoms

Faith A. Mutale, MSN, CRNP, and Cecile B. Miller, MSN, CRNP

I. Definition: Infection and inflammatory changes of the prostate gland; based on clinical and laboratory findings, can be acute or chronic or present as chronic pelvic pain syndrome (Ho, 2017)

II. Physiology/Pathophysiology (Bajic et al., 2019; Ho, 2017; Magri et al., 2019; Ye et al., 2018; Yin et al., 2019)
   A. Normal
      1. Prostate gland surrounds the urethra at the bladder neck. The seminal vesicles extend from the prostate onto the posterior surface of the bladder.
      2. Defense mechanisms protecting the lower urogenital tract from infection include urethral length, micturition, ejaculation, and antimicrobial substances in prostatic fluid.
   B. Pathophysiology
      1. Nonbacterial prostatitis is the most common cause of inflammation without evidence of bacterial infection caused by reflux of sterile urine into ejaculatory ducts because of high-pressure voiding. Reflux may be triggered by spasm of external or internal sphincters.
      2. An autoimmune response to prostate antigens may contribute to chronic nonbacterial prostatitis. This is characterized by presence of cytotoxic T cells in prostatic excretion, which is consistent with an inflammatory etiology.
      3. *Escherichia coli* accounts for most acute bacterial prostatitis infections. Less common organisms include *Proteus, Pseudomonas, Klebsiella,* and *Serratia* species.
      4. Bacteria can infect the prostate gland by ascending the urethra, such as reflux of urine into the prostatic ducts, or hematogenous seeding.

III. Clinical features: Acute prostatitis typically presents as an acute illness with fever and chills, irritative urinary symptoms, and bacteremia. Chronic bacterial prostatitis may present as symptoms from a recurrent UTI with or without a low-grade fever. Prostatitis is the most common prostate infection in men younger than age 50 years (Coker & Dierfeldt, 2016; Górski et al., 2018; Ho, 2017; Magri et al., 2019; Reese et al., 2015; Zaidi et al., 2018).
   A. Classification
      1. Acute bacterial prostatitis (class I): Urinary reflux of bacteria into the prostate via prostatic and ejaculatory ducts and/or ascending infection from urethral meatus occurring most often during sexual intercourse

2. Chronic bacterial prostatitis (class II): Approximately 90% of infections; may follow acute bacterial prostatitis; clinical findings more subtle than in acute prostatitis
3. Chronic prostatitis/chronic pelvic pain syndrome (class III)
    a) IIIA: Inflammatory; defined by presence of leukocytes in semen or post-prostatic massage specimen
    b) IIIB: Noninflammatory
4. Asymptomatic inflammatory prostatitis (class IV): Defined by incidental finding of prostatitis on examination of biopsy specimen, abnormal semen analysis, and elevated prostate-specific antigen

B. Etiology
1. Nonbacterial: May be related to chemicals in the urine, immune system response to a previous UTI, or nerve damage in the pelvic area
2. Bacterial
    a) Bacteria etiology is related to gram-negative bacilli (*E. coli*) or *Enterococcus*, accounting for greater than or equal to 50% of infections.
    b) *Salmonella, Candida,* and *Cryptococcus* organisms are uncommon in prostatitis but occur more frequently in people with HIV.
    c) *Ureaplasma urealyticum* in expressed prostatic secretions and urine voided after prostatic massage accounts for approximately 13% of infections.
    d) Rarely, fungi and *Mycobacterium tuberculosis* may be responsible for the infections. *Enterococcus faecalis* is now the most common organism in chronic bacterial prostatitis.
3. Obstruction may result from edema of prostate already enlarged by BPH.
4. Prostatitis shares some molecular traits with prostatic intraepithelial neoplasia.
5. Somatic alteration of genes involved in defense against inflammatory damage and tissue recovery is being studied.

C. History
1. History of cancer and cancer treatment
2. Current medications: Prescribed, over the counter
3. History of presenting symptoms: Precipitating factors, onset, location, duration
4. Changes in ADLs
5. Past medical history: UTI, prostate disease, STI

D. Signs and symptoms
1. Pelvic tenderness
2. Acute back pain
3. Fever (spiking) or low grade in chronic prostatitis
4. Voiding symptoms
    a) Slow stream or hesitancy
    b) Acute urinary retention
    c) Nocturia
    d) Urgency or urge incontinence
    e) Dribbling
    f) Dysuria
    g) Cloudy urine
    h) Perineal pain or discomfort
    i) Pelvic pain
5. Discomfort with ejaculation
6. Urethral discharge
7. Depressive symptoms and/or anxiety

E. Physical examination

    1. Vital signs: Fever

    2. Prostate

       a) Enlarged prostate: Vigorous examination contraindicated if abscess is suspected, as massage increases risk of bacteremia

       b) Prostate: Tender, enlarged, or boggy suggestive of acute prostatitis

       c) Rectal vault: Smooth without lesions or nodules

       d) Chronic prostatitis: Hypertrophy, tenderness, enlarged prostate, edema, and nodularity; prostate examination frequently normal

    3. Abdominal: May reveal suprapubic pain

    4. Lymph node: Enlarged inguinal nodes in palpitation

    5. Genital

       a) Lesions on scrotum and penis indicating STI or malignancy

       b) Masses and tenderness of testes and spermatic cord on palpitation

       c) Examine penis for drainage indicating STI or urethritis.

IV. Diagnostic tests (Bajic et al., 2019; Coker & Dierfeldt, 2016; Gill & Shoskes, 2016; Magri et al., 2019; Polackwich & Shoskes, 2016)

  A. Laboratory

    1. Urinalysis and urine culture: Almost always positive in chronic bacterial prostatitis; positive growth greater than 100,000 colony-forming units of bacteria

    2. Expressed prostatic secretions (obtained by digital massage): Reveal lipid-laden leukocytes; not routinely performed

    3. Gram stain and culture of expressed prostatic secretions

    4. CBC: Not routine but considered in systemically ill patients; WBC potentially increased with left shift

    5. Blood culture if bacteremia suspected

    6. The four-glass test: Considered to be diagnostic standard in patients suspected to have chronic bacterial prostatitis; lower leukocyte and bacterial count in voided urine in comparison to prostatic massage voided urine or expressed prostatic secretions; not commonly performed because not adequately validated and cumbersome

    7. *Chlamydia trachomatis* testing: Can be cause of chronic prostatitis

  B. Radiology

    1. Ultrasound of prostate to evaluate size and masses

    2. Spinal MRI: In patients with pelvic pain with signs of radiculopathy

    3. Noncontrast pelvic CT scan: If fever persists or no response to treatment

  C. Other: Urodynamic test to assess urinary flow and postvoid residual urine

V. Differential diagnosis (Bajic et al., 2019; Coker & Dierfeldt, 2016; Reese et al., 2015)

  A. Acute cystitis (see Chapter 89)

  B. BPH (see Chapter 87)

  C. Prostate cancer

  D. Urethral stricture

  E. Urological cancers

  F. Neurogenic bladder

  G. Urethritis

  H. Sphincter dyssynergia

  I. Trauma

  J. Foreign body

  K. Urolithiasis, abscess

L. Acute epididymitis

M. STI

N. Diverticulitis (see Chapter 70)

VI. Treatment (Bajic et al., 2019; Coker & Dierfeldt, 2016; Gill & Shoskes, 2016; Górski et al., 2018; Ho, 2017; Magri et al., 2019; Orlin et al., 2017; Polackwich & Shoskes, 2016; Reese et al., 2015; Zaidi et al., 2018)

A. Acute bacterial prostatitis

1. Hydration: Increase oral fluids to 3 L daily.

2. Analgesics

   a) Initiate celecoxib and other NSAIDs unless contraindicated (see Appendix E).

   b) For neurologic symptoms, treat with pregabalin starting dose 50 mg PO two times a day or amitriptyline starting dose 25 mg PO at night.

   c) Opioids usually are not necessary.

3. Stool softeners (see Chapter 55)

4. Antibiotic: First-line therapy should last for six weeks. Shorter duration of therapy is associated with progression to chronic symptoms (see Appendix C).

   a) For gram-negative bacteria, initiate ciprofloxacin 500 mg PO two times a day, levofloxacin 500 mg PO daily, or trimethoprim/sulfamethoxazole one double-strength tablet two times a day (see Appendix C). Tetracyclines may be considered because of their excellent penetration into prostatic fluid.

   b) If cultures not performed, treat as if gram negative.

   c) For gram-positive enterococci, treat with amoxicillin 500 mg PO three times a day.

   d) Parenteral therapy for toxicity or systemically ill patients should be considered. Switch to oral antibiotics if responding well, such as cephalexin 500 mg PO four times a day or dicloxacillin 500 mg PO four times a day for *Staphylococcus* and *Streptococcus*.

B. Chronic prostatitis: Selection of antibiotic agents and duration of therapy have not been studied using comparative trials; however, fluoroquinolones are most commonly used for four to eight weeks.

1. Bacterial: First-line treatment is fluoroquinolones (e.g., ciprofloxacin) 500 mg PO two times a day or levofloxacin 500 mg PO daily. Trimethoprim/sulfamethoxazole 160 mg/800 mg PO two times a day may be considered for recurrent infections. Second-line treatment is azithromycin 500 mg PO daily or doxycycline 100 mg PO two times a day.

2. Nonbacterial: Treat with two weeks of tetracycline 500 mg PO four times a day, azithromycin 500 mg PO daily, or doxycycline 100 mg PO two times a day. This is effective against *Chlamydia trachomatis* and gonorrhea, as these drugs have also shown to be an effective treatment.

3. Surgery for removal of calculi if cause of condition

4. NSAIDs for pain and inflammation (see Appendix E)

5. Alpha-blockers (receptor specific or receptor nonspecific; e.g., tamsulosin 0.4 mg PO daily) in combination with antibiotics for urinary retention

6. Psychosocial specialist (e.g., psychiatrist, psychologist, cognitive behavioral therapist) for patients with clinically relevant level of psychosocial symptoms

VII. Follow-up (Coker & Dierfeldt, 2016; Ho, 2017; Reese et al., 2015)

A. Assess response to therapy in one to two weeks.

B. Repeat urinalysis and culture in seven days; if positive, change antibiotic therapy.

C. Chronic prostatitis requires follow-up to distinguish symptoms from the development of BPH or prostate cancer.
  1. Link between chronic inflammation and cancer continues to be studied.
  2. Relative risk of prostate cancer is increased with certain STIs and prostatitis.
D. Intractable pain, dehydration, or fever greater than 102°F (38.8°C) may require a brief hospital stay.
E. Patients with psychosocial symptoms should stay engaged with psychosocial specialist.

VIII. Referral
  A. Urologist: For no response to appropriate treatment, if abscess suspected, or if complications or malignancy suspected
  B. Physical therapy: For pelvic floor strengthening and exercises

References

Bajic, P., Dornbier, R.A., Doshi, C.P., Wolfe, A.J., Farooq, A.V., & Bresler, L. (2019). Implications of the genitourinary microbiota in prostatic disease. *Current Urology Reports, 20*(7), 34. https://doi.org/10.1007/s11934-019-0904-6

Coker, T.J., & Dierfeldt, D.M. (2016). Acute bacterial prostatitis: Diagnosis and management. *American Family Physician, 93*(2), 114–120. https://www.aafp.org/afp/2016/0115/p114.html

Gill, B., & Shoskes, D.A. (2016). Bacterial prostatitis. *Current Opinion in Infectious Diseases, 29*(1), 86–91. https://doi.org/10.1097/QCO.0000000000000222

Górski, A., Jończyk-Matysiak, E., Łusiak-Szelachowska, M., Międzybrodzki, R., Weber-Dąbrowska, B., Borysowski, J., ... Sfanos, K.S. (2018). Phage therapy in prostatitis: Recent prospects. *Frontiers in Microbiology, 9,* 1434. https://doi.org/10.3389/fmicb.2018.01434

Ho, D.-R. (2017). Prostate inflammation: A brief review. *Urological Science, 28*(3), 113–118. https://doi.org/10.1016/j.urols.2017.04.003

Magri, V., Boltri, M., Cai, T., Colombo, R., Cuzzocrea, S., De Visschere, P., ... Wagenlehner, F.M.E. (2019). Multidisciplinary approach to prostatitis. *Archivio Italiano di Urologia e Andrologia, 90*(4), 227–248. https://doi.org/10.4081/aiua.2018.4.227

Orlin, I., Dekel, Y., Friedman, B., Zriek, R., Boyarsky, L., Mizrahi, G.R., & Stein, A. (2017). Recent developments in chronic prostatitis and pelvic pain syndrome. *Journal of Urology and Research, 4*(3), 1089. https://www.jscimedcentral.com/Urology/urology-4-1089.pdf

Polackwich, A.S., & Shoskes, D.A., (2016). Chronic prostatitis/chronic pelvic pain syndrome: A review of evaluation and therapy. *Prostate Cancer and Prostatic Diseases, 19*(2), 132–138. https://doi.org/10.1038/pcan.2016.8

Reese, J., Abrahams, M., Doble, A., & Cooper, A. (2015). Diagnosis and treatment of chronic bacterial prostatitis and chronic prostatitis/chronic pelvic pain syndrome: A consensus guideline. *BJU International, 116*(4), 509–525. https://doi.org/10.1111/bju.13101

Ye, C., Xiao, G., Xu, J., Qin, S., Luo, Y., Chen, G., ... Zhou, T. (2018). Differential expression of immune factor between patients with chronic prostatitis/chronic pelvic pain syndrome and the healthy volunteers. *International Urology and Nephrology, 50*(3), 395–399. https://doi.org/10.1007/s11255-017-1763-z

Yin, L., Tang, Y., Pan, A., Yang, L., Zhu, X., & Yongang, L. (2019). The application of IL-10 and TNF-α in expressed prostatic secretions and prostatic exosomal protein in urine in diagnosis of patients with chronic prostatitis. *Medicine, 98*(33), e16848. https://doi.org/10.1097/MD.0000000000016848

Zaidi, N., Thomas, D., & Chughtai, B. (2018). Management of chronic prostatitis (CP). *Current Urology Reports, 19*(11), 88. https://doi.org/10.1007/s11934-018-0841-9

CHAPTER 93

Proteinuria

Gary Shelton, DNP, MSN, NP, ANP-BC, AOCNP®, ACHPN

I. Definition: An abnormal excretion of protein greater than 150 mg in 24 hours; differentiate between transient and persistent proteinuria (Hogan et al., 2016; Yang et al., 2016)

II. Physiology/Pathophysiology (Hogan et al., 2016; Smith, 2019; Yang et al., 2016)
   A. Normal
      1. The kidneys are two organs located in the posterior retroperitoneal space.
      2. The kidneys receive 20%–25% of cardiac output to maintain adequate glomerular profusion.
      3. Function of the kidneys
         a) Remove metabolic waste products.
         b) Regulate body fluids and electrolytes.
         c) Process is measured by GFR, a measure of plasma volume that can be cleared of substances.
      4. Urinary proteins normally are composed of filtered proteins from plasma (50%) and proteins that are secreted into the urine from urinary tract cells (50%).
      5. The normal amount of protein excreted daily by healthy adults is 80–150 mg, of which 30% is albumin, 30% is serum globulins, and 40% is tissue proteins.
      6. Glomerular barrier within kidneys is a complex sieve allowing for high filtration rates of water and small- to medium-sized molecules, restricting albumin and larger proteins.
      7. The glomerular filtration barrier consists of endothelial cells, basement membrane, and podocytes.
   B. Pathophysiology
      1. Proteinuria is classified into three major categories.
         a) Overflow proteinuria: Occurs when serum protein exceeds the absorption capacity of proximal tubules because of increased production of low-molecular-weight proteins
         b) Tubular proteinuria: Occurs with renal tubule injury, causing the proximal tubules to fail to completely reabsorb low-molecular-weight proteins filtered by the glomerulus (less than 2 g of protein excreted in 24 hours)
         c) Glomerular proteinuria: Most common; occurs with injury to the glomerulus, causing an increase in the clearance of serum proteins or an increase in glomerular permeability (greater than 2 g of protein in 24 hours)
      2. Proteinuria of any significant degree higher than 100 mg/dl is suggestive of renal disease and parenchymal involvement.
      3. Proteinuria higher than 500 mg in 24 hours suggests significant glomerular disease.
      4. Transient proteinuria may relate to glomerular permeability or decreased tubular reabsorption.

III. Clinical features: Transient or intermittent proteinuria is unlikely to contribute to significant pathology. Proteinuria should be documented on more than one visit prior to performing a complete workup for etiology (Hogan et al., 2016; Parr et al., 2018; Yang et al., 2016).
  A. Etiology
    1. Benign conditions: Exercise, pelvic or lower abdominal trauma, contact sports, stress
    2. Primary renal disease
    3. Secondary to comorbid disease, immune-mediated glomerular disease such as diabetes mellitus, myeloma, or amyloidosis
  B. History
    1. History of cancer and cancer treatment
    2. Current medications: Prescribed, over the counter
    3. History of presenting symptoms: Precipitating factors, onset, location, duration, urinary pattern
    4. Changes in ADLs
    5. Past medical history: Diabetes mellitus, kidney disease, autoimmune disease, amyloidosis, multiple myeloma, CHF, typhus, hepatitis, UTIs, hypertension, vascular or coagulation defects, exposure to toxic agents, drugs that may produce toxic or sensitive reactions
    6. Family history: Diabetes mellitus, kidney disease, tubular metabolic anomalies
    7. Social history: Exercise pattern, sport involvement, stressors
  C. Signs and symptoms
    1. Changes in urinary pattern, hematuria
    2. Flank pain, bone pain
    3. Arthralgia
    4. Skin rash, pallor
    5. Dry eyes: Sjögren syndrome
    6. Edema
  D. Physical examination
    1. Vital signs: Hypertension
    2. Integument: Erythematous rash suggestive of connective tissue disease; pallor indicative of anemia
    3. Ophthalmologic: Potential retinopathy present with diabetes
    4. Cardiac: S_3, JVD, lower extremity edema indicative of CHF
    5. Pulmonary: Rales indicative of CHF
    6. Abdominal
      a) Distended bladder, flank pain suggestive of acute postrenal obstructive renal failure
      b) Enlarged kidneys suggestive of polycystic disease
      c) Abdominal bruits suggestive of renal artery stenosis

IV. Diagnostic tests (Bezinque et al., 2017; Hogan et al., 2016; Smith, 2019; Yang et al., 2016)
  A. Laboratory
    1. Urinalysis (see Figure 93-1): Evaluate for formed elements in urine.
    2. Dipstick urinalysis detects proteinuria only when excretion is greater than 300 mg daily, or greater than 20–30 mg/dl.
      a) Qualitative test should be performed only (1+ to 4+), reflecting progressive increase in urine albumin concentration.
      b) Test cannot detect microalbuminuria.
      c) Positive result occurs if urine is too alkaline-concentrated or contaminated with blood or after IV contrast material.

FIGURE 93-1 Urinalysis Diagnostic Results

Glomerulonephritis
- Gross hematuria
- Proteinuria (2+ to 4+)
- Red blood cell casts (microscopic hematuria may not be of glomerular origin)

Metabolic Disorders: Diabetes Mellitus, Gout, Hyperparathyroidism
- Abnormal urinary chemical constituents
- Glycosuria
- Hematuria
- Proteinuria

Nephrotic Syndrome, Nephrosis, Amyloidosis, Damage From Toxins (Lead, Mercury)
- Double refractile fat globules
- Fatty casts
- Oval fat bodies
- Proteinuria greater than 3.5 g daily

Note. Based on information from Bezinque et al., 2017; McCloskey & Maxwell, 2017; Sharp et al., 2014.

> *d)* False-negative occurs if urine is too diluted. Dipstick can only detect albumin, not other proteins; this is important to note, as Bence-Jones proteins will be missed, such as with multiple myeloma.
>
> 3. A 24-hour urinary protein collection should be performed to analyze total protein and composition of urinary protein and to quantify degree of proteinuria (see Figure 93-2).
>   *a)* The test may not be necessary if urinalysis reveals trace or 1+ protein and no other evidence of renal disease.
>   *b)* Patients with minimal to moderate proteinuria should be checked for postural or orthostatic proteinuria.
>   (1) Orthostatic proteinuria can be differentiated from other etiologies by evaluating a urine sample collected upon arising and another after staying continuously upright for two hours.
>   (2) For patients with postural orthostatic proteinuria, the total urinary protein excretion exceeds 150 mg but is less than 1 g during urine collection; protein excreted during recumbency should not exceed 75 mg.

FIGURE 93-2 24-Hour Collection of Urine

Empty the bladder and discard the first urine on the morning of collection.
Collect all subsequent urine for the next 24 hours.
The final urine at the end of the 24-hour period is kept as part of the collection.

Prerenal Acute Renal Failure	Intrarenal Acute Renal Failure	Chronic Renal Failure
• Urine osmolality greater than 500 mOsm/kg	• Urine osmolality approximately 300 mOsm/kg	• Glomerular filtration tests greater than 30 ml/min
• Specific gravity greater than 1.020	• Specific gravity approximately 1.010	• Normal urine osmolality
• Hyaline casts	• Tubular casts	• Normal specific gravity
	• Tubular cells	
	• Brownish muddy appearance due to brown granular casts	

Note. Based on information from Gounden et al., 2020.

(3) Urine creatinine: Depending on the patient's muscle tone, the total 24-hour creatinine should be 16–26 mg/kg for men (young and middle aged) and 12–24 mg/kg for women; amount will be decreased in older adults or malnourished patients.

4. Simultaneous serum creatinine and 24-hour urine collection for urinary creatinine levels (see Figure 93-2)

    a) Quantify the degree of proteinuria.

    b) Albumin–creatinine ratio could indicate nephrotic syndrome.

5. Serum studies to determine etiology

    a) CBC to evaluate for anemia resulting from renal insufficiency or myeloma

    b) Serum creatinine: Clearance can be determined in conjunction with the urine creatinine to evaluate for renal insufficiency.

    c) BUN to follow renal function: Less sensitive than creatinine clearance

    d) Glucose to evaluate for diabetes mellitus

    e) Serum albumin: Inversely correlates with the severity of proteinuria

    f) SPEP to evaluate for monoclonal gammopathy or multiple myeloma

B. Radiology

1. Renal ultrasound to evaluate for polycystic kidney disease, renal stones, obstruction, and kidney size (small in chronic renal failure)

2. Three-phase CT scan if renal function is adequate to evaluate for lesion or mass

3. Radioisotope studies to evaluate size, structure, blood supply, and function of kidneys, which may clearly identify functional defects or malignancy

C. Renal biopsy to establish diagnosis, determine prognosis, follow progression, and evaluate response to therapy

V. Differential diagnosis (Hogan et al., 2016)

A. Hypertension (see Chapter 47)

B. Medication induced

1. Gold salts: Oral or parenteral; can cause nephropathy

2. Penicillamine

3. NSAIDs (see Appendix E)

4. Lithium

5. Heavy metals

6. Heroin

C. Prerenal diseases: Renal artery stenosis

D. Renal parenchymal diseases

1. Glomerular diseases: Most common cause of pathologic proteinuria

    a) Membranous glomerulonephritis

    b) HIV nephropathy

    c) IgA nephropathy

    d) Diabetic glomerulosclerosis

2. Tubulointerstitial diseases

    a) Drug-induced interstitial nephritis

    b) Chronic pyelonephritis with reflux (see Chapter 94)

    c) Analgesic nephropathy

    d) Radiation nephritis

    e) Sickle cell nephropathy (see Chapter 119)

    f) Uric acid nephropathy

    g) Obstructive uropathy

    h) Myelomatosis

E. Postrenal diseases
    1. Ureteral obstruction
    2. Bladder outlet obstruction
F. Transient proteinuria induced
    1. CHF (see Chapter 42)
    2. Fever (see Chapter 147), heat injury
    3. Heavy exercise
    4. Dehydration
    5. Inflammatory process
    6. Acute illness
G. Overflow proteinuria
    1. Multiple myeloma
    2. Amyloidosis
    3. Lymphoproliferative disorder

VI. Treatment: Treat the underlying etiology (Lee et al., 2017; Tsai et al., 2017; Wang et al., 2017).
    A. Transient and orthostatic proteinuria are benign conditions and require no treatment.
    B. Proteinuria is caused by AKI; remove the nephrotoxin, if involved.
    C. When proteinuria is caused by chronic renal failure, consider the following interventions.
        1. Control hypertension (see Chapter 47).
        2. In glomerular disease, the reduction of urinary protein excretion protects renal function.
            a) Dietary protein restriction
            b) ACE inhibitors, such as lisinopril 10 mg PO daily, to protect the kidney by improving blood flow and reducing protein excretion
            c) Angiotensin II receptor agonists, such as losartan 50 mg PO daily, if cough or angioedema develop
        3. Correct fluid and electrolyte imbalance (see Chapters 152–156).
            a) Hypocalcemia from impaired vitamin D synthesis
            b) Serum phosphorus levels as the excretion of phosphorus is decreased
            c) Hyperphosphatemia with oral phosphate binders such as calcium acetate
            d) Salt/fluid restriction for edema associated with nephrotic syndrome (see Chapter 91)
        4. Anemia results from the inability of the kidney to produce EPO. When hematocrit falls below 30%, as in end-stage renal disease, EPO can be administered (see Chapter 113).
        5. Monitor for glucose intolerance, hypertriglyceridemia, and elevated uric acid.
        6. Control glucose level and blood pressure in patients with diabetes (see Chapter 151).

VII. Follow-up: Dependent on etiology

VIII. Referrals
    A. Nephrologist: If further evaluation is warranted, autoimmune process is suspected, etiology for proteinuria is unknown, or renal biopsy is necessary
    B. Hematologist/oncologist (e.g., Bence-Jones protein): For diagnosis and management of multiple myeloma

References

Bezinque, A., Noyes, S.L., Kirmiz, S., Parker, J., Dey, S., Kahnoski, R.J., & Lane, B.R. (2017). Prevalence of proteinuria and other abnormalities in urinalysis performed in the urology clinic. *Urology, 103,* 34–38. https://doi.org/10.1016/j.urology.2017.02.011

Gounden, V., Bhatt, H., & Jialal, I. (2020). Renal function tests. In *StatPearls*. https://www.ncbi.nlm.nih.gov/books/NBK507821

Hogan, M.C., Reich, H.N., Nelson, P.J., Adler, S.G., Cattran, D.C., Appel, G.B., ... Lieske, J.C. (2016). The relatively poor correlation between random and 24-hour urine protein excretion in patients with biopsy-proven glomerular diseases. *Kidney International, 90*(5), 1080–1089. https://doi.org/10.1016/j.kint.2016.06.020

Lee, S., Oh, H.J., Lee, E.-K., Lee, O., Ha, E., Kim, S.-J., ... Ryu, D.-R. (2017). Blood pressure control during chronic kidney disease progression. *American Journal of Hypertension, 30*(6), 610–616. https://doi.org/10.1093/ajh/hpx017

McCloskey, O., & Maxwell, A.P. (2017). Diagnosis and management of nephrotic syndrome. *Practitioner, 261*(1801), 11–15. https://www.thepractitioner.co.uk//Symposium/Renal-Medicine/9859-/Diagnosis-and-management-of-nephrotic-syndrome

Parr, S.K., Matheny, M.E., Abdel-Kader, K., Greevy, R.A., Jr., Bian, A., Fly, J., ... Siew, E.D. (2018). Acute kidney injury is a risk factor for subsequent proteinuria. *Kidney International, 93*(2), 460–469. https://doi.org/10.1016/j.kint.2017.07.007

Sharp, V.J., Lee, D.K., & Askeland, E.J. (2014). Urinalysis: Case presentations for the primary care physician. *American Family Physician, 90*(8), 542–547. https://www.aafp.org/afp/2014/1015/p542.html

Smith, C.A. (2019). Proteinuria and albuminuria: What's the difference? *Clinician Reviews, 29*(10), 8e–9e. https://www.mdedge.com/clinicianreviews/article/210146/nephrology/proteinuria-and-albuminuria-whats-difference

Tsai, W.-C., Wu, H.-Y., Peng, Y.-S., Yang, J.-Y., Chen, H.-Y., Chiu, Y.-L., ... Chien, K. (2017). Association of intensive blood pressure control and kidney disease progression in nondiabetic patients with chronic kidney disease: A systematic review and meta-analysis. *JAMA Internal Medicine,177*(6), 792–799. https://doi.org/10.1001/jamainternmed.2017.0197

Wang, M., Chou, J., Chang, Y., Lau, W.L., Reddy, U., Rhee, C.M, ... Kalantar-Zadeh, K. (2017). The role of low protein diet in ameliorating proteinuria and deferring dialysis initiation: What is old and what is new. *Panminerva Medica, 59*(2), 157–165. https://doi.org/10.23736/S0031-0808.16.03264-X

Yang, Y., Li, H.-Y., Zhou, Q., Peng, Z.-W., An, X., Li, W., ... Mao, H.-P. (2016). Renal function and all-cause mortality risk among cancer patients. *Medicine, 95*(20), e3728. https://doi.org/10.1097/MD.0000000000003728.

CHAPTER 94

Pyelonephritis

Mary W. Dunn, MSN, RN, OCN®, NP-C

I. Definition: Inflammation or infection of the renal parenchyma involving the upper urinary tract (i.e., renal pelvis, tubules, and interstitial tissue of one or both kidneys) (Johnson & Russo, 2018)
   A. Acute: Clinical syndrome of fevers, chills, and flank pain with bacteriuria and pyuria
   B. Chronic: Shrunken, scarred kidney diagnosed by morphologic, radiologic, or functional evidence of renal disease
   C. Uncomplicated: Infection in a healthy person with normal urinary tract
   D. Complicated: Associated with factors that increase the chance of acquiring bacteria and decrease efficacy of treatment

II. Physiology/Pathophysiology (Choong et al., 2015; Fogo et al., 2016; Keenan et al., 2017)
   A. Normal
      1. The kidneys are responsible for excreting some of the waste products of metabolism, regulating electrolyte balance, and secreting hormones that help regulate renal hemodynamics and RBC production.
      2. The structures of the renal parenchyma are sterile.
   B. Pathophysiology
      1. Bacteria can enter the urinary tract through three pathways.
         a) Ascension from the urethra into the bladder, then up the ureters to the kidneys (most common)
         b) Lymphatic channels from GI or pelvic origin (rare)
         c) Hematogenous route to kidneys (rare in healthy individuals)
      2. Most of the causative microorganisms originate in the GI flora.
      3. Acute
         a) Tubule interstitial inflammation with accumulation of leukocytes
         b) No inflammatory mass or abscess
      4. Chronic
         a) Leukocytes, plasma cells, and macrophages infiltrate the interstitium of the kidney.
         b) Portions of parenchyma may be fibrotic.
         c) Mass or abscess may form in the renal parenchyma.

III. Clinical features: Upper UTIs are less common and more serious than lower UTIs. Most cases develop as a consequence of undiagnosed or inadequately treated lower UTIs (Kolman, 2019; Long & Koyfman, 2018; Nikolaidis et al., 2018).
   A. Etiology
      1. Acute: Generally caused by ascending bacteria, uropathogens, *Escherichia coli* (most common), *Proteus, Klebsiella*

    2. Chronic: Caused by functions or structural urinary tract abnormalities or chronic UTI

  B. History

    1. History of cancer and cancer treatment

    2. Current medications: Prescribed, over the counter

    3. Presenting symptoms: Precipitating factors, onset, location, duration

    4. Changes in ADLs

    5. Past medical history: UTIs, sexual history

  C. Signs and symptoms

    1. Acute

      a) Flank pain

      b) Fever

      c) Pyuria

      d) Bacteriuria

      e) Nausea, vomiting

      f) Costovertebral angle tenderness

      g) Symptoms of cystitis: Dysuria, urinary frequency/urgency, suprapubic pain, hematuria

      h) Fatigue

    2. Chronic

      a) Can be asymptomatic until renal insufficiency occurs, then symptoms are similar to chronic renal failure (e.g., nausea, vomiting, anorexia, fatigue, decreased urine output, myalgias, lower extremity edema, uncontrolled hypertension)

      b) The result of multiple episodes of acute pyelonephritis, intermittent fevers, flank pain, dysuria

  D. Physical examination: Acute and chronic

    1. Vital signs: Fever, tachycardia, hypertension

    2. Abdominal: Suprapubic tenderness, distended bladder

    3. Posterior thorax: Flank or costovertebral angle tenderness

    4. Pelvic (women) if symptoms not convincing for UTI: Cervical motion, uterine tenderness suggestive of pelvic inflammatory disease

    5. Digital rectal (men) if pelvic or perineal pain: Prostate tenderness suggestive of prostatitis or enlargement suggestive of BPH

IV. Diagnostic tests (Long & Koyfman, 2018; Nikolaidis et al., 2018; Pierce et al., 2019; Pietrucha-Dilanchian & Hooton, 2016)

  A. Laboratory

    1. Acute

      a) Urinalysis

        (1) Pyuria, with or without casts: Almost always present

        (2) Other: Nitrites, hematuria typically present

      b) Urine culture and sensitivity: Presence of bacteriuria (greater than or equal to 100,000 colony-forming units/ml; can be fewer)

      c) CBC to assess for leukocytosis

    2. Chronic

      a) Urinalysis

        (1) Pyuria: May or may not be present

        (2) Proteinuria: Common

      b) Chemistry panel: Renal insufficiency with elevation of creatinine and electrolyte imbalance, especially hyperkalemia

3. Blood cultures indicated if patient is acutely ill, appears septic, or immunocompromised

4. Culture for gonorrhea and chlamydia, if suspected

B. Radiology

    1. Rarely performed in acute pyelonephritis unless presence of sepsis, known or suspected urolithiasis, new decrease in GFR to 40 ml/min or lower, or in those who do not respond to treatment within 72 hours

    2. CT scan: Most definitive procedure for chronic pyelonephritis diagnosis

        a) Asymmetry and irregularity of the kidney outlined

        b) Blunting and dilation of greater than or equal to 1 calyces, clubbing

        c) Cortical scars

        d) Hypertrophy of residual normal tissue

        e) Parenchymal thinning

    3. Renal ultrasound to assess for abnormalities

V. Differential diagnosis (Johnson & Russo, 2018; Nikolaidis et al., 2018)

A. Acute

    1. Cystitis (see Chapter 89)

    2. Acute appendicitis

    3. Diverticulitis (see Chapter 70)

    4. Pancreatitis (see Chapter 77)

    5. Cholecystitis (see Chapter 68)

    6. Urolithiasis

    7. Pelvic inflammatory disease

    8. Paraspinous muscle disorders

    9. Acute prostatitis (see Chapter 92)

    10. Acute bacterial nephritis

    11. Renal or perirenal abscess

    12. Emphysematous pyelonephritis

    13. Chemotherapy- or radiation-induced nephrotoxicity

    14. BPH (see Chapter 87)

B. Chronic

    1. Xanthogranulomatous pyelonephritis

    2. Malacoplakia

    3. TB

    4. Urolithiasis

VI. Treatment (Bader et al., 2019; Johnson & Russo, 2018; Keenan et al., 2017; Kolman, 2019; Long & Koyfman, 2018; Pietrucha-Dilanchian & Hooton, 2016)

A. Acute: Outpatient pharmacologic therapy (mild symptoms) based on isolated organisms and risk for multidrug resistant organisms (see Appendix C)

    1. Fluoroquinolones: Five to seven days

        a) Ciprofloxacin: 500 mg PO two times a day

        b) Ciprofloxacin extended release: 1,000 mg PO daily

        c) Levofloxacin: 750 mg PO daily

        d) Ceftriaxone: 1 g IM once pre-fluoroquinolone in communities with high fluoroquinolone resistance

    2. Fluroquinolone-sparing regimens

        a) Trimethoprim/sulfamethoxazole: One double-strength tablet (160 mg/800 mg) PO two times a day for 7–10 days *b)* Amoxicillin/clavulanate: 875 mg PO two times a day for 10–14 days

    c) Cefpodoxime: 200 mg PO two times a day for 10–14 days

    d) Cefdinir: 300 mg PO two times a day for 10–14 days

    e) Ceftriaxone: 1 g IM once before starting any PO therapy

B. Acute: Inpatient pharmacologic therapy; moderate to severe symptoms

  1. Critically ill (antipseudomonal agents): Cefepime 1 g IV every eight hours, imipenem 500 mg IV every six hours, meropenem 1 g IV every eight hours, or doripenem 500 mg IV every eight hours

  2. Not critically ill

    a) No risk factors for resistance: Ceftriaxone 1 g IV daily or piperacillin/tazobactam 3.375 g IV every six hours

    b) Risk factors for resistance: Antipseudomonal carbapenem

  3. Transitioned to PO once clinically stable depending on isolate

C. Chronic

  1. Treat underlying UTI.

  2. Reduce risk factors for UTI (e.g., vesicoureteral reflux).

  3. Control hypertension (see Chapter 47) and other diseases that may affect renal function.

  4. If contralateral kidney is normal, nephrectomy of the affected may be indicated if it is nonfunctioning and causing chronic pain or recurrent UTIs.

VII. Follow-up (Johnson & Russo, 2018)

A. Short term: No follow-up testing is needed if symptoms improve within 72 hours. If no improvement or worsening symptoms, repeat urine culture and obtain imaging (renal ultrasound or CT).

B. Long term

  1. Acute: If recurrent infection, treat with longer course of antibiotics (usually six weeks).

  2. Chronic: Follow-up is dependent on acute treatment.

VIII. Referrals

A. Nephrology: For renal insufficiency

B. Urology: For recurrent UTIs or treatment of any structural abnormality

C. Infectious disease: For recurrent UTIs or multidrug resistant organisms

The author would like to acknowledge Diane G. Cope, PhD, ARNP-BC, AOCNP®, for her contribution to this chapter that remains unchanged from the previous edition of this book.

References

Bader, M.S., Loeb, M., Leto, D., & Brooks, A.A. (2019). Treatment of urinary tract infections in the era of antimicrobial resistance and new antimicrobial agents. *Postgraduate Medicine, 132*(3), 234–250. https://doi.org/10.1080/00325481.2019.1680052

Choong, F.X., Antypas, H., & Richter-Dahlfors, A. (2015). Integrated pathophysiology of pyelonephritis. *Microbiology Spectrum, 3*(5). https://doi.org/10.1128/microbiolspec.UTI-0014-2012

Fogo, A.B., Lusco, M.A., Najafian, B., & Alpers, C.E. (2016). *AJKD* atlas of renal pathology: Chronic pyelonephritis. *American Journal of Kidney Disease, 68*(4), e23–e25. https://doi.org/10.1053/j.ajkd.2016.08.001

Johnson, J.R., & Russo, T.A. (2018). Acute pyelonephritis in adults. *New England Journal of Medicine, 378*(1), 48–59. https://doi.org/10.1056/NEJMcp1702758

Keenan, D.B., O'Rourke, D.M., & Courtney, A.E. (2017). Pyelonephritis can lead to life-threatening complications. *Practitioner, 261*(1801), 17–20.

Kolman, K.B. (2019). Cystitis and pyelonephritis: Diagnosis, treatment, and prevention. *Primary Care: Clinics in Office Practice, 46*(2), 191–202. https://doi.org/10.1016/j.pop.2019.01.001

Long, B., & Koyfman, A. (2018). The emergency department diagnosis and management of urinary tract infection. *Emergency Medicine Clinics of North America, 36*(4), 685–710. https://doi.org/10.1016/j.emc.2018.06.003

Nikolaidis, P., Dogra, V.S., Goldfarb, S., Gore, J.L., Harvin, H.J., Heilbrun, M.E., ... Lockhart, M.E. (2018). ACR Appropriateness Criteria® acute pyelonephritis. *Journal of the American College of Radiology, 15*(11 Suppl.), S232–S239. https://doi.org/10.1016/j.jacr.2018.09.011

Pierce, C., Keniston, A., & Albert, R.K. (2019). Imaging in acute pyelonephritis: Utilization, findings, and effect on management. *Southern Medical Journal, 112*(2), 118–124. https://doi.org/10.14423/SMJ.0000000000000936

Pietrucha-Dilanchian, P., & Hooton, T.M. (2016). Diagnosis, treatment, and prevention of urinary tract infection. *Microbiology Spectrum, 4*(6). https://doi.org/10.1128/microbiolspec.UTI-0021-2015.

CHAPTER 95

Syndrome of Inappropriate Antidiuretic Hormone

Gary Shelton, DNP, MSN, NP, ANP-BC, AOCNP®, ACHPN

I. Definition: Abnormal production and secretion of ADH (e.g., vasopressin), causing water reabsorption in the kidneys and reducing serum osmolality; results in hyponatremia, often a presenting finding (Frazer, 2017; Grant et al., 2015; Verbalis et al., 2016)

II. Physiology/Pathophysiology (Frazer, 2017; Grant et al., 2015; Jain & Nandy, 2019; Verbalis et al., 2016)
   A. Normal
      1. ADH is released from the posterior pituitary gland in response to increased osmolality or decreased plasma volume and acts on the collecting ducts of the kidneys.
      2. Receptors located near the hypothalamus create a feedback control for ADH resecretion.
      3. Changes in extracellular fluid osmolality occur secondary to serum sodium concentrations.
      4. ADH normally causes the kidneys to reabsorb water, thereby concentrating urine and normalizing serum osmolality.
   B. Pathophysiology
      1. Excess production of ADH results in increased water retention by the kidneys, increasing body water and causing moderate expansion of plasma volume.
      2. SIADH
         a) Primary excess of ADH (vasopressin) is present, increasing water retention and causing hyponatremia.
         b) Secondary stimulation of ADH (vasopressin) occurs by four mechanisms.
            (1) Tumors may synthesize and autonomously release ADH.
            (2) Nontumorous tissue may synthesize and release ADH autonomously or stimulated ADH is released by the pituitary gland.
            (3) ADH may be released from the pituitary gland inappropriately because of inflammation, neoplasm, vascular lesions, or drugs (e.g., morphine).
            (4) Limbic system activation from pain, nausea, fear, trauma, and surgery can increase ADH production.

III. Clinical features: SIADH is considered an isovolumic, hypotonic, hyponatremic condition (Babaliche et al., 2017; Cuesta et al., 2016; Frazer, 2017; Grant et al., 2015; Jain & Nandy, 2019; Rondon-Berrios et al., 2018; Sterns, 2018b; Verbalis et al., 2016).
   A. Etiology

    1. CNS disturbances: Stroke, hemorrhage, trauma, psychosis

    2. Malignancies: Most commonly small cell lung cancer

    3. Drug induced

    4. Pneumonia

    5. Adrenal insufficiency

    6. Hypothyroidism

    7. HIV infection

    8. Hereditary SIADH

    9. TB

B. History

    1. History of cancer and cancer treatment

    2. Current medications: Prescribed, over the counter

    3. History of presenting symptoms: Precipitating factors, onset, location, duration

    4. Changes in ADLs

    5. History of fluid intake and output in the past 24 hours

C. Signs and symptoms: Dependent on speed of development and degree of hyponatremia

    1. Mild: Sodium 110–134 mEq/L

        a) Muscle cramps

        b) Anorexia, nausea, vomiting

        c) Fatigue

        d) Headache

        e) Lethargy

    2. Moderate: Sodium 100–110 mEq/L

        a) Irritability

        b) Disorientation, confusion, lethargy

        c) Extrapyramidal effects: Changes in muscle tone, abnormal posturing, tremors

        d) Abdominal cramps, diarrhea

    3. Severe: Sodium less than 100 mEq/L

        a) Seizure

        b) Coma

    4. Other symptoms

        a) Weight gain without edema

        b) Thirst

        c) Headache

        d) Impaired memory

        e) Decreased urine output

D. Physical examination: Neurologic

    1. Change in level of consciousness: Confusion, irritability

    2. Deep tendon reflexes: Hyporeflexia

IV. Diagnostic tests (Babaliche et al., 2017; Frazer, 2017; Grant et al., 2015; Rondon-Berrios et al., 2018; Verbalis et al., 2016)

A. Laboratory

    1. Serum osmolality: Less than 280 mOsm/kg

    2. Serum sodium concentration: Less than 135 mEq/L

    3. Urine sodium: Greater than 30 mEq/L

    4. Urine osmolality: 400–600 mOsm/kg

    5. Urine-specific gravity increased: Greater than 1.032

    6. Renal, thyroid, adrenal, pituitary, and cardiac function: Etiology causing SIADH, typically normal

      7. Plasma creatinine, BUN, uric acid, and phosphate: Low normal in SIADH
  B. Radiology
      1. CT scan of the head to evaluate for anatomic lesions
      2. Chest x-ray to evaluate for pulmonary source, such as pneumonia

V. Differential diagnosis: Focus on identifying the cause of SIADH (Arshad et al., 2016; Cuesta et al., 2016; Grant et al., 2015; Verbalis et al., 2016).
  A. Malignant tumors (see Appendix M)
      1. Small cell lung cancer: Most common
      2. Other: Non-small cell lung, head and neck, esophageal, pancreatic, duodenal, breast, brain, skin, ovarian, GU, and GI cancers; thymoma; leukemia; lymphomas; sarcoma
  B. CNS disorders
      1. Stroke (see Chapter 146), infection, trauma, hemorrhage, psychosis
      2. Hyponatremia associated with cerebral salt wasting (see Chapter 155)
  C. Pulmonary noncancerous conditions: TB (see Chapter 36), pneumothorax (see Chapter 31), pneumonia (see Chapter 30), asthma (see Chapter 28), respiratory failure
  D. Hyperglycemia (see Chapter 151), hyperlipidemia (see Chapter 44), hyperproteinemia, hypothyroidism (see Chapter 158)
  E. Drugs that may potentiate the release or action of ADH
      1. Vinca alkaloids, antifolates, antimetabolites, alkylating agents, platinum compounds
      2. Antipsychotics, antidepressants, monoamine oxidase inhibitors, barbiturates, anticonvulsants
      3. NSAIDs, opiates, hallucinogens
      4. Diuretics, ACE inhibitors, ADH analogs
      5. Theophylline
      6. Amphetamines
      7. IFN-α, IFN-γ
      8. Anesthetic agents
      9. Antidiabetic drugs
      10. Vasopressin analogs
  F. Hereditary SIADH, nephrogenic and hypothalamic syndromes
  G. HIV infection, AIDS

VI. Treatment (Arshad et al., 2016; Cuesta et al., 2016; Frazer, 2017; Grant et al., 2015; Lockett et al., 2019; Rondon-Berrios et al., 2018; Sterns, 2018a, 2018b; Verbalis et al., 2016)
  A. Treatment of SIADH is aimed at disrupting the effects of ADH on the kidneys. Therapy is based on the severity of hyponatremia, symptomatology, and cause of SIADH (see Chapter 155).
  B. Treat the underlying cause. Chronic treatment may be necessary for SIADH caused by cancer.
      1. Hormone replacement in adrenal insufficiency: Hydrocortisone 10–20 mg PO two times a day
      2. Treatment of infections (see Appendix C)
      3. Discontinuation of offending drugs
  C. Fluid restriction of less than 800–1,000 ml/24 hours to treat mild SIADH
  D. IV fluid administration
      1. Administration of isotonic (0.9%) saline is adequate in most cases.
        a) Mild hyponatremia: Serum sodium less than or equal to 120 mEq/L; infuse minimal hydration.

> b) Moderate hyponatremia: Serum sodium less than or equal to 110 mEq/L; may require administration of IV fluids, electrolytes, and diuretics

2. Administration of hypertonic (3%) saline solution may be used for severe symptomatic hyponatremia (serum sodium less than 105 mEq/L). Correct sodium by 0.5–1 mEq/L/hr until normalization of sodium levels occurs and symptoms resolve. Target level is 125 mEq/L.
3. In symptomatic chronic SIADH, the rate of sodium replaced might be 1 mEq/L/hr for approximately five hours, followed by slowing therapy to allow raising the sodium level to 8–12 mEq/L in 24 hours.
4. Too rapid correction of hyponatremia in patients with chronic hyponatremia (longer than two to five days) may lead to central pontine myelinolysis or demyelination, which is caused by rapid loss of brain electrolytes and organic osmolytes. Stop hypertonic solution when level reaches 120 mEq/L.
5. Avoid administration of hypotonic fluids (e.g., IV 5% dextrose), as it could potentiate water retention and hyponatremia.

E. Drug therapy may be initiated if hyponatremia continues despite fluid restriction or IV administration of saline solution.

1. Loop diuretics increase free water excretion rates (not useful in long-term therapies), such as furosemide 20–40 mg PO two times a day.
2. Demeclocycline 600–1,200 mg PO daily is a tetracycline derivative that can cause diabetes insipidus; monitor output.
   a) May take two to three days to become effective
   b) Should be avoided with food
   c) Causes nausea, photosensitivity, nephrotoxicity, and irreversible renal failure
   d) Should be avoided in those who are pregnant
3. Lithium 900–1,200 mg PO daily can cause diabetes insipidus; monitor output.
   a) May take four days to be effective
   b) Causes nausea, vomiting, and anorexia
   c) Monitoring for neurologic status, tremors, weakness
   d) Monitoring for cardiac status
   e) May cause irreversible diabetes insipidus and end-stage renal failure
4. Veno-venous hemodialysis can be used for a gradual correction of sodium.
5. Oral urea (powder formulation, various dosages) is considered a food by FDA.
   a) Daily dose for inpatient use to allow for monitoring
   b) Rarely causes overly rapid correction of plasma sodium
   c) Contraindications
      (1) Patients with hypovolemic hyponatremia
      (2) Patients with hyponatremia associated with adrenal insufficiency
      (3) Patients with drug-induced hyponatremia when the offending medication can be safely discontinued
6. Vasopressin antagonists include vaptans.
   a) Give tolvaptan 15 mg PO. Discontinue fluid restriction to reduce risk of rapid correction of sodium; lower doses have been used but there is a need to repeat, as the half-life is four to six hours.
   b) Vaptans are costly and include safety concerns for the risk of liver injury with continued dosing as well as rapid correction of sodium.
   c) More research is needed for safe outpatient use, as well as safety data.

F. Initiate seizure precautions if severe hyponatremia is present (see Chapter 144).
G. Initiate safety measures if altered mental status is present.

    H. Implement frequent mouth care to minimize dryness and promote integrity of mucous membranes.

    I. Use normal saline to irrigate NG or enteral tubes.

    J. Avoid tap water or saline enemas.

    K. Increase salt intake (e.g., 3 g or ½ teaspoon three times a day).

VII. Follow-up

    A. Frequently monitor serum sodium; frequency is determined by cause.

    B. Schedule outpatient visits for history and physical examination for symptom monitoring.

VIII. Referrals

    A. Nephrologist or endocrinologist: For diagnostic workup of hyponatremia and recommendations for management if etiology is unknown

    B. Hematologist/oncologist: If malignancy is suspected or if cancer workup is needed

    C. Pharmacist: For drug and fluid management recommendations

    D. Nutritionist: For suggestions in food requirements, such as low salt or high protein

    E. Neurologist: For seizure management and input of treatment

References

Arshad, H.M.S., Rodriguez, A., & Suhail, F. (2016). SIADH induced by pharyngeal squamous cell carcinoma: Case report and literature review. *Case Reports in Nephrology, 2016,* 3186714. https://doi.org/10.1155/2016/3186714

Babaliche, P., Madnani, S., & Kamat, S. (2017). Clinical profile of patients admitted with hyponatremia in the medical intensive care unit. *Indian Journal of Critical Care Medicine, 21*(12), 819–824. https://doi.org/10.4103/ijccm.IJCCM _257_17

Cuesta, M., Garrahy, A., & Thompson, C.J. (2016). SIAD: Practical recommendations for diagnosis and management. *Journal of Endocrinological Investigation, 39*(9), 991–1001. https://doi.org/10.1007/s40618-016-0463-3.

Frazer, C.A. (2017). Syndrome of inappropriate antidiuresis. *Medsurg Nursing, 26*(5), 346–348.

Grant, P., Ayuk, J., Bouloux, P.-M., Cohen, M., Cranston, I., Murray, R.D., ... Grossman, A. (2015). The diagnosis and management of inpatient hyponatraemia and SIADH. *European Journal of Clinical Investigation, 45*(8), 888–894. https://doi.org/10.1111/eci.12465

Jain, A.K., & Nandy, P. (2019). Clinico-etiological profile of hyponatremia among elderly age group patients in a tertiary care hospital in Sikkim. *Journal of Family Medicine and Primary Care, 8*(3), 988–994. https://doi.org/10.4103/jfmpc .jfmpc_32_19

Lockett, J., Berkman, K.E., Dimeski, G., Russell, A.W., & Inder, W.J. (2019). Urea treatment in fluid restriction–refractory hyponatremia. *Clinical Endocrinology, 90*(4), 630–636. https://doi.org/10.1111/cen.13930.

Rondon-Berrios, H., Tandukar, S., Mor, M.K., Ray, E.C., Bender, F.H., Kleyman, T.R., & Weisbord, S.D. (2018). Urea for the treatment of hyponatremia. *Clinical Journal of the American Society of Nephrology, 13*(11), 1627–1632. https://doi .org/10.2215/CJN.04020318

Sterns, R.H. (2018a). Tolvaptan for the syndrome of inappropriate secretion of antidiuretic hormone: Is the dose too high? *American Journal of Kidney Diseases, 71*(6), 763–765. https://doi.org/10.1053/j.ajkd.2018.02.355

Sterns, R.H. (2018b). Treatment of severe hyponatremia. *Clinical Journal of the American Society of Nephrology, 13*(4), 641–649. https://doi.org/10.2215/CJN.10440917

Verbalis, J.G., Greenberg, A., Burst, V., Haymann, J.-P., Johannsson, G., Peri, A., ... Dave, J. (2016). Diagnosing and treating the syndrome of inappropriate antidiuretic hormone secretion. *American Journal of Medicine, 129*(5), 537.e9–537.e23. https://doi.org/10.1016/j.amjmed.2015.11.005

Musculoskeletal

SYMPTOMS

MEDICAL DIAGNOSES

CHAPTER 96

Arthralgia

Kimberly A. Noonan, DNP, ANP-BC, AOCN®

I. Definition: Pain or stiffness in a joint or joints (Irwin et al., 2015; Mao et al., 2014)
   A. The term *arthralgia* should only be used when the condition is noninflammatory.
   B. The term *arthritis* is used when the condition is inflammatory.

II. Physiology/Pathophysiology (Bauml et al., 2015; Chen et al., 2017; Faisal et al., 2019; Long et al., 2019; Marks & Marks, 2016; Salva & Merrill, 2018; Smeeton et al., 2016)
   A. Normal
      1. Most joints are freely moving articulations that are enclosed by a capsule of fibrous articular cartilage, ligaments, and cartilage covering the ends of the opposing bones. Joints hold the bones together and maintain skeletal stability and mobility.
      2. Three types of joints
         a) Fibrous joints are found in the flat bone of the skull and permit flexibility during birth.
         b) Cartilaginous joints provide limited mobility in areas such as the vertebrae.
         c) Synovial joints are lubricated joints found in limbs and jaw.
      3. Articular versus nonarticular
         a) Articular structures include synovium, synovial fluid, articular cartilage, intra-articular ligaments, joint capsule, and juxta-articular bone.
         b) Nonarticular structures or periarticular structures include supportive extra-articular ligaments, tendons, bursae, muscle fascia, bone, nerve, and overlying skin.
   B. Pathophysiology: Joint pain usually originates in the activation of free nerve endings. The specific pathophysiology is dependent on the articular finding, and overall, the etiology is not clearly understood.
      1. Estrogen has a protective joint mechanism. Menopause and syndromes caused by a decrease in estrogen are linked to an increase in systemic inflammation. This can cause an increase in joint discomfort.
      2. Increased body temperature (fever) causes a cell-mediated immunity (e.g., infection, inflammation, cancer, immunotherapy, allergic reaction).
         a) Pyrogens trigger the cells of the immune system to release prostaglandins to reset the base temperature.
         b) Muscle contraction and prostaglandins stimulate pain receptors, producing myalgia and arthralgia.
      3. Bacterial and viral infections can induce arthralgia. Large joints usually are affected, especially knees and hips, with septic arthritis. The most common organisms are *Staphylococcus aureus* and *Streptococcus*. Less common organisms are gram-negative such as *Pseudomonas aeruginosa*, *Escherichia coli*, and *Proteus* species, as well as mycobacterial and fungal (rare).

4. Arthralgia can be caused by ectopic hypertrophic differentiation of chondrocytes found on the joint surface that erode the cartilage. As a result, cartilage degenerates or can develop crystal deposits within the joint.

III. Clinical features: Arthralgia is classified as monoarthralgia (involving one joint), oligoarticular or pauciarticular (two to four joints), or polyarthralgia (involving four or more joints) (Almoallim et al., 2017; Bauml et al., 2015; Benfaremo et al., 2018; Boeters et al., 2017; Ghouri & Conaghan, 2019; Molendijk et al., 2018; van Nies et al., 2015; van Steenbergen et al., 2018).
  A. Etiology
    1. Infection: Bacterial, viral, fungal
    2. Fever
    3. Cancer related
      a) Metastases to a joint are rare but can mimic inflammatory arthritis.
      b) Acute leukemic arthritis is caused by leukemic infiltration of synovium.
      c) Myeloma cells can infiltrate synovial tissues.
      d) Sarcomas can involve the joint capsule.
      e) Pancreatic cancer may present with joint pain, panniculitis, and eosinophilia.
    4. Hypersensitivity reactions
    5. Medication induced: Not an all-inclusive listing
      a) Antiretroviral
      b) Hepatitis B vaccines
      c) Vitamin A and the retinoids
      d) Rifabutin
      e) H_2 blockers
      f) PPIs
      g) Procainamide
      h) Bisphosphonates
      i) Chemotherapy agents
        (1) All-trans retinoic acid
        (2) Bleomycin
        (3) Aromatase inhibitors: Anastrozole, letrozole, exemestane
        (4) Ibrutinib
        (5) Dacarbazine
        (6) Topotecan
        (7) Taxanes
        (8) Procarbazine
        (9) L-asparaginase
        (10) Nucleoside antimetabolites: Cladribine, cytarabine, fludarabine, gemcitabine
      j) Monoclonal antibodies
        (1) Alemtuzumab
        (2) Bevacizumab
        (3) Cetuximab
        (4) Gemtuzumab ozogamicin
        (5) Ipilimumab
        (6) Immune checkpoint inhibitors: Nivolumab, atezolizumab, cemiplimab, durvalumab, avelumab
        (7) Pembrolizumab
      k) Arthralgia syndrome: Associated with the use of aromatase inhibitors; characterized as bilateral and symmetric joint pain and stiffness

      l) Growth factor use: Filgrastim, pegfilgrastim, sargramostim

      m) Cancer vaccines that work on cell-mediated immunity

      n) Radiation: Potentially causes necrosis of the bone and joints

      o) IFNs: Commonly cause arthralgia

  6. Disease of the joints: RA, OA

  7. Autoimmune disease

      a) RA

      b) SLE

      c) Sjögren syndrome

      d) Polymyositis

B. History

  1. History of cancer and cancer treatment

  2. Current medications: Prescribed, over the counter

  3. History of presenting symptoms: Precipitating factors, onset, location, duration

  4. Changes in ADLs

  5. Past medical history: RA or OA, rheumatic fever, chronic renal failure, psoriasis, gout, Lyme disease, GVHD, fibromyalgia, SLE, low back pain, prior musculoskeletal injuries, prosthetic joint, kidney stones, psychiatric disorder, significant trauma, soft tissue injury or fracture

  6. Social history: Sexual history, occupation, alcohol use, illicit drug use

  7. Travel history, exposure to wooded areas (increased risk of tick bite)

C. Signs and symptoms

  1. Constitutional symptoms (e.g., fever, chills, sweats, weight loss, malaise) may be present with infection, sepsis, or worsening of cancer.

  2. Neurogenic pain: Asymmetric or symmetric

      a) Radiculopathy, reflex sympathetic dystrophy, myelopathy

      b) Entrapment or peripheral neuropathy: Numbness, tingling or burning sensation

  3. Weakness (focal or diffuse), gait disturbance

  4. Erythema of the joints

  5. Tenosynovitis, tendinopathy, tendinitis

D. Physical examination

  1. Vital signs: Fever or tachycardia suggestive of infectious source

  2. Musculoskeletal

      a) Muscle atrophy: Neuromuscular origin

      b) Muscle strength in all involved joints

      c) Gait

      d) Joint assessment

         (1) Range of motion: Active and passive

         (2) Reduced active range of motion with intact passive range of motion suggestive of bursitis, tendonitis, or muscle injury

         (3) Decreased active and passive range of motion suggestive of contracture, synovitis, or structural abnormality of the joint

         (4) Tenderness, erythema, warmth, effusion, or soft tissue swelling

         (5) Weakness: Can be focal or diffuse suggestive of cord compression, compartment syndrome, entrapment neuropathy, or radiculopathy

  3. Integument

      a) Rash: Multiple etiologies

      b) Nail pitting: Psoriasis, GVHD

      c) Skin nodules: Rheumatoid nodules, tophi

    d) Ecchymosis: Possible coagulopathy

    e) Spinal tenderness: Ankylosing spondylitis

  4. HEENT

    a) Sicca syndrome: Combination of dry eyes and dry mouth suggestive of Sjögren syndrome, RA, SLE, or polymyositis

    b) Uveitis suggestive of SLE, sarcoidosis, or RA

    c) Episcleritis suggestive of rheumatoid illness or GVHD

    d) Mouth sores/ulcers suggestive of SLE, GVHD, Behçet disease, or Reiter syndrome

    e) Jaw and mandibular tenderness suggestive of TMJ syndrome

  5. Cardiac

    a) Heart murmur and pleural rub suggestive of RA or SLE

    b) Decreased peripheral pulses suggestive of vascular disease

  6. Genital: Urethral or cervical discharge suggestive of gonococcal arthritis

IV. Diagnostic tests (Almoallim et al., 2017; Benfaremo et al., 2018; Boeters et al., 2017; Molendijk et al., 2018)

  A. Laboratory

    1. ESR and CRP

      a) Nonspecific indicators of inflammation

      b) Elevated in presence of infection, inflammatory states, and malignancy

      c) Useful in equivocal joint examination; inflammatory arthritis more likely if elevated

    2. Antinuclear antibody: High sensitivity but low specificity for SLE

      a) Negative test essentially rules out SLE.

      b) Positive test may occur in many rheumatic illnesses.

    3. Rheumatoid factor: Limited value, particularly in monoarthritis

      a) It is present in a variety of rheumatic disorders.

      b) Many patients with RA never have a positive rheumatoid factor.

    4. HLA-B27: Can be increased with post-gonoccocal arthritis and spondyloarthropathies

    5. Lyme titer, if indicated

    6. CMV viral load assay in known CMV-positive population and those who are immunocompromised

    7. HIV testing in high-risk patients

    8. Uric acid: Usually elevated in gout

    9. Blood cultures: If sepsis is suspected

    10. PT, PTT, platelet count, and bleeding time

      a) If suspected hemorrhagic synovial fluid

      b) High-risk patients: Anticoagulated, thrombocytopenic

    11. Gonorrhea testing of the synovial fluid analysis, if indicated

  B. Radiology

    1. Plain films

      a) OA: Confirm the diagnosis and assess severity. It may be normal.

      b) RA: Marginal erosions in the joint can be diagnostic.

      c) Chronic gout: Erosions may be visible as an "overhanging edge."

    2. Fluoroscopy can be used to observe the range of motion and to guide proper needle insertion for aspiration of joint fluid.

    3. CT scan has limited value, except in the following cases.

      a) Malignant cause

        b) For better characterization of soft tissue calcifications and bony abnormalities compared to MRI

        c) Patients with metallic implants or pacemakers

    4. MRI is best in detecting changes caused by inflammation, neoplasm, trauma or ischemia, and extraosseous extension of a soft tissue mass through the bone.

    5. Radionuclide bone scan is the most effective screening test for skeletal metastases.

C. Other

    1. Synovial fluid examination: Important in monoarticular joint pain to evaluate whether the effusion has the following characteristics

        a) Inflammatory (cloudy)

        b) Noninflammatory (clear)

        c) Infection

        d) Hemorrhagic (pink/red; caused by Hgb breakdown): Indicates coagulopathy, pseudogout, tumor, trauma, or Charcot joint

        e) Contains crystals

        f) Normal/sterile: Suspected systemic rheumatic disorders

    2. Synovial fluid leukocyte count

        a) Septic arthritis: Most common

            (1) Greater than 90% polymorphonuclear leukocytes

            (2) Leukocyte count: 20,000–150,000/mm^3

        b) Noninflammatory: If less than 2,000 WBCs or less than 75% neutrophils, consider OA, soft tissue injury, or viral infection.

V. Differential diagnosis (Amdekar et al., 2017; Marks & Marks, 2016; Molendijk et al., 2018; van Nies et al., 2015)

A. Monoarthralgias: Infection until proven otherwise

    1. Septic arthritis

        a) Nongonococcal bacterial: High-risk groups

            (1) RA (see Chapter 108)

            (2) Chronic GVHD

            (3) Immune compromise

        b) Gonococcal arthritis

        c) Acute retroviral syndrome: Initial HIV presentation

    2. OA (see Chapter 105)

    3. Internal derangement or trauma

        a) Meniscus injury

        b) Ligament tears

        c) Overuse injury

        d) Fractures (see Chapter 102)

    4. Peripheral neuropathy (see Chapter 143)

    5. Ischemic bone: Avascular necrosis

    6. Neoplasm

    7. Palindromic rheumatism

    8. Gout, pseudogout, other crystal-induced arthritis (see Chapters 103 and 108)

    9. Paget disease

    10. Lyme disease (see Chapter 104)

B. Polyarthralgias

    1. Viruses: Common

        a) CMV

        b) Influenza

        c) Hepatitis B or C (see Chapter 74)

        d) Parvovirus B19

        e) Herpetic viruses

        f) Enterovirus

        g) Mononucleosis

        h) Chikungunya

  2. Adrenal insufficiency

  3. Endocarditis (see Chapter 46)

  4. FMS (see Chapter 101)

  5. Chronic GVHD

  6. Inflammatory bowel disease, ulcerative colitis, Crohn disease

  7. Late-stage Lyme disease (see Chapter 104)

  8. Polymyalgia rheumatica

  9. Psoriatic arthritis

  10. Reiter syndrome

  11. Rheumatic heart disease

  12. RA (see Chapter 108)

  13. Sickle cell disease (see Chapter 119)

  14. Spondyloarthropathies: Associated with the *HLA-B27* gene

  15. SLE (see Chapter 110)

  16. Medication induced

  17. Transfusion reaction

  18. Allergic reaction

  19. Sarcoidosis

  20. Aromatase inhibitor–induced arthralgia

C. Joint pain in general by location

  1. Single: Trauma, infection, gout, pseudogout

  2. Multiple: RA, OA, SLE, GVHD

  3. Migratory: Gonococcal arthritis, rheumatic fever, FMS

    a) Hours to days: Crystal arthritis, infection, septic arthritis

    b) Weeks to months: Rheumatic disease, indolent infection, chronic inflammatory polyarthritis

    c) After rest

      (1) Worse: Inflammatory arthralgias (e.g., RA)

      (2) Improved: Noninflammatory arthritis (e.g., OA)

VI. Treatment (Ghouri & Conaghan, 2019; Henry et al., 2018; Irwin et al., 2015; Mao et al., 2014; Nelson & Churilla, 2017; van Nies et al., 2015)

A. Treatment is based on etiology of the arthralgias.

  1. Treat infection with an antimicrobial as indicated by source.

  2. Remove or alter dose of medication suspected of triggering the arthralgias. Adjust method of administration if related.

  3. Treat chronic GVHD with immunosuppressive agent, as indicated.

B. Symptomatic therapy

  1. Rest involved joints if inflammatory cause.

  2. Refer to physical therapy, as indicated, and initiate appropriate therapy.

    a) Exercise

    b) Weight reduction

    c) Range-of-motion exercise

    d) Warm or cold therapy

3. Undergo acupuncture.
4. Undergo massage therapy.

C. Pharmacologic intervention
   1. NSAIDs (see Appendix E)
   2. Opioids, when indicated (see Appendix F)
   3. Corticosteroids: Dosing is based on etiology (see Appendix K).
   4. Adjuvant therapy: Duloxetine starting dose 30–60 mg PO daily
   5. Immunosuppressants/immunomodulatory agents: May be beneficial (see Chapter 108)

VII. Follow-up
   A. Care is dependent on the etiology of the arthralgias.
   B. Treatment of the underlying cause should improve arthralgias.
   C. Monitor therapeutic intervention to evaluate its effectiveness.
   D. If patient is immunosuppressed, monitor for infection.

VIII. Referrals: Should be considered based on arthralgia etiology

References

Almoallim, H., Abdulaziz, S., Fallatah, E., Alhazmi, H., Meraiani, N., Bazuhair, T., ... Fathaldin, O. (2017). Clinical characteristics and outcomes of cancer patients with post-chemotherapy arthritis: A retrospective case series report. *Open Access Rheumatology: Research and Reviews, 9,* 111–116. https://doi.org/10.2147/OARRR.S134816

Amdekar, S., Parashar, D., & Alagarasu, K. (2017). Chikungunya virus-induced arthritis: Role of host and viral factors in the pathogenesis. *Viral Immunology, 30*(10), 691–701 https://doi.org/10.1089/vim.2017.0052

Bauml, J., Chen, L., Chen, J., Boyer, J., Kalos, M., Li, S.Q., ... Mao, J.J. (2015). Arthralgia among women taking aromatase inhibitors: Is there a shared inflammatory mechanism with co-morbid fatigue and insomnia? *Breast Cancer Research, 17,* 89. https://doi.org/10.1186/s13058-015-0599-7

Benfaremo, D., Manfredi, L., Luchetti, M., & Gabrielli, A. (2018). Musculoskeletal and rheumatic diseases induced by immune checkpoint inhibitors: A review of the literature. *Current Drug Safety, 13*(3), 150–164. https://doi.org/10.2174/1574886313666180508122332

Boeters, D.M., Raza, K., & vander Helm-van Mil, A.H.M. (2017). Which patients presenting with arthralgia eventually develop rheumatoid arthritis? The current state of the art. *RMD Open, 3*(2), e000479. https://doi.org/10.1136/rmdopen-2017-000479

Chen, D., Shen, J., Zhao, W., Wang, T., Han, L., Hamilton, J.L., & Im, H.-J. (2017). Osteoarthritis: Toward a comprehensive understanding of pathological mechanism. *Bone Research, 5,* 16044. https://doi.org/10.1038/boneres.2016.44

Faisal, A.I., Majumder, S., Mondal, T., Cowan, D., Naseh, S., & Deen, M.J. (2019). Monitoring methods of human body joints: State-of-the-art and research challenges. *Sensors, 19*(11), 2629. https://doi.org/10.3390/s19112629

Ghouri, A., & Conaghan, P.G. (2019). Update on novel pharmacological therapies for osteoarthritis. *Therapeutic Advances in Musculoskeletal Disease, 11.* https://doi.org/10.1177/1759720X19864492

Henry, N.L., Unger, J.M., Schott, A.F., Fehrenbacher, L., Flynn, P.J., Prow, D.M., ... Wade, J.L., III. (2018). Randomized, multicenter, placebo-controlled clinical trial of duloxetine versus placebo for aromatase inhibitor–associated arthralgias in early-stage breast cancer: SWOG S1202. *Journal of Clinical Oncology, 36*(4), 326–332. https://doi.org/10.1200/JCO.2017.74.6651

Irwin, M.L., Cartmel, B., Gross, C.P., Ercolano, E., Li, F., Yao, X., ... Ligibel, J. (2015). Randomized exercise trial of aromatase inhibitor–induced arthralgia in breast cancer survivors. *Clinical Journal of Oncology, 33*(10), 1104–1111 https://doi.org/10.1200/JCO.2014.57.1547

Long, B., Koyfman, A., & Gottlieb, M. (2019). Evaluation and management of septic arthritis and its mimics in the emergency department. *Western Journal of Emergency Medicine, 20*(2), 331–341. https://doi.org/10.5811/westjem.2018.10.40974

Mao, J.J., Farrar, J.T., Bruner, D., Zee, J., Bowman, M., Seluzicki, L., ... Xie, S.X. (2014). Electro-acupuncture for fatigue, sleep, and psychological distress in breast cancer patients with aromatase inhibitor–related arthralgia: A randomized trial. *Cancer, 120*(23), 3744–3751. https://doi.org/10.1002/cncr.28917

Marks, M., & Marks, J.L. (2016). Viral arthritis. *Clinical Medicine, 16*(2), 129–134. https://doi.org/10.7861/clinmedicine.16-2-129

Molendijk, M., Hazes, J.M.W., & Lubbert, E. (2018). From patients with arthralgia, pre-RA and recently diagnosed RA: What is the current status of understanding RA pathogenesis? *RMD Open, 4*(1), e000256. https://doi.org/10.1136/rmdopen-2016-000256

Nelson, N.L., & Churilla, J.R. (2017). Massage therapy for pain and function in patients with arthritis: A systematic review of randomized controlled trials. *American Journal of Physical Medicine and Rehabilitation, 96*(9), 665–672. https://doi.org/10.1097/PHM.0000000000000712

Salva, J.E., & Merrill, A.E. (2018). Signaling networks in joint development. *Developmental Dynamics, 246*(4), 262–274. https://doi.org/10.1002/dvdy.24472

Smeeton, J., Askary, A., & Crump, J.G. (2016). Building and maintaining joints by exquisite local control of cell fate. *Wiley Interdisciplinary Reviews Developmental Biology, 6*(1), e245. https://doi.org/10.1002/wdev.245

van Nies, J.A.B., Alves, C., Radix-Bloemen, A.L.S., Gaujoux-Viala, C., Huizinga, T.W.J., Hazes, J.M.W., ... van der Helm-van Mil, A.H.M. (2015). Reappraisal of the diagnostic and prognostic value of morning stiffness in arthralgia and early arthritis: Results from the Groningen EARC, Leiden EARC, ESPOIR, Leiden EAC and REACH. *Arthritis Research and Therapy, 17,* 108. https://doi.org/10.1186/s13075-015-0616-3

van Steenbergen, H.W., Pereira da Silva, J.A., Huizinga, T.W.J., & van der Helm-van Mil, A.H.M. (2018) Preventing progression from arthralgia to arthritis: Targeting the right patients. *Nature Reviews Rheumatology, 14*(1), 32–41. https://doi.org/10.1038/nrrheum.2017.185

CHAPTER 97

Bone Pain

Jeannine M. Brant, PhD, APRN, AOCN®, FAAN

I. Definition: Somatic pain resulting from the activation of peripheral nociceptors (Zajączkow-ska et al., 2019)

II. Physiology/Pathophysiology (Figura et al., 2018; Russo & Sundaramurthi, 2019; Zajączkow-ska et al., 2019)
   A. Normal
      1. The skeletal system has 206 bones, which provide the stability and mobility necessary for physical activity.
      2. Other functions include hematopoiesis within bone marrow; reservoir to maintain homeostasis of calcium, magnesium, phosphorus, and sodium; and protection of vital organs.
      3. The two types of bone are cortical and trabecular. Cortical bone is exterior bone with no bone marrow contact. Trabecular bone is inner bone and has contact with bone marrow.
   B. Pathophysiology
      1. Peripheral nociceptors are activated and sensitized by mechanical (e.g., tumor compression, infiltration), thermal, or chemical (e.g., inflammatory mediators such as epinephrine, serotonin, substance P, bradykinin, prostaglandin, and histamine) stimuli.
      2. Pain arises from primary afferent and sympathetic nerve fibers associated with blood vessels; pain arises predominantly from the periosteum.
      3. Neuropathic and bone pain frequently coexist, especially with encroachment or invasion of nerve roots or the spinal cord (e.g., spinal compression, brachial and lumbosacral plexopathy).

III. Clinical features: Bone is the most common site of cancer pain and is the third leading metastatic site after the lung and liver. Bone pain may be accompanied by a neuropathic component with nerve invasion (Figura et al., 2018; Russo & Sundaramurthi, 2019; van den Beuken-van Everdingen et al., 2016).
   A. Etiology
      1. Fracture
      2. Bone metastasis
      3. Cancer therapies
      4. Arthritis
      5. SCC
      6. Paraneoplastic syndrome
      7. Cancers: Bone, multiple myeloma, osteosarcoma

        8. Acromegaly

        9. Bisphosphonates

       10. Paget disease

   B. History

      1. History of cancer and cancer treatment

      2. Current medications: Prescribed, over the counter

      3. History of presenting symptoms: Precipitating factors, onset, location, pain severity, quality (e.g., sharp, dull, aching, burning, intermittent, continuous), presence of radiculopathy and other potential neuropathic indicators, duration, relieving factors

      4. Changes in ADLs

      5. Past medical history: Paget disease, osteoporosis, arthritis, scoliosis, recent trauma or falls

   C. Signs and symptoms

      1. Pain is often localized if strictly somatic but can be radicular with nerve involvement; multiple types of pain can be present in multiple locations.

      2. It is described as constant aching to a deep, boring sensation accompanied by breakthrough pain. Episodes of stabbing pain occur. With neuropathic involvement, pain is described as shooting, stabbing, radiating, and/or burning.

      3. Pain is often worse at night; sleeping or lying down may provide little relief.

      4. It may occur around joints because of mechanical, chemical, or bony changes.

      5. Symptoms may depend on location, activity (i.e., increasing pain with ambulation in weight-bearing areas, such as hip and femur), and neurologic involvement.

   D. Physical examination

      1. Musculoskeletal

         a) Pain assessment with percussion in painful areas identified by the patient

         b) Identification of the most painful locations if multiple sites are involved

         c) Range of motion and pain associated with movement

         d) Bony enlargement indicating acromegaly

         e) Increased radicular pain with straight leg raises indicating lumbar and thoracic compression

         f) Joint assessment for erythema, warmth, or edema indicating arthritis or gout

      2. Neurologic: Bilateral versus unilateral muscle strength, sensory deficits, and radiculopathy, especially in patients with vertebral pain and suspected nerve root compression or SCC

         a) Numbness and paresthesia that progresses to loss of sensation of light touch, pain, and heat with compression

         b) Pain with neck flexion suggestive of cervical compression

         c) Loss of sensation for light touch, pain, or temperature with disc abnormalities, compression, or fractures

         d) Loss or decrease of positional sense with compression

      3. Back: Percussion over areas of tenderness indicating disc involvement or compression

IV. Diagnostic tests (Russo & Sundaramurthi, 2019)

   A. Laboratory

      1. Alkaline phosphatase increased in bone metastasis, RA, or Paget disease

      2. Calcium possibly increased, and phosphorus inversely decreased in bone metastasis or Paget disease

      3. TSH testing to evaluate for hyperthyroidism or hypothyroidism

   B. Radiology

1. Plain radiograph over painful area of bone
   a) Blastic/lytic metastases often are identified with plain film. It is important in weight-bearing areas (e.g., neck, proximal femur) to evaluate integrity of bone cortex.
   b) Assess for pathologic fractures (impending or actual).
2. Bone scan
   a) To identify bone metastasis; bone scans are most sensitive to blastic lesions.
   b) Lytic bone metastases (e.g., multiple myeloma) rarely absorb tracer, and bone scan will not visualize well; if lytic metastasis is suspected, order plain films first.
   c) Other types of bone lesions or defects (e.g., past trauma, osteoporotic lesions) will be visualized on bone scan.
3. CT and MRI to evaluate extent of bone involvement if metastasis is suspected; will visualize associated soft tissue mass; MRI preferred for evaluation of suspected or impending SCC
4. DEXA scan, as indicated, to evaluate for osteopenia or osteoporosis

V. Differential diagnosis (Beckwée et al., 2017; Moore & Pellegrino, 2017; Portenoy & Ahmed, 2018)
   A. Malignant
      1. Bone metastasis: Axial skeleton is the most common site.
      2. Bone marrow infiltration by tumor
      3. Pathologic fracture (see Chapter 102)
      4. SCC (see Chapter 145)
      5. Hypercalcemia (see Chapter 152)
      6. Hypertrophic osteoarthropathy: Paraneoplastic syndrome (see Appendix M)
      7. Primary bone tumor: Sarcoma
   B. Sequelae from cancer treatment
      1. Growth factor administration: Filgrastim, pegfilgrastim, sargramostim
      2. Arthralgias related to hormone therapy, such as aromatase inhibitors, or chemotherapy, such as docetaxel (see Chapter 96)
      3. Osteonecrosis of the jaw from bone-stabilizing therapy
   C. Arthritis (see Chapters 105 and 108)
   D. Nonmalignant vertebral compression fracture
   E. Osteopenia secondary to drug therapy: Glucocorticoids, post-transplant immunosuppression (see Chapter 106)
   F. Paget disease
   G. Hyper/hypothyroidism (see Chapters 157 and 158)
   H. Benign osteoid osteoma: Most frequent benign bone tumor; may mimic other musculoskeletal conditions because symptoms generally are nonspecific
   I. Acromegaly: Causes bony enlargement and soft tissue thickening of fingers, toes, and scalp

VI. Treatment (Brant et al., 2017; Chiras et al., 2017; Eaton et al., 2017; Filippiadis et al., 2019; Gallicchio et al., 2019; Pin et al., 2018; Shiloh & Krishnan, 2018; Tesfamariam et al., 2019)
   A. Malignant bone pain
      1. Treatment goals
         a) Treatment is dependent on stage of disease, goals of care, and potential success of outcome.
         b) The goals are pain relief, maintenance of function, and prevention of complications.
      2. Pharmacologic management

        a) Opioids: Maximize opioid dosage, as indicated (e.g., primary bone cancer, bone metastasis; see Appendix F)

        b) Coanalgesics: Acetaminophen, NSAIDs (see Appendix E), corticosteroids for short-term relief (see Appendix K), tricyclic antidepressants, SSRIs (see Appendix L), anticonvulsants for neurologic involvement

        c) Bone-stabilizing agents: Bisphosphonates and monoclonal antibodies to prevent skeletal-related events (e.g., pathologic fracture, SCC) that can lead to bone pain

        d) Loratadine: 10 mg PO daily; found to be beneficial in G-CSF–induced bone pain

    3. Radiation therapy

        a) External beam radiation therapy: Targeted to the painful area

        b) Radioisotopes: Bone-targeted agents that extend overall survival while reducing bone pain and symptomatic skeletal events

    4. Radiofrequency ablation: Reduces bone pain by destroying small nerves that carry the pain signal from the bone to spinal cord

    5. Epidural blocks with nerve compression

    6. Surgery: Vertebroplasty, spinal decompression, fixation

  B. Other etiologies: Referral to appropriate medical diagnosis chapter

VII. Follow-up

  A. Follow-up is dependent on diagnosis and treatment plan.

  B. Monitor for potential skeletal-related events.

  C. Monitor pain regimen for relief of pain and for functional improvement. Typically, patients are seen for evaluation within one week after beginning treatment plan.

  D. Monitor for potential neurologic compromise in patients with vertebral metastasis.

VIII. Referrals

  A. Radiation oncologist: For treatment evaluation

  B. Orthopedist: If surgical intervention is required

  C. Interventional radiologist: For radiofrequency ablation, blocks, and vertebroplasty

  D. Physical or occupational therapist: For evaluation of safety issues and mobility and assistance in use of orthotic devices PRN

References

Beckwée, D., Leysen, L., Meuwis, K., & Adriaenssens, N. (2017). Prevalence of aromatase inhibitor-induced arthralgia in breast cancer: A systematic review and meta-analysis. *Supportive Care in Cancer, 25*(5), 1673–1686. https://doi.org/10.1007/s00520-017-3613-z

Brant, J.M., Keller, L., McLeod, K., Yeh, C.H., & Eaton, L.H. (2017). Chronic and refractory pain: A systematic review of pharmacologic management in oncology. *Clinical Journal of Oncology Nursing, 21*(Suppl. 3), 31–59. https://doi.org/10.1188/17.CJON.S3.31-53

Chiras, J., Shotar, E., Cormier, E., & Clarençon, F. (2017). Interventional radiology in bone metastases. *European Journal of Cancer Care, 26*(6), e12741. https://doi.org/10.1111/ecc.12741

Eaton, L.H., Brant, J.M., McLeod, K., & Yeh, C.H. (2017). Nonpharmacologic pain interventions: A review of evidence-based practices for reducing chronic cancer pain. *Clinical Journal of Oncology Nursing, 21*(Suppl. 3), 54–79. https://doi.org/10.1188/17.CJON.S3.54-70

Figura, N., Smith, J., & Yu, H.-H.M. (2018). Mechanisms of, and adjuvants for, bone pain. *Hematology/Oncology Clinics of North America, 32*(3), 447–458. https://doi.org/10.1016/j.hoc.2018.01.006

Filippiadis, D.K., Cornelis, F.H., & Kelekis, A. (2019). Interventional oncologic procedures for pain palliation. *La Presse Médicale, 48* (7–8, Pt. 2), e251–e256. https://doi.org/10.1016/j.lpm.2019.06.006

Gallicchio, R., Mastrangelo, P.A., Nardelli, A., Maienti, P.P., Colasurdo, A.P., Landriscina, M., ... Storto, G. (2019). Radium-223 for the treatment of bone metastases in castration-resistant prostate cancer: When and why. *Tumori, 105*(5), 367–377. https://doi.org/10.1177/0300891619851376

Moore, D.C., & Pellegrino, A.E. (2017). Pegfilgrastim-induced bone pain: A review on incidence, risk factors, and evidence-based management. *Annals of Pharmacotherapy, 51*(9), 797–803. https://doi.org/10.1177/1060028017706373

Pin, Y., Paix, A., Le Fèvre, C., Antoni, D., Blondet, C., & Noël, G. (2018). A systematic review of palliative bone radiotherapy based on pain relief and retreatment rates. *Critical Reviews in Oncology/Hematology, 123,* 132–137. https://doi.org/10.1016/j.critrevonc.2018.01.006

Portenoy, R.K., & Ahmed, E. (2018). Cancer pain syndromes. *Hematology/Oncology Clinics of North America, 32*(3), 371–386. https://doi.org/10.1016/j.hoc.2018.01.002

Russo, M.M., & Sundaramurthi, T. (2019). An overview of cancer pain: Epidemiology and pathophysiology. *Seminars in Oncology Nursing, 35*(3), 223–228. https://doi.org/10.1016/j.soncn.2019.04.002

Shiloh, R., & Krishnan, M. (2018). Radiation for treatment of painful bone metastases. *Hematology/Oncology Clinics of North America, 32*(3), 459–468. https://doi.org/10.1016/j.hoc.2018.01.008

Tesfamariam, Y., Jakob, T., Wöckel, A., Adams, A., Weigl, A., Monsef, I., ... Skoetz, N. (2019). Adjuvant bisphosphonates or RANK-ligand inhibitors for patients with breast cancer and bone metastases: A systematic review and network meta-analysis. *Critical Reviews of Oncology/Hematology, 137,* 1–8. https://doi.org/10.1016/j.critrevonc.2019.02.004

van den Beuken-van Everdingen, M.H.J., Hochstenbach, L.M.J., Joosten, E.A.J., Tjan-Heijnen, V.C.G., & Janssen, D.J.A. (2016). Update on prevalence of pain in patients with cancer: Systematic review and meta-analysis. *Journal of Pain and Symptom Management, 51*(6), 1070–1090.e9. https://doi.org/10.1016/j.jpainsymman.2015.12.340

Zajączkowska, R., Kocot-Kępska, M., Leppert, W., & Wordliczek, J. (2019). Bone pain in cancer patients: Mechanisms and current treatment. *International Journal of Molecular Sciences, 20*(23), 6047. https://doi.org/10.3390/ijms20236047

CHAPTER 98

Low Back Pain

Kathryn R. Waitman, DNP, MSN, FNP-C, AOCNP®

I. Definition: Pain, muscle tension, or stiffness below the costal margin and above the inferior gluteal folds; may be localized to the lumbar area between the inferior ribcage and the waistline, or may include the sciatica, with pain radiating down the posterior–lateral thigh distal to the knee (Traeger et al., 2017; Urits et al., 2019; Will et al., 2018)

   A. Local pain: Caused by injury to pain-sensitive structures that irritate sensory nerve endings

   B. Pain referred from back: Abdominal or pelvic origin

   C. Pain of lower lumbar spine: Restricted to the lower back or referred to lower extremities or buttocks

   D. Radicular back pain: Radiates from spine to leg in specific nerve root

II. Physiology/Pathophysiology (El Sayed et al., 2020; Figura et al., 2018; Russo & Sundaramurthi, 2019)

   A. Normal

   1. The skeletal system has 206 bones, which provide stability and mobility necessary for physical activity.

   2. The lumbar spine forms the caudal flexible portion of an axial structure that supports the head, upper extremities, and internal organs over a bipedal stance. The sacrum forms the foundation of the spine, through which it articulates with the sacroiliac joints to the pelvis.

   3. The lumbar spine is unsupported laterally and has considerable mobility in both the sagittal and coronal planes.

   4. Bony vertebrae act as specialized structures to transport loads through the spine. Vertebral bodies progressively enlarge going down because gravitational loads increase from the cephalic to the caudal segments.

   5. The intervertebral disc consists of the outer annulus fibrosus and the inner nucleus pulposus. The outer portion of the annulus inserts into the vertebral body and accommodates nociceptors and proprioceptive nerve endings. The inner portion of the annulus encapsulates the nucleus, providing the disc with extra strength during compression.

   B. Pathophysiology

   1. Peripheral nociceptors are activated and sensitized by mechanical (e.g., tumor compression, infiltration), thermal, or chemical (e.g., inflammatory mediators such as epinephrine, serotonin, substance P, bradykinin, prostaglandin, histamine) stimuli.

   2. Pain arises from primary afferent and sympathetic nerve fibers associated with blood vessels; pain arises predominantly from the periosteum.

3. Neuropathic and bone pain frequently coexist, especially with encroachment or invasion of nerve roots or the spinal cord (e.g., SCC, brachial and lumbosacral plexopathy).

III. Clinical features: Bone is the most common site of cancer pain and is the third leading metastatic site after lung and liver. Bone pain may be accompanied by a neuropathic component with nerve invasion. Manifestations vary depending on acute (less than 6 weeks), subacute (6–12 weeks), or chronic (greater than 12 weeks) nature. Back pain is the second most common symptom-related reason for clinic visits in the United States. Episodes of back pain typically are self-limited and resolve without therapy; however, recurrent and chronic back pain can interfere with QOL and ADLs (de Oliveira et al., 2019; Figura et al., 2018; Fink et al., 2019; Oliveira et al., 2018; Patel, 2018; Russo & Sundaramurthi, 2019; Urits et al., 2019; van den Beuken-van Everdingen et al., 2016).
   A. Risk factors
       1. Smoking
       2. Obesity
       3. Older age
       4. Female sex
       5. Physically strenuous work
       6. Sedentary work
   B. Etiology
       1. Fracture
       2. Bone metastasis
       3. Trauma
       4. Arthritis
       5. SCC
       6. Vertebral metastasis
       7. Cancers: Bone, multiple myeloma, osteosarcoma
       8. Acromegaly
       9. HZV
      10. Paget disease
      11. Degenerative disc disease
      12. Osteomyelitis
      13. OA
      14. Osteoporosis
   C. History: A complete history will assist in determining potential etiologies of low back pain.
       1. History of cancer and cancer treatment
       2. Current medications: Prescribed, over the counter, corticosteroids
       3. History of presenting symptoms: Precipitating factors, onset, location, duration, associated symptoms (e.g., sciatic pain, weight loss, neurologic deficits)
       4. Changes in ADLs
       5. Past medical history: Radiculopathy, spinal stenosis, trauma, osteoporosis, back pain with failure to improve after four weeks, no relief with bed rest, nonspecific pain
       6. Social history: Illicit drug use
   D. Signs and symptoms
       1. Sciatic pain
       2. Severe leg pain, pseudoclaudication
       3. Gradual onset, morning stiffness, improves with exercise, pain not relieved when supine
       4. Nonspecific pain

5. Numbness and tingling of legs or feet
6. Unilateral pain in distribution of dermatome: Often localized if strictly somatic but can be radicular with nerve involvement; multiple types of pain can be present in multiple locations.
7. Described as constant aching to a deep, boring sensation accompanied by break-through pain; episodes of stabbing pain; with neuropathic involvement, described as shooting, stabbing, radiating, and/or burning

E. Physical examination
    1. Integument: Unilateral dermatomal rash indicating HZV
    2. Musculoskeletal
       a) Decreased spinal range of motion indicating vertebral fracture, lumbar segmental instability, or ankylosing spondylitis
       b) Fever and localized tenderness indicating osteomyelitis or spinal abscess
       c) Localized tenderness indicating malignancy in spine or vertebral fracture with osteoporosis or metastatic bone disease with or without compression fracture
       d) Straight leg raises: Pain with raised leg indicative of herniated disc
       e) Pain over the disease or injured area upon spine palpitation
    3. Neurologic
       a) Presence or absence of and levels (if present) of radiculopathy and myelopathy indicating cerebral or brain stem involvement
       b) Wide-based gait, abnormal Romberg test, and thigh pain after 30 seconds of lumbar extension indicative of potential spinal stenosis
       c) Impaired ankle or patellar reflex; great toe, ankle, or quadriceps weakness; and lower extremity sensory loss indicative of potential degenerative joint disease

IV. Diagnostic tests: Routine imaging or diagnostic testing should not be obtained in patients with nonspecific low back pain. Testing is performed only in select, higher-risk patients who have severe neurologic deficits or the presence of a specific underlying condition (de Oliveira, 2019; Maher et al., 2017; Oliveira et al., 2018; Patel, 2018; Urits et al., 2019).

A. Laboratory
    1. CBC with differential indicating infection or cancer
    2. ESR elevation possibly indicating vertebral infection, cancer, or ankylosing spondylitis
    3. CRP indicating vertebral infection or ankylosing spondylitis
    4. Serum calcium increase possibly indicating cancer or osteoporosis
    5. SPEP to evaluate for multiple myeloma
    6. HLA-B27 elevation indicating ankylosing spondylitis
    7. Increased alkaline and acid phosphatase indicating ankylosing spondylitis

B. Radiology
    1. Plain spine radiograph for initial evaluation of possible vertebral compression fracture in select higher-risk patients, such as those with a history of osteoporosis, osteopenia, or steroid use
    2. MRI (preferred) or CT scan
       a) Useful for visualization of soft tissue and recommended in patients who have severe or progressive neurologic deficits or are suspected of having a serious underlying condition (e.g., vertebral infection, cauda equina syndrome, cancer with impending SCC)
       b) Useful for visualization of bony anatomy and evaluation of patients with persistent back and leg pain who are potential candidates for invasive intervention for possible bulging disc

C. Other: Myelogram or nerve conduction velocity is recommended to detect neuromuscular abnormalities or signs of nerve injury.

V. Differential diagnosis (Patel, 2018; Portenoy & Ahmed, 2018)
   A. Soft tissue strain or sprain
   B. Tumor
   C. Degenerative arthritis of hip
   D. Insufficiency fracture of hip or pelvis (see Chapter 102)
   E. Herniated disc
   F. SCC (see Chapter 145)
   G. Osteoporosis (see Chapter 106)
   H. Spinal stenosis
   I. Spondylosis
   J. Sciatica (see Chapter 109)
   K. Aortic aneurysm

VI. Treatment: Interprofessional modalities should be used to manage low back pain (American Pain Society, 2016; Brant et al., 2017; de Oliveira et al., 2019; Eaton et al., 2017; Figura et al., 2018; Maher et al., 2017; Oliveira et al., 2018; Tagliaferri et al., 2020; Urits et al., 2019).
   A. Restricted activities for one to six weeks: Bed rest for one to two days; ADLs should be resumed as soon as possible.
   B. First-line medications
      1. Acetaminophen: 500–1,000 mg PO every four to six hours PRN; maximum 4,000 mg daily
      2. NSAIDs (see Appendix E)
         a) Ibuprofen: Up to 800 mg PO every six hours PRN; maximum 3,200 mg daily
         b) Naproxen: 500 mg PO two times a day PRN; maximum 1,500 mg daily
      3. Muscle relaxants to relax muscles and relieve pain and discomfort caused by strains, sprains, and other muscle injuries
         a) Cyclobenzaprine: 10 mg PO at bedtime or every eight hours PRN; maximum 30 mg daily
         b) Carisoprodol: 350 mg PO three times a day and at bedtime
         c) Metaxalone: 800 mg PO three to four times a day
      4. Gabapentin for radicular low back pain
   C. Second-line medications: Short-acting opioid analgesics (see Appendix F) should only be considered for moderate to severe pain not controlled with NSAIDs or muscle relaxants.
   D. Epidural blocks with nerve compression
   E. Complementary approaches
      1. Massage
      2. Yoga
      3. Acupuncture
      4. Cold and heat application
      5. Spinal manipulation
      6. Exercise
      7. Change of mattress
   F. Surgery
      1. Spinal interventional procedures
         a) Injection of local anesthetics and corticosteroids into painful soft tissues, facet joints, nerve roots, or epidural spaces
         b) Epidural adhesiolysis to disrupt presumed epidural adhesions

        c) Spinal fusion to manage fracture, infection, progressive deformity, or spondy-lolisthesis leading to instability

        d) Decompression for degenerative disc disease and spondylosis

    2. Spinal laminectomy for herniation

VII. Follow-up (Maher et al., 2017; Urits et al., 2019)

    A. Short term: Estimated duration of care is one to six weeks.

        1. Schedule follow-up at two to four weeks.

        2. Assess the following at each follow-up visit.

            a) Pain

            b) Functional status

            c) Medication-related adverse effects

        3. Reevaluate for possible underlying causes if relief does not occur.

        4. Encourage the patient to maintain normal levels of activity.

        5. Consider ongoing physical therapy.

        6. Educate the patient regarding activity, weight reduction (if applicable), and using medications as prescribed.

    B. Long term: Symptoms can recur in 50%–80% of patients within the first year. Monitor and treat for recurrence.

VIII. Referrals

    A. Neurosurgeon or orthopedist: For intractable pain or severe neurologic deficit

    B. Emergency referral: For patients with cauda equina syndrome

    C. Physical therapist: For exercise

References

American Pain Society. (2016). *Principles of analgesic use in the treatment of acute pain and cancer pain* (7th ed.). APS Press.

Brant, J.M., Keller, L., McLeod, K., Yeh, C.H., & Eaton, L.H. (2017). Chronic and refractory pain: A systematic review of pharmacologic management in oncology. *Clinical Journal of Oncology Nursing, 21*(Suppl. 3), 31–59. https://doi.org/10.1188/17.CJON.S3.31-53

de Oliveira, R.F., Fandim, J.V., Fioratti, I., Fernandes, L.G., Saragiotto, B.T., & Pena Costa, L.O. (2019). The contemporary management of nonspecific lower back pain. *Pain Management, 9*(5), 478–482. https://doi.org/10.2217/pmt-2019-0016

Eaton, L.H., Brant, J.M., McLeod, K., & Yeh, C.H. (2017). Nonpharmacologic pain interventions: A review of evidence-based practices for reducing chronic cancer pain. *Clinical Journal of Oncology Nursing, 21*(Suppl. 3), 54–79. https://doi.org/10.1188/17.CJON.S3.54-70

El Sayed, S.A., Nezwek, T.A., & Varacallo, M. (2020). Physiology, bone. In *StatPearls.* https://www.ncbi.nlm.nih.gov/books/NBK441968

Figura, N., Smith, J., & Yu, H.-H.M. (2018). Mechanisms of, and adjuvants for, bone pain. *Hematology/Oncology Clinics of North America, 32*(3), 447–458. https://doi.org/10.1016/j.hoc.2018.01.006

Fink, R.M., Gates, R.A., & Jeffers, K.D. (2019). Pain assessment. In B.R. Ferrell & J.A. Paice (Eds.), *Oxford textbook of palliative nursing* (5th ed., pp. 98–115). Oxford University Press.

Maher, C., Underwood, M., & Buchbinder, R. (2017). Non-specific low back pain. *Lancet, 389*(10070), 736–747. https://doi.org/10.1016/S0140-6736(16)30970-9

Oliveira, C.B., Maher, C.G., Pinto, R.Z., Traeger, A.C., Lin, C.-W.C., Chenot, J.-F., ... Koes, B.W. (2018). Clinical practice guidelines for the management of non-specific low back pain in primary care: An updated overview. *European Spine Journal, 27*(11), 2791–2803. https://doi.org/10.1007/s00586-018-5673-2

Patel, S.R. (2018). Soft tissue and bone sarcomas and bone metastases. In J.L. Jameson, A.S. Fauci, D.L. Kasper, S.L. Hauser, D.L. Longo, & J. Lossalzo (Eds.), *Harrison's principles of internal medicine* (20th ed.). McGraw-Hill Education. http://accessmedicine.mhmedical.com/content.aspx?bookid=2129&sectionid=192016646

Portenoy, R.K., & Ahmed, E. (2018). Cancer pain syndromes. *Hematology/Oncology Clinics of North America, 32*(3), 371–386. https://doi.org/10.1016/j.hoc.2018.01.002

Russo, M.M., & Sundaramurthi, T. (2019). An overview of cancer pain: Epidemiology and pathophysiology. *Seminars in Oncology Nursing, 35*(3), 223–228. https://doi.org/10.1016/j.soncn.2019.04.002

Tagliaferri, S.D., Miller, C.T., Owen, P.J., Mitchell, U.H., Brisby, H., Fitzgibbon, B., ... Belavy, D.L. (2020). Domains of chronic low back pain and assessing treatment effectiveness: A clinical perspective. *Pain Practice, 20*(2), 211–225 https://doi.org/10.1111/papr.12846

Traeger, A., Buchbinder, R., Harris, I., & Maher, C. (2017). Diagnosis and management of low-back pain in primary care. *CMAJ, 189*(45), E1386–E1395. https://doi.org/10.1503/cmaj.170527

Urits, I., Burshtein, A., Sharma, M., Testa, L., Gold, P.A., Orhurhu, V., ... Kaye, A.D. (2019). Low back pain, a comprehensive review: Pathophysiology, diagnosis, and treatment. *Current Pain and Headache Reports, 23*(3), 23. https://doi.org/10.1007/s11916-019-0757-1

van den Beuken-van Everdingen, M.H.J., Hochstenbach, L.M.J., Joosten, E.A.J., Tjan-Heijnen, V.C.G., & Janssen, D.J.A. (2016). Update on prevalence of pain in patients with cancer: Systematic review and meta-analysis. *Journal of Pain and Symptom Management, 51*(6), 1070–1090.e9. https://doi.org/10.1016/j.jpainsymman.2015.12.340

Will, J.S., Bury, D.C., & Miller, J.A. (2018). Mechanical low back pain. *American Family Physician, 98*(7), 421–428. https://www.aafp.org/afp/2018/1001/p421.html

CHAPTER 99

Muscle Cramps

Kristine Dukart-Harrington, DNP, RN, AGNP-C, ACHPN

I. Definition: Involuntary muscle contractions tending to be localized and abrupt in onset (Katzberg, 2015; Katzberg et al., 2010; Moore, 2016; Swash et al., 2019; Swash & de Carvalho, 2019)

II. Physiology/Pathophysiology (Giuriato et al., 2018; Jahic & Begic, 2018; Katzberg, 2015; Katzberg et al., 2010; Moore, 2016; Rabbitt et al., 2016; Swash et al., 2019; Swash & de Carvalho, 2019)
   A. Normal: Muscle is a type of tissue composed of contractile cells or fibers that affect movement of an organ or body part.
      1. Can contract or shorten to perform functions
      2. Have the properties of irritability, conductivity, and elasticity
      3. Three types of muscles: Smooth, striated, and cardiac
   B. Pathophysiology
      1. Originate in the distal portion of the motor nerves
      2. May reflect spontaneous or elicited neurogenic activity
      3. May be from local muscle fiber damage
      4. Action potentials generated in the motoneuron soma, likely accompanied by an imbalance between the rising excitatory drive from the muscle spindles and the decreasing inhibitory drive from the Golgi tendon organ

III. Clinical features: Muscle cramps are painful and difficult to manage but rarely reflect a serious underlying disease. Cramps can significantly interfere with QOL and frequently occur in neurogenic disorders, such as radiculopathies and polyneuropathies. They are also common in electrolyte imbalances from severe disorders of metabolism. Common triggers are environmental cold or contact with cold surfaces (Hallegraeff & de Greef, 2020; Iwasa et al., 2018; Katzberg et al., 2010; Maisonneuve et al., 2016; Rabbitt et al., 2016; Saguil & Lauters, 2016; Sheehan et al., 2016; Swash et al., 2019; Swash & de Carvalho, 2019).
   A. Etiology
      1. Cancer or cancer treatment related
         a) Chemotherapy
         b) Radiation
         c) Surgery
         d) Compression or infiltration by tumor
         e) Paraneoplastic syndromes
         f) Leptomeningeal disease
      2. Vitamin deficiency: B_1, B_{12}
      3. Diabetes mellitus

    4. Hypothyroidism

    5. Uremia

    6. Previous injury

    7. Guillain-Barré syndrome

    8. Peripheral neuropathy

    9. Amyotrophic lateral sclerosis

    10. Dystonia, writer's cramp

    11. Electrolyte imbalance: Sodium, potassium, magnesium, calcium

    12. Dehydration: Heat induced

    13. Hemodialysis induced: Volume and electrolyte shifts

    14. Drug induced

        a) Hormone therapy

        b) Chemotherapy

        c) Diuretics

        d) Amphotericin B

        e) Cimetidine

        f) Lithium

        g) Clofibrate

        h) Statins

        i) Beta-blockers

        j) Beta-agonists: Inhaled and oral

    15. Nocturnal leg cramps of unknown etiology: More common after age 50 years

    16. Vigorous exercise

    17. Cirrhosis

  B. History

    1. History of cancer and cancer treatment

    2. Current medications: Prescribed, over the counter, especially diuretics and statins

    3. History of presenting symptoms: Precipitating factors, onset, location, duration (e.g., nocturnal pain), associated symptoms (e.g., cold or heat intolerance, profuse sweating, vomiting, diarrhea)

    4. Changes in ADLs

    5. Past medical history: Leptomeningeal disease, renal disease (more common with dialysis), thyroid disease, neuropathies, polio, diabetes, hypothyroidism

    6. Social history: Occupation that affects fine motor activity; vigorous or sustained exercise routine, especially without hydration

    7. Family history: Hereditary myopathy

  C. Signs and symptoms

    1. Acute onset of severe muscle pain: Most commonly occurs in the gastrocnemius muscle

    2. Pain with residual tenderness, even after release of the cramp

    3. Local pain after a severe cramping muscular contraction that persists for several days

    4. Twitching at the start and end of the cramp

    5. May occur after trivial movement or at rest

    6. Alleviated by passive stretching of the muscle

    7. Palpable hardening of affected muscles

    8. Muscle tightness

  D. Physical examination

    1. Vital signs: Postural signs of dehydration

    2. Musculoskeletal

        a) Muscle assessment for spasm, tightness, erythema, warmth, or tenderness

        b) Easily palpable or visibly hardened muscle

        c) Focal weakness in muscle group

    3. Neurologic

        a) Complete neurologic examination to assess for neurologic causes

        b) Absent or abnormal deep tendon reflexes

        c) Trousseau sign indicating tetany (see Appendix D)

        d) Sensory: Distribution of sensory changes

            (1) Position and vibration sense decreased with large fiber loss

            (2) Loss of hot/cold and pain sensation with small fiber loss

        e) Decreased muscle strength or weakness with myopathy

IV. Diagnostic tests (Aldulaimi. 2017; Moore, 2016; Tipton & Wszolek, 2017)

    A. Laboratory

        1. Glucose to evaluate for hypoglycemia

        2. Sodium to evaluate for hyponatremia

        3. Magnesium to evaluate for hypomagnesemia

        4. Calcium to evaluate for hypocalcemia

        5. TSH level to evaluate for hypothyroidism

        6. Vitamin B_{12} level to evaluate for deficiency

    B. Radiology: Typically not helpful

    C. Other: Nerve conduction study may show a high-frequency, high-amplitude discharge of potentials that resemble motor unit potentials. This is frequently preceded or accompanied by fasciculation in the same muscle.

V. Differential diagnosis (Aldulaimi, 2017; Katzberg et al., 2010; Swash et al., 2019; Swash & de Carvalho, 2019)

    A. Neurologic

        1. Peripheral neuropathy (see Chapter 143)

        a) Chemotherapy induced

        b) Vitamin deficiency: B_1, B_{12}

        c) Diabetes mellitus (see Chapter 151)

        d) Hypothyroidism (see Chapter 158)

        e) Paraneoplastic syndrome (see Appendix M)

        2. Nerve root or plexus pathology

        a) Leptomeningeal disease

        b) Compression or infiltration by tumor

        c) Radiation induced

        d) Surgery induced

        e) Guillain-Barré syndrome

        3. Anterior horn disorders: Amyotrophic lateral sclerosis

        4. Dystonia (see Chapter 135)

    B. Myalgias (see Chapter 100)

    C. Dehydration

    D. Contractures

    E. Peripheral vascular disease (see Chapter 51)

    F. Compartment syndrome

    G. Restless legs syndrome (see Chapter 107)

    H. Raynaud syndrome

    I. Opioid withdrawal

    J. Nonalcoholic cirrhosis (see Chapter 69)

    K. Hemodialysis-induced with electrolyte imbalances

VI. Treatment: No clear evidence supports that nonpharmacologic measures prevent or treat severe cramping, but they can be helpful. Pharmacologic treatments have not been well studied in controlled trials (Abd-Elsalam et al., 2019; Chan et al.,1998; El-Tawil et al., 2015; Garrison et al., 2012; Hallegraeff & de Greef, 2020; Jahic & Begic, 2018; Katzberg, 2015; Katzberg et al., 2010; Moledina & Wilson, 2015; Moore, 2016; Rabbitt et al., 2016; Saguil & Lauters, 2016; Sheehan et al., 2016).

A. Treat the underlying cause.

B. Cancer treatment protocol may require dose adjustment or alternative regimen for debilitating cramping.

C. Teach the patient to stretch the cramped muscle (e.g., pointing heel downward for cramping of the calf).

D. Massage the involved muscle.
   1. Passive stretching of contracting muscle
   2. Walking

E. Apply ice locally.

F. Compression garments can be used.

G. Administer pharmacologic agents for relief of cramps. These may have highly variable success and significant side effects.
   1. Quinine sulfate may reduce cramp intensity (200–500 mg PO every night). It is not recommended for routine use or use for more than 60 days because of limited evidence about risk of serious adverse events with longer-term use. It is reserved for most severe cases in which risks of side effects are clearly understood for the relatively low benefit.
      a) Tonic water contains variable amounts of quinine. Monitor for severe side effects such as nausea, vomiting, tinnitus, dysrhythmias, and ITP.
      b) Avoid prescribing with QT-prolonging agents, as quinine can affect cardiac conduction pathways.
      c) Caution should be used. Side effects can include GI upset, abdominal pain, tinnitus, and vertigo. Acute intoxication can lead to serious adverse events, such as dysrhythmias, convulsions, and respiratory arrest.
   2. Gabapentin, vitamin E, and magnesium supplements were found to be equivalent to placebo in relieving cramps in controlled trials. No evidence has been found for the prophylactic benefit of magnesium supplementation to prevent muscle cramps in older adults.
   3. Limited data are available about role of the supplement L-carnitine in reducing muscle cramps.
   4. Diltiazem hydrochloride 30 mg PO daily has been found to be helpful, but note use of other calcium channel blockers before prescribing.
   5. Methocarbamol has shown efficacy in reducing frequency and duration and decreasing pain for muscle cramps in patients with cirrhosis.
   6. B-complex vitamins may reduce the frequency, intensity, and duration of nocturnal leg cramps.

H. Administer targeted electrolyte replacement for documented electrolyte imbalances (see Chapters 152–156), and follow up with appropriate laboratory tests (e.g., ionized calcium, magnesium).

I. Encourage fluid replacement during exercise.

J. Rapidly expand volume with hypertonic dextrose or saline solutions if patient is undergoing hemodialysis.

K. If patient is hypoglycemic, adjust insulin regimen as appropriate (see Chapter 151).

VII. Follow-up
- A. Dependent on the cause of the muscle cramp
- B. Frequent (every month) monitoring of pharmacologic therapy and side effects (e.g., metabolic panels, LFTs, platelet count)

VIII. Referrals
- A. Dependent on cause of muscle cramps
- B. Admittance for severe electrolyte imbalances, such as tetany presentation

The author would like to acknowledge Miriam Rogers, EdD, APRN, AOCN®, CNS, for her contribution to this chapter that remains unchanged from the previous edition of this book.

References

Abd-Elsalam, S., Arafa, M., Elkadeem, M., Elfert, A., Soliman, S., Elkhalawany, W., & Badawi, R. (2019). Randomized-controlled trial of methocarbamol as a novel treatment for muscle cramps in cirrhotic patients. *European Journal of Gastroenterology and Hepatology, 31*(4), 499–502. https://doi.org/10.1097/MEG.0000000000001310

Aldulaimi, S. (2017). Muscle cramps/pain, weakness, muscle twitching, Dx? *Journal of Family Practice, 66*(2), 100–102. https://www.mdedge.com/node/129922/path_term/51948

Chan, P., Huang, T.Y., Chen, Y.J., Huang, W.P., & Liu, Y.C. (1998). Randomized, double-blind, placebo-controlled study of the safety and efficacy of vitamin B complex in the treatment of nocturnal leg cramps in elderly patients with hypertension. *Journal of Clinical Pharmacology, 38*(12), 1151–1154.

El-Tawil, S., Al Musa, T., Valli, H., Lunn, M.P.T., Brassington, R., El-Tawil, T., & Weber, M. (2015). Quinine for muscle cramps. *Cochrane Database of Systematic Reviews, 2015*(4). https://doi.org/10.1002/14651858.CD005044.pub3

Garrison, S.R., Allan, G.M., Sekhon, R.K., Musini, V.M., & Khan, K.M. (2012). Magnesium for skeletal muscle cramps. *Cochrane Database of Systematic Reviews, 2012*(9). https://doi.org/10.1002/14651858.CD009402.pub2

Giuriato, G., Pedrinolla, A., Schena, F., & Venturelli, M. (2018). Muscle cramps: A comparison of the two-leading hypothesis. *Journal of Electromyography and Kinesiology, 41,* 89–95. https://doi.org/10.1016/j.jelekin.2018.05.006

Hallegraeff, J., & de Greef, M. (2020). Pilot testing a stretching regimen for prevention of night time nocturnal leg pain. *Geriatric Nursing, 41*(2), 105–109. https://doi.org/10.1016/j.gerinurse.2019.07.010

Iwasa, M., Karino, Y., Kawaguchi, T., Nakanishi, H., Miyaaki, H., Shiraki, M., ... Koike, K. (2018). Relationship of muscle cramps to quality of life and sleep disturbance in patients with chronic liver diseases: A nationwide study. *Liver International, 38*(12), 2309–2316. https://doi.org/10.1111/liv.13745

Jahic, D., & Begic, E. (2018). Exercise-associated muscle cramp—Doubts about the cause. *Materia Socio-Medica, 30*(1), 67–69. https://doi.org/10.5455/msm.2018.30.67-69

Katzberg, H.D. (2015). Neurogenic muscle cramps. *Journal of Neurology, 262*(8), 1814–1821. https://doi.org/10.1007/s00415-015-7659-x

Katzberg, H.D., Khan, A.H., & So, Y.T. (2010). Assessment: Symptomatic treatment for muscle cramps (an evidence-based review): Report of the therapeutics and technology assessment subcommittee of the American Academy of Neurology. *Neurology, 74*(8), 691–696. https://doi.org/10.1212/WNL.0b013e3181d0ccca

Maisonneuve, H., Chambe, J., Delacour, C., Muller, J., Rougerie, F., Haller, D.M., & Leveque, M. (2016). Prevalence of cramps in patients over the age of 60 in primary care: A cross sectional study. *BMC Family Practice, 17,* 111. https://doi.org/10.1186/s12875-016-0509-9

Moledina, D.G., & Wilson, F.P. (2015). Pharmacologic treatment of common symptoms in dialysis patients: A narrative review. *Seminars in Dialysis, 28*(4), 377–383. https://doi.org/10.1111/sdi.12378

Moore, C. (2016). Evaluation and management of insomnia, muscle cramps, fatigue, and itching in cirrhotic patients. *Clinical Liver Disease, 7*(1), 5–7. https://doi.org/10.1002/cld.516

Rabbitt, L., Mulkerrin, E.C., & O'Keeffe, S.T. (2016). A review of nocturnal leg cramps in older people. *Age and Ageing, 45*(6), 776–782. https://doi.org/10.1093/ageing/afw139

Saguil, A., & Lauters, R. (2016). Quinine for leg cramps. *American Family Physician, 93*(3), 177–178. https://www.aafp.org/afp/2016/0201/p177.html

Sheehan, E.T., Frizzell, J.D., Gabaldon, J., & West, M.B. (2016). Quinine and the ABCs of long QT: A patient's misfortune with arthritis, (alcoholic) beverages, and cramps. *Journal of General Internal Medicine, 31*(10), 1254–1257. https://doi.org/10.1007/s11606-016-3738-7

Swash, M., Czesnik, D., & de Carvalho, M. (2019). Muscular cramp: Causes and management. *European Journal of Neurology, 26*(2), 214–221. https://doi.org/10.1111/ene.13799

Swash, M., & de Carvalho, M. (2019). Testing electrolyte supplementation for muscle cramp. *Muscle and Nerve, 60*(5), 499–500. https://doi.org/10.1002/mus.26686

Tipton, P.W., & Wszolek, Z.K. (2017). Restless legs syndrome and nocturnal leg cramps: A review and guide to diagnosis and treatment. *Polish Archives of Internal Medicine, 127*(12), 865–872. https://doi.org/10.20452/pamw.4148

CHAPTER 100

Myalgia

Kimberly A. Noonan, DNP, ANP-BC, AOCN®

I. Definition (Gerdle et al., 2014; Taylor & Thompson, 2018)
   A. Muscle pain can be associated with spasms, cramping, stiffness, rigidity, or contractures of muscles, which are often described as myalgia.
   B. The true meaning of myalgia is muscle aches, weakness, or tenderness.

II. Physiology/Pathophysiology (Brewer et al., 2016; Keskin et al., 2019; Mammen, 2016; Owens et al., 2019; Queme et al., 2017; Selva-O'Callaghan et al., 2018; Taylor & Thompson, 2018)
   A. Normal
      1. Muscle tissue that attaches to bone is called skeletal muscle. Skeletal muscle consists of elongated cylindrical cells called muscle fibers.
      2. These fibers lie parallel to each other.
      3. Skeletal muscle fibers reveal thread-like structures called myofibrils.
      4. The normal muscle contraction happens by the myofilaments sliding and causing shortening of the muscle.
   B. Pathophysiology: Differs with the cause of myalgia
      1. Fever
         a) Body temperature is controlled in the hypothalamic brain center, and a feedback mechanism is dependent on peripheral sensory input.
         b) Pyrogenic pathogens, drugs, or toxins stimulate the release of cytokines to release prostaglandins and attempt to reset body temperature.
         c) Feedback mechanisms attempt to increase body temperature and generate heat by involuntary muscle contractions.
         d) This may strain the large muscle groups of the body.
      2. Medication induced
         a) Paclitaxel is hypothesized to damage microtubules and, in turn, affects axonal transport in nerves.
         b) Aromatase inhibitors cause an acute decrease in estrogen, which can cause arthralgia and myalgia.
         c) Statin-induced toxicity may be caused by mitochondrial dysfunction, oxidative stress, and impaired mevalonate metabolism. A depletion of intracellular cholesterol occurs, which could potentially affect intracellular signaling and depletion of coenzyme Q10. This cellular interaction reduces mitochondrial respiratory function. Genetic factors may also play a role in statin-related myalgias.
         d) Myalgias and arthralgias may be an early manifestation of peripheral nerve injury caused by many chemotherapy agents.
      3. Cancer related: Bone and soft tissue tumors can involve and penetrate muscle and contiguous tissue, inducing myalgia.

    4. Decreased blood flow to muscle tissue from peripheral vascular disease can cause myalgia.

    5. Autoimmune myopathies are associated with specific autoantibodies, and clinical phenotypes induce myalgias from inflammatory cell infiltrates into the muscle tissue.

III. Clinical features (Amato & Brown, 2020; Cush, 2020; Gerdle et al., 2014; Gunton & Girgis, 2018; Keskin et al., 2019; Owens et al., 2019; Pasnoor et al., 2014; Queme et al., 2017; Taylor & Thompson, 2018)

  A. Etiology

    1. Infection (e.g., viral, spirochetal, bacterial) causing fever

    2. Several medications have the potential to cause myalgia, including the following.

      a) Bisphosphonates: Alendronate, pamidronate, zoledronic acid

      b) Chemotherapy agents: Azacitidine, bortezomib, docetaxel, paclitaxel

      c) Antirheumatic drugs: Azathioprine

      d) Antidysrhythmic: Amiodarone

      e) Monoclonal antibodies: Pembrolizumab, nivolumab, rituximab, durvalumab, atezolizumab

      f) Antimalarial: Chloroquine

      g) Gout medications: Colchicine

      h) Antibiotic: Fluoroquinolones

      i) Immunosuppressant: Cyclosporine, tacrolimus

      j) Growth factors: Colony-stimulating factor, G-CSF

      k) Cytokine therapy: IFN, IL, ipilimumab, cemiplimab, avelumab

      l) Antifungals: Ketoconazole, itraconazole, voriconazole

      m) Dyslipidemia: Niacin, statins

      n) PPIs: Omeprazole

      o) Antiviral: Zidovudine

      p) Vitamin E

    3. Rheumatic or autoimmune disease

      a) Polymyalgia rheumatica

      b) Dermatomyositis

      c) Polymyositis

      d) Arthritis

      e) Multiple sclerosis

    4. Exercise-related or overuse injury

    5. Trauma

    6. Electrolyte imbalances

      a) Hypokalemia

      b) Hypomagnesemia

      c) Hypophosphatemia

    7. Rhabdomyolysis

    8. Drug withdrawal

      a) Antidepressants

      b) Opioids

    9. Liver disease

      a) Hepatitis C

      b) Hepatitis B

      c) Alcoholism

    10. Endocrine disorders

      a) Thyroid disease

   b) Adrenal insufficiency

   c) Long-term glucocorticoid use

  11. FMS

  12. HSCT survivors

  13. Vitamin D deficiency

  14. Depression

  15. Peripheral vascular disease

  16. Joint disease with inflammation

  17. Alcoholism

  18. Chronic fatigue syndrome

B. History

  1. History of cancer and cancer treatment

  2. Current medications: Prescribed, over the counter

  3. History of presenting symptoms: Precipitating factors, onset, location, duration

  4. Changes in ADLs

  5. Social history: Occupation-related injury, alcohol use, exercise pattern

  6. Past medical history: Depression, thyroid disease, hepatitis, trauma, arthralgia, trauma

C. Signs and symptoms

  1. Location of myalgia: Localized, generalized

  2. Diffuse or referred pain: Cramps, aches, spasm, tearing

  3. Fever suggestive of infection

  4. Warmth at the site of myalgia or generalized body warmth

  5. Joint pain or swelling

  6. Paresthesia

  7. Fatigue

  8. Constipation

  9. Weight gain

  10. Depression

D. Physical examination

  1. Vital signs: Tachycardia, increase in temperature, tachypnea

   a) Fever suggestive of viral infection, pyomyositis, endocarditis, or impending sepsis

   b) Hypotension and/or tachycardia suggestive of sepsis

  2. Musculoskeletal

   a) Erythematous or inflamed muscle suggestive of trauma

   b) Point tenderness or referred pain

   c) Presence of muscle spasm

   d) Muscle weakness unilateral/bilateral

   e) Range of motion bilaterally, typically normal

   f) Warmth of muscle

  3. Neurologic

   a) Sensory and motor deficits affecting muscles

   b) Coordination and gait

   c) Reflexes that are delayed, slowed speech, or hoarse voice suggestive of hypothyroidism

   d) Flat affect suggestive of depression

  4. Integument

   a) Rash, lesions, ecchymosis, swelling or decubitus in the region described

   b) Hyperpigmentation indicative of possible adrenal insufficiency

   c) Cutaneous lesions found in SLE, Lyme disease, or psoriasis

IV. Diagnostic tests (Cush, 2020; Gerdle et al., 2014; Taylor & Thompson, 2018)
  A. Laboratory
     1. Electrolytes: Abnormalities are most consistent with muscle cramping or muscle weakness but could be described by the patient as a myalgia.
     2. Blood cultures or viral titers to determine infectious process
     3. Sputum and/or nasal washing to identify bacterial or viral agent
     4. TSH or thyroid panel to assess for hypothyroidism
     5. Creatinine phosphatase kinase to monitor muscle inflammation or muscular damage
     6. Creatinine and GFR to evaluate renal status
     7. ESR or CRP to identify inflammatory process
     8. Urinalysis to identify presence of RBCs, which may indicate rhabdomyolysis
     9. Autoantibodies
        a) Antinuclear antibodies
        b) Antineutrophillic cytoplasmic antibodies
        c) Rheumatoid factor
        d) Anticyclic citrullinated peptide
  B. Radiology: MRI of affected area showing mass or cancer is of concern.
  C. Others
     1. Electromyography to differentiate an inflammatory or metabolic myopathy from neuropathy
     2. Muscle biopsy, as indicated, to determine etiology

V. Differential diagnosis (Amato & Brown, 2020; Cush, 2020; Greenberg & Amato, 2020; Mensch & Zierz, 2020)
  A. Generalized myalgia
     1. FMS (see Chapter 101)
     2. Dermatomyositis: Often associated with malignancy; cancer highly considered
     3. Polymyositis: Associated with malignancy to a lesser degree
     4. Polymyalgia rheumatica
     5. Fabry disease
     6. Guillain-Barré syndrome
     7. Parkinson disease
     8. Amyotrophic lateral sclerosis
     9. Fever (see Chapter 147)
     10. Lyme disease (see Chapter 104)
     11. Electrolyte imbalances (see Chapters 152–156)
     12. Drug-induced myalgia
     13. Chronic fatigue syndrome (see Chapter 163)
     14. Charcot-Marie-Tooth disease
     15. Spinal muscular atrophy
  B. Localized myalgia
     1. Metastatic or bone malignancy
     2. Muscle strain from exertion or tendon damage
     3. Steroid withdrawal
     4. Sarcoidosis
     5. Muscular infarction: Cardiac or diabetic (see Chapters 49 and 151)
     6. DVT (see Chapter 43)

VI. Treatment (Gunton & Girgis, 2018; Owens et al., 2019; Taylor & Thompson, 2018)
  A. Treat underlying disease.

B. Treat infection with appropriate antimicrobial (see Appendix C). If fever-induced myalgia, minimize exposure to chills/rigors by giving antipyretics and warm the body (see Chapter 147).

C. Treat electrolyte imbalance (see Chapters 152–156).

D. Identify medication that has potential to cause myalgia, and educate the patient to the appropriate treatment and length of time myalgia will continue.

E. Massage therapy of a localized muscle may help.

F. Ice or heat, if indicated to localized muscle pain, may alleviate discomfort.

G. Pharmacologic interventions

1. NSAIDs (see Appendix E)
2. Opioids: If NSAIDs do not provide adequate relief (see Appendix F)
3. Neuropathic pain medications: May be used if inflamed muscle is thought to have a neuropathic component (see Appendix L)
4. Vitamin supplementation PRN
   a) Calcium: 1,000–1,200 mg daily
   b) Magnesium: 280 mg for women and 350 mg for men daily
   c) Vitamin D: 1,000 units of vitamin D_3 daily

VII. Follow-up: The patient should be monitored according to specific etiology. Interventions should significantly improve symptoms.

VIII. Referrals: If symptoms of myalgia do not improve with treatment, referral to rheumatology, orthopedics, neurology, or infectious disease consults may be indicated.

References

Amato, A.A., & Brown, R.H. (2020). Muscular dystrophies and other muscle diseases. In J. Jameson, A.S. Fauci, D.L. Kasper, S.L. Hauser, D.L. Longo, & J. Loscalzo (Eds.), *Harrison's principles of internal medicine* (20th ed., pp. 3239–3254). McGraw-Hill.

Brewer, J.R., Morrison, G., Dolan, M.E., & Fleming, G.F. (2016). Chemotherapy-induced peripheral neuropathy: Current status and progress. *Gynecologic Oncology, 140*(1), 176–183. https://doi.org/10.1016/j.ygyno.2015.11.011

Cush, J.J. (2020). Approach to articular and musculoskeletal disorders. In J. Jameson, A.S. Fauci, D.L. Kasper, S.L. Hauser, D.L. Longo, & J. Loscalzo (Eds.), *Harrison's principles of internal medicine* (20th ed., pp. 2614–2631). McGraw-Hill.

Gerdle, B., Ghafouri, B., Emberg, M., & Larsson, B. (2014). Chronic musculoskeletal pain: Review of mechanisms and biochemical biomarkers as assessed by the microdialysis technique. *Journal of Pain Research, 7*, 313–326. https://doi.org/10.2147/JPR.S59144

Greenberg, S.A., & Amato, A.A. (2020). Inflammatory myopathies. In J. Jameson, A.S. Fauci, D.L. Kasper, S.L. Hauser, D.L. Longo, & J. Loscalzo (Eds.), *Harrison's principles of internal medicine* (20th ed., pp. 460–482) McGraw-Hill.

Gunton, J.E., & Girgis, C.M. (2018). Vitamin D and muscle. *Bone Reports, 8*, 163–167. https://doi.org/10.1016/j.bonr.2018.04.004

Keskin, H., Cadirci, K., Demirkazik, A., Akbulut, H., & Yalcin, B. (2019). Following chemotherapy: Serum cytokine (tumor necrosis factor, interleukin-2, interleukin-11), immunoglobulin, complement, vascular endothelial growth factor levels, and the systemic symptoms like capillary leak syndrome. *Biomarkers in Cancer, 11*. https://doi.org/10.1177/1179299X19854447

Mammen, A.L. (2016). Autoimmune myopathies. *Continuum, 22*(6), 1852–1870. https://doi.org/10.1212/01.CON.0000511070.50715.ab

Mensch, A., & Zierz, S. (2020). Cellular stress in the pathogenesis of muscular disorders: From cause to consequence. *International Journal of Molecular Sciences, 21*(16), 5830. https://doi.org/10.3390/ijms21165830

Owens, D.J., Twist, C., Cobley, J.N., Howatson, G., & Close, G.L. (2019). Exercise-induced muscle damage: What it is, what causes it and what are the nutritional solutions? *European Journal of Sport Science, 19*(1), 71–85. https://doi.org/10.1080/17461391.2018.1505957

Pasnoor, M., Barohn, R.J., & Dimachkie, M.M. (2014). Toxic myopathies. *Neurologic Clinics, 32*(3), 647–670. https://doi.org/10.1016/j.ncl.2014.04.009

Queme, L.F., Ross, J.L., & Jankowski, M.P. (2017). Peripheral mechanisms of ischemic myalgia. *Frontiers in Cellular Neuroscience, 11,* 419. https://doi.org/10.3389/fncel.2017.00419

Selva-O'Callaghan, A., Alvarado-Cardenas, M., Pinal-Fernández, I., Trallero-Araguás, E., Millsenda, J.C., Martínez, M.A., ... Grau-Junyent, J.M. (2018). Statin-induced myalgia and myositis: An update on pathogenesis and clinical recommendations. *Expert Review in Clinical Immunology, 14*(3), 215–224. https://doi.org/10.1080/1744666X.2018.1440206

Taylor, B.A., & Thompson, P.D. (2018). Statin-associated muscle disease: Advances in diagnosis and management. *Neurotherapeutics, 15*(4), 1006–1017. https://doi.org/10.1007/s13311-018-0670-z

CHAPTER 101

Fibromyalgia Syndrome

Marlon Garzo Saria, PhD, RN, FAAN, and Santosh Kesari, MD, PhD, FANA, FAAN

I. Definition: Chronic disorder defined by widespread musculoskeletal pain, often accompanied by fatigue, cognitive dysfunction, and sleep disturbance (Arnold et al., 2016; Borchers & Gershwin, 2015; Chinn et al., 2016; Duque & Fricchione, 2019; Stournaras & Petrovic, 2019)

II. Physiology/Pathophysiology (Arnold et al., 2016; Borchers & Gershwin, 2015; Chinn et al., 2016)
   A. Normal
      1. Acute pain sensation is the result of noxious stimuli affecting normal tissue.
         a) Nociception involves transduction, transmission, perception, and modulation.
         b) Nociceptors (A-delta and C fibers) are present in somatic and visceral structures.
      2. Noxious stimuli (i.e., mechanical, thermal, and chemical) cause the release of chemical mediators (e.g., prostaglandin, bradykinin, serotonin, substance P, potassium, histamine) from damaged cells.
      3. The pain impulse from noxious stimuli is transmitted via A-delta and C fibers, which terminate at the dorsal horn of the spinal cord. The pain impulse is next transmitted to the nociceptive dorsal horn neurons by the release of neurotransmitters. The pain impulse then ascends to the brain.
      4. Perception of pain activates multiple areas of the brain.
         a) Reticular system: Automatic and motor responses
         b) Somatosensory cortex: Perception and interpretation of pain
         c) Limbic system: Emotional and behavioral response to pain
      5. Modulation of pain either leads to an increased or decreased transmission of pain impulses in the spinal cord. The release of neurotransmitters produces analgesia and includes the following.
         a) Endorphins
         b) 5-HT (5-hydroxytryptamine)
         c) Gamma-aminobutyric acid
         d) Neurotensin
         e) Acetylcholine
         f) Oxytocin
   B. Pathophysiology: Cause is unknown; however, studies suggest genetic predisposition and possible triggering events.
      1. Dysfunction in CNS pain processing mechanisms including central sensitization or central augmentation of pain contribute to the development of chronic pain in patients with FMS.
         a) Results in the "volume control" for pain being turned up
         b) Allodynia: A heightened sensitivity to stimuli that are not normally painful

        c) Hyperalgesia: An increased response to painful stimuli

    2. The theory of central sensitization or central augmentation explains both the heterogeneous clinical aspects of FMS and several of the associated symptoms.

    3. Many of the same neurotransmitters that control pain and sensory sensitivity also control sleep, mood, memory, and alertness.

III. Clinical features: FMS is the second most common musculoskeletal disorder after OA and is considerably more common than RA or other autoimmune disorders. It is often associated with other symptoms or comorbid conditions (Arnold et al., 2016; Borchers & Gershwin, 2015; Chinn et al., 2016; Clauw, 2014; Clauw et al., 2018; Duque & Fricchione, 2019; Stournaras & Petrovic, 2019; Tan et al., 2019).

  A. Risk factors

    1. Pain-prone phenotype: Manifested as having many discrete episodes of chronic pain

    2. Environmental

      a) Psychiatric or affective spectrum disorders: Depression, anxiety

      b) Prior acute or chronic medical illness

      c) Can be triggered by certain types of infections: Epstein-Barr virus, Lyme disease, Q fever, viral hepatitis

      d) Trauma to skeletal system or trunk

      e) Military deployment to war inducing emotional or traumatic stress

    3. Genetic factors: First-degree relatives of patients with FMS have an eightfold increased likelihood of developing FMS.

    4. Female sex: Women outnumber men by an average of 3:1 worldwide.

    5. Lower education level and other indicators of lower social status

    6. Peak prevalence rates in the sixth or seventh decade of life

  B. Etiology: Centralized pain state with an unknown etiology is a lifelong disorder, beginning in adolescence or young adulthood, and is manifested by pain experienced in different body regions at different times.

  C. History

    1. History of cancer and cancer treatment

    2. Current medications: Prescribed, over the counter

    3. History of presenting symptoms: Precipitating factors, onset, location, duration

    4. Changes in ADLs

    5. Past medical history: Rheumatic disease, psychiatric disorders, migraine, TMJ, chronic fatigue syndrome, IBS, endometriosis, thyroid disorders

    6. Social history: Military service, stress level

    7. Family history: Fibromyalgia

  D. Signs and symptoms

    1. Chronic multifocal or diffuse pain is the defining feature of FMS. Core symptom is chronic, widespread pain. It occurs most frequently in the shoulders, arms, lower back, buttocks, and thighs as throbbing, aching, or tender pain.

    2. At least 75% of patients report fatigue.

    3. Approximately 70%–90% report poor sleep quality.

    4. At least 76% report concentration difficulties, forgetfulness, mental confusion, or a combination of these complaints.

    5. Mood disorders

      a) Major depression: 20%–86%

      b) Anxiety disorders: 27%–60%

      c) Post-traumatic stress disorder: 3%–57%

  E. Physical examination

1. Vital signs: Self-report pain measures (e.g., body pain diagram, assessment of symptoms)
2. Neurology: Evaluation may yield normal examination or a decrease or increase in neurologic findings.
    a) Cranial nerves (see Appendix A)
    b) Cerebellar: Presence of tremor, dysdiadochokinesia, dysmetria
    c) Sensory deficits: Analgesia, anesthesia
    d) Dissociated sensory loss and impaired proprioception
    e) Vibration, temperature, or pinprick sensation
    f) Dorsal columns: Romberg sign
    g) Motor: Weakness, impaired fine motor control, decreased or increased tone, atrophy
    h) Reflex testing: Hyperreflexia or hyporeflexia, Babinski sign, clonus, trophic joint changes
    i) Gait: Ataxia, tandem maneuvers, stance
    j) Neuropsychological: Mini-Mental State Examination
3. Extremities
    a) Joints for the presence of inflammation
    b) Tenderness or pain by palpation

F. Diagnostic criteria
1. Widespread pain index (WPI) greater than or equal to 7 and symptom severity (SS) scale greater than or equal to 5, or WPI 3–6 and SS greater than or equal to 9
    a) WPI is obtained by summing the body areas (out of a possible 19 sites) in which the patient indicates having experienced pain during the preceding week.
    b) SS scale consists of two parts.
        (1) Patient grades the severity of three somatic symptoms (waking unrefreshed, disturbed cognition, and fatigue) over the past week on a scale of 0–3 (maximum score of 9).
        (2) Provider rates the overall extent of somatic symptoms on a four-point scale (0—absent; 1—slight; 2—moderate; 3—severe).
2. Symptoms have been present at a similar level for at least three months.
3. No other etiology exists to explain the pain.

IV. Diagnostic tests (Arnold et al., 2016; Clauw, 2014)
A. Laboratory: Laboratory testing is not useful for establishing a diagnosis of FMS but allows assessment of potential causes.
1. CBC to assess for anemia or infection
2. Serum chemistries to assess for electrolyte imbalance and renal function
3. ESR and CRP for potentially useful evaluation of inflammatory, arthritic, or myalgia conditions
4. Vitamin D to assess for deficiency
5. LFTs to assess for liver disease: Hepatitis, cirrhosis
6. Thyroid function test to assess for hypothyroidism
7. Detailed serologic studies (e.g., antinuclear antibody, rheumatoid factor assays) often not necessary unless an autoimmune or other condition is suspected
B. Radiology: Not routinely performed

V. Differential diagnosis (Chinn et al., 2016; Stournaras & Petrovic, 2019)
A. Inflammatory and autoimmune disorders: RA (see Chapter 108), SLE (see Chapter 110), Sjögren syndrome, polymyalgia rheumatica, spondylarthritis

    B. Muscle disorders and myalgias (see Chapter 100)

    C. Endocrinopathies: Hypothyroidism (see Chapter 158), hyperparathyroidism

    D. Neurologic disorders: Peripheral neuropathies (see Chapter 143), nerve entrapment syndromes, multiple sclerosis, myasthenia gravis

    E. Myofascial pain syndrome, TMJ dysfunction, low back pain (see Chapter 98)

    F. Headache disorders (see Chapter 137)

VI. Treatment: Lack of consensus on management often results in patients seeing multiple specialists, exhaustive investigations, prescription of multiple drugs to treat different symptoms, increased disability, and increased healthcare resource utilization (Arnold et al., 2016; Borchers & Gershwin, 2015; Chinn et al., 2016; Clauw, 2015; Clauw et al., 2018; Kim et al., 2019; Lian et al., 2020).

    A. Current treatment options focus on symptom-based management to improve function and QOL rather than disease modification. Even minor symptomatic improvements may improve patient function.

    B. Integration of pharmacologic and nonpharmacologic treatments will give the best outcomes. This requires a multimodal approach consisting of education, cognitive behavioral therapy, exercise, and pharmacologic therapy.

    C. Nonpharmacologic measures

        1. Patient education: Provide core information about diagnosis, treatment, and prognosis; manage expectations.

        2. Exercise: Start low, go slow. Build up to moderate activity over time, including aerobic exercise, resistance training, or flexibility training.

        3. Cognitive behavioral therapy: Methods include face-to-face counseling, online self-help courses, books, audio CDs, and websites.

        4. Sleep hygiene: Optimize sleep environment and prioritize relaxing sleep routine.

        5. Complementary and alternative medicine: Examples include tai chi, yoga, massage, diet, balneotherapy, and acupuncture.

        6. Mind and body therapy/meditative movement therapy: Examples include qigong.

    D. Pharmacologic measures

        1. NSAIDs are commonly prescribed for FMS despite limited evidence of efficacy (see Appendix E).

        2. FDA-approved drugs

            a) Pregabalin: Starting dose of 150 mg PO daily, titrated to maximum of 450 mg PO daily

            b) Duloxetine: 60–120 mg PO daily

            c) Milnacipran: Starting dose of 12.5 mg PO daily, titrated to maximum of 100 mg PO two times a day

            d) Increases the activity of inhibitory neurotransmitters to decrease the pain sensation

            e) Reduces the activity of facilitatory neurotransmitters

        3. Medications not approved but have demonstrated efficacy in randomized controlled trails

            a) Amitriptyline: 10 mg PO nightly, increased to 25–50 mg nightly

            b) Cyclobenzaprine: 5–10 mg PO three times a day, titrated as tolerated to maximum dose of 30 mg PO daily; not recommended to use longer than two to three weeks in older adults

            c) Gabapentin: 300 mg PO at night, titrated up to 3,600 mg PO daily

        4. Short-acting strong opioids: Commonly prescribed treatment (both before and after diagnosis); limited evidence of efficacy (see Appendix F)

   a) Opioids have demonstrated no efficacy in FMS and are associated with potentially severe side effects.
   b) Patients who receive opioids may experience poorer outcomes.
   c) Opioids may be considered for refractory pain when other agents have failed.
   5. Drugs with more limited evidence of efficacy: Older SSRIs (e.g., fluoxetine, paroxetine, sertraline; see Appendix L), low-dose naltrexone, esreboxetine (an SSRI not available in the United States), cannabinoids, memantine
   E. Trigger point injections, chiropractic manipulation, and myofascial release therapy have some evidence of efficacy and are among the more commonly used modalities.
   F. Neurostimulatory therapies, such as transcutaneous electrical nerve stimulation, can be effective.

VII. Follow-up
   A. Short term: Schedule regular visits initially to evaluate therapy.
   B. Long term: Schedule every three to six months to monitor symptoms and therapy.

VIII. Referrals: If the symptom or medical diagnosis warrants a referral to a specialist (Clauw, 2014, 2015; Clauw et al., 2018)
   A. Individuals with FMS should not readily be referred to proceduralists because this type of CNS pain will not respond to peripherally directed injections and surgical procedures.
   B. Referral to specialists should be necessary only for patients in whom the diagnosis is uncertain (e.g., to a rheumatologist or neurologist, depending on symptoms) or for patients refractory to therapy (e.g., interprofessional pain clinics) or with significant comorbid psychiatric issues (e.g., psychiatrist, psychologist).
   C. Psychological, behavioral, and social issues can both contribute to the underlying pathogenesis of FMS and complicate its treatment.

The authors would like to acknowledge Deanna Sanchez Yamamoto, RN, MS, ANP, for her contribution to this chapter that remains unchanged from the previous edition of this book.

References

Arnold, L.M., Gebke, K.B., & Choy, E.H.S. (2016). Fibromyalgia: Management strategies for primary care providers. *International Journal of Clinical Practice, 70*(2), 99–112. https://doi.org/10.1111/ijcp.12757

Borchers, A.T., & Gershwin, M.E. (2015). Fibromyalgia: A critical and comprehensive review. *Clinical Reviews in Allergy and Immunology, 49*(2), 100–151. https://doi.org/10.1007/s12016-015-8509-4

Chinn, S., Caldwell, W., & Gritsenko, K. (2016). Fibromyalgia pathogenesis and treatment options update. *Current Pain and Headache Reports, 20*(4), 25. https://doi.org/10.1007/s11916-016-0556-x

Clauw, D.J. (2014). Fibromyalgia: A clinical review. *JAMA, 311*(15), 1547–1555. https://doi.org/10.1001/jama.2014.3266

Clauw, D.J. (2015). Fibromyalgia and related conditions. *Mayo Clinical Proceedings, 90*(5), 680–692. https://doi.org/10.1016/j.mayocp.2015.03.014

Clauw, D.J., D'Arcy, Y., Gebke, K., Semel, D., Pauer, L., & Jones, K.D. (2018). Normalizing fibromyalgia as a chronic illness. *Postgraduate Medicine, 130*(1), 9–18. https://doi.org/10.1080/00325481.2018.1411743

Duque, L., & Fricchione, G. (2019). Fibromyalgia and its new lessons for neuropsychiatry. *Medical Science Monitor Basic Research, 25,* 169–178. https://doi.org/10.12659/MSMBR.915962

Kim, S.Y., Busch, A.J., Overend, T.J., Schachter, C.L., van der Spuy, I., Boden, C., … Bidonde, J. (2019). Flexibility exercise training for adults with fibromyalgia. *Cochrane Database of Systematic Reviews, 2019*(9). https://doi.org/10.1002/14651858.CD013419

Lian, Y.-N., Wang, Y., Zhang, Y., & Yang, C.-X. (2020). Duloxetine for pain in fibromyalgia in adults: A systematic review and a meta-analysis. *International Journal of Neuroscience, 130*(1), 71–82. https://doi.org/10.1080/00207454.2019.1664510

Stournaras, D., & Petrovic, K. (2019). Fibromyalgia treatment and management considerations for nurse practitioners. *Journal of the American Association of Nurse Practitioners, 31*(6), 371–377. https://doi.org/10.1097/JXX.0000000000000178

Tan, A.C., Jaaniste, T., & Champion, D. (2019). Chronic widespread pain and fibromyalgia syndrome: Life-course risk markers in young people. *Pain Research and Management, 2019,* 6584753. https://doi.org/10.1155/2019/6584753

CHAPTER 102

Fractures

Kimberly A. Noonan, DNP, ANP-BC, AOCN®

I. Definition: A break in the continuity of bone that occurs when stress placed on the bone exceeds biologic loading capacity (Baker et al., 2018; Morgan et al., 2014; Singaram & Naidoo, 2019)

II. Physiology/Pathophysiology (Baker et al., 2018; Jha et al., 2019; Lewiecki et al., 2016; Loi et al., 2016; Morshed, 2014; Ottanelli, 2015; Tarantino et al., 2017; Tins et al., 2015; Tsuzuki et al., 2016)
   A. Normal: Composed of two types of bone—cortical and trabecular
      1. Cortical bone is located on the outer part of the bone and is responsible for the strength of the bone.
      2. Trabecular bone located in the inner aspect of the bone has direct contact with the blood supply.
      3. Normal bone can withstand considerable compression, shearing, and tension forces.
      4. Under normal conditions, bone undergoes remodeling, a process that allows the bone to break down and build back up, providing the strength in bones.
      5. There are four types of bone cells.
         a) Osteoblasts are the cells in the bone responsible for bone replacement and building.
         b) Osteoclasts are the cells in the bone responsible for bone resorption or break-down of mature bone.
         c) Osteoprogenitor cells are undifferentiated cells found in the periosteum, endosteum, and epiphyseal plate of developing bone. These cells differentiate into osteoblasts and are activated during normal growth, healing fractures, or when mature bone requires replacement.
         d) Osteocytes are mature bone cells involved in maintaining the bony matrix. They are responsible for releasing calcium into the blood.
      6. Bone healing is typically divided into three stages: inflammatory, reparative, and remodeling. Healing rates vary widely according to age and comorbidities.
   B. Pathophysiology
      1. Fracture of the bone occurs when more stress is placed on the bone and the bone is unable to accommodate.
      2. Nonmalignant bone fractures
         a) Sudden injury by direct force (e.g., from falling) or indirect force caused by a massive muscle contraction from trauma is the most common type of fracture.
         b) Stress fractures or fatigue are caused by repeated wear on the bone and overuse by exercise.
      3. Pathologic fractures are certain conditions that change the normal physiology of bone. The bones are weakened by disease or tumors caused by tumors, infections,

or cysts. The underlying problem can be generalized (e.g., aging population, Paget disease).

4. Osteoporosis is a systemic skeletal disease caused by a decrease in bone density and a deterioration in bone quality associated with hormonal and age-related changes in the bone microarchitecture.

   a) Osteoporosis causes a decline in bone mineral density, an increase in bone fragility, and a propensity to develop bone fractures.

   b) Osteoclastic activity is enhanced while a decrease in osteoblast activity occurs, causing bones to thin in certain areas.

5. Malignant bone fractures

   a) Metastatic disease that spreads to the bone is common. Sites of metastatic disease are the long bones. The spine is the most common site of metastatic bone.

   b) Lesions caused by osteoblasts (bone-building cells), known as osteosclerotic lesions, are prevalent in certain cancers (e.g., prostate, small cell lung) and weaken the bone.

      (1) Tumor cells express multiple osteoclast-stimulating factors.

      (2) Marrow stromal cells express messenger RNA to stimulate osteoclastogenesis and cause thickened bone.

   c) Lesions caused by osteoclasts (osteolytic lesions) are bone resorption cells that breakdown bone, are prevalent in certain types of malignancies (e.g., multiple myeloma, breast, renal cell, non-small cell lung), and weaken the bone.

      (1) Osteoclast precursors express receptor activator of nuclear factor kappa-B (RANK) on the cell surface.

      (2) RANK allows the osteoclast precursors to respond to the respective ligand.

      (3) RANK ligand (RANKL) is expressed on the surfaces of osteoblasts, which secrete osteoprotegerin. Osteoprotegerin is the decoy receptor that sequesters RANKL and blocks its action.

      (4) RANKL is the master osteoclastogenic mediator controlling formation and function of mature osteoclasts.

III. Clinical features: An estimated 12–15 million fractured bones occur annually in the United States (Jha et al., 2019; Loi et al., 2016; Ottanelli, 2015; Pollak & Watkins-Castillo, 2014; Tarantino et al., 2017; Tins et al., 2015; Tsuzuki et al., 2016).

A. Etiology

1. Nonpathogenic: Trauma

   a) Direct contact with an object

   b) Twisting motion that is usually sudden

   c) Crushing force

2. Pathogenic

   a) Metastatic disease: Breast, lung, prostate, melanoma, thyroid

   b) Primary malignancy: Multiple myeloma, sarcoma

3. Osteoporosis

4. Medications: Not an all-inclusive listing

   a) Glucocorticoids

   b) Aromatase inhibitors

   c) Long-term bisphosphonate use causing atypical femur fractures

   d) Gonadotropin-releasing hormone agonists and antagonists

   e) Thiazolidinediones

   f) PPIs

      g) SSRIs
- 5. Lifestyle or indirect effects of cancer therapies affecting bone health
    - *a)* Decrease in dietary calcium or calcium supplementation
    - *b)* Decrease in vitamin D from poor nutrition, lack of supplementation, or limited sun exposure
    - *c)* Sedentary lifestyle with limited weight-bearing physical activity
    - *d)* Postmenopausal or ovarian ablation: Medically or surgically induced
    - *e)* Cachexia
- 6. Severe muscle contraction

B. Classification of fractures: Appearance, general description, anatomic location
- 1. Appearance
    - *a)* Burst: Multiple pieces of bone located at the end of the bone
    - *b)* Comminuted: More than one fracture line and more than two fragments
    - *c)* Complete: Break across entire section of bone
    - *d)* Displaced: Fracture out of normal position
    - *e)* Incomplete: Fracture through only one cortex
    - *f)* Longitudinal: Fracture line extends in the direction of longitudinal axis
    - *g)* Nondisplaced: Fragments in normal position of fracture site
    - *h)* Oblique: Fracture approximately 45° angle across longitudinal axis of bone
    - *i)* Spiral: Fracture line encircles bone
    - *j)* Stellate: Fracture line radiated from central point
    - *k)* Transverse: Fracture at 90° angle to longitudinal axis of bone
    - *l)* Open: Bone exposed through the skin
        - (1) Puncture wound less than 1 cm with minimal contamination and muscle injury
        - (2) Laceration greater than 1 cm with moderate soft tissue injury
        - (3) Extensive soft tissue damage with sever crush injury of muscle and massive contamination
    - *m)* Closed: Bone not exposed through the skin
- 2. General description
    - *a)* Avulsion: Fragments (e.g., ligaments, tendons) that tear away from bone
    - *b)* Compression: Bone buckles and cracks; unusual loading force on longitudinal axis
    - *c)* Greenstick: Incomplete fracture in which one side of the cortex is broken and the other side is flexed but intact; occurs most often in children
    - *d)* Impact: One bone fragment driven into the other
    - *e)* Pathologic: Bone weakened by an underlying illness
    - *f)* Stress: Repeated stress on a bone (e.g., from running, bone overuse)
- 3. Anatomic location or eponym
    - *a)* Colles fracture: Occurs within the last inch of the distal radius with distal fragments displaced in position of dorsal and medial deviation
    - *b)* Pott fracture: Occurs in distal fibula where the internal and lateral ligaments rupture; often causes chips in the medial malleolus
- 4. Types of long bone deformities caused by a fracture
    - *a)* Angulation: Fragments may be felt at the fracture site and may push up against the soft tissue, which may cause a tenting effect on the skin.
    - *b)* Shortened: Bone fragments slide and override each other because of the pull of the muscles on the long axis of the extremity.
    - *c)* Rotation: The fracture fragments rotate out of their normal longitudinal axis, which can cause a rotational strain.

C. History
1. History of cancer and cancer treatments
2. Current medications: Prescribed, over the counter
3. History of presenting symptoms: Precipitating factors, onset, location, duration
4. Changes in ADLs
5. Past medical history: Osteoporosis, osteopenia, neurologic disease, musculoskeletal abnormalities, recent falls, trauma
6. Social history
    a) Tobacco use, alcohol use
    b) Low BMI
7. Family history of osteoporosis or osteopenia

D. Signs and symptoms
1. Pain at fracture site: Approximately 60%–84% develop pain.
2. Point tenderness
3. Inability to bear weight; significantly diminished mobility
4. Loss of bony or limb contour
5. Edema or joint effusion
6. Ecchymosis or discoloration
7. Limb shortening
8. Diminished range of motion
9. Open wound and bone exposure

E. Physical examination
1. Vital signs: Signs of shock (e.g., hypotension) caused by blood loss, especially if caused by trauma
2. Cardiac: Assessment for adequate tissue perfusion, extremity palpitation for pulses bilaterally
3. Musculoskeletal
    a) Deformity or crepitus on palpitation: Caused by bone fragments
    b) Assessment of range of motion of extremity after radiologic assessment to prevent exacerbating fracture displacement, soft tissue damage, or neurovascular compromise
    c) Inability to bear weight, gait abnormalities, loss of function
    d) Assessment of soft tissue injury to determine microvascular and inflammatory responses that could cause tissue hypoxia and acidosis
        (1) Superficial abrasions or contusions
        (2) Skin contusion or crush with severe damage to underlying muscle
    e) Tenderness of site on palpitation
    f) Edema and deformity of affected bone
4. Integument: Skin abrasions, ecchymosis, fracture blisters, bleeding
5. Neurologic
    a) Mental status for symptoms of shock: Confusion, lethargy
    b) Loss of sensation in the affected extremity

IV. Diagnostic tests (Loi et al., 2016; Ottanelli, 2015; Tarantino et al., 2017, Tins et al., 2015; Tsuzuki et al., 2016)
A. Laboratory: Indicated if surgery required
1. CBC including platelets to evaluate need for blood products
2. PT, PTT, INR
3. Chemistries to evaluate renal status and electrolytes
4. Wound culture if open fracture and wound at risk for contamination

     5. Tumor markers to determine status of disease if suspected pathologic fracture (see Appendix O)

B. Radiology

    1. Anterior–posterior and lateral x-ray: Used most often to diagnose fracture

    2. MRI: May be helpful to evaluate complicated fracture, stress fractures, and scaphoid fractures

    3. CT scan: Used to assess small bones and stress fractures

    4. Bone scans: If metastasis is suspected

    5. PET-CT: Used to evaluate for metastases with pathological fracture

C. Other

    1. Arthroscopy: Used to identify intra-articular fractures

    2. DEXA scan

       a) Used to identify osteoporosis or osteopenia.

       b) Directly measures bone mineral mass and indirectly measures bone strength

V. Differential diagnosis (Jha et al., 2019; Ottanelli, 2015; Subbiah & West, 2016)

A. Multiple myeloma

B. Bone metastasis

C. Osteosarcoma

D. Osteoporosis (see Chapter 106)

E. Osteopenia (see Chapter 106)

F. Muscle destruction

    1. Sprain

    2. Strain

G. Dislocation

H. Subluxation

I. Hematoma

J. Paget disease

K. Osteomalacia

L. Benign tumor: Osteochondromas, enchondromas, giant cell tumor

VI. Treatment (Geusens et al., 2019; Halvachizadeh et al., 2019; Jha et al., 2019; Loi et al., 2016; Morgan et al., 2014; Singaram & Naidoo, 2019; Subbiah & West, 2016; Tins et al., 2015)

A. Determined by the following

    1. Cause of fracture

    2. Extent of injury

    3. Ability to align bone fragments

    4. Ability to immobilize fracture

    5. Complications of fracture caused by trauma

       a) Fracture blisters

       b) Compartment syndrome

       c) Reflex sympathetic dystrophy and causalgia

       d) Fat embolism syndrome

       e) Osteomyelitis

B. Pathologic fracture from malignancy

    1. Consider treatment options and QOL.

    2. Radiation should be used for radiosensitive tumors and pain control.

    3. Consider chemotherapy as a single agent or combination.

    4. Consider medication to strengthen the bone and prevent future fracture.

       a) Bisphosphonate therapy if bone metastasis or osteoporosis is the cause (see Chapter 106)

       b) Denosumab, a monoclonal antibody and antagonist of RANKL, if osteoporosis or bone metastasis is the cause (see Chapter 106)

       c) Diet with adequate calcium, vitamin D, and supplementation

  C. Nonpathologic fracture

    1. Immobilization of bone

    2. Bed rest: Vertebrae or pelvis

    3. Immobilization devices: Closed reduction

       a) Casts: Most effective method to immobilize bone; hard or soft cast

       b) Collars

       c) Splints

       d) Slings/swathes

  D. External fixation and surgical interventions

    1. Used to penetrate fracture fragments and attach to universal joints

       a) Kirschner wires

       b) Steinmann pins

    2. Comminuted fractures with extensive tissue injury

    3. Neurovascular injury

  E. Traction

    1. Less popular intervention with improved surgical techniques

    2. Skeletal traction used for multiple trauma victims who are not immediate surgical candidates

    3. Pulling force applied to achieve reduction at fracture site

  F. Continuous passive movement: Machine that places joint through repeated extension and flexion; used as adjunctive therapy

  G. Electrical bone stimulation

    1. Device used when fracture healing is delayed

    2. Designed to go over cast or can be implanted near the site of the fracture

  H. Progressive range of motion and muscle strengthening requiring physical therapy: Necessary after immobilization period to aid in regaining joint and muscle function

  I. Devices to support fractured limb: Crutches, walker, cane

  J. Pain management (see Appendices E and F)

VII. Follow-up (Halvachizadeh et al., 2019)

  A. In malignancy-induced fracture, follow up with medical oncology for treatment.

  B. Physical therapy is often required after a fracture to regain mobilization and bone strength.

  C. Follow up with an orthopedic specialist if bone strength or mobilization is not restored.

VIII. Referrals

  A. Radiation oncologist or medical oncologist: For treatment of cancer

  B. Orthopedic specialist: For mobilization of fracture

  C. Physical therapy: For strengthening exercises and training

  D. Occupational or physical therapy: To assess functional status and physical status

References

Baker, C.E., Moore-Lotridge, S.N., Hysong, A.A., Posey, S.L., Robinette, J.P., Blum, D.M., … Schoenecker, J.G. (2018). Bone fracture acute phase response—A unifying theory of fracture repair: Clinical and scientific implications. *Clinical Reviews in Bone and Mineral Metabolism, 16*(4), 142–158. https://doi.org/10.1007/s12018-018-9256-x

Geusens, P., Lems, W.F., Bours, S., & van den Bergh, J.P. (2019). Secondary fracture prevention: Drug treatment, fall prevention and nutrition requirements. *Best Practice and Research Clinical Rheumatology, 33*(2), 290–300. https://doi.org/10.1016/j.berh.2019.04.005

Halvachizadeh, S., Teuber, H., Pape, H.-C., & Allemann, F. (2019). Principles and current concepts in the surgical treatment of fragility fractures in the elderly. *Best Practice and Research Clinical Rheumatology, 33*(2), 264–277. https://doi.org/10.1016/j.berh.2019.03.018

Jha, S., Chapman, M., & Roszko, K. (2019). When low bone mineral density and fractures is not osteoporosis. *Current Osteoporosis Reports, 17*(5), 324–332. https://doi.org/10.1007/s11914-019-00529-7

Lewiecki, E.M., Baron, R., Bilezikian, J.P., Gagel, R.E., Leonard, M.B., Leslie, W.D., ... Miller, P.D. (2016). Proceedings of the 2015 Santa Fe Bone Symposium: Clinical applications of scientific advances in osteoporosis and metabolic bone disease. *Journal of Clinical Densitometry, 19*(1), 102–116. https://doi.org/10.1016/j.jocd.2015.11.003

Loi, F., Córdova, L.A., Pajarinen, J., Lin, T.-H., Yao, Z., & Goodman, S.B. (2016). Inflammation, fracture, and bone repair. *Bone, 86,* 119–130. https://doi.org/10.1016/j.bone.2016.02.020

Morgan, E.F., De Giacomo, D., & Gerstenfeld, L.C. (2014). Overview of skeletal repair (fracture healing and its assessment). In M.J. Hilton (Ed.), *Methods of molecular biology: Vol. 1130. Skeletal development and repair: Methods and protocols* (pp. 13–31). Springer. https://doi.org/10.1007/978-1-62703-989-5_2

Morshed, S. (2014). Current opinions in determining fracture unions. *Advances in Medicine, 2014,* 708574. https://doi.org/10.1155/2014/708574

Ottanelli, S. (2015). Prevention and treatment of bone fragility in cancer patient. *Clinical Cases in Mineral and Bone Metabolism, 12*(2), 116–129. https://doi.org/10.11138/ccmbm/2015.12.2.116

Pollak, A.N., & Watkins-Castillo, S.I. (2014). Fracture trends. In *The burden of musculoskeletal diseases in the United States* (3rd ed.). United States Bone and Joint Initiative. https://www.boneandjointburden.org/2014-report/via23/fracture-trends

Singaram, S., & Naidoo, M. (2019). The physical, psychological and social impact of long bone fractures on adults: A review. *African Journal of Primary Health Care and Family Medicine, 11*(1), a1908. https://doi.org/10.4102/phcfm.v11i1.1908

Subbiah, V., & West, H.L. (2016). Bone complications in patients with cancer. *JAMA Oncology, 2*(5), 695. https://doi.org/10.1001/jamaoncol.2015.3495

Tarantino, U., Iolascon, G., Cianferotti, L., Masi, L., Marcucci, G., Giusti, F., ... Brandi, M.L., (2017). Clinical guidelines for the prevention and treatment of osteoporosis: Summary statements and recommendations from the Italian Society for Orthopaedics and Traumatology. *Journal of Orthopaedics and Traumatology, 18*(Suppl. 1), 3–36. https://doi.org/10.1007/s10195-017-0474-7

Tins, B.J., Garton, M., Cassar-Pullicino, V.N., Tyrrell, P.N.M., Lalam, R., & Singh, J. (2015). Stress fracture of the pelvis and lower limbs including atypical femoral fractures—A review. *Insights Into Imaging, 6*(1), 97–110. https://doi.org/10.1007/s13244-014-0371-z

Tsuzuki, S., Park, S.H., Eber, M.R., Peters, C.M., & Shiozawa, Y. (2016). Skeletal complications in cancer patients with bone metastases. *International Journal of Urology, 23*(10), 825–832. https://doi.org/10.1111/iju.13170

CHAPTER 103

Gout

Kimberly A. Noonan, DNP, ANP-BC, AOCN®

I. Definition: A chronic systemic disease caused by the deposition of monosodium urate crystals in joints and bones and characterized by symptomatic hyperuricemia (Benn et al., 2018; Dowell et al., 2017; Pisaniello et al., 2018; Ragab et al., 2017; Wallace et al., 2016)

II. Physiology/Pathophysiology (Bardin & Richette, 2017; Benn et al., 2018; Dalbeth et al., 2019; Dowell et al., 2017; Landgren et al., 2017; Ragab et al., 2017)
   A. Normal
      1. Uric acid is broken down into urate and is the final breakdown product of unwanted purine nucleotides.
         a) Purine (adenine and guanine) catabolism is broken down into uric acid.
         b) Uric acid has a beneficial effect because it scavenges potential harmful radicals within the body.
         c) Uric acid is freely filtered at the glomerulus, and most is reabsorbed in the S1 segment of the proximal tubule.
      2. The musculoskeletal system is a bony structure with joints held together by ligaments, attached to muscles by tendons, and cushioned by cartilage.
      3. Most joints are diarthrodial, move freely, and are enclosed by a capsule of fibrous articular cartilage, ligaments, and cartilage covering the ends of the opposing bones.
   B. Pathophysiology
      1. Gout is a disorder of purine metabolism and occurs when its final metabolite, uric acid, crystallizes in the form of monosodium urate, precipitating in joints, on tendons, and in the surrounding tissue called micro-tophi. Micro-tophi will form particularly in cooler areas of the body, such as distal extremities.
      2. Uric acid is a weak acid with a pH of 5.8. Urate crystal deposition in tissues occurs when uric acid levels increase. Monosodium urate crystals trigger an immune-mediated inflammatory reaction.
         a) Crystals are thought to be released either by some metabolic change or by mechanical trauma.
         b) In the joint space, synovial lining cells appear to be the first to phagocytize the crystals.
         c) Once the inflammatory cascade is triggered, the release of chemokines, cytokines, prostaglandins, and other proinflammatory molecules occurs.
         d) The chemokines attract neutrophils into the synovial tissue.
         e) Monosodium urate crystals induce the release of IL-1, IL-6, and TNF from monocytes resulting in inflammation.
         f) IL-1β and the activation of receptor activator of nuclear factor kappa-B and its ligand pathways are triggered and form bone erosion.

III. Clinical features: Gout is a systemic metabolic disease and the most common inflammatory arthritis in the United States. Prevalence is on the rise and increases with age, with 3%–6% of men and 1%–2% of women developing gout. Approximately 20% of people with sustained hyperuricemia develop gout. Acute gouty arthritis most commonly begins with involvement of a single joint or multiple joints in the lower extremities. Common joints affected are metatarsophalangeal, midtarsal, ankle, or knee joints. Gout can become more serious with time and become polyarthritic (Bardin & Richette, 2017; Dalbeth et al., 2019; Dowell et al., 2017; Evans et al., 2018; Hutton et al., 2018; Landgren et al., 2017; Liu et al., 2015; Ragab et al., 2017; Vargas-Santos et al., 2016).

A. Stages of gout

   1. Asymptomatic: Hyperuricemia exists for several years before the first clinical attack.
   2. Acute attack: First attack is usually monoarticular and frequently begins at night.
      a) One-half of first attacks occur in the first metatarsophalangeal, referred to as *podagra.*
      b) People with OA in fingers may experience the first gout attack in fingers.
   3. Intercritical period: This time is between gout attacks.
      a) Additional attacks typically occur within two years of the first.
      b) They may occur more frequently after the first attack and may involve multiple joints as more attacks occur.
      c) If left untreated, attacks may occur more frequently and become more severe.
   4. Chronic gouty arthritis or chronic tophaceous gout: Frequent recurrent attacks cause chronic tophi deposits of monosodium urate crystals in soft tissue.
      a) When left untreated, tophaceous gout may lead to joint erosion and destruction.
      b) Occurrence of chronic tophaceous gout is approximately 50% despite medication and is most often associated with noncompliance with diet and alcohol use.

B. Risk factors

   1. Obesity
   2. Male gender
   3. Postmenopausal women
   4. Hypertriglyceridemia
   5. Hypertension
   6. Increase in fructose intake
   7. Diet high in red meat and fish high in purines
   8. Increased intake of beer and hard liquor but not wine
   9. Recent surgery
   10. Fasting or malnutrition
   11. Exacerbation of psoriasis
   12. Cirrhosis
   13. Medications: Cyclosporine, low-dose ASA, diuretics (e.g., loop, thiazide), antivirals (e.g., ritonavir, darunavir, didanosine), levodopa, nicotinic acid, pancreatic enzymes, sildenafil

C. Etiology

   1. Enzyme defect
   2. Hereditary kidney disease: Familial juvenile hyperuricemic nephropathy, autosomal dominant medullary cystic kidney disease, autosomal dominant polycystic kidney disease
   3. Impaired renal excretion of uric acid
   4. Metabolic syndrome: Combination of abdominal obesity, hypertension, insulin resistance, and dyslipidemia; associated with an increased risk of MI

D. History
 1. History of cancer and cancer treatment
 2. Current medications: Prescribed, over the counter
 3. History of presenting symptoms: Precipitating factors, onset, location, duration
 4. Changes in ADLs
 5. Past medical history: Organ transplant, lymphoproliferative disorder, myeloprolif-
    erative disorder, cardiac disease, renal impairment, diabetes
 6. Social history: Alcohol use, diet history
 7. Family history of gout
E. Signs and symptoms
 1. Severe joint pain, swelling, and erythema typically occurring in the morning
 2. Decreased mobility due to inflamed joints
 3. Fever and/or chills
 4. Tophi are visible in chronic gout and usually are not tender.
    a) Helix of ear
    b) Olecranon process
    c) Interphalangeal joint
 5. Dactylitis (sausage digits): The affected digit may appear dusky and reddish pur-
    ple in color, leading to desquamation. Dactylitis can take one or two months
    to resolve.
F. Physical examination
 1. Vital signs
    a) Increased blood pressure: Hypertension is a risk factor for gout.
    b) Increased temperature
 2. Musculoskeletal
    a) Inflamed, erythematous, warm, and tender joints
    b) Presence of tophi in the fingers, hands, knees, feet, ulna, sides of forearms, helix
       of ear, and Achilles tendon
    c) Range of motion decrease in gouty joint
    d) Dactylitis

IV. Diagnostic tests (Bardin & Richette, 2017; Dowell et al., 2017; Landgren et al., 2017; Liu et
    al., 2015; Neogi et al., 2015; Ragab et al., 2017; Vargas-Santos et al., 2016)
 A. Laboratory
  1. Uric acid: Typically elevated but can be normal
  2. ESR or CRP: May be elevated
  3. Lipid panel: Potential increased LDL and cholesterol in presence of dyslipidemia
  4. Synovial fluid analysis: Presence of monosodium urate crystals
     a) Gram stain and culture if septic arthritis is suspected
     b) Tophi confirmed with visualization of crystals
  5. RA and antinuclear antibody: As indicated but typically normal
  6. CBC: Potential elevated WBC count; elevated hematocrit suggestive of polycythemia
  7. Creatinine to evaluate renal function
 B. Radiology
  1. X-ray of affected area may be helpful to evaluate for chondrocalcinosis seen in
     pseudogout. Late destructive gout changes may reveal overhanging edges, erosions,
     and bone cysts, which would distinguish it from RA.
  2. Ultrasound of area is helpful in diagnosing tophaceous deposits without needle
     aspiration.
  3. MRI and CT can be used to diagnose gout and particularly tophaceous deposits.

C. Diagnostic criteria: Updated diagnostic criteria adopted by the American College of Rheumatology and the European League Against Rheumatism Gout Classification System
   1. At least one episode of swelling, pain, or tenderness in a peripheral joint or bursa
   2. Presence of monosodium urate crystals in a symptomatic joint or bursa (i.e., in synovial fluid) or tophus
   3. Ankle or mid-foot (as part of monoarticular or oligoarticular episode without involvement of the first metatarsophalangeal joint); involvement of the first metatarsophalangeal joint (as part of monoarticular or oligoarticular episode)
   4. Erythema overlying affected joint; patient reported or physician observed
      a) Unable to touch or apply pressure to affected joint
      b) Great difficulty with walking or inability to use affected joint
   5. Clinical evidence of tophus
      a) Draining or chalk-like subcutaneous nodule under transparent skin, often with overlying vascularity
      b) Located in typical locations: joints, ears, olecranon bursae, finger pads, tendons (e.g., Achilles)

V. Differential diagnosis (Dowell et al., 2017; Golenbiewski & Keenan, 2019)
   A. Pseudogout: Calcium pyrophosphate deposition disease
   B. Acute septic arthritis
   C. Stress fracture (see Chapter 102)
   D. Tumor lysis syndrome
   E. RA (see Chapter 108)
   F. Cellulitis (see Chapter 19)
   G. Lymphoproliferative disorder
   H. Myeloproliferative disorder
   I. Multiple myeloma
   J. Drug induced
   K. Bursitis
   L. Polycythemia vera (see Chapter 128)
   M. Psoriasis

VI. Treatment: Maximum severity of disease is reached over hours with complete resolution in five to seven days, even if untreated. Goal is to decrease pain and inflammation quickly and safely (Bardin & Richette, 2017; Benn et al., 2018; Dalbeth et al., 2019; Day et al., 2017; Dowell et al., 2017; Morris et al., 2016; Proudman et al., 2019; Qaseem et al., 2017; Rainer et al., 2016; Tatlock et al., 2017).
   A. Recommended gout practices
      1. Therapy should begin as soon as flare symptoms occur and is associated with more rapid and complete symptom resolution.
      2. Low dose anti-inflammatory therapy treatment should be continued during the early months of urate lowering treatment to reduce additional flares.
      3. Urate lowering therapy (e.g., allopurinol, febuxostat, probenecid, lesinurad, peglotkicase, benzbromarone) should be continued without interruption.
      4. Oral or injected steroids can be administered.
      5. Avoid salicylates.
   B. Acute gout: Treatment modalities
      1. Ice applied for 20–30 minutes several times a day decreases pain.
      2. NSAIDs are first-line treatment for gout. No specific agent is significantly more or less effective (see Appendix E).

       a) NSAIDs should not be used with many existing comorbidities, such as renal disease, GI bleeding, or heart failure.

       b) Indomethacin 50 mg PO every eight hours for 4–10 days is most commonly used.

       c) Avoid salicylates.

          (1) Low doses can cause renal uric acid retention.

          (2) High doses can cause uricosuria.

  3. Colchicine

       a) Mechanism of action is unknown but thought to reduce leukocyte lactic acid production and decrease deposits of uric acid. Colchicine also is an anti-inflammatory drug.

       b) Dose

          (1) For acute attack, administer 1–2 mg PO initially, then 0.5–1.2 mg every one to two hours until pain subsides, with a maximum of 8 mg in 24 hours.

          (2) Decrease dosing for creatinine clearance less than 50 ml/min.

       c) Use caution with combination P-glycoprotein inhibitors (e.g., amiodarone, macrolide antibiotics) or cytochrome P450 3A4 inhibitors (e.g., clarithromycin, azole antifungals), which increase colchicine levels.

  4. Steroids

       a) Intra-articular steroid injection using methylprednisolone

       b) Oral steroids: Prednisone 20–40 mg PO for two to three days, tapered over 10 days; discontinued with resolution of flare

C. Antihyperuricemia medications are prophylaxis to decrease serum urate to 5–6 mg/dl to cure the disease. Initiation is usually one to two weeks after an acute attack has resolved. It is not recommended until a person has had two attacks of gout or if destructive joint changes, tophi, or urate nephropathy exists.

  1. Colchicine: 0.6 mg PO one or two times a day is usual dose.

  2. Allopurinol

       a) Drug inhibits an enzyme, xanthine oxidase, to prevent the conversion of oxypurine to uric acid.

       b) Use with caution in patients taking ampicillin or patients with renal disease. Dose is based on creatinine clearance.

       c) Dose is 100–300 mg PO daily. Minimal effective dose is 100–200 mg daily.

  3. Probenecid

       a) Mechanism of action is resorption of uric acid at proximal convoluted tubules and increased urinary excretion of uric acid.

       b) Dose is 250 mg PO two times a day. It may be titrated to 1–2 g daily.

  4. Febuxostat

       a) Xanthine oxidase inhibitor is used for chronic gout.

       b) Dose is 40–80 mg PO daily.

       c) Use with caution in patients with hepatic impairment.

  5. Pegloticase

       a) Pegylated uricase dose is 8 mg IV every two weeks. It is typically given under care of a rheumatologist.

       b) Refractory gout treatment is used as a third-line treatment.

       c) Use with caution in patients with glucose-6-phosphate dehydrogenase deficiency.

D. Surgery

  1. Surgery is indicated if tophaceous deposits compress the cauda equina or spinal cord.

  2. Chronic ulcer may develop from tophaceous deposits, and wound may require debridement.

E. Lifestyle changes
  1. Educate patients about risk factors and lifestyle changes.
  2. Implement dietary changes that are known to decrease uric acid levels.
     a) Low-fat dairy products such as yogurt and skim milk
     b) Vitamin C: May lower uric acid levels
     c) Weight loss
  3. Limit dietary intake of the following.
     a) Red meat and fish rich in purines
     b) Fructose: Soft drinks
     c) Beer and alcohol
  4. Decrease weight-bearing activities during acute attacks.
  5. Instruct patients that without treatment and lifestyle changes, episodes of acute gout may develop into chronic gout with destruction of joint surfaces, joint deformity, and painless tophi.

VII. Follow-up (Tatlock et al., 2017)
  A. Patients with acute gout should return to the clinic 24–48 hours after initiating treatment to assess pain relief, then again in four weeks to discuss prophylactic therapy.
  B. Patients with chronic gout should have uric acid levels checked biannually.

VIII. Referrals
  A. Dietitian: For diet recommendations
  B. Rheumatologist: If intra-articular corticosteroid injections are required or with the development of chronic tophaceous gout intolerant or unresponsive to current therapies

References

Bardin, T., & Richette, P. (2017). Impact of comorbidities on gout and hyperuricaemia: An update on prevalence and treatment options. *BMC Medicine, 15,* 123. https://doi.org/10.1186/s12916-017-0890-9

Benn, C.L., Dua, P., Gurrell, R., Loudon, P., Pike, A., Storer, R.I., & Vangjeli, C. (2018). Physiology of hyperuricemia and urate-lowering treatments. *Frontiers in Medicine, 5,* 160. https://doi.org/10.3389/fmed.2018.00160

Dalbeth, N., Choi, H.K., Joosten, L.A.B., Khanna, P.P., Matsuo, H., Perez-Ruiz, F., & Stamp, L.K. (2019). Gout. *Nature Reviews Disease Primers, 5,* 69. https://doi.org/10.1038/s41572-019-0115-y

Day, R.O., Frensham, L.J., Nguyen, A.D., Baysari, M.T., Aung, E., Lau, A.Y.S., ... Westbrook, J.I. (2017). Effectiveness of an electronic patient-centered self-management tool for gout sufferers: A cluster randomised controlled trial protocol. *BMJ Open, 7*(10), e017281. https://doi.org/10.1136/bmjopen-2017-017281

Dowell, A., Morris, C., Macdonald, L., & Stubbe, M. (2017). "I can't bend it and it hurts like mad": Direct observation of gout consultations in routine primary health care. *BMC Family Practice, 18,* 91. https://doi.org/10.1186/s12875-017-0662-9

Evans, P.L., Prior, J.A., Belcher, J., Mallen, C.D., Hay, C.A., & Roddy, E. (2018). Obesity, hypertension and diuretic use as risk factors for incident gout: A systematic review and meta-analysis of cohort studies. *Arthritis Research and Therapy, 20,* 136. https://doi.org/10.1186/s13075-018-1612-1

Golenbiewski, J., & Keenan, R.T. (2019). Moving the needle: Improving the care of the gout patient. *Rheumatology and Therapy, 6*(2), 179–193. https://doi.org/10.1007/s40744-019-0147-5

Hutton, J., Fatima, T., Major, T.J., Topless, R., Stamp, L.K., Merriman, T.R., & Dalbeth, N. (2018). Mediation analysis to understand genetic relationships between habitual coffee intake and gout. *Arthritis Research and Therapy, 20,* 135. https://doi.org/10.1186/s13075-018-1629-5

Landgren, A.J., Jacobsson, L.T.H., Lindström, U., Sandström, T.Z.S., Drivelegka, P., Björkman, L., ... Dehlin, M. (2017). Incidence of and risk factors for nephrolithiasis in patients with gout and the general population, a cohort study. *Arthritis Research and Therapy, 19,* 173. https://doi.org/10.1186/s13075-017-1376-z

Liu, S.-C., Xia, L., Zhang, J., Lu, X.-H., Hu, D.-K., Zhang, H.-T., & Li, H.-J. (2015). Gout and risk of myocardial infarction: A systematic review and meta-analysis of cohort studies. *PLOS ONE, 10*(7), e0134088. https://doi.org/10.1371/journal.pone.0134088

Morris, C., Macdonald, L., Stubbe, M., & Dowell, A. (2016). "It's complicated"—Talking about gout medicines in primary care consultations: A qualitative study. *BMC Family Practice, 17,* 114. https://doi.org/10.1186/s12875-016-0515-y

Neogi, T., Jansen, T.L.T.A., Dalbeth, N., Fransen, J., Schumacher, H.R., Berendsen, D., ... Taylor, W.J. (2015). 2015 gout classification criteria: An American College of Rheumatology/European League Against Rheumatism collaborative initiative. *Annals of the Rheumatic Diseases, 74*(10), 1789–1798. https://doi.org/10.1136/annrheumdis-2015-208237

Pisaniello, H.L., Lester, S., Gonzalez-Chica, D., Stocks, N., Longo, M., Sharplin, G.R., ... Hill, C.L. (2018). Gout prevalence and predictors of urate-lowering therapy use: Results from a population-based study. *Arthritis Research and Therapy, 20,* 143. https://doi.org/10.1186/s13075-018-1633-9

Proudman, C., Lester, S.E., Gonzalez-Chica, D.A., Gill, T.K., Dalbeth, N., & Hill, C.L. (2019). Gout, flares, and allopurinol use: A population-based study. *Arthritis Research and Therapy, 21,* 132. https://doi.org/10.1186/s13075-019-1918-7

Qaseem, A., Harris, R.P., & Forciea, M.A. (2017). Management of acute and recurrent gout: A clinical practice guideline from the American College of Physicians. *Annals of Internal Medicine, 166*(1), 58–68 https://doi.org/10.7326/M16-0570

Ragab, G., Elshahaly, M., & Bardin, T. (2017). Gout: An old disease in new perspective—A review. *Journal of Advanced Research, 8*(5), 495–511. https://doi.org/10.1016/j.jare.2017.04.008

Rainer, T.H., Cheng, C.H., Janssens, H.J.E.M., Man, C.Y., Tam, L.S, Choi, Y.F., ... Graham, C.A. (2016). Oral prednisolone in the treatment of acute gout: A pragmatic, multicenter, double blind, randomized trial. *Annals of Internal Medicine, 164*(7), 464–471. https://doi.org/10.7326/M14-2070

Tatlock, S., Rüdell, K., Panter, C., Arbuckle, R., Harrold, L.R., Taylor, W.J., & Symonds, T. (2017). What outcomes are important for gout patients? In-depth qualitative research into the gout patient experience to determine optimal endpoints for evaluating therapeutic interventions. *The Patient—Patient-Centered Outcomes Research, 10*(1), 65–79. https://doi.org/10.1007/s40271-016-0184-x

Vargas-Santos, A.B., Taylor, W.J., & Neogi, T. (2016). Gout classification criteria: Update and implications. *Current Rheumatology Reports, 18*(7), 46. https://doi.org/10.1007/s11926-016-0594-8

Wallace, B., Khanna, D., Aquino-Beaton, C., Singh, J.A., Duffy, E., Elashoff, D., & Khanna, P.P. (2016). Performance of gout impact scale in a longitudinal observational study of patients with gout. *Rheumatology, 55*(6), 982–990. https://doi.org/10.1093/rheumatology/kew007

CHAPTER 104

Lyme Disease

Marlon Garzo Saria, PhD, RN, FAAN, and Santosh Kesari, MD, PhD, FANA, FAAN

I. Definition: Immune-mediated disease secondary to exposure to *Borrelia burgdorferi*; also known as Lyme borreliosis (Chomel, 2015; Halperin, 2019; Van Hout, 2018)

II. Physiology/Pathophysiology (Aguirre et al., 2019; Hu, 2016; Pujalte et al., 2018)
   A. Normal: Multisystem infection that enters the bloodstream at tick exposure
   B. Pathophysiology: *B. burgdorferi*, a spirochete, is transmitted by the bite of infected *Ixodes* ticks (black-legged deer ticks).
      1. The ticks have a three-stage lifecycle—larvae, nymph, and adult.
      2. Ticks become infected after feeding on an infected wild animal, typically white-footed mice, voles, chipmunks, or birds.
      3. The infection is sustained during the tick molting process to the nymphal stage and is transmitted to other animals.
      4. Humans can be infected by either nymphal or adult *Ixodes* ticks.

III. Clinical features: In the United States, white-tailed deer serve as an important host. In 2015, approximately 95% of Lyme disease cases were reported from 14 states—Connecticut, Delaware, Maine, Maryland, Massachusetts, Minnesota, New Hampshire, New Jersey, New York, Pennsylvania, Rhode Island, Vermont, Virginia, and Wisconsin. Lyme disease has been reported in all 48 continental states. It is one of the most frequently diagnosed vector-borne diseases worldwide. Acrodermatitis chronica atrophicans, lymphocytoma, chronic arthritis, encephalomyelitis, or chronic neuroborreliosis may present months or years after infection. Fleas, flies, or mosquitoes cannot transmit Lyme disease (Aguirre et al., 2019; CDC, 2020; Chomel, 2015; Halperin, 2019; Hu, 2016; Pujalte et al., 2018; Randolph, 2016; Ross Russell et al., 2018; Sanchez, 2015).
   A. Risk factors
      1. Exposure to infected *Ixodes* ticks is the essential condition for the risk for Lyme disease.
      2. Ticks are active in the months of April through October and peak in the summer months of June through August.
      3. Ticks must be attached to the human body for 36–48 hours to transmit disease.
   B. History
      1. History of cancer and cancer treatment
      2. Current medications: Prescribed, over the counter
      3. History of presenting symptoms: Precipitating factors, onset, location, duration
      4. Changes in ADLs
      5. Social history: Gardening, recreational exposure, recent travel
   C. Signs and symptoms: Manifested in three stages (localized erythema migrans, disseminating, persistent infection)

     1. Localized: Erythema migrans or "bull's-eye" rash
        a) Rash or patch on the skin about 10 cm across that may expand peripherally as a palpable band; may or may not be itchy
        b) Develops in 60%–80% of cases several days or weeks after a tick bite
        c) Appears 7–10 days after inoculation and usually resolves spontaneously
        d) Rashes that are hot, itchy, and resolve within 48 hours are more likely to be caused by an allergy.
     2. Early infection: May be completely asymptomatic
     3. Disseminating: Days or weeks after infection
        a) Influenza-like symptoms: Fever, malaise, fatigue, headaches, chills, muscle or joint pain
        b) Lymphadenopathy
        c) Neuroborreliosis
            (1) Occurs in 10%–20% of symptomatic patients in the United States
            (2) Causes all or part of a triad, including meningoradiculitis, meningitis, or meningoencephalitis
            (3) Facial palsy or Bell's palsy unilateral or bilateral (e.g., cranial neuropathy)
                (a) Arthralgia: Joint pain especially in large joints, typically the knees; Lyme arthritis is more common than neuroborreliosis in the United States.
                (b) Borrelial lymphocytoma
                (c) Multiple erythema migrans
                (d) Syncope indicating Lyme carditis inducing heart block
     4. Late or persistent post-Lyme syndrome: Chronic fatigue, arthralgia, headache
   D. Physical examination
     1. Vital signs: Fever
     2. Integument: Area of bite for "bull's-eye" rash
     3. Neurology: For motor or sensory radiculopathies; potential palsy in later stage
     4. Lymph node: Regional lymphadenopathy (see Appendix D)
     5. Extremity: Joint pain, particularly large joints and knees, on palpitation and with use of passive range of motion

IV. Diagnostic tests: Patients presenting with typical erythema migrans require no laboratory confirmation because approximately 30% will have positive Lyme serology during early phase of infection (Aguirre et al., 2019; Chomel, 2015; Halperin, 2019; John & Taege, 2019; Pujalte et al., 2018; Ross Russell et al., 2018; Yeung & Baranchuk, 2019).
   A. Laboratory: Serological assays
     1. Two-tiered testing remains the gold standard.
        a) Enzyme immunoassay or indirect immunofluorescence assay
        b) Followed by immunoblotting assay: Western blot
     2. Detection of IgM has a low specificity.
     3. False-positive enzyme immunoassays can be caused by the following.
        a) Alternative infections
            (1) Syphilis
            (2) Leptospirosis
            (3) *Helicobacter pylori*
            (4) Epstein-Barr virus
            (5) Infective endocarditis
            (6) Non-UK tick-borne relapsing fever
        b) Autoimmune disorders: SLE
        c) IVIg administration

        4. ESR will be increased with inflammation present.

   B. Radiology: MRI can show clinically relevant inflammatory or neurovascular changes in the brain or spinal cord.

   C. Other

        1. Lumbar puncture: CSF should be tested if there is any diagnostic doubt and may help in the acute setting while waiting for serology.

        2. ECG: Assess for heart block, as warranted.

V. Differential diagnosis (Hu, 2016; Ross Russell et al., 2018; Sanchez, 2015)

   A. Cellulitis (see Chapter 19)

   B. Urticaria

   C. Rocky Mountain spotted fever

   D. Cutaneous fungal infections

   E. Local reaction to tick bites

   F. Southern tick–associated rash illness

   G. Febrile viral illnesses, particularly enteroviruses during summer

   H. Facial nerve palsy

   I. Viral meningitis (see Chapter 141)

   J. Heart block (see Chapter 45)

   K. Inflammatory arthritis: Reactive arthritis, gout (see Chapter 103), pseudogout, RA (see Chapter 108)

   L. Peripheral neuropathy (see Chapter 143)

   M. Radiculoneuropathy

   N. Encephalomyelitis

   O. VZV infection

   P. Spider bite

VI. Treatment (Chomel, 2015; Halperin, 2019; Hu, 2016; Ross Russell et al., 2018; Yeung & Baranchuk, 2019)

   A. Erythema migrans should be treated empirically without waiting for serologic confirmation. Antibodies to *B. burgdorferi* may take four to eight weeks to be detected.

   B. Nonpharmacologic measures

        1. Ticks that have not attached and are moving on the skin cannot transmit Lyme disease and can be brushed off.

        2. Ticks that have attached to a host and started feeding should be removed by grasping the tick at the point nearest to the attachment site with a pair of flat tweezers or fingers and applying gentle, constant tugging.

        3. Methods such as burning with a flame, dousing the tick in strong solvents, or covering it with an occlusive agent are not recommended and can lead to further injury.

   C. Pharmacologic measures

        1. Doxycycline: 100 mg PO two times a day; recommended antibiotic

        2. Alternative oral antibiotics: Amoxicillin 500 mg PO three times a day; cefuroxime 500 mg PO two times a day; or erythromycin 250 mg PO four times a day

        3. Neurologic or cardiac manifestations: Ceftriaxone 2 g IV daily for 14–28 days

        4. Infections: Local treated for 14 days; disseminated treated for 21 days

   D. Other

        1. Patients with a high-degree heart block may require hospitalization.

        2. Lyme disease typically resolves without further intervention after antibiotic therapy.

   E. Prevention

1. Avoid tick-infested areas, wear long-sleeved shirts and long trousers, and tuck trousers into socks.
2. Apply tick repellents containing DEET (N,N-diethyl-meta-toluamide) directly to skin and spray or treat clothes with acaricides (permethrin).
3. Assess self and pets regularly for ticks. Removal of ticks before 48 hours of attachment significantly decreases the likelihood of transmission of *B. burgdorferi* from an infected tick.

VII. Follow-up (Ross Russell et al., 2018)
    A. Most patients fully recover with treatment, although this can take several months.
    B. Warn patients that there may be an exacerbation in their symptoms after starting antibiotic therapy due to a Jarisch-Herxheimer reaction.
        1. Usually starts within 12 hours of antibiotic treatment and is due to rapid destruction of multiple bacteria
        2. Does not usually require treatment to be discontinued
    C. Late Lyme disease
        1. Clinical symptoms lasting more than six months with evidence of active infection
        2. Rare and comprises less than 2% of cases
        3. May not be self-limiting; antibiotic treatment necessary for recovery
    D. Chronic Lyme disease
        1. Persistent symptoms following laboratory-confirmed and treated neuroborreliosis
        2. Atypical symptoms that occur in the setting of positive serology, which may be due to asymptomatic past infection
        3. Symptoms attributed to borreliosis but with persistently negative, equivocal, or inconsistent serology results

VIII. Referrals: If symptoms persist or post-Lyme syndrome, refer to appropriate specialist (e.g., immunologist, infectious disease).

References

Aguirre, L.E., Chueng, T., Lorio, M., & Mueller, M. (2019). Anchoring bias, Lyme disease, and the diagnosis conundrum. *Cureus, 11*(3), e4300. https://doi.org/10.7759/cureus.4300

Centers for Disease Control and Prevention. (2020). Lyme disease. https://www.cdc.gov/ticks/tickbornediseases/lyme.html

Chomel, B. (2015). Lyme disease. *Revue Scientifique et Technique, 34*(2), 569–576. https://doi.org/10.20506/rst.34.2.2380

Halperin, J.J. (2019). A neurologist's view of Lyme disease and other tick-borne infections. *Seminars in Neurology, 39*(4), 440–447. https://doi.org/10.1055/s-0039-1692143

Hu, L.T. (2016). Lyme disease. *Annals of Internal Medicine, 164*(9), ITC65–ITC80. https://doi.org/10.7326/aitc201605030

John, T.M., & Taege, A.J. (2019). Appropriate laboratory testing in Lyme disease. *Cleveland Clinic Journal of Medicine, 86*(11), 751–759. https://doi.org/10.3949/ccjm.86a.19029

Pujalte, G.G.A., Marberry, S.T., & Libertin, C.R. (2018). Tick-borne illnesses in the United States. *Primary Care: Clinics in Office Practice, 45*(3), 379–391. https://doi.org/10.1016/j.pop.2018.05.011

Randolph, S.A. (2016). Lyme disease. *Workplace Health and Safety, 64*(1), 40. https://doi.org/10.1177/2165079915616398

Ross Russell, A.L., Dryden, M.S., Pinto, A.A., & Lovett, J.K. (2018). Lyme disease: Diagnosis and management. *Practical Neurology, 18*(6), 455–464. https://doi.org/10.1136/practneurol-2018-001998

Sanchez, J.L. (2015). Clinical manifestations and treatment of Lyme disease. *Clinics in Laboratory Medicine, 35*(4), 765–778. https://doi.org/10.1016/j.cll.2015.08.004

Van Hout, M.C. (2018). The controversies, challenges and complexities of Lyme disease: A narrative review. *Journal of Pharmacy and Pharmaceutical Sciences, 21*(1), 429–436. https://doi.org/10.18433/jpps30254

Yeung, C., & Baranchuk, A. (2019). Diagnosis and treatment of Lyme carditis: JACC review topic of the week. *Journal of American College of Cardiology, 73*(6), 717–726. https://doi.org/10.1016/j.jacc.2018.11.035

Osteoarthritis

Marlon Garzo Saria, PhD, RN, FAAN, and Santosh Kesari, MD, PhD, FANA, FAAN

I. Definition (Fu et al., 2018; Malfait & Schnitzer, 2013; Schmidt, 2018)
   A. A disease of the whole joint, not only involving changes in the articular cartilage but also the subchondral bone, ligaments, capsule, synovial membrane, and periarticular muscles
   B. Historically, defined as a degenerative, noninflammatory arthritis with cartilage loss and joint space narrowing

II. Physiology/Pathophysiology (Ghouri & Conaghan, 2019; Schmidt, 2018; Vincent, 2019; Zeddou, 2019)
   A. Normal
      1. The joint is composed of bone, cartilage, tendons, ligaments, and a synovial lining that function synchronously.
      2. The musculoskeletal system is a bony structure with joints held together by ligaments attached to muscle by tendons and cushioned with cartilage.
      3. Most joints are freely moving articulations (diarthrodial) enclosed by a capsule of fibrous articular cartilage and ligaments.
      4. Synovial membrane lines the articular cavity and secretes serous lubricating synovial fluid.
      5. Hyaline articular cartilage, lining the bony ends of all synovial joints, is made of type II collagen fibers, proteoglycans, chondrocytes, and water.
   B. Pathophysiology: Mechanical, genetic, metabolic, and inflammatory mechanisms result in disruption in the bone, cartilage, tendons, and ligaments and a synovial lining interaction that triggers a cascade of pathologic events.
      1. Previously described as a passive degenerative disease, OA is now thought of as an active dynamic alteration arising from an imbalance between repair and destruction of joint tissues.
      2. The subchondral bone breaks down, resulting in hypertrophic repair. This results in sclerotic changes and the formation of osteophytes.
      3. Cartilage injury in conjunction with proinflammatory cytokines and metalloproteinases propagate the development of OA.
      4. Patients with an injured joint have higher levels of proinflammatory cytokines TNF-α, IL-1β, and IL-6 compared to healthy controls.

III. Clinical features: OA is a common chronic disease that occurs in synovial joints (e.g., knees, hips, hands, spine) and causes pain, stiffness, and reduced motion. It is a complex, heterogeneous condition and the most common cause of pain and disability in older adults. OA is considered a major cause of disability around the world and is the most common type of arthritic condition. It ranges from an asymptomatic, incidental finding on a clinical or radiographic examination to progressive joint failure (Choi et al., 2019; Fu et al., 2018; Ghouri & Conaghan, 2019; Schmidt, 2018; Vincent, 2019; Zeddou, 2019).

A. Risk factors
   1. Old age: Greatest risk factor
   2. Female gender: Higher prevalence and more severe OA
   3. High BMI (greater than 30 kg/m^2) or obesity: Increase in joint loading and general metabolic disturbance
   4. Genetic: Genes that encode for vitamin D receptor, insulin-like growth factor 1, type II collagen, and growth differentiation factor 5
   5. Environmental factors: Smoking, alcohol use
   6. Prior joint injury or trauma: Malaligned joints, abnormal loading of the joints

B. Etiology
   1. Joint pain associated with OA has a strong mechanical component that is triggered by specific activities (e.g., climbing stairs) and relieved by rest.
   2. Traditional classification has separated OA into primary or secondary.
      a) Primary OA is joint damage that occurs without an inciting cause.
      b) Secondary OA is the result of a proceeding insult (e.g., trauma, infection, metabolic, inflammatory, other conditions).

C. History
   1. History of cancer and cancer treatment
   2. Current medications: Prescribed, over the counter
   3. History of presenting symptoms: Precipitating factors, onset, location, duration, associated symptoms (e.g., morning stiffness; warm, painful joints
   4. Changes in ADLs
   5. Past medical history: Diabetes, trauma, hypothyroidism
   6. Social history: Smoking, alcohol use, occupational, sports activities

D. Signs and symptoms
   1. Pain is the most common OA symptom that prompts patients to seek medical care.
      a) Two types of manifestation in hip/knee OA
         (1) Intermittent but severe: Greatest impact on QOL, especially when unpredictable
         (2) Constant background pain or aching
      b) OA pain mainly occurs during the day and typically during movement or physical activities. Resting pain at night may be associated with advanced stages of disease.
         (1) Early-stage OA is characterized by predictable episodes of pain triggered by an activity.
         (2) Middle stage OA is often characterized by constant pain, particularly at night.
         (3) Advanced stages of OA have more constant pain, with episodes of unpredictable pain.
      c) Pain becomes more constant over time and has been described as "dull, aching, throbbing, punctuated increasingly with shorter episodes of a more intense, often unpredictable, and emotionally draining pain" (Hawker et al., 2008, p. 417).
      d) Neuropathic traits can be present, such as a burning sensation and "pins and needles," in advanced disease.
   2. Joint stiffness
   3. Reduced joint function
   4. Reduced joint range of motion
   5. Joint instability
   6. Swelling

7. Crepitus
8. Muscle weakness
9. Pain-related psychological distress
10. Chronic fatigue leading to heightened pain awareness and depression
E. Physical examination
1. Extremities: When examining the area of concern, where a patient says it hurts and the actual anatomic location of pain may differ. The involved joint may show range of motion loss, cracking, or crepitus. The joint is typically cool to touch, but an effusion, particularly in the knee, may be present.
2. Various joints may be involved.
   a) Distal interphalangeal and proximal interphalangeal joints: To assess for Heberden and Bouchard nodes
   b) First carpometacarpal joints: May have decreased grip
   c) Hips (for internal rotation), knees, cervical and lumbar spine (for pain, paresthesia, and limited range of motion of spine)
   d) First metatarsophalangeal: For enlargement, decreased range of motion
3. Bony enlargement and overgrowth from osteophyte formation may be present.
4. Deformity of joints with malalignment may be present.
F. OA assessment tools: Questionnaire to assess pain, stiffness, and physical function in patients with hip/knee OA
1. Mobile Western Ontario and McMaster Index (m-WOMAC)
2. Appropriate Use Criteria: Osteoarthritis of the Knee (AUC OAK)

IV. Diagnostic tests (Schmidt, 2018)
A. Laboratory: If the history, physical examination, and imaging are consistent with OA, additional laboratory testing is not necessary.
1. Immunologic markers commonly used in the evaluation of other rheumatic diseases are not associated with OA (e.g., rheumatoid factor, antinuclear antibody).
2. Nonspecific markers of inflammation (e.g., ESR, CRP) are generally low.
3. Assess hepatic and renal function as baseline prior to therapy.
4. Synovial fluid analysis, when available, is characteristically viscous, clear, noninflammatory (WBC count less than 2,000/mm^3), and absent of crystals.
B. Radiology
1. Plain radiographs remain the most used imaging technique. Radiographic evidence of OA includes joint space narrowing, osteophyte formation, subchondral cysts, and sclerosis.
   a) Severity of OA has historically been based on Kellgren and Lawrence grade values from 0–4, with a score of greater than or equal to 2 consistent with radiographic OA.
   b) This grading has been used to evaluate hand, knee, and hip OA.
2. MRI can add three-dimensional detail, better evaluate soft tissue defects, uncover synovitis, accurately measure cartilage thickness, and detect effusions. It can also identify OA at earlier stages before radiographic changes become apparent.
3. Ultrasound is also being incorporated into practice. Advantages of ultrasound are portability, quick examination of several anatomic locations, and low cost, but it remains user dependent and can detect only superficial structures. Ultrasound can be useful in detecting synovial inflammation, effusion, and osteophytosis.

V. Differential diagnosis (Schmidt, 2018)
A. Tendonitis

B. RA (see Chapter 108)

C. Seronegative spondyloarthropathy: Psoriatic arthritis, reactive arthritis

D. Crystalline arthritis: Gout (see Chapter 103), pseudogout

E. Septic arthritis or infectious arthritis: Bacterial, viral, fungal, Lyme disease (see Chapter 104)

F. Avascular necrosis

G. Foreign body synovitis

VI. Treatment (DiRenzo & Finan, 2019; Ghouri & Conaghan, 2019; Hagen & Alchin, 2019; Malfait & Schnitzer, 2013; Miller et al., 2018; Rees, 2020; Schmidt, 2018)

A. OA management has largely focused on arresting or slowing structural disease progression of joint damage; however, from the patient perspective, pain control remains the most significant unmet need in OA treatment.

B. Nonpharmacologic measures

1. Education: Patients should be familiarized with the type of arthritis they are experiencing, risk factors for the development of OA, available treatment options, and expectations.

2. Weight loss: Weight reduction can off-load the forces of the joint, lessen pain, and slow the progression or disability associated with OA.

3. Exercise: Physical or occupational therapy should be encouraged.

4. Bracing, orthotics, and assistive devices: These devices address joint malalignment.

C. Pharmacologic measures

1. NSAIDs: Celecoxib, naproxen, ibuprofen, meloxicam (see Appendix E)

   a) Clinical studies have repeatedly demonstrated efficacy, compared with placebo, in relieving pain and increasing function in people with OA.

   b) Adverse effects, including dyspepsia, nausea, vomiting, diarrhea, and rash, are a common reason to discontinue use of these drugs.

2. SSRIs for patients with OA in multiple joints: Duloxetine, venlafaxine, milnacipran

   a) Duloxetine: 60 mg PO daily

   b) Venlafaxine: Starting dose of 37.5 mg PO daily, titrated to a maximum of 225 mg PO daily

   c) Milnacipran: Starting dose of 12.5 mg PO daily, titrated to a maximum of 100 mg PO two times a day

3. Topical options: NSAIDs, capsaicin, anesthetics (e.g., lidocaine), compounded agent

4. Acetaminophen: It is commonly used to treat OA; it is relatively safe if taken at recommended amounts (less than 4,000 mg daily); has no anti-inflammatory effect and offers analgesia only.

5. Tramadol: This additional analgesic is used to treat OA. It generally is reserved for patients who have not achieved adequate pain relief with acetaminophen or NSAIDs, or for those who cannot tolerate those medications. The usual dose is 50–100 mg PO four times a day with a maximum dose of 400 mg daily.

6. Glucosamine and chondroitin: It is not recommended by the American College of Rheumatology for the treatment of OA.

7. Hydroxychloroquine: It has been used in clinical practice in patients with inflammatory hand OA with anecdotal evidence of benefit.

8. Injectable (intra-articular) corticosteroids: Although patients experience substantial improvement in pain scores, symptomatic improvement tends to be short lived, with no associated benefit seen at six months.

9. Intra-articular triamcinolone acetonide extended release: A study showed significant improvement over placebo. It is licensed by FDA for managing OA-related knee pain.

10. IM corticosteroid: A study found this to be significantly superior to placebo at reducing pain on walking at 4, 6, and 12 weeks.

11. Strontium ranelate: A study demonstrated a significant reduction in joint space width degradation with both strontium doses compared to placebo.

12. Therapies in advanced trial development
    a) Intra-articular capsaicin
    b) Antinerve growth factor monoclonal antibodies: Tanezumab, fasinumab, fulranumab
        (1) Rapidly progressive OA is the most serious adverse effect reported with tanezumab and fulranumab.
        (2) It is a painful condition diagnosed radiographically by rapid joint space narrowing and severe progressive atrophic bone and has been reported in approximately 1% of patients who received tanezumab.
        (3) Combination tanezumab and NSAIDs appears to increase the risk of rapidly progressive OA compared with tanezumab alone.
    c) Potential disease-modifying OA drugs
        (1) Sprifermin (rhFGF18) is a recombinant fibroblast growth factor 18 that is administered via intra-articular route and acts on FGFR3 receptors in cartilage.
        (2) SM04690 is an inhibitor of the Wnt signaling pathway, a signal transduction pathway thought to play a role in cartilage degeneration and the pathogenesis of OA.
        (3) Anakinra is a recombinant form of an IL-1 receptor antagonist (IL-1Ra); elevated IL-1 levels are associated with increased expression of markers of OA pathophysiology.
        (4) Lutikizumab (formerly ABT-981) is a novel human dual variable domain Ig that binds and inhibits the actions of IL-1α and IL-1β.
        (5) Canakinumab is a monoclonal antibody targeting IL-1β.
        (6) MIV-711 is a potent, selective, and reversible inhibitor of cathepsin K which aims to prevent degradation of cartilage; cathepsin K is a cysteine protease involved in bone resorption.

D. Surgery: Patients who have failed conservative and medical options may benefit from surgical consultation.

E. Cryoneurolysis (also termed *cryoneuroablation, cryoanalgesia, cryogenic nerve blockade*, or *cryolesioning*): This technique exposes peripheral nerves to local freezing, which causes axonal damage and blocks nerve conduction.

F. Prevention
    1. Modifiable risk factors include weight and injury. Sport-specific conditioning can also be of benefit.
    2. Additional interventions have focused on biomechanics.
    3. Neuromuscular training and high intensity plyometrics.

VII. Follow-up (DiRenzo & Finan, 2019; Schmidt, 2018)
    A. Periodic assessment is needed every three to six months to assess effects of treatment on symptoms, function, and muscle strength.
    B. Follow-up chemistry profile with liver function values should be obtained one to two weeks after initiating treatment and then every three to six months to detect any renal or hepatic toxicity.

VIII. Referrals (Schmidt, 2018)
   A. Surgical consultation: Patients who have failed conservative and medical options may benefit from this service.
   B. Physical or occupational therapist: Refer upon diagnosis to assess function, recommend assistive devices and exercises, and teach joint-preserving body mechanics.
   C. Self-management programs: Patients participating in self-help groups have less joint pain, fewer office visits, increased physical activity, and overall improvement in QOL.

The authors would like to acknowledge Deanna Sanchez Yamamoto, RN, MS, ANP, for her contribution to this chapter that remains unchanged from the previous edition of this book.

References

Choi, W., Zheng, H., Franklin, P., & Tulu, B. (2019). mHealth technologies for osteoarthritis self-management and treatment: A systematic review. *Health Informatics Journal, 25*(3), 984–1003. https://doi.org/10.1177/1460458217735676

DiRenzo, D., & Finan, P. (2019). Self-efficacy and the role of non-pharmacologic treatment strategies to improve pain and affect in arthritis. *Current Treatment Options in Rheumatology, 5*(2), 168–178. https://doi.org/10.1007/s40674-019-00123-z

Fu, K., Robbins, S.R., & McDougall, J.J. (2018). Osteoarthritis: The genesis of pain. *Rheumatology, 57*(Suppl. 4), iv43–iv50. https://doi.org/10.1093/rheumatology/kex419

Ghouri, A., & Conaghan, P.G. (2019). Update on novel pharmacological therapies for osteoarthritis. *Therapeutic Advances in Musculoskeletal Disease, 11*. https://doi.org/10.1177/1759720x19864492

Hagen, M., & Alchin, J. (2019). Nonprescription drugs recommended in guidelines for common pain conditions. *Pain Management, 10*(2), 117–129. https://doi.org/10.2217/pmt-2019-0057

Hawker, G.A., Stewart, L., French, M.R., Cibere, J., Jordan, J.M., March, L., ... Gooberman-Hill, R. (2008). Understanding the pain experience in hip and knee osteoarthritis—An OARSI/OMERACT initiative. *Osteoarthritis and Cartilage, 16*(4), 415–422. https://doi.org/10.1016/j.joca.2007.12.017

Malfait, A.-M., & Schnitzer, T.J. (2013). Towards a mechanism-based approach to pain management in osteoarthritis. *Nature Reviews Rheumatology, 9*(11), 654–664. https://doi.org/10.1038/nrrheum.2013.138

Miller, R.E., Block, J.A., & Malfait, A.-M. (2018). What is new in pain modification in osteoarthritis? *Rheumatology, 57*(Suppl. 4), iv99–iv107. https://doi.org/10.1093/rheumatology/kex522

Rees, H.W. (2020). Management of osteoarthritis of the hip. *Journal of the American Academy of Orthopaedic Surgeons, 28*(7), e288–e291. https://doi.org/10.5435/JAAOS-D-19-00416

Schmidt, T.W. (2018). Approach to osteoarthritis management for the primary care provider. *Primary Care: Clinics in Office Practice, 45*(2), 361–378. https://doi.org/10.1016/j.pop.2018.02.009

Vincent, T.L. (2019). Mechanoflammation in osteoarthritis pathogenesis. *Seminars in Arthritis and Rheumatism, 49*(3 Suppl.), S36–S38. https://doi.org/10.1016/j.semarthrit.2019.09.018

Zeddou, M. (2019). Osteoarthritis is a low-grade inflammatory disease: Obesity's involvement and herbal treatment. *Evidence-Based Complementary and Alternative Medicine, 2019*, 2037484. https://doi.org/10.1155/2019/2037484

CHAPTER 106

Osteoporosis

Marlene SanFilippo, MSN, ARNP, FNP-C, AOCNP®

I. Definition: A chronic, metabolic skeletal disorder characterized by low bone mass, deterioration of bone tissue with disruption of architecture, and increased skeletal fragility (Cosman et al., 2014; Crowther-Radulewicz & McCance, 2017a; Nicholson & Kapur, 2020)

    A. Primary (postmenopausal) osteoporosis is bone loss as a result of decline in gonadal function secondary to aging.

    B. Secondary osteoporosis is bone loss secondary to other conditions such as endocrine and metabolic imbalances, systemic diseases, medications, and nutritional deficiencies.

    C. Osteopenia is defined as low bone mass of spinal or hip bone mineral density (BMD), which increases risk of osteoporosis.

II. Physiology/Pathophysiology (Crowther-Radulewicz & McCance, 2017a, 2017b; French & Emanuele, 2019; Shapiro et al., 2019)

    A. Normal

        1. The skeleton is composed of 206 bones that provide a framework for support and protection of the body's soft tissue structure.

        2. Two types of osseous tissue compose every bone.

            a) Cortical (compact) bone is composed of densely packed layers of mineralized collagen, which provides rigidity and protection to the total body. It composes 85% of the skeleton and is a major component of the appendicular skeleton, including the extremities, shoulder girdle, and pelvic girdle. Cortical bone is on the exterior portion of the bone.

            b) Cancellous (spongy or trabecular) bone provides strength and elasticity to the total body. It composes 15% of the skeleton and is the major component of the axial skeleton, including the skull, vertebral column, and thorax. The space between the trabeculae are filled with bone marrow.

        3. The formation, maintenance, and remodeling of bone is affected by multiple factors, with balance between two key factors—receptor activator of nuclear factor kappa-B ligand (RANKL) and osteoprotegerin. Balance is regulated by cytokines and hormones.

            a) The cytokine known as RANKL stimulates osteoclast precursor cells and activates intracellular signaling pathways to promote osteoclast differentiation and activation, which increases resorption and bone loss.

            b) Osteoblasts secrete the glycoprotein receptor antagonist osteoprotegerin, which inhibits bone remodeling and resorption. It is the key interaction between osteoblasts and osteoclasts. It is considered a decoy receptor and blocks RANKL binding, which reduces bone resorption and loss.

B. Pathophysiology
  1. Osteoporosis results from an accelerated imbalance in the normal cycle of bone resorption and formation.
    a) Resorption (osteoclastic activity) exceeds bone formation (osteoblastic activity), resulting in thinner and more porous bones.
    b) Individual trabecular plates of bone are lost, resulting in an architecturally weakened structure.
  2. Several different biochemical factors may contribute to the imbalance, resulting in decreased bone mass.
    a) Malabsorption or insufficient intake of vitamins and minerals
      (1) Vitamin D deficiency decreases intestinal absorption of calcium.
      (2) Decreased plasma concentration of calcium activates PTH secretion.
      (3) Increased circulation of PTH increases plasma calcium concentration and clearance of phosphate.
      (4) Decreased phosphate in bone results in decreased mineralization.
      (5) Osteoclastic activity is increased, resulting in increased resorption of bone.
    b) Declining levels of estrogen and androgens result in decreased apoptosis and increased activity and survival of osteoclasts, increasing bone resorption.
    c) Glucocorticoid excess (endogenous or pharmacologically induced) stimulates osteoblast and osteocyte apoptosis and prolongs the life span of osteoclasts. Glucocorticoids increase expression of RANKL and inhibit production of osteoprotegerin by osteoblasts.

III. Clinical features: Osteoporosis is a major health problem for an estimated 10 million Americans. Decreased bone mass leads to an increased incidence of fractures, which most commonly occur in the vertebral column, hip, humerus, and wrist. The majority of postmenopausal women will have osteoporosis caused by estrogen deficiency and/or age. Early diagnosis and bone loss evaluation are important precursors to therapy that can slow or reverse progression of osteoporosis (Aggarwal & Masuda, 2018; Cosman et al., 2014; French & Emanuele, 2019; Handforth et al., 2018; Jeremiah et al., 2015; Larson & Kosteocke, 2020; McCarthy & Davis, 2016; Nicholson & Kapur, 2020; Shapiro et al., 2019).
  A. Etiology and risk factors: The more risk factors present, the greater the risk of fractures.
    1. Age older than 65 years
    2. Cancer therapies
      a) Antiandrogen and antiestrogen therapy: Result in hormone deprivation
      b) Chemotherapy: Induce premature ovarian failure and can also have a direct effect on bone turnover by affecting cell division of osteoclast and osteoblast precursors
      c) Surgical interventions resulting in hormone deprivation: Oophorectomy, orchiectomy
    3. Smoking
    4. Excessive alcohol use
    5. Ethnicity: Caucasian or Asian race
    6. Excessive caffeine intake: More than 2.5 cups of coffee daily
    7. Family history of osteoporosis
    8. Female gender
    9. Inactivity: Prolonged bed rest, lack of weight-bearing exercise
    10. Low body weight: Less than 58 kg or BMI less than 21 kg/m^2
    11. Medications
      a) Anticonvulsants
      b) Corticosteroids: Equivalent to 5 mg prednisone daily for longer than three months

      c) Heparin

      d) Immunosuppressants: Tacrolimus, cyclosporine

      e) PPIs

      f) SSRIs

      g) Thyroid hormone replacement: Beyond euthyroid state

  12. Menopause: Natural or induced

  13. Personal history of atraumatic fractures

  14. Systemic medical conditions: Acute or chronic

      a) Allogeneic HSCT

      b) Celiac disease

      c) COPD

      d) Cushing syndrome

      e) Diabetes mellitus

      f) Hemochromatosis

      g) Hematologic disorders: Hemophilia, sickle cell disease, multiple myeloma, thalassemia

      h) HIV

      i) Hyperparathyroidism

      j) Hyperthyroidism

      k) Inflammatory bowel disease

      l) Malabsorption syndrome

      m) Musculoskeletal disease: Parkinson disease, muscular dystrophy, multiple sclerosis

      n) Organ transplantation

      o) Primary biliary cirrhosis

      p) Renal insufficiency or renal failure

      q) RA

      r) SLE

  15. Vitamin D or calcium deficiency

B. History

  1. History of cancer and cancer treatment

  2. Current medications: Prescribed, over the counter

  3. History of presenting symptoms: Precipitating factors, onset, location, duration, associated symptoms (e.g., chronic back pain, loss of height)

  4. Changes in ADLs

  5. Past medical history: Chronic or acute systemic disease

  6. Family history of osteoporosis and spinal fractures

  7. Social history: Tobacco, alcohol, or caffeine use

  8. Nutritional history: Intake of calcium and vitamin D

  9. Menstrual and menopausal history

C. Signs and symptoms

  1. Backache

  2. Loss of height: May indicate vertebral compression

  3. Pain and bone deformity from fracture

  4. Kyphosis

D. Physical examination: May include no physical findings unless a fracture is present

  1. Vital signs: Measure height and compare to previous measurements. Height loss greater than 1.5 cm is considered significant.

  2. Musculoskeletal

      a) Back assessment for kyphosis (hunchback) as a result of vertebral collapse *b)* Spinal point tenderness and pain upon palpation or percussion indicative of compression

       c) Gait and mobility

    3. Neurologic: Signs and symptoms of spinal cord or root compression from bone fragments (rare)

       a) Increased radicular pain with straight leg raises with lumbar and thoracic compression

       b) Neck flexion resulting in pain with cervical compression

       c) Reduced proprioception

       d) Variable sensory changes below level of injury

IV. Diagnostic tests (Cosman et al., 2014; Nicholson & Kapur, 2020)

  A. Laboratory

    1. Initially, evaluate for common secondary causes.

       a) Chemistry panel

          (1) Alkaline phosphatase: Elevated in Paget disease, vitamin D deficiency, GI malabsorption, hyperparathyroidism, and liver/biliary disease

          (2) Calcium: Low levels in vitamin D deficiency and GI malabsorption; high levels in hyperparathyroidism

          (3) Creatinine: Elevated in renal dysfunction

       b) CBC to evaluate for anemia: May indicate multiple myeloma, nutritional deficiency, or renal insufficiency

       c) 25-hydroxyvitamin D: Low in under supplementation, GI malabsorption, and celiac disease

       d) TSH: Low in hyperthyroidism; high in hypothyroidism

       e) Total testosterone (male): Low in hypogonadism

    2. Additional tests are based on clinical suspicion for secondary causes.

       a) Estradiol (pre- and perimenopausal women): Hypogonadism

       b) PTH: Hyperparathyroidism

       c) SPEP: Multiple myeloma

       d) Urinary free cortisol: Cushing disease

    3. Consider biochemical markers of bone remodeling to assess rapidity of bone loss, risk of fracture, or response to treatment

       a) Resorption markers: Serum C-telopeptide, urinary N-telopeptide

       b) Formation markers: Serum bone-specific alkaline phosphatase, osteocalcin, aminoterminal propeptide of type I procollagen

  B. Radiology (Cosman et al., 2014; Handforth et al., 2018; McCarthy & Davis, 2016)

    1. Lateral thoracic and lumbar x-ray to determine if vertebral compression deformities or fractures are present

       a) For women aged 70 years or older and men aged 80 years or older, if T-score less than or equal to −1

       b) For women aged 65–69 years and men aged 70–79 years, if T-score less than or equal to −1.5

       c) For postmenopausal women and men aged 50 years or older with at least one of the following

          (1) Low trauma fracture

          (2) Historical height loss (difference between current height and peak height at age 20 years) of 1.5 inches or more

          (3) Prospective height loss (difference between current height and a previously documented height measurement) of 0.8 inch or more

(4) Recent or current long-term glucocorticoid treatment
2. Quantitative CT scan: Improved sensitivity over plain film
   a) Measures volumetric trabecular and cortical bone density of the spine and hip
   b) Skeletal coverage limited secondary to relatively high radiation dose, making it unsuitable as a screening tool
3. Quantitative ultrasound densitometry: No radiation exposure
   a) Does not measure BMD directly; uses speed of sound and/or broadband ultrasound attenuation
   b) Measures heel, tibia, patella, or other peripheral skeletal sites
   c) May predict fractures in postmenopausal women and men older than 65 years
4. Central DEXA scan
   a) This technique is considered the gold standard for measuring BMD for diagnosing osteoporosis and monitoring effects of therapy
   b) Scan provides measurement of bone mineral content in spine, hip, or forearm.
   c) Results may vary with the machine; serial BMD monitoring should be performed on the same piece of equipment.
   d) OA or calcification of aorta may lead to falsely high BMD.
   e) T-score is a measurement of patient's grams of mineral per square centimeter compared to "young normal" adult of same sex. Difference in score is expressed in standard deviation above or below the mean.
   f) T-score of less than or equal to –2.5 is diagnostic for osteoporosis. T-score between –1 and –2.5 is diagnostic for osteopenia.
   g) T-score is not considered reliable for premenopausal women or men younger than 50 years. Z-scores (comparison of BMD with average person of same age, sex, and ethnicity) are recommended for these patients.
5. Peripheral DEXA scan: More portable and affordable than central DEXA
   a) Scan measures BMD in the heel, finger, and forearm.
   b) Results do not correlate with central DEXA to use diagnostically.
   c) Scan not useful in monitoring BMD after treatment for osteopenia.
   d) Scan may be used as a screening tool for fracture risk in postmenopausal women.

V. Differential diagnosis (Nicholson & Kapur, 2020)
   A. Metastatic bone disease
   B. Multiple myeloma
   C. Osteomalacia
   D. Osteogenesis imperfecta
   E. Type I collagen mutations
   F. OA (see Chapter 105)
   G. Osteopenia

VI. Treatment: Goals of treatment are to increase BMD and decrease the risk of osteoporotic fractures (Aggarwal & Masuda, 2018; De Iuliis et al., 2014; Eastell et al., 2019; Hadji et al., 2017; Handforth et al., 2018; Jeremiah et al., 2015; Nicholson & Kapur, 2020; Shapiro et al., 2019).
   A. Nonpharmacologic
      1. Exercise: Weight-bearing exercise 30 minutes or more at least three times a week
      2. Smoking cessation
      3. Avoidance of excessive alcohol use: Fewer than three drinks a day
      4. Fall risk assessment and modification of environment to reduce risk of falls
   B. Pharmacologic
      1. Indications for pharmacologic treatment

    a) Postmenopausal women and men aged 50 years or older with hip or vertebral fracture

    b) T-score less than or equal to –2.5 with no risk factors

    c) T-score between –1 and –2.5 and a 10-year probability of a hip fracture of at least 3%, or a 10-year probability of a major osteoporosis-related fracture of at least 20% based on World Health Organization fracture risk algorithm (www.shef .ac.uk/FRAX); the risk algorithm is intended for postmenopausal women and men aged 50 years or older and does not include cancer treatment as a risk factor.

    d) T-score between –1.5 and –2.5 with one additional risk factor suggesting an increased risk of fracture, such as patients on aromatase inhibitors or long-term glucocorticoids

2. Supplements

    a) Calcium to equal total calcium intake (including diet) 1,000–1,200 mg PO daily

    b) Vitamin D 800–1,000 IU PO daily

3. Bisphosphonates: Decrease risk of fracture by 40%–70%

    a) Bisphosphonates are a first-line medication.

    b) They inhibit activity of osteoclasts, shortening their life span and reducing bone resorption.

    c) No current evidence-based recommendations exist regarding optimal duration of bisphosphonate therapy, as it should be individualized based on response and adverse effects. A comprehensive review of therapy should be performed at three to five years. Discontinuation should be considered at five years if no personal history of fracture.

    d) Osteonecrosis of the jaw is rare and most commonly occurs following high-dose IV bisphosphonates for patients with cancer. Incidence increases with treatment beyond five years. For general patients with osteoporosis, the incidence is thought to be 0.3%–4.3%. For patients with malignancy, incidence is 1%–12%.

    e) Atypical fractures (femur fracture) are low risk (less than 0.5%) and most often associated with long-term use for more than five years.

    f) Bisphosphonates can affect renal function and should be avoided in patients with GFR less than 30–35 ml/min.

        (1) Alendronate

            (a) 10 mg PO daily or 70 mg PO weekly to treat osteoporosis in men and postmenopausal women

            (b) 5 mg PO daily or 35 mg PO weekly as osteoporosis prevention

        (2) Ibandronate

            (a) 150 mg PO monthly to prevent or treat osteoporosis in postmenopausal women

            (b) 3 mg IV every three months to treat osteoporosis in postmenopausal women

        (3) Risedronate: 5 mg PO daily, 35 mg PO weekly, 35 mg PO weekly delayed release, 75 mg PO on two consecutive days each month, or 150 mg PO monthly to treat osteoporosis in men or postmenopausal women; also approved for prevention of steroid-induced osteoporosis in men and women

        (4) Zoledronic acid

            (a) 5 mg IV over at least 15 minutes once yearly to treat osteoporosis in postmenopausal women, men with osteoporosis, or patients with steroid-induced osteoporosis

    (b) 5 mg IV over at least 15 minutes every two years to prevent osteoporosis in postmenopausal women

  4. Calcitonin: 200 IU intranasal spray one puff daily, alternating nostrils for treatment of osteoporosis in postmenopausal women unable to take other treatments

  5. Hormone replacement therapy: Approved for prevention of osteoporosis

  6. PTH: Teriparatide

    a) 20 mcg subcutaneous daily for no more than two years in patient lifetime

    b) Approved for treatment of osteoporosis in postmenopausal women, patients with steroid-induced osteoporosis, and men with osteoporosis

    c) Not recommended for patients with skeletal metastases, malignancy-associated hypercalcemia, unexplained elevated alkaline phosphatase, Paget disease, or history of skeletal radiation

  7. Estrogen agonist/antagonist (selective estrogen receptor modulator): Raloxifene 60 mg PO daily for prevention and treatment of osteoporosis in postmenopausal women; added benefit of decreased risk of invasive breast cancer

  8. RANKL inhibitor: Denosumab 60 mg subcutaneous every six months

    a) Approved for treatment of osteoporosis in postmenopausal women at high risk for fracture, prevention in women with breast cancer on aromatase inhibitor, for men with osteoporosis at high risk of fracture, and to treat bone loss in men on gonadotropin-reducing hormone treatment for prostate cancer

    b) Small risk of osteonecrosis of the jaw (approximately 2%)

    c) Fewer renal side effects compared to bisphosphonates

VII. Follow-up (Cosman et al., 2014)

  A. Repeat bone mass testing one to two years after initiating therapy and every two years thereafter.

  B. Follow up within one month after initiation of pharmacologic therapy to determine tolerance.

VIII. Referrals (Chandra et al., 2018; Cosman et al., 2014; Nicholson & Kapur, 2020)

  A. Endocrinologist: For progressive bone loss or fracture despite treatment of osteoporosis, or to evaluate and treat possible secondary causes

  B. Orthopedist, neurosurgeon, or interventional radiologist: For treatment of vertebral fracture for vertebroplasty or kyphoplasty

  C. Neurologist or neurosurgeon: Emergent referral if patient exhibits dorsal or lumbar neurologic deficits secondary to vertebral fracture or signs or symptoms of SCC

  D. Physical and/or occupational therapy: For evaluation of need for walking aids or other assistive devices

References

Aggarwal, L., & Masuda, C. (2018). Osteoporosis: A quick update. *Journal of Family Practice, 67*(2), 59–62, 64–65. https://www.mdedge.com/clinicianreviews/article/157318/rheumatology/osteoporosis-quick-update

Chandra, R.V., Maingard, J., Asadi, H., Slater, L.-A., Mazwi, T.-L., Marcia, S., ... Hirsch, J.A. (2018). Vertebroplasty and kyphoplasty for osteoporotic vertebral fractures: What are the latest data? *American Journal of Neuroradiology, 39*(5), 798–806. https://doi.org/10.3174/ajnr.A5458

Cosman, F., de Beur, S.J., LeBoff, M.S., Lewiecki, E.M., Tanner, B., Randall, S., & Lindsay, R. (2014). Clinician's guide to prevention and treatment of osteoporosis. *Osteoporosis International, 25*(10), 2359–2381. https://doi.org/10.1007/s00198-014-2794-2

Crowther-Radulewicz, C.L., & McCance, K.L. (2017a). Alterations of musculoskeletal function. In S.E. Huether & K.L. McCance (Eds.), *Understanding pathophysiology* (6th ed., pp. 991–1037). Elsevier.

Crowther-Radulewicz, C.L., & McCance, K.L. (2017b). Structure and function of the musculoskeletal system. In S.E. Huether & K.L. McCance (Eds.), *Understanding pathophysiology* (6th ed., pp. 968–990). Elsevier.

De Iuliis, F., Taglieri, L., Amoroso, L., Vendittozzi, S., Blasi, L., Slerno, G., … Scarpa, S. (2014). Prevention of osteonecrosis of the jaw in patients with bone metastasis treated with bisphosphonates. *Anticancer Research, 34*(5), 2477–2480. http://ar.iiarjournals.org/content/34/5/2477.long

Eastell, R., Rosen, C.J., Black, D.M., Cheung, A.M., Murad, M.H., & Shoback, D. (2019). Pharmacological management of osteoporosis in postmenopausal women: An Endocrine Society clinical practice guideline. *Journal of Clinical Endocrinology and Metabolism, 104*(5), 1595–1622. https://doi.org/10.1210/jc.2019-00221

French, K.D., & Emanuele, D. (2019). Osteoporosis: Increasing screening and treatment for postmenopausal women. *Journal for Nurse Practitioners, 15*(5), 347–350. https://doi.org/10.1016/j.nurpra.2019.02.014

Hadji, P., Aapro, M.S., Body, J.-J., Gnant, M., Brandi, M.L., Reginstor, J.Y., … Coleman, R.E. (2017). Management of aromatase inhibitor–associated bone loss (AIBL) in postmenopausal women with hormone sensitive breast cancer: Joint position statement of the IOF, CABS, ECTS, IEG, ESCEO, IMS, and SIOG. *Journal of Bone Oncology, 7*, 1–12. https://doi.org/10.1016/j.jbo.2017.03.001

Handforth, C., D'Oronzo, S., Coleman, R., & Brown, J. (2018). Cancer treatment and bone health. *Calcified Tissue International, 102*(2), 251–264. https://doi.org/10.1007/s00223-017-0369-x

Jeremiah, M.P., Unwin, B.K., & Greenwalk, M.H. (2015). Diagnosis and management of osteoporosis. *American Family Physician, 92*(4), 261–268. https://www.aafp.org/afp/2015/0815/p261.html

Larson, S.L., & Kosteocke, R.A. (2020). Cervical hyperextension injuries. In F.J. Domino, R.A. Baldor, J. Golding, & M.B Stephens (Eds.), *The 5-minute clinical consult 2020* (28th ed., pp. 716–717). Wolters Kluwer.

McCarthy, J., & Davis, A. (2016). Diagnosis and management of vertebral compression fractures. *American Family Physician, 94*(1), 44–50. https://www.aafp.org/afp/2016/0701/p44.html

Nicholson, C., & Kapur, R. (2020). Osteoporosis and osteopenia. In F.J. Domino, R.A. Baldor, J. Golding, & M.B. Stephens (Eds.), *The 5-minute clinical consult 2020* (28th ed., pp. 726–727). Wolters Kluwer.

Shapiro, C.L., Van Poznak, C., Lacchetti, C., Kirshner, J., Eastell, R., Gagel, R., … Neuner, J. (2019). Management of osteoporosis in survivors of adult cancers with nonmetastatic disease: ASCO clinical practice guideline. *Journal of Clinical Oncology, 37*(31), 2916–2946. https://doi.org/10.1200/JCO.19.01696

CHAPTER 107

Restless Legs Syndrome

Marlon Garzo Saria, PhD, RN, FAAN, and Santosh Kesari, MD, PhD, FANA, FAAN

I. Definition (Allen et al., 2014; Alonso-Navarro et al., 2019; Jiménez-Jiménez et al., 2018)
   A. Restless legs syndrome, also known as Willis-Ekbom disease, is an overwhelming urge to move the legs associated with an unpleasant sensation.
   B. Chronic persistent restless legs syndrome is frequent and troublesome enough to require daily treatment.

II. Physiology/Pathophysiology (Connor et al., 2017; During & Winkelman, 2019; Gonzalez-Latapi & Malkani, 2019; Muth, 2017)
   A. Normal: The lower extremity is the portion of the lower limb that extends from the knee to the ankle.
   B. Pathophysiology
      1. Restless legs syndrome remains incompletely understood, although studies have identified a variety of both central and PNS abnormalities in patients with this disorder.
      2. It has been attributed to abnormal regulation of dopamine.
      3. A state of brain iron deficiency could play a central role and be upstream to a series of dysfunctions that are not limited to the dopaminergic system.
      4. Several genetic risk loci have been described including *MEIS1*, which is currently considered to be the strongest genetic risk factor for restless legs syndrome. Other variants identified include *PTPRD, BTBD9, MEIS1, MAP2K5/SKOR1,* and *TOX3* genes.
      5. Pathologies associated with classical neurodegenerative processes do not explain cause of restless legs syndrome.

III. Clinical features: Restless legs syndrome is a common neurologic sensorimotor disorder. Clinically significant symptoms are reported in 2%–3% of adults in the United States and Europe. Restless legs syndrome has a high prevalence in the older adult population and can impact sleep quality and sleep quantity, reduce QOL, and increase the risk of falls during episodes of nighttime ambulation. Restless legs syndrome is a treatable condition that generally responds well to pharmacologic treatment; however, if left untreated, it can cause exhaustion and fatigue, which are often associated with issues with daytime concentration, memory, and depression. Approximately 60%–85% of patients with idiopathic restless legs syndrome reported a positive family history of restless legs syndrome (Allen et al., 2014; Alonso-Navarro et al., 2019; During & Winkelman, 2019; Gonzalez-Latapi & Malkani, 2019; Jiménez-Jiménez et al., 2018; Klingelhoefer et al., 2016; Muth, 2017; Wijemanne & Ondo, 2017).
   A. Risk factors
      1. Gender: In adults aged 35 years or older, it occurs twice as frequently in women. No difference in occurrence exists in genders for those younger than 35 years.

2. Sleep disturbance: Approximately 75% of patients with restless legs syndrome likely to seek treatment will report sleep disturbance characterized by waking disrupting sleep onset and/or sleep maintenance.

3. Degree of pain versus discomfort for restless legs syndrome symptoms: One-half of patients with restless legs syndrome report symptoms as painful, not only uncomfortable.

4. Association with other movement disorders: Restless legs syndrome is associated with Parkinson disease, other parkinsonian syndromes, essential tremor, choreic and dystonic syndromes, Tourette syndrome, and heredodegenerative ataxias.

B. Etiology

1. Primary: Idiopathic

   a) Considerable evidence suggests genetic factors have a role.

   b) Autosomal dominant (most frequent), autosomal recessive, and non-Mendelian patterns of inheritance of restless legs syndrome have been reported.

2. Secondary

   a) Iron deficiency anemia

   b) Pregnancy

   c) End-stage renal disease

   d) Vitamin B_{12}/folate deficiency

   e) Peripheral neuropathy associated with diabetes mellitus

   f) RA

   g) Spinal disorders such as spinal nerve root irritation

   h) Parkinson disease

   i) FMS

   j) Spinocerebellar ataxia, particularly type 3

   k) Charcot-Marie-Tooth disease

   l) Alcoholism

C. History

1. History of cancer and cancer treatment

2. Current medications: Prescribed, over the counter

3. History of presenting symptoms: Precipitating factors, onset, location, duration

4. Changes in ADLs

5. Past medical history: Iron, vitamin B_{12}, or folate deficiency; RA; Parkinson disease; FMS

6. Family history: Restless legs syndrome, neurodegenerative disease

7. Social history: Sleep patterns, alcohol use

D. Signs and symptoms

1. Symptoms are worse at night, with a distinct symptom-free period in the early morning. This is a classic feature.

2. Uncontrollable urge to move occurs because of uncomfortable, sometimes painful sensations in the legs.

3. Sensations can be difficult to describe but include burning, aching, tingling, cramping, creeping, pulling, electric, itching, prickly, or crawling.

4. Symptoms are typically felt deep inside the muscles, in the middle portions of the lower limbs, especially the calves; feet or joints may be involved.

5. Symptoms tend to become more frequent and last longer with age.

E. Physical examination

1. Neurologic: Typically, normal sensory, coordination, reflex and fine motor skills

2. Extremities: Normal muscle strength examination in restless legs syndrome

IV. Diagnostic criteria (Allen et al., 2014; Gonzalez-Latapi & Malkani, 2019; Jiménez-Jiménez et al., 2018; Klingelhoefer et al., 2016; Trotti, 2017)

    A. Rapid screening of restless legs syndrome: "When you try to relax in the evening or sleep at night, do you ever have unpleasant, restless feelings in your legs that can be relieved by walking or movement?"

        1. This single standard question is validated by the International Restless Legs Syndrome Study Group.

        2. It has high sensitivity and specificity for the diagnosis of restless legs syndrome.

    B. First diagnostic criteria established by the International Restless Legs Syndrome Study Group in 1995; updated in 2003 and 2014

        1. An urge to move the legs usually but not always accompanied by, or felt to be caused by, uncomfortable and unpleasant sensations in the legs

        2. The beginning or worsening of the urge to move the legs and an unpleasant sensation during periods of rest or inactivity (sitting or lying down)

        3. The partial or total relief of the urge to move and unpleasant sensations by movement (including walking or stretching) as long as the movement is maintained

        4. The occurrence or worsening of the urge to move and unpleasant sensations during rest in the evening or at night

        5. The exclusion of other medical or behavioral conditions that can mimic these symptoms, such as myalgia, leg cramps, leg edema, venous stasis, arthritis, positional discomfort, or habitual foot tapping

    C. URGED: Mnemonic for diagnostic criteria

        1. **U**rge to move the legs, often accompanied by leg discomfort

        2. **R**est worsens the urge to move

        3. **G**etting up and moving improves the urge

        4. **E**vening or night worsens symptoms

        5. **D**isorders that mimic restless legs syndrome have been excluded

    D. Clinical course

        1. Chronic persistent restless legs syndrome: Symptoms, when not treated, would occur on average at least two times weekly for the past year.

        2. Intermittent restless legs syndrome: Symptoms, when not treated, would occur, on average, less than two times a week for the past year, with at least five lifetime events.

    E. Clinical features supporting the diagnosis of restless legs syndrome

        1. Periodic limb movements: Presence of periodic leg movements in sleep or resting wake at rates or intensity greater than expected for age or medical/medication status

        2. Dopaminergic treatment response: Reduction in symptoms at least initially with dopaminergic treatment

        3. Family history of restless legs syndrome among first-degree relatives

        4. Lack of profound daytime sleepiness

V. Diagnostic tests (Connor et al., 2017; Klingelhoefer et al., 2016)

    A. Laboratory

        1. Iron studies, specifically serum ferritin level, to evaluate for deficiency

        2. CBC to exclude anemia

        3. Serum vitamin B_{12} and folate to evaluate for deficiency

        4. Serum glucose and Hgb A1c to evaluate for diabetes

        5. Electrolytes to evaluate for imbalances

        6. Serum creatinine and urea to evaluate for renal insufficiency

        7. Thyroid function tests to evaluate for hypothyroidism

B. Radiology: Not indicated
C. Other
  1. Best-established neurobiologic abnormality in restless legs syndrome is low brain iron despite normal peripheral iron.
  2. Levodopa in a test dose can be used as a clinical "challenge test" for restless legs syndrome diagnosis.
  3. Sleep studies, such as polysomnography or immobilization tests, can be performed for patients with severe restless legs syndrome and insomnia.
  4. Electrophysiologic examination can be performed if peripheral neuropathy is suspected.

VI. Differential diagnosis (Allen et al., 2014; Klingelhoefer et al., 2016)
  A. Common conditions
    1. Nocturnal leg cramps
    2. Positional discomfort
    3. Local leg injury
    4. Arthritis (see Chapter 108)
    5. Leg edema (see Chapter 39)
    6. Vascular disease: Varicose veins, venous stasis, DVT (see Chapter 43)
    7. Intermittent claudication: Vascular/neurogenic
    8. Peripheral neuropathy (see Chapter 143)
    9. Radiculopathy
    10. Habitual foot tapping/leg rocking
    11. Painful legs/moving toes syndrome
    12. Anxiety (see Chapter 161)
    13. Myalgia (see Chapter 100)
    14. Drug-induced akathisia
  B. Less common
    1. Myelopathy
    2. Myopathy
    3. Vascular or neurogenic claudication
    4. Hypotensive akathisia
    5. Orthostatic tremor
    6. Sleep apnea (see Chapter 34)

VII. Treatment (During & Winkelman, 2019; Gonzalez-Latapi & Malkani, 2019; Klingelhoefer et al., 2016; Trenkwalder et al., 2018; Walters et al., 2003)
  A. Goal of treatment is to improve QOL by reducing nighttime sleep disturbance and daytime somnolence.
  B. Symptomatic treatment is dependent on the severity and frequency of restless legs syndrome symptoms and considers age, concomitant diseases, and medication.
    1. Restless Legs Syndrome Severity Scale scores disease burden from mild to very severe.
    2. Mild restless legs syndrome may be managed with reassurance and lifestyle changes, whereas severe restless legs syndrome may require drug therapy.
    3. Secondary causes and exacerbating factors should be identified and corrected.
      a) Iron supplementation can be used for anemia and low serum ferritin levels (less than 50 mcg/L); ferritin needs to be rechecked after iron supplementation (see Chapter 118).

        b) Concomitant medications that can induce or worsen restless legs syndrome symptoms include antidepressants, neuroleptics, beta-blockers, dopamine antagonists, antinausea drugs, antihistamines, anticonvulsants, L-thyroxine, and lithium.

    C. Nonpharmacologic measures
       1. Lifestyle changes
          a) Avoid high intake of caffeine or alcohol before bedtime.
          b) Sleep in a quiet, comfortable, cool environment, and keep regular bed and wake hours.
       2. Behavioral strategies during an attack: Allows patients to cope with symptoms
          a) Walking and stretching
          b) Massaging affected limbs
          c) Bathing in hot or cold water
          d) Relaxation exercises: Biofeedback, yoga
          e) Distracting the mind

    D. Pharmacologic measures: Pharmacologic treatment is only symptomatic and not preventive.
       1. Use in a step-by-step approach; consider patient age and concomitant diseases.
       2. Treatment is only required when the symptoms are clinically significant, such as with impairment of nighttime sleep, daytime alertness, and QOL.
       3. Keep dosages as low as possible and administer as a single evening dose.
       4. First-line treatment is dopaminergic agents.
          a) Nonergot dopamine agonists: Pramipexole 0.25–0.5 mg PO daily, ropinirole 0.5–4 mg daily, rotigotine 1 mg daily as transdermal patch applied nightly
          b) Levodopa: Levodopa/carbidopa or levodopa/benserazide starting dose of 50 mg/12.5 mg PO daily
       5. Second-line treatment for refractory cases
          a) Alpha-2-delta calcium channel ligands: Starting dose of pregabalin 25 mg PO nightly; starting dose of gabapentin 300 mg PO nightly (see Appendix Q)
          b) Benzodiazepines: Clonazepam 0.5–2 mg PO nightly
          c) Opioids: If indicated (see Appendix F)

    E. Treatment-related adverse effects
       1. Augmentation
          a) Most common treatment-related adverse effect
          b) Characterized by an overall increase in the severity of restless legs syndrome symptoms
          c) A paradoxical response to treatment: Symptoms get worse with increasing dose of the medication and improve following decrease in dose.
       2. Early morning rebound: Reappearance of restless legs syndrome symptoms in the morning as medication effects are wearing off
       3. Impulse control disorders from dopaminergic agents
          a) Incidence estimated to be 3%–17%
          b) Includes obsessive-compulsive behavior, hypersexuality, binge eating, pathologic gambling, and compulsive shopping

VIII. Follow-up (Klingelhoefer et al., 2016)
    A. Follow up in one to two weeks to evaluate effects of medication.
    B. Frequent follow-up may be needed for lifetime pharmacologic treatment; restless legs syndrome is a chronic disorder.

IX. Referrals: If the symptoms are not improving with treatment, refer to neurologist.

References

Allen, R.P., Picchietti, D.L., Garcia-Borreguero, D., Ondo, W.G., Walters, A.S., Winkelman, J.W., ... Lee, H.B. (2014). Restless legs syndrome/Willis-Ekbom disease diagnostic criteria: Updated International Restless Legs Syndrome Study Group (RLSSG) consensus criteria—History, rationale, description, and significance. *Sleep Medicine, 15*(8), 860–873. https://doi.org/10.1016/j.sleep.2014.03.025

Alonso-Navarro, H., García-Martín, E., Agúndez, J.A.G., & Jiménez-Jiménez, F.J. (2019). Association between restless legs syndrome and other movement disorders. *Neurology, 92*(20), 948–964. https://doi.org/10.1212/wnl.0000000000007500

Connor, J.R., Patton, S.M., Oexle, K., & Allen, R.P. (2017). Iron and restless legs syndrome: Treatment, genetics and pathophysiology. *Sleep Medicine, 31,* 61–70. https://doi.org/10.1016/j.sleep.2016.07.028

During, E.H., & Winkelman, J.W. (2019). Drug treatment of restless legs syndrome in older adults. *Drugs and Aging, 36*(10), 939–946. https://doi.org/10.1007/s40266-019-00698-1

Gonzalez-Latapi, P., & Malkani, R. (2019). Update on restless legs syndrome: From mechanisms to treatment. *Current Neurology and Neuroscience Reports, 19*(8), 54. https://doi.org/10.1007/s11910-019-0965-4

Jiménez-Jiménez, F.J., Alonso-Navarro, H., García-Martín, E., & Agúndez, J.A.G. (2018). Genetics of restless legs syndrome: An update. *Sleep Medicine Reviews, 39,* 108–121. https://doi.org/10.1016/j.smrv.2017.08.002

Klingelhoefer, L., Bhattacharya, K., & Reichmann, H. (2016). Restless legs syndrome. *Clinical Medicine, 16*(4), 379–382. https://doi.org/10.7861/clinmedicine.16-4-379

Muth, C.C. (2017). Restless legs syndrome. *JAMA, 317*(7), 780. https://doi.org/10.1001/jama.2016.21375

Trenkwalder, C., Allen, R., Högl, B., Clemens, S., Patton, S., Schormair, B., & Winkelmann, J. (2018). Comorbidities, treatment, and pathophysiology in restless legs syndrome. *Lancet Neurology, 17*(11), 994–1005. https://doi.org/10.1016/s1474-4422(18)30311-9

Trotti, L.M. (2017). Restless legs syndrome and sleep-related movement disorders. *Continuum, 23*(4), 1005–1016. https://doi.org/10.1212/con.0000000000000488

Walters, A.S., LeBrocq, C., Dhar, A., Hening, W., Rosen, R., Allen, R.P., ... Trenkwalder, C. (2003). Validation of the International Restless Legs Syndrome Study Group rating scale for restless legs syndrome. *Sleep Medicine, 4*(2), 121–132. https://doi.org/10.1016/s1389-9457(02)00258-7

Wijemanne, S., & Ondo, W. (2017). Restless legs syndrome: Clinical features, diagnosis and a practical approach to management. *Practice Neurology, 17*(6), 444–452. https://doi.org/10.1136/practneurol-2017-001762

CHAPTER 108

Rheumatoid Arthritis

Marlon Garzo Saria, PhD, RN, FAAN, and Santosh Kesari, MD, PhD, FANA, FAAN

I. Definition: Chronic inflammatory disease characterized by inflammation and swelling of the synovium of the joint, with subsequent destruction of articular structures (Alpay-Kanıtez et al., 2019; Gibofsky, 2014; Schett, 2019)

II. Physiology/Pathophysiology (Gibofsky, 2014; Schett, 2019; Sharif et al., 2018)
   A. Normal: The musculoskeletal system is a bony structure with its joints held together by ligaments attached to muscles by tendons and cushioned with cartilage.
      1. Most joints are freely moving articulations (diarthrodial) enclosed by a capsule of fibrous articular cartilage and ligaments.
      2. Synovial membrane lines the articular cavity and secretes lubricating synovial fluid.
      3. The synovial joint is the most common type of joint in the body and is characterized by the synovial cavity. The articular capsule, a fibrous connective tissue, attaches to the periarticular bones and encloses the synovial cavity within it.
      4. The bones in the synovial joint, in contrast to other joint types, are protected from direct contact by the articular cartilage, a highly specialized hyaline connective tissue that provides a lubricating surface for efficient articulation to facilitate free locomotion.
   B. Pathophysiology: RA is the result of complex autoimmune and inflammatory processes that involve components of both the innate and adaptive immune systems.
      1. The nature of these interactions is greatly affected by the local cytokine and chemokine environment of the synovium.
      2. In established RA, the synovial membrane is populated by a variety of inflammatory cell types that work together to cause joint destruction.
      3. Dendritic cells and helper T17 cells are pivotal in disease pathogenesis.
         a) Dendritic cells increase the release of IL-1, IL-6, IL-23, TNF-α, and other factors.
         b) Activation of dendritic cells results in the stimulation and selective differentiation of specific T-cell subsets.
         c) Helper T17 cells are notable for secreting the cytokine IL-17, which effects a wide array of functions by affecting multiple cell lines, including monocytes, fibroblasts, osteoclasts, and chondrocytes.
         d) IL-17 orchestrates chronic inflammation and joint destruction through its influence on cytokine release from those activated cells, including IL-1, IL-6, TNF-α, prostaglandin E2, metalloproteinases, and other molecules.
         e) Upregulated expression of receptor activator of nuclear factor kappa-B ligand on osteoblasts has been shown to follow IL-17 secretion. This upregulation promotes the formation of osteoclasts, the agents of bone dissolution.

III. Clinical features: RA is a chronic systemic disease of unknown etiology. It typically leads to deformity through the stretching of tendons and ligaments and to the destruction of joints through the erosion of cartilage and joints. Patients with active RA also experience systemic inflammation associated with a variety of comorbidities, most importantly cardiovascular disease, which contributes to increased morbidity and mortality. Patients with RA have an increased propensity toward infection, even without the addition of immunomodulatory therapies. They also have markedly increased risk of hematologic malignancies. For example, their risk of lymphoma is up to 26 times higher than the general population (Alpay-Kanıtez et al., 2019; Brown & Isaacs, 2014; Gibofsky, 2014; Kay & Upchurch, 2012; Schett, 2019; Smolen et al., 2018; Srivastava et al., 2019; van der Woude & van der Helm-van Mil, 2018).

A. Risk factors
   1. Gender: Approximately twice as prevalent in females than males
   2. Genetic factors: Differences in *HLA-DRB1* alleles, rheumatoid factor, anticitrullinated protein antibody, common amino acid motif
   3. Environment: Infectious agents (e.g., Epstein-Barr virus, CMV, *Proteus* species, *Escherichia coli*) and their products (e.g., heat-shock proteins), smoking, silica exposure, vitamin D deficiency, obesity, and changes in the microbiota
   4. Genetic–environmental interactions: Increased incidence of RA in individuals with certain *HLA-DRB1* alleles who smoke cigarettes

B. Etiology
   1. Exact cause of RA is unknown, but initiation of disease seems to result from an interaction among genetic susceptibility, environmental triggers, and chance.
   2. The local and systemic fallout from the inflammatory process drives the excess morbidity and mortality in patients with RA.
      a) In early disease, the process of inflammation causes thickening of the synovium and exudation of fluid into the joint. Synovitis occurs as a consequence of leukocyte infiltration into the synovium.
      b) Left unchecked, this synovitis underpins joint damage and destruction, which becomes evident in serial radiographs as joint space narrowing and erosions.
      c) Patients with RA have an excess cardiovascular risk that is equivalent to that of diabetes. They have double the risk of having a MI and an approximately 70% increased risk of stroke compared with non-RA matched controls.

C. History
   1. History of cancer and cancer treatment
   2. Current medications: Prescribed, over the counter
   3. History of presenting symptoms: Precipitating factors, onset, location, duration, associated symptoms (e.g., painful joints, morning stiffness, fever, weight loss, sleep disturbances)
   4. Changes in ADLs
   5. Past medical history: Cardiac disease, COPD, depression, vitamin D deficiency
   6. Social history: Smoking

D. Signs and symptoms
   1. The classic presentation of RA is a symmetrical polyarthritis involving hand and foot joints that has a chronic, persistent course.
   2. RA can affect all synovial-lined joints but has a predilection for the small joints of the hands and feet before it affects larger joints, including the knees, shoulders, hips, and others.
   3. Musculoskeletal symptoms
      a) Symmetric joint pain
      b) Morning stiffness lasting one hour or longer for six weeks

    c) Pain occurring with movement and rest

    d) Swelling involving wrist or metacarpophalangeal, proximal interphalangeal, ankle, or metatarsophalangeal joints

    e) Swelling of three or more joints for six or more weeks

    f) Muscle weakness

  4. Constitutional symptoms

    a) Rest interrupted by pain

    b) Depression

    c) Anorexia, weight loss

    d) Malaise

    e) Fatigue

    f) Low-grade fever

  5. Extra-articular manifestations

    a) Subcutaneous nodules

    b) Shortness of breath

E. Physical examination: Although some patients can be asymptomatic, others can present with severe symptoms including paralysis.

  1. Neurologic

    a) Gait assessment for ambulation difficulties

    b) Myelopathy: Babinski sign, Romberg sign, Lhermitte sign, clonus

  2. Pulmonary: Decrease in breath sounds and dullness indicating pleural effusion, interstitial lung disease, or fibrosis

  3. Cardiac: Extra or distant heart sounds or rub indicating pericarditis or pericardial effusion

  4. Extremities

    a) Joint deformities including swan neck deformity, boutonniere deformity of the hands, flexion deformity of the wrist, or lesser toe deformities

    b) Soft synovial joint swelling (a key clinical feature of RA) typically with tenderness

F. Classification criteria: Any patient who has active synovitis in at least one joint not explained by a non-RA diagnosis

  1. Numerical scores are assessed in four domains: joint involvement, serology, acute phase reactants, and duration of symptoms.

    a) Joint involvement and distribution (0–5 points): This variable includes any swollen or tender joint on clinical examination, excluding the distal interphalangeal joints of hands and feet, the first metatarsophalangeal joints, and the first carpometacarpal joints. Additional evidence from MRI or ultrasonography may be used to identify additional joints.

      (1) 1 large joint (e.g., shoulder, elbow, hip, knee, ankle): 0 points

      (2) 2–10 large joints: 1 point

      (3) 1–3 small joints (e.g., metacarpophalangeal joint, proximal interphalangeal joint, the second to fifth metatarsophalangeal joints, the interphalangeal joint of the thumb and the wrist): 2 points

      (4) 4–10 small joints: 3 points

      (5) Greater than 10 joints (of which greater than or equal to 1 is a small joint): 5 points

    b) Symptom duration (0–1 points): This variable refers to the patient's self-report on the maximum duration of signs and symptoms of any joint that is clinically involved at the time of assessment.

      (1) Less than six weeks: 0 points

      (2) Greater than or equal to six weeks: 1 point

    c) Serology (0–3 points)
        (1) Negative for rheumatoid factor and negative for anticitrullinated protein antibody: 0 points
        (2) Low positive for rheumatoid factor or low positive for anticitrullinated protein antibody: 2 points
        (3) High positive for rheumatoid factor or high positive for anticitrullinated protein antibody: 3 points
    d) Acute phase reactants (0–1 points)
        (1) Normal CRP and ESR levels: 0 points
        (2) Abnormal CRP levels or abnormal ESR: 1 point
  2. A score of greater than or equal to 6 points out of 10 can be classified as having RA.

IV. Diagnostic tests: RA is generally a diagnosis based on history taking and physical examination (Allard-Chamard & Boire, 2019; Alpay-Kanıtez et al., 2019; England et al., 2019; Gibofsky, 2014; Sharif et al., 2018).
  A. Laboratory
    1. Rheumatoid factor and anticitrullinated protein antibodies: Markers of autoimmune dysfunction
      a) Normal: Less than ULN
      b) Low positive: Between ULN and less than 3 times ULN
      c) High positive: Greater than 3 times ULN
    2. ESR and CRP levels typically elevated but not diagnostic of RA
    3. Baseline chemistries to assess hepatic and renal function
    4. CBC to assess anemia and thrombocytosis consistent with chronic inflammation
  B. Radiology
    1. Plain films: Bone erosions are usually detected. The number and size of bone erosions constitute a key measure of disease severity, progression, and disease response to therapeutic measures.
    2. MRI: Imaging is not needed to diagnose RA but is useful in detecting early signs of inflammation, joint effusion, and bone marrow edema.
  C. Other: Synovial fluid analysis to determine if joint effusion is present to evaluate for gout, pseudogout, or infection

V. Differential diagnosis (Alpay-Kanıtez et al., 2019; Smolen et al., 2018)
  A. Trauma
  B. Acute inflammatory events: Gout (see Chapter 103), pseudogout, septic arthritis
  C. Psoriatic arthritis
  D. OA (see Chapter 105)
  E. FMS (see Chapter 101)
  F. Lyme arthritis
  G. Osteoarthropathy (see Appendix M)

VI. Treatment (DiRenzo & Finan, 2019; Law & Taylor, 2019; Mian et al., 2019; Owens, 2014; Smolen et al., 2018; Srivastava et al., 2019)
  A. Management is focused on preventing disease progression and improving patient health status and productivity that can result from optimal disease control.
  B. The current treatment strategy for RA involves a treat-to-target approach based on tight monitoring of disease activity and change of management if a treatment target is not reached.
  C. Nonpharmacologic measures

1. Hot and cold therapy
   a) Cold packs help to reduce inflammation and swelling; instruct patients to avoid applying directly to skin.
   b) Heat therapy is ideal as a hot bath or shower. Advise patients on safety measures with heating pad or hot pack use.
2. Occupational therapy
   a) Appropriate for patients with joint deformity and functional difficulties
   b) Can recommend assistive devices for fine motor activities
3. Exercise, specifically aquatic exercise, is beneficial for reducing pain and disability in many musculoskeletal conditions, including RA.
D. Pharmacologic measures
   1. Early disease: Daily NSAIDs (see Appendix E)
   2. Synthetic disease-modifying antirheumatic drugs
      a) Conventional
         (1) Unknown target
            (a) Methotrexate: 7.5–25 mg PO weekly
            (b) Sulfasalazine: 500 mg PO two times a day, up to 1.5 g two times a day
         (2) Hydroxychloroquine: 200–400 mg PO daily, not to exceed 6.5 mg/kg daily
         (3) Known target of dihydroorotate dehydrogenase: Leflunomide 20 mg PO daily
         (4) CBC, chemistries, and eye examinations prior to initiating therapy, laboratory monitoring at least monthly, eye examination yearly
      b) Targeted
         (1) Janus kinase (JAK)1 and JAK2: Baricitinib 2 mg PO daily
         (2) JAK1, JAK2, and JAK3: Tofacitinib 5 mg PO two times a day, or tofacitinib extended release 100 mg PO daily
   3. Biologic (see Table 108-1)
E. Prevention
   1. Smoking cessation
   2. Oral health programs
   3. Weight loss
   4. Increased fish consumption

VII. Follow-up (Smolen et al., 2018; van der Woude & van der Helm-van Mil, 2018)
   A. Patient-reported outcomes and status free of disease-modifying antirheumatic drugs are novel important outcome measures.
   B. An effective treat-to-target approach relies on frequent monitoring of disease activity and prompt treatment adaptations.
   C. When starting medications or during an exacerbation, see patient every two or three weeks.
   D. Obtain laboratory tests based on drug therapy.

VIII. Referrals
   A. Rheumatologist: For consultation at the time of diagnosis prior to beginning therapy or if the patient appears to need second-line therapy
   B. Physical therapist: For initial consultation upon diagnosis to counsel on body mechanics, devices to assist with ADLs, range-of-motion exercises, and thermal modalities (e.g., paraffin baths)
   C. Ophthalmologist: For eye examination annually for patients receiving hydroxychloroquine therapy

TABLE 108-1		Immunotherapy for Rheumatoid Arthritis	
Drug and Classification	**Trade Name**	**Dose**	**Laboratory Monitoring**
Abatacept T-cell inhibitor	Orencia®	IV regimen based on patient's weight; given weeks 0, 2, and 4 followed by once-a-month infusion Subcutaneous: a single IV loading dose, then 125 mg subcutaneous injection given the following day, followed by 125 mg subcutaneous injection once a week	Obtain baseline CBC and LFTs, and repeat every 3 months for the first 6–12 months.
Adalimumab TNF inhibitor	Humira®	40 mg subcutaneous every other week if used in combination with methotrexate, or 40 mg weekly if used as single agent	Obtain baseline CBC and LFTs, and repeat every 3 months for the first 6–12 months.
Certolizumab pegol TNF inhibitor	Cimzia®	400 mg subcutaneous weeks 0, 2, and 4, then 200 mg subcutaneous every 2 weeks	Obtain baseline CBC and LFTs, and repeat every 3 months for the first 6–12 months.
Etanercept TNF inhibitor	Enbrel®	50 mg subcutaneous once a week	Obtain baseline CBC and LFTs, and repeat every 3 months for the first 6–12 months.
Golimumab TNF inhibitor	Simponi®	50 mg subcutaneous once a month	Obtain baseline CBC and LFTs, and repeat every 3 months for the first 6–12 months.
Infliximab TNF inhibitor	Remicade®	3 mg/kg IV on weeks 0, 2, and 6, then every 8 weeks	Obtain baseline CBC and LFTs, and repeat every 3 months for the first 6–12 months.
Rituximab Anti-CD20 monoclonal antibody	Rituxan®	A single course of 1,000 mg IV infusion given at weeks 0 and 2; used only for patients who have failed TNF inhibitor therapy	Obtain baseline CBC and LFTs, and repeat every 3 months for the first 6–12 months.
Tocilizumab IL-6 receptor inhibitor	Actemra®	IV infusion based on patient's weight; used only for patients who have failed TNF inhibitor therapy	Obtain baseline CBC and LFTs, then repeat every 4–8 weeks. Perform lipid panel 4–8 weeks following the initiation of tocilizumab, then repeat every 24 weeks.
Tofacitinib citrate Inhibitor of Janus kinases	Xeljanz®	5 mg PO two times a day 11 mg PO daily extended release 5 mg PO once daily for moderate to severe renal insufficiency or moderate hepatic impairment	Obtain baseline CBC, next obtain CBC and lipid panel 4–8 weeks after initiation, then repeat CBC every 3 months

CBC—complete blood count; CD20—cluster of differentiation 20; IL-6—interleukin 6; IV—intravenous; LFTs—liver function tests; PO—by mouth; TNF—tumor necrosis factor

Note. Based on information from Law & Taylor, 2019; Mian et al., 2019.

The authors would like to acknowledge Deanna Sanchez Yamamoto, RN, MS, ANP, for her contribution to this chapter that remains unchanged from the previous edition of this book.

References

Allard-Chamard, H., & Boire, G. (2019). Serologic diagnosis of rheumatoid arthritis. *Clinics in Laboratory Medicine, 39*(4), 525–537. https://doi.org/10.1016/j.cll.2019.07.002

Alpay-Kanıtez, N., Çelik, S., & Bes, C. (2019). Polyarthritis and its differential diagnosis. *European Journal of Rheumatology, 6*(4), 167–173. https://doi.org/10.5152/eurjrheum.2019.19145

Brown, P.M., & Isaacs, J.D. (2014). Rheumatoid arthritis: From palliation to remission in two decades. *Clinical Medicine, 14*(Suppl. 6), s50–s55. https://doi.org/10.7861/clinmedicine.14-6-s50

DiRenzo, D., & Finan, P. (2019). Self-efficacy and the role of non-pharmacologic treatment strategies to improve pain and affect in arthritis. *Current Treatment Options in Rheumatology, 5*(2), 168–178. https://doi.org/10.1007/s40674-019-00123-z

England, B.R., Tiong, B.K., Bergman, M.,J., Curtis, J.R., Kazi, S., Mikuls, T.R., ... Michaud, K. (2019). 2019 update of the American College of Rheumatology recommended rheumatoid arthritis disease activity measures. *Arthritis Care and Research, 71*(12), 1540–1555. https://doi.org/10.1002/acr.24042

Gibofsky, A. (2014). Epidemiology, pathophysiology, and diagnosis of rheumatoid arthritis: A synopsis. *American Journal of Managed Care, 20*(Suppl. 7), S128–S135. https://www.ajmc.com/view/ace017_may14_ra-ce_gibofsky1_s128

Kay, J., & Upchurch, K.S. (2012). ACR/EULAR 2010 rheumatoid arthritis classification criteria. *Rheumatology, 51*(Suppl. 6), vi5–vi9. https://doi.org/10.1093/rheumatology/kes279

Law, S.T., & Taylor, P.C. (2019). Role of biological agents in treatment of rheumatoid arthritis. *Pharmacological Research, 150,* 104497. https://doi.org/10.1016/j.phrs.2019.104497

Mian, A., Ibrahim, F., & Scott, D.L. (2019). A systematic review of guidelines for managing rheumatoid arthritis. *BMC Rheumatology, 3,* 42. https://doi.org/10.1186/s41927-019-0090-7

Owens, G.M. (2014). Managed care implications in managing rheumatoid arthritis. *American Journal of Managed Care, 20*(7 Suppl.), S145–S152. https://www.ajmc.com/view/ace017_may14_ra-ce_owens_s145tos152

Schett, G. (2019). Resolution of inflammation in arthritis. *Seminars in Immunopathology, 41*(6), 675–679. https://doi.org/10.1007/s00281-019-00768-x

Sharif, K., Sharif, A., Jumah, F., Oskouian, R., & Tubbs, R.S. (2018). Rheumatoid arthritis in review: Clinical, anatomical, cellular and molecular points of view. *Clinical Anatomy, 31*(2), 216–223. https://doi.org/10.1002/ca.22980

Smolen, J.S., Aletaha, D., Barton, A., Burmester, G.R., Emery, P., Firestein, G.S., ... Yamamoto, K. (2018). Rheumatoid arthritis. *Nature Reviews Disease Primers, 4,* 18001. https://doi.org/10.1038/nrdp.2018.1

Srivastava, S.B., Fluegel, N., & Mansukhani, R.P. (2019). Pharmacologic management of rheumatoid arthritis. *Orthopedic Nursing, 38*(6), 390–395. https://doi.org/10.1097/NOR.0000000000000610

van der Woude, D., & van der Helm-van Mil, A.H.M. (2018). Update on the epidemiology, risk factors, and disease outcomes of rheumatoid arthritis. *Best Practice and Research Clinical Rheumatology, 32*(2), 174–187. https://doi.org/10.1016/j.berh.2018.10.005

CHAPTER 109

Sciatica

Marlon Garzo Saria, PhD, RN, FAAN, and Santosh Kesari, MD, PhD, FANA, FAAN

I. Definition (Di Mattia et al., 2018; Jensen et al., 2019; Koes et al., 2007; Stynes et al., 2018; Troutner & Battaglia, 2020)
   A. A disease of the PNS that is consistent with lumbar radiculopathy
   B. An arcane term universally used by clinicians and the public to refer to back-related leg pain
   C. Neither diagnostically nor epistemologically accurate
      1. No consensus over a universally accepted definition
      2. Absence of widely accepted diagnostic criteria
   D. Also referred to as lumbosacral radicular syndrome, ischia, nerve root pain, and nerve root entrapment

II. Physiology/Pathophysiology: Poor understanding of the underlying pathophysiology (Ropper & Zafonte, 2015; Troutner & Battaglia, 2020)
   A. Normal
      1. Lumbar spine consists of five movable lumbar vertebral bodies (L1–L5).
      2. Sacrum is made up of five developmentally fused vertebral levels terminating in the coccyx.
      3. Commonly, this region is referred to as the lumbosacral spine.
      4. Spinal nerve root passes below each level. On each side are five lumbar, five sacral, and one coccygeal spinal nerve roots.
      5. The fourth and fifth lumbar nerve roots and the first two sacral nerve roots join in the lumbosacral plexus to form the peroneal and tibial nerves that leave the pelvis in an ensheathed single trunk as the sciatic nerve.
   B. Pathophysiology
      1. Disturbances anywhere along the course of the sciatic nerve can give rise to sciatica.
         a) Most common areas are at the sites of disc rupture and OA change at the L4–L5 and L5–S1 levels.
         b) Less frequently, there is compression of the root below the corresponding disc at the L3–L4 level.
         c) Other sites of sciatic injury are in the lower pelvic cavity, buttock, gluteal fold, and proximal biceps femoris muscle.
      2. Symptoms may be caused by distortion of the nerve root or its sensory ganglion.
      3. Pain may also be related to the effect of local inflammatory cytokines.

III. Clinical features: The diagnosis of sciatica and its management vary considerably within and between countries (Ferreira & McLachlan, 2016; Jensen et al., 2019; Koes et al., 2007; Ropper & Zafonte, 2015; Stynes et al., 2018; Troutner & Battaglia, 2020).

A. Risk factors
   1. Personal factors
      a) Age: Peak 45–64 years
      b) Increasing risk with height
      c) Smoking
      d) Mental stress
      e) Obesity
   2. Occupational factors
      a) Strenuous physical activity: Frequent lifting, especially while bending and twisting
      b) Driving: Vibration of whole body
B. Etiology
   1. Herniated disc with nerve root compression
   2. Lumbar stenoses
   3. Tumors of the spine
   4. Infection of the spine
C. History
   1. History of cancer and cancer treatment
   2. Current medications: Prescribed, over the counter
   3. History of presenting symptoms: Precipitating factors, onset, location, duration
   4. Changes in ADLs
   5. Past medical history: Trauma to back, herniated disc
   6. Social history: Smoking, occupational
D. Signs and symptoms
   1. Radiating pain most commonly at the leg and below the knee
   2. Characterized by radiating pain that follows a dermatomal pattern (see Appendix B)
   3. Pain beginning suddenly with physical activity or slowly
      a) Described as aching or sharp
      b) Usually unilateral; bilateral pain in central disc herniation, lumbar stenosis, and spondylolisthesis
      c) Radiates along a broad line from the middle or lower buttock, proceeding dorsolaterally in the thigh in cases of compression of the L5 nerve root, and posteriorly in cases of compression of S1
      d) With L4 compression, anterolateral pain in the thigh that may be misattributed to hip disease
      e) Increased back and sciatic pain with coughing, sneezing, straining, or other forms of the Valsalva maneuver suggestive of disc rupture
      f) Pain potentially radiating to foot or toes
      g) Pain around the buttocks area that occurs suddenly or develops gradually
   4. Sensory symptoms (e.g., numbness, tingling, burning) in the involved lower leg
E. Physical examination
   1. Neurologic: Nerve root tension or neurologic deficits; in cases with a dermatomal pattern, positive result on straight leg raising test, or loss of strength or sensibility disorders, perform the following.
      a) Reflexes (Achilles or knee tendon): Positive dorsiflexion of ankle, decrease or loss of deep tendon reflexes on the affected leg
      b) Sensitivity of lateral and medial sides of feet and toes decreased; light touch pinprick and two-point discrimination decreased or not present on the affected leg with sciatica
      c) Strength of great toe during extension decreased

    d) Walking on toes and heel: Left–right differences

  2. Extremities

    a) Lasègue sign (straight leg raising test): Positive test consists of reproduction or marked worsening of the patient's initial pain and firm resistance to further elevation of the leg; sciatica induces more leg pain. Back pain indicates herniated disc.

    b) Fajersztajn test (crossed, straight leg raising test): When raising the unaffected leg, positive test consists of pain elicited in the opposite (affected) leg.

    c) Unilateral leg pain greater than low back pain

IV. Diagnostic tests (Bernstein et al., 2017; Jensen et al., 2019; Koes et al., 2007; Stynes et al., 2018)

  A. Laboratory: Not indicated

  B. Radiology

    1. Imaging should be done only in specialist care settings and only if the result is likely to change management.

    2. Imaging is indicated if there are red flags that the condition may be caused by an underlying disease (e.g., infections, malignancies) rather than disc herniation.

    3. Diagnostic imaging may also be indicated in patients with severe symptoms who fail to respond to conservative care for six to eight weeks.

    4. Some experts favor MRI above other imaging techniques because CT has a higher radiation dose and soft tissues are better visualized; however, both are equally accurate at diagnosing lumbar disc herniation.

  C. Other: Needle electromyography and nerve conduction studies can reveal a topographic distribution of muscular denervation corresponding to a nerve root.

V. Differential diagnosis: Alternative diagnoses should be considered when examining patients with low back pain, particularly if they develop new or changed symptoms (Bernstein et al., 2017).

  A. Cancer of spine

  B. Infection of spine

  C. Trauma

  D. Inflammatory disease: Spondylarthritis

  E. Compression fracture (see Chapter 102)

  F. Bony osteophytes

  G. Peripheral neuropathy (see Chapter 143)

  H. Degenerative spinal stenosis

  I. Herniated disc

  J. Cauda equina syndrome

VI. Treatment (Bernstein et al., 2017; Di Mattia et al., 2018; Ferreira & McLachlan, 2016; Jensen et al., 2019; Koes et al., 2007; Mathieson et al., 2017; Rasmussen-Barr et al., 2016; Shiri et al., 2019)

  A. Conservative treatment for sciatica is primarily aimed at pain reduction. Surgical intervention focuses on removal of disc herniation with the purpose of eliminating the suspected cause of the sciatica.

  B. Exercise programs, activity, and participation in work and everyday life form the basis of the treatment because they are effective and can be continued beyond the episode of low back pain to improve long-term outcomes.

  C. Avoiding bed rest is recommended in numerous clinical practice guidelines pertaining to the management of acute, nonspecific low back pain in a primary care setting.

D. Risk stratification (e.g., STarT Back Screening Tool) should be considered at the first encounter with a healthcare professional for each new episode of low back pain with or without sciatica.

1. Less intensive support for patients with low back pain with or without sciatica who are likely to improve quickly and have a good outcome
   a) Reassurance
   b) Advice to stay active
   c) Guidance on self-management

2. More complex and intensive support for patients with low back pain with or without sciatica at higher risk of a poor outcome
   a) Exercise programs with or without manual therapy
   b) Psychological approach

E. Nonpharmacologic measures

1. Individual exercise programs with psychological and/or manual therapy
   a) Manual therapy: Manipulation, mobilization, soft tissue techniques such as massage
   b) Psychological therapies: Cognitive behavioral approach
   c) Educational components
      (1) Inform patients of the nature, causes, and expected prognosis of low back pain and sciatica.
      (2) Encourage to continue normal activities.

2. Group exercise programs: Biomechanical, aerobic, mind–body, or a combination of approaches

F. Pharmacologic measures: Prescribe drugs, if necessary, according to four steps.

1. NSAIDs (see Appendix E)
2. Tramadol, paracetamol, or NSAIDs in combination with codeine
3. Opioids (see Appendix F) in patients with severe pain inadequately controlled with NSAIDs
4. Muscle relaxants (e.g., cyclobenzaprine 10 mg PO daily up to three times a day) for short-term use
5. Gabapentin and pregabalin for neuropathic pain (see Appendix Q)

G. Other

1. Epidural injections of local anesthetic and steroid can be used in patients with acute and severe sciatica.
2. Spinal decompression may be considered for people with sciatica when nonsurgical treatment has not improved pain or function and their radiological findings are consistent with sciatic symptoms.
3. Cauda equina syndrome (symptoms of urinary retention or decreased anal sphincter tone) is an absolute indication for immediate surgery.
4. Elective surgery is the choice for unilateral sciatica.
5. Radiofrequency denervation is effective for people with severe localized low back pain arising from structures innervated by the medial branch nerves, where other nonsurgical treatments have not worked for them.

VII. Follow-up (Bernstein et al., 2017; Koes et al., 2007)

A. Short term: Evaluate interventions prescribed within two weeks of presentation. Clinical course of acute sciatica is favorable, and most pain and related disability resolves within two weeks.

B. Long term: Approximately 20% of patients are still symptomatic, and approximately 3% remain off work a year after an episode of low back pain. Continue to monitor and refer as warranted.

VIII. Referrals (Bernstein et al., 2017; Koes et al., 2007)
  A. Neurosurgeon: Immediately in cases of cauda equina syndrome or acute severe paresis or progressive paresis (within a few days)
  B. Neurologist, neurosurgeon, or orthopedic surgeon: For consideration of surgery in cases of intractable radicular pain (not responding to morphine) or if pain does not diminish after six to eight weeks of conservative care
  C. Primary care with pain clinic support: PRN
  D. Physical and/or occupational therapy: For evaluation, treatment, and exercise program

References

Bernstein, I.A., Malik, Q., Carville, S., & Ward, S. (2017). Low back pain and sciatica: Summary of NICE guidance. *BMJ, 356,* i6748. https://doi.org/10.1136/bmj.i6748

Di Mattia, F., Tejani, S., & Hall, T. (2018). Bed rest for sciatica: A closer look at the evidence. *Journal of Orthopaedic and Sports Physical Therapy, 48*(6), 436–438. https://doi.org/10.2519/jospt.2018.0609

Ferreira, M.L., & McLachlan, A. (2016). The challenges of treating sciatica pain in older adults. *Drugs and Aging, 33*(11), 779–785. https://doi.org/10.1007/s40266-016-0404-z

Jensen, R.K., Kongsted, A., Kjaer, P., & Koes, B. (2019). Diagnosis and treatment of sciatica. *BMJ, 367,* l6273. https://doi.org/10.1136/bmj.l6273

Koes, B.W., van Tulder, M.W., & Peul, W.C. (2007). Diagnosis and treatment of sciatica. *BMJ, 334*(7607), 1313–1317. https://doi.org/10.1136/bmj.39223.428495.BE

Mathieson, S., Maher, C.G., McLachlan, A.J., Latimer, J., Koes, B.W., Hancock, M.J., ... Lin, C.-W.C. (2017). Trial of pregabalinn for acute and chronic sciatica. *New England Journal of Medicine, 376*(12), 1111–1120. https://doi.org/10.1056/NEJMoa1614292

Rasmussen-Barr, E., Held, U., Grooten, W.J.A., Roelofs, P.D.D.M., Koes, B.W., van Tulder, M.W., & Wertli, M.M. (2016). Non-steroidal anti-inflammatory drugs for sciatica. *Cochrane Database of Systematic Reviews, 2016*(10). https://doi.org/10.1002/14651858.CD012382

Ropper, A.H., & Zafonte, R.D. (2015). Sciatica. *New England Journal of Medicine, 372*(13), 1240–1248. https://doi.org/10.1056/NEJMra1410151

Shiri, R., Falah-Hassani, K., Heliövaara, M., Solovieva, S., Amiri, S., Lallukka, T., ... Viikari-Juntura, E. (2019). Risk factors for low back pain: A population-based longitudinal study. *Arthritis Care and Research, 71*(2), 290–299. https://doi.org/10.1002/acr.23710

Stynes, S., Konstantinou, K., Ogollah, R., Hay, E.M., & Dunn, K.M. (2018). Clincial diagnositic model for sciatica developed in primary care patients with low back–related leg pain. *PLOS ONE, 13*(4), e0191852. https://doi.org/10.1371/journal.pone.0191852

Troutner, A.M., & Battaglia, P.J. (2020). The ambiguity of sciatica as a clinical diagnosis: A case series. *Journal of the American Association of Nurse Practitioners, 32*(8), 589–593. https://doi.org/10.1097/JXX.0000000000000288

Systemic Lupus Erythematosus

Marlon Garzo Saria, PhD, RN, FAAN, and Santosh Kesari, MD, PhD, FANA, FAAN

I. Definition (Fairley et al., 2020; Kado, 2018)
   A. Autoimmune condition with variable and often extensive manifestations; characterized by autoantibodies to nuclear components and immune complex deposition
   B. Discoid lupus erythematous: Affects the skin
   C. SLE: Attacks body organs and systems; can be life threatening
   D. Drug induced: Symptoms usually disappear when medicine is discontinued.

II. Physiology/Pathophysiology (Kokosi et al., 2019; Oparina et al., 2019)
   A. Normal
      1. The immune system provides the body's defense against infections and malignant diseases.
      2. Autoimmunity results in antibodies being produced against the body's own tissues.
   B. Pathophysiology
      1. Loss of tolerance in the immune system leads to the presence of autoantibodies and the deposition of immune complexes in various tissues, causing a diversity of symptoms.
      2. This process is initiated by polyclonal B-cell activation leading to hyperglobulinemia, which, in turn, leads to autoantibody production and immune complex formation, resulting in inflammation and damage to organ systems.

III. Clinical features: SLE causes irreversible damage to organ systems. Although it is an autoantibody and immune complex disease, most organ manifestations are inflammatory. Lupus nephritis is the most common organ-threatening manifestation of SLE, whereas the most common cardiac manifestation is pericarditis (Ahn et al., 2020; Aringer, 2020; Fairley et al., 2020; Gatto et al., 2019; Heinlen & Chakravarty, 2019; Illescas-Montes et al., 2019; Kado, 2018; Kokosi et al., 2019; Lam et al., 2016; Oparina et al., 2019; Zielinski et al., 2019; Zucchi et al., 2019).
   A. Risk factors
      1. Gender: Ten times more common in females than in males
      2. Race/ethnicity: Two times as prevalent in African Americans than Caucasians
   B. Etiology
      1. SLE is a systemic autoimmune disease with a complex multifactorial etiology and a broad spectrum of clinical manifestations.
      2. Multiple genome-wide and candidate–gene association studies identified over 80 SLE susceptibility loci, explaining about 30% of narrow-sense SLE heritability.
      3. Pathogens most frequently associated with SLE are viruses, including endogenous retrovirus, Epstein-Barr virus, parvovirus B19, CMV, and HIV type 1.

4. Drug-induced etiology includes procainamide, hydralazine, isoniazid, methyldopa, and minocycline.

C. History
1. History of cancer and cancer treatment
2. Current medications: Prescribed, over the counter
3. History of presenting symptoms: Precipitating factors, onset, location, duration, associated symptoms (e.g., painful joints, skin rashes or lesions, oral ulcers, Raynaud syndrome, arthralgias, alopecia, chest pain, photosensitivity)
4. Changes in ADLs
5. Family history: Autoimmune disorders
6. Past medical history: DVT, PE, recurrent and spontaneous abortions

D. Signs and symptoms: Symptoms are nonspecific, overlap with those of more common conditions, and vary with organ involvement.
1. Most common presenting symptoms are constitutional (e.g., fatigue, weight loss, fever without a focal infection).
2. Arthralgia, myalgia
3. Malar rash over cheeks and nose, or "butterfly rash"
4. Photosensitivity
5. Pleuritic chest pain
6. New-onset Raynaud phenomenon
7. Mouth sores
8. Seizures
9. Numbness and tingling of extremities
10. Fatigue

E. Manifestations in organs
1. Renal disease is present in one-third of patients with SLE.
   a) Active urine sediment indicates nephritis.
   b) Proteinuria indicates nephropathy.
2. Cardiovascular
   a) Pericarditis
   b) Accelerated atherosclerosis
   c) Valvular abnormalities
   d) Endocarditis and myocarditis
   e) Raynaud phenomenon
   f) Palpitations
3. Pulmonary
   a) Pleurisy
   b) PH
   c) Pulmonary parenchymal disease
4. Hematologic
   a) Anemia
   b) Thrombocytopenia
   c) Leukopenia
5. Neurologic
   a) Seizures
   b) Mononeuritis multiplex
   c) Peripheral and cranial neuropathy
   d) Cognitive impairment: Most common
   e) Transverse myelitis: Rare
   f) Headaches

        g) Vision changes

        h) Dizziness

    6. Serous membrane manifestations: Serositis

    7. Reticuloendothelial

        a) Lymphadenopathy

        b) Splenomegaly

        c) Hepatomegaly

F. Physical examination

    1. Integument

        a) Acute cutaneous lupus erythematosus: Photosensitive malar or macular rash

        b) Subacute cutaneous lupus erythematosus: Photosensitive papulosquamous or annular lesions

        c) Chronic cutaneous lupus erythematosus: Discoid lupus erythematosus, lupus profundus/panniculitis, chilblain lupus, lupus tumidus

        d) Cutaneous vasculitis, urticarial vasculitis, livedo reticularis, Raynaud phenomenon, periungual telangiectasias, erythema multiforme, calcinosis

    2. Neurologic: For patients complaining of neurologic symptoms or deficits, which are exhibited as memory loss or decreased cognitive function, peripheral neuropathy, and acute confusion

    3. Pulmonary: Pleural rub, decreased breath sounds, or dullness to percussion indicating fibrosis, pleural effusion, pleuritis with or without pleural effusion, acute pneumonitis, or interstitial lung disease

    4. Cardiac

        a) Pericardial rub suggestive of pericarditis, pericardial effusion

        b) Murmurs suggestive of valvular abnormalities

    5. Extremities: Joint pain and swelling

G. Systemic Lupus International Collaborating Clinics classification system: Must meet four criteria, including one clinical and one immunologic

    1. Clinical

        a) Acute cutaneous lupus: One or more of the following

            (1) Malar rash

            (2) Bullous lupus

            (3) Maculopapular rash

            (4) Photosensitive rash

        b) Chronic cutaneous lupus: One or more of the following

            (1) Classic discoid: Localized versus generalized

            (2) Hypertrophic lupus

            (3) Lupus panniculitis

            (4) Mucosal lupus

            (5) Lupus erythematosus tumidus

            (6) Chilblains lupus

            (7) Discoid lupus/lichen planus overlap

                (a) Oral or nasal ulcers

                (b) Nonscarring alopecia

                (c) Synovitis or tendonitis: Two or more joints with morning stiffness

                (d) Serositis: Pleural or pericardial

                (e) Renal

                    i. Urine protein-to-creatinine ratio with more than 500 mg protein in 24 hours *or*

                    ii. RBC casts

   c) Neurologic: One or more of the following
    (1) Seizures
    (2) Psychosis
    (3) Mononeuritis multiplex
    (4) Myelitis
    (5) Neuropathy
    (6) Acute confusion state
   d) Hematologic
    (1) Hemolytic anemia *or*
    (2) Leukopenia less than 4,000/mm³ at least once *or*
    (3) Lymphopenia less than 1,000/mm³ at least once *or*
    (4) Thrombocytopenia less than 100,000/mm³
  2. Immunologic criteria
   a) Antinuclear antibody (ANA) positivity
   b) Anti-dsDNA (double-stranded DNA) positivity
   c) Anti-Smith positivity
   d) Antiphospholipid antibody positivity
   e) Low complement
   f) Direct Coombs in absence of hemolytic anemia
 H. 1997 Update of the 1982 American College of Rheumatology Criteria for Classification of SLE: Must meet 4 of 11 criteria
  1. Malar rash
  2. Discoid rash
  3. Photosensitivity
  4. Oral or nasal ulcers
  5. Nonerosive arthritis: Two or more joints
  6. Serositis: Pleural or pericardial
  7. Renal disorder
   a) Persistent proteinuria: Greater than 0.5 g daily *or* greater than 3+ if quantification not performed (dipstick) *or*
   b) Cellular cast: Red cell, Hgb, granular, tubular, or mixed
  8. Neurologic disorder
   a) Seizure *or*
   b) Psychosis
  9. Hematologic disorder
   a) Hemolytic anemia with reticulocytosis *or*
   b) Leukopenia less than 4,000/mm³ on more than two occasions *or*
   c) Lymphopenia less than 1,500/mm³ on more than two occasions *or*
   d) Thrombocytopenia less than 100,00/mm³
  10. Antinuclear antibody positivity
  11. Anti-DNA, anti-Smith, *or* antiphospholipid antibody positivity

IV. Diagnostic tests (Aringer, 2020; Gatto et al., 2019; Kado, 2018; Lam et al., 2016; Zucchi et al., 2019)
 A. Laboratory
  1. Serologic testing can be useful before evaluation in rheumatology. The presence of specific autoantibodies correlates with particular organ involvement and prognosis.
   a) Positive antinuclear antibody is necessary but not sufficient for a diagnosis of SLE.
   b) Do not test antinuclear antibody sub-serologies without a positive and clinical suspicion of immune-mediated disease.

       c) Anti-Smith and anti-dsDNA antibodies are specific for systemic lupus and rarely found to be positive in people without SLE.

       d) Anti-RNP antibody is associated with mixed connective tissue.

       e) Anti-SSA/SSB antibody is associated with Sjögren syndrome.

       f) Antiphospholipid antibodies are present with lupus anticoagulant, IgM cardiolipin antibody, and IgG and IgM anti-beta2-glycoprotein (B2GP1).

  2. CBC

       a) Leukopenia indicating immune involvement

       b) Thrombocytopenia indicating chronic inflammation

       c) Autoimmune hemolytic anemia indicating immune injury to RBC

       d) ACD indicating chronic inflammation

  3. Lupus nephritis

       a) Manifestation is persistent proteinuria greater than 0.5 g daily or 3+ on dipstick, and/or RBCs, Hgb, granular, tubular, or mixed casts on examination of urine.

       b) Spot urine protein-to-creatinine ratio greater than 0.5 and an active urinary sediment with greater than 5 RBCs, greater than 5 WBCs/high-power field (without infection), WBC casts, or RBC casts serving as surrogate markers for proteinuria and casts.

  4. Complement C3 and C4: Decreased in SLE

  5. Vitamin D: Deficiency noted in SLE

 B. Radiology

  1. MRI of the brain in patients with headache or seizure to evaluate for white matter lesions common in neuropsychiatric SLE

  2. Chest x-ray to evaluate for pleural effusion

  3. DEXA scan to evaluate for osteopenia or osteoporosis with long-term steroid use

 C. Other

  1. Renal biopsy to evaluate for lupus nephritis

  2. Skin biopsy to evaluate for vasculitis

  3. ECG to evaluate chest pain due to pericarditis or ischemia

V. Differential diagnosis (Kokosi et al., 2019; Lam et al., 2016; Zielinski et al., 2019)

 A. Adult-onset Still disease

 B. Behçet syndrome

 C. Chronic fatigue syndrome (see Chapter 163)

 D. Endocarditis (see Chapter 46)

 E. FMS (see Chapter 101)

 F. HIV infection

 G. Inflammatory bowel disease

 H. Lyme disease (see Chapter 104)

 I. Mixed connective tissue disease

 J. Psoriatic arthritis

 K. Reactive arthritis

 L. RA (see Chapter 108)

 M. Sarcoidosis

 N. Systemic sclerosis

 O. Sjögren syndrome

VI. Treatment (Aringer et al., 2019; Fairley et al., 2020; Heinlen & Chakravarty, 2019; Kokosi et al., 2019; Lam et al., 2016; Zucchi et al., 2019)

A. Treatment of SLE should aim at ensuring long-term survival, preventing organ damage, and optimizing QOL.

1. For SLE, remission implicates absence of active joint disease, active skin disease, active kidney disease, and absence of hemolytic anemia.
2. Leukopenia, lymphopenia, or thrombocytopenia are manifestations that may lead to untoward consequences only if they reach a certain level. They do not always need immunomodulatory treatment and may be acceptable in remission.

B. Nonpharmacologic measures: All patients with SLE should receive education, counseling, and support.

1. Counsel patients to reduce traditional cardiovascular risk factors (e.g., smoking, healthy diet, maintain or lose weight) and to have routine screenings for diabetes mellitus, hypertension, and dyslipidemia.
2. Use sunscreens of SPF 15 or higher.

C. Pharmacologic measures

1. Hydroxychloroquine reduces disease flares and other constitutional symptoms and is considered the cornerstone of treatment.
   a) Dose is 200–400 mg PO daily.
   b) Hydroxychloroquine is favored over chloroquine because it is less toxic.
2. Low-dose glucocorticoids can be used to treat most manifestations (e.g., prednisone 5–30 mg PO daily; see Appendix K).
3. NSAIDs can be used as adjunctive therapy to treat joint pain (see Appendix E).
4. Immunosuppressive drugs
   a) Azathioprine: 2 mg/kg PO one or two times a day, then decreased to 1.5 mg/kg PO daily as tolerated
   b) Cyclophosphamide for lupus nephritis: 500 mg IV once every two weeks for six doses, or 500–1,000 mg/m^2 once every month for six doses, or 500–1,000 mg/m^2 every month for six months then every three months for a total of at least 2.5 years
   c) Methotrexate for vasculitis, arthritis, and skin conditions: 7.5–20 mg PO weekly
   d) Rituximab for refractory lupus nephritis: 375 mg/m^2 IV weekly for four weeks
5. Biologic agents
   a) Belimumab: 10 mg/kg IV every two weeks for three doses, then every four weeks for mild to moderate involvement
   b) Mycophenolate used instead of cyclophosphamide for SLE nephritis: 500–1,000 mg PO two times a day
6. Topical corticosteroids or calcineurin inhibitors for skin lesions (see Appendix K)
7. Replace vitamin D if deficient

D. Immunization

1. For patients with CKD who are receiving long-term immunosuppressive therapy, immunization with 13-valent pneumococcal conjugate vaccine followed by 23-valent pneumococcal polysaccharide vaccine should be considered.
2. Live vaccines should not be given to patients with SLE when they are receiving immunosuppressive therapy, and they should be delayed for at least one month after completion of the therapy.

VII. Follow-up (Lam et al., 2016)

A. Family practitioners can monitor disease activity and therapy in patients with moderate to severe SLE.
B. Measurement of anti-dsDNA antibodies, complements, and creatinine; CBC; and urinalysis should be performed every three to six months to monitor disease activity.
C. Annual eye examinations are required for patients receiving hydroxychloroquine.

    D. Screening for dyslipidemia, diabetes, and osteoporosis should be performed regularly in patients receiving glucocorticoids.

VIII. Referrals (Lam et al., 2016)
    A. Rheumatologist: For patients with increased disease activity, complications, or adverse effects from treatment
    B. Ophthalmologist: For retinal toxicity as a potential side effect and for patients with SLE who have ocular pain and visual impairment requiring urgent evaluation
    C. Renal biopsy: For patients with proteinuria of at least 1 g in 24 hours, or at least 0.5 g in 24 hours with hematuria or cellular casts
    D. Nephrologist: For lupus nephritis

The authors would like to acknowledge Deanna Sanchez Yamamoto, RN, MS, ANP, for her contribution to this chapter that remains unchanged from the previous edition of this book.

References

Ahn, G.Y., Lee, J., Won, S., Ha, E., Kim, H., Nam, B., ... Bae, S.-C. (2020). Identifying damage clusters in patients with systemic lupus erythematosus. *International Journal of Rheumatic Diseases, 23*(1), 84–91. https://doi.org/10.1111/1756-185x.13745

Aringer, M. (2020). Inflammatory markers in systemic lupus erythematosus. *Journal of Autoimmunity, 110,* 102374. https://doi.org/10.1016/j.jaut.2019.102374

Aringer, M., Leuchten, N., & Schneider, M. (2019). Treat to target in systemic lupus erythematosus. *Rheumatic Diseases Clinics of North America, 45*(4), 537–548. https://doi.org/10.1016/j.rdc.2019.07.004

Fairley, J.L., Oon, S., Saracino, A.M., & Nikpour, M. (2020). Management of cutaneous manifestations of lupus erythematosus: A systematic review. *Seminars in Arthritis and Rheumatism, 50*(1), 95–127. https://doi.org/10.1016/j.semarthrit.2019.07.010

Gatto, M., Saccon, F., Zen, M., Iaccarino, L., & Doria, A. (2019). Preclinical and early systemic lupus erythematosus. *Best Practice and Research Clinical Rheumatology, 33*(4), 101422. https://doi.org/10.1016/j.berh.2019.06.004

Heinlen, L., & Chakravarty, E.F. (2019). Lupus nephritis: Duration of therapy and possibility to withdrawal. *Advances in Chronic Kidney Disease, 26*(5), 387–392. https://doi.org/10.1053/j.ackd.2019.08.010

Illescas-Montes, R., Corona-Castro, C.C., Melguizo-Rodriguez, L., Ruiz, C., & Costela-Ruiz, V.J. (2019). Infectious processes and systemic lupus erythematosus. *Immunology, 158*(3), 153–160. https://doi.org/10.1111/imm.13103

Kado, R. (2018). Systemic lupus erythematosus for primary care. *Primary Care: Clinics in Office Practice, 45*(2), 257–270. https://doi.org/10.1016/j.pop.2018.02.011

Kokosi, M., Lams, B., & Agarwal, S. (2019). Systemic lupus erythematosus and antiphospholipid antibody syndrome. *Clinics in Chest Medicine, 40*(3), 519–529. https://doi.org/10.1016/j.ccm.2019.06.001

Lam, N.-C.V., Ghetu, M.V., & Bieniek, M.L. (2016). Systemic lupus erythematosus: Primary care approach to diagnosis and management. *American Family Physician, 94*(4), 284–294. https://www.aafp.org/afp/2016/0815/p284.html

Oparina, N., Martínez-Bueno, M., & Alarcón-Riquelme, M.E. (2019). An update on the genetics of systemic lupus erythematosus. *Current Opinion in Rheumatology, 31*(6), 659–668. https://doi.org/10.1097/bor.0000000000000654

Zielinski, M.R., Systrom, D.M., & Rose, N.R. (2019). Fatigue, sleep, and autoimmune and related disorders. *Frontiers in Immunology, 10,* 1827. https://doi.org/10.3389/fimmu.2019.01827

Zucchi, D., Elefante, E., Calabresi, E., Signorini, V., Bortoluzzi, A., & Tani, C. (2019). One year in review 2019: Systemic lupus erythematosus. *Clinical and Experimental Rheumatology, 37*(5), 715–722. https://www.clinexprheumatol.org/abstract.asp?a=14436

Lymph

CHAPTER 111

Lymphadenopathy

Christina Ferraro, MSN, APRN-CNP, BMTCN®

I. Definition: Lymph nodes that are abnormal secondary to size (greater than 1 cm or palpable supraclavicular, popliteal, epitrochlear, and iliac nodes), number, or consistency; may be primary or secondary manifestations of infective, benign, or malignant processes (Deosthali et al., 2019; Gaddey & Riegel, 2016; Tzankov & Dirnhofer, 2018)

   A. Generalized lymphadenopathy involves enlarged lymph nodes in two or more noncontiguous areas.

   B. Localized lymphadenopathy is confined to one area of involvement.

II. Physiology/Pathophysiology (Aulino et al., 2019; Gaddey & Riegel, 2016; Gru & O'Malley, 2018; Newton et al., 2017; Randolph et al., 2017)

   A. Normal

      1. Highly organized centers of immune cells that filter antigens from extracellular fluid

         a) Approximately 600 lymph nodes are located throughout the body.

         b) In healthy people, nodes in the submandibular, axillary, or inguinal regions may be palpable.

         c) Associated lymphoid organs include the spleen, tonsils, adenoids, thymus gland, and ileum, referred to as Peyer patches (small masses of lymphatic tissue located in the submucosa layer of the ileum).

         d) Aggregates are found in the bone marrow, lung, GI mucosa, and appendiceal mucosa.

      2. Functions

         a) Transport of lymph fluids and proteins: Lymphatics retain filtered protein and fluid to the systemic circulation via the thoracic duct.

         b) Maturation of lymphocytes: B and T cells

         c) Production of antibodies in response to microorganisms

         d) Phagocytosis

         e) Absorption of fat from the intestine; filtration of debris or dead cells from general circulation

      3. Lymph enters the node through afferent vessel and leaves through efferent vessel.

      4. Major mechanisms

         a) An extensive vascular network drains lymph fluid from body tissues and returns it to the venous circulation.

         b) It is important in the body's immune system. Cells within the lymph nodes engulf cellular debris and bacteria and produce antibodies.

      5. Only superficial lymph nodes are accessible to physical examination.

   B. Pathophysiology

      1. Lymphadenopathy represents infiltration of benign or malignant aggregates, causing swelling of affected lymph nodes.

2. Enlarged lymph nodes are secondary to nodal accumulation of inflammatory cells in response to an infection, neoplastic lymphocytes or macrophages, or metabolite-laden macrophages in storage diseases.

3. Exposure to antigen through a break in the skin or mucosa results in antigen being absorbed by an antigen-presenting cell and carried through lymphatic channels to the nearest lymph node.

III. Clinical features: Lymphadenopathy may be a primary or secondary manifestation of infective, benign, or malignant processes. Edema, erythema, or discomfort in a limb distal to previous lymph node removal may indicate lymphedema or lymphadenopathy; it may be transient or permanent. Lymphadenopathy is common, often benign, and self-limiting. If the lymph node is hard, nontender, and fixed to surrounding tissue, this could be a sign of metastatic cancer. Benign nodes are most often tender (Ammar et al., 2017; Deosthali et al., 2019; Scasso et al., 2018; Tzankov & Dirnhofer, 2018; Uddin et al., 2019).

A. Etiology
1. Small lymph nodes palpable in the neck, axilla, or groin that measure less than 1 cm are typically benign. Similar findings on radiographic studies (e.g., mammogram, chest x-ray, scans) are likewise typically benign.
2. Palpable lymph nodes greater than 2 cm or similar findings on radiographic studies are often indicative of bacterial, viral, or neoplastic etiology. Inguinal lymph nodes less than or equal to 2 cm can present in healthy patients.
3. Palpable lymph nodes greater than 3 cm or similar findings on radiographic studies indicate neoplastic disease unless proved negative with adequate tissue sampling.
4. Enlarged lymph nodes with concomitant erythema, pain, warmth, and erythematous streaks along a lymphatic chain (lymphangitis) typically are associated with an infected wound or area of cellulitis and suggest acute inflammation, infection, or obstructive processes secondary to neoplasm.
   a) Frequent etiology is secondary to viral, bacterial, or fungal organisms.
   b) Typically, this presents distal to the involved lymphatic basin.
5. Medication induced etiology includes allopurinol, captopril, cephalosporins, hydralazine, imatinib, penicillin, phenytoin, and sulfonamides.

B. History
1. History of cancer and cancer treatment
2. Current medications: Prescribed, over the counter
3. History of presenting symptoms: Precipitating factors, location, duration, associated symptoms (e.g., recent illness, recent ill contacts, fever, fatigue, rash, sore throat, weight loss, pain in nodes, night sweats)
4. Changes in ADLs
5. Social history: Pet or animal exposure, recent international travel, infectious process, sexual behavior, occupation, drug use including IV drugs (e.g., diphenylhydantoin), exposure to TB, recent body piercing or tattoo

C. Signs and symptoms
1. Weight loss or gain
2. Fever, chills, malaise
3. Inflammation
4. Unusual sweating, particularly night sweats
5. Skin changes: Rash, erythema, inflammation, abrasions
6. Sternal tenderness: May signify mediastinal pressure from node enlargement
7. Coughing or shortness of breath indicative of mediastinal lymph node enlargement
8. Abdominal swelling secondary to hepatosplenomegaly

9. Edema or swelling of extremity

10. Arthralgia, myalgia

D. Physical examination

    1. Integument: Includes all areas adjacent to the lymphadenopathy; edema distal to the involved nodes often indicative of obstruction

    2. Lymph node (see Appendix D)

       a) Location and symmetry

       b) Size (e.g., dimensions in centimeters, shape): Matted nodes usually indicative of malignancy or metastasis

       c) Surface characteristics: Smooth, nodular, irregular

       d) Consistency: Hard, firm, soft, resilient, spongy, cystic

          (1) Soft, rubbery nodes often indicative of non-Hodgkin lymphoma

          (2) Firm, hard nodes indicative of Hodgkin lymphoma or metastasis

       e) Fixation or mobility of underlying or overlying tissue: Fixed usually indicative of malignancy

       f) Tenderness or pain (e.g., direct, referred, rebound) indicative of acute inflammation or excessive manipulation

       g) Erythema or warmth indicative of infection

       h) Increased vascularity and transillumination (i.e., of scrotum): May be useful in distinguishing among tumor, lymphadenopathy, or infection

    3. Abdominal: Splenomegaly suggesting mononucleosis, lymphoma, or leukemia

IV. Diagnostic tests (Aulino et al., 2019; Gaddey & Riegel, 2016; Newton et al., 2017; Sher-Locketz et al., 2017; Uddin et al., 2019)

A. Laboratory

    1. CBC with differential to evaluate for leukocytosis, leukopenia, anemia, elevated Hgb, thrombocytosis, and thrombocytopenia

       a) Increased granulocytes indicative of pyogenic infection or myeloproliferative condition

       b) Increased eosinophils indicative of possible hypersensitivity/allergic reaction, parasitism, or underlying neoplastic condition

       c) Left shift indicative of infection

       d) Increase in lymphocytes indicative of viral process or lymphoproliferative condition.

    2. Throat culture if symptoms of pharyngitis or cervical or submandibular adenopathy

    3. Urethral or cervical culture and sensitivity with symptoms of genital disease or inguinal adenopathy (e.g., lymphogranuloma venereum, granuloma inguinale)

    4. Serologic tests for syphilis, HIV, antibody titers (dependent on suspected causative agent), Epstein-Barr virus, antinuclear antibodies, rheumatoic factor; testing for tuberculosis, histoplasmosis, toxoplasmosis, and Lyme disease to evaluate for other infectious causes

    5. Blood chemistries including LDH: Specifically, liver and renal panels if malignancy is suspected; in the presence of unexplained lymphadenopathy, an elevated uric acid and LDH level possibly indicative of lymphoma or other hematologic cancer

    6. Peripheral smear review: May be useful in indicating other tests to order

B. Radiology

    1. Chest x-ray (posterior–anterior and lateral) to evaluate for evidence of infection or hilar lymphadenopathy

    2. CT scan if generalized lymphadenopathy or organomegaly is present or clinical correlation with plain films

      3. PET scan if CT scan is inconclusive

      4. MRI if CT/PET scans are inconclusive and clinical correlation is necessary

  C. Other

      1. Lymph node biopsy via needle aspiration or excisional biopsy for tissue confirmation for benign and malignant etiology

      2. Bone marrow aspiration and biopsy if leukemia or lymphoma is suspected

      3. Protein derivative/Mantoux test with mumps control to evaluate for TB

V. Differential diagnosis (Ammar et al., 2017; Deosthali et al., 2019; Gaddey & Riegel, 2016; Gru & O'Malley, 2018; Newton et al., 2017; Scasso et al., 2018; Tzankov & Dirnhofer, 2018)

  A. Infectious diseases

      1. Viral: Infectious mononucleosis syndromes (e.g., Epstein-Barr virus, CMV), infectious hepatitis, HSV, human herpesvirus-6, VZV, rubella, measles, adenovirus, HIV, epidemic keratoconjunctivitis, vaccinia, human herpesvirus-8

      2. Bacterial: Streptococci, staphylococci, cat-scratch disease, brucellosis, tularemia, plague, chancroid, melioidosis, glanders, TB (see Chapter 36), atypical mycobacterial infection, primary and secondary syphilis, diphtheria, leprosy

      3. Fungal: Histoplasmosis, coccidioidomycosis, paracoccidioidomycosis

      4. Chlamydial: Lymphogranuloma venereum, trachoma

      5. Parasitic: Toxoplasmosis, leishmaniasis, trypanosomiasis, filariasis

      6. Rickettsial: Scrub typhus, rickettsial pox, Q fever

  B. Immunologic diseases

      1. RA (see Chapter 108)

      2. Serum sickness

      3. Mixed connective tissue disease

      4. SLE (see Chapter 110)

      5. Dermatomyositis

      6. Sjögren syndrome

      7. Angioimmunoblastic lymphadenopathy

      8. Drug hypersensitivity: Diphenylhydantoin, hydralazine, allopurinol, primidone, gold, carbamazepine

      9. Primary biliary cirrhosis (see Chapter 69)

    10. GVHD after HSCT

    11. Autoimmune lymphoproliferative syndrome

    12. Silicone associated

  C. Malignant diseases

      1. Hematologic: Hodgkin lymphoma, non-Hodgkin lymphomas, acute or chronic lymphocytic leukemia, hairy cell leukemia, malignant histiocytosis, amyloidosis

      2. Metastatic disease from primary tumor

  D. Lipid storage diseases: Gaucher, Niemann-Pick, Fabry, or Tangier disease

  E. Endocrine diseases: Hyperthyroidism (see Chapter 157)

  F. Other disorders

      1. Castleman disease: Giant lymph node disorder

      2. Sarcoidosis

      3. Dermatopathic lymphadenitis

      4. Lymphomatoid granulomatosis

      5. Histiocytic necrotizing lymphadenitis: Kikuchi disease

      6. Sinus histiocytosis with massive lymphadenopathy: Rosai-Dorfman disease

      7. Mucocutaneous lymph node syndrome: Kawasaki disease

      8. Histiocytosis X

9. Familial Mediterranean fever
10. Severe hypertriglyceridemia
11. Vascular transformation of sinuses
12. Inflammatory pseudotumor of lymph node
13. CHF (see Chapter 42)

VI. Treatment: Dependent on etiology and extent of lymphadenopathy (Tzankov & Dirnhofer, 2018)
   A. Observation: Resolution with time
   B. Antibiotic therapy: For *Streptococcus* coverage or hemolytic *Streptococcus* (e.g., broad-spectrum penicillin, cephalosporin depending on organism isolated) (see Appendix C)
   C. Antiviral agents (e.g., acyclovir): For known viral infection (see Appendix J)
   D. Appropriate cancer treatment: Surgery, chemotherapy, or radiation, depending on histology

VII. Follow-up
   A. Short term: Based on the etiology and treatment of lymphadenopathy
      1. For viral or infectious condition, marked resolution should occur within 48–72 hours of treatment initiation; progression of symptoms warrants further investigation.
      2. Patients should be rechecked two to three weeks after end of treatment for resolution of adenopathy; if not, tissue biopsy is warranted.
   B. Long term: Dependent on etiology

VIII. Referrals (Ammar et al., 2017)
   A. Surgeon: For patients with persistent lymphadenopathy for a tissue biopsy
   B. Oncologist: Referral of patients exhibiting symptoms of a malignancy to the appropriate specialist for evaluation and treatment

The author would like to acknowledge Joanne Lester, PhD, CNP, AOCN®, for her contribution to this chapter that remains unchanged from the previous edition of this book.

References

Ammar, M.I., Oeppen, R.S., Bowles, C., & Brennan, P.A. (2017). Hard neck lumps: A review of uncommon and sometimes overlooked causes of these worrying presentations. *British Journal of Oral and Maxillofacial Surgery, 55*(9), 899–903. https://doi.org/10.1016/j.bjoms.2017.06.008

Aulino, J.M., Kirsch, C.F.E., Burns, J., Busse, P.M., Chakraborty, S., Choudhri, A.F., ... Bykowski, J. (2019). ACR Appropriateness Criteria® neck mass-adenopathy. *Journal of the American College of Radiology, 16*(5 Suppl.), S150–S160. https://doi.org/10.1016/j.jacr.2019.02.025

Deosthali, A., Donches, K., DelVecchio, M., & Aronoff, S. (2019). Etiologies of pediatric cervical lymphadenopathy: A systematic review of 2687 subjects. *Global Pediatric Health, 6.* https://doi.org/10.1177/2333794X19865440

Gaddey, H.L., & Riegel, A.M. (2016). Unexplained lymphadenopathy: Evaluation and differential diagnosis. *American Family Physician, 94*(11), 896–903. https://www.aafp.org/afp/2016/1201/p896.html

Gru, A.A., & O'Malley, D.P. (2018). Autoimmune and medication-induced lymphadenopathies. *Seminars in Diagnostic Pathology, 35*(1), 34–43. https://doi.org/10.1053/j.semdp.2017.11.015

Newton, M.V., Ramesh, R.S., Manjunath, S., ShivaKumar, K., Nanjappa, H.G., Damuluri, R., ... Prasad, C. (2017). Histological surprises in benign cytologies after lymph node biopsy—Surgeon's knife improving patient care. *Indian Journal of Surgical Oncology, 8*(2), 113–118. https://doi.org/10.1007/s13193-016-0577-2

Randolph, G.J., Ivanov, S., Zinselmeyer, B.H., & Scallan, J.P. (2017). The lymphatic system: Integral roles in immunity. *Annual Review of Immunology, 35*, 31–52. https://doi.org/10.1146/annurev-immunol-041015-055354

Scasso, F., Ferrari, G., De Vincentiis, G.C., Arosio, A., Bottero, S., Carretti, M., ... Viaggi, B. (2018). Emerging and re-emerging infectious disease in otorhinolaryngology. *Acta Otorhinolaryngologica Italica, 38*(Suppl. 1), S1–S106. https://doi.org/10.14639/0392-100X-suppl.1-38-2018

Sher-Locketz, C., Schubert, P.T., Moore, S.W., & Wright, C.A. (2017). Successful introduction of fine needle aspiration biopsy for diagnosis of pediatric lymphadenopathy. *Pediatric Infectious Disease Journal, 36*(8), 811–814. https://doi.org/10.1097/INF.0000000000001521

Tzankov, A., & Dirnhofer, S. (2018). A pattern-based approach to reactive lymphadenopathies. *Seminars in Diagnostic Pathology, 35*(1), 4–19. https://doi.org/10.1053/j.semdp.2017.05.002

Uddin, M.J., Rahim, M.A., Hasan, M.N., Mazumder, M.K., Haq, M.M., Rahman, M.A., ... Billah, M.M. (2019). Etiological evaluation of patients with lymphadenopathy by clinical, histopathological and microbiological assessment. *Mymensingh Medical Journal, 28*(4), 854–861.

CHAPTER 112

Lymphedema

Diane G. Cope, PhD, APRN, BC, AOCNP®

I. Definition: Obstruction of the lymphatic system that causes collection of excess water, interstitial fluid, plasma proteins, bacteria, and cellular waste products in the interstitial spaces (Grada & Phillips, 2017)

II. Physiology/Pathophysiology (Grada & Phillips, 2017; Hutchison, 2018; Tandra et al., 2019)
   A. Normal
      1. Lymphatic fluid travels into major regional lymph node groups via subcutaneous collectors or deep lymphatics.
      2. Major groups of lymph nodes at the base of each lymphatic vessel facilitate lymphatic drainage from the local limb.
      3. The lymphatics return filtered protein and fluid to the systemic circulation via the thoracic duct.
   B. Pathophysiology
      1. Lymphedema results from an imbalance between the rate of lymph production, which reflects fluid movement out of the capillary, and the rate of return of the lymphatic fluid to systemic circulation.
      2. Blockage or destruction of the lymphatic vessels causes an increase in the interstitial hydrostatic fluid and colloid oncotic pressures.
      3. Increased pressure causes leaking of fluid and proteins into interstitial spaces.
      4. Collagen accumulation and fibrosclerosis cause brawny skin changes with edema.

III. Clinical features: Lymphedema is a chronic condition caused by an abnormality in the lymphatic system, often involving one limb, and is generally irreversible (Grada & Phillips, 2017; Hutchison, 2018; Levenhagen et al., 2017; Schaverien & Coroneos, 2019; Tandra et al., 2019).
   A. Etiology
      1. Primary lymphedema occurs without any obvious etiology.
        a) More common in women
        b) More common in lower extremities
        c) May be familial or congenital: Congenital lymphedema occurs at birth; lymphedema praecox occurs late in life; lymphedema tarda occurs after age 35.
      2. Secondary lymphedema is caused by injury, scarring, or excision of the lymph nodes.
        a) Injury: Vascular access device placement, other causes
        b) Lymph node dissection for malignancy
        c) Scarring from a vesicant extravasation
        d) Burns
        e) Radiation to lymph nodes
   B. History

1. History of cancer and cancer treatment
2. Current medications: Prescribed, over the counter
3. History of presenting symptoms: Precipitating factors, location, duration, associated symptoms (e.g., pain, onset of swelling, extent of edema, skin changes, muscle strength, range of motion, sensory deficits)
4. Changes in ADLs: Exercise, activity level
5. Past medical history: Burns, extravasation, chronic inflammation, cellulitis, diabetes mellitus, CHF, cardiovascular disease, cerebrovascular disease, venous thromboembolism, hypertension, obesity, lymph node irradiation
6. Past surgical history: Lymphatic dissection, lymphadenectomy

C. Signs and symptoms

1. Sudden onset: May occur for the first time after traumatic injury, infection, excessive physical exertion, or airplane travel (especially with suboptimal pressurization of cabin)
2. Gradual onset: Usually begins in the distal portion of the extremity and later involves the proximal area, occurring over a three-month period
   a) Edema
   b) Tightness of clothing, watch, or jewelry
   c) Weakness of the involved extremity
   d) Decreased range of motion
   e) Stiffness
   f) Pain
   g) Numbness or paresthesia of the extremity
   h) Erythema
   i) Weight gain
   j) Heavy extremity: Subjective finding

D. Physical examination

1. Vital signs: Fever indicating infection
2. Integument
   a) Thickening, pitting, and erythema; usually unilateral but can be bilateral
   b) Chronic lymphedema indurated with nonpitting edema
   c) Hyperpigmentation
   d) Stasis dermatitis
   e) Superficial veins
   f) Peau d'orange changes of the skin
   g) Positive Stemmer sign; inability to grasp the skin of the dorsum of the second digit of the feet
3. Extremities: Measurements compared to contralateral unaffected extremity
   a) Mild lymphedema: 1–3 cm discrepancy
   b) Moderate lymphedema: 3–5 cm discrepancy
   c) Severe lymphedema: For greater than 5 cm discrepancy, measure upper extremities 10 cm above or below olecranon process; for lower extremities, measure instep, ankle, calf, knee, lower thigh, and upper thigh.
4. Lymph node: Enlargement; noting size, tenderness, and consistency (see Appendix D)

IV. Diagnostic tests (Hutchison, 2018; International Society of Lymphology, 2016; Levenhagen et al., 2017; McLaughlin et al., 2017; Tandra et al., 2019)

A. Laboratory: Not indicated
B. Radiology
1. Lymphoscintigraphy: High sensitivity and specificity

    2. CT scan or MRI to evaluate bulky tumor involvement or obstruction; both studies demonstrate high sensitivity and specificity.

    3. Doppler ultrasound to evaluate venous patency

C. Other: Bioelectric impedance spectroscopy is used to determine arm volume by comparing the composition of fluid compartments using resistance to electric current.

V. Differential diagnosis

  A. Disease recurrence: Lymphoma

  B. Tumor involvement

  C. Lymphangitis

  D. Cellulitis (see Chapter 19)

  E. DVT (see Chapter 43)

  F. Superficial thrombosis

  G. Phlebitis (see Chapter 164)

  H. Cardiac failure (see Chapter 42)

  I. Renal failure (see Chapter 86)

  J. Chronic venous insufficiency

  K. Myxedema

  L. Inflammatory arthritis

  M. Obesity

  N. Lipedema

  O. Hypothyroidism (see Chapter 158)

  P. Peripheral edema (see Chapter 39)

VI. Treatment (International Society of Lymphology, 2016; Schaverien & Coroneos, 2019; Tandra et al., 2019)

  A. Prevention

    1. Patient should avoid the following.

      a) Weight gain

      b) Laceration, abrasion, and injury to extremity

      c) Constricting clothing and jewelry on affected extremity

      d) Heat: Saunas, hot baths, overexposure to sunlight

      e) Lifting or moving objects heavier than 15 pounds with affected extremity

      f) Strenuous exercise of affected extremity

      g) Prolonged dependency of affected extremity

      h) Crossing the legs

    2. The unaffected arm should be preferred for blood draws, injections, IV administration, vaccinations, and blood pressure monitoring, if possible.

  B. Maintenance nonpharmacologic therapy

    1. Elevation of extremity for 45 minutes two to three times a day

    2. Regular, light aerobic exercise daily or several times weekly

    3. Elastic garment (requires measuring by a physical or occupational therapist) to compress fluid

    4. Elevation of extremity or wearing a well-fitted garment when traveling by air

    5. Weight management counseling

    6. Massage therapy to affected extremity or manual lymphatic drainage; massage therapy is contraindicated in the following situations.

      a) Active cellulitis

      b) Active neoplasia

      c) Acute DVT

     d) CHF

     e) Local massage over irradiated soft tissue

   7. Intermittent pneumatic compression devices

   8. Complete decongestive physiotherapy: Manual lymphatic drainage

   9. Use of compression sleeve during air travel

  10. Meticulous skin hygiene and nail care

C. Pharmacologic therapy: No chronic medications are recommended for patients with lymphedema.

   1. Antibiotic therapy for *Staphylococcus* and hemolytic *Streptococcus* includes the following.

     a) Cephalexin: 500 mg PO every 12 hours for 7–14 days

     b) Any agent directed against gram-positive organisms (see Appendix C)

     c) Antibiotics early in course to decrease scarring of lymphatic channels, which increases the risk for lymphedema

   2. Diuretics are not recommended and can cause more harm.

D. Surgical intervention as warranted for lymphovenous bypass, debulking, or direct excisional procedures for conditions such as recurrent cellulitis, leakage of lymph into body cavities or organs, or for limitation of function

VII. Follow-up: Every one to two weeks during acute phase for patients undergoing massage therapy or if cellulitis occurs

VIII. Referral

A. Skilled lymph drainage therapist: May be necessary for decongestive physiotherapy

B. Physical or occupational therapist: For measurement of elastic garment

C. Surgeon: For surgical correction of lymphedema

IX. Resources

A. American Cancer Society: www.cancer.org

B. National Cancer Institute: www.cancer.gov/cancerinformation

C. National Lymphedema Network: www.lymphnet.org

D. Susan G. Komen: www.komen.org

References

Grada, A.A., & Phillips, T.J. (2017). Lymphedema: Pathophysiology and clinical manifestations. *Journal of the American Academy of Dermatology, 77*(6), 1009–1020. https://doi.org/10.1016/j.jaad.2017.03.022

Hutchison, N.A. (2018). Diagnosis and treatment of edema and lymphedema in the cancer patient. *Rehabilitation Nursing, 43*(4), 229–242. https://doi.org/10.1097/rnj.0000000000000177

International Society of Lymphology. (2016). The diagnosis and treatment of peripheral lymphedema: 2016 consensus document of the International Society of Lymphology. *Lymphology, 49,* 170–184.

Levenhagen, K., Davies, C., Perdomo, M., Ryans, K., & Gilchrist, L. (2017). Diagnosis of upper quadrant lymphedema secondary to cancer: Clinical practice guideline from the Oncology Section of the American Physical Therapy Association. *Physical Therapy, 97*(7), 729–745. https://doi.org/10.1093/ptj/pzx050

McLaughlin, S.A., Staley, A.C., Vicini, F., Thiruchelvam, P., Hutchison, N.A., Mendez, J., ... Feldman, S.M. (2017). Considerations for clinicians in the diagnosis, prevention, and treatment of breast cancer–related lymphedema: Recommendations from a multidisciplinary expert ASBrS panel: Part 1: Definitions, assessments, education, and future directions. *Annals of Surgical Oncology, 24*(10), 2818–2826. https://doi.org/10.1245/s10434-017-5982-4

Schaverien, M.V., & Coroneos, C.J. (2019). Surgical treatment of lymphedema. *Plastic and Reconstructive Surgery, 144*(3), 738–758. https://doi.org/10.1097/PRS.0000000000005993

Tandra, P., Kallam, A., & Krishnamurthy, J. (2019). Identification and management of lymphedema in patients with breast cancer. *Journal of Oncology Practice, 15*(5), 255–262. https://doi.org/10.1200/JOP.18.00141

SECTION IX

Hematologic

CHAPTER 113

Anemia of Chronic Disease

Mailey Wilks, DNP, MSN, APRN, NP-C,
and Beth Faiman, PhD, MSN, APRN-BC, AOCN®, FAAN

I. Definition: Anemia is a decrease in Hgb, hematocrit, or RBCs (Cullis, 2011).
   A. ACD is characterized by normocytic, normochromic, hypoproliferative anemia with low reticulocyte count.
   B. Iron-deficiency anemia is the most prevalent type of anemia, although this often coexists with ACD.

II. Physiology/Pathophysiology (Cullis, 2011; Gangat & Wolanskyj, 2013; Lee et al., 2019; Schop et al., 2018; Suega & Widiana, 2019; Weiss et al., 2019)
   A. Normal: Erythrocytes, or RBCs, are manufactured in the bone marrow.
      1. RBCs carry Hgb, which delivers oxygen and nutrients to body tissues and returns carbon dioxide to the lungs for elimination.
      2. EPO stimulates the production of RBCs.
      3. Oxygen attaches to Hgb, the iron-containing substance of RBCs.
      4. Normal Hgb amounts to 15 g/dl of blood. It is composed of a simple protein called *globin* and a red component called *heme*, which contains iron and porphyrin.
   B. Pathophysiology
      1. Primarily, ACD is a reduction in RBC production by bone marrow, as with iron-deficiency anemia or as a result of inadequate hematopoiesis from cancer invading the bone marrow environment.
      2. Hepcidin, a component of the innate immune response to infection, appears to be directly involved in iron availability. Increased hepcidin production, increased urinary excretion of hepcidin, and increased serum levels of hepcidin have been noted in patients with infections, malignancy, or inflammatory states. An increase in hepcidin levels is characterized by an immune activation with an increase in inflammatory cytokines.
      3. The normal RBC life span of 120 days is shortened in ACD.
      4. Iron is not released from storage but remains in the reticuloendothelial system (often seen in inflammatory conditions and myelodysplasia).
      5. EPO is inadequately released from the kidneys in response to the degree of anemia (usually seen in patients with chronic renal insufficiency).
      6. EPO fails to stimulate RBC production with mild hemolysis.
      7. ACD can be caused by immune activation in reaction to foreign antigens in the production of cytokines that directly inhibit action and production of EPO.

III. Clinical features: Despite the term *chronic disease,* the characteristics of ACD may occur very quickly (e.g., following an acute infection, blood loss, or trauma). ACD is considered the second most common form of anemia worldwide. Also known as *anemia of chronic inflammation*, ACD can be seen in heart failure, cancer, renal failure, diabetes mellitus, severe trauma, infection, and acute or chronic immune activation. Anemia is an indication of an underlying disorder. Even mild anemia should be investigated to determine the primary problem (Gangat & Wolanskyj, 2013; Lanier et al., 2018; Lee et al., 2019; NCCN, 2021; Schop et al., 2018).

A. Etiology
1. Chronic infection
2. Inflammatory disease: RA, connective tissue disease, celiac disease
3. Neoplastic disease: More severe with widespread metastases
4. Cancer treatments
5. Severe trauma
6. Heart disease or heart failure
7. Diabetes mellitus
8. Renal failure

B. History
1. History of cancer and cancer treatment
2. Current medications: Prescribed, over the counter
3. History of presenting symptoms: Precipitating factors, onset, duration
4. Changes in ADLs
5. Past medical history: Infection, inflammation (e.g., HIV, hepatitis C, malaria, collagen vascular disorders), trauma, diabetes, kidney disease, other contributory conditions, chronic blood losses (e.g., GI, hematuria, vaginal, epistaxis, hemoptysis, surgical)

C. Signs and symptoms: Fewer and milder symptoms than most anemias
1. Fatigue
2. Weakness, light-headedness, dizziness
3. Dyspnea on exertion
4. Other signs and symptoms related to underlying disease: Infection, trauma
5. Palpitations
6. Pallor

D. Physical examination: Although the physical examination is important to determine the underlying cause of anemia, findings are nonspecific.
1. Vital signs: Tachycardia and tachypnea with moderate to severe anemia
2. Integument: Pallor
3. HEENT: Pale conjunctivae

IV. Diagnostic tests (Cullis, 2011; Lanier et al., 2018; NCCN, 2021; Schop et al., 2018; Weiss et al., 2019)
A. Laboratory (see Tables 113-1 and 113-2)
1. CBC with differential
   a) Mildly decreased Hgb: If less than 9 g/dl, consider other causes.
   b) RBC indices: If normochromic or normocytic but hypochromic, microcytic features develop as ACD progresses and are associated with defective utilization of iron.
   c) Anemia, thrombocytopenia, and neutropenia suggest aplastic anemia.
2. Reticulocyte count decreased
3. Serum iron decreased
4. Total iron-binding capacity decreased or normal
5. Serum ferritin normal or increased
6. EPO levels normal to low

TABLE 113-1	Laboratory Assessment of Anemia: Normal Values (Adults)
Laboratory Test	**Normal Value**
Coombs test (direct and indirect)	Negative
Ferritin	Male: 20–300 ng/ml; female: 15–120 ng/ml
Hemoglobin	Male: 13.5–18 g/dl; female: 12–16 g/dl
Hematocrit	Male: 42%–52%; female: 37%–47%
Mean corpuscular volume	78–100 fl
Mean corpuscular hemoglobin	27–31 pg/cell
Red blood cell count	Male: 4.7–6 million/mm^3; female: 4.2–5.4 million/mm^3
Red cell distribution width	11.5%–14%
Reticulocyte count	0.5%–1.85% of erythrocytes
Serum vitamin B$_{12}$	190–900 pg/ml
Serum erythropoietin level	Male: 17.2 mU/ml; female: 18.8 mU/ml
Serum folate	> 3.5 mcg/L
Serum iron	Male: 75–175 mcg/dl; female: 65–165 mcg/dl
Total iron-binding capacity	250–450 mcg/dl

Note. Based on information from Cullis, 2011; National Comprehensive Cancer Network, 2020; Weiss et al., 2019.

     7. Creatinine increased with renal insufficiency
     8. TSH to evaluate thyroid disorders
     9. Viral studies, as indicated, such as HIV
    10. ESR and CRP elevated with inflammatory state
  B. Radiology: Not indicated

V. Differential diagnosis (Cullis, 2011; Lanier et al., 2018; Lee et al., 2019)
  A. Aplastic anemia (see Chapter 114)
  B. Pure red cell aplasia: May be associated with signs and symptoms of parvovirus infection (e.g., rash, arthralgia)
  C. Malignant invasion of the bone marrow caused by myelodysplasia: Distinguished by the presence of teardrop cells for myelodysplasia and leukoerythroblastic changes
  D. Drug-induced marrow suppression or hemolysis
  E. Anemia of chronic renal failure
  F. Endocrine disorders: Hyperthyroidism, hypothyroidism, hyperparathyroidism (see Chapters 157 and 158)
  G. Inflammatory bowel disease
  H. Heart failure (see Chapter 42)
  I. Renal insufficiency (see Chapter 86)

VI. Treatment (Bohlius et al., 2019; Lanier et al., 2018; Madu & Ughasoro, 2017; NCCN, 2021; Schop et al., 2018; Thavarajah & Choi, 2019; Weiss et al., 2019)
  A. No treatment may be necessary.

| TABLE 113-2 | Laboratory Assessment of Anemia: Results of Tests | | | | | | | |

Type of Anemia	Mean Corpuscular Volume	Retic	Ferritin	Iron	Total Iron-Binding Capacity	Bilirubin	B₁₂	Folate
Acute blood loss	N	NA	NA	NA	NA	NA	NA	NA
Anemia of chronic disease[a]	D/N	I/N	I/N	D	D	N	N	N/D
Aplastic anemia[a]	N	NA	NA	NA	NA	NA	NA	NA
Folate deficiency[a]	I	I	I	I	N	N	N	D
G6PD deficiency	N	NA	NA	NA	NA	NA	NA	NA
Hemolytic: Cold	N	NA	NA	NA	NA	NA	NA	NA
Hemolytic: Warm	N	NA	NA	NA	NA	NA	NA	NA
Iron deficiency[a]	D	D	D	D/N	I	N	N	N
Sickle cell[a]	N	NA	NA	NA	NA	NA	NA	NA
Sideroblastic anemia	D	I	I	NA	NA	NA	NA	NA
Thalassemia	D	I/N	I/N	I/N	N	I	N	N/D
Vitamin B₁₂ deficiency[a]	I	I	I	I	N	N	D	N

[a] Located in this section of the manual

D—decreased; G6PD—glucose-6-phosphate dehydrogenase; I—increased; N—normal; NA—not applicable

Note. Based on information from Cullis, 2011.

1. ACD is often a mild anemia.
2. Progressive anemia requires a thorough evaluation.
B. Preferred therapy is to correct underlying disease or disorder.
C. Medications
1. Erythropoiesis-stimulating agents (ESAs) can raise blood Hgb if the underlying disorder is not reversible or if anemia persists. Agents are only indicated for patients without cancer.
   a) Currently, the American Society of Hematology and American Society of Clinical Oncology recommend against the use of ESAs in patients with cancer based on the results of three clinical trials.
   b) These trials suggested that ESAs increase mortality in patients with cancer not receiving chemotherapy or radiation when administered to a target Hgb greater than 12 g/dl.
   c) However, patients with malignancy and CKD-related anemia (not related to chemotherapy-induced anemia) may benefit from ESAs to maintain a maximum Hgb greater than 10 g/dl. In this setting, the lowest dose of an ESA should be used, and EPO levels should be monitored during ESA therapy.
2. EPO 20,000–40,000 units subcutaneous weekly may effectively raise blood Hgb concentration greater than 10 g/dl.
   a) It may take two to four weeks to increase RBCs. If no increase in four weeks, increase the dose by 10,000 units.
   b) Reticulocyte count should increase in two to four weeks. Hgb should increase in four to six weeks.

c) If no increase in hematocrit in seven to eight weeks after increasing the dose, EPO usually will not be helpful and should be discontinued.

3. Darbepoetin alfa 2.25 mcg/kg subcutaneous can be given as a biweekly alternative to EPO.

   a) If after six weeks the Hgb correction is less than 1 g/dl, the dose should be increased to 4.5 mcg/kg subcutaneously.

   b) Dose should be stopped if Hgb exceeds 13 g/dl.

4. Once treatment with EPO growth factor has begun, ferritin usually decreases quickly, and the patient becomes iron deficient; therefore, ferrous sulfate (e.g., 325 mg PO three times a day) usually is started along with EPO.

5. Iron replacement can be accomplished through oral and parenteral routes to achieve target levels of greater than 100 mg/ml (see Chapter 118).

   a) Ferrous sulfate 325 mg administered after meals is used to avoid GI side effects and decreased compliance.

   b) Vitamin C 250 mg PO daily or acidic environment (orange juice) can be taken with iron supplementation for optimal absorption.

D. Blood transfusions: Performed only if patient is symptomatic; usually not necessary unless the patient has poor cardiac reserve

E. Patient education

1. Patients should be instructed on the importance of adequate nutritional intake and rest, as well as instruction on self-injection for EPO if necessary.

2. All patients who receive ESAs must be educated about the increased risk of MI, thromboembolism, and mortality.

VII. Follow-up (Lanier et al., 2018; Weiss et al., 2019)

A. Short term: Repeat Hgb when underlying process has resolved. Hgb should correct itself within a few months.

B. Long term

1. When underlying process cannot be resolved, monitor Hgb monthly unless blood transfusions are required for symptomatic anemia.

2. For patients receiving ESAs, monitor reticulocyte count and Hgb monthly. Reticulocyte count should increase within two to four weeks; Hgb should increase within six weeks. Patients with cancer should not receive ESAs except in specific instances (e.g., CKD).

   a) Continue EPO if observed to be effective in a seven-week therapeutic trial.

   b) Ensure that the patient has adequate iron; iron stores must be normal or increased for EPO to be effective. Vitamin C (approximately 60 mg daily) is necessary for iron absorption.

VIII. Referrals: Refer to appropriate specialist for treatment when workup reveals underlying inflammatory, infectious, or neoplastic disease.

References

Bohlius, J., Bohlke, K., Castelli, R., Djulbegovic, B., Lustberg, M.B., Martino, M., ... Lazo-Langner, A. (2019). Management of cancer-associated anemia with erythropoiesis-stimulating agents: ASCO/ASH clinical practice guidelines update. *Journal of Clinical Oncology, 37*(15), 1336–1351. https://doi.org/10.1200/JCO.18.02142

Cullis, J.O. (2011). Diagnosis and management of anaemia of chronic disease: Current status. *British Journal of Haematology, 154*(3), 289–300. https://doi.org/10.1111/j.1365-2141.2011.08741.x

Gangat, N., & Wolanskyj, A.P. (2013). Anemia of chronic disease. *Seminars in Hematology, 51*(3), 232–238. https://doi.org/10.1053/j.seminhematol.2013.06.006

Lanier, J.B., Park, J.J., & Callahan, R.C. (2018). Anemia in older adults. *American Family Physician, 98*(7), 437–442. https://www.aafp.org/afp/2018/1001/p437.html

Lee, Y.-G., Chang, Y., Kang, J., Doo, D.-H., Lee, S.-S., Ryu, S., & Oh, S. (2019). Risk factors for incident anemia of chronic diseases: A cohort study. *PLOS ONE, 14*(5), e0216062. https://doi.org/10.1371/journal.pone.0216062

Madu, A.J., & Ughasoro, M.D. (2017). Anaemia of chronic disease: An in-depth review. *Medical Principles and Practice, 26*(1), 1–9. https://doi.org/10.1159/000452104

National Comprehensive Cancer Network. (2021). *NCCN Clinical Practice Guidelines in Oncology (NCCN Guidelines®): Hematopoietic growth factors* [v.4.2021]. https://www.nccn.org/professionals/physician_gls/pdf/growthfactors.pdf

Schop, A., Stouten, K., van Houten, R., Riedl, J., van Rosmalen, J., Bindels, P.J., & Levin, M.-D. (2018). Diagnostics in anaemia of chronic disease in general practice: A real-world retrospective cohort study. *BJGP Open, 2*(3). https://doi.org/10.3399/bjgpopen18X101597

Suega, K., & Widiana, G.R. (2019). Predicting hepcidin level using inflammation markers and iron indicators in patients with anemia of chronic disease. *Hematology, Transfusion and Cell Therapy, 41*(4), 342–348. https://doi.org/10.1016/j.htct.2019.03.011

Thavarajah, S., & Choi, M.J. (2019). The use of erythropoiesis-stimulating agents in patients with CKD and cancer: A clinical approach. *American Journal of Kidney Diseases, 74*(5), 667–674. https://doi.org/10.1053/j.ajkd.2019.04.022

Weiss, G., Ganz, T., & Goodnough, L.T. (2019). Anemia of inflammation. *Blood, 133*(1), 40–50. https://doi.org/10.1182/blood-2018-06-856500

Aplastic Anemia

Heather T. Mackey, MSN, RN, ANP-BC, AOCN®

I. Definition: A nonmalignant acquired or hereditary condition characterized by a markedly hypocellular and ineffective bone marrow secondary to marrow failure resulting in pancytopenia (Shallis et al., 2018)

II. Physiology/Pathophysiology (Moore & Krishnan, 2020; Mufti & Marsh, 2018; Shallis et al., 2018; Young, 2018)
  A. Normal hematopoiesis
    1. Production of blood components in adults occurs in the bone marrow through a process of differentiation derived from the hematopoietic stem cell.
    2. Two main lineages (myeloid and lymphoid) are further differentiated, resulting in the normal production of the cellular components of the blood.
    3. Myeloid lineage results in the production of granulocytes/monocytes, erythrocytes (RBCs), and megakaryocytes/platelets.
    4. Lymphoid lineage results in the production of mature lymphocytes (T and B cells).
  B. Pathophysiology
    1. The reduction in functional marrow mass by either direct or indirect damage to the bone marrow is initiated by multiple forms of injury to the marrow stem cells or their microenvironment and bone marrow architecture.
    2. Damaged hematopoietic stem cells can mature into helper T cells that release cytokines to kill and suppress other hematopoietic stem cells.
    3. Stem cells with inherent defects can lose their capacity to differentiate and proliferate, which can lead to clonal evolution into hematologic neoplasms.
    4. These processes result in a marrow lacking the morphologic precursors to form granulocytes, erythrocytes, and platelets, leading to pancytopenia secondary to the failure of the bone marrow to replace normal blood cells.

III. Clinical features: Aplastic anemia is a life-threatening form of bone marrow failure characterized by pancytopenia. Most cases of aplastic anemia are idiopathic. Incidence is estimated to be 0.6–6.1 cases per million population. The male to female ratio is 1:1 and occurs more commonly in children or young adults (Boddu et al., 2017; Moore & Krishnan, 2020; Solomou, 2017; Shallis et al., 2018; Young, 2018).
  A. Etiology
    1. Hereditary causes: Fanconi anemia, dyskeratosis congenita, telomerase defects, germline mutations such as in *GATA2* and *CTLA-4*
    2. Idiopathic: Occurring in about 65% of patients (e.g., stem cell defects)
    3. Acquired
      a) Autoimmune: Antibody induced, GVHD, SLE

       b) Chemicals: Benzene and related compounds, insecticides, toluene

       c) Drug induced: Gold salts, penicillamine, phenylbutazone, carbamazepine, indomethacin, chloramphenicol, linezolid, NSAIDs, phenytoin, sulfonamides, valproic acid, phenytoin, nifedipine, antineoplastics (dose dependent)

       d) Ionizing radiation

       e) Infections: HIV, Epstein-Barr virus, seronegative hepatitis, sepsis

       f) Miscellaneous: Malnutrition, hypopituitarism, pregnancy, thymoma

  B. History

    1. History of cancer and cancer treatment

    2. Current medications: Prescribed, over the counter

    3. History of presenting symptoms: Precipitating factors, onset, duration

    4. Changes in ADLs

    5. Social history: Occupational or environmental exposure to ionizing radiation, benzene, insecticides

    6. Past medical history: Exposure to viruses or bacteria; history of anorexia nervosa, bulimia, SLE

  C. Signs and symptoms: Onset may be insidious or sudden and related to the absent cell lineage.

    1. Fatigue

    2. Weakness

    3. Dyspnea

    4. Mucosal bleeding: Bleeding from nose, gums, or GI tract; increased menstrual flow

    5. Easy bruising

    6. Frequent or persistent infections: Bacterial, viral

    7. Congenital aplastic anemia: Short stature, café-au-lait spots (Fanconi anemia)

  D. Physical examination

    1. Vital signs: Fever present with infection

    2. Integument

       a) Pallor: Not usually visible until Hgb less than 8 g/dl

       b) Petechiae

       c) Purpura

    3. HEENT

       a) Pale conjunctiva

       b) Retinal or scleral hemorrhages

    4. Cardiovascular: May reveal resting tachycardia or murmur if Hgb and hematocrit are low

    5. Abdominal: Hepatomegaly and splenomegaly not present

IV. Diagnostic tests (Boddu et al., 2017; Moore & Krishnan, 2020; Shallis et al., 2018; Young, 2018)

  A. Diagnostic criteria include the presence of hypocellularity of the bone marrow and two or more cytopenias.

  B. Laboratory: See Tables 113-1 and 113-2 for common diagnostic testing and normal values.

    1. CBC

       a) Pancytopenia: Lymphocytes often normal

       b) Elevated mean corpuscular volume

       c) Low ANC

    2. Peripheral blood smear

       a) Anisopoikilocytosis: Varying shapes and sizes of erythrocytes

       b) Toxic granulation of neutrophils

       c) Reduction in number and size of platelets

3. Vitamin B$_{12}$ and folate levels: Deficiency can present as macrocytic anemia or pancytopenia and should be corrected prior to diagnosis of aplastic anemia.

4. Bone marrow aspirate and biopsy (profoundly hypocellular) with cytogenetic studies may be difficult in hypocellular marrow but should be attempted.

   a) Marrow may be fat replaced, making aspiration difficult if not impossible.

   b) Flow cytometry and fluorescence in situ hybridization help exclude malignancies resulting in pancytopenia.

5. Reticulocyte count: Usually low

6. Peripheral blood flow cytometry to rule out paroxysmal nocturnal hemoglobinuria: Present in approximately 60% of patients with aplastic anemia

7. EPO: Increased level

8. Liver function and viral serologies, if indicated: Hepatitis A, B, and C, Epstein-Barr virus, CMV

C. Radiology: Not indicated

V. Differential diagnosis (Moore & Krishnan, 2020; Shallis et al., 2018; Young, 2018)

A. Hypoplastic myelodysplastic syndrome/acute myeloid leukemia

B. Paroxysmal nocturnal hemoglobinuria

C. Hypoplastic acute lymphoblastic leukemia

D. Hairy cell leukemia

E. Lymphoma: Hodgkin, non-Hodgkin

F. Myelofibrosis

G. Metastatic cancer

H. Fanconi anemia

I. Mycobacterial infection

J. Anorexia nervosa/starvation (see Chapter 66)

VI. Treatment (Boddu et al., 2017; Chen et al., 2018; Hwang et al., 2018; Messa et al., 2017; Moore & Krishnan, 2020; Peslak et al., 2017; Scheinberg, 2018; Shallis et al., 2018; Young, 2018)

A. Untreated patients with severe aplastic anemia have a median survival of three to six months.

B. Management should be aimed at underlying cause with correction when possible (e.g., remove offending medication, treat infection, resection of thymoma, delivery of child).

C. Allogeneic HSCT is the only curative treatment when other treatment is not possible or ineffective.

   1. HLA-matched sibling donor is preferred.

   2. Approximately 50% survival rate exists for those older than age 40 years.

D. Immunosuppressive therapy is frequently administered as combination therapy and can be undertaken in those who are older or not candidates for HSCT; however, it is not curative. It should be administered by those familiar with its use.

   1. Indications: Patients ineligible for HLA-matched sibling transplantation (i.e., age older than 40 years, nonsevere aplastic anemia dependent on transfusions, with profound neutropenia, or without HLA-matched sibling donor)

   2. Antithymocyte globulin: Derived from horse antibodies

      a) Dose and duration are dependent on the protocol and institution.

      b) A 40%–50% response rate if given by itself; this increases to 60%–70% when given with cyclosporine.

      c) Significant risk of adverse reactions exists, including immediate allergic reactions or delayed reactions such as serum sickness 7–14 days after administration.

      d) Administration requires hospitalization.

3. Cyclosporine is given daily with antithymocyte globulin therapy for four to six months at a dose of 10 mg/kg PO daily in divided doses, with dose adjustments to maintain trough blood levels of 200–400 ng/ml.
4. Eltrombopag, a thrombopoietin nonpeptide agonist, can be used in monotherapy or in combination in those who fail other immunosuppressive agents for treatment of severe aplastic anemia.
   a) Dose is 150 mg PO daily concurrently with immunosuppressive therapy with reductions PRN based on platelet count and toxicity.
   b) Dose should be taken on an empty stomach one hour before or two hours after a meal.

E. Supportive care
   1. Instruct the patient on measures to reduce risk of infection and bleeding.
   2. Transfusion support, if indicated
      a) Do not use family members as donors, as potential antibodies can develop and increase the risk for the patient to become refractory to blood products.
      b) Use of irradiated blood products may reduce alloimmunization.
      c) Use single-donor platelets to decrease development of antibodies.
   3. Antiviral and/or antifungal prophylaxis (see Appendix J)
      a) Antiviral: Acyclovir 400 mg PO two times a day or valacyclovir 1 g PO daily
      b) Antifungal: Fluconazole 200 mg PO daily or voriconazole 200 mg PO two times a day
   4. Promptly institute broad-spectrum antibiotics for fever (see Chapter 147 and Appendix C).
   5. Use of hematopoietic growth factors to stimulate WBC count is controversial (e.g., G-CSF, granulocyte macrophage–colony-stimulating factor) and is usually avoided.
   6. Iron chelation therapy for ferritin greater than 1,000 mcg/L: Deferasirox 10–20 mg/kg PO daily based on transfusion requirements

VII. Follow-up (Moore & Krishnan, 2020; Shallis et al., 2018; Young, 2018)
   A. Short term: Aplastic anemia requires frequent visits to check blood counts, check liver function, and evaluate for signs and symptoms of infection or bleeding.
   B. Long term: Follow-up is required with the transplant team following HSCT.

VIII. Referrals
   A. Aplastic anemia should always be managed in collaboration with an oncologist or hematologist.
   B. Refer patient and potential sibling donors to transplant center for evaluation immediately following diagnosis and once patient is stabilized.

The author would like to acknowledge Andrea B. Moran, APRN, MSN, for her contribution to this chapter that remains unchanged from the previous edition of this book.

References

Boddu, P., Garcia-Manero, G., Ravandi, F., Borthakur, G., Jabbour, E., DiNardo, C., ... Kadia, T. (2017). Clinical outcomes in adult patients with aplastic anemia: A single institution experience. *American Journal of Hematology, 92*(12), 1295–1302. https://doi.org/10.1002/ajh.24897

Chen, M., Liu, C., Qiao, X., Zhou, D., Zhuang, J., & Han, B. (2018). Comparative study of porcine anti–human lymphocyte immunoglobulin and rabbit anti–human thymocyte immunoglobulin as a first-line treatment of acquired severe aplastic anemia. *Leukemia Research, 65,* 55–60. https://doi.org/10.1016/j.leukres.2018.01.001

Hwang, Y.-Y., Gill, H., Chan, T.S.Y., Leung, G.M.K., Cheung, C.Y.M., & Kwong, Y.-L. (2018). Eltrombopag in the management of aplastic anaemia: Real-world experience in a non-trial setting. *Hematology, 23*(7), 399–404. https://doi.org/10.1080/10245332.2017.1422306

Messa, E., Biale, L., Castiglione, A., Lunghi, M., Bonferroni, M., Salvi, F., ... Cilloni, D. (2017). Erythroid response during iron chelation therapy in a cohort of patients affected by hematologic malignancies and aplastic anemia with transfusion requirement and iron overload: A FISM Italian multicenter retrospective study. *Leukemia and Lymphoma, 58*(11), 2752–2754. https://doi.org/10.1080/10428194.2017.1312385

Moore, C.A., & Krishnan, K. (2020). Aplastic anemia. In *StatPearls.* https://www.ncbi.nlm.nih.gov/books/NBK534212

Mufti, G.J., & Marsh, J.C.W. (2018). Somatic mutations in aplastic anemia. *Hematology/Oncology Clinics of North America, 32*(4), 595–607. https://doi.org/10.1016/j.hoc.2018.03.002

Peslak, A., Olson, T., & Babushok, D. (2017). Diagnosis and treatment of aplastic anemia. *Current Treatment Options in Oncology, 18*(12), 70. https://doi.org/10.1007/s11864-017-0511-z

Scheinberg, P. (2018). Activity of eltrombopag in severe aplastic anemia. *Blood Advances, 2*(21), 3054–3062. https://doi.org/10.1182/bloodadvances.2018020248

Shallis, R.M., Ahmad, R., & Zeidan, A.M. (2018). Aplastic anemia: Etiology, molecular pathogenesis, and emerging concepts. *European Journal of Haematology, 101*(6), 711–720. https://doi.org/10.1111/ejh.13153

Solomou, E. (2017). An update on acquired aplastic anemia. *Hematology and Transfusion International Journal, 4*(2), 57–58. https://doi.org/10.15406/htij.2017.04.00080

Young, N.S. (2018). Aplastic anemia. *New England Journal of Medicine, 379*(17), 1643–1656. https://doi.org/10.1056/NEJMra1413485

CHAPTER 115

Cobalamin (Vitamin B$_{12}$) Deficiency

Mailey Wilks, DNP, MSN, APRN, NP-C,
and Beth Faiman, PhD, MSN, APRN-BC, AOCN®, FAAN

I. Definition: A megaloblastic, macrocytic, normochromic anemia caused by a deficiency of cobalamin (vitamin B$_{12}$), which may be the result of a dietary deficiency or an inability of the body to absorb cobalamin from ingested food (Oo & Rojas-Hernandez, 2017; Salinas et al., 2018)

II. Physiology/Pathophysiology (Langan & Goodbred, 2017; Mikkelsen & Apostolopoulos, 2018; Oo & Rojas-Hernandez, 2017; Pavlov et al., 2019; Wolffenbuttel et al., 2019)
   A. Normal
      1. Cobalamin is necessary for proper functioning of the neurologic and hematologic systems.
      2. Cobalamin is a cofactor necessary for DNA synthesis and nuclear maturation, which leads to normal maturation and division of RBCs as well as other rapidly dividing cells.
      3. It is a coenzyme needed for the metabolism of MMA and homocysteine.
      4. Cobalamin is required for the production of myelin-based proteins. Cobalamin prevents the development of abnormal fatty acids from being incorporated into neuronal lipids, which has been associated with myelin breakdown and linked to neurologic complications.
      5. Pepsin, transcobalamin, and pancreatic proteases help cobalamin bind to intrinsic factor, a glycoprotein secreted from the parietal cells of the stomach.
      6. Intrinsic factor is necessary for cellular transport of cobalamin. After cobalamin–intrinsic factor complex is absorbed in the distal ileum, cobalamin is released into the plasma.
      7. This water-soluble vitamin is required for formation of hematopoietic cells.
   B. Pathophysiology
      1. Interference with DNA synthesis is caused by the lack of cobalamin, which is required for metabolism of folate.
      2. Cobalamin deficiency can result from an autoimmune attack on gastric intrinsic factor in the gastric juices produced by the stomach or from atrophy of gastric mucosa.
      3. Deficiency usually results from impaired absorption of cobalamin or deficiency of intrinsic factor.
      4. Deficiency of cobalamin results in a demyelinating condition, causing mixed motor and sensory peripheral neuropathy.

5. Pernicious anemia refers to cobalamin deficiency caused by autoantibodies that interfere with vitamin cobalamin absorption by targeting intrinsic factor and/or gastric parietal cells.

III. Clinical features: Common in Caucasian people of northern European descent, cobalamin deficiency usually occurs in the sixth decade of life. It can occur in younger patients, especially those with vegan diets. Cobalamin deficiency increases with age and manifests with greater risk of sensory disturbances, neurologic abnormalities, and cognitive decline. Increased incidence is seen in those with other immunologic diseases (Langan & Goodbred, 2017; Mikkelsen & Apostolopoulos, 2018; Miller, 2018; Oo & Rojas-Hernandez, 2017; Pavlov et al., 2019; Salinas et al., 2018; Simonson, 2018; Wolffenbuttel et al., 2019).

A. Etiology
1. Pernicious anemia: Atrophy causes gastric mucosa to fail to secrete intrinsic factor.
2. Gastrectomy syndrome: After a partial or total gastrectomy, intrinsic factor ceases to secrete within five to six years.
3. Insufficient diet: Although rare, it usually is experienced by vegans or vegetarians who avoid dairy products and eggs and do not take supplemental cobalamin.
4. Chronic atrophic gastritis
5. Autoimmune disorders: Thyroid abnormalities, Sjögren syndrome, Addison disease, Graves disease
6. Drug induced: PPIs, colchicine, H_2 receptor agonists, metformin, cholestyramine, nitrous oxide
7. Gastric bypass surgery
8. Pancreatic disease
9. Bacterial or parasitic competition for cobalamin: Blind loops of intestine, fish tapeworms, diverticulosis
10. Alcoholism

B. History
1. History of cancer and cancer treatment
2. Current medications: Prescribed, over the counter, drugs that suppress gastric acid secretion
3. History of presenting symptoms: Precipitating factors, onset, duration
4. Changes in ADLs
5. Past medical history: Pancreatic disease, gastritis, current or past *Helicobacter pylori* infection
6. Past surgical history: Partial or total gastrectomy, gastric bypass, resection of ileum
7. Dietary intake: Diet recall (e.g., vegan diet)

C. Signs and symptoms: Patients with subclinical cobalamin deficiency may not exhibit symptoms.
1. Weakness/fatigue
2. Sore throat
3. Swelling of legs
4. Dizziness
5. Dementia in advanced stages of cobalamin deficiency
6. Shortness of breath: If one becomes anemic
7. Neuropathy: Symmetric and affects legs more than arms
8. Paresthesia of extremities: Numbness, tingling, burning
9. Glossitis
10. Cheilosis
11. Unsteady or shuffling gait

12. Mental sluggishness
13. Irritability
14. Insomnia
15. Visual disturbances: May be associated with optic atrophy
16. Restless legs syndrome

D. Physical examination
1. HEENT
   a) Vision changes
   b) Skin and sclera becoming slightly icteric
   c) Smooth, beefy, red tongue
2. Cardiovascular: Systolic murmur with decreased hematocrit
3. Neurologic
   a) Decreased position sense
   b) Poor or absent vibratory sense in lower extremities
   c) Ataxia: Uncontrolled falling
   d) Increased or decreased deep tendon reflexes
   e) Mental status changes: Confusion, lethargy, memory loss
   f) Lhermitte sign: A form of myelopathy in which patients complain of an unpleasant electrical shock sensation when looking downward; can radiate to the extremities
   g) Romberg sign: Positive with loss of balance
   h) Proprioception: A pinprick or light touch; can be decreased with sensory loss
   i) Two-point discrimination or vibration: Decreased with sensory loss
4. Integument: Yellow tone or hyperpigmentation

IV. Diagnostic tests (Oo & Rojas-Hernandez, 2017; Pavlov et al., 2019; Salinas et al., 2018; Simonson, 2018)
A. Laboratory (see Tables 113-1 and 113-2)
1. CBC: Increased mean corpuscular volume (greater than 100 fl), presence of hyper-segmented neutrophils; possible pancytopenia
2. Decreased or normal reticulocyte count
3. Decreased cobalamin levels less than 200 pg/L (less than 148 pmol/L) or less than 250 pg/L; common, especially among older adults
4. Normal or increased serum folate
5. Increased LDH and total bilirubin
6. Increased homocysteine or elevated MMA levels
   a) Homocysteine and MMA are more sensitive than the Schilling test, which is rarely used.
   b) Elevated MMA levels appear superior to homocysteine in detecting cobalamin deficiency.
   c) Homocysteine and MMA assays reliably detect elevated homocysteine and MMA levels. These are known substrates of cobalamin-mediated reactions.
   d) Laboratory cutoff values for elevated MMA levels vary by laboratory. Elevated MMA can range from 210–480 nmol/L.
   e) Elevated MMA and low or normal cobalamin constitutes a diagnosis of subclinical cobalamin deficiency.
   f) Patients can be diagnosed with subclinical cobalamin deficiency if they exhibit macrocytic anemia, elevated mean corpuscular volume and MMA, and neurologic symptoms despite an elevated cobalamin level.
7. Other blood tests may be ordered to further delineate diagnosis.
   a) Increased holotranscobalamin II level: Can detect early cobalamin deficiency

       b) Increased serum or urine MMA levels with normal cobalamin
       c) Anti-intrinsic factor antibodies
       d) Schilling test: Measures urinary radioactivity after ingestion of oral dose of radio-active cobalamin; detects lack of intrinsic factor to rule out pernicious anemia or malabsorption disorders; if Schilling test is normal, consideration for non-malabsorptive disorders; not used as first-line diagnostic test
    8. Potassium level: Hypokalemia
    9. Thyroid-stimulating factor to evaluate for thyroid disorders
   10. *H. pylori* testing, if suspected
  B. Radiology: Not indicated
  C. Other
    1. Bone marrow aspiration and biopsy will reveal hypercellular marrow and mega-loblastic erythroid hyperplasia; however, it generally is not recommended for the diagnosis of cobalamin deficiency.
    2. EGD should be performed for suspected gastritis.

V. Differential diagnosis (Mikkelsen & Apostolopoulos, 2018; Miller, 2018)
  A. Folate deficiency (see Chapter 116)
  B. ACD (see Chapter 113)
  C. Myelodysplastic syndrome
  D. Hypogammaglobulinemia
  E. Iron-deficiency anemia (see Chapter 118)
  F. Cirrhosis (see Chapter 69)
  G. Hemolytic anemia (see Chapter 117)
  H. Thyroid disorders (see Chapters 157 and 158)
  I. ITP (see Chapter 124)
  J. Pancreatic insufficiency
  K. Thalassemia
  L. Drug induced: Metformin, histamine receptor antagonists, PPI, methotrexate
  M. Alcoholism

VI. Treatment (Langan & Goodbred, 2017; Oo & Rojas-Hernandez, 2017; Simonson, 2018; Wang et al., 2018; Wolffenbuttel et al., 2019)
  A. Urgency of correction
    1. Repletion of cobalamin can be instituted over a period of weeks when deficiency is asymptomatic, with an incidental laboratory finding, or with slow symptom development.
    2. Urgent correction and intensive monitoring is warranted with symptomatic ane-mia and neurologic findings due to risk of adverse events and irreversibility of neu-rologic deficits.
  B. Cobalamin replacement
    1. Cobalamin is administered 100–1,000 mcg IM daily over two weeks, then weekly until Hgb normalizes.
    2. Initial treatment with IM cobalamin will overcome oral absorption issues and pre-vent delay in normalization of cobalamin levels.
  C. Oral, sublingual, and nasal formulations are available but require a high level of patient adherence.
    1. Patients with impaired intrinsic factor function will have selective impaired absorp-tion of vitamin cobalamin; however, a second cobalamin transport system exists and does not require intrinsic factor or a functioning terminal ileum.

2. Oral doses of 1–2 mg cobalamin daily are effective in most individuals. This is 200 times higher than the maximum recommended daily dose found in standard multivitamins (usually less than 100 mcg daily).

3. Sublingual and nasal routes of administration are not currently recommended because of lack of evidence.

D. Transfusion: If prompt alleviation of anemia symptoms is necessary to mitigate hemodynamic instability

E. Patient education: The nature of the disease, need for lifelong replacement, injection technique, diet

    1. If neuropathy is present, encourage patient to wear well-fitting shoes, pay attention to hot and cold temperatures, and implement fall precautions (e.g., remove throw rugs and objects within the home; see Chapter 143).

    2. Encourage intake of meat, fish, dairy products, and eggs for natural sources of cobalamin.

    3. Encourage adherence to treatment plan.

    4. Caution patients that potassium supplements and vitamin C may inhibit the absorption of cobalamin.

F. Cobalamin deficiency, if untreated, remains a public health concern because neurologic decline may result.

VII. Follow-up (Oo & Rojas-Hernandez, 2017; Wang et al., 2018)

A. Short term

    1. Reticulocyte count should increase in three to five days, indicating marrow response to cobalamin replacement; recovery phase may be associated with a temperature spike.

    2. Hgb should normalize in one to two months.

    3. Neurologic improvement begins within the first week but is less reliable than hematologic improvement. This is complete within three to six months, but long-standing lesions may be irreversible.

B. Long term

    1. Once levels are replete, patient takes cobalamin for life.

    2. Cobalamin can be given at a dose of 1,000–2,000 mcg PO daily or 1,000 mcg IM monthly for maintenance. This will accommodate variations in diffusion, absorption, and retention in patients who are deficient.

    3. Conduct appropriate follow-up for increased risk of gastric cancer in patients with pernicious anemia.

VIII. Referrals

A. Gastroenterologist: If gastric analysis, EGD, or GI radiographic studies are indicated

B. Neurologist: May be helpful if patient presents with unusual neurologic manifestations

C. Physical or occupational therapist: For improvement of gait, balance, and strength

D. Hematologist: For bone marrow biopsy if anemia persists despite normalization of serum cobalamin levels

E. Nutritionist: As warranted regarding diet

References

Langan, R.C., & Goodbred, A.J. (2017). Vitamin B$_{12}$ deficiency: Recognition and management. *American Family Physician, 96*(6), 384–389. https://www.aafp.org/afp/2017/0915/p384.html

Mikkelsen, K., & Apostolopoulos, V. (2018). B vitamins and ageing. In J. Harris & V. Korolchuk (Eds.), *Subcellular biochemistry: Vol. 90. Biochemistry and cell biology of ageing: Part I biomedical science* (pp. 451–470). Springer. https://doi.org/10.1007/978-981-13-2835-0_15

Miller, J.W. (2018). Proton pump inhibitors, H_2-receptor antagonists, metformin, and vitamin B-12 deficiency: Clinical implications. *Advances in Nutrition, 9*(4 Suppl.), 511S–518S. https://doi.org/10.1093/advances/nmy023

Oo, T.H., & Rojas-Hernandez, C.M. (2017). Challenging clinical presentations of pernicious anemia. *Discovery Medicine, 24*(131), 107–115. https://www.discoverymedicine.com/Thein-H-Oo/2017/09/challenging-clinical-presentations-of-pernicious-anemia

Pavlov, C.S., Damulin, I.V., Shulpekova, Y.O., & Andreev, E.A. (2019). Neurological disorders in vitamin B_{12} deficiency. *Terapeuticheskii Arkhv, 91*(4), 122–129. https://doi.org/10.26442/00403660.2019.04.000116

Salinas, M., Flores, E., López-Garrigós, M., & Leiva-Salinas, C., (2018). Vitamin B_{12} deficiency and clinical laboratory: Lessons revisited and clarified in seven questions. *International Journal of Laboratory Hematology, 40*(Suppl. 1), 83–88. https://doi.org/10.1111/ijlh.12833

Simonson, W. (2018). Vitamin B_{12} deficiency: Detection and treatment considerations. *Geriatric Nursing, 39*(4), 477–478. https://doi.org/10.1016/j.gerinurse.2018.06.013

Wang, H., Li, L., Qin, L.L., Song, Y., Vidal-Alaball, J., & Liu, T.H. (2018). Oral vitamin B_{12} versus intramuscular vitamin B_{12} for vitamin B_{12} deficiency. *Cochrane Database of Systematic Reviews, 2018*(3). https://doi.org/10.1002/14651858.CD004655.pub3

Wolffenbuttel, B.H.R., Wouters, H.J.C.M., Heiner-Fokkema, M.R., & van der Klauw, M.M. (2019). The many faces of cobalamin (vitamin B_{12}) deficiency. *Mayo Clinic Proceedings: Innovations, Quality and Outcomes, 3*(2), 200–214. https://doi.org/10.1016/j.mayocpiqo.2019.03.002

CHAPTER 116

Folate (Vitamin B₉) Deficiency

Heather T. Mackey, MSN, RN, ANP-BC, AOCN®

I. Definition: Inadequate intake or poor absorption of the micronutrient folate (vitamin B₉) that may result in a macrocytic, normochromic, megaloblastic anemia and congenital abnormalities (Antony, 2019; Green & Mitra, 2017; Khan & Jialal, 2020)

II. Physiology/Pathophysiology (Antony, 2019; Devalia et al., 2014; Green & Mitra, 2017; Hwang et al., 2019; Khan & Jialal, 2020; Mikkelsen & Apostolopoulos, 2018)
   A. Normal
   1. Folate is a water-soluble B vitamin (B₉) needed for DNA synthesis, RBC maturation, maintenance of gastric mucosa, and normal cell proliferation.
   2. Absorption of folate primarily occurs in the proximal jejunum and duodenum.
   3. Serum folate levels reflect the recent oral intake of folate.
   4. The synthesized form of folate is folic acid, which is found in fortified foods and supplements. Its bioavailability is higher than that of naturally occurring folate.
   B. Pathophysiology
   1. Inadequate dietary intake of folic acid or inadequate absorption of folic acid results in deficiency.
   2. Within five weeks of inadequate oral folate intake, serum folate levels will decline to the subnormal range.

III. Clinical features: Folate reserves are small; deficiency can develop rapidly. Signs and symptoms closely resemble vitamin B₁₂ (cobalamin) deficiency without the presence of neurologic symptoms. It is far less common today as a result of dietary fortification. Women of childbearing age and those at risk for malnourishment are particularly at risk. Folate deficiency is the most common cause of megaloblastic anemia in patients with cancer. In aging populations, B vitamin deficiency has been linked to cardiovascular disorders, cognitive dysfunction, osteoporosis, and risk of developing degenerative disease (Antony, 2019; Devalia et al., 2014; Green & Mitra, 2017; Hesdorffer & Longo, 2015; Khan & Jialal, 2020; Komorniak et al., 2019; Lanier et al., 2018; Mikkelsen & Apostolopoulos, 2018).
   A. Etiology
   1. Inadequate diet is the principal cause of folate deficiency because folate is absorbed from food throughout the small intestine.
   2. Impaired absorption from celiac disease, sprue, inflammatory bowel disease, short bowel syndrome, or gastric bypass

3. Increased requirements due to marked cellular proliferation during pregnancy, infancy, or chronic hemolytic anemia
4. Increased excretion or loss due to vitamin B_{12} deficiency leading to folate trapping, chronic alcohol intake, or hemodialysis
5. Congenital deficiencies of required enzymes to metabolize folate
6. Long-term hemodialysis
7. Medications that may impair folate absorption
   a) Metformin
   b) Cholestyramine
8. Medications that may cause decreased folate metabolism
   a) Phenytoin
   b) Antimalarial agents
   c) Oral contraceptives
   d) Chloramphenicol
   e) Phenobarbital
   f) Methotrexate
   g) Antibiotics: Ampicillin, erythromycin, nitrofurantoin, tetracycline, trimethoprim/sulfamethoxazole
   h) Pemetrexed

B. History
1. History of cancer and cancer treatment
2. Current medications: Prescribed, over the counter
3. History of presenting symptoms: Precipitating factors, onset, duration
4. Changes in ADLs
5. Past medical history: Celiac disease, sprue, bowel disease, gastric bypass surgery, pregnancy
6. Social history: Alcohol use, dietary history, types of food, food processing

C. Signs and symptoms: Often asymptomatic, dependent on degree and rapidity of onset
1. Fatigue
2. Shortness of breath, dyspnea on exertion
3. Dizziness
4. Pallor
5. Weakness
6. Headache
7. Angina pectoris
8. Light-headedness
9. Brittle nails

D. Physical examination
1. No overt findings if anemia is mild
2. Integument
   a) Pallor: Not usually visible until Hgb less than 8 g/dl
   b) Brittle nails
   c) Fine hair
3. Oral
   a) Angular cheilitis
   b) Red, beefy tongue
   c) Stomatitis
4. Cardiovascular: Potential for resting tachycardia or systolic murmur with low hematocrit
5. Neurologic: Typically normal

IV. Diagnostic tests (Devalia et al., 2014; Green & Mitra, 2017; Khan & Jialal, 2020; Lanier et al., 2018)
  A. Laboratory (see Tables 113-1 and 113-2)
    1. CBC
      a) Decreased Hgb and hematocrit
      b) Increased mean corpuscular volume
      c) Leukopenia and thrombocytopenia
    2. Normal or decreased reticulocyte count
    3. Decreased serum folate level
    4. Normal serum vitamin B$_{12}$
    5. Peripheral smear: Presence of megaloblastic cells and oval macrocytes, hypersegmented neutrophils
    6. Increased homocysteine level
    7. Normal MMA
    8. Increased unconjugated bilirubin and LDH if hemolysis present
    9. Bone marrow evaluation: Not required
    10. Homocysteine level elevated in folate deficiency
  B. Radiology: Not indicated

V. Differential diagnosis (Devalia et al., 2014; Green & Mitra, 2017; Hesdorffer & Longo, 2015; Khan & Jialal, 2020; Komorniak et al., 2019)
  A. Pernicious anemia (see Chapter 115)
  B. Myelodysplastic syndrome
  C. Drug-induced megaloblastic anemia
    1. Methotrexate
    2. Pyrimethamine
    3. Trimethoprim
    4. Sulfasalazine
    5. Triamterene
    6. Acyclovir
    7. 5-Fluorouracil
    8. Zidovudine
    9. Hydroxyurea
    10. Cytarabine
    11. Phenytoin
    12. Phenobarbital
    13. Pemetrexed disodium

VI. Treatment (Antony, 2019; Devalia et al., 2014; Green & Mitra, 2017; Hwang et al., 2019; Khan & Jialal, 2020)
  A. Give folate 1 mg PO daily, up to 5 mg PO daily, for one to two months. Duration is dependent on etiology of deficiency.
    1. Dose may be given via IV or subcutaneously if a patient is unable to tolerate oral medications.
    2. Symptoms should resolve quickly.
  B. When possible, eliminate underlying cause. Those with malabsorption or short bowel syndrome may require long-term therapy.
  C. Teach patients dietary sources of folate (e.g., asparagus, bananas, fish, green leafy vegetables, peanut butter, oatmeal, red beans, beef liver, wheat bran).
    1. Encourage daily intake of these foods.
    2. Instruct patients in food preparation (i.e., overcooking can destroy folate).

VII. Follow-up (Lanier et al., 2018)
   A. Short term
      1. Check Hgb and reticulocyte count for response (increase) in one to two weeks.
      2. Evaluate for vitamin B_{12} deficiency; failure to assess B_{12} status can result in delayed identification and treatment of B_{12} deficiency and result in progressive cognitive impairment and neuropathy.
   B. Long term
      1. Check Hgb and reticulocyte count every 6–12 months while on treatment.
      2. Check folate level in four months to evaluate repletion.

VIII. Referral: Consult hematologist if treatment is refractory or if a coexisting iron deficiency, vitamin B_{12} deficiency, or other hemoglobinopathy is suspected.

The author would like to acknowledge Andrea B. Moran, APRN, MSN, for her contribution to this chapter that remains unchanged from the previous edition of this book.

References

Antony, A.C. (2019). Vitamin B_{12} (cobalamin) and folate deficiency. In H. Lazarus & A. Schmaier (Eds.), *Concise guide to hematology* (2nd ed, pp. 37–48). Springer. https://doi.org/10.1007/978-3-319-97873-4_6

Devalia, V., Hamilton, M.S., & Molloy, A.M. (2014). Guidelines for the diagnosis and treatment of cobalamin and folate disorders. *British Journal of Haematology, 166*(4), 496–513. https://doi.org/10.1111/bjh.12959

Green, R., & Mitra, A.D. (2017). Megaloblastic anemias: Nutritional and other causes. *Medical Clinics of North America, 101*(2), 297–317. https://doi.org/10.1016/j.mcna.2016.09.013

Hesdorffer, C.S., & Longo, D.L. (2015). Drug-induced megaloblastic anemia. *New England Journal of Medicine, 373*(17), 1649–1658. https://doi.org/10.1056/NEJMra1508861

Hwang, S.Y., Sung, B., & Kim, N.D. (2019). Roles of folate in skeletal muscle cell development and functions. *Archives of Pharmacal Research, 42*(4), 319–325. https://doi.org/10.1007/s12272-018-1100-9

Khan, K.M., & Jialal, I. (2020). Folic acid deficiency. In *StatPearls*. https://www.ncbi.nlm.nih.gov/books/NBK535377

Komorniak, N., Szczuko, M., Kowalewski, B., & Stachowska, E. (2019). Nutritional deficiencies, bariatric surgery, and serum homocysteine level: Review of current literature. *Obesity Surgery, 29*(11), 3735–3742. https://doi.org/1010.1007/s11695-019-04100-2

Lanier, J.B., Park, J.J., & Callahan, R.C. (2018). Anemia in older adults. *American Family Physician, 98*(7), 437–442. https://www.aafp.org/afp/2018/1001/p437.html

Mikkelsen, K., & Apostolopoulos, V. (2018). B vitamins and ageing. In J. Harris & V. Korolchuk (Eds.), *Subcellular biochemistry: Vol. 90. Biochemistry and cell biology of ageing: Part I biomedical science* (pp. 451–470). Springer. https://doi.org/10.1007/978-981-13-2835-0_15

CHAPTER 117

Hemolytic Anemia

Heather T. Mackey, MSN, RN, ANP-BC, AOCN®

I. Definition: A condition representing a group of hematologic conditions characterized by the premature destruction or shortened life span of mature RBCs in the bloodstream (Michel, 2020; Phillips & Henderson, 2018)

II. Physiology/Pathophysiology (Alder & Tambe, 2020; Baldwin & Olarewaju, 2020; Berentsen et al., 2019; Michel, 2020; Phillips & Henderson, 2018; Siddon & Tormey, 2019)
   A. Normal adult RBCs are characterized by their biconcave shape and absent nucleus.
      1. RBCs are pliable and pass through the circulatory system in diameters one-half their size.
      2. They are durable cells that remain in the circulatory system for approximately 120 days.
      3. Haptoglobin is a protein in the plasma produced by the liver and is responsible for binding to Hgb from a damaged RBC and safely removing it from the circulation.
      4. Three major components of RBCs
         a) Hgb transports oxygen to the body tissue.
         b) The RBC membrane protects the cell.
         c) Enzymes within the RBC are responsible for the uptake and release of oxygen and for cell protection.
      5. When natural hemolysis occurs, the degree of anemia is minimized by a compensatory increase in the secretion of EPO, which enhances RBC production. This response manifests initially as an increase in the reticulocyte percentage and absolute reticulocyte count followed by an increase in Hgb concentration.
      6. Reticulocytosis requires adequate iron and vitamin (B_{12} and folate), functioning bone marrow, and adequate EPO for RBC production.
   B. Pathophysiology
      1. An abnormality or damage to one of the three components of RBCs can lead to a process of hemolysis occurring sporadically or continuously.
      2. This change can be intracorpuscular (i.e., the defect occurs within the RBC) or extracorpuscular (i.e., the defect is external to the RBC).
      3. Hemolysis can be a result of an immune-related condition, where RBCs are destroyed by antibodies, or a nonimmune condition.
      4. Damage or abnormality in RBCs can occur intravascularly or extravascularly.
         a) Intravascular hemolysis/microangiopathic hemolysis
            (1) Destruction of RBCs occurs within the bloodstream.
            (2) Haptoglobin binds with the free Hgb molecule, and the complex is removed from the bloodstream to the liver.
            (3) When haptoglobin levels become depleted, Hgb can accumulate in the kidney and be seen in the urine.

    b) Extravascular hemolysis: More common

       (1) This occurs when RBCs are destroyed by macrophages in the spleen, liver, and bone marrow.

       (2) Because RBCs are not lysed into the bloodstream, haptoglobin is not depleted, LDH is not elevated, and schistocytes are not seen.

  5. Hemolysis can result from physical or chemical injury to RBCs, infections from microorganisms, immune injury to RBCs, or congenital alterations in RBC molecules.

  6. Anemia results when the rate of hemolysis exceeds the bone marrow's ability to produce adequate cells despite significant reticulocytosis.

III. Clinical features: Incidence varies depending on the underlying cause of hemolysis. There are numerous causes of hemolytic anemia, including inherited and acquired conditions. Hemolytic anemia can be acute and chronic and a mild to potentially life-threatening condition. Autoimmune hemolytic anemia, glucose-6-phosphate dehydrogenase (G6PD) deficiency, and hereditary spherocytosis tend to occur more commonly than other causes of hemolytic anemia. Incidence is an equal distribution between men and women (Alder & Tambe, 2020; Al Qahtani, 2018; ARUP Laboratories, 2020; Baldwin & Olarewaju, 2020; Berentsen et al., 2019; Guo et al., 2018; Michel, 2020; Phillips & Henderson, 2018; Renard & Rosselet, 2017; Siddon & Tormey, 2019).

  A. Etiology

    1. Hemolysis from physical injury to RBCs

      a) Malignancy

      b) Fragmentation of RBCs over prosthetic valve

      c) Eclampsia/preeclampsia and HELLP syndrome (**H**emolysis, **E**levated **L**iver function tests, and **L**ow **P**latelets)

      d) Mechanical trauma–induced hemolysis: March hemoglobinuria, footstrike hemolysis

    2. Hemolysis from infection

      a) Malaria

      b) Babesiosis

      c) Clostridium perfringens syndrome

    3. Hemolysis from immune injury to RBCs

      a) Warm antibody autoimmune hemolytic anemia

        (1) Primary causes: Idiopathic

        (2) Secondary causes: Lymphoproliferative disorders, autoimmune disorders, acute leukemia, solid malignancy (ovarian cancer)

      b) Cold agglutinin hemolytic anemia

        (1) Primary causes: Idiopathic; often seen in occult lymphoma

        (2) Secondary causes: Lymphoproliferative disorders, *Mycoplasma/* Epstein-Barr virus infection

      c) Drug-induced immune hemolytic anemia

        (1) Antineoplastic agents: Fludarabine, oxaliplatin, mitomycin, bleomycin, daunorubicin with cytosine arabinoside, cisplatin, IFN-α

        (2) Antibiotics: Penicillins, cephalosporins, dapsone, ciprofloxacin, rifampin, sulfonamides

        (3) Antihypertensives: ACE inhibitors, methyldopa

        (4) Antiseizure agents: Phenytoin, phenobarbital

        (5) PPIs: Lansoprazole, omeprazole

        (6) Ig therapy

      4. Hereditary causes of hemolytic anemia
        a) Hereditary spherocytosis
        b) Hereditary stomatocytosis/xerocytosis
        c) Sickle cell disease
        d) G6PD deficiency

B. History
    1. History of cancer and cancer treatment
    2. Current medications: Prescribed, over the counter
    3. History of presenting symptoms: Precipitating factors, onset, duration
    4. Changes in ADLs
    5. Past medical history: Splenectomy, recent infections, cardiac valve replacement, autoimmune disease, recent transfusion history
    6. Family history: Hemolytic anemia, hereditary blood disorders

C. Signs and symptoms: Related to the underlying process
    1. Fatigue
    2. Shortness of breath, dyspnea on exertion
    3. Chest pain
    4. Weakness
    5. Oliguria or anuria or dark urine
    6. Bleeding: Oral cavity, nose, ears, urethra, rectum, vagina
    7. Palpitations: Associated with sudden onset
    8. Jaundice

D. Physical examination: Related to the underlying process
    1. Integument: Indicating low levels of RBCs or degree of hemolysis
        a) Petechiae
        b) Pallor: Not usually visible until Hgb less than 8 g/dl
        c) Edema
        d) Jaundice
        e) Icterus
    2. HEENT: Pale conjunctiva
    3. Abdominal: Hepatomegaly and splenomegaly in chronic hemolytic anemia
    4. Lymph node: Lymphadenopathy in chronic hemolytic anemia (see Appendix D)

IV. Diagnostic tests (Alder & Tambe, 2020; ARUP Laboratories, 2020; Baldwin & Olarewaju, 2020; Michel, 2020; Phillips & Henderson, 2018; Siddon & Tormey, 2019)
  A. Laboratory evidence of intravascular hemolysis: See Tables 113-1 and 113-2 for common diagnostic tests and normal values.
    1. Anemia with hematocrit less than 25% and Hgb less than 8 g/dl
    2. Reticulocyte count increased
    3. Serum LDH increased
    4. Indirect bilirubin increased
    5. Serum haptoglobin level decreased
    6. Peripheral smear: Reveals red cell fragmentation with presence of schistocytes (helmet cells), spherocytes, and blister or bite cells
    7. Ferritin decreased secondary to iron deficiency because of urinary blood loss
    8. Direct Coombs (or antiglobulin) test positive in immune causes of hemolysis
    9. Renal failure/acute tubular necrosis with increased creatinine
    10. ADAMTS-13 assay: May assist in diagnosis of thrombotic thrombocytopenic purpura

11. Urine for Hgb, hemosiderin (evident in paroxysmal nocturnal hemoglobinuria), and urobilinogen
    B. Laboratory evidence of extravascular hemolysis: See Tables 113-1 and 113-2 for common diagnostic tests and normal values.
        1. Anemia with hematocrit less than 25% and Hgb less than 8 g/dl
        2. Reticulocyte count increased
        3. Normal serum LDH
        4. Normal haptoglobin
        5. Peripheral smear revealing depleted RBC count and showing spherocytosis, elliptocytosis, or sickled RBCs in sickle cell disease; teardrop RBCs or circulating nucleated RBCs suggestive of bone marrow involvement; acanthocytes (spur cells) indicative of hepatic dysfunction
    C. Radiology: Ultrasound for evaluation of splenomegaly; other imaging to evaluate for occult malignancy; high suspicion of lymphoma if immune hemolytic anemia suspected

V. Differential diagnosis (Alder & Tambe, 2020; Al Qahtani, 2018; Baldwin & Olarewaju, 2020; Berentsen et al., 2019; Michel, 2020; Phillips & Henderson, 2018; Renard & Rosselet, 2017)
    A. Paroxysmal nocturnal hemoglobinuria
    B. Paroxysmal cold hemoglobinuria
    C. Autoimmune hemolytic anemia
    D. DIC (see Chapter 120)
    E. Malignant hypertension (see Chapter 47)
    F. Thrombotic thrombocytopenic purpura (normal coagulation studies; see Chapter 130)
    G. Hemolytic uremic syndrome (normal coagulation studies)
    H. Hypersplenism
    I. Warm antibody hemolytic anemia
    J. Cold antibody disease
    K. G6PD deficiency
    L. Infection
    M. Hereditary spherocytosis or other congenital RBC membrane disorder
    N. Sickle cell disease (see Chapter 119)

VI. Treatment (Alder & Tambe, 2020; Al Qahtani, 2018; Baldwin & Olarewaju, 2020; Dierickx et al., 2015; Michel, 2020; Phillips & Henderson, 2018; Renard & Rosselet, 2017)
    A. Understanding the underlying cause of hemolysis is critical because treatment should be directed toward management of the underlying process.
    B. Folate 1 mg PO daily should be administered for those experiencing chronic hemolysis.
    C. Corticosteroids should be given to manage autoimmune hemolytic anemia as first-line therapy. If ineffective, rituximab or splenectomy can be considered.
    D. If thrombotic thrombocytopenic purpura is confirmed, plasmapheresis or prednisone can be beneficial (see Chapter 130).
    E. RBC transfusions may be required when anemia is severe; however, transfusions to manage anemia in general should be avoided unless absolutely necessary.
    F. In drug-induced hemolytic anemia, immediate drug discontinuation is necessary and corticosteroid administration be considered.

VII. Follow-up (Renard & Rosselet, 2017)
    A. Short term: Repeat CBC and reticulocyte count one to two weeks after initiating treatment, then monthly until corrected or underlying process is corrected.
    B. Long-term: Follow up as indicated by etiology.

VIII. Referrals
   A. Hematologist: For management of hemolysis
   B. Appropriate specialist: For treatment of underlying process

The author would like to acknowledge Andrea B. Moran, APRN, MSN, for her contribution to this chapter that remains unchanged from the previous edition of this book.

References

Alder, L., & Tambe, A. (2020). Acute anemia. In *StatPearls*. https://www.ncbi.nlm.nih.gov/books/NBK537232

Al Qahtani, S.A. (2018). Drug-induced megaloblastic, aplastic, and hemolytic anemias: Current concepts of pathophysiology and treatment. *International Journal of Clinical and Experimental Medicine, 11*(6), 5501–5512.

ARUP Laboratories. (2020). Hemolytic anemias. In *ARUP Consult*. https://arupconsult.com/content/hemolytic-anemias

Baldwin, C., & Olarewaju, O. (2020). Hemolytic anemia. In *StatPearls*. https://www.ncbi.nlm.nih.gov/books/NBK558904

Berentsen, S., Hill, A., Hill, Q.A., Tvedt, T.H.A., & Michel, M. (2019). Novel insights into the treatment of complement-mediated hemolytic anemias. *Therapeutic Advances in Hematology, 10*. https://doi.org/10.1177/2040620719873321

Dierickx, D., Kentos, A., & Delannoy, A. (2015). The role of rituximab in adults with warm antibody autoimmune anemia. *Blood, 125*(21), 3223–3229. https://doi.org/10.1182/blood-2015-01-588392

Guo, Y., Tian, X., Wang, X., & Xiao, Z. (2018). Adverse effects of immunoglobulin therapy. *Frontiers in Immunology, 9*, 1299. https://doi.org/10.3389/fimmu.2018.01299

Michel, M. (2020). Autoimmune and intravascular hemolytic anemias. In L. Goldman & A. Cecil (Eds.), *Goldman-Cecil medicine* (26th ed., pp. 1040–1045). Elsevier.

Phillips, J., & Henderson, A.C. (2018). Hemolytic anemia: Evaluation and differential diagnosis. *American Family Physician, 98*(6), 354–361. https://www.aafp.org/afp/2018/0915/p354.html

Renard, D., & Rosselet, A. (2017). Drug-induced hemolytic anemia: Pharmacological aspects. *Transfusion Clinique et Biologique, 24*(3), 110–114. https://doi.org/10.1016/j.tracli.2017.05.013

Siddon, A.J., & Tormey, C.A. (2019). The chemical and laboratory investigation of hemolysis. In G.S. Makowski (Ed.), *Advances in clinical chemistry: Vol. 89* (pp. 215–258). Elsevier. https://doi.org/10.1016/bs.acc.2018.12.006

CHAPTER 118

Iron-Deficiency Anemia

Heather T. Mackey, MSN, RN, ANP-BC, AOCN®

I. Definition: A condition resulting from low levels of iron associated with a decrease in Hgb and the presence of microcytic, hypochromic RBCs (Boone et al., 2019; Camaschella, 2015)

II. Physiology/Pathophysiology (Camaschella, 2019; Lopez et al., 2016; Rishi & Subramaniam, 2017; Warner & Kamran, 2020)
   A. Normal: Approximately 20–25 mg of daily iron is needed by the bone marrow to maintain adequate erythropoiesis and cellular metabolism. Iron levels are maintained at a relatively constant level by the following mechanisms.
      1. Regulation of hepcidin, a peptide hormone, which is affected by erythropoiesis, hypoxia, inflammation, and iron stores
      2. The release of iron from senescent RBCs stored in the liver and spleen ("iron recycling")
         a) Hgb breaks down into globin (polypeptide chains) and heme (iron and porphyrin) fractions.
         b) Iron and heme fractions return to the liver, spleen, and bone marrow to be reused for Hgb.
      3. Small amount from dietary sources
         a) Dietary iron is absorbed by luminal cells in the small intestine and released into the circulation where it binds to transferrin.
         b) The transferrin–iron complex is brought to the bone marrow for erythropoiesis.
      4. Erythrocytes, or RBCs, are manufactured in the bone marrow through a process of hematopoietic stem cell differentiation. RBCs carry Hgb, which delivers oxygen and nutrients to the body tissue.
   B. Pathophysiology
      1. Iron losses or requirements exceed the rate of iron absorption, resulting in a decreased production of Hgb. This is largely a result of excessive loss of iron (i.e., blood loss) or inadequate intake of iron.
      2. Inadequate absorption of dietary iron (e.g., from interference of gastric contents, abnormal mucosa, alteration in intestinal transit time) leads to a decrease in iron availability.
         a) Delayed intestinal transit time increases iron absorption.
         b) Ascorbic acid promotes the absorption of nonheme iron (iron derived from plant and dairy foods).
         c) Helicobacter pylori infection reduces iron absorption.
      3. When iron supply is decreased, stores of iron are first depleted, followed by a reduction in Hgb formation.
      4. In an effort to compensate for iron deficiency, the body increases production of EPO and suppresses the transcription of hepcidin.

III. Clinical features: Iron deficiency frequently occurs in young children, women during child-bearing years, and older adults. Vegetarians and blood donors are also at risk. Iron deficiency is the most frequent cause of anemia worldwide. Onset usually is slow. Iron deficiency in older adults is also more prominent than in the general population (Busti et al., 2019; Camaschella, 2015, 2019; DeLoughery, 2017; Lopez et al., 2016; Warner & Kamran, 2020).

A. Etiology
1. Inadequate intake: Less than 1–2 mg daily
2. Inadequate absorption (after partial gastrectomy), celiac disease (sprue), infection (*H. pylori*)
3. Excessive loss of iron
   a) Uterine bleeding
   b) GI bleeding: Causes can include gastric or duodenal ulcers, diverticula, angiodysplasia, hemorrhoids, and ulcerative colitis.
   c) Hematuria, melena, hematemesis
   d) Excessive blood loss from surgery or trauma
4. Lead exposure: High blood levels of lead impair iron uptake and use, preventing Hgb formation.
5. Drug related: NSAIDs, PPIs, salicylates

B. History
1. History of cancer and cancer treatment
2. Current medications: Prescribed, over the counter (e.g., iron supplements, vitamins containing iron)
3. History of presenting symptoms: Precipitating factors, onset, duration, associated symptoms (e.g., black tarry stools, pica)
4. Changes in ADLs
5. Menstrual blood loss (if appropriate): Type and number of pads used (i.e., super vs. light pads)
6. Past medical history: Gastric surgery, ulcers, gastritis
7. Social history: Frequency of voluntary blood donation

C. Signs and symptoms: Dependent on etiology, degree, and rapidity of onset of anemia
1. Fatigue
2. Shortness of breath, dyspnea on exertion
3. Pica (including ice craving)
4. Burning or pain of the tongue
5. Paresthesia
6. Brittle nails
7. Exercise intolerance
8. Angina pectoris
9. Palpitations: Associated with sudden onset
10. Intolerance to cold
11. Restless legs syndrome/restless legs
12. Headache
13. Light-headedness
14. Difficulty in concentration

D. Physical examination
1. Integument
   a) Pallor: Not usually visible until Hgb less than 8 g/dl
   b) Koilonychia: Spoon nails
2. HEENT
   a) Pale conjunctiva

      b) Oral

         (1) Papillary atrophy of the tongue

         (2) Glossitis

         (3) Angular cheilitis

         (4) Plummer-Vinson syndrome: Cervical esophageal webs on diagnostic imaging

   3. Cardiovascular: May reveal resting tachycardia or murmur if Hgb and hematocrit are low

IV. Diagnostic tests (Boone et al., 2019; Busti et al., 2019; DeLoughery, 2017; Lopez et al., 2016; Warner & Kamran, 2020)

   A. Laboratory: See Tables 113-1 and 113-2 for common diagnostic tests and normal values.

      1. CBC

         a) Decreased Hgb and hematocrit, mean corpuscular volume, mean corpuscular Hgb concentration, and/or reticulocyte count

         b) Increased RBC distribution width

      2. Iron studies

         a) Decreased ferritin

         b) Low or normal serum iron concentration

         c) Increased total iron-binding capacity

      3. Stool for occult blood

   B. Radiology: Not indicated

   C. Other

      1. Bone marrow biopsy to check iron stores if diagnosis is not clear; evaluation for any concurrent processes

      2. Upper and lower endoscopy in men or postmenopausal women to evaluate for GI malignancy or ulcer; capsule endoscopy

V. Differential diagnosis (Hempel & Bollard, 2016)

   A. Thalassemia

   B. ACD (see Chapter 113)

   C. Sideroblastic anemia

   D. Lead toxicity

   E. Anemia of renal failure

   F. Hypothyroidism and hyperthyroidism (see Chapters 157 and 158)

   G. Folate deficiency (see Chapter 116)

   H. Sickle cell disease (see Chapter 119)

   I. Hemolytic anemia (see Chapter 117)

   J. Traumatic hemorrhage

VI. Treatment (Boone et al., 2019; Busti et al., 2019; Camaschella, 2015, 2019; DeLoughery, 2017; Jimenez et al., 2015; Lopez et al., 2016; Short & Domagalski, 2013; Warner & Kamran, 2020)

   A. Treat the underlying cause; stop the bleeding.

   B. Replete with ferrous sulfate 200–325 mg PO two times a day for six months.

      1. Side effects of iron therapy include nausea, constipation, diarrhea, and black stools.

      2. If side effects are significant, consider starting iron daily for one week, two times a day for the next week, and three times a day the following week.

      3. It may take up to six months to measure normal iron stores after the Hgb has normalized.

      4. Dose should be given two hours before or four hours after ingestion of antacids.

C. RBC transfusions usually are not needed.

D. Ascorbic acid 250–500 mg PO is needed to promote iron absorption.

E. Encourage foods high in iron, including organ and lean meats, egg yolks, shellfish, apricots, peaches, potatoes, prunes, grapes, raisins, green leafy vegetables, iron-fortified breads and cereals, and dried beans.

F. Parenteral iron replacement can be considered for patients not responding or intolerant or noncompliant with oral iron. Parenteral therapy may be used for those who have undergone gastrectomy, gastrojejunostomy, bariatric surgery, or other small bowel surgeries. Optimal dose and schedule of these preparations requires more research. Infusion reactions and anaphylaxis are possible; however, they occur less frequently with newer products available today.

    1. Calculation of parenteral dose: Elemental iron (mg) = 50 × (0.442 [desired Hgb level in g per L – observed Hgb level in g per L] × lean body weight + 0.26 × lean body weight)

    2. IV iron therapy dose is based on weight and amount of desired change in Hgb. Product examples include the following.

       a) Ferric gluconate: 12.5 mg/ml

       b) Iron sucrose: 20 mg/ml

       c) Low-molecular-weight iron dextran: 50 mg/ml

VII. Follow-up (Camaschella, 2015, 2019; Jimenez et al., 2015; Lopez et al., 2016; Warner & Kamran, 2020)

A. Short term

    1. Repeat CBC and reticulocyte count in two weeks and monthly until corrected.

    2. Response is indicated by increase in reticulocyte count in one to two weeks, correction of anemia in two to four months, and reaccumulation of iron stores in four to six months.

    3. Consider IV iron infusion if no response to PO iron supplementation.

    4. Repeat endoscopy or further investigations warranted if inadequate response to iron therapy or if Hgb and RBC indices cannot be maintained.

B. Long term

    1. Iron supplementation may be withdrawn when Hgb and ferritin have normalized, provided the underlying source of iron deficiency has been treated.

    2. Patients may need long-term or lifetime iron replacement if cause of the iron deficiency cannot be resolved.

VIII. Referrals

A. Gastroenterologist: If positive fecal occult blood or other GI cause of iron deficiency is suspected

B. Hematologist: If patient fails to respond to iron supplementation

C. Urologist: If hematuria is present

The author would like to acknowledge Andrea B. Moran, APRN, MSN, for her contribution to this chapter that remains unchanged from the previous edition of this book.

References

Boone, S., Powers, J.M., Goodgame, B., & Peacock, W.F. (2019). Identification and management of iron deficiency anemia in the emergency department. *Journal of Emergency Medicine, 57*(5), 637–645 https://doi.org/10.1016/j.jemermed.2019.08.052

Busti, F., Marchi, G., Lira Zidanes, A., Castagna, A., & Girelli, D. (2019). Treatment options for anemia in the elderly. *Transfusion and Apheresis Science, 58*(4), 416–421. https://doi.org/10.1016/j.transci.2019.06.018

Camaschella, C. (2015). Iron-deficiency anemia. *New England Journal of Medicine, 372*(19), 1832–1843. https://doi.org/10.1056/NEJMra1401038

Camaschella, C. (2019). Iron deficiency. *Blood, 133*(1), 30–39. https://doi.org/10.1182/blood-2018-05-815944

DeLoughery, T.G. (2017). Iron deficiency anemia. *Medical Clinics of North America, 101*(2), 319–332. https://doi.org/10.1016/j.mcna.2016.09.004

Hempel, E.V., & Bollard, E.R. (2016). The evidence-based evaluation of iron deficiency anemia. *Medical Clinics of North America, 100*(5), 1065–1075. https://doi.org/10.1016/j.mcna.2016.04.015

Jimenez, K., Kulnigg-Dabsch, S., & Gasche, C. (2015). Management of iron deficiency anemia. *Gastroenterology and Hepatology, 11*(4), 241–250. https://www.gastroenterologyandhepatology.net/archives/april-2015/management-of-iron-deficiency-anemia

Lopez, A., Cacoub, P., Macdougall, I.C., & Peyrin-Biroulet, L. (2016). Iron deficiency anemia. *Lancet, 387*(10021), 907–916. https://doi.org/10.1016/S0140-6736(15)60865-0

Rishi, G., & Subramaniam, V.N. (2017). The relationship between systemic iron homeostasis and erythropoiesis. *Bioscience Reports, 37*(6). https://doi.org/10.1042/BSR20170195

Short, M.W., & Domagalski, J.E. (2013). Iron deficiency anemia: Evaluation and management. *American Family Physician, 87*(2), 98–104. https://www.aafp.org/afp/2013/0115/p98.html

Warner, M.J., & Kamran, M.T. (2020). Iron deficiency anemia. In *StatPearls.* https://www.ncbi.nlm.nih.gov/books/NBK448065

CHAPTER 119

Sickle Cell Disease

Heather T. Mackey, MSN, RN, ANP-BC, AOCN®

I. Definition: An inherited hemoglobinopathy characterized by chronic RBC hemolysis resulting in tissue hypoxia, vaso-occlusion, acute and chronic multiorgan damage, and shortened life span (Howard, 2020; Mangla et al., 2020; Piel et al., 2017; Ware et al., 2017)

II. Physiology/Pathophysiology (Azar & Wong, 2017; Houwing et al., 2019; Howard, 2020; Mangla et al., 2020; Piel et al., 2017; Pinto et al., 2019; Ware et al., 2017)
   A. Normal adult RBCs are characterized by their biconcave shape and absent nucleus.
      1. RBCs are pliable and pass through the circulatory system in diameters one-half their size.
      2. They are durable cells that remain in the circulatory system for approximately 120 days.
      3. Their major function is to transport Hgb.
      4. Hgb A1 is the major component and Hgb A2 is a minor component of Hgb in the normal RBC.
      5. Hgb F is the major Hgb in the fetus, yet it exists in only minimal quantities in a typical adult.
   B. Pathophysiology
      1. Sickle-shaped RBCs result from a Hgb molecule abnormality.
      2. It is an autosomal recessive genetic disorder, homozygous for Hgb S.
      3. Abnormal Hgb (Hgb S) develops in place of normal Hgb (Hgb A) in the beta-globin gene.
      4. Patients with sickle cell trait are heterozygous (only one beta-globin gene mutated) and have approximately 30%–40% Hgb in abnormal form (Hgb S).
      5. Vaso-occlusive pain and tissue injury result from the following.
         a) Increased adhesion of the Hgb S molecule to the RBC vessel wall, obstructing capillary blood flow
         b) Hemolytic anemia: Intravascular and extravascular
      6. Higher risk of infection occurs as a result of functional hyposplenism early in life and altered neutrophil response.

III. Clinical features: Alternating periods of wellness occur despite moderate anemia interspersed with episodes of deterioration; severity of symptoms varies widely among patients and are often referred to as "crises." Life expectancy is reduced by approximately 30 years with often-times poor QOL. Infarction and ischemia in the lung, bone, spleen, retina, brain, and other organs lead to symptoms and dysfunction. Individuals with sickle cell disease are at high risk for bacterial and viral infections from asplenia that develops early in childhood. Common infections include bacteremia, meningitis, and pulmonary infections (pneumonia and acute chest). Common organisms of bacterium include encapsulated organisms (e.g., *Streptococcus pneumoniae, Haemophilus influenza*). It is the most common genetic disease in United States. Its highest prevalence is in people from Sub-Saharan African, South Asian, Mediterranean, and Middle Eastern ancestries (Houwing et al., 2019; Howard, 2020; Mangla et al., 2020; Piel et al., 2017; Pinto et al., 2019; Shah et al., 2019; Ware et al., 2017).

A. Etiology: Autosomal recessive genetic disorder with mutation in beta-globin chain, in which glutamic acid is substituted with valine at position six on chromosome 11

B. History
  1. History of cancer and cancer treatment
  2. Current medications: Prescribed, over the counter
  3. History of presenting symptoms: Precipitating factors (e.g., pain), onset, duration, associated symptoms (e.g., presence of fever, other signs and symptoms of infection)
  4. Changes in ADLs
  5. Past medical history: Hemolytic anemia, dehydration, previous sickle cell crisis, infections, pregnancy, alcohol use
  6. Family history: Sickle cell disease or trait, malaria exposure

C. Signs and symptoms
  1. Patients with sickle cell trait are essentially asymptomatic except in cases of severe hypoxia, such as vigorous exercise, heat overexposure, or high altitudes.
  2. Acute pain episodes or crisis
    a) Episodes are caused by microvascular occlusion precipitated by hypoxia, exposure to cold or sudden change in temperature, infection, high altitudes, stress, surgery, blood loss, pregnancy, and dehydration. They occasionally occur spontaneously.
    b) This occlusion can progress to tissue and vascular damage, with release of inflammatory mediators that activate nociceptors. Reperfusion can intensify the inflammation and worsen pain.
    c) Symptoms may last hours to days.
    d) Episodes are associated with sudden onset of acute pain, often skeletal (e.g., long bones) in nature but can occur in any organ.
  3. Acute and chronic complications
    a) Acute chest syndrome: New pulmonary infiltrate involving one lung segment accompanied by fever, chest pain, or new pulmonary symptoms (e.g., tachypnea, wheeze, cough, hypoxia)
    b) Cardiovascular: Symptoms suggestive of CHF and cardiomegaly
      (1) Peripheral edema
      (2) Shortness of breath or dyspnea on exertion
      (3) PE incidence higher in those with sickle cell disease
    c) Pulmonary: Exertional dyspnea, fatigue, and syncope suggestive of PH
    d) CNS: Symptoms suggestive of stroke (e.g., vision disturbances, muscle weakness, slurred speech)
    e) GU: Symptoms suggestive of renal failure or other complications
      (1) Hematuria
      (2) Priapism
      (3) Decreased output
      (4) Peripheral edema
    f) Musculoskeletal pain
      (1) Joint pain, low back pain, skeletal in origin
      (2) Dactylitis
    g) Ophthalmologic: Visual changes suggestive of retinal detachment, retinal artery occlusion, vitreous hemorrhage

D. Physical examination
   1. Acute: May present without physical findings
   2. Cardiac: Tachycardia and/or flow murmurs secondary to anemia
   3. Chronic
      a) Integument: Skin ulcers, usually involve malleolus of ankles
      b) Abdominal
         (1) Splenomegaly: Unusual in homozygous sickle cell disease because of auto-infarction of spleen during childhood
         (2) Hepatomegaly
         (3) Positive Murphy sign in gallbladder disease (see Appendix D)
      c) Eye: Visual loss and retinopathy
      d) Neurologic
         (1) Muscle strength: Hemiplegia with stroke
         (2) Cranial nerves: Cranial nerve palsies from occlusion of major intracranial vessels (see Appendix A)

IV. Diagnostic tests (Howard, 2020; Mangla et al., 2020; Piel et al., 2017; Ware et al., 2017)
   A. Laboratory: See Tables 113-1 and 113-2 for common diagnostic tests and normal values.
      1. CBC
         a) Normocytic, normochromic hemolytic anemia: Hgb usually 5–11 g/dl
         b) Leukocytosis present with infection
      2. Peripheral smear
         a) Variation in RBC size and shape
         b) Sickle cells and target cells on smear
      3. Elevated reticulocyte count: If not elevated and hematocrit dropped, suspected aplastic crisis
      4. Hgb electrophoresis: Presence of Hgb S in sickle cell disease; presence of Hgb S and Hgb A in sickle cell trait
      5. Evidence of hemolysis: Indirect bilirubinemia, elevated LDH, reduced haptoglobin
      6. Urinalysis: Proteinuria or hematuria present in renal insufficiency
      7. BUN and creatinine increased with renal insufficiency
      8. Ferritin level increased with iron overload from multiple transfusions
   B. Radiology
      1. Chest x-ray to evaluate for chest syndrome or pneumonia
      2. Plain films or MRI to evaluate for avascular necrosis or osteomyelitis of bones, as indicated
      3. DEXA scan to evaluate for osteopenia or osteoporosis
   C. Other
      1. Sleep study to evaluate for sleep apnea
      2. Pulmonary function tests to evaluate for asthma, as indicated

V. Differential diagnosis (Howard, 2020; Mangla et al., 2020; Piel et al., 2017; Ware et al., 2017)
   A. Acute pulmonary infection (see Chapter 37)
   B. Acute hepatitis (see Chapter 74)
   C. Cholecystitis (see Chapter 68)
   D. Stroke (see Chapter 146)
   E. Osteoporosis (see Chapter 106)
   F. AKI (see Chapter 86)
   G. Osteomyelitis

H. Acute splenic sequestration

I. Acute hepatic sequestration

VI. Treatment (Azar & Wong, 2017; Houwing et al., 2019; Howard, 2020; Kassim & Sharma, 2017; Mangla et al., 2020; Matthie & Jenerette, 2015; Piel et al., 2017; Pinto et al., 2019; Shah et al., 2019; Ware et al., 2017; Zassman et al., 2019)

  A. Therapy for vaso-occlusive crisis includes supportive care.

    1. IV fluids: The optimal solution and rate of infusion remain unclear.

    2. Analgesics (see Appendices E and F)

      a) Regimen and medication should be based on patient's prior response/intolerance to therapy.

      b) Opioid therapy should be initiated rapidly upon presentation.

      c) Doses should be repeated frequently (every 15–30 minutes) PRN.

      d) Consideration should be given to continuous infusion with available bolus of opioid to control pain (see Appendix F).

      e) Once pain is controlled, a transitional plan to oral agents should be in place.

    3. Adjuvant medications to control side effects

      a) Diphenhydramine: 25–50 mg PO every four to six hours for pruritus

      b) NSAIDs (see Appendix E)

      c) Antiemetics for nausea (see Appendix P)

      d) Laxatives for bowel regimen with opioids (see Chapter 55)

      e) Anxiolytics for anxiety (see Chapter 161)

    4. Antibiotics, as indicated, for infectious source (see Appendix C) or empirically if acute chest syndrome is suspected

    5. Oxygen needed only if hypoxic

    6. RBC transfusion to replace prematurely destroyed RBCs and to diminish percentage of Hgb S in circulation in presence of severe anemic complications

    7. Incentive spirometer to expand lung capacity to potentially prevent chest syndrome

    8. Nonpharmacologic: Heat, adequate hydration, nutrition, rest, avoiding alcohol and drugs, prayer, social support

  B. General therapy for sickle cell disease

    1. Hydroxyurea

      a) Only FDA-approved medication for sickle cell disease with newer agents in development

      b) 10–15 mg/kg/day PO daily as initial dose; dose escalation by 5 mg/kg every four to six weeks to maximum of 35 mg/kg daily; goal ANC 2,000–3,000/mm³

      c) Works by enhancing fetal Hgb (Hgb F) production, resulting in improved red cell survival and decreased sickling

    2. Other treatments

      a) Allogeneic HSCT: Offers curative therapy for those who are appropriate candidates

      b) Transfusion therapy: Simple transfusions, manual exchange transfusions, erythrocytapheresis procedures

      c) Iron chelation: Deferasirox 10–20 mg/kg PO daily based on transfusion requirements

      d) Folate supplementation

  C. Patient education

    1. Pain control with NSAIDs (see Appendix E) and opioids (see Appendix F)

    2. Genetic counseling for individuals with sickle cell trait

    3. Adherence to treatment plan with iron chelation therapy and hydroxyurea

VII. Follow-up (Shet & Thein, 2019)
  A. Short term: Perform in approximately three to six months to monitor CBC, reticulocyte count, and ferritin; side effects of medications; and transfusion needs.
  B. Long term: Lifelong management of the disease is required to assess for complications (e.g., stroke, osteoporosis, iron overload, avascular necrosis).

VIII. Referral: Sickle cell specialist or hematologist for evaluation and treatment

The author would like to acknowledge Andrea B. Moran, APRN, MSN, for her contribution to this chapter that remains unchanged from the previous edition of this book.

References

Azar, S., & Wong, T.E. (2017). Sickle cell disease: A brief update. *Medical Clinics of North America, 101*(2), 375–393. https://doi.org/10.1016/j.mcna.2016.09.009

Houwing, M.E., de Pagter, P.J., van Beers, E.J., Biemond, B.J., Rettenbacher, E., Rijneveld, A.W., ... Cnossen, M.H. (2019). Sickle cell disease: Clinical presentation and management of a global health challenge. *Blood Reviews, 37,* 100580. https://doi.org/10.1016/j.blre.2019.05.004

Howard, J. (2020). Sickle cell disease and other hemoglobinopathies. In L. Goldman & A. Cecil (Eds.), *Goldman-Cecil medicine* (26th ed., pp. 1061–1069). Elsevier.

Kassim, A.A., & Sharma, D. (2017). Hematopoietic stem cell transplantation for sickle cell disease: The changing landscape. *Hematology/Oncology and Stem Cell Therapy, 10*(4), 259–266. https://doi.org/10.1016/j.hemonc.2017.05.008

Mangla, A., Ehsan, M., & Maruvada, S. (2020). Sickle cell anemia. In *StatPearls.* https://www.ncbi.nlm.nih.gov/books/NBK482164

Matthie, N., & Jenerette, C. (2015). Sickle cell disease in adults: Developing an appropriate care plan. *Clinical Journal of Oncology Nursing, 19*(5), 562–567. https://doi.org/10.1188/15.CJON.562-567

Piel, F., Steinberg, M.H., & Rees, D.C. (2017). Sickle cell disease. *New England Journal of Medicine, 376*(16), 1561–1573. https://doi.org/10.1056/NEJMra1510865

Pinto, V.M., Balocco, M., Quintino, S., & Forni, G.L. (2019). Sickle cell disease: A review for the internist. *Internal and Emergency Medicine, 14*(7), 1051–1064. https://doi.org/10.1007/s11739-019-02160-x

Shah, N., Bhor, M., Xie, L., Paulose, J., & Yuce, H. (2019). Sickle cell disease complications: Prevalence and resource utilization. *PLOS ONE, 14*(7), e0214355. https://doi.org/10.1371/journal.pone.0214355

Shet, A.S., & Thein, S.L. (2019). A growing population of older adults with sickle cell disease. *Clinics in Geriatric Medicine, 35*(3), 349–367. https://doi.org/10.1016/j.cger.2019.03.006

Ware, R.E., de Montalembert, M., Tshilolo, L., & Abboud, M.R. (2017). Sickle cell disease. *Lancet, 390*(10091), 311–323. https://doi.org/10.1016/S0140-6736(17)30193-9

Zassman, S.M., Zamora, F.J., & Roberts, J.D. (2019). Inpatient pain management in sickle cell disease. *American Journal of Health-System Pharmacy, 76*(23), 1965–1971. https://doi.org/10.1093/ajhp/zxz228

CHAPTER 120

Disseminated Intravascular Coagulation

Deborah Kirk, DNP, FNP-BC, NP-C, AOCN®, FAANP

I. Definition: DIC is a systemic thrombohemorrhagic disorder seen in association with well-defined clinical situations and laboratory evidence of procoagulant activation, fibrinolytic activation, inhibitor consumption, and biochemical evidence of end-organ damage. Systemic intravascular activation of the coagulation cascade occurs with fibrin formation and deposition in the microvasculature (Toh et al., 2016; Wada et al., 2014).

II. Physiology/Pathophysiology (Levi, 2019; Liaw et al., 2016; Papageorgiou et al., 2018; Toh et al., 2016; Wada et al., 2014)
   A. Normal
      1. Intrinsic (i.e., endothelial cell damage) and extrinsic (i.e., tissue injury) coagulation pathways are responsible for formation of fibrin clots and blood clotting, thereby maintaining hemostasis.
      2. Under normal conditions, a balance of coagulation and fibrinolysis occurs to maintain hemostasis.
   B. Pathophysiology
      1. Several mechanisms of pathophysiologic insult may lead to the pathway of DIC, including endothelial damage, antigen–antibody complexes, endotoxemia, tissue damage, platelet damage or release, and RBC damage.
      2. Circulation of plasmin and thrombin may be stimulated by many pathways because of activation of the coagulation system.
      3. Systemic circulation of plasmin leads to hemorrhage, and systemic circulation of thrombin leads to clot formation or thrombosis.
      4. Platelet dysfunction and coagulation factor depletion occur with stimulation of fibrinolysis.
      5. Cytokines TNF-α, IL-1, and IL-6 may induce vascular endothelial damage, leading to end-organ damage.
      6. The inflammatory cascade and coagulation pathway both are activated and perpetuate each other.
      7. Protein C deficiency in sepsis promotes thrombin formation in the microvasculature and may augment inflammation and endothelial cell dysfunction.

III. Clinical features: DIC may be fulminant or low grade depending on the disease associated with triggering the syndrome. Acute DIC is a serious complication with a high mortality rate (Cope, 2016; Feinstein, 2015; Gando et al., 2016; Gobel, 2018; Iba et al., 2019;

Levi, 2019; National Heart, Lung, and Blood Institute, 2019; Toh et al., 2016; Wada et al., 2014).

A. Etiology (see Table 120-1)

1. The intrinsic pathway can be activated by septicemia, UTI, hypotension, and acidosis.

2. The extrinsic pathway can be activated by tissue injury caused by obstetric complications, trauma, and hematologic or solid tumors.

3. DIC occurs in patients with solid tumor malignancies, which include the lung, pancreas, prostate, stomach, colon, ovary, gallbladder, breast, and kidney.

4. The most common leukemia in which DIC occurs is acute promyelocytic leukemia.

5. DIC can manifest as acute or chronic.

   a) Acute: Bleeding occurs simultaneously from at least three sites and is associated with shock, respiratory failure, or renal failure.

TABLE 120-1	**Clinical Conditions and Mechanisms Associated With Development of Disseminated Intravascular Coagulation**	
Clinical Condition	**Mechanisms**	**Type of DIC**
Sepsis/severe infection • Bacterial infections (gram-negative or gram-positive organisms) • Viral infections (varicella, hepatitis, cytomegalovirus) • Parasitic infections	Activation of factor XII (factor XIIa) by endo-toxins Platelet release reaction (release of ADP from platelets induces platelet aggregation) Release of TNF-α, IL-1, and complement activation Inflammatory response Proinflammatory cytokines Results in endothelial damage, endothelial permeability, and multiorgan damage	Acute
Trauma • Polytrauma • Neurotrauma • Fat embolism	Activation of coagulation Release of tissue material (e.g., fat, phospholipids, enzymes) into circulation Hemolysis Endothelial damage Cytokine release	Acute
Burns	Microhemolysis Release of red cell membrane phospholipids or red cell ADP Release of tissue materials or cellular enzymes into systemic circulation	Acute
Solid tumors: mucin-secreting adeno-carcinomas • Prostate • Lung • Breast • Stomach	Activation of coagulation Expression of procoagulant materials (e.g., tissue factor, cysteine protease with factor X–activating properties) by tumor cells Severe hyperfibrinolysis	Chronic
Hematologic malignancies • Acute promyelocytic leukemia • Myeloproliferative diseases • Lymphoproliferative disease	Severe hyperfibrinolysis Activation of coagulation Bleeding and thrombosis	Acute and chronic

(Continued on next page)

TABLE 120-1	Clinical Conditions and Mechanisms Associated With Development of Disseminated Intravascular Coagulation *(Continued)*	
Clinical Condition	**Mechanisms**	**Type of DIC**
Hematologic disease • Polycythemia rubra vera • Paroxysmal nocturnal hemoglobinuria	Underlying compensated DIC process Thrombosis Thromboembolism	Chronic
Obstetric conditions • Acute fatty liver of late pregnancy	Rare, life-threatening buildup of fat in liver cells Associated with preeclampsia High mortality rates in liver failure with coagulopathy (e.g., thrombocytopenia, very low fibrinogen levels), encephalopathy, and DIC	Acute
• Amniotic fluid emboli	Activation of coagulation by amniotic fluid in circulation	Acute
• Placental abruption	Activation of coagulation due to leakage of thromboplastin-like material into bloodstream from placental separation	Acute
• Preeclampsia: HELLP syndrome	Activation of coagulation in preeclampsia A variant of preeclampsia Endothelial damage, platelet aggregation, thrombin formation, and impaired fibrinolysis	Acute
• Retained dead fetus syndrome	Fibrinogen depletion, coagulopathy, and chronic DIC due to presence of dead fetus for > 4–5 weeks	Acute
Intravascular hemolysis • Any etiology • Transfusion reaction	Triggers intravascular coagulation Activation of coagulation Induction of platelet aggregation due to release of ADP from red cells Release of red cell membrane phospholipoprotein	Acute
Vascular disorders • Aortic aneurysms • Hemangiomas • Kasabach-Merritt syndrome	Activation of coagulation Consumption of coagulation proteins and platelets Overflow of coagulation factors to systemic circulation	Chronic
Microangiopathic hemolytic anemias	Thrombocytopenic thrombotic purpura Hemolytic uremic syndrome Chemotherapy-induced microangiopathic hemolytic anemia Malignant hypertension	Acute and chronic
Organ destruction	Activation of coagulation Fibrin deposition in small and midsize blood vessels Ischemia and necrosis within organs	Acute
Severe acute pancreatitis	Activation of coagulation secondary to circulating pancreatic enzymes (particularly trypsin) or vascular injury Consumption of coagulation factors	Acute
Severe hepatic failure	Intrahepatic or extrahepatic cholestasis	Acute

(Continued on next page)

TABLE 120-1	Clinical Conditions and Mechanisms Associated With Development of Disseminated Intravascular Coagulation *(Continued)*	
Clinical Condition	**Mechanisms**	**Type of DIC**
Metabolic acidosis	Endothelial sloughing Activation of factor XII (factor XIIa) Activation of factor XI (factor XIa) Platelet activation Clinical state of acidosis Activation of coagulation pathway and down-regulation of thrombomodulin due to release of inflammatory cytokines (TNF-α, IL-1, IL-6, and IFN-γ) Thrombus formation End-organ damage	Acute
Severe toxic or immunologic reactions • Snakebites • Recreational drugs • Transfusion reactions • Transplant rejection	Endothelial damage Circulating antigen–antibody complexes Endotoxemia Tissue damage Platelet or red cell damage	Acute

ADP—adenosine diphosphate; DIC—disseminated intravascular coagulation; HELLP—hemolysis, elevated liver enzymes, and low platelet count; IFN—interferon; IL—interleukin; TNF—tumor necrosis factor

Note. Based on information from Cope, 2016; Gando et al., 2016; Gobel, 2018; Levi & Schmaier, 2016.

From "Disseminated Intravascular Coagulation," by D.G. Cope, in M. Kaplan (Ed.), *Understanding and managing oncologic emergencies: A resource for nurses* (3rd ed., pp. 180–182), 2018, Oncology Nursing Society. Copyright 2018 by Oncology Nursing Society. Reprinted with permission.

    b) Chronic: It is usually manifested with minimal bleeding and frequently seen in malignancy-induced condition.

B. History
    1. History of cancer and cancer treatment
    2. Current medications: Prescribed, over the counter
    3. History of presenting symptoms: Precipitating factors, onset, duration
    4. Changes in ADLs
    5. Past medical history: Hepatitis, HIV, recent viral infection, recent burn, cardiovascular disease, autoimmune disease, renal disorder, coagulation disorder

C. Signs and symptoms: Relates to underlying disease and whether it is acute or chronic
    1. Petechiae, purpura, ecchymosis
    2. Gingival bleeding
    3. Epistaxis
    4. Hemoptysis
    5. Blood in urine and stool
    6. Heavy prolonged vaginal bleeding
    7. Peripheral edema secondary to fluid overload
    8. Headaches
    9. Chest pain
    10. Shortness of breath

D. Physical examination: Focus on hemodynamic stability and instability.
    1. Vital signs
        a) Tachycardia; weak, thready pulse
        b) Hypotension
        c) Narrow pulse pressure

        d) Tachypnea
- 2. Integument
  - *a)* Wounds, IV sites, vascular access devices for bleeding
  - *b)* Ecchymosis, petechiae, purpura, skin breakdown
  - *c)* Sluggish capillary refill
  - *d)* Cool, clammy skin
- 3. HEENT
  - *a)* Scleral hemorrhage
  - *b)* Gingival or mucosal bleeding from oral cavity
  - *c)* Epistaxis
- 4. Pulmonary: Abnormal sounds in lungs (e.g., rales) indicating signs of pulmonary edema from hemorrhage; respiratory compromise (e.g., accessory muscle use)
- 5. Cardiac: Decreased peripheral pulses
- 6. Neurologic: Every two to four hours
  - *a)* Altered mental status, changes in level of consciousness
  - *b)* Sluggish pupil reaction or dilated pupil
- 7. Abdominal: Tenderness and distention from abdominal bleeding

IV. Diagnostic tests (Arruda & High, 2015; Cope, 2016; Feinstein, 2015; Gando & Otomo, 2015; Gobel, 2018; Iba et al., 2019; Levi, 2019; Toh et al., 2016; Wada et al., 2014; see Table 120-2)
- A. Laboratory
  - 1. CBC: Leukocytosis with a shift to the immature WBCs may be present with infection. Bleeding may be present with abnormal platelet numbers.
  - 2. Increased reticulocyte count indicating presence of immature RBCs: This is important because it suggests the bone marrow's ability to produce in response to blood loss or destruction.
  - 3. Additional coagulation studies
    - *a)* Protamine sulfate test positive for fibrin
    - *b)* Decreased plasminogen: Measure of fibrinolytic system activation by immunologic methods (normal = 10–20 mg/dl)
  - 4. Other: Guaiac stool, emesis, and NG tube secretions
- B. Radiology: Chest radiography to rule out acute respiratory distress syndrome

TABLE 120-2	Laboratory Data in Disseminated Intravascular Coagulation	
Laboratory Test	**Result**	**Comments**
Prothrombin time	Prolonged	Prolonged, shortened, or normal Nonspecific in disseminated intravascular coagulation (DIC); may be prolonged because of liver disease, vitamin K deficiency, obstructive biliary disease, or warfarin therapy
Activated partial thromboplastin time	Prolonged	Prolonged, shortened, or normal Decreased quantity of coagulation factors Nonspecific in DIC; may be caused by heparin therapy, increased fibrin degradation products, and consumption of clotting factors
International normalized ratio	Prolonged	Prolonged, shortened, or normal Nonspecific in DIC Evaluates overall coagulation

(Continued on next page)

TABLE 120-2	Laboratory Data in Disseminated Intravascular Coagulation *(Continued)*	
Laboratory Test	**Result**	**Comments**
Platelet count	Decreased	Frequent finding, but nonspecific in DIC Decreasing trend in serial platelet counts; may show steep drop Absolute platelet count < 100,000/mm^3
Fibrin degradation products	Elevated	Indicates breakdown of fibrin and fibrinogen Elevated levels possible with surgery, obstetric complication, inflammation, and venous thromboembolism
D-dimer	Elevated	Indicates hyperfibrinolysis Common in DIC, trauma, recent surgery, inflammation, and venous thromboembolism
Antithrombin	Decreased	Anticoagulant activity inhibited Accelerated coagulation
Protein C	Decreased	Anticoagulant activity inhibited Accelerated coagulation
Thrombin time	Elevated	Estimate of plasma fibrinogen Prolonged with heparin, streptokinase, or urokinase therapy Prolonged in DIC, liver disease, or fibrinogen deficiency
Fibrinogen	Decreased	Plasma concentration of fibrinogen decreases very slowly; seen only in severe cases of DIC Nonspecific in DIC; may be low because of congenital or acquired hypofibrinogenemia, fibrinolysis, severe liver disease, malignant disease, or obstetric trauma
Peripheral smear	Schistocytes (red cell fragments) present	Nonspecific finding in DIC
Plasminogen levels	Decreased	Hyperfibrinolysis
Alpha-2 antiplasmin levels	Decreased	Hyperfibrinolysis
Fibrinopeptide A level	Elevated	Indicates accelerated rate of fibrin formation and coagulation
Thrombin–antithrombin complex	Elevated	Indicates accelerated rate of fibrin formation and coagulation

Note. Based on information from Arruda & High, 2015; Cope, 2016; Gando et al., 2016; Gobel, 2018; Levi & Schmaier, 2020.

From "Disseminated Intravascular Coagulation," by D.G. Cope, in M. Kaplan (Ed.), *Understanding and managing oncologic emergencies: A resource for nurses* (3rd ed., pp. 199–200), 2018, Oncology Nursing Society. Copyright 2018 by Oncology Nursing Society. Reprinted with permission.

V. Differential diagnosis: DIC always is considered secondary to an underlying disorder (see Table 120-1).

VI. Treatment (Cope, 2016; Feinstein, 2015; Gobel, 2018; Levi, 2019; Murao & Yamakawa, 2019; Papageorgiou et al., 2018; Thachil, 2016; Wada et al., 2014)
   A. Treat underlying cause or disease process (e.g., infection, malignancy).
   B. Eliminate the triggering cause (e.g., septicemia, shock, chemotherapy, other therapies), such as with antibiotic therapy for treatment of sepsis.

   C. Avoid medications that interfere with platelet function (e.g., ASA-containing products, NSAIDs).

   D. Monitor hemodynamic status and vital signs frequently.

   E. Monitor daily weight, intake, and output to avoid dehydration or fluid overload.

   F. Drug therapy

      1. Heparin therapy may be used to treat DIC to inhibit intravascular fibrin formation and reduce the consumption of clotting factors.

         a) Heparin therapy should be used with caution in all patients with DIC but especially in those with acute promyelocytic leukemia because of increased risk of bleeding.

         b) Contraindications for heparin therapy include CNS disorders, open wounds, or recent surgery because of the increased risk of hemorrhage.

         c) Maintain a PTT 1–2 times normal levels.

      2. Antithrombin III may be used to supplement the low levels found during DIC. Supplementation is thought to prevent endothelial cell injury and coagulation, as well as act as an anti-inflammatory agent.

      3. Plasma protein C supplementation may be used as an anti-inflammatory mediator and inhibitor of coagulation.

      4. Tissue factor pathway inhibitor therapy may be used to reduce endotoxin-induced activation of coagulation. Use with caution because of the risk of hemorrhage.

   G. Blood component therapy

      1. Platelet transfusions are administered to maintain a platelet count of 10,000–20,000/mm^3 without active bleeding and to maintain a platelet count of 50,000/mm^3 if active bleeding is evident.

      2. Packed RBCs may be transfused if Hgb less than 8 g/dl, the patient is symptomatic, or active bleeding is present.

      3. Fresh frozen plasma, purified fibrinogen concentrates, or cryoprecipitate may be used to correct the coagulation defect.

      4. Careful consideration must be given to the use of prothrombin complex concentrates.

VII. Follow-up

   A. Patients most often require hospitalization for close monitoring of signs and symptoms of acute bleeding or thrombosis.

   B. Patients with chronic DIC may be closely monitored in the outpatient setting through PT, PTT, fibrinogen, and antithrombin levels.

VIII. Referrals: Consult hematologist if the follow occur.

   A. Bleeding persists despite interventions

   B. DIC diagnosed during initial evaluation; referral based on underlying condition

References

Arruda, V.R., & High, K.A. (2015). Coagulation disorders. In D.L. Kasper, A.S. Fauci, S.L. Hauser, D.L. Longo, J.L. Jameson, & J. Loscalzo (Eds.), *Harrison's principles of internal medicine* (19th ed., pp. 732–740). McGraw-Hill Medical.

Cope, D.G. (2016). Metabolic emergencies. In B.H. Gobel, S. Triest-Robertson, & W.H. Vogel (Eds.), *Advanced oncology nursing certification review and resource manual* (2nd ed., pp. 643–692). Oncology Nursing Society.

Feinstein, D.I. (2015). Disseminated intravascular coagulation in patients with solid tumors. *Oncology, 29*(2), 96–102. https://www.cancernetwork.com/view/disseminated-intravascular-coagulation-patients-solid-tumors

Gando, S., Levi, M., & Toh, C.-H. (2016). Disseminated intravascular coagulation. *Nature Reviews Disease Primers, 2,* 16037. https://doi.org/10.1038/nrdp.2016.37

Gando, S., & Otomo, Y. (2015). Local hemostasis, immunothrombosis, and systemic disseminated intravascular coagulation in trauma and traumatic shock. *Critical Care, 19,* 72. https://doi.org/10.1186/s13054-015-0735-x

Gobel, B.H. (2018). Disseminated intravascular coagulation. In C.H. Yarbro, D. Wujcik, & B.H. Gobel (Eds.), *Cancer nursing: Principles and practice* (8th ed., pp. 1095–1106). Jones and Bartlett Learning.

Iba, T., Watanabe, E., Umemura, Y., Wada, T., Hayashida, K., Kushimoto, S., ... Wada, H. (2019). Sepsis-associated disseminated intravascular coagulation and its differential diagnosis. *Journal of Intensive Care, 7,* 32. https://doi.org/10.1186/s40560-019-0387-z

Levi, M. (2019). Disseminated intravascular coagulation in cancer: An update. *Seminars in Thrombosis and Hemostasis, 45*(4), 342–347. https://doi.org/10.1055/s-0039-1687890

Levi, M.M., & Schmaier, A.H. (2020). Disseminated intravascular coagulation. http://emedicine.medscape.com/article/199627-overview

Liaw, P.C., Ito, T., Iba, T., Thachil, J., & Zeerleder, S. (2016). DAMP and DIC: The role of extracellular DNA and DNA-binding proteins in the pathogenesis of DIC. *Blood Reviews, 30*(4), 257–261. https://doi.org/10.1016/j.blre.2015.12.004

Murao, S., & Yamakawa, K. (2019). A systematic summary of systematic reviews on anticoagulant therapy in sepsis. *Journal of Clinical Medicine, 8*(11), 1869. https://doi.org/10.3390/jcm8111869

National Heart, Lung, and Blood Institute. (2019). Disseminated intravascular coagulation. https://www.nhlbi.nih.gov/health-topics/disseminated-intravascular-coagulation

Papageorgiou, C., Jourdi, G., Adjambri, E., Walborn, A., Patel, P., Fareed, J., ... Gerotziafas, G.T. (2018). Disseminated intravascular coagulation: An update on pathogenesis, diagnosis, and therapeutic strategies. *Clinical and Applied Thrombosis/Hemostasis, 24*(9 Suppl.), 8S–28S. https://doi.org/10.1177/1076029618806424

Thachil, J. (2016). Disseminated intravascular coagulation: A practical approach. *Anesthesiology, 125*(1), 230–236. https://doi.org/10.1097/ALN.0000000000001123

Toh, C.H., Alhamdi, Y., & Abrams, S.T. (2016). Current pathological and laboratory considerations in the diagnosis of disseminated intravascular coagulation. *Annals of Laboratory Medicine, 36*(6), 505–512. https://doi.org/10.3343/alm.2016.36.6.505

Wada, H., Matsumoto, T., & Yamashita, Y. (2014). Diagnosis and treatment of disseminated intravascular coagulation (DIC) according to four DIC guidelines. *Journal of Intensive Care, 2,* 15. https://doi.org/10.1186/2052-0492-2-15.

CHAPTER 121

Hemochromatosis

Deborah Kirk, DNP, FNP-BC, NP-C, AOCN®, FAANP

I. Definition: A group of disorders in which excessive intestinal iron absorption, either alone or in combination with parenteral loading, leads to an increase in total body iron stores (Fitzsimons et al., 2018; Hollerer et al., 2017; Palmer et al., 2018; Radford-Smith et al., 2018)

II. Physiology/Pathophysiology (Asimakopoulou et al., 2017; Fitzsimons et al., 2018; Golfeyz et al., 2018; Waldvogel-Abramowski et al., 2014)
   A. Normal: Healthy individuals have 4–5 g of total body iron, with 35% stored in macrophages of the liver, spleen, and bone marrow in the form of ferritin, which is mobilized when needed.
      1. Most adults ingest 10–15 mg of iron daily as organic iron from grains and vegetables and heme iron from meats. Only 10% of this iron is absorbed into the circulation via the duodenum or jejunum.
      2. For those with normal iron metabolism, daily loss of iron (menstrual losses, stool, and sweat) roughly equals absorption.
      3. No physiologic mechanism exists in the body for excreting iron in substantial quantities. Intestinal absorption of iron is regulated only by replacing amounts lost from exfoliated cells of the GI tract, skin, and menstrual blood; males excrete 1 mg daily, and females excrete 1.5 mg daily.
      4. Inorganic ferric irons are transported by transferrin, a beta globulin in the plasma, from the GI tract to reticulocytes and tissue stores and from tissue stores to bone marrow.
      5. The rate of synthesis of transferrin from the liver is regulated by total body iron stores, not Hgb.
      6. The low transferrin levels in hemochromatosis are attributable to increased total body iron stores. Total iron-binding capacity levels reflect the amount of iron contained in transferrin, usually approximately 30%.
      7. Ferritin is an intracellular protein containing inorganic iron at its core. It is found in macrophages, reticulocytes, intestinal mucosa, skeletal muscle, and placenta, as well as the testes, kidneys, heart, and pancreas.
         a) Serum and tissue ferritin are regulated by total body iron stores.
         b) Approximately 1 mg/ml of serum ferritin is the equivalent of 8–10 mg of stored tissue iron.
      8. Hemosiderin contains multiple forms of ferritin, a stable form of iron storage, which can be mobilized by venesection.
   B. Pathophysiology: Iron is deposited in the tissues of the liver, heart, pancreas, skin, and endocrine organs, leading to cell damage, cell death, and fibrosis.

1. Hereditary hemochromatosis refers to an inherited autosomal-recessive disorder (most commonly C282Y and H63D on the hemochromatosis [*HFE*] gene on chromosome 6) of iron metabolism, leading to inappropriate intestinal iron absorption with subsequent tissue iron deposits.
2. Hepcidin, a hormone mostly in hepatocytes, is responsible for iron absorption. When a malfunction occurs in the expression of hepcidin, iron absorption is affected.
3. Crypt cells of the duodenum are unable to retain iron, which leads to iron overload. Excess iron is deposited in tissues such as the myocardium, pancreas, and other organs, usually sparing the bone. Eventually, this process leads to end-organ damage.
4. In secondary hemochromatosis, excess iron is stored in reticuloendothelial system cells of the bone marrow, the spleen, and in Kupffer cells of the liver as hemosiderin, a less destructive form of iron. Reticuloendothelial system cells have a storage capacity of 10 g of iron or approximately 40 units of blood. Once this capacity is exceeded, iron is accumulated in the same destructive manner as hereditary hemochromatosis.

III. Clinical features: Hereditary hemochromatosis is the most common autosomal recessive disease in people of Northern European ancestry, occurring in approximately 1 in 250 people. Because of genetic testing, the number of men and women identified are relatively equal, but men have more symptoms of the disease. Hemochromatosis is rarely diagnosed before middle age. Risk of infection is heightened in hemochromatosis. Severe bacterial infections, particularly with *Yersinia enterocolitica,* enteric gram-negative bacteria, *Staphylococcus aureus,* and *Listeria monocytogenes,* may cause sepsis, meningitis, enterocolitis, peritonitis, and intra-abdominal abscesses. Increased availability of iron is used for bacterial growth (Asimakopoulou et al., 2017; Fitzsimons et al., 2018; Hollerer et al., 2017; Milman et al., 2019; Palmer et al., 2018).
   A. Etiology
      1. Primary hereditary hemochromatosis: Inherited disorder of iron metabolism
      2. Secondary hemochromatosis
         a) Parenteral hemochromatosis: Result of multiple RBC transfusions given in chronic anemic states, such as myelodysplasia
         b) Erythropoietic hemochromatosis: An ineffective erythropoiesis in the bone marrow, as seen in thalassemia major, sideroblastic anemia, and aplastic anemia
         c) Dietary iron overload
         d) Chronic liver disease: Alcoholic liver disease, hepatitis
   B. History
      1. History of cancer and cancer treatment
      2. Current medications: Prescribed, over the counter, iron supplementation
      3. History of presenting symptoms: Precipitating factors, onset, location, duration
      4. Changes in ADLs
      5. Family history of hemochromatosis
      6. Past medical history: Multiple blood transfusions, diabetes, cardiac failure (accounts for one-third of deaths associated with hemochromatosis), cirrhosis, hormonal disorders
   C. Signs and symptoms: Nonspecific, usually occurring in late stage
      1. Fatigue
      2. Nonspecific abdominal pains
      3. Enlarged metacarpophalangeal joints, usually second and third joints
      4. Bronze hyperpigmented skin
      5. Impotence: Pituitary hypofunction

6. Loss of libido
7. Arthralgia
8. Malaise
9. Symptoms of diabetes: Polydipsia, polyphagia, polyuria
10. Cardiac failure symptoms: Shortness of breath, peripheral edema

D. Physical examination: Vague signs with early disease; symptoms worsen with advanced disease.
    1. Vital signs: Fever present with infection, weight loss
    2. Integument
        a) Loss of body hair
        b) Dry skin
        c) Atrophic skin
        d) Hyperpigmentation
        e) Palmar erythema
        f) Spider angiomas
        g) Dark metallic hue (because of melanin deposits in the dermis), darker on face, neck, exterior surface of the lower arms, dorsal hand surface, in genital folds, lower legs, and in scar tissue; pigmented oral mucosa
        h) Gynecomastia
    3. Abdominal: Hepatomegaly, splenomegaly, ascites
    4. Cardiac: Symptoms of heart failure
        a) Tachycardia
        b) Irregular heart rate
        c) Altered heart sounds
    5. External male genitalia: Testicular atrophy
    6. Musculoskeletal: Enlarged joints involving metacarpophalangeal and proximal interphalangeal joints of the hands; knees, hips, wrists, and shoulders may be involved in advanced disease.

IV. Diagnostic tests: Most diagnoses of hemochromatosis are incidental findings when ferritin level is ordered in a patient with fatigue. Criteria are based on demonstration of excessive iron studies in the absence of other causes of iron overload, such as refractory anemia, thalassemia, and alcoholic cirrhosis (Asimakopoulou et al., 2017; Fitzsimons et al., 2018; Hollerer et al., 2017; Kowdley et al., 2019; Palmer et al., 2018).

A. Laboratory
    1. CBC to assess for anemia
    2. LFTs to assess for abnormalities
    3. Iron studies: Serum iron, serum ferritin level, and transferrin saturation; transferrin saturation = serum ferritin ÷ total iron-binding capacity
        a) Normal range for serum iron is 50–150 mg/dl. If greater than 180 mg/dl, serum iron should be rechecked one month after iron supplements are discontinued.
        b) Serum iron and percent saturation of iron: Elevated (more than 45%) in early disease, but specificity is reduced by false positives and false negatives in young patients or patients with other illnesses.
        c) Serum ferritin (normal 30–300 ng/ml) reflects hepatic and total body iron stores.
            (1) Normal levels may be found in those with latent hemochromatosis or precirrhotic hemochromatosis.
            (2) Ascorbic acid deficiency will show false low serum ferritin concentrations.
        d) Elevated serum ferritin in absence of iron overload can be attributable to infection or acute/chronic liver disease.

4. Genetic testing: Family screening is recommended for all first-degree relatives of a patient with hereditary hemochromatosis.

   a) Approximately 90% of patients who are genetically tested and found to have hemochromatosis are homozygous for C282Y mutation of the *HFE* gene; familial iron overload is rare in absence of *HFE* mutations.

   b) Compound heterozygotes (C282Y mutation and H63D mutation) and H63D homozygotes have lower risk for iron overload and may show normal iron studies.

   c) Presence of C282Y homozygote may alleviate the need for liver biopsy.

B. Radiology

   1. Ultrasound of the abdomen may be needed to evaluate hepatomegaly.
   2. MRI of the liver is used for quantification of hepatic iron deposition, eliminating need for liver biopsy.

C. Other

   1. Genetic testing has become more available, and liver biopsy has assumed less importance.
   2. Liver biopsy provides the iron content of the liver, iron distribution in the liver, and presence of tissue damage, most particularly cirrhosis. Liver biopsy is indicated in the following cases.

      a) To document the degree of fibrosis in hereditary hemochromatosis homozygotes in people older than age 40 years with elevated ALT and clinical evidence of liver disease

      b) In individuals with increased serum ferritin level greater than 1,000 ng/ml, which is associated with increased likelihood of significant hepatic cirrhosis or fibrosis

      c) In individuals who are compound heterozygotes (C282Y/H63D) or C282Y heterozygotes, or for non-*HFE*–mutated individuals who have indirect markers or iron overload, particularly if they have elevated liver enzymes or evidence of liver disease

      d) For further testing in patients with a negative genetic test in the presence of iron overload

   3. ECG: Changes are often seen with dilated cardiomyopathy, such as sick sinus syndrome.

V. Differential diagnosis (Waldvogel-Abramowski et al., 2014)

   A. Alcoholic cirrhosis (see Chapter 69)
   B. Inflammatory liver disease
   C. Nonalcoholic fatty liver disease
   D. Hepatitis (see Chapter 74)
   E. Alpha antitrypsin deficiency
   F. Bacterial infection
   G. Refractory anemia
   H. Thalassemia
   I. Hepatocellular carcinoma

VI. Treatment: Prognosis of hemochromatosis primarily is dependent on the presence of cirrhosis at the time of diagnosis (Asimakopoulou et al., 2017; de Lima et al., 2019; Fitzsimons et al., 2018; Hollerer et al., 2017; Kowdley et al., 2019; Milman et al., 2019; Radford-Smith et al., 2018).

   A. Phlebotomy is the primary treatment for hereditary hemochromatosis. Treatment usually consists of a series of induction phlebotomies followed by maintenance phlebotomy to prevent reaccumulation of excess iron and to prevent or minimize further organ damage.

1. Provide pre- and postphlebotomy hydration, if needed.
2. Take precautions to protect patients from orthostatic hypotension after phlebotomy.
3. In general, men require more phlebotomies than women, and older patients are phlebotomized more frequently than younger patients.
4. Effective initial treatment goal is to remove 5–20 g of iron for most patients. Therapeutic phlebotomy initially is done weekly, depending upon Hgb level, removing 500 ml of whole blood, which is equal to 200–250 mg of iron.
5. Continue until serum ferritin reaches 50–100 ng/ml or until hematocrit and Hgb are unable to recover before the next phlebotomy.
6. It is not necessary for patients to become anemic, only depleted of their iron stores. However, a mild form of iron deficiency may be required to bring iron levels to adequate control.
7. Once the initial series of therapeutic phlebotomies is completed, frequency will depend on serum ferritin levels. Goal should be to keep ferritin between 50–100 ng/ml. Most patients require maintenance therapy every three months, removing one unit of blood.
8. In few individuals, for reasons unknown, iron does not reaccumulate, and they require no maintenance therapy.

B. Patients should ingest only moderate amounts of iron-rich foods, such as red or organ meats, foods cooked in iron containers, and black tea.

C. Alcohol use should be discouraged in any patient with liver disease because it can increase iron absorption.

D. Patients should strictly avoid iron supplements.

E. Chelating agents may be used for treatment of secondary hemochromatosis related to dyserythropoietic syndromes or in patients who cannot tolerate phlebotomy, such as those with cardiac failure or severe anemia. These agents remove approximately 10–20 mg of iron daily.

1. These agents are less effective than phlebotomy and ideally require daily dosing.
2. Chelating agents can be used as a single agent or prior to RBC transfusions to decrease iron load.
3. Drugs

    a) Deferoxamine infusion is 20–60 mg/kg daily. Dosing recommendations are usually determined by the patient's serum ferritin levels.

        (1) Serum ferritin less than 2,000 ng/ml requires approximately 25 mg/kg daily.

        (2) Serum ferritin of 2,000–3,000 ng/ml may require 35 mg/kg daily.

        (3) Higher serum ferritin levels may require greater than 55 mg/kg daily.

        (4) It is not advised to regularly exceed an average daily dose of 50 mg/kg daily, except in instances requiring intense chelation therapy in patients who have completed growth and development.

        (5) As ferritin level drops below 1,000 ng/ml, the risk of deferoxamine toxicity increases, such as respiratory distress and neurotoxicity.

        (6) Patients must be monitored closely to lower total weekly dose if necessary.

            (a) Routes of administration

                i. Subcutaneous infusion via portable pump: Slow subcutaneous infusion by means of a portable pump over 8–12 hours is effective and convenient for ambulatory patients. Weekly dosage must be calculated in terms of how frequently the pump is worn.

                ii. IV during blood transfusion: Dosage and mode of administration are individually based and adapted during the course of therapy according to the patient's iron burden. Lowest effective dose should be used. Effectiveness is measured by 24-hour urinary iron excretion on a daily basis, and dosage then is monitored accordingly. It can be given prior to transfusion.

 iii. Continuous IV infusion: It is indicated in patients who cannot tolerate subcutaneous infusion or those with cardiac problems secondary to iron overload. Implanted IV systems can be used. Care is advised when flushing lines as not to "bolus" a patient with residual deferoxamine, as it can lead to complete vascular collapse—hypotension, shock, flushing, tachycardia, and urticaria.
- IV route is preferable because rate can be controlled.
- In hypotensive patients, IV route is recommended.

 iv. IM injection: Because subcutaneous injections are more effective, IM injection is used only if subcutaneous access is not feasible.

 v. In normotensive patients, deferoxamine can be given in a single IM dose of 2 g for adults.

 vi. Whatever route is selected, the individual maintenance dose should be based on the patient's iron excretion rate.

 b) Deferasirox is an oral chelating therapy
  (1) It may be used for iron overload related to blood transfusions.
  (2) Dose is dependent on formulation (e.g., 14 mg/kg daily, 20 mg/kg PO daily).
  (3) Use with extreme caution in patients with hepatic and renal impairment.

4. Patients with iron overload usually become vitamin C deficient, as iron oxidizes this vitamin.

 a) As an adjunct to chelation therapy, vitamin C in divided doses up to 200 mg daily can be given starting one month after the initial chelation.

 b) Vitamin C increases availability of iron for chelation. High doses should be avoided.

VII. Follow-up
 A. Short term: Careful monitoring of iron levels every month during phlebotomy or chelation therapy
 B. Long term: Every three to six months, then annually depending on stabilization of iron levels

VIII. Referrals
 A. Rheumatologist: For management of arthritis and degenerative OA from iron deposits
 B. Diabetic management: Diabetes is a late complication because of iron deposits on pancreatic islet cells; patients usually become insulin resistant.
 C. Cardiologist: For management of cardiac failure and dysrhythmias from iron deposits
 D. GI: For liver biopsy
 E. Endocrinologist: For management of diabetes or pituitary failure
 F. Hematologist: For phlebotomy
 G. Long term: Referral to subspecialty practice to prevent and manage long-term complications (e.g., gastroenterology, renal, cardiac, respiratory, dermatology)

References

Asimakopoulou, A., Weiskirchen, S., & Weiskirchen, R. (2017). Pathogenesis, diagnostics, and treatment of hereditary haemochromatosis: A 150-year-long understanding of an iron overload disorder. *European Medical Journal, 2*(4), 122–133.

de Lima, T.G., Benevides, F.L.N., Esmeraldo Filho, F.L., Farias, I.S., Dourado, D.X.C., Fontenele, E.G.P., ... Quidute, A.R.P. (2019). Treatment of iron overload syndrome: A general review. *Revista da Associação Médica Brasileira, 65*(9), 1216–1222. https://doi.org/10.1590/1806-9282.65.9.1216

Fitzsimons, E.J., Cullis, J.O., Thomas, D.W., Tsochatzis, E., & Griffiths, W.J.H. (2018). Diagnosis and therapy of genetic haemochromatosis (review and 2017 update). *British Journal of Haematology, 181*(3), 293–303. https://doi.org/10.1111/bjh.15164

Golfeyz, S., Lewis, S., & Weisberg, I.S. (2018). Hemochromatosis: Pathophysiology, evaluation, and management of hepatic iron overload with a focus on MRI. *Expert Review of Gastroenterology and Hepatology, 12*(8), 767–778. https://doi.org/10.1080/17474124.2018.1496016

Hollerer, I., Bachmann, A., & Muckenthaler, M.U. (2017). Pathophysiological consequences and benefits of HFE mutations: 20 years of research. *Haematologica, 102*(5), 809–817. https://doi.org/10.3324/haematol.2016.160432

Kowdley, K.V., Brown, K.E., Ahn, J., & Sundaram, V. (2019). ACG clinical guideline: Hereditary hemochromatosis. *American Journal of Gastroenterology, 114*(3), 1202–1218. https://doi.org/10.14309/ajg.0000000000000315

Milman, N.T., Schioedt, F.V., Junker, A.E., & Magnussen, K. (2019). Diagnosis and treatment of genetic *HFE*-hemochromatosis: The Danish aspect. *Gastroenterology Research, 12*(5), 221–232. https://doi.org/10.14740/gr1206

Palmer, W.C., Vishnu, P., Sanchez, W., Aqel, B., Riegert-Johnson, D., Seaman, L.A.K., ... Rivera, C.E. (2018). Diagnosis and management of genetic iron overload disorders. *Journal of General Internal Medicine, 33*(12), 2230–2236. https://doi.org/10.1007/s11606-018-4669-2

Radford-Smith, D.E., Powell, E.E., & Powell, L.W. (2018). Haemochromatosis: A clinical update for the practising physician. *Internal Medicine Journal, 48*(5), 509–516. https://doi.org/10.1111/imj.13784

Waldvogel-Abramowski, S., Waeber, G., Gassner, C., Buser, A., Frey, B.M., Favrat, B., & Tissot, J.-D. (2014). Physiology of iron metabolism. *Transfusion Medicine and Hemotherapy, 41*(3), 213–221. https://doi.org/10.1159/000362888

CHAPTER 122

Hypercoagulable State

Mailey Wilks, DNP, MSN, APRN, NP-C,
and Beth Faiman, PhD, MSN, APRN-BC, AOCN®, FAAN

I. Definition: *Hypercoagulable state, thrombophilia*, and *thrombotic disorders* are terms used to describe a hereditary or acquired predisposition to thromboembolism (Dautaj et al., 2019; Favaloro, 2019).
  A. *Thrombophilia* is a generic term that defines an increased propensity toward thrombosis and associated morbidity.
  B. Thrombophilias are hereditary and/or acquired conditions.

II. Physiology/Pathophysiology (Campello et al., 2019; Dautaj et al., 2019; Singh et al., 2018)
  A. Normal: The purpose of the clotting cascade is to prevent blood loss and repair blood vessel damage.
    1. Primary hemostasis occurs when activated platelets become attached to damaged endothelium to form a clot. Multiple clotting mediators interact with platelets to form a clot, including negatively charged phospholipids that activate the intrinsic pathway.
    2. Secondary hemostasis changes soluble fibrinogen into fibrin strands via two pathways.
      a) The intrinsic pathway is initiated when collagen inside the damaged endothelium or phospholipids on activated platelets change inactive factor XII to active, thus activating factors XI, IX, and then VIII.
      b) The extrinsic pathway is activated when factor VII becomes active and contacts tissue factor released by the endothelium.
      c) Both pathways lead to the common pathway, in which factor X becomes active with factor V present (factor Xa), which activates factor II and changes prothrombin to thrombin. Factor I is then activated, which changes fibrinogen to fibrin. Activated factor XII causes cross-linking of fibrin strands to form a stable clot.
  B. Pathophysiology
    1. Slow blood flow, increased proclotting components, and lack of anticlotting factors and endothelial injury (Virchow triad) can all result in a hypercoagulable state.
    2. Anticlotting factors include antithrombin III, protein C, protein S, and tissue factor pathway inhibitor, which block the clotting cascade at different sites. Endogenous heparin increases the activity of antithrombin II to block thrombin production and block factors XII, XI, and IX in the intrinsic pathway.
    3. Cancer cells activate the clotting system and stimulate platelets, endothelial cells, and leukocytes to express procoagulant activity.

III. Clinical features: An inherited thromboembolic defect is present in 1%–2% of patients presenting with initial DVT. Factor V Leiden and the prothrombin gene mutation are the most common genetic associations with thrombosis (Campello et al., 2019; Carroll & Piazza, 2018; Dautaj et al., 2019; Favaloro, 2019; Linnemann & Hart, 2019; Rybstein & DeSancho, 2018; Singh et al., 2018).

A. Classification
  1. Classifications of inherited thrombophilias
      a) Procoagulant protein abnormalities
          (1) Activated protein C resistance: factor V Leiden
          (2) Prothrombin G20210A mutation
          (3) Selected dysfibrinogenemia variants
      b) Anticoagulant protein deficiencies
          (1) Antithrombin
          (2) Protein C
          (3) Protein S
  2. Other
      a) Homocystinuria
      b) Increased procoagulant proteins: Factor II, III, IX, and XI, fibrinogen
      c) Factor XIII polymorphisms
      d) Hyperhomocysteinemia
      e) Reduced tissue factor pathway inhibitor
      f) Deficiency of protein Z
      g) Elevated levels: Plasminogen activator inhibitor-1, thrombin-activatable fibrinolysis inhibitor
B. Risk factors for recurrent thromboembolism
  1. Smoking
  2. Obesity
  3. Hypercholesterolemia
  4. Heparin use
  5. Estrogen use: Oral contraceptives
  6. Advancing age
C. Etiology
  1. Inherited
      a) Family history of DVT, PE, stroke, or hypercoagulable state
      b) Inherited thrombophilias
  2. Acquired
      a) Cancer
      b) Immobility
      c) Trauma
      d) Surgery
  3. Other causes
      a) Diabetes
      b) SLE
      c) Thyroid disease
      d) Sepsis
      e) Sickle cell disease/thalassemia
      f) CHF
      g) Renal failure
      h) Polycythemia vera
      i) Pregnancy and postpartum
      j) Warfarin-induced skin necrosis
      k) Purpura fulminans: Neonatalis or adult

   D. History
1. History of cancer and cancer treatment
2. Current medications: Prescribed, over the counter
3. History of presenting symptoms: Precipitating factors, onset, location, duration
4. Changes in ADLs
5. Past medical history of DVT/PE, miscarriage, risk factors for hypercoagulable state
6. Family history of DVT/PE, hypercoagulable state, miscarriage

   E. Signs and symptoms
1. Dull ache, tight feeling, or frank pain in the calf or upper extremity
2. Distention of the superficial venous collateral vessels
3. Mild fever possible
4. Tenderness over involved vein

   F. Physical examination
1. Vital signs: Fever, tachycardia, hypertension
2. Integument: Skin assessment for paleness, coolness, necrosis, purpura fulminans (neonatalis or adult), and cyanosis depending on degree of obstruction
3. Pulmonary: Pleural friction rubs or rales possible with PE
4. Cardiac: Right-sided gallop suggesting right ventricular failure
5. Abdominal
    a) Splenomegaly noted with splenic infarction
    b) Hepatomegaly often seen with polycythemia vera or other myeloproliferative diseases
6. Extremities
    a) Unilateral edema of involved extremity
    b) Warmth and erythema of involved extremity
    c) Tender palpable venous cord of involved vein
    d) Thigh or calf tenderness of involved vein
    e) Positive Homan sign (see Appendix D)
7. Neurologic
    a) Ataxia
    b) Level of consciousness
    c) Extraocular movement
    d) Facial palsy
    e) Unilateral weakness of extremities

IV. Diagnostic tests (Carroll & Piazza, 2018; Cohn et al., 2008; Favaloro, 2019; Kwang et al., 2019; Linnemann & Hart, 2019; Pruthi, 2017; Stevens et al., 2016)
   A. Laboratory
1. The goal of testing is to determine which patients require long-term anticoagulation.
2. No consensus has been established on whether to screen patients with DVT for a hypercoagulable state. No randomized controlled trials have shown that testing decreases risk of recurrence. The presence of a thrombophilia does not change the treatment of an initial DVT, and screening is not routinely recommended.
3. Patients should not be screened in the following situations.
    a) Recent major surgery, trauma, or immobilization
    b) Active malignancy
    c) SLE
    d) Inflammatory bowel disease
    e) Myeloproliferative disorders
    f) Heparin-induced thrombocytopenia with thrombosis

    g) Preeclampsia at term

    h) Retinal vein thrombosis

    i) Upper limb DVT

4. Consider screening for protein C and S deficiency and antithrombin deficiency if the patient has first DVT before age 50 years, a family history of DVT, recurrent DVT, or DVT occurring with oral contraceptives or pregnancy.

5. Consider screening for factor V Leiden, prothrombin gene mutation, and antiphospholipid antibodies in Caucasian patients if first DVT occurred before age 50 years, or in women with DVT associated with hormones. In non-Caucasian patients, the incidence of factor V Leiden and prothrombin gene mutation is less than 1%, so routine screening is not recommended.

6. Consider testing for *JAK2* mutations if myeloproliferative disorders are suspected in the presence of mesenteric vein thrombosis.

7. Consider flow cytometry in suspected cases of paroxysmal nocturnal hemoglobinuria with pancytopenia and intravascular hemolysis/thrombosis.

8. An acute thrombosis can decrease the plasma concentration of antithrombin, protein C, and protein S. Heparin can decrease antithrombin concentration by approximately 30%, and warfarin causes a marked reduction in functional activity of protein C and S. Therefore, testing is preferred at least two weeks after completing the initial three to six months of anticoagulation therapy.

9. The presence of liver disease and a history of liver or stem cell transplantation can influence the results of testing.

10. Testing may result in psychological distress.

11. Testing is very costly, so the decision to test should not be taken lightly.

    a) CBC, chemistry panel, lipid panel, and TSH for baseline and to evaluate for underlying causes

    b) PT: A value of 11–16 seconds indicates the extrinsic pathway is functioning normally.

    c) aPTT: A value of 33–45 seconds indicates the intrinsic coagulation system is functioning normally.

    d) Specific testing for causes of hypercoagulable state

        (1) Protein C

        (2) Protein S

        (3) Antithrombin III assay

        (4) Factor V Leiden mutation: Functional and nucleic acid

        (5) Prothrombin 20210A mutation

        (6) Homocysteine level

        (7) Anticardiolipin antibodies

        (8) Antinuclear antibodies

        (9) Antiphospholipid antibodies

        (10) Lupus anticoagulant

        (11) Fibrinogen level

V. Differential diagnosis (Campello et al., 2019)

  A. Diabetes mellitus (see Chapter 151)

  B. SLE (see Chapter 110)

  C. Thyroid disorders (see Chapters 157 and 158)

  D. Sepsis

  E. Sickle cell disease (see Chapter 119)

  F. Thalassemia

G. CHF (see Chapter 42)

H. Renal failure (see Chapter 86)

I. Polycythemia vera (see Chapter 128)

VI. Treatment (Campello et al., 2019; Serrao et al., 2019; Skeith, 2018)

A. Reduce risk factors for clotting.

1. Encourage smoking cessation.

2. Emphasize the importance of weight reduction.

3. Manage hyperlipidemia.

4. Use alternatives to oral contraceptives.

5. Avoid hormone replacement.

6. Optimize disease management for conditions known to contribute to risk.

7. Avoid immobility.

8. Use compression stockings and pneumatic compression devices.

B. Follow recommended guidelines for treatment of initial venous thromboembolic events (see Chapter 43).

C. Heterozygote factor V Leiden or prothrombin mutation alone does not justify long-term anticoagulation.

D. Patients with lupus anticoagulant deficiency, deficiency of protein C or S, antithrombin double heterozygous mutation, and homozygous mutation for factor V Leiden require long-term anticoagulant and periodic reassessment of bleeding risk.

VII. Follow-up (Rybstein & DeSancho, 2018; Serrao et al., 2019)

A. Short term

1. Perform frequent follow-up if the patient is on active anticoagulation therapy (see Chapter 43).

2. Monitor closely for adverse reactions to medications and bleeding risk.

B. Long term

1. Monitor for recurrence of DVT.

2. If testing has not been done for hypercoagulable state and no new inciting factor is present, consider testing.

VIII. Referrals

A. Hematologist: For guidance on appropriate testing and treatment

B. Genetic counselor: For consideration of screening of first-degree relatives

The authors would like to acknowledge Kristine Turner Story, RN, MSN, APRN, BC, for her contribution to this chapter that remains unchanged from the previous edition of this book.

References

Campello, E., Spiezia, L., Adamo, A., & Simioni, P. (2019). Thrombophilia, risk factors, and prevention. *Expert Review of Hematology, 12*(3), 147–158. https://doi.org/10.1080/17474086.2019.1583555

Carroll, B.J., & Piazza, G. (2018). Hypercoagulable states in arterial and venous thrombosis: When, how, and who to test? *Vascular Medicine, 23*(4), 388–399. https://doi.org/10.1177/1358863X18755927

Cohn, D.M., Vansenne, F., Kaptein, A.A., de Borgie, C.A.J.M., & Middeldorp, S. (2008). The psychological impact of testing for thrombophilia: A systematic review. *Journal of Thrombosis and Haemostasis, 6*(7), 1099–1104. https://doi.org/10.1111/j.1538-7836.2008.03005.x

Dautaj, A., Krasi, G., Bushati, V., Precone, V., Gheza, M., Fioretti, F., ... Bertelli, M. (2019). Hereditary thrombophilia. *Acta Biomedica, 90*(Suppl. 10), 44–46. https://doi.org/10.23750/abm.v90i10-s.8758

Favaloro, E.J. (2019). Genetic testing for thrombophilia-related genes: Observations of testing patterns for factor V Leiden (G1691A) and prothrombin gene "mutation" (G20210A). *Seminars in Thrombosis and Hemostasis, 45*(7), 730–742. https://doi.org/10.1055/s-0039-1694772

Kwang, H., Mou, E., Richman, I., Kumar, A., Berube, C., Kaimal, R., ... Hom, J. (2019). Thrombophilia testing in the inpatient setting: Impact of an educational intervention. *BMC Medical Informatics and Decision Making, 19,* 167. https://doi.org/10.1186/s12911-019-0889-6

Linnemann, B., & Hart, C. (2019). Laboratory diagnostics in thrombophilia. *Hämostaseologie, 39*(1), 49–61. https://doi.org/10.1055/s-0039-1677840

Pruthi, R. (2017). Optimal utilization of thrombophilia testing. *International Journal of Laboratory Hematology, 39*(Suppl. 1), 104–110. https://doi.org/10.1111/ijlh.12672

Rybstein, M.D., & DeSancho, M.T. (2018). Hypercoagulable states and thrombophilias: Risks relating to recurrent venous thromboembolism. *Seminars in Interventional Radiology, 35*(2), 99–104. https://doi.org/10.1055/s-0038-1642037

Serrao, A., Lucani, B., Mansour, D., Ferretti, A., Baldacci, E., Santoro, C., ... Chistolini, A. (2019). Direct oral anticoagulants in patients affected by major congenital thrombophilia. *Mediterranean Journal of Hematology and Infectious Diseases, 11*(1), e2019044. https://doi.org/10.4084/MJHID.2019.044

Singh, D., Natarajan, A., Nand, S., & Mai, H.P. (2018). Genetics of hypercoagulable and hypocoagulable states. *Neurosurgery Clinics of North America, 29*(4), 493–501. https://doi.org/10.1016/j.nec.2018.06.002

Skeith, L. (2018). Anticoagulating patients with high-risk acquired thrombophilias. *Blood, 132*(21), 2219–2229. https://doi.org/10.1182/blood-2018-05-848697

Stevens, S.M., Woller, S.C., Bauer, K.A., Kasthuri, R., Cushman, M., Streiff, M., ... Douketis, J.D. (2016). Guidance for the evaluation and treatment of hereditary and acquired thrombophilia. *Journal of Thrombosis and Thrombolysis, 41*(1), 154–164. https://doi.org/10.1007/s11239-015-1316-1

CHAPTER 123

Essential Thrombocythemia

Kristine Deano Abueg, RN, MSN, OCN®, CBCN®

I. Definition: Myeloproliferative neoplasm resulting in an increased peripheral platelet count greater than or equal to 450,000/mm³ (Arber et al., 2016; Rumi & Cazzola, 2017; Tefferi & Barbui, 2021)
   A. Also referred to as ET, essential hemorrhagic thrombocythemia, essential thrombocytosis, idiopathic thrombocythemia, idiopathic thrombocytosis, or primary thrombocythemia
   B. Not to be confused with reactive thrombocythemia, an elevated platelet count resulting from a secondary cause, such as inflammation, infection, or injury
   C. Characterized as myeloproliferative neoplasm, along with polycythemia vera, primary myelofibrosis, and chronic myeloid leukemia

II. Physiology/Pathophysiology (Barbui et al., 2016; Rumi & Cazzola, 2016, 2017; Tefferi & Barbui, 2021; Tefferi et al., 2018)
   A. Normal: Platelet count in adults range 150,000–400,000/mm³.
      1. Most platelets are formed from megakaryocytes in the extravascular spaces of the bone marrow. Tissues such as the lungs can retain megakaryocytes and also produce platelets.
      2. The megakaryocytes produce 35,000 platelets/mm³ of blood per day. During stress, they can produce up to eight times the normal number of platelets.
      3. The hormone thrombopoietin promotes megakaryocyte production and maturation. Platelets are found in circulation and in the spleen with approximately two-thirds of the total platelet count in circulation. The average life span of platelets is 8–12 days. As platelets age, they are destroyed by the spleen, liver, and bone marrow.
   B. Pathophysiology: Underlying cause is a noninherited, somatic mutation in one of the three known mutually exclusive driver genes.
      1. *JAK2* (V617F) is found in approximately 55% of patients with ET and involves the highest risk of thrombosis compared to the other myeloproliferative neoplasm–defining mutations.
      2. *CALR* exon 9 is found in approximately 25% of patients with ET and is associated with a lower risk of thrombosis but higher risk of myelofibrosis progression.
      3. *MPL* exon 10 is the least common, occurring in only 3% of ET cases, and is associated with an intermediate prognosis of thrombosis.
      4. Triple-negative ET, or ET in the absence of any of the known driver mutations, occurs in approximately 17% of patients and carries a low risk of aggressive transformation and low incidence of vascular events.
      5. Progression of disease pathophysiology
         a) During early phases of disease, patients with ET are generally asymptomatic with an incidental laboratory finding of elevated platelets.

    b) Thrombosis and hemorrhage are common and due to qualitative and quantitative aberrations in platelet aggregation.

    c) Some studies suggest ET is associated with changes in von Willebrand factor, antithrombin III, protein C, and protein S.

    d) Worsening disease may present with splenomegaly, leukocytosis, and bleeding and clotting abnormalities that cause microvascular symptoms.

    e) Late-stage disease and death are due to leukemic transformation or fibrotic progression.

III. Clinical features: ET incidence is 2.5 cases per 100,000 people annually, with an average onset of age 68 years. Early stages of the disease are associated with normal life expectancy, but increased mortality occurs because of transformation into a more aggressive myeloid neoplasm (leukemia), myelofibrosis, or cardiovascular complications arising from abnormal blood clotting. ET is usually noninherited; therefore, it is unlikely to pass to progeny (Arber et al., 2016; Cozzani et al., 2015; Emanuel et al., 2012; Fowlkes et al., 2018; Gisslinger et al., 2016; Mesa et al., 2016; NCCN, 2021; Rumi & Cazzola, 2016, 2017; Swerdlow et al., 2017; Tefferi & Barbui, 2021; Trifa et al., 2014).

A. Etiology
1. Thrombocytosis with platelet counts greater than 600,000/mm^3
    a) Infection
    b) Postsplenectomy
    c) Postacute blood loss
    d) Recovery from marrow injury
    e) Recovery after nutritional deficiency
    f) Drug induced
2. Female predominance
3. Comorbid conditions: Renal disease, hematologic disorders

B. History
1. History of cancer and cancer treatment
2. Current medications: Prescribed, over the counter
3. History of presenting symptoms: Precipitating factors, onset, location, duration, associated symptoms (e.g., headache, bruising, bleeding, weakness)
4. Changes in ADLs
5. Prior medical history: Thrombocytosis, bleeding, vascular disorders, diabetes, hypertension, arterial/venous thrombosis, dyslipidemia
6. Surgical history: Splenectomy
7. Family history: Thrombocytosis, other hematologic disorders
8. Social history: Diet, smoking, exercise

C. Signs and symptoms: Severity of symptom burden is a major component in determining treatment initiation or intensification.
1. Thrombotic events
    a) Headache, vertigo, light-headedness
    b) Weakness
    c) Bruising or bleeding
    d) Pain or swelling in extremities, acral paresthesia, erythromelalgia
    e) Cutaneous ulcers
    f) Atypical chest pain
    g) Transient visual disturbances
2. Constitutional events
    a) Persistent fatigue not relieved by rest

        b) Impaired activity level

        c) Difficulty with concentration

        d) Insomnia and sleeping quality

    3. The Myeloproliferative Neoplasm Symptom Assessment Form Total Symptom Score (MPN-SAF TSS) is a validated assessment tool for patient self-report of pertinent and representative myeloproliferative neoplasm symptoms with results that can be tracked over time.

  D. Physical examination

    1. Vital signs: Temperature to rule out infection, blood pressure to assess hypertension

    2. Integument: Hematomas, ecchymosis, petechiae, or purpura indicating bleeding

    3. HEENT: Ocular disturbances

    4. Abdominal: Tenderness, pain, hepatomegaly, splenomegaly

    5. Extremities Erythromelalgia, ecchymosis, or unilateral edema indicative of thrombosis

IV. Diagnostic tests (Arber et al., 2016; Barbui et al., 2016; Rumi & Cazzola, 2017; Swerdlow et al., 2017; Tefferi & Barbui, 2021; Tefferi et al., 2018)

  A. Laboratory: Assays are conducted to first rule out other causes of thrombocytosis (e.g., reactive thrombocytosis, iron deficiency, infection) and other myeloproliferative neoplasms and to assess for ET-defining driver mutations.

    1. CBC

        a) A consistently elevated platelet count greater than 450,000/mm³ is required for definitive diagnosis.

        b) WBC count and differential are typically normal to mildly increased.

        c) RBC indices are typically within normal limits.

    2. Peripheral blood smear

        a) Expected findings in ET are clusters of giant platelets, abnormal platelet morphology, and mild reticulin fibrosis.

        b) Increased leukoerythroblastic cells suggest myelofibrosis.

    3. Iron studies: Normal iron stores and serum ferritin

        a) Increased serum ferritin is indicative of reactive thrombocytosis.

        b) Decreased serum iron and ferritin levels are indicative of iron deficiency.

    4. LDH increase indicative of worsening bone marrow fibrosis

    5. Inflammatory assays to rule of reactive thrombocytosis

        a) CRP and ESR are typically normal.

        b) CRP and ESR are typically elevated in reactive thrombocythemia.

    6. Screening for *BCR-ABL1* rearrangement via peripheral blood to rule out chronic myeloid leukemia

    7. Sequential testing of the disease-defining genetic mutations of myeloproliferative neoplasms via peripheral blood

        a) Testing sequence is based on mutation frequency assessing first *JAK2* exon 9, followed by *CALR*, *JAK2* exon 12, and *MPL*.

        b) Absence of mutations does not rule ET out, as approximately 17% of affected patients will test negative ("triple negative"), in which case a bone marrow biopsy may be required to meet World Health Organization (WHO) Diagnostic Criteria.

    8. Bone marrow

        a) Bone marrow examination (e.g., morphology, histology, flow cytometry) is indicated as Criterion 2 of the WHO criteria. Confirmatory findings include the following.

        (1) Normal or hypercellular with proliferation of enlarged, mature megakaryocytes with hyperlobulated nuclei

        (2) No significant increase or left shift in neutrophil granulopoiesis or erythropoiesis

        (3) Mild to absent myelofibrosis

        (4) Normal erythroid and granulocyte proliferation

      b) Findings that suggest an alternative diagnosis include increased myeloblasts, myelodysplastic features, significant reticulin, or collagen fibrosis.

  B. Radiology: Not indicated

  C. Diagnostic criteria: In 2016, WHO revised its diagnostic criteria for ET to improve and standardize bone marrow morphology. An ET diagnosis requires meeting either all four major diagnostic criteria, or alternatively, the first three major diagnostic criteria and the minor diagnostic criterion.

    1. Major diagnostic criteria

      a) Criterion 1: Platelet count greater than or equal to 450,000/mm³

      b) Criterion 2: Bone marrow biopsy showing megakaryocyte proliferation with large and mature morphology and hyper-lobulated nuclei; reticulin fibrosis of grade 1 or lower

      c) Criterion 3: Does not meet WHO criteria for *BCR-ABL1*–positive chronic myeloid leukemia, polycythemia vera, or primary myelofibrosis; myelodysplastic syndromes; or other myeloid neoplasms

      d) Criterion 4: Detection of somatic mutations in one of the three mutually exclusive driver genes: *JAK2*, *CALR*, or *MPL*

    2. Minor diagnostic criteria: Presence of a clonal marker (e.g., abnormal karyotype) or absence of evidence for reactive thrombocytosis

  V. Differential diagnosis (Cozzani et al., 2015; Rumi & Cazzola, 2017; Tefferi & Barbui, 2021)

    A. Chronic myeloid leukemia

    B. Polycythemia vera (see Chapter 128)

    C. Primary myelofibrosis

    D. Prefibrotic myelofibrosis

    E. Myelodysplastic syndrome

    F. Iron-deficiency anemia (see Chapter 118)

    G. Surgical or functional asplenia

    H. Metastatic cancer

    I. Trauma

    J. Acute bleeding or hemolysis

    K. Infection

    L. Inflammatory process

    M. Renal disorders

    N. Hemolytic anemia (see Chapter 117)

    O. Familial ET

  VI. Treatment (NCCN, 2021; Rumi & Cazzola, 2016, 2017; Tefferi & Barbui, 2021; Tefferi et al., 2018)

    A. Goals

      1. Pharmacologic treatment may be indicated for prevention and treatment of thrombosis.

      2. Treatment does not alter the natural course of disease or prevent leukemic or fibrotic progression.

    3. Treatment considerations must balance risks of thrombosis, with the incurred risk of increased bleeding due to antithrombotic therapy.

B. Thrombotic risk algorithm guides pharmacologic management of ET.

    1. The four identified high-risk factors for thrombosis in ET are age 60 years or older, presence of *JAK2* mutation, history of thrombosis, and cardiovascular risk factors (e.g., diabetes, hypertension, hyperlipidemia).

    2. Risk categories stratify patients into tiers according to their risk of developing a thrombosis (see Table 123-1).

    3. Treatments are designed to prevent thrombosis and applied according to the patient's measured risk tier (see Table 123-2).

    4. Platelet count is not considered in risk stratification, as extreme thrombocytosis does not independently increase thrombosis risk.

C. Mortality/morbidity of ET largely from cardiovascular or thrombotic events

    1. Provide education on early signs and symptoms of thrombotic events.

    2. Emphasize management of modifiable risk factors (e.g., smoking cessation, healthy weight, blood pressure, cholesterol, moderate routine exercise).

D. Assessment of response has been developed for use in clinical trials; however, response assessment should be based on improvement of disease-related symptoms.

    1. Complete response: Durable resolution (at least 12 weeks) of disease-related symptoms, normalization of hematologic values (e.g., platelet count less than or equal to $400,000/mm^3$, WBC count less than or equal to $10,000/mm^3$), absence of hemorrhagic and thrombotic events, and absence of megakaryocytic hyperplasia and reticulin fibrosis on bone marrow examination

    2. Partial remission: Durable resolution of disease-related symptoms, normalization of hematologic values, and absence of hemorrhagic and thrombotic events

    3. Progressive disease: Transformation into polycythemia vera, post-ET myelofibrosis, myelodysplastic syndrome, or acute leukemia

E. Specific pharmacologic agents are initiated to prevent or treat cardiovascular complications from thrombosis.

    1. ASA

        a) Recommended initial dose is 81 mg PO daily, referred to as low-dose ASA.

        b) Low-dose ASA is effective in preventing recurrent vascular events of headache, transient neurologic disturbances, and paresthesia. ASA should be avoided with extreme thrombocytosis or acquired von Willebrand disease because of risk of bleeding.

TABLE 123-1　　**Essential Thrombocythemia Risk Stratification**

Risk Stratification	Use in Treatment Considerations
Very low risk	No history of thrombosis, age ≤ 60 years, no *JAK2* mutation
Low risk	No history of thrombosis, age ≤ 60 years, *JAK2* mutation
Intermediate risk	No history of thrombosis, age ≥ 60 years, no *JAK2* mutation
High risk	History of thrombosis or age ≥ 60 years with *JAK2* mutation
Refractory disease	Cardiovascular symptoms, thrombosis, and/or fibrosis despite prior therapy
Progressive disease	Confirmed transformation to myelofibrosis or acute leukemia

Note. Based on information from Barbui et al., 2012; Rumi & Cazzola, 2017.

TABLE 123-2	Algorithm for Initiation of Essential Thrombocythemia Therapy
Risk	**Recommended Therapies**
In all risk groups	Monitor for signs of thrombosis, bleeding, and acquired von Willebrand disease. Manage modifiable cardiovascular risk factors. Evaluate for indications of cytoreductive therapy every 3–6 months.
Very low risk	Consider low-dose (81 mg), once-daily aspirin.
Low risk	Use low-dose (81 mg), once-daily aspirin. Consider twice-daily aspirin for patients with significant cardiovascular risk factors. Avoid aspirin in very low–risk and low-risk disease with concurrent extreme thrombocytosis or acquired von Willebrand syndrome.
Intermediate risk	Use low-dose (81 mg), once- or twice-daily aspirin. Consider hydroxyurea.
High-risk disease	Use hydroxyurea with once- or twice-daily aspirin. Consider systemic anticoagulation if there is history or risk of arterial thrombosis.
Refractory	Patient may require initiation of hydroxyurea (if not previously used), busulfan, pipobroman, interferons, or anagrelide.
Progressive disease	Initiation of cytoreductive therapy may be appropriate for the new diagnosis.

Note. Based on information from Haider et al., 2016; Tefferi & Barbui, 2021.

    2. Hydroxyurea

       a) Recommended initial dose is 15 mg/kg PO daily in divided doses. Doses are then adjusted depending on the balance between the desired effects on the platelet count.

       b) Treatment goal is platelet count less than $100,000/mm^3$.

       c) The patient's RBC mean corpuscular volume should rise during therapy with hydroxyurea. If it does not rise, the patient is not taking the medication as prescribed. A rising mean corpuscular volume is indicative of appropriate drug action and is not a reason to modify the dose of hydroxyurea.

       d) Onset of action is rapid, usually within three to five days of initiation of therapy. Effect is short once medication is withdrawn; therefore, patients should be educated to avoid missing doses.

       e) Dose adjustments should not be made more frequently than once a week.

       f) Toxicity is usually minimal.

          (1) Neutropenia and anemia, oral ulcers, hyperpigmentation, skin rash, nail changes

          (2) Rare: Leg ulcers, nausea, diarrhea, alopecia, fever, abnormal LFTs

       g) Indications of intolerance to hydroxyurea include persistent platelet count greater than $400,000/mm^3$ with anemia (Hgb less than 10 g/dl) and/or WBC count less than $2,500/mm^3$; leg ulcers; other mucocutaneous symptoms; or fever.

    3. Agents indicated for persistent thrombocytosis despite hydroxyurea include the following.

       a) IFN: Starting dose is 3–5 million units subcutaneous daily.

       b) Busulfan: Starting dose is 2–4 mg PO daily.

    c) Anagrelide: Starting dose is 0.5 mg PO taken three to four times daily. Dose is adjusted according to platelet count, response, and symptoms.

        (1) Not commonly used because of increased arterial thrombosis, major hemorrhage, and progression to myelofibrosis compared to hydroxyurea

        (2) Toxicity: Headache, palpitations/tachycardia, diarrhea, fluid retention, reduction of Hgb, idiopathic cardiomyopathy

    4. Thrombosis: Clinically appropriate anticoagulation therapy is recommended (see Chapter 43).

    5. Plateletpheresis is often used in the acute setting if platelet count is greater than 800,000/mm^3 or there is an acute serious thrombotic or hemorrhagic event.

VII. Follow-up: ET is a chronic disease requiring lifetime monitoring. Ongoing monitoring is every three to six months, or as clinically indicated. Focus should be on treatment tolerance, early identification of thrombosis or bleeding diathesis, cardiovascular compromise, and leukemic or fibrotic transformation (Tefferi & Barbui, 2021).

  A. Thrombosis

  B. Bleeding and hemorrhagic sources that require emergent attention: Acquired von Willebrand disease

    1. ASA should be withheld until bleeding is controlled.

    2. Perform coagulation tests to evaluate for acquired von Willebrand disease.

    3. Refer to appropriate specialist for organ-specific hemorrhage.

  C. Indications of progression to post-ET thrombocythemia myelofibrosis

    1. Worsening bone marrow fibrosis

    2. Anemia with decrease of greater than or equal to 2 g/dl from baseline Hgb level

    3. Detection of peripheral blasts

    4. Worsening or new splenomegaly

    5. Increased LDH

    6. Worsening constitutional symptoms: Fatigue, pain, fever, weight loss

VIII. Referrals: Hematologist for management of ET

The author would like to acknowledge Barbara Barnes Rogers, CRNP, MN, AOCN®, ANP-BC, for her contribution to this chapter that remains unchanged from the previous edition of this book.

References

Arber, D.A., Orazi, A., Hasserjian, R., Thiele, J., Borowitz, M.J., Le Beau, M.M., ... Vardiman, J.W. (2016). The 2016 revision to the World Health Organization classification of myeloid neoplasms and acute leukemia. *Blood, 127*(20), 2391–2405. https://doi.org/10.1182/blood-2016-03-643544

Barbui, T., Finazzi, G., Carobbio, A., Thiele, J., Passamonti, F., Rumi, E., ... Tefferi, A. (2012). Development and validation of an international prognostic score of thrombosis in World Health Organization–essential thrombocythemia (IPSET-thrombosis). *Blood, 120*(26), 5128–5133. https://doi.org/10.1182/blood-2012-07-444067

Barbui, T.T., Thiele, J., Gisslinger, H., Finazzi, G., Vannucchi, A.M., & Tefferi, A. (2016). The 2016 revision of WHO classification of myeloproliferative neoplasms: Clinical and molecular advances. *Blood Reviews, 30*(6), 453–459. https://doi.org/10.1016/j.blre.2016.06.001

Cozzani, E., Iurlo, A., Merlo, G., Cattaneo, D., Burlando, M., Pierri, I., ... Parodi, A. (2015). Essential thrombocythemia: The dermatologic point of view. *Clinical Lymphoma, Myeloma and Leukemia, 15*(12), 739–747. https://doi.org/10.1016/j.clml.2015.08.086

Emanuel, R.M., Dueck, A.C., Geyer, H.L., Kiladjian, J.-J., Slot, S., Zweegman, S., ... Mesa, R.A. (2012). Myeloproliferative neoplasm (MPN) symptom assessment form total symptom score: Prospective international assessment of an abbreviated symptom burden scoring system among patients with MPNs. *Journal of Clinical Oncology, 30*(33), 4098–4103. https://doi.org/10.1200/JCO.2012.42.3863

Fowlkes, S., Murray, C., Fulford, A., De Gelder, T., & Siddiq, N. (2018). Myeloproliferative neoplasms (MPNs)—Part 2: A nursing guide to managing the symptom burden of MPNs. *Canadian Oncology Nursing Journal, 28*(4), 276–281. https://doi.org/10.5737/23688076284276281

Gisslinger, H., Jeryczynski, G., Gisslinger, B., Wölfler, A., Burgstaller, S., Buxhofer-Ausch, V., … Thiele, J. (2016). Clinical impact of bone marrow morphology for the diagnosis of essential thrombocythemia: Comparison between the BCSH and the WHO criteria. *Leukemia, 30*(5), 1126–1132. https://doi.org/10.1038/leu.2015.360

Haider, M., Gangat, N., Lasho, T., Abou Husseun, A., Elala, Y., Hanson, C., & Tefferi, A. (2016). Validation of the revised International Prognostic Score of Thrombosis for Essential Thrombocythemia (IPSET-thrombosis) in 585 Mayo Clinic patients. *American Journal of Hematology, 91*(4), 390–394. https://doi.org/10.1002/ajh.24293

Mesa, R., Miller, C.B., Thyne, M., Mangan, J., Goldberger, S., Fazal, S., … Mascarenhas, J.O. (2016) Myeloproliferative neoplasms (MPNs) have a significant impact on patients' overall health and productivity: The MPN landmark survey. *BMC Cancer, 16,* 167. https://doi.org/10.1186/s12885-016-2208-2

National Comprehensive Cancer Network. (2021). *NCCN Clinical Practice Guidelines in Oncology (NCCN Guidelines®): Myeloproliferative neoplasms* [v.2.2021]. https://www.nccn.org/professionals/physician_gls/pdf/mpn.pdf

Rumi, E., & Cazzola, M. (2016). How I treat essential thrombocythemia. *Blood, 128*(20), 2403–2414. https://doi.org/10.1182/blood-2016-05-643346

Rumi, E., & Cazzola, M. (2017). Diagnosis, risk stratification, and response evaluation in classical myeloproliferative neoplasm. *Blood, 129*(6), 680–692. https://doi.org/10.1182/blood-2016-10-695957

Swerdlow, S., Campo, E., Harris, N.L., Jaffe, E.S., Pileri, S.A., Stein, H., & Thiele, J. (Eds). (2017). *WHO classification of tumours of haematopoietic and lymphoid tissues* (4th ed.). International Agency for Research on Cancer.

Tefferi, A., & Barbui, T. (2021). Polycythemia vera and essential thrombocythemia: 2021 update on diagnosis, risk-stratification and management. *American Journal of Hematology, 95*(12), 1599–1613. https://doi.org/ 10.1002/ajh.26008

Tefferi, A., Vannucci, A.M., & Barbui, T. (2018). Essential thrombocythemia treatment algorithm 2018. *Blood Cancer Journal, 8,* 2. https://doi.org/10.1038/s41408-017-0041-8

Trifa, A., Cucuianu, A., & Popp, R.A. (2014). Familial essential thrombocythemia associated with *MPL* W515L mutation in father and *JAK2* V617F mutation in daughter. *Case Reports in Hematology, 2014,* 841787. https://doi.org/10.1155/2014/841787

CHAPTER 124

Immune Thrombocytopenia

Mailey Wilks, DNP, MSN, APRN, NP-C,

and Beth Faiman, PhD, MSN, APRN-BC, AOCN®, FAAN

I. Definition (Cooper & Ghanima, 2019; Lambert & Gernsheimer, 2017; Neunert & Cooper, 2018; Zainal et al., 2019)
   A. ITP is an immune-mediated disorder characterized by isolated thrombocytopenia and decreased platelet count (less than 100,000/mm³) with no obvious underlying cause. It can be acute, chronic, or acute on chronic in nature. Typically, normal production or overproduction of megakaryocytes occurs in the bone marrow.
   B. *Immune thrombocytopenia* was previously referred to as *idiopathic thrombocytopenia purpura*. *Immune thrombocytopenia* (ITP) continues to be used in medical practice, although it was changed to *primary immune thrombocytopenia* (IT) because of a better understanding of the immune-mediated mechanism of the disease.
   C. Corticosteroid-dependent immune thrombocytopenia is defined as the need for ongoing or repeated administration of corticosteroids to control platelet count less than 30,000/mm³.

II. Physiology/Pathophysiology (Audia et al., 2017; Cooper & Ghanima, 2019; Lambert & Gernsheimer, 2017; Marini & Bakchoul, 2019)
   A. Normal
      1. Platelets, or thrombocytes, develop in the bone marrow from megakaryocytes.
      2. Platelets function in hemostasis, initiating the clotting mechanisms in conjunction with numerous clotting factors in the blood.
   B. Pathophysiology: Decreased platelet count occurs from two main physiologic processes. Suboptimal plasma levels of endogenous thrombopoietin inhibit the repletion of platelets when there is inadequate levels of platelets.
      1. Platelets undergo premature destruction as a result of autoantibody or immune complex deposition on their membranes.
         a) The site of destruction is usually the reticuloendothelial system of the spleen or, less commonly, the liver.
         b) Platelets are coated with IgG antibodies (found in approximately 50%–60% of patients with ITP) and are recognized by tissue macrophage receptors and destroyed.
         c) Antibody production appears to be driven by cluster of differentiation 4–positive helper cells reacting to platelet surface glycoproteins.
      2. Suboptimal platelet production arises from megakaryocytes in the bone marrow.
      3. Secondary ITP is associated with another condition inducing platelet destruction.

III. Clinical features: Yearly incidence is 3.3 per 100,000 adults and is more common in older adults. Patients may be asymptomatic at presentation or present with mild mucocutaneous to life-threatening bleeding. Refractory ITP is the presence of severe ITP occurring after splenectomy. Diagnosis is by exclusion. The adult form is usually chronic (longer than 12 months) and seldom follows a viral infection. Long-term morbidity and mortality is from hemorrhage (Cooper & Ghanima, 2019; Marini & Bakchoul, 2019; Neunert & Cooper, 2018; Zainal et al., 2019).

A. Classification of ITP
   1. Acute: Less than three to six months, resolving spontaneously with incidence peaks in winter and spring or following a viral infection
   2. Persistent: 3–12 months
   3. Chronic: 6–12 months, requiring therapy and occurring most commonly in adults; may spontaneously improve
B. Etiology
   1. May occur in isolation (primary) or in association with other disorders (secondary)
   2. Secondary causes
      a) Antiphospholipid antibody syndrome
      b) Rheumatologic or autoimmune thrombocytopenia: Evans syndrome
      c) Infections: CMV, *Helicobacter pylori*, hepatitis C, HIV, VZV, Zika virus
      d) Drugs: Quinidine, quinine, sulfonamides, gold compounds, heparin, acetaminophen, naproxen, cimetidine
      e) Lymphoproliferative disorders
      f) Malignancies
      g) HSCT side effect
      h) Vaccination side effect
      i) SLE
      j) Pregnancy
      k) Chronic alcoholism
      l) Sepsis
C. History
   1. History of cancer and cancer treatment
   2. Current medications: Prescribed, over the counter, recent new medications, herbal supplements, recreational drug use
   3. History of presenting symptoms: Precipitating factors, onset, duration
   4. Changes in ADLs
   5. Past medical history: Prior transfusions with marked thrombocytopenia occurring 5–10 days after a routine RBC transfusion or the presence of antiplatelet antibody; prior infection; autoimmune history; recent immunization; recent trauma such as surgery; dental work; recent pregnancy; cirrhosis; sexual encounters; bleeding history
   6. Family history: Low platelets or easy bruising, autoimmune history
D. Signs and symptoms: Vary widely at presentation
   1. Presence of fevers, bone or joint pain
   2. Petechiae, wet purpura, and ecchymosis
   3. Potential for serious bleeding
      a) GI tract
      b) Intracranial hemorrhage
      c) Mucosal
      d) Menstrual
   4. Fatigue
E. Physical examination
   1. HEENT

       a) Oral cavity: Gingival bleeding/wet purpura
       b) Funduscopic: Retinal bleeding
    2. Lymph: Lymphadenopathy indicating infection (see Appendix D)
    3. Integument
       a) Nonpetechial rash
       b) Petechiae: Chest, arms, legs, back, especially in dependent regions
       c) Purpura and ecchymosis
    4. Abdominal: Splenomegaly, which strongly indicates ITP yet is not the cause of platelet destruction
    5. Neurologic: Confusion suggestive of CNS bleeding

IV. Diagnostic tests: No gold standard exists for diagnostic workup. Multiple tests are used for patient evaluation and are supported by the American Society of Hematology 2018 guidelines and "International Consensus Report on the Investigation and Management of Immune Thrombocytopenia" (Cooper & Ghanima, 2019; Neunert & Cooper, 2018; Umakanthan et al., 2019; Zainal et al., 2019).
  A. Laboratory
    1. CBC with differential
       a) Thrombocytopenia will be present.
       b) An abnormal WBC count is not typical in ITP and should prompt additional testing for other causes.
       c) Anemia from blood loss may be present.
    2. Peripheral blood smear
       a) It may demonstrate abnormalities that are not consistent with ITP, such as schistocytes, as in thrombotic thrombocytopenic purpura–hemolytic uremic syndrome (referred to as TTP-HUS).
       b) Excessive numbers of giant or small platelets may indicate inherited thrombocytopenia.
       c) Evaluate for pseudothrombocytopenia, a laboratory phenomenon caused by clumping of platelets and ethylenediaminetetraacetic acid, the preservative found in blood tubes.
       d) Large platelets are often noted. Absence of large platelets does not exclude diagnosis of IT.
    3. Ig testing: Low levels may reveal conditions such as common variable immunodeficiency or selective IgA deficiency.
    4. Bone marrow biopsy
       a) It is recommended if CBC or blood smear is abnormal.
       b) It is recommended if patient is older than 60 years and has systemic symptoms.
       c) Megakaryocytes usually are increased in size and are increased or normal in number.
       d) Flow cytometry may be particularly helpful in identifying patients with ITP secondary to chronic lymphocytic leukemia.
       e) When a patient does not respond to multiple lines of therapy or diagnosis is in question, bone marrow biopsy should be considered.
    5. HIV and Epstein-Barr virus testing, if indicated
    6. Screening for hepatitis C, which can cause low platelets
    7. *H. pylori* testing, if indicated
    8. Antiplatelet antibody test: Positive with autoantibodies against platelets
    9. Viral panel or influenza, if indicated
  B. Radiology: CT scan of head if patient is complaining of headaches/neurologic symptoms to assess for bleed

V. Differential diagnosis (Cooper & Ghanima, 2019; Zainal et al., 2019)
   A. Infection
      1. CMV
      2. *H. pylori* (see Chapter 78)
      3. Hepatitis C (see Chapter 74)
      4. HIV
      5. VZV (see Chapter 22)
      6. Zika virus
   B. Lymphoproliferative disorders
   C. Autoimmune/immunodeficiency disorders: SLE (see Chapter 110)
   D. Liver disease: Alcoholic liver cirrhosis (see Chapter 69)
   E. Drug induced or exposure to toxins: Chemotherapy, heparin, quinine, sulfonamides, gold compounds
   F. Bone marrow diseases: Myelodysplastic syndromes, leukemia
   G. Recent transfusions or immunizations
   H. Inherited thrombocytopenic disorders
   I. Antiphospholipid syndrome
   J. Chronic DIC (see Chapter 120)
   K. Aplastic anemia (see Chapter 114)

VI. Treatment (Audia et al., 2017; Cooper & Ghanima, 2019; Deshayes & Godeau, 2020; Dou & Yang, 2019; Lambert & Gernsheimer, 2017; Neunert & Cooper, 2018; Umakanthan et al., 2019; Witkowski et al., 2019; Worrest et al., 2019; Zainal et al., 2019)
   A. Primary goal is to achieve a platelet count that will prevent major bleeding and attain a sustained increase of the platelet count to be hemostatic for the individual patient.
   B. Factors on which to base treatment
      1. Presence and severity of bleeding
      2. How rapid platelet counts need to rise
      3. Other individual patient issues
         a) Bleeding risk based on previous bleeding episodes
         b) Comorbidities that predispose patient to bleeding, such as history of stroke and antiplatelet therapy
         c) Complications of specific therapies and tolerance of side effects
         d) Activity level and lifestyle
         e) Patient preference, expectations, and worries
   C. Pharmacologic measures: Platelet transfusions do not help raise platelet counts and should only be given if active bleeding is an issue.
      1. Acute
         a) Treat patients with a platelet count less than 30,000/mm³.
         b) First-line therapy with corticosteroids (e.g., dexamethasone, prednisone, solumedrol): Prednisone 1 mg/kg PO daily for two to four weeks with gradual taper, or dexamethasone 40 mg PO daily for four days with 10-day break, and repeated PRN (see Appendix K)
            (1) Longer courses of corticosteroids are preferred over shorter courses of corticosteroids or IVIg as first-line therapy.
            (2) IVIg can be used with corticosteroids when a more rapid increase in platelet count is required.
            (3) IVIg can be used as first-line therapy if corticosteroids are contraindicated.
            (4) If IVIg is used, the typical dose is 2 g/kg, typically given in divided doses (0.4 g/kg for five days, 1 g/kg for two days). IVIg is favored when ITP

is severe, when a rapid increase in platelet count is desired, or when an adequate response is not achieved with steroid therapy. Response should occur within 24–48 hours. Side effects may include hypotension, headache, and chills.

2. Chronic or refractory IT

   a) High-dose corticosteroids are given typically with dexamethasone 40 mg PO daily for four days every four weeks; other steroids have also been used, either IV or PO (see Appendix K).

   b) Splenectomy is considered for patients who have failed corticosteroid therapy.

   c) Thrombopoietin receptor agonist might be used for patients at risk for bleeding who relapse after splenectomy or have a contraindication to undergoing splenectomy.

      (1) Romiplostim: 1 mcg/kg subcutaneous weekly to maximum of 10 mcg weekly based on platelet count response

      (2) Eltrombopag: 50 mg PO once daily to a maximum dose of 75 mg; discontinued if platelet count does not respond to a level sufficient to avoid clinically important bleeding after four weeks of therapy

      (3) Avatrombopag: 20 mg PO daily

   d) Anti-Rh(D), a plasma-derived Ig, has been used successfully in managing ITP.

   e) Rituximab 375 mg/m² IV may be considered for patients at risk of bleeding who have failed corticosteroids, IVIg, or splenectomy. It can be repeated weekly for four doses.

   f) Immunosuppressive agents: Overall effectiveness of these drugs is variable, with short remissions achieved.

      (1) Cyclophosphamide: 1–2 mg/kg PO daily

      (2) Azathioprine: 1–4 mg/kg PO daily

      (3) Cyclosporin A: 5–6 mg/kg PO daily

   g) Fostamatinib is an orally bioavailable small molecule spleen TKI that leads to reduced antibody-mediated platelet destruction. Initial dose is 100 mg PO two times a day. Dose may be increased to 150 mg PO two times a day if platelets do not increase to at least 50,000/mm³ within the first month.

3. Secondary ITP, hepatitis C associated

   a) Antiviral therapy can be administered (see Chapter 74, Appendix J).

   b) Closely monitor platelet count because of risk of worsening thrombocytopenia attributable to IFN therapy.

   c) If treatment for ITP is required, initial treatment should be IVIg.

4. Secondary ITP, HIV related

   a) Treatment of the HIV infection with antiviral therapy should be considered before other treatments unless patient has significant bleeding complications.

   b) If treatment for ITP is required, initial treatment should consist of corticosteroids, IVIg, or anti-Rh(D) and splenectomy.

5. Secondary ITP, H. pylori associated: Eradication therapy should be administered (see Chapter 78).

D. Surgical therapy: Splenectomy usually is second-line therapy to reduce the destruction of antibody-sensitized platelets and to possibly reduce antibody production.

   1. Splenectomy should be delayed for at least 12 months unless patient has severe disease.

   2. It is recommended for adult patients who have failed corticosteroid therapy or having complications related to medication use.

   3. Both laparoscopic and open splenectomy offer similar efficacy.

4. Because of risk of septicemia, pneumococcal vaccine, *Haemophilus influenza* type B vaccine, and meningococcal polysaccharide vaccine should be administered at least two weeks before elective splenectomy.

E. Plasma exchange therapy with fresh frozen plasma as replacement fluid has been used to manage acute and chronic ITP.

F. Patient education

1. Restrict physical activity to minimize risk from trauma, particularly head injury.
2. Avoid drugs that impair platelet function, such as NSAIDs and ASA (see Appendix E).

VII. Follow-up

A. Perform ongoing monitoring of CBC to assess platelet count.

B. Consider retreatment if bleeding occurs with recurrent thrombocytopenia.

VIII. Referral: See hematologist for appropriate diagnostic workup and treatment plan. Patient will require close follow-up by hematology.

The authors would like to acknowledge Barbara Barnes Rogers, CRNP, MN, AOCN®, ANP-BC, for her contribution to this chapter that remains unchanged from the previous edition of this book.

References

Audia, S., Mahévas, M., Samson, M., Godeau, B., & Bonnotte, B. (2017). Pathogenesis of immune thrombocytopenia. *Autoimmunity Reviews, 16*(6), 620–632. https://doi.org/10.1016/j.autrev.2017.04.012

Cooper, N., & Ghanima, W. (2019). Immune thrombocytopenia. *New England Journal of Medicine, 381*(10), 945–955. https://doi.org/10.1056/NEJMcp1810479

Deshayes, S., & Godeau, B. (2020). Second-line and beyond: Treatment options for primary persistent and chronic immune thrombocytopenia. *Platelets, 30*(3), 291–299. https://doi.org/10.1080/09537104.2019.1636018

Dou, X., & Yang, R. (2019). Current and emerging treatments for immune thrombocytopenia. *Expert Review of Hematology, 12*(9), 723–732. https://doi.org/10.1080/17474086.2019.1636644

Lambert, M.P., & Gernsheimer, T.B. (2017). Clinical updates in adult immune thrombocytopenia. *Blood, 129*(21), 2829–2835. https://doi.org/10.1182/blood-2017-03-754119

Marini, I., & Bakchoul, T. (2019). Pathophysiology of autoimmune thrombocytopenia: Current insight with a focus on thrombopoiesis. *Hämostaseologie, 39*(3), 227–237. https://doi.org/10.1055/s-0039-1678732

Neunert, C.E., & Cooper, N. (2018). Evidence-based management of immune thrombocytopenia: ASH guideline update. *Hematology: American Society of Hematology Education Program Book, 2018,* 568–575. https://doi.org/10.1182/asheducation-2018.1.568

Umakanthan, J.M., Dhakal, P., Gundabolu, K., Kallam, A., Almquist, D.R., & Bhatt, V.R. (2019). Initial management of immune thrombocytopenia in adults based on risk stratification. *Postgraduate Medical Journal, 95*(1128), 558–562. https://doi.org/10.1136/postgradmedj-2019-136636

Witkowski, M., Witkowska, M., & Robak, T. (2019). Autoimmune thrombocytopenia: Current treatment options in adults with a focus on novel drugs. *European Journal of Haematology, 103*(6), 531–541. https://doi.org/10.1111/ejh.13319

Worrest, T., Cunningham, A., Dewey, E., Delougherty, T.G., Gilbert, E., Sheppard, B.C., & Fischer, L.E. (2019). Immune thrombocytopenic purpura splenectomy in the context of new medical therapies. *Journal of Surgical Research, 245,* 643–648. https://doi.org/10.1016/j.jss.2019.06.092

Zainal, A., Salama, A., & Alweis, R. (2019). Immune thrombocytopenia purpura. *Journal of Community Hospital Internal Medicine Perspectives, 9*(1), 59–61. https://doi.org/10.1080/20009666.2019.1565884

CHAPTER 125

Leukocytosis

Heather T. Mackey, MSN, RN, ANP-BC, AOCN®

I. Definition: A condition exhibited by the elevation of WBC count in excess of 11,000/mm³ in nonpregnant adults of one or more subsets of circulating WBCs (Flanagan et al., 2019; Korkmaz, 2018; Riley & Ruppert, 2015)

II. Physiology/Pathophysiology (Berliner, 2020; Chabot-Richards & George, 2014; Riley & Ruppert, 2015; Widick & Winer, 2016)
   A. Normal
      1. The two main types of leukocytes are granulocytes and agranulocytes.
      2. Granulocytes include neutrophils, basophils, and eosinophils.
         a) Neutrophils attach to and destroy bacteria and viruses in the circulating blood.
         b) Eosinophils contain toxic granules that participate in repeated and persistent tissue inflammatory response.
         c) Basophils release histamine, heparin, bradykinin, and serotonin into circulation to mediate the inflammatory response.
      3. Agranulocytes include lymphocytes and monocytes.
         a) Lymphocytes enter the circulatory system continually, along with the drainage of lymph from the lymph nodes. They differentiate into T and B lymphocytes and natural killer cells.
            (1) T lymphocytes perform cell-mediated immunity with the aid of memory cells (remember the antigen), killer cells (destroy the antigen), helper cells (activate humoral immunity), and suppressor cells (inhibit the immune response).
            (2) B lymphocytes perform humoral immunity. Upon activation, B cells secrete plasma cells which, in turn, produce antibodies. These antibodies (Igs) have the ability to bind to surface receptors on antigens, either neutralizing the antigen or activating additional components of the immune system such as complement.
            (3) Natural killer cells kill cancer cells and prevent development of autoimmune disease.
         b) Monocytes (macrophages) are very effective in removing cellular debris. They play a role in adaptive immunity responses.
   B. Pathophysiology
      1. Alterations can occur genetically with the production of abnormal Igs or cellular alterations.
      2. A secondary response to a disease or toxin, such as infection or hemorrhage, can cause WBC overproduction.

III. Clinical features: Leukocytosis is one of the most common laboratory abnormalities in medicine and one of the most frequent reasons for hematologic consultation. It is most commonly reactive and a result of nonhematologic disorders (Berliner, 2020; Chabot-Richards & George, 2014; Flanagan et al., 2019; Korkmaz, 2018; Lynch et al., 2018; Riley & Ruppert, 2015; Widick & Winer, 2016).

A. Etiology

1. Lymphocytosis can occur from lymphoproliferative disease, lymphoma, hairy cell leukemia, chronic lymphocytic leukemia, thymoma, or genetic alterations. It can commonly be present in the general population as monoclonal B-cell lymphocytosis.

2. Neutrophilia can be indicative of Down syndrome, infection, chronic inflammation, congenital neutropenia syndromes, MI, myeloproliferative neoplasms, smoking, or stress. It can also be drug induced.

3. Eosinophilia is most commonly due to secondary causes such as from allergic conditions, parasitic infections, malignancies, or immune disorders (e.g., Sjögren syndrome), as well as a result of certain medications.

4. Basophilia can occur from an inflammatory response, from a hypersensitivity reaction to drugs or food, or in association with chronic myeloid leukemia.

5. Monocytosis is associated with certain myeloproliferative neoplasms (e.g., chronic myeloid leukemia), acute myelomonocytic leukemia, lymphoma, solid tumors, autoimmune disease (e.g., SLE), or chronic infections with enhanced T-lymphocyte activity (e.g., TB, syphilis).

B. History

1. History of cancer and cancer treatment

2. Current medications: Prescribed, over the counter, herbal products

3. History of presenting symptoms: Precipitating factors, onset, location, duration, associated symptoms (e.g., fevers, sweats, weight loss)

4. Changes in ADLs

5. Past medical history: Chronic conditions (e.g., ulcerative colitis, arthritis, vasculitis), CAD, frequent infections

6. Social history: Travel history, smoking, stress

C. Signs and symptoms: Dependent on etiology

1. Fever
2. Chills
3. Rash
4. Fatigue
5. Sore throat
6. Night sweats
7. Weight loss
8. Cough
9. Myalgias
10. Rhinitis
11. Abdominal discomfort
12. Lymphadenopathy

D. Physical examination

1. Vital signs: Fever

2. HEENT: Oral cavity assessment for erythema of throat; oral mucosa observation for petechial rash on palate, enlarged tonsils, and presence of exudates

3. Abdominal: Hepatomegaly, splenomegaly

4. Lymph: Lymphadenopathy (see Appendix D)

IV. Diagnostic tests (Berliner, 2020; Chabot-Richards & George, 2014; Flanagan et al., 2019; Lynch et al., 2018; Malek & Chen, 2019; Riley & Ruppert, 2015; Widick & Winer, 2016)

    A. Laboratory

        1. CBC with differential: WBC and subset will be elevated; anemia or thrombocytopenia may be present in leukemia conditions.

        2. Peripheral smear

            a) Confirm automated counts and rule out spurious leukocytosis.

            b) Evaluate for blasts and dysplastic cells.

            c) Increased bands, vacuolation, Döhle bodies, or toxic granulations in neutrophils indicate infection or inflammation.

            d) Review of smear can confirm basophilia or monocytosis.

            e) In lymphocytosis, look for evidence of reactive lymphocytosis associated with infection, large granular lymphocytes associated with large granular lymphocytic leukemia, smudge cells associated with chronic lymphocytic leukemia, or blasts associated with acute leukemia.

        3. Viral titers: HIV, Epstein-Barr virus, hepatitis, CMV, influenza

        4. Peripheral blood for flow cytometry for characterizing lymphocytes

        5. Fluorescence in situ hybridization or cytogenetics to rule out chronic myeloid leukemia

        6. LDH: Elevated in hemolytic anemia and possibly in lymphoma

        7. Antinuclear antibody and rheumatoid factor, if indicated

        8. Uric acid: Elevated in gout

        9. Bone marrow biopsy if leukemia suspected

        10. In eosinophilia

            a) Stool for ova and parasites, culture

            b) Vitamin B_{12}, serum tryptase, and IgE level

        11. *JAK2* testing if myeloproliferative disease suspected

        12. Blood, wound, and urine cultures, as appropriate

    B. Radiology

        1. Chest x-ray to evaluate for pneumonia

        2. CT scan of the chest, abdomen, and pelvis if lymphadenopathy noted

V. Differential diagnosis: Increases in absolute numbers of lymphocytes, eosinophils, monocytes, or basophils are less common than neutrophilia, and this distinction directs the differential (Berliner, 2020; Chabot-Richards & George, 2014; Flanagan et al., 2019; Lynch et al., 2018; Riley & Ruppert, 2015; Widick & Winer, 2016).

    A. Leukocytosis

        1. Infection

        2. Burns

        3. Inflammation due to arthritis, infarction, or tissue necrosis

        4. Stress: Overexertion, anxiety (see Chapter 161), seizures (see Chapter 144)

        5. Trauma: Splenectomy, hemolytic anemia

        6. Drugs: Corticosteroids, lithium, beta-agonists, colony-stimulating factors, epinephrine

        7. Leukemia or myeloproliferative neoplasm

    B. Neutrophilia

        1. False reading with pseudothrombocytopenia or in the presence of cryoglobulins

        2. Hereditary: Neutrophilia

        3. Familial syndromes

    4. Myeloproliferative neoplasm: Chronic myeloid leukemia, polycythemia vera, primary myelofibrosis

    5. Leukocyte adhesion deficiency

    6. Infection

    7. Tobacco use

    8. Chronic inflammation: RA (see Chapter 108), inflammatory bowel disease

    9. Stress

    10. Exercise

    11. Medications: G-CSF; glucocorticoids, beta-agonists, lithium

C. Eosinophilia

    1. Myeloid and lymphoid neoplasms

    2. Chronic eosinophilic leukemia

    3. Idiopathic hypereosinophilic syndrome

    4. Medications: Allopurinol, antiepileptic agents (e.g., carbamazepine, phenytoin), antibiotics (e.g., sulfa, dapsone, vancomycin)

    5. Parasitic infections

D. Lymphocytosis

    1. Leukemia

    2. Other malignancies: Thymoma

    3. Infection: Epstein-Barr virus, CMV, HSV, HIV, rubella, *Toxoplasma*, adenovirus, VZV, human herpesvirus, *Bordetella bronchiseptica*

    4. Stress lymphocytosis: Surgery, MI, septic shock, sickle cell crisis

    5. Hypersensitivity reactions: Insect bites and drugs

    6. Tobacco use

VI. Treatment (Berliner, 2020; Flanagan et al., 2019; Korkmaz, 2018; Ruggiero et al., 2016)

    A. Treat underlying etiology.

    B. Treat infection with appropriate medication, such as antibiotics, antivirals, and antifungals (see Appendices C and J).

    C. For patients with extremely high WBC counts (i.e., hyperleukocytosis), especially when accompanied by neurologic or respiratory symptoms, leukapheresis may be an option as well as hydration, allopurinol, or urate oxidase to prevent tumor lysis.

VII. Follow-up

    A. Monitor blood counts as indicated.

    B. Monitor response to therapy.

VIII. Referral

    A. Specialists: As indicated for management of disorders

    B. Hematology/oncology: For acute leukemia management

The author would like to acknowledge Barbara Barnes Rogers, CRNP, MN, AOCN®, ANP-BC, for her contribution to this chapter that remains unchanged from the previous edition of this book.

References

Berliner, N. (2020). Leukocytosis and leukopenia. In L. Goldman & A.I. Schafer (Eds.), *Goldman-Cecil medicine* (26th ed., pp. 1094–1103). Elsevier.

Chabot-Richards, D.S., & George, T.I. (2014). Leukocytosis. *International Journal of Laboratory Hematology, 36*(3), 279–288. https://doi.org/10.1111/ijlh.12212

Flanagan, B., Keber, B., Mumford, J., & Lam, L. (2019). Hematologic conditions: Leukocytosis and leukemia. *FP Essentials, 485,* 17–23.

Korkmaz, S. (2018). The management of hyperleukocytosis in 2017: Do we still need leukapheresis? *Transfusion and Apheresis Science, 57*(1), 4–7. https://doi.org/10.1016/j.transci.2018.02.006

Lynch, D.T., Hall, J., & Foucar, K., (2018). How I investigate monocytosis. *International Journal of Laboratory Hematology, 40*(2), 107–114. https://doi.org/10.1111/ijlh.12776

Malek, T., & Chen, L. (2019). Spurious laboratory values in patients with leukocytosis. *Critical Care Nursing Quarterly, 42*(1), 44–46. https://doi.org/10.1097/CNQ.0000000000000236

Riley, L.K., & Ruppert, J. (2015). Evaluation of patients with leukocytosis. *American Family Physician, 92*(11), 1004–1011. https://www.aafp.org/afp/2015/1201/p1004.html

Ruggiero, A., Rizzo, D., Amato, M., & Riccardi, R. (2016). Management of hyperleukocytosis. *Current Treatment Options in Oncology, 17,* 7. https://doi.org/10.1007/s11864-015-0387-8

Widick, P., & Winer, E. (2016). Leukocytosis and leukemia. *Primary Care: Clinics in Office Practice, 43*(4), 575–587. https://doi.org/10.1016/j.pop.2016.07.007

CHAPTER 126

Monoclonal Gammopathy of Undetermined Significance

Beth Faiman, PhD, MSN, APRN-BC, AOCN®, FAAN

I. Definition (Atkin et al., 2018; Khouri et al., 2019; Mouhieddine et al., 2019; Rajkumar et al., 2014)
  A. Monoclonal gammopathies (paraproteinemias or dysproteinemias) are a group of disorders characterized by the overproliferation of a single clone of plasma cells.
  B. They are defined by the presence of a serum monoclonal protein (M protein) at a concentration less than 3 g/dl and bone marrow with less than 10% monoclonal plasma cells in the absence of end-organ damage (e.g., hypercalcemia, renal insufficiency, anemia, bone lesions) that can be attributed to the plasma cell proliferative disorder.
  C. MGUS is a clinically asymptomatic, premalignant clonal plasma cell or lymphoplasmacytic proliferative disorder.

II. Physiology/Pathophysiology (Faiman et al., 2018; Mouhieddine et al., 2019)
  A. Normal
    1. When the immune system is challenged by a foreign substance (antigen), the activated B lymphocytes differentiate into plasma cells. The plasma cells then produce Igs, which are Y-shaped proteins with identical antigen-binding sites on each arm of the "Y." Antigenic stimulation leading to antibody formation is critical to a normal immune response.
    2. The Y-shaped structure of an intact Ig is composed of a light-chain amino acid covalently linked to a heavy-chain amino acid. An M protein is comprised of two heavy and two light chains (a clone of a normal protein).
    3. The light and heavy determinations are based on the number of amino acids in each chain. The heavy chain has more amino acids than the light chain; therefore, it is longer and has a higher molecular weight than the light chain.
      a) Both chains have a variable region and a constant region. The variable region contains the antigen-binding site.
      b) Igs have identical constant regions in their heavy chains, which determine the class.
    4. Five classes of Igs exist: IgA, IgG, IgM, IgE, and IgD.
  B. Pathophysiology
    1. Monoclonal gammopathies produce an immunologically homogeneous protein commonly referred to as *paraprotein* or *monoclonal protein* (M protein) in the serum or urine in people without evidence of multiple myeloma, Waldenström macroglobulinemia, amyloidosis, or other myeloproliferative diseases.

2. An M protein is a monoclonal Ig secreted by an abnormally expanded clone of plasma cells in an amount that can be detected by immunofixation or by the serum-free light-chain assay.

3. A protein can be produced that is malignant and associated with disease infiltrating bone, lymph nodes, liver, spleen, or other organs (e.g., multiple myeloma, solitary plasmacytoma, Waldenström macroglobulinemia).

4. Polyclonal gammopathy is the presence of a broad-based peak or band most often due to an infectious, inflammatory, or reactive process.

5. IgA or IgG M proteins (rarely IgE or IgD) most commonly are associated with a monoclonal proliferation of plasma cells in the bone marrow.

III. Clinical features: MGUS is often found incidentally during comprehensive evaluation of peripheral neuropathy, unexplained anemia or kidney disease, or if an elevated total protein is present in serum or urine. MGUS represents two-thirds of all plasma cell dyscrasias. The incidence increases with age. MGUS is present in roughly 3%–4% of the general population aged older than 50 years and is considered for most to be a benign condition. In the majority of patients, M proteins are never associated with complications or evolution to malignancy (Amaador et al., 2019; Atkin et al., 2018; González-Calle & Mateos, 2018; Khouri et al., 2019; Landgren et al., 2017; Mouhieddine et al., 2019; Pascual-Goñi et al., 2019; Rajkumar et al., 2014).

A. Classifications: Broad range of diseases that vary in severity by disease entity

1. IgG or IgA monoclonal gammopathy can progress to multiple myeloma, primary amyloidosis, or smoldering myeloma. Patients with small fiber polyneuropathy may have a paraprotein associated neuropathy.

2. IgM gammopathy can progress to Waldenström macroglobulinemia, lymphoma, and (rarely) multiple myeloma.

3. Light-chain MGUS (kappa or lambda) is characterized by an increase in serum-free light chains or urine Bence Jones proteins. Patients with light-chain MGUS rarely have an overproduction of an intact paraprotein detected on SPEP (e.g., IgG kappa, IgA lambda).

4. Monoclonal gammopathy of renal significance is an entity in which the B-cell clone causes kidney damage. The plasma cell clone must be treated to prevent further renal damage.

5. Three distinct types of MGUS
   a) Non-IgM MGUS
   b) IgM MGUS
   c) Light-chain MGUS

B. Risk factors: Chronic antigen stimulation, often due to illness, pesticide exposure, and obesity, has been associated with increased risk of MGUS.

C. Etiology

1. Etiology is associated with several nonmalignant disorders, some of which are rare, and with autoimmune disorders (e.g., SLE, IT).

2. Prevalence remains about twice as high among African Americans and in obese individuals despite age group.

3. Patients with malignant lymphoproliferative disorders, such as lymphoma, can have a coexisting MGUS.

D. History

1. History of cancer and cancer treatment

2. Current medications: Prescribed, over the counter

3. History of presenting symptoms: Precipitating factors, onset, duration, associated symptoms indicative of multiple myeloma, amyloidosis, or Waldenström macro-

globulinemia (e.g., bone pain, recent infections, weight loss, fever, night sweats, changes in urination, foamy urine)
4. Changes in ADLs
5. Social history: Exposure to Agent Orange, occupational exposure to pesticides or chemicals
E. Signs and symptoms
   1. Patients with MGUS should exhibit no symptoms.
   2. If symptoms are exhibited, such as with bone pain or anemia, patients either have another plasma cell disorder or another underlying unrelated disease.
F. Physical examination: Typically, normal findings in MGUS
   1. HEENT
      a) Possible macroglossia present in amyloidosis
      b) Possible periorbital ecchymosis present in amyloidosis
   2. Abdominal: Hepatomegaly or splenomegaly, which can be present in lymphoma, POEMS syndrome (polyneuropathy, organomegaly, endocrinopathy, monoclonal gammopathy, skin changes), and other disorders that may have an underlying M protein
   3. Extremities: Edema present with CHF in cardiac or renal amyloidosis in patients with low serum albumin, often due to renal glomerular damage and excess loss of protein in urine
   4. Posterior thorax: Percussion tenderness of spine, joints, or sternum suggestive of possible multiple myeloma

IV. Diagnostic tests (Amaador et al., 2019; Kurtin et al., 2016; NCCN, 2021; Rajkumar et al., 2014)
A. Laboratory
   1. CBC with differential and platelets: Typically, this is normal in MGUS. Anemia can be present in multiple myeloma or monoclonal gammopathy of renal significance.
   2. Peripheral smear: This is usually normal. Rouleaux formation occurs when RBCs take on the appearance of a stack of coins in diluted suspensions of blood. It is often associated with high serum paraprotein levels and a diagnosis of multiple myeloma.
   3. Comprehensive metabolic panel: Elevated total protein can be noted in MGUS but is not diagnostic of myeloma. BUN, serum creatinine, electrolytes, calcium, and albumin are typically normal.
      a) Patients with amyloidosis may demonstrate renal insufficiency or hypoalbuminemia reflective of nephrotic syndrome.
      b) Patients with multiple myeloma may have abnormal renal function secondary to cast neuropathy.
   4. Beta-2 microglobulin is often normal in MGUS and elevated in multiple myeloma. It is a nonspecific marker of inflammation and is often elevated in CKD or acute infection.
   5. SPEP shows a spike that is commonly referred to as the *monoclonal spike* or *M spike.*
      a) After a spike has been recognized on SPEP, immunofixation must be performed to determine the type of M protein causing a spike in the patient's peripheral blood.
      b) A monoclonal spike is seen as a discrete band that usually migrates to the gamma (IgG or IgM) or beta region (usually IgA) of the electrophoresis.
      c) The presence of two M proteins (biclonal gammopathy) occurs in 8%–9% of cases.

6. Immunofixation
   a) This determines the type of M protein.
   b) It may be performed when a B-cell or plasma cell neoplasm is suspected but no monoclonal spike is apparent. This is frequently the case in amyloidosis or non-secretory multiple myeloma.
7. 24-hour urine collection for urine protein electrophoresis with monoclonal spike and immunofixation
   a) Both heavy and light chains may be excreted in serum; however, only monoclonal light chains are common in the urine.
   b) Traditionally, the excretion of light chains in the urine has been referred to as Bence-Jones proteinuria.
   c) The presence of Bence-Jones proteinuria alone does not indicate a diagnosis of multiple myeloma. It can occur in up to 30% of patients with MGUS.
   d) If patients have measurable monoclonal Igs in the serum, or if multiple myeloma or amyloidosis is suspected, a 24-hour urine collection should be performed to quantify the amount of total protein excreted, as well as the amount of M protein excretion.
   e) Patients with a pattern of nonselective proteinuria (i.e., albumin predominance) are more likely to have amyloidosis with kidney involvement.
   f) Nephrotic-range proteinuria (greater than 4 g/24 hrs of total protein) occurs in a variety of disorders, including multiple myeloma and renal amyloidosis.
8. Quantitative Igs
   a) This may determine the serum concentration of the M protein affected.
   b) It can detect a decrease in uninvolved immunoglobulins in smoldering myeloma or multiple myeloma.
      (1) Not as useful when the concentration of the M protein is low
      (2) Should not compare quantitative Ig results with SPEP because of the inherent technical differences in the techniques
      (3) Serum concentration of IgG: May be falsely elevated with IV administration
9. Hepatitis panel to evaluate for hepatitis C, which has been associated with Waldenström macroglobulinemia
10. Serum viscosity
    a) It should be performed in any patient with a monoclonal gammopathy and signs and symptoms suggesting the hyperviscosity syndrome found in Waldenström macroglobulinemia or multiple myeloma, such as confusion or mental status changes.
    b) Normal value is 1.5 cP (centipoise).
11. Myelin-associated glycoprotein antibody: Expensive and only indicated if a patient has an IgM paraprotein and progressive polyneuropathy
12. Tests for polyclonal gammopathy may include rheumatoid factor, antinuclear factors, and other autoantibodies. In addition, tests for infectious and inflammatory disease may be needed.
13. HIV testing in patients with non-neoplastic or neoplastic plasma cell disorders
14. The presence of M protein may interfere with other laboratory tests that are performed on liquid-based automated analyzers. This occurs either by precipitating during the analysis of the test or because of the specific binding properties. Tests that can be affected by the presence of M protein include the following.
    a) HDL, LDL, and cholesterol decreased
    b) Bilirubin elevated

        c) Altered measurement of inorganic phosphate—elevated or decreased

        d) CRP increased

        e) Antistreptolysin-O increased

        f) Creatinine decreased or elevated; BUN decreased

        g) Glucose decreased

        h) Sodium, chloride, and bicarbonate decreased

        i) Iron elevated

        j) Inorganic calcium elevated

        k) Albumin decreased

    15. Bone marrow aspirate/biopsy to evaluates the amount of clonal plasma cell infiltration; should be performed if high suspicion of multiple myeloma, monoclonal gammopathy of renal significance, amyloidosis, lymphoma, or Waldenström macroglobulinemia

  B. Radiology

    1. Skeletal survey to evaluate for lytic lesions in asymptomatic patients

    2. CT scan of the chest, abdomen, and pelvis to exclude organomegaly and bulky lymphadenopathy with IgM MGUS

V. Differential diagnosis (Khouri et al., 2019; Rajkumar et al., 2014)

  A. IgM type

    1. IgM MGUS

    2. Smoldering Waldenström macroglobulinemia

    3. Waldenström macroglobulinemia

    4. Other: Lymphoma and IgM multiple myeloma

  B. Non-IgM type: IgG, IgA kappa, IgA lambda

    1. Non-IgM MGUS: May be biclonal

    2. Smoldering multiple myeloma

    3. Multiple myeloma

    4. Plasma cell leukemia

  C. Amyloidosis

  D. Miscellaneous monoclonal gammopathy–associated conditions

    1. Osteosclerotic multiple myeloma with peripheral neuropathy (POEMS syndrome)

    2. Cryoglobulinemia type I

    3. Peripheral neuropathy–associated MGUS (see Chapter 143)

    4. Fanconi syndrome

    5. Castleman disease

    6. Scleromyxedema

    7. Necrobiotic xanthogranuloma

    8. Systemic capillary leak syndrome (see Chapter 35)

    9. Angioimmunoblastic lymphadenopathy with M protein

    10. SLE (see Chapter 110)

    11. IT (see Chapter 124)

VI. Treatment: No therapy is needed for MGUS; however, if M protein is due to alternate diagnosis, treat underlying cause (Amaador et al., 2019; Atkin et al., 2018; González-Calle & Mateos, 2018).

  A. Nonpharmacologic measures to manage the increased risk for fracture, osteoporosis, renal disease, infection, and DVT

    1. Management of bone fractures (see Chapter 102)

    2. Monitoring for DVT (see Chapter 43)

  3. Assessment for osteoporosis (see Chapter 106), calcium with vitamin D supplementation
  B. Pharmacologic measures: Not recommended

VII. Follow-up (Atkin et al., 2018; González-Calle & Mateos, 2018; Khouri et al., 2019; Landgren et al., 2017; Mouhieddine et al., 2019)
  A. Monitor for signs of progression to myeloma by monitoring monoclonal gammopathy.
  B. Patients with low-risk MGUS should be monitored with SPEP in six months, and if stable, can be followed every two to three years or if symptoms arise.
  C. Patients with intermediate- or high-risk MGUS
    1. SPEP in six months and then annually for life
    2. CBC in six months and then annually for life

VIII. Referrals
  A. Alternate specialists: If cause of gammopathy is due to nonmalignant cause
  B. Neurologist/hematologist: For patients with polyneuropathy and IgM MGUS to test for antimyelin-associated glycoprotein, which may be related to the clonal paraprotein

The author would like to acknowledge Barbara Barnes Rogers, CRNP, MN, AOCN®, ANP-BC, for her contribution to this chapter that remains unchanged from the previous edition of this book.

References

Amaador, K., Peeters, H., Minnema, M.C., Nguyen, T.Q., Dendooven, A., Vos, J.M.I., ... Abrahams, A. (2019). Monoclonal gammopathy of renal significance (MGRS): Histopathologic classification, diagnostic workup, and therapeutic options. *Netherlands Journal of Medicine, 77*(7), 243–254. http://www.njmonline.nl/article.php?a=2137&d=1405&i=228

Atkin, C., Richter, A., & Sapey, E. (2018). What is the significance of monoclonal gammopathy of undetermined significance? *Clinical Medicine, 18*(5), 391–396. https://doi.org/10.7861/clinmedicine.18-5-391

Faiman, B., Richards, T., & Tariman, J.D. (2018). Multiple myeloma. In C.H. Yarbro, D. Wujcik, & B.H. Gobel (Eds.), *Cancer nursing: Principles and practice* (8th ed., pp. 1753–1791). Jones and Bartlett Learning.

González-Calle, V., & Mateos, M.V. (2018). Monoclonal gammopathies of unknown significance and smoldering myeloma: Assessment and management of the elderly patients. *European Journal of Internal Medicine, 58,* 57–63. https://doi.org/10.1016/j.ejim.2018.05.029

Khouri, J., Samaras, C., Valent, J., Mejia Garcia, A., Faiman, B., Mathur, S., ... Kalaycio, M. (2019). Monoclonal gammopathy of undetermined significance: A primary care guide. *Cleveland Clinic Journal of Medicine, 86*(1), 39–46. https://doi.org/10.3949/ccjm.86a.17133

Kurtin, S., Bertolotti, P., Brigle, K., & Vernia, D. (2016). Updates in the diagnosis and monitoring of multiple myeloma. *Journal of the Advanced Practitioner in Oncology, 7*(Suppl. 2), 59–70. https://doi.org/10.6004/jadpro.2016.7.2.15

Landgren, O., Graubard, B.I., Kumar, S., Kyle, R.A., Katzmann, J.A., Murata, K., ... Rajkumar, S.V. (2017). Prevalence of myeloma precursor state monoclonal gammopathy of undetermined significance in 12372 individuals 10–49 years old: A population-based study from the National Health and Nutrition Examination Survey. *Blood Cancer Journal, 7*(10), e618. https://doi.org/10.1038/bcj.2017.97

Mouhieddine, T.H., Weeks, L.D., & Ghobrial, I.M. (2019). Monoclonal gammopathy of undetermined significance. *Blood, 133*(23), 2484–2494. https://doi.org/10.1182/blood.2019846782

National Comprehensive Cancer Network. (2021). *NCCN Clinical Practice Guidelines in Oncology (NCCN Guidelines®): Multiple myeloma* [v.1.2022]. https://www.nccn.org/professionals/physician_gls/pdf/myeloma.pdf

Pascual-Goñi, E., Martín-Aguilar, L., Lleixà, C., Martínez-Martínez, L., Simón-Talero, M.J., Díaz-Manera, J., ... Querol, L. (2019). Clinical and laboratory features of anti-MAG neuropathy without monoclonal gammopathy. *Scientific Reports, 9*(1), 6155. https://doi.org/10.1038/s41598-019-42545-8

Rajkumar, S.V., Dimopoulos, M.A., Palumbo, A., Blade, J., Merlini, G., Mateos, M.-V., ... San Miguel, J.F. (2014). International Myeloma Working Group updated criteria for the diagnosis of multiple myeloma. *Lancet Oncology, 15*(12), e538–e548. https://doi.org/10.1016/s1470-2045(14)70442-5

CHAPTER 127

Neutropenia

Christina Ferraro, MSN, APRN-CNP, BMTCN®

I. Definition (Afzal et al., 2017; NCCN, 2021a, 2021b)
   A. A significant reduction in the absolute number of circulating neutrophils in the blood; usually defined as an ANC less than 1,500/mm³
   B. Neutropenia is classified and defined by levels.
      1. Mild: ANC is less than 1,500/mm³.
      2. Moderate: ANC equals 1,000–500/mm³.
      3. Severe: ANC is less than 500/mm³.
   C. Chronic neutropenia: Neutropenia lasting longer than three months

II. Physiology/Pathophysiology (Afzal et al., 2017; NCCN, 2021a, 2021b)
   A. Normal
      1. Neutrophils are produced from the myeloid stem cell. Eosinophils, basophils, and monocytes arise from the same stem cell. Collectively, they are called *granulocytes.*
      2. Lymphoid stem cells produce T lymphocytes and B lymphocytes, which are responsible for specific, cell-mediated immunity and humoral immunity, respectively.
      3. The primary role of granulocytes is to ingest and destroy microorganisms and release chemical mediators that enhance and prolong the inflammatory response.
      4. The normal range for WBC count is 4,000–10,000/mm³. Five percent of the normal population may fall outside the normal reference range.
      5. Neutrophils make up 50%–60% of all circulating WBCs and are vital in the non-specific immune response.
   B. Pathophysiology: Decrease of neutrophils impairs nonspecific immunity.
      1. Decreased production of neutrophils from bone marrow
      2. Ineffective granulopoiesis
      3. Increased margination of neutrophils to peripheral pools
      4. Increased peripheral destruction of neutrophils by circulating antibodies

III. Clinical features: Neutropenia is a common reason for hematology consult in the inpatient and outpatient settings. Neutropenia varies in severity, with more profound neutropenia being associated with higher rates of infections and infection-related deaths. Risk of infection increases when ANC is less than 1,000/mm³ (Afzal et al., 2017; Lalami & Klastersky, 2017; Lehrnbecher et al., 2017; NCCN, 2021a, 2021b; O'Brien et al., 2014; Smith et al., 2015).
   A. Risk factors
      1. Treatment related

    a) Previous chemotherapy
    b) Planned relative dose intensity of chemotherapy
    c) Concurrent or prior irradiation of bone marrow
    d) Preexisting neutropenia
    e) Multimodal treatment
2. Comorbidities
    a) COPD
    b) Cardiovascular disease
    c) Liver disease
    d) Renal insufficiency
    e) Diabetes mellitus
3. Patient related
    a) Age older than 65 years
    b) Female
    c) Poor performance status
    d) Poor nutritional status
    e) Decreased immune function
    f) Decreased body surface area
4. Cancer related
    a) Bone marrow involvement of tumor
    b) Advanced cancer
    c) Type of malignancy: Leukemia, lymphoma, myelodysplastic syndrome, lung cancer
5. High- and low-risk patients with fever and neutropenia
    a) High risk
        (1) Anticipated prolonged (longer than seven days) duration of neutropenia
        (2) Profound neutropenia: ANC less than or equal to 100/mm^3
        (3) Significant medical comorbid conditions: Hypotension, pneumonia, new-onset abdominal pain, neurologic changes
        (4) Alteration in physical barriers: Oral mucosa, skin
    b) Low risk
        (1) Anticipated brief (fewer than seven days) neutropenic period
        (2) No or few comorbidities and no history of fungal infection
        (3) Age younger than 60 years, asymptomatic or mild to moderate symptoms, and stable vital signs

B. Etiology
1. Bacterial infection: Noted in the earlier phases of neutropenia
2. Fungal infection: Generally seen in patients with severe and prolonged neutropenia and in those receiving multiple courses of broad-spectrum antibiotics
3. Viral and parasitic infection
4. Certain drugs have a higher risk of causing neutropenia.
    a) Drug and toxin exposure usually follows a temporal course.
    b) Mechanisms of drug-induced neutropenia include the following.
        (1) Antibody mediated
        (2) Direct toxic effect on marrow

C. History
1. History of cancer and cancer treatment
2. Current medications: Prescribed, over the counter, herbal products
3. History of presenting symptoms: Precipitating factors, onset, duration

    4. Changes in ADLs

    5. Past medical history: TB exposure, comorbid illnesses, history of prior infections, HIV status, recurrent episodes of neutropenia

    6. Social history: Tobacco use, alcohol use, recent travel, exposure to people with illness, occupational exposure to toxic agents

    7. Family history: Recent infections, unexplained sudden deaths

D. Signs and symptoms: Fever is often the only sign of infection in patients with neutropenia. Neutropenia is technically asymptomatic with associated symptoms.

    1. Fever

    2. Chills or rigors: Uncontrolled violent shaking or trembling

    3. Confusion or somnolence

    4. Productive cough

    5. Headache

    6. Dysuria

    7. Vaginal discharge

    8. Skin lesions with swelling, tenderness, and heat at the site; rashes, ulcerations, abscesses, or wounds that are not healing

    9. Diarrhea

    10. Sore throat

    11. Discomfort at site of implanted access device

    12. Neck stiffness

    13. Mucositis

    14. Fatigue

E. Physical examination

    1. Vital signs

       a) Temperature elevation: Single temperature greater than 100.4°F–101°F (38°C–38.3°C) over one hour in patients with ANC less than or equal to 500/mm³ is considered urgent.

       b) Hypotension and tachycardia suggesting sepsis

    2. HEENT

       a) Oral mucosa for signs of erythema and inflammation

       b) Possible sinus tenderness

    3. Lymph: Palpate for lymphadenopathy in the area of predicted lymphatic drainage from the suspected site of infection (see Appendix D).

    4. Integument

       a) Open lesions

       b) Edema, erythema, and tenderness of the skin, especially at biopsy sites and venous access sites

       c) Evidence of pallor

       d) Rash

    5. Pulmonary

       a) Decreased breath sounds suggesting pneumonia

       b) Crackles and wheezing indicating pulmonary edema or CHF

       c) Egophony or increased fremitus suggesting pneumonia

       d) Bronchial breath sounds over affected area suggesting lobar pneumonia

    6. Abdominal

       a) Distention with gas

       b) Tenderness on palpation indicating infection

       c) Costovertebral angle tenderness suggestive of kidney infection

       d) Splenomegaly

7. Neurologic: Subtle changes in mental status (e.g., restlessness, irritability, somnolence, confusion) indicating sepsis
8. Rectal: Perineum and perianal areas for evidence of mucosal irritation and inflammation; digital examination contraindicated

IV. Diagnostic tests (Afzal et al., 2017; Dale, 2016; Dale & Bolyard, 2017; NCCN, 2021a, 2021b)
  A. Laboratory
    1. CBC with differential
      a) Screen for cyclic neutropenia with serial CBC.
      b) Calculate ANC: Total WBC times (% segmented plus % bands).
      c) Increased bands or shift to the left suggests bacterial infection.
    2. Creatinine, BUN, electrolytes, hepatic transaminase enzymes, and total bilirubin to evaluate renal status, electrolytes, and liver status
    3. Blood cultures with fever for bacteria, fungi, and viruses
      a) Obtain one set of aerobic and one set of anaerobic cultures from at least two different peripheral sites or a vascular access device.
      b) If vascular access device is double or triple lumen, obtain blood culture set from each lumen along with a peripheral set of cultures.
    4. Urine, wound, stool, and sputum cultures, as indicated
    5. Peripheral blood smear to evaluate for atypical lymphocytes and abnormal cells depressing neutrophil count
    6. Bone marrow biopsy and aspiration for persistent neutropenia without known cause
      a) Intrinsic marrow defects via morphology, flow cytometry, or cytogenetics
      b) Myelokathexis: Retention of neutrophils in bone marrow
      c) Severe congenital neutropenia: Maturation arrest at promyelocyte stage
      d) Benign congenital neutropenia: Maturation arrest at metamyelocyte stage
      e) Morphologic identification of fungal infection
      f) Evidence of megaloblastosis: Vitamin B_{12} or folate
      g) Leukemia, myelodysplasia, other atypical cells
    7. Antineutrophil antibody screen: Autoimmune or isoimmune neutropenia
    8. HIV testing, as indicated
    9. Other studies: Copper, vitamin B_{12}, and folate levels
    10. Viral titers, as indicated, for CMV, HIV, herpes, and parvovirus
  B. Radiology
    1. Radiographs of long bones to evaluate for phenotypic forms of neutropenia
    2. Chest x-ray to evaluate for pneumonia
    3. Kidneys, ureters, bladder x-ray to assess bowel gas pattern if patient is symptomatic
      a) Typhlitis may occur in patients with prolonged neutropenia.
      b) Diagnosis is suggested by gaseous distention or the presence of gas in the bowel wall.
  C. Other
    1. Lumbar puncture if CNS is suspected source
    2. Pulse oximetry to evaluate oxygen level if pulmonary source is suspected
    3. ABGs to assess for metabolic acidosis

V. Differential diagnosis (Afzal et al., 2017; Dale, 2016; Dale & Bolyard, 2017)
  A. Primary hematologic disorders
    1. Congenital/inherited
      a) Severe congenital neutropenia: Kostmann syndrome
      b) Cyclic neutropenia

   c) Familial benign neutropenia
   d) Diamond-Blackfan syndrome
   e) Shwachman-Diamond syndrome
   f) Chédiak-Higashi syndrome
   g) Glycogen storage disease type Ib
   h) Fanconi anemia
  2. Acquired
   a) Acute leukemia
   b) Myelodysplastic syndromes
   c) Chronic lymphocytic leukemia
   d) Hodgkin lymphoma
   e) Non-Hodgkin lymphoma
   f) Aplastic anemia (see Chapter 114) and pure white cell aplasia
   g) Chronic idiopathic neutropenia
   h) Nutritional disorders
    (1) Anorexia/cachexia (see Chapter 66)
    (2) Deficiencies: Copper, vitamin B_{12} (see Chapter 115), folate (see Chapter 116)
B. Secondary disorders
  1. Viral illnesses: Most common cause of neutropenia (e.g., Epstein-Barr virus, parvovirus, HIV)
  2. Drug induced: Second most common etiology of neutropenia
   a) Analgesics and anti-inflammatory agents
   b) Antibiotics: Cephalosporin, chloramphenicol, penicillin, sulfonamide, trimethoprim/sulfamethoxazole
   c) Anticonvulsants: Phenytoin, carbamazepine
   d) Antidepressants: Amitriptyline, imipramine
   e) Antihistamines and H_2 blockers: Cimetidine
   f) Antimalarials: Dapsone, quinine, chloroquine
   g) Antithyroid drugs: Carbimazole, methimazole, propylthiouracil
   h) Cardiovascular drugs: Captopril, hydralazine, propranolol
   i) Diuretics: Hydrochlorothiazide, acetazolamide
   j) Hypnotics and sedatives: Chlordiazepoxide, benzodiazepines
   k) Atypical antipsychotics: Chlorpromazine, olanzapine, clozapine
   l) Other drugs: Allopurinol, colchicine, penicillamine, ticlopidine
  3. Antineutrophil antibodies causing neutropenia
   a) Splenic sequestration
   b) Complement-mediated neutrophil lysis
  4. Autoimmune-mediated conditions
   a) Wegener granulomatosis
   b) RA (see Chapter 108)
   c) SLE (see Chapter 110)
   d) Chronic hepatitis (see Chapter 74)
   e) Hypersplenism
   f) Felty syndrome triad: RA, splenomegaly, neutropenia
   g) Sjögren syndrome
  5. Pseudoneutropenia
   a) Automated counter error
   b) Prolonged time from blood draw to testing
   c) Asymmetric distribution of circulating neutrophils to the marginated pool

VI. Treatment (Aapro et al., 2017; Afzal et al., 2017; Botteri et al., 2018; Dale & Bolyard, 2017; Hill et al., 2018; Lalami & Klastersky, 2017; Lehrnbecher et al., 2017; Marty et al., 2017; Mehta et al., 2015; NCCN, 2021a, 2021b; Smith et al., 2015; Taplitz, Kennedy, Bow, et al., 2018; Taplitz, Kennedy, & Flowers, 2018; van Dalen et al., 2016)
  A. Guided by underlying etiology and severity of neutropenia
  B. Ranges from close observation in patients with benign neutropenia to growth factor support and antibiotics in patients with neutropenic fevers
  C. Prophylactic antibiotics in patients with malignancy
    1. Antibacterial prophylaxis
      a) Indications
        (1) Anticipated prolonged neutropenia for more than 7–10 days
        (2) Significant comorbid conditions
        (3) Receiving induction or consolidation therapy for acute leukemia, patients with lymphoma, multiple myeloma, chronic lymphocytic leukemia, or receiving purine analog therapy
        (4) Undergoing HSCT (either autologous or allogeneic)
        (5) Receiving alemtuzumab therapy
        (6) GVHD being treated with high-dose steroids
        (7) Patients undergoing CAR T-cell immunotherapy
          (a) FDA approved for the treatment of refractory or relapsed B-cell malignancies
          (b) Under investigative study for other hematologic and solid tumor malignancies
      b) Example: Typically quinolone; levofloxacin 500 mg PO daily
    2. Antifungal prophylaxis
      a) Indications
        (1) Allogeneic HSCT
        (2) Induction therapy for acute leukemia/myelodysplastic syndromes with expected long periods of neutropenia
        (3) Autologous HSCT with mucositis
        (4) Therapy for acute lymphoblastic leukemia
        (5) Significant GVHD
        (6) CAR T-cell immunotherapy
          (a) FDA approved for the treatment of refractory or relapsed B-cell malignancies
          (b) Under investigative study for other hematologic and solid tumor malignancies
      b) Examples: Fluconazole 100 mg PO daily; posaconazole 300 mg PO daily
    3. Antiviral prophylaxis (see Appendix J)
      a) Increased risk of VZV or HSV reactivation
        (1) Patients with acute leukemia undergoing induction or consolidation; patients with lymphoma, multiple myeloma, or chronic lymphocytic leukemia undergoing therapy with anticipated neutropenia
        (2) Treatment with proteasome inhibitors, purine analogs
        (3) Autologous or allogeneic HSCT
        (4) CAR T-cell immunotherapy
          (a) FDA approved for the treatment of refractory or relapsed B-cell malignancies
          (b) Under investigative study for other hematologic and solid tumor malignancies

(5) Examples to prevent varicella reactivation: Acyclovir 400 mg PO two times a day; valacyclovir 500 mg PO daily

   b) Patients with increased risk of hepatitis reactivation: Entecavir 0.5 mg PO daily

   c) Patients with increased risk of CMV reactivation after receiving allogeneic HSCT: Letermovir 240 mg PO daily

  4. *Pneumocystis jirovecii* pneumonia prophylaxis

   a) Indications

    (1) Autologous or allogeneic HSCT

    (2) Induction therapy for acute lymphoblastic leukemia

    (3) Treatment with alemtuzumab

    (4) Prolonged corticosteroid use or therapy with temozolomide and radiation therapy

    (5) Prolonged high-dose corticosteroid therapy (greater than or equal to 20 mg prednisone equivalents daily for more than or equal to one month)

    (6) Treatment with purine analogs

    (7) CAR T-cell immunotherapy

     (a) FDA approved for the treatment of refractory or relapsed B-cell malignancies

     (b) Under investigative study for other hematologic and solid tumor malignancies

   b) Trimethoprim/sulfamethoxazole

    (1) One single-strength tablet PO daily or one double-strength tablet PO two or three times weekly

    (2) If sulfa allergic: Dapsone 100 mg PO daily or aerosolized pentamidine

D. Growth factors to decrease prolonged nadir from drug-induced neutropenia

  1. Primary prophylaxis is recommended for all patients with cancer undergoing chemotherapy with greater than 20% risk of febrile neutropenia.

  2. Secondary prophylaxis is recommended for patients who experienced neutropenia with a prior chemotherapy treatment cycle.

  3. G-CSF (filgrastim): 5 mcg/kg subcutaneous daily

   a) Filgrastim biosimilar: 5 mcg/kg subcutaneous daily; may be used in place of filgrastim

   b) Should be given 24–72 hours after the completion of chemotherapy

  4. Long acting (pegfilgrastim): 6 mg/dose subcutaneous; should not be given between 14 days before and 24 hours after administration of cytotoxic chemotherapy

   a) Pegfilgrastim biosimilar: 6 mcg subcutaneous; can be used in place of pegfilgrastim

   b) Should be given 24–72 hours after the completion of chemotherapy

E. Nonpharmacologic measures

  1. Practice good hand washing.

  2. Maintain good oral hygiene, including cleaning and attention to and correction of dental problems.

  3. Avoid placement of venous access catheters when patient is neutropenic.

  4. Encourage nutritional intake. Enteral nutrition is preferred to parenteral route.

  5. Little evidence exists to support neutropenic diet. Consideration for Safe Food Handling Approach as outlined by the U.S. Department of Agriculture, which focuses on safe handling of food and less on which foods patients should avoid, as little evidence supports the benefit of a neutropenic diet.

  6. Protect perirectal area.

   a) Avoid trauma, such as rectal temperatures and examinations.

      b) If constipation is of concern, administer stool softeners (see Chapter 55).

      c) Educate patients to report perirectal pain or irritation.

  7. Protect skin: Skin abrasions or cuts need prompt cleaning and topical antibacterial therapy.

  8. Immunizations

      a) Influenza vaccine annually

      b) Pneumococcal polysaccharide vaccine

F. Empiric antibiotic therapy: High-risk patients with febrile neutropenia

VII. Follow-up (NCCN, 2021b; Taplitz, Kennedy, & Flowers, 2018)

  A. Follow-up will be determined by the cause of the neutropenia.

  B. For inpatients, evaluate daily, and review vital signs, physical examination, laboratory values, fever curve, culture results, and CBC.

  C. For outpatients, call patients daily and recommend an office visit at least two to three times per week for physical examination, laboratory values, culture results, and antibiotic levels, if appropriate.

VIII. Referral

  A. Hematologist: If the patient has not been under the care of a physician; if the patient has leukemic blasts, abnormal findings on the peripheral smear, or agranulocytosis (ANC less than 200/mm³)

  B. Infectious disease specialist: For fevers that do not respond to therapy

The author would like to acknowledge Barbara Barnes Rogers, CRNP, MN, AOCN®, ANP-BC, for her contribution to this chapter that remains unchanged from the previous edition of this book.

References

Aapro, M., Boccia, R., Leonard, R., Camps, C., Campone, M., Choquet, S., ... Valero, V. (2017). Refining the role of pegfilgrastim (a long-acting G-CSF) for prevention of chemotherapy-induced febrile neutropenia: Consensus guidance recommendations. *Supportive Care in Cancer, 25*(11), 3295–3304. https://doi.org/10.1007/s00520-017-3842-1

Afzal, W., Owlia, M.B., Hasni, S., & Newman, K.A. (2017). Autoimmune neutropenia updates: Etiology, pathology, and treatment. *Southern Medical Journal, 110*(4), 300–307. https://doi.org/10.14423/SMJ.0000000000000637

Botteri, E., Krendyukov, A., & Curigliano, G. (2018). Comparing granulocyte colony–stimulating factor filgrastim and peg-filgrastim to its biosimilars in terms of efficacy and safety: A meta-analysis of randomised clinical trials in breast cancer patients. *European Journal of Cancer, 89,* 49–55. https://doi.org/10.1016/j.ejca.2017.10.034

Dale, D.C. (2016). How I diagnose and treat neutropenia. *Current Opinion in Hematology, 23*(1), 1–4. https://doi.org/10.1097/MOH.0000000000000208

Dale, D.C., & Bolyard, A.A. (2017). An update on the diagnosis and treatment of chronic idiopathic neutropenia. *Current Opinion in Hematology, 24*(1), 46–53. https://doi.org/10.1097/MOH.0000000000000305

Hill, J.A., Li, D., Hay, K.A., Green, M.L., Cherian, S., Chen, X., ... Turtle, C.J. (2018). Infectious complications of CD19-targeted chimeric antigen receptor–modified T-cell immunotherapy. *Blood, 131*(1), 121–130. https://doi.org/10.1182/blood-2017-07-793760

Lalami, Y., & Klastersky, J. (2017). Impact of chemotherapy-induced neutropenia (CIN) and febrile neutropenia (FN) on cancer treatment outcomes: An overview about well-established and recently emerging clinical data. *Critical Reviews in Oncology/Hematology, 120,* 163–179. https://doi.org/10.1016/j.critrevonc.2017.11.005

Lehrnbecher, T., Robinson, P., Fisher, B., Alexander, S., Ammann, R.A., Beauchemin, M., ... Sung, L. (2017). Guideline for the management of fever and neutropenia in children with cancer and hematopoietic stem-cell transplantation recipients: 2017 update. *Journal of Clinical Oncology, 35*(18), 2082–2094. https://doi.org/10.1200/JCO.2016.71.7017

Marty, F.M., Ljungman, P., Chemaly, R.F., Maertens, J., Dadwal, S.S., Duarte, R.F., ... Badshah, C. (2017). Letermovir prophylaxis for cytomegalovirus in hematopoietic-cell transplantation. *New England Journal of Medicine, 377*(25), 2433–2444. https://doi.org/10.1056/NEJMoa1706640

Mehta, H.M., Malandra, M., & Corey, S.J. (2015). G-CSF and GM-CSF in neutropenia. *Journal of Immunology, 195*(4), 1341–1349. https://doi.org/10.4049/jimmunol.1500861

National Comprehensive Cancer Network. (2021a). *NCCN Clinical Practice Guidelines in Oncology (NCCN Guidelines®): Hematopoietic growth factors* [v. 4.2021]. https://www.nccn.org/professionals/physician_gls/pdf/growthfactors.pdf

National Comprehensive Cancer Network. (2021b). *NCCN Clinical Practice Guidelines in Oncology (NCCN Guidelines®): Prevention and treatment of cancer-related infections* [v.1.2021]. https://www.nccn.org/professionals/physician_gls/pdf/infections.pdf

O'Brien, C., Dempsey, O., & Kennedy, M.J. (2014). Febrile neutropenia risk assessment tool: Improving clinical outcomes for oncology patients. *European Journal of Oncology Nursing, 18*(2), 167–174. https://doi.org/10.1016/j.ejon.2013.11.002

Smith, T.J., Bohlke, K., & Armitage, J.O. (2015). Recommendations for the use of white blood cell growth factors: American Society of Clinical Oncology clinical practice guideline update. *Journal of Oncology Practice, 11*(6), 511–513. https://doi.org/10.1200/JOP.2015.006742

Taplitz, R.A., Kennedy, E.B., Bow, E.J., Crews, J., Gleason, C., Hawley, D.K., … Flowers, C.R. (2018). Antimicrobial prophylaxis for adult patients with cancer-related immunosuppression: ASCO and IDSA clinical practice guideline update. *Journal of Clinical Oncology, 36*(30), 3043–3054. https://doi.org/10.1200/JCO.18.00374

Taplitz, R.A., Kennedy, E.B., & Flowers, C.R. (2018). Outpatient management of fever and neutropenia in adults treated for malignancy: American Society of Clinical Oncology and Infectious Diseases Society of America clinical practice guideline update summary. *Journal of Oncology Practice, 14*(4), 250–255. https://doi.org/10.1200/JOP.18.00016

van Dalen, E.C., Mank, A., Leclercq, E., Mulder, R.L., Davies, M., Kersten, M.J., & van de Wetering, M.D. (2016). Low bacterial diet versus control diet to prevent infection in cancer patients treated with chemotherapy causing episodes of neutropenia. *Cochrane Database of Systematic Reviews, 2016*(4). https://doi.org/10.1002/14651858.CD006247.pub3

CHAPTER 128

Polycythemia Vera

Heather T. Mackey, MSN, RN, ANP-BC, AOCN®

I. Definition: A myeloproliferative neoplasm characterized by clonal proliferation of a multipotent stem cell with trilineage hyperplasia primarily affecting the red cell line, but potentially involving the WBCs and platelets, associated with increased thrombotic events, leukemic transformation, and myelofibrosis (Tefferi & Barbui, 2021)

II. Physiology/Pathophysiology (Bose & Verstovsek, 2019; Cuthbert & Stein, 2019; Lu & Chang, 2020; Pillai et al., 2020; Tefferi & Barbui, 2021; Vannuchhi et al., 2018)
   A. Normal: Hematopoiesis is the complex process of blood cell production in the bone marrow. A primitive pluripotent stem cell in the bone marrow is the progenitor for all blood cell lines.
      1. WBCs are the body's primary defense against infection and are composed of granulocytes, monocytes, and lymphocytes.
      2. Platelets are involved in hemostasis and in initiating the clotting mechanism in conjunction with numerous clotting factors.
      3. RBCs carry Hgb, which delivers oxygen to body tissues and returns carbon dioxide to the lungs for elimination.
   B. Pathophysiology
      1. Causes of polycythemia
         a) Polycythemia vera: Primary polycythemia
         b) Secondary polycythemia due to decreased oxygen: Respiratory disorders, smoking, living in high altitudes
      2. Polycythemia vera is driven by *JAK2* mutations involving either exon 12 (*JAK2*) or exon 14 (*JAK2V617F*) that activate the Janus kinase/signal transducer and activator of transcription (JAK/STAT) pathway of the thrombopoietin receptor and the G-CSF receptor.
         a) The presence of *JAK2* mutation is neither specific for polycythemia vera nor necessary for the development of polycythemia vera.
         b) *JAK2V617F* mutation has been noted in almost all patients with polycythemia vera (up to 90%) and can lead to proliferation of multiple cell lines (e.g., RBCs, WBCs, platelets). Its presence does not appear to impact survival or leukemic transformation.
         c) JAK2 is an essential kinase in the EPO receptor signal transduction pathway and its activity results in EPO-independent proliferation of erythrocyte precursors.
      3. Polycythemia vera is characterized by growth factor–independent erythroid proliferation producing an elevated RBC mass.
      4. Phases
         a) Prodromal/prepolycythemic phase: Generally asymptomatic with isolated increase in platelets or RBCs

        b) Overt polycythemic phase: Characterized by erythrocytosis as well as increased WBCs and platelets; may last for a number of years

        c) Postpolycythemic/spent phase: Late polycythemia vera in which the bone marrow eventually fails, and the patient becomes severely anemic

    5. Polycythemia vera is one of the myeloproliferative neoplasms. Others are chronic myeloid leukemia, chronic neutrophilic leukemia, chronic eosinophilic leukemia, myeloproliferative neoplasm (unclassified), ET, and primary myelofibrosis.

III. Clinical features: Incidence is approximately 2.5–10 in 100,000 people, with a median age of 60 years and male predominance among all races and ethnicities (more common in Eastern European Jewish population). Although longevity can usually be expected, venous and arterial thrombosis is a leading cause of mortality in those affected with polycythemia vera. Patients can have significant symptoms as the disease progresses (Lu & Chang, 2020; Pillai et al., 2020; Spivak, 2018; Tefferi & Barbui, 2021).

  A. Etiology: Underlying cause is unknown, but *JAK2* mutations frequently exist.

  B. History
    1. History of cancer and cancer treatment
    2. Current medications: Prescribed, over the counter
    3. History of presenting symptoms: Precipitating factors, location, duration
    4. Changes in ADLs
    5. Past medical history: Hypertension, stroke, DVT, PE, dyslipidemia
    6. Social history: Tobacco use

  C. Signs and symptoms: Often asymptomatic
    1. Pruritus, typically after bathing
    2. Evidence of ulcers on fingers and toes
    3. Burning sensation of fingers: Erythromelalgia caused by microarteriolar occlusion
    4. Joint pain
    5. Evidence of bleeding: Epistaxis, easy bruising, gingival bleeding, melena
    6. Weight changes in recent months
    7. Abdominal pain due to organomegaly
    8. Headache
    9. Weakness
    10. Transient visual disturbances: Blurred vision or vision loss
    11. Vertigo
    12. Tinnitus
    13. Ruddy cyanosis of face

  D. Physical examination
    1. Vital signs: Hypertension
    2. HEENT
        a) Facial plethora: Red face
        b) Ophthalmologic: Engorged retinal veins
        c) Altered visual acuity
    3. Integument
        a) Ruddy cyanosis
        b) Ulcers on fingers and toes
        c) Petechiae
        d) Ecchymosis
        e) Dry skin, excoriation from itching
    4. Abdominal

a) Palpable splenomegaly in 70% of patients
b) Possible hepatomegaly

IV. Diagnostic tests (see Table 128-1; Arber et al., 2016; Lu & Chang, 2020; Maffioli et al., 2017; NCCN, 2021; Pillai et al., 2020; Tefferi & Barbui, 2021)
  A. Diagnostic criteria: Either all three major criteria must be present, or the first two major criteria must be present along with the minor criterion.
    1. Major criteria
      a) Hgb greater than 16.5 g/dl in men; greater than 16 g/dl in women, or hematocrit greater than 49% in men or greater than 48% in women, or increased RBC mass
      b) Bone marrow showing hypercellularity for age with trilineage proliferation with pleomorphic mature megakaryocytes
      c) Presence of *JAK2V617F* or *JAK2* exon 12 mutation
    2. Minor criterion: Low serum EPO level
  B. Laboratory: See Tables 113-1 and 113-2 for common diagnostic tests and normal values.
    1. CBC
      a) Elevated hematocrit, WBCs, or platelets
      b) RBC morphology: Normal in early disease; late disease presenting with marked anisocytosis, poikilocytosis, and increased numbers of nucleated RBCs
      c) Mild basophilia
    2. Reticulocyte count: Slightly increased
    3. PT, PTT, and INR: May appear prolonged if the amount of anticoagulant used in the test is not adjusted for the increase in hematocrit
    4. Peripheral blood smear
      a) Smear may show microcytic hypochromic RBCs with anisocytosis and poikilocytosis, reflecting exhaustion of iron stores due to increased Hgb synthesis.
      b) WBCs generally have normal morphology.
      c) Basophils, eosinophils, and immature forms are often increased.
      d) Platelets often have abnormal morphology.
    5. *JAK2* molecular testing: *JAK2V617F* or *JAK2* exon 12 mutations commonly present; may be absent
    6. EPO level: Low and often undetectable

TABLE 128-1 Features of Primary Versus Secondary Polycythemia Vera

Finding	Primary	Secondary
Arterial oxygen saturation	Normal	Decreased
Bone marrow	Panhyperplasia	Erythroid hyperplasia
Erythropoietin level	Decreased	Increased
Leukocytosis	Present	Not present
Red cell volume	Increased	Increased
Splenomegaly	Present	Not present
Thrombocytosis	Present	Not present
Vitamin B$_{12}$	Increased	Normal

Note. Based on information from Pillai et al., 2020; Tefferi & Barbui, 2021.

    7. Bone marrow biopsy: Not diagnostic for polycythemia; performed to evaluate fibrosis and cytogenetics

       a) Hypercellularity with trilineage hyperplasia

       b) Atypical megakaryocyte hyperplasia and clustering megakaryocytes

       c) Possible positive *JAK2* mutation, either involving exon 14 or 12

       d) Abnormal karyotype in 10%–20% of patients, commonly trisomy 9, trisomy 8, trisomy 1q, del(5q) and del(7q), and del(13q)

       e) Fluorescence in situ hybridization testing for *BCR-ABL1* negative

       f) Decreased stainable iron

    8. LDH: Elevated

    9. Uric acid: Elevated

    10. Serum vitamin B_{12}: Elevated

    11. ABGs: Typically normal

    12. Potential Von Willebrand panel

    13. Ferritin and iron: Decreased

    14. Liver and kidney function studies: Typically normal

    15. Blood carboxyhemoglobin level: Should be less than 5%; increased in smokers

    16. Cytogenetics of peripheral blood abnormalities: Trisomy 8, trisomy 9, del(20q); *BCR-ABL1* negative

  C. Radiology: Not indicated unless abdominal ultrasound obtained to evaluate spleen

V. Differential diagnosis (Arber et al., 2016; Lu & Chang, 2020; Maffioli et al., 2017; NCCN, 2021; Pillai et al., 2020; Tefferi & Barbui, 2021)

  A. Other myeloproliferative neoplasms: ET, chronic myeloid leukemia, myelofibrosis

  B. Secondary polycythemia from conditions causing RBC overproduction secondary to hypoxia

    1. COPD (see Chapter 28)

    2. High altitude

    3. Smoking: Carboxyhemoglobin

    4. Cyanotic heart disease

    5. Methemoglobinemia

    6. High oxygen affinity Hgb

    7. Cobalt

  C. Pure erythrocytosis

    1. Tumors: Renal, brain, hepatoma, uterine fibroids, pheochromocytoma, adrenal

    2. Renal artery stenosis

    3. Inappropriate EPO secretion

    4. Bartter syndrome

    5. Renal cysts, hydronephrosis

  D. Other causes

    1. EPO receptor hypersensitivity

    2. Congenital erythrocytosis

    3. Androgen therapy

    4. Autotransfusion (blood doping), self-injection of EPO

VI. Treatment (Aruch & Mascarenhas, 2016; Bose & Verstovsek, 2019; Griesshammer et al., 2019; Lu & Chang, 2020; Maffioli et al., 2017; NCCN, 2021; Pillai et al., 2020; Spivak, 2018; Tefferi & Barbui, 2021; Vannuchhi et al., 2018)

  A. Goals of therapy

    1. Relieve clinical symptoms

    2. Decrease thrombotic risk

    3. Slow or prevent leukemic transformation

B. Risk stratification: To estimate likelihood of recurrent thrombosis

    1. Low risk: Age 60 years or younger and no history of thrombosis

    2. High risk: Age older than 60 years or history of thrombosis

C. Nonpharmacologic measures: Phlebotomy for most low- and high-risk patients

    1. Hematocrit should be maintained at less than 45% in men and women.

    2. Initiation of phlebotomy is transiently associated with an increase in thrombotic risk, which is highest in older adults.

    3. Phlebotomy induces iron deficiency, but iron supplementation may result in rapid reappearance of polycythemia; therefore, it should not be undertaken.

D. Pharmacologic measures

    1. Low-risk patients

        a) Give low-dose ASA 81 mg PO daily unless contraindicated or in those with acquired von Willebrand disease.

            (1) Measure alleviates microvascular sequelae, including headache, vertigo, visual disturbances, distal paresthesia, and erythromelalgia.

            (2) Consider two times a day dosing if there is inadequate control of microvascular symptoms, presence of cardiovascular risk factors, or leukocytosis.

        b) Management of refractory symptoms

        c) Cytoreductive agents typically are reserved for those with uncontrolled symptoms, progressive increases in WBC or platelet counts, symptomatic or progressive splenomegaly, or in those whom phlebotomy is poorly tolerated.

    2. High-risk patients

        a) Give low-dose ASA 81 mg PO daily unless contraindicated or in those with acquired von Willebrand disease.

            (1) Measure alleviates microvascular sequelae, including headache, vertigo, visual disturbances, distal paresthesia, and erythromelalgia.

            (2) Consider two times a day dosing if there is inadequate control of microvascular symptoms, presence of cardiovascular risk factors, or leukocytosis.

            (3) Consider two times a day dosing in those with arterial thrombosis if older, those who have *JAK2* mutation, or in those with cardiovascular disease.

        b) Management of refractory symptoms

        c) Cytoreductive agents

            (1) Hydroxyurea 15–30 mg/kg PO daily can be used as a first-line therapy. It is used in divided doses initially, with dose adjustments no more often than weekly. The goals are to achieve a platelet count of 100,000–400,000/mm^3 and to limit anemia and neutropenia.

                (a) Controls blood counts

                (b) Reduces rate of thromboembolic events

                (c) May alleviate cytopenia due to splenomegaly

                (d) Side effects: Fever, rash, stomatitis, GI upset, leg ulcers, jaundice, elevated creatinine

            (2) Ruxolitinib can be considered in those who are refractory after hydroxyurea treatment or intolerant to hydroxyurea.

            (3) Pegylated IFN or busulfan are acceptable alternatives for patients who are intolerant of hydroxyurea or fail to achieve adequate control of symptoms or hematocrit.

E. Supportive care
   1. Antihistamines: Diphenhydramine 25–50 mg PO every four to six hours PRN or hydroxyzine 25–50 mg PO every six hours PRN can be used to treat pruritus (see Appendix H and Chapter 16).
   2. Other agents that may help pruritus include cholestyramine 4 g PO daily or SSRIs, such as paroxetine 20 mg daily or fluoxetine 10 mg PO daily.
   3. PUVA (psoralen with ultraviolet A light therapy) may be helpful in eliminating pruritus.
   4. Topical corticosteroids can be beneficial (see Appendix K).
F. Patient education
   1. Refer for smoking cessation therapy.
   2. Promote healthy lifestyle to maintain weight, healthy diet, and exercise for patients at risk for cardiovascular disease.

VII. Follow-up (Cuthbert & Stein, 2019; Griesshammer et al., 2019; NCCN, 2021; Tefferi & Barbui, 2021)
   A. Monitor CBC at least every three to six months (or more frequently if clinically indicated), and monitor for complications.
      1. Major complication is thrombosis due to increase in hematocrit and leukocytosis.
      2. Monitor for DVT and stroke-like symptoms.
   B. Monitor for side effects of pharmacologic therapy.
   C. Monitor closely for transformation to acute leukemia. Incidence of transformation is approximately 5%–10%.

VIII. Referrals
   A. Orthopedist: For evaluation and intervention for management of bleeding into joints
   B. Hematologist: For complete evaluation and treatment plan

The author would like to acknowledge Barbara Barnes Rogers, CRNP, MN, AOCN®, ANP-BC, for her contribution to this chapter that remains unchanged from the previous edition of this book.

References

Arber, D.A., Orazi, A., Hasserjian, R., Thiele, J., Borowitz, M.J., Le Beau, M.M., … Vardiman, J.W. (2016). The 2016 revision to the World Health Organization classification of myeloid neoplasms and acute leukemia. *Blood, 127*(20), 2391–2405. https://doi.org/10.1182/blood-2016-03-643544

Aruch, D., & Mascarenhas, J. (2016). Contemporary approach to essential thrombocythemia and polycythemia vera. *Current Opinion in Hematology, 23*(2), 150–160. https://doi.org/10.1097/MOH.0000000000000216

Bose, P., & Verstovsek, S. (2019). Updates in the management of polycythemia vera and essential thrombocythemia. *Therapeutic Advances in Hematology, 10.* https://doi.org/10.1177/2040620719870052

Cuthbert, D., & Stein, B.L. (2019). Polycythemia vera–associated complications: Pathogenesis, clinical manifestations, and effects on outcomes. *Journal of Blood Medicine, 10,* 359–371. https://doi.org/10.2147/JBM.S189922

Griesshammer, M., Kiladjian, J.-J., & Besses, C. (2019). Thromboembolic events in polycythemia vera. *Annals of Hematology, 98*(5), 1071–1082. https://doi.org/10.1007/s00277-019-03625-x

Lu, X., & Chang, R. (2020). Polycythemia vera. In *StatPearls.* https://www.ncbi.nlm.nih.gov/books/NBK557660

Maffioli, M., Mora, B., & Passamonti, F. (2017). Polycythemia vera: From new, modified diagnostic criteria to new therapeutic approaches. *Clinical Advances in Hematology and Oncology, 15*(9), 700–707.

National Comprehensive Cancer Network. (2021). *NCCN Clinical Practice Guidelines in Oncology (NCCN Guidelines®): Myeloproliferative neoplasms* [v.2.2021]. https://www.nccn.org/professionals/physician_gls/pdf/mpn.pdf

Pillai, A., Fazal, S., & Babiker, H. (2020). Polycythemia. In *StatPearls.* https://www.ncbi.nlm.nih.gov/books/NBK526081

Spivak, J.L. (2018). Polycythemia vera. *Current Treatment Options in Oncology, 19,* 12. https://doi.org/10.1007/s11864-018-0529-x

Tefferi, A., & Barbui, T. (2021). Polycythemia vera and essential thrombocythemia: 2021 update on diagnosis, risk-stratification and management. *American Journal of Hematology, 95,* 1599–1613. https://doi.org/ 10.1002/ajh.26008

Vannuchhi, A.M., Guglielmelli, P., & Tefferi, A. (2018). Polycythemia vera and essential thrombocythemia: Algorithmic approach. *Current Opinions in Hematology, 25*(2), 112–199. https://doi.org/10.1097/MOH.0000000000000402

CHAPTER 129

Thrombocytopenia

Kristine Deano Abueg, RN, MSN, OCN®, CBCN®

I. Definition: A decrease in the normal number of circulating platelets, typically below 140,000/mm³ (Abrams, 2019; Musson et al., 2019)
   A. Mild: 100,000–150,000/mm³
   B. Moderate: 50,000–90,000/mm³
   C. Severe: Less than 50,000/mm³

II. Physiology/Pathophysiology (Abrams, 2019; Danese et al., 2020; Gremmel et al., 2016; Hvas, 2016; Kaushansky, 2016; Mariri & Bakchoul, 2019; Musson et al., 2019)
   A. Normal
      1. Platelets are anucleated cell fragments of megakaryocytes derived from the common myeloid progenitor cell.
      2. Platelets have an average life span of nine days and are stored in the spleen. They are ultimately destroyed by phagocytosis in the liver and spleen.
      3. In hemostasis, platelets initiate the coagulation cascade by secreting chemicals (e.g., prostaglandins) that promote adhesion with other platelets.
      4. Platelet clumps block small breaks in blood vessels and capillaries, ultimately stopping blood loss.
      5. Platelets function in numerous physiologic processes, including inflammation, atherogenesis, antimicrobial host defense, as well as tumor growth and metastasis via activation of multiple molecular pathways (e.g., von Willebrand factor, thrombin, adenosine diphosphate).
      6. Thrombopoietin is the primary regulator of megakaryocyte growth, platelet differentiation, and maturation.
         a) It is produced primarily in the liver at a constant rate, with additional production by the kidney, spleen, and bone marrow.
         b) Serum levels are controlled via negative feedback, with suppression during high platelet and megakaryocyte volumes.
   B. Pathophysiology
      1. Decreased peripheral platelet volumes: Associated with a wide variety of conditions, which can be grossly divided into decreased production, increased sequestration, or increased destruction
      2. Decreased platelet production: Occurs as a result of tumor invasion of bone marrow (e.g., leukemia, myelodysplastic syndromes), chemotherapy drugs, and radiation to bone marrow, aplastic anemia, or after viral infections
      3. Abnormal pooling (sequestration) of platelets in the spleen: The spleen may sequester up to 90% of platelets, resulting in an enlarged spleen. Congestive splenomegaly can result in splenic vein obstruction, as seen with portal hypertension.

4. Increased peripheral platelet destruction

    a) An abnormal proliferation of autoreactive T cells is formed against the patient's platelets, resulting in immune-mediated thrombocytopenia. This may be idiopathic, drug induced, or disease induced.

    b) Acute processes, such as DIC, sepsis, thrombotic thrombocytopenic purpura, hemolytic–uremic syndrome, preeclampsia or eclampsia, cardiopulmonary bypass, and giant cavernous hemangioma, increase consumption of circulating platelets.

III. Clinical features: Thrombocytopenia is the most common cause of abnormal bleeding and frequently complicates critical illness with organ dysfunction, sepsis, and renal failure. It is often the first sign of an underlying hematologic malignancy. Emergent presentations require accelerated assessment and intervention to prevent hemodynamic instability due to bleeding or thrombosis. Spontaneous bleeding is unusual unless count less than 20,000/mm³; less than 10,000/mm³ is often associated with serious hemorrhage (Cooper, 2017; Curtis, 2014; Danese et al., 2020; Izak & Bussel, 2014; Mariri & Bakchoul, 2019; Musson et al., 2019; Neunert & Cooper, 2018; Tan et al., 2016).

  A. Risk factors

    1. Patient related

      a) Hereditary thrombocytopenia: Wiskott-Aldrich syndrome

      b) Splenomegaly, disorders of the spleen

    2. Comorbidities

      a) Thrombotic microangiopathies: DIC, thrombotic thrombocytopenic purpura, hemolytic–uremic syndrome

      b) Splenomegaly, hypothermia

      c) Aplastic anemia

      d) Infection

    3. Treatment related

      a) Chemotherapy drugs: IFN, alkylating agents, antimetabolites

      b) Radiation to bone marrow

      c) Drug sensitivity

      d) Multiple blood transfusions

    4. Cancer related

      a) Tumor invasion of bone marrow

      b) Splenomegaly: Platelet sequestration

  B. Etiology: Refer to Pathophysiology section for discussion on underlying causes.

    1. Pseudothrombocytopenia: Laboratory sampling problem caused by anticoagulant-dependent platelet agglutinins of IgG, IgA, or IgM subtypes; occurs when blood is collected into ethylenediaminetetraacetic acid anticoagulant, falsely mimicking a low platelet count

    2. Overt bleeding

    3. Platelet consumption in intravascular thrombi or on damaged endothelial surfaces: DIC, thrombotic thrombocytopenic purpura, heparin-induced thrombocytopenia, microangiopathic processes

    4. Deficient platelet production

      a) Acute hematologic malignancy

      b) Bone marrow suppression from cancer treatments

      c) Liver abnormalities

      d) Acquired: Aplastic anemia

    5. Peripheral platelet clearance

      a) Drug induced (see Table 129-1): Mean onset is one to two weeks after the patient's exposure to the drug.

         (1) Variability in the time frame response is determined by whether the patient has preexisting antibodies from prior exposure to the drug.

         (2) If the patient has never been exposed to the drug, the time frame is two to three weeks to undergo primary alloimmunization.

      b) Autoimmune process

         (1) Idiopathic

         (2) Secondary: Infections, pregnancy, collagen vascular disorders, lymphoproliferative disorders

      c) Nonimmunologic processes

         (1) Thrombotic microangiopathies: DIC, thrombotic thrombocytopenic purpura, hemolytic–uremic syndrome

         (2) Platelet dilution after blood transfusions

         (3) Abnormal pooling of platelets associated with splenomegaly

C. History

  1. History of cancer and cancer treatment

  2. Current medications: Prescribed, over the counter, herbal preparations, exposure to quinine

  3. History of presenting symptoms: Precipitating factors, onset, duration

  4. Changes in ADLs

  5. Past medical history: Bleeding history, recent viral and bacterial infections, vaccinations

  6. Social history: Exposure to toxins

  7. Family history: Bleeding and bruising, hereditary thrombocytopenia

TABLE 129-1   **Examples of Drugs That Induce Thrombocytopenia**

Category	Drug
Anticancer agents	Gemcitabine, oxaliplatin, leucovorin, checkpoint inhibitors
Anticoagulation agents	Heparin, warfarin
Anticonvulsants	Carbamazepine, phenytoin, valproic acid
Antidysrhythmias	Procainamide
Antiemetics	Ondansetron
Anti-infectives	Vancomycin, trimethoprim/sulfamethoxazole, piperacillin, quinine, rifampin, acyclovir
Antiplatelets	Abciximab, dipyridamole, eptifibatide, ticlopidine, tirofiban
Antiulcer agents	Cimetidine
Diuretics	Thiazide
Gold compounds	Gold salts
Nonsteroidal anti-inflammatory drugs	Aspirin
Steroids	Prednisone

Note. Based on information from Abrams, 2019; Calvo, 2019; Mitta et al., 2019; Weycker et al., 2019.

D. Signs and symptoms
1. Cutaneous bleeding: Petechiae, ecchymosis
2. Epistaxis or gingival bleeding
3. Vaginal bleeding
4. Hematuria
5. GI bleeding: Melena, hematemesis
6. Prolonged bleeding from injection sites
7. Headache or change in level of consciousness: Emergent sign
E. Physical examination
1. Integument: Petechiae, purpura, ecchymoses
2. HEENT: Blood blisters in oral mucosa, vitreous hemorrhage, nose bleeds, gingival bleeding, icterus
3. Abdominal
   a) Splenomegaly
   b) Hepatomegaly: Uncommon
4. Lymph: Enlarged lymph nodes indicating infection (see Appendix D)
5. Neurologic: Changes in mental status indicating intracranial bleed

IV. Diagnostic tests (Cooper, 2017; Izak & Bussel, 2014; Mariri & Bakchoul, 2019; Musson et al., 2019; NCI CTEP, 2017; Tan et al., 2016)
A. Laboratory
1. CBC
   a) Repeated CBC using non–ethylenediaminetetraacetic acid collection tubes to rule out pseudothrombocytopenia if false reading suspected
   b) Concomitant abnormal WBC count suggestive of an underlying infectious process
   c) Concomitant anemia suggestive of active bleeding
   d) Pancytopenia suggestive of bone marrow suppression, as seen in malignancies or with medications
   e) Isolated thrombocytopenia suggestive of immune-mediated or inherited disorders
2. Peripheral smear
   a) Platelet clumping
   b) Schistocytes (RBC fragments) indicating intravascular hemolysis
   c) Abnormalities of platelet size and morphologic characteristics: Giant forms, bizarre shapes, deeply stained forms
3. Blood cell morphology revealing atypical shapes indicative of underlying disease states
4. AST, alkaline phosphatase, bilirubin, and alanine transaminase: Elevation in liver enzymes suggestive of concomitant or underlying liver disease
5. Coagulation studies
   a) Normal coagulation studies with uncomplicated thrombocytopenia
   b) DIC causing thrombocytopenia, revealing an increase in fibrin split products or D-dimer, prolonged PT and PTT, prolonged thrombin time, and decreased fibrinogen
6. Increased LDH if large volume of RBC loss
7. Platelet antibody testing for drug-induced thrombocytopenia
8. Haptoglobin decreased with hemolytic anemia or transfusion reaction
9. Viral panels: HIV, hepatitis, as indicated
10. Heparin antibody
11. Bone marrow biopsy indicated in slowly evolving cases or those not associated with drug exposure

B. Radiology: Not indicated

C. The Common Terminology Criteria for Adverse Events from NCI CTEP is a useful tool for grading of thrombocytopenia.

V. Differential diagnosis: Clinicians must address emergent bleeding or thrombosis risks, then identify and address possible underlying causative diseases (Curtis, 2014; Danese et al., 2020; Izak & Bussel, 2014; Mariri & Bakchoul, 2019; Mitta et al., 2019; Musson et al., 2019; Palta & Dhiman, 2016).

A. Inherited platelet abnormalities

1. Bernard-Soulier syndrome
2. May-Hegglin anomaly
3. Paris-Trousseau thrombocytopenia
4. Mediterranean macrothrombocytopenia

B. Disorders of increased destruction

1. Autoimmune platelet destruction: IT (see Chapter 124), thrombotic thrombocytopenia purpura (see Chapter 130), hemolytic–uremic syndrome
2. Drug-induced thrombocytopenia: Most commonly associated with heparin (see Table 129-1)

C. Disorders of decreased production

1. Malignancies due to both underlying disease and treatments: Leukemia, myelodysplastia syndromes, liver involvement
2. Congenital or acquired primary bone marrow failure: Fanconi anemia, megakaryocytic thrombocytopenia, paroxysmal nocturnal hemoglobinuria

D. Disorders of platelet sequestration or consumption

1. HELLP (hemolysis, elevated liver enzymes, and low platelets) syndrome
2. DIC (see Chapter 120)
3. Splenic sequestration

E. Infection: HIV, hepatitis C (see Chapter 74), parvovirus, varicella, rubella, mumps)

F. Metabolic deficiencies

1. Vitamin deficiencies: B_{12}, Folate, iron (see Chapters 115, 116, and 118)
2. Alcohol induced

G. SLE (see Chapter 110)

VI. Treatment: Dependent on the underlying cause of the thrombocytopenia (Neunert & Cooper, 2018)

A. Platelet transfusion

1. Transfusion is generally administered when platelet count is less than 10,000/mm³ or if the patient is actively bleeding.
2. Typically, one unit of platelets should increase the platelet count by 10,000/mm³.

B. Drug-induced thrombocytopenia

1. Offending agents should be discontinued.
2. Oprelvekin can be used after chemotherapy to reduce the need for platelet transfusion at a dose of 50 mcg/kg subcutaneous daily for approximately 10–21 days.
3. Heparin-induced thrombocytopenia
   a) Avoid heparin preparations until the platelet count is normalized. Patients may need to permanently avoid heparin depending on etiology.
   b) Thrombosis is the primary risk; therefore, platelet transfusion is not indicated.
   c) Consider initiation of a direct thrombin inhibitor (e.g., lepirudin, bivalirudin, argatroban).

C. IT (see Chapter 124)

   1. For asymptomatic or mild thrombocytopenia (platelet count greater than 30,000/ mm³), monitor platelet count.
   2. Assess indications for immunosuppressive glucocorticoid therapy, IVIg, and or rituximab.
   3. Hospital admission is required for adults with platelet count less than 20,000/mm³ or mucocutaneous bleeding.
   4. Splenectomy is a last resort for refractory IT.
D. Thrombotic thrombocytopenia purpura (see Chapter 130)
   1. Exchange plasmapheresis and plasma infusions.
   2. Give steroids with prednisone 1 mg/kg PO daily.
   3. Splenectomy is a last resort for refractory thrombotic thrombocytopenia purpura.
E. DIC (see Chapter 120)
   1. Remove the precipitating factor or underlying cause.
   2. Take supportive measures to control active bleeding with blood products.
F. Inherited thrombocytopenia: Educate patients regarding risk reduction behaviors, especially prophylaxis before surgical or medical interventions.

VII. Follow-up
   A. Short term
      1. Response to platelet infusions usually occurs within six hours of transfusion; however, it may last only for a short time.
      2. Monitor platelet counts closely.
   B. Long term: Mild to moderate asymptomatic thrombocytopenia
      1. Check counts every six to eight weeks.
      2. Instruct patients to call if bleeding occurs.

VIII. Referrals
   A. Gastroenterologist: If the site of bleeding is in the GI tract
   B. Hematologist: For diagnostic workup and treatment plan
   C. Geneticist: For workup for inherited thrombocytopenia

The author would like to acknowledge Barbara Barnes Rogers, CRNP, MN, AOCN®, ANP-BC, for her contribution to this chapter that remains unchanged from the previous edition of this book.

References

Abrams, C.S. (2019). Thrombocytopenia. In L. Goldman & A.I. Schafer (Eds.), *Goldman-Cecil medicine* (26th ed., pp. 1123–1132). Elsevier.

Calvo, R. (2019) Hematological side effects of immune checkpoint inhibitors: The example of immune-related thrombocytopenia. *Frontiers in Pharmacology, 10,* 454. https://doi.org/10.3389/fphar.2019.00454

Cooper, N. (2017). State of the art—How I manage immune thrombocytopenia. *British Journal of Haematololgy, 177*(1), 39–54. https://doi.org/10.1111/bjh.14515

Curtis, B.R. (2014). Drug-induced immune thrombocytopenia: Incidence, clinical features, laboratory testing, and pathogenic mechanisms. *Immunohematology, 30*(2), 55–65.

Danese, E., Montagnana, M., Favaloro, E.J., & Lippi, G. (2020). Drug-induced thrombocytopenia: Mechanisms and laboratory diagnostics. *Seminars in Thrombosis and Hemostasis, 46*(3), 264–274. https://doi.org/10.1055/s-0039-1697930

Gremmel, T., Felinger, A.J., III, & Michelson, A.D. (2016). Platelet physiology. *Seminars in Thrombosis and Hemostasis, 42*(3), 191–204. https://doi.org/10.1055/s-0035-1564835

Hvas, A.-M. (2016). Platelet function in thrombosis and hemostasis. *Seminars in Thrombosis and Hemostasis, 42*(3), 183–184. https://doi.org/10.1055/s-0036-1572329

Izak, M., & Bussel, J.B. (2014). Management of thrombocytopenia. *F1000Prime Reports, 6,* 45. https://doi.org/10.12703/P6-45

Kaushansky, K. (2016). Thrombopoietin and its receptor in normal and neoplastic hematopoiesis. *Thrombosis Journal, 14*(Suppl. 1), 40. https://doi.org/10.1186/s12959-016-0095-z

Mariri, I., & Bakchoul, T. (2019). Pathophysiology of autoimmune thrombocytopenia: Current insight with a focus on thrombopoiesis. *Hämostaseologie, 39*(3), 227–237. https://doi.org/10.1055/s-0039-1678732

Mitta, A., Curtis, B.R., Reese, J.A., & George, J.N. (2019). Drug-induced thrombocytopenia: 2019 update of clinical and laboratory data. *American Journal of Hematology, 94*(3), E76–E78. https://doi.org/10.1002/ajh.25379

Musson, E.N., Lomas, O., & Murphy, M.F. (2019). Acute thrombocytopenia: picking a way through a paucity of platelets. *British Journal of Hospital Medicine, 80*(9), 507–512. https://doi.org/10.12968/hmed.2019.80.9.507

National Cancer Institute Cancer Therapy Evaluation Program. (2017). *Common terminology criteria for adverse events*[v. 5.0]. https://ctep.cancer.gov/protocoldevelopment/electronic_applications/docs/CTCAE_v5_Quick_Reference _8.5x11.pdf

Neunert, C.E., & Cooper, N. (2018). Evidence-based management of immune thrombocytopenia: ASH guideline update. *Hematology: American Society of Hematology Education Program Book, 2018,* 568–575. https://doi.org/10.1182/asheducation-2018.1.568

Palta, A., & Dhiman, P. (2016). Thrombocytopenia in pregnancy. *Journal of Obstetrics and Gynecology, 36*(2), 146–152. https://doi.org/10.3109/01443615.2015.1041893

Tan, G.C., Stalling, M., Dennis, G., Nunez, M., & Kahwash, S.B. (2016). Pseudothrombocytopenia due to platelet clumping: A case report and brief review of the literature. *Case Reports in Hematology, 2016,* 3036476. https://doi.org/10.1155/2016/3036476

Weycker, D., Hatfiled, M., Grossman, A., Hanau, A., Lonshteyn, A., Sharma, A., & Chandler, D. (2019). Risk and consequences of chemotherapy-induced thrombocytopenia in US clinical practice. *BMC Cancer, 19*(1), 151. https://doi.org/10.1186/s12885-019-5354-5

CHAPTER 130

Thrombotic Thrombocytopenia Purpura

Mailey Wilks, DNP, MSN, APRN, NP-C,
and Beth Faiman, PhD, MSN, APRN-BC, AOCN®, FAAN

I. Definition: A rare and life-threatening disorder of blood clotting in which microscopic clots form in smaller blood vessels; characterized by microangiopathic hemolytic anemia, consumption thrombocytopenia, and organ injury (Joly et al., 2019; Scully, 2019)

II. Physiology/Pathophysiology (Brierley & Pavord, 2018; Chiasakul & Cuker, 2018; Sadler, 2017; Scully, 2019; Tsai, 2019)
   A. Normal
      1. Platelets are small, irregular cells produced by bone marrow megakaryocytes.
      2. Platelets have the ability to recruit cells in the process of hemostasis and induce clotting when damage to the vascular bed occurs.
      3. Normal platelet count is 150,000–450,000/mm³. A diagnosis of thrombocytopenia can be made when platelet count is less than 150,000/mm³.
   B. Pathophysiology: Thrombocytopenia is usually a result of decreased production (low bone marrow megakaryocytes) or increased peripheral destruction (breakdown of blood platelets once they exit the bone marrow). Endothelial cells form the inner layer of blood vessels. Injury to endothelial cells can occur as a result of many factors or conditions such as cancer, drugs, or autoimmune disorders (see Table 130-1). Endothelial injury results in the deposition of platelets (thrombi), mechanical destruction of RBCs, and organ ischemia. Lesions occur at high density in the heart, pancreas, kidney, and brain.
      1. Congenital: Metalloproteinases are groups of enzymes that play a key role in physiologic processes such as cell migration, tissue remodeling, and growth factor regulation. Patients with congenital thrombotic thrombocytopenia purpura (TTP) have a severe deficiency (less than 5%) of the metalloproteinase ADAMTS13, an enzyme that cleaves von Willebrand factor, a blood protein essential to promote blood homeostasis. Congenital TTP (Upshaw-Schulman syndrome) can manifest at any age. Hereditary TTP is an autosomal recessive condition.
      2. Idiopathic: It is usually the result of an acquired deficiency of ADAMTS13.
      3. Nonidiopathic or secondary: The sequela of anemia, thrombocytopenia (with or without renal or neurologic abnormalities) occurs secondary to an immunologic or other health condition (see Table 130-1). People with secondary forms of TTP may not have severe ADAMTS13 deficiency and will not always respond to treatment such as plasmapheresis. Acquired TTP is due to an autoantibody inhibitor.

TABLE 130-1	Factors or Conditions That Can Lead to Thrombotic Thrombocytopenia Purpura
Category	**Disease/Disorder**
Autoimmune disorders	Systemic lupus erythematosus, antiphospholipid antibody syndrome, scleroderma, Wegener granulomatosis, Sjögren syndrome
Infections	Sepsis
Malignancy	Allogeneic hematopoietic stem cell transplantation, lymphoma
Medications	Gemcitabine, carmustine, mitomycin C, pentostatin, cyclosporine, alendronate, clopidogrel, cocaine, ticlopidine, trimethoprim/sulfamethoxazole, vancomycin
Pregnancy	Postpartum
Systemic disease	Malignant hypertension, systemic vasculitis

Note. Based on information from Brierley & Pavord, 2018; Joly et al., 2017.

III. Clinical features: Three types of TTP exist: congenital, idiopathic, and nonidiopathic (also called secondary). Incidence of TTP in the United States is approximately 4–10 per every 1 million people. Acquired TTP is more common than hereditary. TTP is a medical emergency that can be fatal if treatment is not initiated promptly (Brierley & Pavord, 2018; Chiasakul & Cuker, 2018; Poullin et al., 2019; Sadler, 2017; Scully, 2019; Tsai, 2019).
   A. Etiology
       1. Autoimmune disorders
       2. Pregnancy
       3. Infections
       4. Malignancy
       5. Malignant hypertension
       6. Medication induced
   B. History
       1. History of cancer and cancer treatment
       2. Current medications: Prescribed, over the counter (e.g., quinine, chemotherapy)
       3. History of presenting symptoms: Precipitating factors, onset, duration, associated symptoms (e.g., easy bruising, bleeding)
       4. Changes in ADLs
       5. Past medical history: SLE or other autoimmune disorders, pregnancy/postpartum, inflammatory conditions such as infections or surgery, recent blood transfusions
       6. Family history: TTP
   C. Signs and symptoms
       1. Easy bruising or bleeding
       2. Dizziness, confusion, change in mental status
       3. Fever
       4. Chest pain, dyspnea
       5. GI symptoms of nausea, vomiting, diarrhea, or abdominal pain
       6. Shortness of breath and/or weakness correlating with the degree of anemia
   D. Physical examination
       1. Vital signs: Tachycardia present with anemia

2. Integument: Petechiae or purpura indicating low platelets, pale skin indicating anemia, jaundice secondary to hemolysis, hyperbilirubinemia
3. HEENT: Pale conjunctiva indicating anemia
4. Neurologic: Orientation and cognitive functioning assessment; cognitive abnormalities (common) such as slight confusion, easy forgetfulness, and trouble concentrating; most patients report that these symptoms never disappear.

IV. Diagnostic tests (Brierley & Pavord, 2018; Chiasakul & Cuker, 2018; Fogarty & Dunbar, 2013)
   A. Laboratory: See Table 130-2 for possible results.
      1. CBC with differential
      2. Comprehensive metabolic panel: Elevated creatinine and LFTs
      3. Serum ADAMTS13: Assays of inhibitor and activity; diagnostic of less than 10% is severe deficiency
      4. Peripheral blood smear with presence of schistocytes and RBC fragments
      5. Indirect/unconjugated bilirubin: Elevated due to hemolysis
      6. Serum haptoglobin: Typically undetectable (less than 10 mg/dl)
      7. Coagulation testing: PT, aPTT, fibrinogen, D-dimer
      8. Direct antiglobulin test (DAT; Coombs test): Negative
      9. LDH: Typically, elevated
      10. Reticulocyte: Typically elevated
   B. Radiology: MRI of the brain would be appropriate for patients with TTP who have any neurologic abnormalities due to possibility of small silent brain infarctions.
   C. Diagnostic criteria of TTP should be considered if patient exhibits one of five findings.
      1. Microangiopathic hemolytic anemia
      2. Thrombocytopenia
      3. Renal failure
      4. Change in neurologic status: Mental confusion, seizures, coma
      5. Fever
   D. PLASMIC score: Validated tool to predict the likelihood of ADAMTS13 activity less than 10% in adults (see Table 130-3 for scoring system); patient scores: low risk (0–4); intermediate risk (5); high risk (6–7)

TABLE 130-2   Laboratory Evaluation of Thrombotic Thrombocytopenia Purpura

Laboratory Value	Normal	Result Expected
Hemoglobin/hematocrit	12–16 g/dl	Low
Lactate dehydrogenase	0–250 U/L	Elevated
Platelets	150,000–400,000/mm³	Low
Serum ADAMTS13 activity	≥ 67%	Less than 5% normal; if low, ADAMTS13 may distinguish thrombotic thrombocytopenia purpura from hemolytic uremic syndrome. A low serum ADAMTS13 level is not required for the diagnosis of thrombotic thrombocytopenia purpura if patients exhibit the normal pentad of symptoms.
Serum bilirubin	0–1.3 mg/dl	Elevated
Serum creatinine	0.7–1.4 mg/dl	Elevated

Note. Based on information from Joly et al., 2017, 2019.

TABLE 130-3	PLASMIC Score of Thrombotic Thrombocytopenia Purpura	
Parameter	**Result**	**Score[a]**
Absence of active cancer	–	1
Creatinine	< 2 mg/dl	1
International normalized ratio	< 1.5	1
Mean corpuscular volume	< 90 fl	1
No prior stem cell or organ transplant	–	1
Platelet count	< 30,000/mm³	1
Presence of hemolysis	Either • Retic > 2.5%, or • Undetectable haptoglobin, or indirect bilirubin > 2 mg/dl	1

[a] Scores can be low risk (0–4), intermediate risk (5), or high risk (6–7).

Note. Based on information from Jamme & Rondeau, 2017.

V. Differential diagnosis (see Table 130-4)

VI. Treatment (Dane & Chaturvedi, 2018; Estcourt, 2019; Joly et al., 2019; Poullin et al., 2019; Tsai, 2019)
  A. The mainstay of treatment for TTP is plasma exchange as soon as possible in the acute phase, a procedure in which the patient's plasma is exchanged with donor plasma.
    1. If the procedure is performed early, a majority of patients will enter into remission.
    2. Plasma exchange reverses the platelet consumption responsible for the thrombus formation and symptoms characteristic of this disorder.
    3. Treatment should be continued daily until platelet count maintains at least 150,000/mm³ for three days.
  B. Corticosteroids (e.g., high-dose methylprednisolone 1,000 mg daily for three days or prednisone 1 mg/kg daily) are used to suppress autoantibodies, inhibiting ADAMTS13. The dose of prednisone varies and is titrated according to platelet recovery (see Appendix K).
  C. Immunosuppressants (e.g., rituximab, cyclosporine, vincristine) may be added to plasma exchange for patients with severe ADAMTS13 deficiency who are at high risk for relapse or if platelet counts fail to increase with plasma exchange.
  D. Caplacizumab (formerly ALX-0081) is an anti–von Willebrand factor monoclonal antibody that inhibits the interaction between ultra-large von Willebrand factor multimers and platelets, preventing the consumption of platelets and the development of microvascular thrombi.
    1. It has been shown to reduce the amount of time that patients are thrombocytopenic and has been shown to reduce TTP-related mortality.
    2. It is often reserved for patients who present with severe features of TTP, such as neurologic abnormalities and high PLASMIC score.
  E. Platelet transfusions: It is unclear whether donor platelet infusions will harm patients, yet platelet transfusions should be avoided after the diagnosis is confirmed.
    1. Platelet transfusion may lead to new or worsening neurologic symptoms and AKI.
    2. AKI is caused by the production of new or expanding microvascular thrombi as the infused platelets are consumed.

   3. However, a platelet transfusion may be necessary if bleeding is noted.
F. Patient education: Patients are at risk for spontaneous bleeding because of thrombocytopenia and should take appropriate precautions, including the following.
   1. Avoid contact sports or activities.
   2. Avoid heavy lifting.
   3. Avoid over-the-counter medications such as ASA and NSAIDs (e.g., ibuprofen,
      naproxen sodium), which may interfere with normal platelet function (see Appen-
      dix E).
   4. Assess whether the patient is at risk for falls, and discuss precautions.
      a) Wear well-fitting shoes; remove throw rugs and obstructive objects within the
         home.
      b) Walk cautiously and change positions slowly.

VII. Follow-up (Dane & Chaturvedi, 2018)
   A. Short term
      1. Hgb, hematocrit, and platelet counts need to be monitored on a daily basis during
         acute phase. Once these levels begin to stabilize, the patient can be monitored twice
         weekly.
      2. Plasmapheresis will be tapered after two days of normal platelet counts.
   B. Long term
      1. Relapses occur most often within the first year of initial treatment; subsequently,
         patients need to be monitored closely with platelet counts.
         a) Patients with ADAMTS13 deficiency are more likely to relapse than those who
            do not have ADAMTS13 deficiency.
         b) The estimated relapse rate in ADAMTS13 deficiency is approximately 41% at
            7.5 years.

TABLE 130-4   Differential Diagnosis of Thrombotic Thrombocytopenia Purpura

Disorder	Description
Autoimmune disorders	Patients with systemic lupus erythematosus and antiphospholipid antibody syndrome may have anemia and thrombocytopenia.
Hemolytic uremic syndrome	A similar thrombotic microangiopathy occurs in which patients have hemolytic anemia, thrombocytopenia, and renal failure. It usually occurs in older adults and younger children (< 5 years). Patients most commonly have symptoms of abdominal pain and diarrhea (from hemorrhagic enterocolitis) caused by Shiga toxin–producing bacteria (most commonly *Escherichia coli*).
Heparin-induced thrombocytopenia	Thrombosis occurs in large veins, thrombocytopenia.
Immune thrombocytopenic purpura	Patients develop thrombocytopenia (without anemia or hemolysis) through the production of antibodies against platelets.
Paroxysmal nocturnal hemoglobinuria	It is a hematopoietic stem cell disorder in which complement regulatory proteins are lacking; thrombosis occurs in large vessels.
Systemic blood infection	Patients with sepsis may develop microangiopathic anemia, thrombocytopenia, and fever that may never convert to thrombotic thrombocytopenia purpura, which requires treatment.

Note. Based on information from Joly et al., 2017, 2019; Scully, 2019.

VIII. Referrals
   A. Hematologists and advanced practice nurses are well poised to diagnose, treat, and monitor patients with TTP. Prompt referrals can expedite appropriate diagnosis and treatment.
   B. Neurologists should be considered to evaluate neurologic findings.

References

Brierley, C.K., & Pavord, S. (2018). Autoimmune cytopenias and thrombotic thrombocytopenic purpura. *Clinical Medicine, 18*(4), 335–339. https://doi.org/10.7861/clinmedicine.18-4-335

Chiasakul, T., & Cuker, A. (2018). Clinical and laboratory diagnosis of TTP: An integrated approach. *Hematology: American Society of Hematology Educational Program Book, 2018,* 530–538. https://doi.org/10.1182/asheducation-2018.1.530

Dane, K., & Chaturvedi, S. (2018). Beyond plasma exchange: Novel therapies for thrombotic thrombocytopenic purpura. *Hematology: American Society of Hematology Educational Program Book, 2018,* 539–547. https://doi.org/10.1182/asheducation-2018.1.539

Estcourt, L.J. (2019). Caplacizumab treatment for acquired thrombotic thrombocytopenic purpura (HERCULES trial). *Transfusion Medicine, 29*(3), 146–148. https://doi.org/10.1111/tme.12615

Fogarty, P.F., & Dunbar, C.E. (2013). Thrombocytopenia. In G.P. Rodgers, & N.S. Young (Eds.), *The Bethesda handbook of clinical hematology* (3rd ed., pp. 269–284). Lippincott Williams and Wilkins.

Jamme, M., & Rondeau, E. (2017). The PLASMIC score for thrombotic thrombocytopenic purpura. *Lancet Haematology, 4*(4), e148–e149. https://doi.org/10.1016/S2352-3026(17)30024-8

Joly, B.S., Coppo, P., & Veyradier, A. (2017). Thrombotic thrombocytopenic purpura. *Blood, 129*(21), 2836–2846. https://doi.org/10.1182/blood-2016-10-709857

Joly, B.S., Coppo, P., & Veyradier, A. (2019). An update on pathogenesis and diagnosis of thrombotic thrombocytopenic purpura. *Expert Review in Hematology, 12*(6), 383–395. https://doi.org/10.1080/17474086.2019.1611423

Poullin, P., Bornet, C., Veyradier, A., & Coppo, P. (2019). Caplacizumab to treat immune-mediated thrombotic thrombocytopenic purpura. *Drugs Today, 55*(6), 367–376. https://doi.org/10.1358/dot.2019.55.6.2989843

Sadler, J.E. (2017). Pathophysiology of thrombotic thrombocytopenic purpura. *Blood, 130*(10), 1181–1188. https://doi.org/10.1182/blood-2017-04-636431

Scully, M. (2019). Hereditary thrombotic thrombocytopenic purpura. *Haematologica, 104*(10), 1916–1918. https://doi.org/10.3324/haematol.2019.225896

Tsai, H.-M. (2019). Thrombotic thrombocytopenic purpura: Beyond empiricism and plasma exchange. *American Journal of Medicine, 132*(9), 1032–1037. https://doi.org/10.1016/j.amjmed.2019.03.009

Neurologic

CHAPTER 131

Ataxia/Incoordination

Christa Seligman, MSN, APRN, AGNP-C

I. Definitions (Akbar & Ashizawa, 2015; Buckley et al., 2018; López et al., 2019; Marcus et al., 2019)
   A. Ataxia: Impairment of gait, hand incoordination, tremors with movement without weakness
   B. Incoordination: Inability to produce voluntary, harmonious, rhythmic muscular coordination

II. Physiology/Pathophysiology (Akbar & Ashizawa, 2015; Ashizawa & Xia, 2016; Delatycki & Bidichandani, 2019; Jahn et al., 2019; Kelly & Shanley, 2016; Kuo, 2019)
   A. Normal
      1. The corticospinal (i.e., cerebral cortex and spinal cord) and corticobulbar (i.e., cerebral cortex and upper portion of brain stem) tracts are the most important pathways used in the initiation of voluntary motor movements. The corticospinal and corticobulbar tracts are referred to as the *pyramidal system* because these tracts are present in the medullary pyramid.
      2. The extrapyramidal system comprises portions of the brain that contribute to motor control, which are not part of the corticospinal–pyramidal tract. These involve the reticular formation of the brain stem, vestibular nuclei, and red nuclei.
      3. Voluntary movements require contraction and relaxation of muscles in proper sequence.
         a) The mechanisms for programming these complex events include the posterior parietal lobe, supplementary motor cortex, and the premotor cortex.
         b) The total integration of these movements is called *coordination*, partially mediated through efferent and afferent tracts of the cerebellum.
      4. The pattern generator for locomotion is contained within the neural circuitry of the spinal cord.
         a) Separate pattern generators exist for each limb.
         b) The activity of these generators allows for coordinated and precise movements of limbs.
      5. Sensory subsystems involved with coordinated movements include the vestibular apparatus and proprioceptive mechanisms.
   B. Pathophysiology
      1. The hierarchic organization of the motor system can be demonstrated by the effects of lesions at different levels of the neuroaxis (i.e., brain and spinal cord).
      2. A lesion can result in a particular effect by abolishing functions or allowing an action to occur by removing an inhibitory influence.
      3. Genetic abnormalities may involve mitochondrial dysfunction, oxidative stress, abnormal mechanisms of DNA repair, and abnormal cytoskeletal proteins.

III. Clinical features: Ataxia are a group of neurodegenerative disorders characterized by cerebellar dysfunction causing irregularities in voluntary movements. Cerebellar lesions produce symptoms on the ipsilateral (same) side of the lesion, in contrast to cerebral lesions, which produce contralateral effects. Inherited ataxia may be autosomal dominant, autosomal recessive, or maternal inheritance, with more than 30 disorders recognized. Acute ataxia occurring over a period of minutes to hours is considered a medical emergency. The most common causes are toxins, medications, infections, or ischemic stroke. Subacute ataxia occurs over days to weeks. Chronic ataxia occurs over years and is the most common presentation of hereditary forms (Akbar & Ashizawa, 2015; Baker, 2018; Delatycki & Bidichandani, 2019; Kuo, 2019; Marcus et al., 2019; O'Riordan et al., 2017; Pfieffer et al., 2019; Tan et al., 2019).

A. Etiology
   1. Malignancy
   2. Vestibular disorders
   3. Fluid and electrolyte imbalance
   4. Infection of CNS
   5. Chronic disease affecting CNS: Stroke, diabetes
   6. Drug induced
   7. Aging
   8. Metabolic disorders
   9. Genetic disorders

B. History
   1. History of cancer and cancer treatment
   2. Current medications: Prescribed, over the counter
   3. History of presenting symptoms: Precipitating factors, onset, location, duration, associated symptoms (e.g., change in hearing or vision, headaches, paresthesia, hemiparesis, weakness of extremities)
   4. Changes in ADLs
   5. Recent or past trauma

C. Signs and symptoms
   1. Disequilibrium: Sensation of feeling drunk, unsteady when standing, imbalance, sensation of "room spinning"
   2. Vomiting that may not be preceded by nausea, especially with positional change
   3. Dysarthria: Lack of coordination to advance and adjust intensity and the speed of sounds, resulting in unintelligible speech (i.e., defective speech)
   4. Hemiparesis: One-sided paralysis
   5. Diplopia: Double vision
   6. Cerebellar nystagmus: Tremor of the eyes when asked to fix the sight to one side or the other
   7. Blurred vision
   8. Light headedness

D. Physical examination
   1. Vital signs: Assess blood pressure for orthostatic hypotension (i.e., decreased systolic blood pressure) by at least 20 mm Hg or an increase of diastolic blood pressure by 10 mm Hg with positional change from lying to sitting to standing; allow three minutes in the changed position to allow stabilization of the blood pressure prior to rechecking.
   2. HEENT
      a) Tympanic membrane observation for bulging, erythema, or loss of landmarks to rule out OM, cerumen impaction, and foreign body

       b) Visual field defects, presence of nystagmus, extraocular muscle function, and ophthalmoscopic evaluation with attention to presence of papilledema that may be indicative of increased ICP

       c) Dix-Hallpike test to evaluate for benign paroxysmal positional vertigo if clinical suspicion.

   3. Neurologic: To determine location of lesion causing ataxia

       a) Mental status: Patient's awareness, orientation, and cognitive abilities

       b) Motor (see Appendices A and D)

          (1) Strength: All muscle groups for symmetry and tremor

          (2) Coordination: Cadence and tremor

             (a) Dysdiadochokinesia: The inability to perform rapid, rhythmic, alternating hand movements

             (b) Dysmetria: Characterized by past pointing; motor control system fails to predict where the body parts are during rapid movements causing poor coordination.

                i. Finger-to-finger test

                ii. Finger-to-nose test

                iii. Heel-to-shin test

             (c) Gait for shuffling, widely placed feet, or toe walking and ability to execute tandem gait

                i. Cerebellar ataxia: Feet wide-based, staggering, swaying of the trunk, unsteady wide gait

                ii. Sensory ataxia: Wide-based gait, feet forward and outward, which brings heels down first, then toes; positive Romberg test

                iii. Ataxia: Uncontrolled falling

          (3) Balance

             (a) Romberg test

             (b) Heel-to-toe test: Tandem gait

       c) Sensory: Loss of proprioception

          (1) Pinprick sensation or light touch

          (2) Two-point discrimination or vibration

       d) Evaluation of cortical sensory function or stereognosis: Place a familiar object in the patient's hand to assess ability to recognize objects by touch.

       e) Reflexes

          (1) Test each reflex, comparing response to corresponding side.

          (2) Absent reflex indicates neuropathy or lower motor neuron disorder.

          (3) Hyperactive reflex indicates upper motor neuron disorder.

IV. Diagnostic tests (Ashizawa & Xia, 2016; Jahn et al., 2019; Kuo, 2019; López et al., 2019; Tan et al., 2019)

   A. Laboratory

      1. Comprehensive metabolic panel, including calcium and magnesium, BUN, and creatinine, to assess for dehydration or electrolyte imbalance that can result in neurologic and muscular dysfunction

      2. CBC to assess for anemia

      3. Vitamin B_{12} level to assess for deficiency

      4. Coagulation profile (e.g., cardiolipin, antithrombin III, fibrinogen) if cerebral thrombosis is suspected

      5. Iron dysregulation (ferritin): Increased iron in the brain has been implicated in some movement disorders.

6. Syphilis titers, if indicated
7. Lyme disease, if indicated
   B. Radiology: CT and MRI
1. If brain metastases are suspected, a head CT scan/MRI is appropriate.
2. If another condition (e.g., superior sulcus tumor) is causing weakness, CT scan of the neck and chest will be helpful.
3. Spine imaging should be considered if weakness is present with associated loss of reflexes to affected area.
   C. Other
1. Audiologic evaluation if vestibular cause is suspected
2. Angiography if vascular etiology is suspected
3. Lumbar puncture, if indicated, for bacteria, fungal, or viral cultures
4. Genetic testing, as indicated
5. Electrooculography to evaluate for ataxia disorder

V. Differential diagnosis (Akbar & Ashizawa, 2015; Ashizawa & Xia, 2016; Baker, 2018; Delatycki & Bidichandani, 2019; Marcus et al., 2019; Tan et al., 2019)
   A. Malignancy related
1. Brain or spinal cord metastasis
2. Bone or soft tissue metastases causing nerve root compression in spine
3. Paraneoplastic syndromes (see Appendix M)
   a) SIADH (see Chapter 95)
   b) Hypercalcemia (see Chapter 152)
   c) Eaton-Lambert syndrome (see Appendix M)
   d) Hypercoagulable state causing thrombosis of cerebral vascular structures (see Chapter 122)
4. Primary malignancy of the nervous system
   B. Vestibular disorders, including acoustic neuroma
   C. Fluid and electrolyte imbalance
1. Dehydration
2. Hypernatremia (see Chapter 155), hypophosphatemia (see Chapter 156), hypo/hyperkalemia (see Chapter 153)
   D. Iatrogenic
1. Drug induced: Steroids (e.g., proximal muscle weakness), opioids, antibiotics (e.g., aminoglycosides), antiseizure medications (e.g., phenytoin, phenobarbital, carbamazepine)
2. Chemotherapy: High-dose cytarabine, ifosfamide, 5-fluorouracil (rare), vinca alkaloids, busulfan
   E. Chronic illness and disorders: It is more prominent in older adults. Multiple etiologies can cause balance disorders or promote degeneration of the CNS (e.g., hypertension, diabetes, heart disease, joint/muscle problems causing generalized weakness).
   F. Infectious disorders of the nervous system
1. Meningitis (see Chapter 141)
2. Encephalitis
3. Reye syndrome
   G. Hypothyroidism (see Chapter 158)
   H. Alcoholic cerebellar degeneration
   I. Postviral complications; status post-HZV (see Chapter 22)
   J. Drug abuse
   K. Tabes dorsalis: Sclerosis of posterior columns of the spinal cord caused by *Treponema pallidum* (tertiary syphilis)

L. Connective tissue disease: RA (see Chapter 108), SLE (see Chapter 110), cerebral vasculitis
M. Vitamin deficiencies: Vitamin B_1, vitamin B_{12} (see Chapter 115), vitamin E
N. Whipple disease: Multisystem infectious disorder; suspected in patients with AIDS
O. Cerebral vascular accident (see Chapter 146)
P. Cerebral palsy
Q. Neurodegenerative diseases: Multiple sclerosis, Parkinson disease, Alzheimer disease
R. Inherited genetic disorders: Friedreich ataxia (most common hereditary ataxia), ataxia–telangiectasia, Huntington disease
S. Traumatic brain injury

VI. Treatment (Baker, 2018; Jahn et al., 2019; Stephen et al., 2019; Tan et al., 2019)
A. Refer to appropriate medical diagnosis chapter for treatment options.
B. Prednisone may be used for immune-mediated or drug-induced ataxia.
C. Educate patients regarding safety to prevent falls and maintain mobility.
   1. Canes and walkers have been shown to improve balance and mobility.
   2. A qualified physical therapist will evaluate the patient for the proper type of assistive device needed and will train on the use of the device.

VII. Follow-up: Management is etiology dependent. Refer to appropriate medical diagnosis chapter.

VIII. Referrals (Kelly & Shanley, 2016; Kuo, 2019; Stephen et al., 2019)
A. Physical or occupational therapist: For evaluation of assistive devices and rehabilitation
B. Exercise program: Focusing on balance, mobility, and exercise; beneficial for effects persisting for more than one year after the intervention
C. Genetic counselor: For suspected inherited ataxia
D. Neurologist: If ataxia caused by cerebrovascular accident or neurodegenerative disease

The author would like to acknowledge Laurie Rice, RN, MSN, ANP-BC, for her contribution to this chapter that remains unchanged from the previous edition of this book.

References

Akbar, U., & Ashizawa, T. (2015). Ataxia. *Neurologic Clinics, 33*(1), 225–248. https://doi.org/10.1016/j.ncl.2014.09.004

Ashizawa, T., & Xia, G. (2016). Ataxia. *Continuum, 22*(4), 1208–1226. https://doi.org/10.1212/CON.0000000000000362

Baker, J.M. (2018). Gait disorders. *American Journal of Medicine, 131*(6), 602–607. https://doi.org/10.1016/j.amjmed.2017.11.051

Buckley, E., Mazzà, C., & McNeill, A. (2018). A systematic review of the gait characteristics associated with cerebellar ataxia. *Gait and Posture, 60,* 154–163. https://doi.org/10.1016/j.gaitpost.2017.11.024

Delatycki, M.G., & Bidichandani, S.I. (2019). Friedreich ataxia—Pathogenesis and implications for therapies. *Neurobiology of Disease, 132,* 104606. https://doi.org/10.1016/j.nbd.2019.104606

Jahn, K., Freiberger, E., Eskofier, B.M., Bollheimer, C., & Klucken, J. (2019). Balance and mobility in geriatric patients: Assessment and treatment of neurological aspects. *Zeitschrift für Gerontologie und Geriatrie, 52*(4), 316–323. https://doi.org/10.1007/s00391-019-01561-z

Kelly, G., & Shanley, J. (2016). Rehabilitation of ataxic gait following cerebellar lesions: Applying theory to practice. *Physiotherapy Theory and Practice, 32*(6), 430–437. https://doi.org/10.1080/09593985.2016.1202364

Kuo, S.-H. (2019). Ataxia. *Continuum, 25*(4), 1036–1054. https://doi.org/10.1212/CON.0000000000000753

López, A., Ferrero, F., & Postolache, O. (2019). An affordable method for evaluation of ataxic disorders based on electrooculography. *Sensors, 19*(17), 3756. https://doi.org/10.3390/s19173756

Marcus, H.J., Paine, H., Sargeant, M., Wolstenholme, S., Collins, K., Marroney, N., … Seemungal, B.M. (2019). Vestibular dysfunction in acute traumatic brain injury. *Journal of Neurology, 266*(10), 2430–2433. https://doi.org/10.1007/s00415-019-09403-z

O'Riordan, S., Vasilakis, N., Hussain, L., Schoo, R., Whitney, J., Windsor, J., ... Martin, F. (2017). Measurement of lying and standing blood pressure in hospital. *Nursing Older People, 29*(8), 20–26. https://doi.org/10.7748/nop.2017.e961

Pfeffer, M.L., Anthamatten, A., & Glassford, M. (2019). Assessment and treatment of dizziness and vertigo. *Nurse Practitioner, 44*(10), 29–36. https://doi.org/10.1097/01.NPR.0000579744.73514.4b

Stephen, C.D., Brizzi, K.T., Bouffard, M.A., Gomery, P., Sullivan, S.L., Mello, J., ... Schmahmann, J.D. (2019). The comprehensive management of cerebellar ataxia in adults. *Current Treatment Options in Neurology, 21*(3), 9. https://doi.org/10.1007/s11940-019-0549-2

Tan, Y.Y., Rannikmäe, K., & Steele, N. (2019). Case report: Immune-mediated cerebellar ataxia secondary to anti-PD-L1 treatment for lung cancer. *International Journal of Neuroscience, 129*(12), 1223–1225. https://doi.org/10.1080/00207454.2019.1655013

CHAPTER 132

Blurred Vision

Tracy C. Wyant, DNP, AOCN®, CHPN, GERO-BC, CPPS, EBP-C

I. Definition: Loss of sharpness of vision and the inability to see fine details (Medline Plus, 2018)

II. Physiology/Pathophysiology (Chang, 2018; Riordan-Eva, 2018; Sen, 2017)
   A. Normal
      1. As light enters the eye through the pupil, it passes through the lens and is projected on the retina at the back of the eye.
      2. Extraocular muscles move the eyeball in the orbits and allow the image to be focused on the central retina or fovea.
      3. Visual acuity is the eye's ability to detect fine details and is the quantitative measure of the eye's ability to see an in-focus image at a certain distance.
      4. The standard for normal visual acuity is scored as a fraction based on the testing distance (generally 20/20) and refers to the ability to resolve a spatial pattern separated by a visual angle of one minute of arc.
   B. Pathophysiology: The result of disorders along the visual neurologic pathway that may affect the ocular muscle, cranial nerves, or retinal function, resulting in refractive error or opacification of the usually transparent ocular media due to edema, bleeding, or cataract formation

III. Clinical features: Blurred vision is considered underreported, not frequently assessed, and associated with many cancer therapies and other diseases. Some agents cause drying of the eye, which can result in blurred vision (Chang, 2018; Dhingra et al., 2019; Heckmann et al., 2018; Kunkler et al., 2018; Rowland & Lee, 2019).
   A. Etiology
      1. Ocular trauma
      2. Hereditary diseases
      3. Hematologic and vascular diseases
      4. Ischemic and inflammatory diseases
      5. Stroke
      6. Demyelinating disease
      7. Brain tumor
   B. History
      1. History of cancer and cancer treatment
      2. Current medications: Prescribed, over the counter, supplements
      3. History of presenting symptoms: Location, precipitating factors, onset, duration, frequency, associated symptoms (e.g., diplopia, unstable visual images [floaters], headache, facial sensations, weakness, ataxia, aphasia)
      4. Changes in ADLs

     5. Past medical and family history: Ocular trauma or surgery; demyelinating disease; ischemic, hematologic, vascular, or inflammatory disorders; trauma to eye

     6. Social history: Exposure to toxic substances, tobacco use, alcohol use, illicit drug use

  C. Signs and symptoms

     1. Blurred vision in central or peripheral vision; unilateral or bilateral (monocular or binocular)

     2. Headache, dizziness

     3. May be reported as mild, moderate, or severe

  D. Physical examination: Visual deficit evaluation using a comprehensive neuro-ophthalmology examination

     1. Eye

        a) Visual acuity testing: Snellen chart to identify approximate visual acuity deficit without visual apparatus (e.g., glasses, contacts)

        b) Visual field testing to evaluate central and peripheral visual loss

        c) Ophthalmoscopy to detect primary ocular abnormalities, such as cataract, papilledema (caused by active inflammation or passive congestion; associated with increased ICP), or optic atrophy

     2. Neurologic (see Appendix A)

        a) Oculomotor (cranial nerve III): Lesions result in partial adduction (i.e., inability to adduct, elevate, and depress the eye); ptosis and nonreactive pupil may occur.

        b) Trochlear (cranial nerve IV): Lesions result in defective depression of the adducted eye.

        c) Abducens (cranial nerve VI): Lesions result in lateral rectus palsy with impaired abduction of the affected eye.

IV. Diagnostic tests (Chang, 2018; Foroozan, 2018)

  A. Laboratory: Hematologic studies depend on suspected cause of the blurred vision.

  B. Radiology

     1. MRI or CT scan of the head to evaluate for tumor or lesion of the brain

     2. MRI of the eye/orbit to evaluate for tumor or lesion of optical apparatus

  C. Other: Angiography, venography, and ultrasonography may be helpful. Diagnostic vitrectomy may be considered if infiltrates are suspected.

V. Differential diagnosis (Dhingra et al., 2019; Foroozan, 2018; Heckmann et al., 2018; NCCN, 2021; Yust-Katz et al., 2020)

  A. Hereditary disease

     1. Optic atrophy

     2. Leber disease

  B. Demyelinating disease

     1. Optic neuritis

     2. Multiple sclerosis

     3. Neuromyelitis

  C. Ischemic disease

     1. Hypotension (see Chapter 48)

     2. Transient ischemic attacks in adults and children

     3. Temporal arteritis

     4. Systemic disease–related ischemia: Diabetes mellitus (see Chapter 151)

     5. Fibromuscular dysplasia

     6. Dysautonomia

  D. Hematologic and vascular disease

      1. Chronic anemia (see Chapter 113)

      2. Vascular hypotension

      3. Blood dyscrasia

      4. Cortical blindness caused by arteriosclerosis, carbon monoxide poisoning, trauma, neoplasm, or infection

      5. Intracranial aneurysm

      6. Migraine headaches (see Chapter 137)

E. Inflammatory disease

      1. Intraocular or orbital inflammation

      2. HIV/AIDS

      3. Lyme disease (see Chapter 104)

      4. Radiation retinopathy

      5. Intracranial inflammation

      6. Toxoplasmosis

      7. Uveitis

F. Tumor

      1. Benign intraocular tumor

         a) Uveal nevus

         b) Melanocytoma

         c) Choroidal hemangioma or osteoma

      2. Malignant intraocular tumor

         a) Uveal melanoma

         b) Uveal lymphoma

         c) Uveal metastasis

      3. Leukemia and multiple myeloma: Increased blood viscosity results in vascular occlusive disease.

      4. Extraocular tumor

         a) May cause increased ICP or optic chiasma compression

         b) Epidermal neoplasms (e.g., seborrheic or actinic keratosis, melanoma, basal or squamous cell carcinoma) near eye with structural obstruction or disturbance

      5. Paraneoplastic syndrome (see Appendix M): May result in peripheral neuropathy, cerebellar degeneration, or brain stem and limbic encephalitis

G. Toxic agents

      1. Tobacco

      2. Alcohol and methyl alcohol

      3. Cocaine

      4. Lead

      5. Ketogenic diets

      6. Drug induced

         a) Anticholinergics

         b) Antiepileptics

         c) First-generation antihistamines

         d) Antimalarials

         e) Corticosteroids

         f) Cyclooxygenase-2 inhibitors

         g) Ethambutol

         h) Indomethacin

         i) Phenothiazines

         j) Thiazide diuretics

    k) Chemotherapy, targeted therapy, and immunotherapy drugs
        (1) Bexarotene
        (2) Busulfan
        (3) Capecitabine
        (4) Carmustine
        (5) Cisplatin
        (6) Epirubicin
        (7) 5-Fluorouracil
        (8) IFN
        (9) Isotretinoin
        (10) Methotrexate
        (11) Mitomycin C
        (12) Protein kinase inhibitors: Mitogen-activated protein kinase, ALK
        (13) Tamoxifen
        (14) Trastuzumab
        (15) Tretinoin

  7. Trauma
  8. Computer vision syndrome (digital eye strain): Ocular (surface conditions or accommodative spasms) or extraocular (ergonomic) etiologies
  9. Opacities of the transparent ocular media
  10. Cataracts (see Chapter 7)
  11. Dislocation of the lens
  12. Vitreous degeneration
  13. Hemorrhage
  14. Corneal opacities and ulcer
  15. Retinal disease
  16. Foreign body in the eye

VI. Treatment: Dependent on accurate diagnosis and treatment of the underlying cause

VII. Follow-up: Dependent on underlying cause of the blurred vision and its treatment

VIII. Referral: Ophthalmologist for complete ophthalmologic evaluation

The author would like to acknowledge Giselle J. Moore-Higgs, ARNP, PhD, AOCN®, for her contribution to this chapter that remains unchanged from the previous edition of this book.

References

Chang, D.F. (2018). Ophthalmologic examination. In P. Riordan-Eva & J.J. Augsburger (Eds.), *Vaughan and Asbury's general ophthalmology* (19th ed., pp. 27–64). McGraw-Hill Education.

Dhingra, D., Kaur, S., & Ram, J. (2019). Illicit drugs: Effects on eye. *Indian Journal of Medical Research, 150*(3), 228–238. https://doi.org/10.4103/ijmr.IJMR_1210_17

Foroozan, R. (2018). Neuroimaging. In R. Foroozan & M. Vaphiades (Eds.), *Kline's neuro-ophthalmology review manual* (8th ed., pp. 273–279). Slack.

Heckmann, J.G., Vachalova, I., Lang, C.J.G., & Pitz, S. (2018). Neuro-ophthalmology at the bedside: A clinical guide. *Journal of Neurosciences in Rural Practice, 9*(1), 561 573. https://doi.org/10.4103/jnrp.jnrp_145_18

Kunkler, A.L., Binkley, E.M., Mantopoulos, D., Hendershot, A.J., Ohr, M.P., Kendra, K.L., ... Cebulla, C.M. (2018). Known and novel ocular toxicities of biologics, targeted agents, and traditional chemotherapeutics. *Graefe's Archive for Clinical and Experimental Ophthalmology, 257*(8), 1771–1781. https://doi.org/10.1007/s00417-019-04337-8

Medline Plus. (2018, August 28). Vision problems. https://medlineplus.gov/ency/article/003029.htm

National Comprehensive Cancer Network. (2021). *NCCN Clinical Practice Guidelines in Oncology (NCCN Guidelines®): Management of immunotherapy-related toxicities* [v.3.2021]. https://www.nccn.org/professionals/physician_gls/pdf/immunotherapy.pdf

Riordan-Eva, P. (2018). Optics and refraction. In P. Riordan-Eva & J.J. Augsburger (Eds.), *Vaughan and Asbury's general ophthalmology* (19th ed., pp. 403–471). McGraw-Hill Education.

Rowland, C.J., & Lee, L.R. (2019). Ocular causes of visual distortions. *Australian Journal of General Practice, 48*(8), 525–530. https://doi.org/10.31128/AJGP-04-19-4904

Sen, N. (2017). An insight into the vision impairment following traumatic brain injury. *Neurochemistry International, 111*, 103–107. https://doi.org/10.1016/j.neuint.2017.01.019

Yust-Katz, S., Khagi, S., & Gilbert, M.R. (2020). Neurologic complications. In J.E. Niederhuber, J.O. Armitage, J.H. Doroshow, M.B. Kastan, & J.E. Tepper (Eds.), *Abeloff's Clinical Oncology* (6th ed., pp. 688–706). Elsevier.

CHAPTER 133

Confusion/Delirium

Elena C. Prendergast, DNP, APRN, FNP-C, ACHPN,
and Constance Dahlin, MSN, ANP-BC, ACHPN, FPCN, FAAN

I. Definition (American Psychiatric Association, 2013; NCCN, 2021)
   A. An alteration in attention that includes reduced ability to sustain, direct, focus, or shift attention and diminished awareness or orientation to environment
   B. Acute confusional state with auditory and visual hallucinations or delusions
   C. Disturbance of consciousness accompanied by a change in cognition that cannot be better accounted for by a preexisting or evolving dementia
   D. Imprecise terminology; may be referred to as *acute confusion* or *agitation*

II. Physiology/Pathophysiology (American Psychiatric Association, 2013; Bush et al., 2018; Caplan, 2018; Fernandez-Robles et al., 2018; Mulkey et al., 2018)
   A. Normal: Balanced levels of neurotransmitters are present within the brain. Three types of delirium exist.
      1. Hypoactive: Patient is quiet.
      2. Hyperactive: Patient is agitated or restless.
      3. Mixed: Patient may fluctuate in activity and agitation.
   B. Pathophysiology
      1. Pathophysiology is not well understood, but delirium signals serious illness. In delirium, disturbances occur in the balance of neurotransmitters.
      2. Delirium is thought to involve increased levels of neurotransmitters in the cortical and subcortical areas of the brain.
      3. Neurotransmitters involved include dopamine, serotonin, gamma-aminobutyric acid, beta-endorphins, and acetylcholine.
      4. It may result from an excess of cytokines, cortisol, or glutamates stimulated by body system failure.

III. Clinical features: Confusion and delirium are common in patients with cancer, with incidence ranging widely at 8%–45% in ambulatory patients and up to 88% at end of life. Delirium is one of the most prevalent and disabling conditions impacting older adults in hospitals and long-term care facilities. Confusion and delirium are associated with many complex underlying medical conditions and can be difficult to recognize (Blazer, 2018; Burhenn, 2016; Bush et al., 2018; Caplan, 2018; Folstein et al., 1975; Hshieh et al., 2018; Loving & Dahlin, 2019; Mulkey et al., 2019; Mulkey et al., 2018; NCCN, 2021; Nasreddine et al., 2005).
   A. Risk factors
      1. Cancer
      2. Cancer therapies
      3. Electrolyte imbalances

      4. Polypharmacy

      5. Immobility

      6. Stress

B. Etiology: Numerous potential causes; may be multifactorial

      1. Uncontrolled pain

      2. Infections: Sepsis, UTI, respiratory infection, brain involvement

      3. Electrolyte imbalances and dehydration: Potassium, sodium, calcium

      4. Nutritional deficiencies: Thiamine, folate, vitamin B_{12}

      5. Cancer process: Metastasis to brain or brain lesion

      6. Neurologic process: Seizures, encephalopathy

      7. Medication induced: Steroids, opioids, anticholinergics, antihistamines, sedatives, benzodiazepines, voriconazole

      8. Substance overdose or withdrawal: Opioids, benzodiazepines, alcohol, amphetamines

      9. Chemotherapy- and immunotherapy-induced examples: Vincristine, ifosfamide, methotrexate IFN

     10. Organ failure: Hepatic encephalopathy

     11. Endocrine issues related to diabetes, hypothyroidism

     12. Sleep deprivation

     13. Sensory deprivation

     14. Changes in environment

     15. Constipation/obstruction

     16. Hypoxia

     17. Fever

     18. End of life

C. History

      1. History of cancer and cancer treatment

      2. Current medications: Prescribed, over the counter

      3. History of presenting delirium symptoms: Precipitating and alleviating factors, onset, duration, associated symptoms (e.g., sleep changes, behavioral changes)

      4. Changes in ADLs

      5. Past medical history: Depressive episodes, insomnia, psychiatric problems

D. Signs and symptoms

      1. Acute onset with a fluctuating course indicative of the presence of an underlying organic cause

      2. Reduced sensorium and disorientation

      3. Attention deficit: Distractibility

      4. Anxiety

      5. Emotional lability

      6. Restlessness, agitation

      7. Hypersensitivity to light and sound

      8. Cognitive or perceptual disturbances: Delusions, hallucination, paranoia

      9. Memory changes

     10. Personality changes: Frequent

     11. Sleep–wake cycle alteration

     12. Hyperactive: Increased activity; restlessness, pacing, picking

     13. Hypoactive: Decreased activity; slowing, increased somnolence

     14. Mixed hyperactive with hypoactive

E. Physical examination

      1. General observation of movement, behavior, and appearance

2. Vital signs: Fever with infection
3. Integument: Sepsis, cardiac failure (e.g., cold, clammy skin), anticholinergic reaction (e.g., hot, flushed skin)
4. HEENT
   a) Chvostek sign indicating hypocalcemia (see Appendix D)
   b) Eye inspection
      (1) Scleral icterus indicating liver failure
      (2) Pinpointed pupils indicating opioid toxicity
      (3) Dilated pupils indicating anticholinergic toxicity
      (4) Papilledema indicating ICP
   c) Oral: Red, shiny tongue indicating nutritional deficits
5. Cardiac: Dysrhythmias with irregular heartbeat and heart failure
6. Pulmonary: Rales from heart failure and dullness from pneumonia
7. Abdominal
   a) Abdomen palpitation for stool indicating constipation
   b) Bladder palpitation to assess for urinary retention
   c) Rectum evaluation for impaction
8. Extremities
   a) Trousseau sign with hypocalcemia (see Appendix D)
   b) Tender, swollen calves with thiamine deficiency
   c) Asterixis with liver failure
9. Neurologic: To evaluate cognitive changes
   a) Gross motor examination to assess for cerebrovascular accident
   b) Ataxia from thiamine or vitamin B_{12} deficiency
   c) Myoclonus, tremor
10. Mental status
    a) Visuospatial/executive function: Have the patient draw a clock and connect dots.
    b) Orientation: Ask the patient to identify the day, month, year, season, and setting.
    c) Memory/recall: Name three items for the patient. Have the patient repeat to remember for later.
    d) Attention/calculation: Instruct the patient to count backward from 100 by serial 7s, and name patterns of numbers or pictures.
    e) Abstraction: Ask the patient to identify commonality between two words, such as banana and apple, sandal and boot, plane and train.
    f) Language: Instruct the patient to perform the following tasks.
       (1) Identify objects.
       (2) Follow a command.
       (3) Write a sentence.
       (4) Copy a sentence.

IV. Diagnostic studies (American Psychiatric Association, 2013; Blazer, 2018; Breitbart et al., 1997; Bush et al., 2018; Hshieh et al., 2018; Inouye et al., 1990; Loving & Dahlin, 2019; Mulkey et al., 2019; NCCN, 2021; Treacy et al., 2001)
   A. Laboratory
      1. CBC to evaluate for infection, anemia, and thrombocytopenia
      2. Electrolytes to evaluate for sodium, potassium, or calcium imbalances
      3. Folate and vitamin B_{12} to evaluate for nutritional deficiencies
      4. LFTs to evaluate for liver failure or insufficiency
      5. Urine culture to evaluate for infection
      6. BUN and creatinine to evaluate for renal failure and insufficiency

      7. Elevated ammonia level indicating encephalopathy

      8. Drug and alcohol screening to evaluate for toxic levels of illicit substances, alcohol, digoxin, lithium, tricyclic medications, or antiseizure medications

      9. Thyroid and adrenal function tests to evaluate for metabolic or endocrine cause

     10. Venereal Disease Research Laboratory test, nucleic acid hybridizations, nucleic acid amplification test, and cultures to evaluate for STIs

     11. HIV testing, as indicated

     12. PT, PTT, and INR to evaluate for DIC

     13. Glucose level to evaluate for hyperglycemia and hypoglycemia

  B. Radiology

      1. Chest x-ray to review for pneumonia, effusion, and heart abnormalities

      2. Head CT scan to evaluate for brain metastases or brain tumor if new onset

      3. Abdominal CT scan for severe nausea and vomiting and no bowel movements with question of obstruction

  C. Other

      1. Oxygen saturation to evaluate for hypoxia

      2. Lumbar puncture to determine CNS involvement or meningitis

  D. Assessment tools

      1. Confusion Assessment Measurement: 10-item scale administered by the clinician to assess nine domains of cognitive function

      2. Delirium Rating Scale: 10-item scale administered by the clinician to assess 10 elements of cognitive impairment

      3. Memorial Delirium Assessment Scale: 10-item scale administered by the clinician to assess cognition and measure severity of delirium

V. Differential diagnosis (American Psychiatric Association, 2013; Bush et al., 2018; Hshieh et al., 2018; Loving & Dahlin, 2019; NCCN, 2021)

  A. Uncontrolled pain or symptoms

  B. Medication induced: Opioids, steroids

  C. Medication withdrawal: Stimulants, alcohol, benzodiazepines

  D. Electrolyte imbalances: Sodium (see Chapter 155), potassium (see Chapter 153), calcium (see Chapter 152)

  E. Disease progression/process

  F. Neurologic condition: Brain lesion, meningitis (see Chapter 141), seizure (see Chapter 144), cerebrovascular accident (see Chapter 146), paraneoplastic neurologic syndrome (see Appendix M)

  G. Liver failure: Cirrhosis (see Chapter 69), liver metastasis

  H. Renal failure (see Chapter 86)

  I. Heart failure (see Chapter 42)

  J. Infection: Pneumonia (see Chapter 30), UTI (see Chapter 89)

  K. Sepsis

  L. DIC (see Chapter 120)

  M. Constipation/obstruction (see Chapters 55 and 67)

  N. Nutritional deficiencies: Vitamin B_{12} deficiency (see Chapter 115)

  O. Cancer therapy induced

  P. Sensory deprivation

  Q. Actively dying from system failure of advanced disease process

  R. Dehydration

  S. Fever (see Chapter 147)

  T. Hyperglycemia (see Chapter 151)

VI. Treatment (Boland et al., 2019; Burhenn, 2016; Bush et al., 2018; Caplan, 2018; Hshieh et al., 2018; Loving & Dahlin, 2019; NCCN, 2021)

 A. Recognize the emergent condition as frightening for patient and family.

 B. Correct underlying factors such as electrolyte imbalances with appropriate measures, including hydration (see Chapters 152–156).

 C. Discontinue problematic medications.

 D. Treat underlying pain. Consider opioid rotation (see Appendix F).

 E. Treat constipation (see Chapter 55).

 F. Treat infections, as appropriate (see Appendix C).

 G. Consider nutrition and hydration issues and manage based on the values and preferences of the patient and the stage of disease.

 H. Specific suggestions for the three types of delirium include the following.

  1. Hypoactive

   a) Treat reversible causes.

   b) Evaluate for metastases.

   c) Treat sepsis.

   d) Consider opioid rotation or decrease in opioids for older patients.

  2. Hyperactive: Pharmacologic treatment (see Table 133-1)

   a) Systematically discontinue all potential medications inducing delirium.

   b) Treat reversible causes.

TABLE 133-1 Common Medications for Delirium

Drug	Common Dosage and Route	Dose Range	Nursing Considerations
Anesthetic			
Propofol	1–3 mg/kg/hr is equivalent to about 10–70 mg/hr IV. Sedation may be initiated by infusing propofol at 100–150 mcg/kg/min (6–9 mg/kg/hr) for a period of 3–5 minutes and titrating to the desired clinical effect while closely monitoring respiratory function.	–	Work with interprofessional team of physicians, pharmacy, and advanced practice providers with competency in the administration of propofol. Propofol may cause an elevation of triglycerides; monitor for dyslipidemia.
Atypical Neuroleptics			
Aripiprazole	2–10 mg every 24 hrs PO Oral solution can be substituted for tablets on a per mg basis up to the 25 mg dose level. Patients receiving 30 mg tablets should receive 25 mg of the solution.	20–30 mg daily	Aripiprazole is used in hypoactive delirium.
Olanzapine	2.5–20 mg every 12–24 hrs PO	2.5–40 mg daily; 20 mg daily for treatment of schizophrenia; no well-established maximum for other approved indications	Olanzapine may worsen dementia.

(Continued on next page)

TABLE 133-1	Common Medications for Delirium *(Continued)*		
Drug	**Common Dosage and Route**	**Dose Range**	**Nursing Considerations**
Quetiapine	25–200 mg every 12–24 hrs PO	25–400 mg daily	Quetiapine is used in sleep disturbances.
Risperidone	1–3 mg every 12–24 hrs PO	1–6 mg daily	Monitor for hypotension.
Benzodiazepines			
Lorazepam	0.5–2 mg every 1–4 hrs PO, IV, or IM	0.5–12 mg daily	Lorazepam may cause delirium.
Midazolam	30–100 mg every 24 hrs IV or subcutaneous For maintenance of sedation by infusion, the usual dose is 0.02–0.1 mg/kg/hr (1–7 mg/hr). The lowest effective dose should be used in those receiving other sedatives or opioids.	30–100 mg daily	Midazolam may cause delirium, anxiety, or agitation.
Neuroleptics			
Chlorpromazine	10–75 mg every 4–8 hrs PO Use lower dose with older adult patients.	30–600 mg daily	Use if haloperidol fails or more sedation desired. Chlorpromazine may worsen delirium.
Haloperidol	0.5–5 mg every 2–24 hrs PO, IV, or IM Use lower dose in older adult or frail patients (0.25–0.5 mg and titrate slowly).	0.5–60 mg daily	Monitor serial electrocardiogram for potential QT interval changes. Avoid in the presence of Parkinson disease or Lewy body dementia. Haloperidol is not effective for hypoactive delirium.
Thioridazine	10–75 mg every 4–8 hrs PO	30–600 mg daily	Monitor for extrapyramidal adverse effects.

hr—hour; IM—intramuscular; IV—intravenous; PO—by mouth

Note. Based on information from Bush et al., 2018; Caplan, 2018; Loving & Dahlin, 2019.

      c) Evaluate for cancer progression for potential metastasis.
      d) Treat sepsis and infections.
      e) Consider opioid rotation and/or change from benzodiazepines.
   3. Mixed
      a) Review medications for polypharmacy.
      b) Follow treatment for both hypoactive and hyperactive delirium.
 I. Pharmacologic therapy (see Table 133-1)
 J. Nonpharmacologic therapy (see Figure 133-1)
   1. Provide family education, including the following.
      a) Predisposing factors to delirium and its effects
      b) Short course and often reversible

       c) Explanation that personality changes may be upsetting for family to observe

       d) Potential for communication barriers because the patient is confused

  2. Continue family discussion when delirium is present at the end of life.

       a) Clarify physical versus psychological issues (e.g., existential distress).

       b) Explain treatment options, including palliative sedation and the process of its use.

          (1) Medications, benzodiazepines, or anesthetics should only be used with the support of a palliative care or pain team.

          (2) Palliative sedation should not be done without consultation with pain or palliative care services.

VII. Follow-up

  A. First 24–48 hours

    1. Reassess interventions for effectiveness, including pharmacologic interventions, within the first 24 hours.

    2. Institute around-the-clock therapy instead of PRN doses to promote adherence and effectiveness.

    3. Evaluate the need for ongoing therapy.

  B. After 48 hours

    1. Evaluate the need for ongoing therapy if other corrective measures have cleared the delirium.

    2. For terminal delirium, discuss the goals of care with the family. This includes continued treatment of delirium as a comfort measure and the possible need for aggressive treatment, such as palliative sedation, if delirium is resistant to medications.

FIGURE 133-1   **Management of Environment**

- Create a safe environment.
  - Location of a call bell within reach
  - Availability of glasses, hearing aids, and dentures
  - Provision of cognitive devices such as calendars and clocks
  - Avoidance of restraints
  - Assistance with positioning, toileting, and any ambulation
  - Promotion of supervised ambulation or range of motion
- Reduce stimuli.
  - Audio—Reduce sound and noise from radios, cell phones, telephones, too much conversation, crowds, alarms from equipment, and overhead paging systems.
  - Visual—Reduce input from television and pictures. Soft lighting is best to prevent hallucinations.
  - Sensory—Reduce interruptions to the patient with constant care. Organize care needs to occur together.
- Provide reassurance.
  - Clear communication with verbal cues of day, time, and location, as well as identity of clinician
  - Clear simple explanations of any interventions or care tasks
  - Consistent staff as possible
  - Familiar objects from home
  - Familiar family, friends, and consistent caregivers
  - Use of sitters
- Promote rest.
  - Sleep protocol with rituals, relaxation
  - Noise reduction
  - Adjusting activities to allow long periods of rest at night
  - Reduction or muting of monitors

Note. Based on information from Bush et al., 2018; Caplan, 2018; Loving & Dahlin, 2019.

VIII. Referrals

    A. Psychiatrist: For input about the nature of the confusion and if there is a psychiatric history

    B. Other specialists: To consider alternative etiologies, such as neurologic, endocrine, or infectious disease, depending on the nature of the underlying delirium

    C. Social worker: To support the family

    D. Chaplain or psychologist: For counseling to support the patient if existential distress is apparent

    E. Pain and palliative care teams: To assist with palliative sedation, if necessary or appropriate

    F. Hospice: If the patient is in the terminal stage of cancer and the family needs hospice support

References

American Psychiatric Association. (2013). *Diagnostic and statistical manual of mental disorders* (5th ed.).

Blazer, D.G. (2018). Advancing our diagnostic tools and treatment options for delirium. *International Psychogeriatrics, 30*(4), 447–449. https://doi.org/10.1017/S1041610218000601

Boland, J.W., Lawlor, P.G., & Bush, S.H. (2019). Delirium: Non-pharmacological and pharmacological management. *BMJ Supportive and Palliative Care, 9*(4), 482–484. https://doi.org/10.1136/bmjspcare-2019-001966

Breitbart, W., Rosenfeld, B., Roth, A., Smith, M.J., Cohen, K., & Passik, S. (1997). The Memorial Delirium Assessment Scale. *Journal of Pain and Symptom Management, 13*(3), 128–137. https://doi.org/10.1016/S0885-3924(96)00316-8

Burhenn, P.S. (2016). Delirium. In C. Dahlin, P.J. Coyne, & B.R. Ferrell (Eds.), *Advanced practice palliative nursing* (pp. 311–318). Oxford University Press.

Bush, S.H., Lawlor, P.G., Ryan, K., Centeno, C., Lucchesi, M., Kanji, S., ... Ripamonti, C.I. (2018). Delirium in adult cancer patients: ESMO clinical practice guidelines. *Annals of Oncology, 29* (Suppl. 4), iv143–iv165. https://doi.org/10.1093/annonc/mdy147

Caplan, J.P. (2018). Delirious patients. In T.A. Stern, O. Freudenreich, F.A. Smith, G.L. Fricchione, & J.F. Rosenbaum (Eds.), *Massachusetts General Hospital handbook of general hospital psychiatry* (7th ed., pp. 83–93). Elsevier.

Fernandez-Robles, C.G., Irwin, K.E., Pirl, W.F., & Greenberg, D.B. (2018). Patients with cancer. In T.A. Stern, O. Freudenreich, F.A. Smith, G.L. Fricchione, & J.F. Rosenbaum (Eds.), *Massachusetts General Hospital handbook of general hospital psychiatry* (7th ed., pp. 349–358). Elsevier.

Folstein, M.F., Folstein, S.E., & McHugh, P.R. (1975). "Mini-mental state": A practical method for grading the cognitive state of patients for the clinician. *Journal of Psychiatric Research, 12*(3), 189–198. https://doi.org/10.1016/0022-3956(75)90026-6

Hshieh, T.T., Inouye, S.K., & Oh, E.S. (2018). Delirium in the elderly. *Psychiatric Clinics of North America, 41*(1), 1–17. https://doi.org/10.1016/j.psc.2017.10.001

Inouye, S.K., van Dyck, C.H., Alessi, C.A., Balkin, S., Siegal, A.P., & Horwitz, R.I. (1990). Clarifying confusion: The confusion assessment method: A new method for detection of delirium. *Annals of Internal Medicine, 113*(12), 941–948. https://doi.org/10.7326/0003-4819-113-12-941

Loving, N.G., & Dahlin, C.M. (2019). Anxiety, depression, and delirium. In M. Matzo & D.W. Sherman (Eds.), *Palliative care nursing: Quality care to the end of life* (5th ed., pp. 545–578). Springer.

Mulkey, M.A., Hardin, S.R., Munro, C.L., Everhart, D.E., Kim, S., Schoemann, A.M., & Olson, D.M. (2019). Methods of identifying delirium: A research protocol. *Research in Nursing and Health, 42*(4), 246–255. https://doi.org/10.1002/nur.21953

Mulkey, M.A., Hardin, S.R., Olson, D.M., & Munro, C.L. (2018). Pathophysiology review: Seven neurotransmitters associated with delirium. *Clinical Nurse Specialist, 32*(4), 195–211. https://doi.org/10.1097/NUR.0000000000000384

Nasreddine, Z.S., Phillips, N.A., Bédirian, V., Charbonneau, S., Whitehead, V., Collin, I., & Chertkow, H. (2005). The Montreal Cognitive Assessment, MoCA: A brief screening tool for mild cognitive impairment. *Journal of the American Geriatrics Society, 53*(4), 941–948. https://doi.org/10.1111/j.1532-5415.2005.53221.x

National Comprehensive Cancer Network. (2021). *NCCN Clinical Practice Guidelines in Oncology (NCCN Guidelines®): Palliative care* [v.2.2021]. https://www.nccn.org/professionals/physician_gls/pdf/palliative.pdf

Treacy, P.T., Mittall, D., Torres, R., Kanary, K., Norton, J., & Jimerson, N. (2001). Validation of the Delirium Rating Scale-Revised-98: Comparison with the Delirium Rating Scale and the Cognitive Test for Delirium. *Journal of Neuropsychiatry and Clinical Neuroscience, 13*(2), 229–242. https://doi.org/10.1176/appi.neuropsych.13.2.229

CHAPTER 134

Dizziness/Vertigo

Catherine Reavis, EdD, FNP-BC, FAANP

I. Definition: *Dizziness* and *vertigo* are interchangeable terms used by patients and providers that are different in both their symptoms and management (Pfieffer et al., 2019; Walker & Daroff, 2018).
   A. Dizziness is described by patients as light-headedness and imbalance that occur when assuming an upright position. Clinically, it is presyncope usually attributed to cerebral hypoperfusion.
   B. Vertigo is a subjective movement sensation (i.e., feeling as though one is revolving in space or as though objects in the environment are moving). It may be accompanied by nausea, postural unsteadiness, and gait ataxia. Vertigo may be provoked or worsened by head movement.

II. Physiology/Pathophysiology (Argaet et al., 2019; Butterfield, 2018; Walker & Daroff, 2018; Welgampola et al., 2019)
   A. Normal
      1. The inner ear is a series of osseous labyrinths filled with fluid or perilymph. The labyrinth is divided into the cochlea (partially responsible for hearing), vestibule, and semicircular canals (controlling balance).
      2. Suspended in the perilymph is a membranous labyrinth filled with a thicker fluid called *endolymph.*
      3. The semicircular canals and vestibule contain equilibrium receptors. Within each semicircular canal is the crista ampullaris, composed of a tuft of hair cells covered by gelatinous cupula. When the head is rotated, the endolymph in the canal slows and moves in the opposite direction of the head's movement.
      4. When the hair cells are stimulated, impulses are transmitted through the vestibular nerve to the cerebellum.
      5. Static equilibrium is controlled in a complex process involving the maculae within the vestibule. As the head moves, otoliths (small calcium salt particles) move in a gel-like material in response to the pull of gravity.
      6. The otoliths pull on the gel that, in response, pulls on the hair cells in the maculae. Nerve cells are again stimulated, and impulses are transmitted to the cerebellum.
      7. Vertigo can be a normal physiologic response to the following.
         a) After spinning around
         b) A mismatch among vestibular, visual, and somatosensory input, with head movements to which the vestibular system is not conditioned (such as with motion sickness or seasickness)
         c) Exaggerated head and neck movements (staring up for a period of time)

B. Pathophysiology
    1. Vertigo is due to lesions of the visual, somatosensory, or vestibular systems. It is a result of inflammation of the semicircular canals and may be classed as peripheral (outside the CNS) or central (origins within the CNS).
    2. Malfunction of the vestibular system results in the symptom of dizziness.

III. Clinical features: Dizziness and vertigo are common symptoms seen in the clinical setting. Clinical features are dependent on the type of vertigo and underlying pathophysiology. Patient description is critical in classifying the etiology of dizziness. Vertigo is the predominant symptom of vestibular dysfunction (Argaet et al., 2019; Bickley, 2020; Pfieffer et al., 2019; Spiegel et al., 2017; Welgampola et al., 2019).

  A. Etiology
    1. Peripheral vertigo: Accounts for greater than 90% of cases in primary care and most commonly caused by benign paroxysmal positional vertigo (BPPV), vestibular neuritis or labyrinthitis, and Ménière disease
    2. Central vertigo: Accounts for less than 10% of cases seen in primary care and includes strokes, migraines, tumors, trauma, and demyelinating diseases (e.g., multiple sclerosis)
    3. Psychogenic vertigo (phobic postural vertigo): May be a manifestation of anxiety progressing to panic attacks or phobias (e.g., agoraphobia); defined as chronic subjective dizziness with diagnostic criteria of more than three months of chronic hypersensitivity to one's own motion or the movement of objects
    4. Viral infection (HSV is most common), cerebrovascular accident, trauma, and rarely bacterial labyrinthitis (serous OM) can induce dizziness.

  B. History: The history may be sensitive to differentiate the etiology among vertigo, presyncope, psychiatric disorders, and disequilibrium. Patients should describe "dizzy" without using this term to elucidate what they mean by the symptoms experienced.
    1. History of cancer and cancer treatment
    2. Current medications: Prescribed, over the counter
    3. History of presenting symptoms: Precipitating factors, onset, location, duration, associated symptoms (e.g., surroundings at time of occurrence, light-headedness [presyncope] or the environment spinning around the individual [vertigo], first episode of experiencing the symptom, nausea, tinnitus)
    4. Changes in ADLs
    5. Past medical history: Migraines, Ménière disease, cardiovascular disease, anemia, recent head trauma, injury to neck
    6. Social history: Tobacco use, alcohol use, recent travel
    7. Family history: Vertigo
    8. Viral history: HSV infections

  C. Signs and symptoms
    1. BPPV: History of minor head trauma
      a) Onset of vertigo when rolling in bed
      b) Vertigo reproducible by changing head position
      c) Vertigo improving after 10–60 seconds without head movement
      d) Nausea common; vomiting less common
    2. Vestibular neuritis/labyrinthitis: May have preceding viral infection
      a) Acute sudden onset with gradual improvement over days
      b) Nonpositional vertigo
      c) Sustained vertigo
      d) Nausea and vomiting common

   3. Ménière disease: Must have first three characteristics to confirm diagnosis
      a) Chronic intermittent paroxysmal vertigo
      b) Tinnitus
      c) Sensorineural hearing loss
      d) Aural pressure before onset of vertigo
   4. Migraine-associated vertigo: Rarely the only symptom
      a) Headache
      b) Photophobia/phonophobia
   5. Chronic subjective dizziness (formerly psychogenic dizziness)
      a) Persistent nonspecific dizziness that cannot be explained by active medical conditions
      b) Light-headedness or heavy-headedness present on most days
      c) Exacerbated with complex visual stimuli, such as using a computer
      d) Anxiety with possible hyperventilation
D. Physical examination: Does not make but confirms the diagnosis
   1. Vital signs: Orthostatic blood pressures
   2. HEENT
      a) Tympanic membrane for loss of landmarks, erythema, cerumen impaction, or cholesteatoma
      b) Hearing (see Appendix D)
         (1) Rinne test to assess bone and air conduction
         (2) Whisper test to assess for hearing acuity
         (3) Weber test to assess lateralization of sound
            (a) With normal hearing, sound is heard in both ears.
            (b) With sensorineural hearing loss, sound localizes to normal ear.
            (c) With conductive loss, sound localizes to affected ear.
      c) Nystagmus (rhythmic oscillation of the eyes) and extraocular movement: Nystagmus is assessed in the five positions of gaze. Minimal nystagmus movement is normal in the lateral gaze; however, nystagmus should not occur on elevation and depression of the eyes, even at gaze extremes.
         (1) Spontaneous nystagmus is an attempt by the vestibular system to maintain gaze during head movement through the vestibular ocular reflexes. Acute unilateral vestibular lesions can cause an asymmetry in vestibular activity. The result is a slow drift of the eyes away from the visual target in one direction, followed by a rapid corrective movement in the reverse direction. Thus, the eyes appear to "beat" in the corrective gaze until the asymmetry of vestibular activity is restored or until the CNS adapts to the vestibular lesion.
         (2) Typical nystagmus patterns and the characteristics of short latency, limited duration, reversal on returning to the upright position, and fatigability on repeated provocation suggest dizziness diagnosis.
            (a) Rotary nystagmus usually occurs within 3–10 seconds, reaching a maximum within a few seconds and lasting 10–60 seconds. When the patient returns to a sitting position, nystagmus is in the opposite direction, suggesting BPPV.
            (b) Horizontal or vertical nystagmus or both suggests brain stem lesions or vestibular neuritis.
            (c) Central nystagmus occurs in disorders of the lower brain stem and cerebellum, including ischemia, demyelination, migraine, and rarely neoplasm.

(3) Nystagmus can be reproduced with Hallpike maneuver (also called Dix-Hallpike). The Hallpike maneuver is the diagnostic test for BPPV.

    (a) Perform the Hallpike test with the patient sitting upright with the legs extended. The patient's head is then rotated by approximately 45°.

    (b) Help the patient to lie down backward quickly with the head held in approximately 20° of extension. This extension may either be achieved by supporting the patient's head as it hangs off the table or by placing a pillow under his or her upper back.

    (c) Observe the patient's eyes for about 45 seconds, as there is a characteristic 5–10-second period of latency prior to nystagmus onset.

    (d) If rotational nystagmus occurs, the test is considered positive for BPPV. During a positive test, the fast phase of the rotatory nystagmus is toward the affected ear, which is the ear closest to the ground. The direction of the fast phase is defined by the rotation of the top of the eye, either clockwise or counterclockwise.

    (e) Home devices are available to assist in the performance of the Hallpike maneuver for patients with a diagnosis of BPPV.

3. Cardiac: Auscultation for carotid bruits suggestive of stenosis or blockage; irregularity of heartbeat suggestive of cerebrovascular disease or dysrhythmias

4. Neurologic: Central lesion, primarily of the cerebellum and brain stem

    a) Cranial nerve evaluation (see Appendix A): Cranial nerve deficit or dysfunction may indicate a lesion of the brain stem; acoustic neuroma can affect nerves V, VII, and X.

    b) Romberg test: This test is used to assess cerebellar function; it is positive in sensory ataxia.

        (1) Decreased conduction of sensory impulses alters proprioception.

        (2) Postural instability may occur with central or vestibular pathology.

        (3) Vertigo with central origin impairs gait and posture to a greater degree than vertigo of a peripheral origin, which may result in the patient's inability to walk without falling.

5. Unilateral peripheral disorders resulting in gait instability in the direction of the lesion

6. Neck: Relationship between symptoms and neck range of motion; deficits possibly from vestibular or visual etiology or cervical spine integrity

7. If examination is normal, an attempt to reproduce symptoms should be made through hyperventilation: The patient should hyperventilate for two minutes; if vertigo results, it is probably psychogenic in etiology.

IV. Diagnostic tests (Nair et al., 2018; Slattery et al., 2011; Spiegel et al., 2017; Walker & Daroff, 2018; Welgampola et al., 2019)

    A. Laboratory: Typically not necessary; used to evaluate for unclear etiology

        1. TSH to assess for thyroid disorders

        2. CBC to assess for anemia

        3. Serum glucose to assess for hypoglycemia

    B. Radiology

        1. Cervical spine x-rays to assess vertebral integrity and evaluate for pathologic fracture, compression fracture, or abnormality (e.g., disc protrusion, tumor) that may cause nerve compression

        2. MRI if central origin is suspected and more comprehensive imaging is indicated based on patient's history and physical examination; CT scan not definitive in evaluating for posterior fossa ischemia

C. Other
1. Audiometry tests to detect hearing abnormalities with acoustic neuroma and Ménière disease: Most sensitive test, especially in low frequencies or hertz
2. Doppler examination of carotid and vertebral arteries if clinical picture suggests transient ischemic attack or stenosis
3. Vestibular function tests
   a) Electronystagmography: Battery of tests designed to assess central and vestibular pathways of brain stem and cerebellum lesions
   b) Vestibular evaluation tests: Provide quantitative information regarding vestibular reflexes, central oculomotor function, and postural control strategies
      (1) Caloric stimulation: Stimulates the inner ear and nearby nerves by delivering cold and warm water to the ear canal at different times to evaluate differences in temperature to evaluate ear nerve damage
      (2) Video-oculography: Noninvasive technology for evaluating eye movement to distinguish nystagmus etiology
      (3) Rotational chair positioning: Multiple method test to analyze vestibular responses by observation of the eye movements during rotation
      (4) Computerized dynamic posturography: Noninvasive specialized clinical assessment technique used to quantify the CNS adaptive mechanisms (sensory, motor, and central) involved in the control of posture and balance

V. Differential diagnosis (Choi et al., 2013; Dyhrfjeld-Johnsen & Attali, 2019; Lindell et al., 2018; Pfieffer et al., 2019; Spiegel et al., 2017; Walker & Daroff, 2018; Welgampola et al., 2019)
  A. Peripheral vestibular disorders: BPPV most common
  B. Acute unilateral labyrinthine dysfunction: Vestibular neuritis
    1. Acute bilateral labyrinthine dysfunction secondary to toxins, drugs (e.g., aminoglycoside antibiotics), or alcohol
    2. Recurrent unilateral labyrinthine dysfunction: Ménière disease
    3. Vestibular nerve vertigo: Acoustic neuroma, acoustic Schwannoma, meningioma
  C. Central vertigo lesions affecting the brain stem pathways from the vestibular end organs to the supranuclear ocular motor integrations in the midbrain or the vestibulocerebellum
    1. Ischemia: Wallenberg syndrome
    2. Hemorrhage
    3. Transient ischemic attacks of posterior cerebral circulation
    4. Vestibular migraine
  D. Chronic subjective dizziness: Psychogenic vertigo
    1. Depression, anxiety, personality disorders (see Chapters 161 and 162)
    2. Acrophobia
    3. Phobic postural vertigo
  E. Physiologic vertigo
    1. Physiologic height vertigo
    2. Motion sickness
  F. Cerebrovascular disease other than vertebrobasilar ischemia
    1. Dysrhythmias (see Chapter 45)
    2. Orthostatic hypotension (see Chapter 48)
    3. Small cerebellar/brain stem strokes (see Chapter 146)
    4. Rare: Central causes such as neoplasms (e.g., cerebellopontine tumors) or disorders affecting the fourth ventricle

G. Demyelinating diseases such as multiple sclerosis often presenting with vertigo

H. Cervical OA (see Chapter 105), spondylosis

I. Visual disturbances, especially cataracts (see Chapter 7)

J. Medication induced: Opioids, benzodiazepines, certain antiepileptics

K. Sinusitis (see Chapter 11)

L. Diabetes mellitus (see Chapter 151)

M. Dehydration, hypovolemia, electrolyte imbalance (see Chapters 152–156)

VI. Treatment (Albu et al., 2015; Cousins et al., 2014; Dyhrfjeld-Johnsen & Attali, 2019; Gupta et al., 2019; Hall et al., 2016; Jung et al., 2012; Meldrum et al., 2012; Nada et al., 2019; Nair et al., 2018; Pfieffer et al., 2019; Shea et al., 2012)

A. Nonpharmacologic measures

1. Vestibular rehabilitation therapy is an exercise-based treatment approach designed to promote vestibular adaptation and substitution.

   a) It originated as a physical therapy to improve vertigo, dizziness, and balance disorders.

   b) Most rehabilitative innovations incorporate tai chi and virtual games that improve balance and behavioral health.

2. Treatment for BPPV may include canalith repositioning interventions that promote remission of symptoms and increase postural control.

   a) Maneuvers may be performed in the office, the patient's home, or a combination for treatment of BPPV with and without nystagmus. Techniques include the Epley or Semont maneuvers.

   b) The maneuvers reposition the canaliths in the semicircular canals to relieve vertigo. Each maneuver takes about 15 minutes to complete.

   c) The Epley maneuver is most widely used. Patients are in a supine position and their head is rotated from side to side.

   d) The Semont maneuver (liberatory maneuver) is a similar procedure in which the patient is rapidly moved from lying on one side to lying on the other. It is effective in approximately 86.8% of patients.

   e) Repositioning maneuvers depend on rapidly moving the head through various planes in space and can be effective. Many patients suffer residual dizziness after successful canalith repositioning interventions and may respond to a short course of anxiolytics.

3. Low-salt diets and elimination of tobacco and caffeine may be beneficial.

B. Pharmacologic measures (see Table 134-1): Many patients improve spontaneously; however, supportive medications may be beneficial in managing symptoms.

1. Antiemetics may be necessary to treat nausea (see Appendix P).

2. Vestibular suppressants are useful in treating symptoms.

C. Other

1. Surgical procedures, such as labyrinthectomy or tenotomy, may be alternatives to refractory Ménière disease.

2. Cochlear implants may be useful to assist patients who suffer deafness due to surgical interventions or progressive disease.

3. Newer procedures, such as tenotomy of the middle ear muscles, promise to improve symptoms.

VII. Follow-up

A. Short term: For peripheral etiologies, the patient should be rechecked in three to six weeks.

TABLE 134-1	Antivertiginous Drugs	
Drug	**Dosage**	**Action**
Anticholinergic		
Scopolamine	1 transdermal patch every 3 days	Muscarine antagonist
Antiemetics		
Ondansetron	8–24 mg PO as single dose or 8 mg every 8–12 hours or 4 mg IM as a single dose	Selective 5-hydroxytryptamine-3 (5-HT$_3$) receptor antagonist
Prochlorperazine	5–10 mg PO 3–4 times a day or 5 mg IM every 6 hours or 25 mg suppository every 12 hours	Muscarine antagonist Dopamine (D$_2$) antagonist
Promethazine	25–50 mg PO every 8 hours or IM every 6–8 hours or 25 mg suppository every 6–8 hours	Histamine (H$_1$) antagonist Muscarine antagonist Dopamine (D$_2$) antagonist
Antihistamines		
Dimenhydrinate	50 mg PO every 4–6 hours or IM every 4–6 hours	Histamine (H$_1$) antagonist Muscarine antagonist
Meclizine	25–50 mg PO every 6–8 hours	Histamine (H$_1$) antagonist Muscarine antagonist
Benzodiazepines		
Clonazepam	0.25 mg PO 3 times a day PRN	GABA$_A$ agonist
Diazepam	2.5 mg PO 3 times a day PRN or IM every 4–6 hours or IV every 4–6 hours	GABA$_A$ agonist
Glucocorticoid		
Prednisone	100 mg PO daily for 3 days tapered by 20 mg every 3 days	Anti-inflammatory

GABA$_A$—gamma-aminobutyric acid A; IM—intramuscular; IV—intravenous; PO—by mouth; PRN—as needed

Note. Based on information from Dyhrfjeld-Johnsen & Attali, 2019; Walker & Daroff, 2018.

B. Long term: For central etiologies, appropriate medical referral for further evaluation and intervention may be required.

VIII. Referrals
   A. Neurologist: For management of chronic migraine
   B. Otolaryngologist: For management of Ménière disease or for vestibular rehabilitation
   C. Surgeon: For surgical management or implants
   D. Psychiatrist: For help in coping with chronic symptoms
   E. Rehabilitation services
      1. For vestibular rehabilitation
      2. Physical or occupational therapist: For evaluation for exercise and activity programs to provide strengthening, gait training, and identification of specific activities (triggers) that cause symptoms; for evaluation for assistive devices

References

Albu, S., Babighian, G., Amadori, M., & Trabalzini, F. (2015). Endolymphatic sac surgery versus tenotomy of the stapedius and tensor tympani muscles in the management of patients with unilateral definite Meniere's disease. *European Archives of Oto-Rhino-Laryngology, 272*(12), 3645–3650. https://doi.org/10.1007/s00405-014-3428-1

Argaet, E.C., Bradshaw, A.P., & Welgampola, M.S. (2019). Benign positional vertigo, its diagnosis, treatment and mimics. *Clinical Neurophysiology Practice, 4,* 97–111. https://doi.org/10.1016/j.cnp.2019.03.001

Bickley, L.S. (2020). *Bates' guide to physical examination and history taking* (13th ed.). Wolters Kluwer.

Butterfield, R. (2018). Structure and function of the neurologic system. In K.L. McCance, S.E. Huether, V.L. Brashers, & N.S. Rote (Eds.), *Pathophysiology: The biologic basis for disease in adults and children* (8th ed., pp. 434–465). Elsevier.

Choi, K.-D., Lee, H., & Kim, J.-S. (2013). Vertigo in brainstem and cerebellar strokes. *Current Opinions in Neurology, 26*(1), 90–95. https://doi.org/10.1097/WCO.0b013e32835c5edd

Cousins, S., Cutfield, N.J., Kaski, D., Palla, A., Seemungal, B.M., Golding, J.F., ... Bronstein, A.M. (2014). Visual dependency and dizziness after vestibular neuritis. *PLOS ONE, 9*(9), e105426. https://doi.org/10.1371/journal.pone.0105426

Dyhrfjeld-Johnsen, J., & Attali, P. (2019). Management of peripheral vertigo with antihistamines: New options on the horizon. *British Journal of Clinical Pharmacology, 85*(10), 2255–2263. https://doi.org/10.1111/bcp.14046

Gupta, A.K., Sharma, K.G., & Sharma, P. (2019). Effect of Epley, Semont maneuvers and Brandt-Daroff exercise on quality of life in patients with posterior semicircular canal benign paroxysmal positional vertigo (PSCBPPV). *Journal of Otolaryngology and Head and Neck Surgery, 71*(1), 99–103. https://doi.org/10.1007/s12070-018-1322-7

Hall, C.D., Herdman, S.J., Whitney, S.L., Cass, S.P., Clendaniel, R.A., Fife, T.D., ... Woodhouse, S.N. (2016). Vestibular rehabilitation for peripheral vestibular hypofunction: An evidence-based clinical practice guideline: From the American Physical Therapy Association Neurology Section. *Journal of Neurologic Physical Therapy, 40*(2), 124–155. https://doi.org/10.1097/NPT.0000000000000120

Jung, H.J., Koo, J.-W., Kim, C.S., Kim, J.S., & Song, J.-J. (2012). Anxiolytics reduce residual dizziness after successful canalith repositioning maneuvers in benign paroxysmal positional vertigo. *Acta Oto-Laryngologica, 132*(3), 277–284. https://doi.org/10.3109/00016489.2011.637179

Lindell, E., Finizia, C., Johansson, M., Karlsson, T., Nilson, J., & Magnusson, M. (2018). Asking about dizziness when turning in bed predicts examination findings for benign paroxysmal positional vertigo. *Journal of Vestibular Research, 28*(3–4), 339–347. https://doi.org/10.3233/VES-180637

Meldrum, D., Glennon, A., Herdman, S., Murray, D., & McConn-Walsh, R. (2012). Virtual reality rehabilitation of balance: Assessment of the usability of the Nintendo Wii® Fit Plus. *Disability and Rehabilitation: Assistive Technology, 7*(3), 205–210. https://doi.org/10.3109/17483107.2011.616922

Nada, E.H., Ibraheem, O.A., & Hassaan, M.R. (2019). Vestibular rehabilitation therapy outcomes in patients with persistent postural-perceptual dizziness. *Annals of Otology, Rhinology and Laryngology, 128*(4), 323–329. https://doi.org/10.1177/0003489418823017

Nair, M.A., Mulvara, A.P., Bloomberg, J., Sangi-Haghpeykar, H., & Cohen, H.S. (2018). Visual dependence and spatial orientation in benign paroxysmal positional vertigo. *Journal of Vestibular Research, 27*(5–6), 279–286. https://doi.org/10.3233/VES-170623

Pfieffer, M.L., Anthamatten, A., & Glassford, M. (2019). Assessment and treatment of dizziness and vertigo. *Nurse Practitioner, 44*(10), 29–36. https://doi.org/10.1097/01.NPR.0000579744.73514.4b

Shea, P.F., Richey, P.A., Wan, J.Y., & Stevens, S.R. (2012). Hearing results and quality of life after streptomycin/dexamethasone perfusion for Meniere's disease. *Laryngoscope, 122*(1), 204–211. https://doi.org/10.1002/lary.22362

Slattery, E.L., Sinks, B.C., & Goebel, J.A. (2011). Vestibular tests for rehabilitation: Applications and interpretation. *NeuroRehabilitation, 29*(2), 143–151. https://doi.org/10.3233/NRE-2011-0688

Spiegel, R., Kirsch, M., Rosin, C., Rust, H., Baumann, T., Sutter, R., ... Mantokoudis, G. (2017). Dizziness in the emergency department: An update on diagnosis. *Swiss Medical Weekly, 147,* w14565. https://doi.org/10.4414/smw.2017.14565

Walker, M.F., & Daroff, R.B. (2018). Dizziness and vertigo. In J.L. Jameson, A.S. Fauci, D.L. Kasper, S.L. Hauser, D.L. Longo, & J. Loscalzo (Eds.), *Harrison's principles of internal medicine* (20th ed., pp. 178–180). McGraw-Hill Education.

Welgampola, M.S., Young, A.S., Pogson, J.M., Bradshaw, A.P., & Halmagyi, G.M. (2019). Dizziness demystified. *Practical Neurology, 19*(6), 492–501. https://doi.org/10.1136/practneurol-2019-002199

CHAPTER 135

Dystonia

Dawn Camp-Sorrell, MSN, CRNP, AOCN®

I. Definition (Albanese et al., 2019; Chirumamilla et al., 2019; Ferreira Camargo & Ghizoni Teive, 2019; Mainka et al., 2019; Richardson & Jinnah, 2019; Ugawa, 2020)
   A. Dystonia is a disorder characterized by involuntary muscle contractions that cause slow repetitive movements, abnormal postures, or both. The movements may be painful.
   B. Torsion is the condition of being twisted. It is usually present with dystonic movement.
   C. In isolated dystonia, dystonia is the sole symptom.
   D. In combined dystonia, it is present with other neurologic symptoms.

II. Physiology/Pathophysiology (Albanese et al., 2019; Balint et al., 2018; Mainka et al., 2019; Marsili et al., 2019; Richardson & Jinnah, 2019; Ugawa, 2020)
   A. Normal
      1. The cerebellum and the motor cortex send information to a set of structures within the brain's deep subcortical gray matter called basal ganglia.
      2. These structures help to control involuntary components of movement.
      3. The basal ganglia send output messages to the motor cortex, helping to initiate movements, regulate repetitive or patterned movements, and control muscle tone.
      4. Any movements are caused by an activation of muscles, which usually occurs following the impulses from the motor nerve. Motor neurons are usually activated by a descending tract. Several descending common pathways carry the impulse from the brain to the spinal cord, including the corticospinal, reticulospinal, rubrospinal, tectospinal, and vestibulospinal tracts.
   B. Pathophysiology: Dystonia is a group of movement disorders that result from an abnormality in or damage to the basal ganglia or other brain regions that control movement.
      1. Abnormalities may exist in the brain's ability to process neurotransmitters that help cells in the brain communicate with each other or in the way the brain processes information and generates commands to move.
      2. Primary dystonia is characterized by enhanced excitability and loss of inhibition at several anatomical levels, which include the sensorimotor cortex, brain stem, and spinal cord.
      3. In secondary dystonia, loss of intracortical inhibition has been demonstrated in basal ganglia lesions.
      4. In isolated dystonia, several genes have been identified, accounting for a very small percentage of cases overall. Examples of these genes include the following.
         a) *TOR1A* (DYT1): Typically presents as a childhood onset and lower limb dystonia, which generalizes throughout the body
         b) *THAP1*: Presents as focal or segmental dystonia, mostly in the upper limbs, neck, and face

    c) *CIZ1*: Linked to familial cervical dystonia
    d) *ANO3*: Linked to familial-dominant cervical dystonia
    e) *GNAL*: Familial linked with onset in the head and neck area

III. Clinical features: Dystonia usually occurs without an identifiable precipitant and at any age. It is associated with poor QOL, pain, and reduced ability to work. Dopamine receptor blocking agents (e.g., metoclopramide, haloperidol) are the most common cause of drug-induced movement disorders, including dystonia. Dystonia varies greatly in clinical presentation, affecting almost any area of the skeletal muscle. The most common presentation in adults is focal movement, with the most common sites being the neck and eye region. Dystonia is not easy to recognize and often misdiagnosed (Albanese et al., 2019; Chirumamilla et al., 2019; Duma & Fung, 2019; Ferreira Camargo & Ghizoni Teive, 2019; Jinnah & Factor, 2015; Mainka et al., 2019; Marsili et al., 2019; Nath et al., 2019; Richardson & Jinnah, 2019; Ugawa, 2020; van der Stouwe et al., 2019).

 A. Classification
  1. Axis 1
   a) Age at onset
   b) Body distribution
   c) Temporal pattern, disease course, variability
   d) Associated features
    (1) Isolated or combined
    (2) Other neurologic symptoms
  2. Axis 2
   a) Nervous system anatomy
    (1) Structural abnormality
    (2) Acquired lesion
    (3) None of the above
   b) Inherited or acquired
 B. Etiology
  1. Isolated: Dystonia is the only phenotypic manifestation with no identifiable cause.
  2. Secondary: Dystonia is inherited or acquired as a consequence of external factors (e.g., toxins, other diseases causing brain damage).
  3. Heredodegenerative: Neurodegenerative disease with dystonia is commonly the major feature. Many patients have a proven or possible genetic basis.
  4. Dystonia syndromes: Dystonia and neurologic symptoms occur. A neurochemical basis is found but no evidence of degeneration exists.
  5. Drug induced: Antiemetics or antipsychotics can cause dystonia.
 C. History
  1. History of cancer and cancer treatment
  2. Current medications: Prescribed, over the counter
  3. History of presenting symptoms: Precipitating factors, onset, location, duration, associated symptoms (sensory or motor behaviors such as tics, tremors, and paresthesia)
  4. Changes in ADLs
  5. Social history: Alcohol use, illicit drug use
  6. Family history: Neurodegenerative disease
 D. Signs and symptoms
  1. Dystonia frequently is associated with other forms of adventitious movements and can seriously affect gait, which may be the first manifestation, and progress to other regions.

2. Some symptoms tend to occur after periods of exertion and fluctuate over the course of the day.

3. Adult-onset dystonia usually is located in one or adjacent parts of the body. Dystonia may progress through various stages. Initially, dystonic movements may be intermittent and appear only during voluntary movements or stress. Later, individuals may show dystonic postures and movements while walking and ultimately even at rest.

   a) Blepharospasm: Focal dystonia of eyelid

   b) Spasmodic: Focal dystonia of vocal cords

   c) Oromandibular: Dystonia of face, lips, tongue, and jaw

   d) Cervical: Dystonia of the neck (e.g., torticollis)

   e) Limb: Often task specific (e.g., writer's cramp)

4. Movement descriptors

   a) Movements usually are of a twisting nature.

   b) Brisk movements occur from the beginning to the peak of the contraction.

   c) Movements can be phasic, rapid, and repetitive.

   d) Dystonic positions can be prolonged but usually only, at most, for one second.

   e) As dystonia worsens, involuntary contractions appear during rest and may lead to permanent deformity.

   f) Lateralized dystonia may relate to focal intracranial disease.

5. Other signs

   a) Muscle weakness

   b) Spasticity

   c) Ataxia

   d) Cognitive impairment

E. Physical examination: Complete neurologic examination to evaluate for coexisting disorders

   1. Cognitive function: Orientation, concentration, memory, language, altered speech depending on etiology

   2. Cranial nerve: Visual fields (see Appendix A)

      a) Motor: Gait and stance; describes dystonic movements

      b) Generalized dystonia: Affects most or all of the body

      c) Focal dystonia: Localized to a specific body part

      d) Multifocal dystonia: Involves two or more unrelated body parts

      e) Segmental dystonia: Affects two or more adjacent body parts

      f) Hemidystonia: Involves the arm and leg on the same side of the body

   3. Deep tendon reflexes: Increased or decreased movement depending on etiology

   4. Sensory: Decreased or increased awareness

IV. Diagnostic studies: Diagnosis is largely based on clinical signs (Albanese et al., 2019; Chirumamilla et al., 2019; Jinnah & Factor, 2015).

   A. Laboratory: Choice of diagnostic studies will depend on the suspected cause of the dystonia.

      1. Vitamin B_{12} to evaluate for deficiency

      2. Drug panel if suspected illicit drug use

      3. Genetic testing if suspected or family history

   B. Radiology: MRI of the brain is performed to evaluate for degenerative disease or structural lesion.

   C. Other: Electromyography mapping may be useful as a complement to examination findings.

V. Differential diagnosis (Albanese et al., 2019; Balint et al., 2018; Duma & Fung, 2019; Jinnah & Factor, 2015; Mainka et al., 2019; Marsili et al., 2019; Nath et al., 2019; Richardson & Jinnah, 2019; van der Stouwe et al., 2019)
   A. Idiopathic dystonia: No known cause
   B. Genetic
      1. Wilson disease
      2. Huntington disease
      3. Parkinson disease
   C. Acquired (secondary dystonia): Results from environmental or other brain damage; often plateaus and does not spread to other body parts
      1. Hypoxia
      2. Perinatal injury: Cerebral palsy
      3. Trauma
      4. Reye syndrome
      5. Encephalitis
      6. Opportunistic infections: HIV/AIDS
      7. Multiple sclerosis
      8. Focal vascular disease
      9. Hypoparathyroidism
      10. Stroke (see Chapter 146)
      11. Exposure to heavy metal
      12. Neoplasm: Paraneoplastic syndrome (see Appendix M), intracranial mass
      13. Drug induced: Not an all-inclusive list
         a) H_2 receptor antagonists
         b) Levodopa
         c) Bromocriptine
         d) Ergot alkaloids
         e) Anticonvulsants
         f) Antipsychotics
         g) Tricyclic antidepressants
         h) Antiemetics: Phenothiazine, metoclopramide
         i) Illicit drugs: Cocaine, amphetamines
         j) Withdrawal phase of illicit drugs or opioid
      14. Chemicals: Methane, carbon monoxide
      15. Vitamin B_{12} deficiency (see Chapter 115)

VI. Treatment: The type of treatment is dependent on an accurate diagnosis and treatment of the underlying cause. Often, due to lifelong duration of dystonia, treatment becomes long term (Albanese et al., 2019; Balint et al., 2018; Duma & Fung, 2019; Ferreira Camargo & Ghizoni Teive, 2019; Jinnah & Factor, 2015; Krack et al., 2019; Marsili et al., 2019; Richardson & Jinnah, 2019).
   A. Eliminate causative agent. Stop offending drug.
   B. Treatment is directly related to the underlying disorder.
   C. Nonpharmacologic
      1. Educate and counsel patients. Frequently, dystonia is misdiagnosed for several years, and many are told dystonia is due to a psychiatric problem.
      2. Institute fall precautions or other safety measures depending on the area of dystonia.
      3. Physical therapy may be beneficial.
   D. Pharmacologic: Several drugs, including anticholinergic agents, GABAergic agents, dopaminergic agents, benzodiazepines, and catecholamine agonists and antagonists, have been

used with varying success in decreasing symptoms. A local injection of botulinum toxin type A has been used for focal dystonia.

1. Benztropine mesylate: 0.5–2 mg PO one or two times a day
2. Levodopa: 250 mg PO two to four times a day with food, increased by 100–750 mg for three to seven days until optimum dosage is reached, not to exceed 8 g daily
3. Carbidopa/levodopa: 10 mg/100 mg PO three to four times a day, increased by a single tablet every one to two days, as tolerated, until total dose is eight tablets daily, using the lowest dose that produces the desired clinical response
4. Baclofen: 5 mg PO three times a day, titrated upward PRN, not to exceed 20 mg four times a day
5. Trihexyphenidyl: 1 mg PO daily, increased in 2 mg increments every three to five days until a total dose of 6–10 mg daily; initial dose low and then increased gradually, especially in patients older than 60 years
6. Benzodiazepines: May be beneficial (e.g., clonazepam)
7. Depression and anxiety treated PRN (see Chapters 161 and 162)

E. Surgery: Procedure may be considered when individuals are no longer responding to other treatments. Surgery is performed to interrupt the pathways responsible for abnormal movements. Types of surgery include anterior cervical rhizotomy, thalamotomy, pallidotomy, and deep brain stimulation.

F. Botulinum toxin injections into the muscle for focal dystonia: Injection is often given in combination with oral medication.

VII. Follow-up
A. Frequency of follow-up is related to the underlying cause and treatment.
B. Follow up on medication use, adverse effects, and outcomes of therapy.

VIII. Referrals: Dependent on the suspected underlying cause
A. Neurologist: To evaluate neurologic deficits
B. Physical therapist: To assist with ambulation, stretching of dystonic area, or exercise to area
C. Occupational therapist: To assist with learning alternative methods to conduct ADLs
D. Speech therapist: To assist with speech deficits and alternative communication tools with oromandibular or cervical dystonia
E. Psychiatrist: To assist with anxiety and depression management

The author would like to acknowledge Giselle J. Moore-Higgs, ARNP, PhD, AOCN®, for her contribution to this chapter that remains unchanged from the previous edition of this book.

References

Albanese, A., Di Giovanni, M., & Lalli, S. (2019). Dystonia: Diagnosis and management. *European Journal of Neurology, 26*(1), 5–17. https://doi.org/10.1111/ene.13762

Balint, B., Mencacci, N.E., Valente, E.M., Pisani, A., Rothwell, J., Jankovic, J., ... Bhatia, K.P. (2018). Dystonia. *Nature Reviews Disease Primers, 4,* 25. https://doi.org/10.1038/s41572-018-0023-6

Chirumamilla, V.C., Dresel, C., Koirala, N., Gonzalez-Escamilla, G., Deuschl, G., Zeuner, K., ... Groppa, S. (2019). Structural brain network fingerprints of focal dystonia. *Therapeutic Advances in Neurological Disorders, 12.* https://doi.org/10.1177/1756286419880664

Duma, S.R., & Fung, V.S.C. (2019). Drug-induced movement disorders. *Australian Prescriber, 42*(2), 56–61. https://doi.org/10.18773/austprescr.2019.014

Ferreira Camargo, C.H., & Ghizoni Teive, H.A. (2019). Use of botulinum toxin for movement disorders. *Drugs in Context, 8,* 212586. https://doi.org/10.7573/dic.212586

Jinnah, H.A., & Factor, S.A. (2015). Diagnosis and treatment of dystonia. *Neurologic Clinics, 33*(1), 77–100. https://doi.org/10.1016/j.ncl.2014.09.002

Krack, P., Volkmann, J., Tinkhauser, G., & Deuschl, G. (2019). Deep brain stimulation in movement disorders: From experimental surgery to evidence-based therapy. *Movement Disorders, 34*(12), 1795–1806. https://doi.org/10.1002/mds.27860

Mainka, T., Erro, R., Rothwell, J., Kühn, A.A., Bhatia, K.P., & Ganos, C. (2019). Remission in dystonia—Systematic review of literature and meta-analysis. *Parkinsonism and Related Disorders, 66,* 9–15. https://doi.org/10.1016/j.parkreldis.2019.02.020

Marsili, L., Bologna, M., Kojovic, M., Berardelli, A., Espay, A.J., & Colosimo, C. (2019). Dystonia in atypical parkinsonian disorders. *Parkinsonism and Related Disorders, 66,* 25–33. https://doi.org/10.1016/j.parkreldis.2019.07.030

Nath, S., Mishra, B.R., Mishra, S., & Pattnaik, J.I. (2019). Acute dystonia following opioid withdrawal: An uncommon presentation. *Indian Journal of Psychological Medicine, 41*(6), 591–593. https://doi.org/10.4103/IJPSYM.IJPSYM_422_18

Richardson, S.P., & Jinnah, H.A. (2019). New approaches to discovering drugs that treat dystonia. *Expert Opinion on Drug Discovery, 14*(9), 893–900. https://doi.org/10.1080/17460441.2019.1623785

Ugawa, Y. (2020). Voluntary and involuntary movements: A proposal from a clinician. *Neuroscience Research, 156,* 80–87. https://doi.org/10.1016/j.neures.2019.10.001

van der Stouwe, A.M.M., Everlo, C.S.J., & Tijssen, M.A.J. (2019). Which disease features run in essential tremor families? A systematic review. *Parkinsonism and Related Disorders, 69,* 71–78. https://doi.org/10.1016/j.parkreldis.2019.10.017

CHAPTER 136

Foot Drop

Corazon Lauren Delumpa, MSN, RN, FNP-C

I. Definition: Loss of ankle and toe dorsiflexion because of weakness or paralysis of the anterior muscles of the lower leg (Carolus et al., 2019; Macki et al., 2018)

II. Physiology/Pathophysiology (Carolus et al, 2019; Dolev et al., 2018; Poage et al., 2016; Stevens et al., 2015)
   A. Normal
      1. Fibers from the L4–L5 and S1–S4 nerves form the lumbosacral plexus, which is located in the pelvis on the anterior surface of the sacrum on the piriformis muscle.
      2. The common peroneal (fibular) nerve innervates the peroneus longus muscle that performs the following.
         a) Motor function: Ankle dorsiflexion
         b) Sensory function: Lateral surface of leg and dorsal surface of foot
      3. Motor control of foot and ankle dorsiflexors includes the anterior tibialis, extensor hallucis longus, and extensor digitorum longus.
         a) The peroneus longus muscle originates at the upper fibula and lateral condyle of the tibia and inserts at the internal cuneiform and first metatarsal.
         b) This muscle controls ankle dorsiflexion, eversion, and abduction.
         c) The anterior tibialis is innervated by the common peroneal nerve, which branches from the sciatic nerve. The sciatic nerve exits the lumbar plexus, with its root arising from the fifth lumbar nerve space.
   B. Pathophysiology: Damage or injury along the course of the peroneal (fibular) nerve from the sciatic insertion to the terminal branches can cause foot drop. With acute compression (trauma or compartment syndrome), ischemia may cause a nerve conduction block; in chronic entrapment, an inflammatory response occurs resulting in a scar tissue (neuroma). Axonal (Wallerian) degeneration can occur after four weeks, causing progressive muscle weakness and atrophy.
      1. The most common compression is at the lateral fibular head.
      2. Entrapment of the L5 nerve root presenting as isolated foot drop is rare.
      3. A lesion in the brain or spinal cord rarely presents as isolated foot drop, but cases have been reported.

III. Clinical features: Bilateral foot drop, in general, is from neuromuscular disorders, whereas unilateral foot drop is from a focal disorder. Foot drop usually occurs without pain; it may occur with sensory changes such as tingling or burning. Systemic diseases with peripheral neuropathy may increase risk for foot drop. Foot drop may be the result of muscular, skeletal, or nervous system disorders (Bowley & Doughty, 2019; Krishnamurthy & Ibrahim, 2019; Macki et al., 2018; Stevens et al., 2015).

A. Etiology
 1. Iatrogenic
  a) Drugs
  b) Surgery
 2. Neurologic
  a) Cord or nerve compression
  b) Brain lesion
 3. Diseases
  a) Systemic
  b) Metabolic
  c) Neuromuscular
 4. Fracture or trauma
 5. Vitamin deficiency
B. History
 1. History of cancer and cancer treatment: Chemotherapy, radiation to lower spine or lower extremity
 2. Current medications: Prescribed, over the counter
 3. History of presenting symptoms: Precipitating factors, onset, location, duration, aggravating and relieving factors
 4. Changes in ADLs: Use of assistive devices
 5. Past medical history: Diabetes, neuropathy, neuromuscular disease, stroke, HZV
 6. History of trauma or recent surgery: Prolonged hospital stay (e.g., total knee arthroplasty, bariatric surgery with weight loss)
 7. Social history: Occupational, habits (e.g., prolonged leg crossing, squatting, kneeling)
C. Signs and symptoms: Categorized as motor weakness or incoordination secondary to sensory dysfunction
 1. Dragging of toes and high lifting of knees
 2. Slapping of foot to the ground when walking
 3. Decreased sensation of plantar surface of foot or extremity
 4. Lumbosacral back pain with radicular component in peroneal nerve distribution
 5. Atrophy of foot and/or distal extremity
D. Physical examination
 1. Neurologic: Sensory and motor evaluation of lumbosacral area, guided by specific symptoms and signs; may be diagnostic
  a) Gait observation for dragging of toes, high lifting of knees, or slapping of foot; irregular wear of patient's shoe
  b) Inability to heel-walk and steppage gait with an exaggerated lifting of the hip and knee to prevent the foot from catching on the ground
  c) Sensory examination of affected extremity compared to unaffected extremity
   (1) Two-point discrimination unrecognizable
   (2) Unable to distinguish hot, cold, sharp, or dull
   (3) Unable to distinguish location of stimuli
   (4) Unable to distinguish position of toe joint (altered proprioception)
   (5) Deep peroneal nerve lesion (reduced pinprick in first web space of great toe and second toe) versus superficial peroneal nerve lesion (reduced sensation in anterolateral lower leg and foot dorsum sparing the first web space or great toe and second toe)
  d) Deep tendon reflexes
   (1) Depressed or absent Achilles deep tendon reflexes

(2) Hyperactive reflexes and positive Babinski response suggestive of a central, not peripheral, etiology

e) Positive Tinel sign at fibular head: Used to detect peroneal (fibular) nerve entrapment; tap over the anterior tarsal tunnel on the proximal dorsum of the foot; test is positive if tapping produces paresthesia in the fibular nerve distribution.

2. Musculoskeletal

a) Muscle strength in foot dorsiflexion and eversion; planter flexion and inversion

b) Hip abduction to differentiate lumbar radiculopathy from peroneal neuropathy; hip weakness suggestive of lumbar radiculopathy as cause for foot drop

c) Supine single leg raise test: Pain with raised leg indicative of possible herniated disc

d) Muscle atrophy indicative of weakness of the extremity and loss of function

3. Integument: Erythema or edema around the knee or fibular head

IV. Diagnostic tests (Daniels et al., 2018)

A. Laboratory tests

1. Comprehensive metabolic panel to evaluate for renal insufficiency
2. Hgb A1c to evaluate for diabetes mellitus
3. Serum and urine protein electrophoresis to check for paraproteinemia
4. Vitamin B_{12}, MMA, and folate to assess for deficiency
5. ESR and CRP to evaluate for inflammation
6. Thyroid function test to assess for hypothyroidism

B. Radiology

1. Plain films or ultrasound of lower extremity if trauma or fracture suspected
2. CT scan and MRI for suspected intracranial, vertebral, or spinal cord pathology to evaluate for herniation or lateral neuroforaminal encroachment
3. Magnetic resonance neurography: More specific imaging of peripheral nerves and intra- and extraneural lesions

C. Other

1. Electromyogram and nerve conduction studies to evaluate site of lesion, estimate extent of injury, and classify chronicity
2. Lumbar puncture to obtain cytology, cell count, glucose, and cultures
3. Muscle or nerve biopsy, as indicated: Can be diagnostic for Charcot-Marie-Tooth disease

V. Differential diagnosis (Bowley & Doughty, 2019; Lomaglio & Canale, 2017; Macki et al., 2018; Rallis et al., 2015)

A. Drug neurotoxicity

1. Chemotherapy: Vinca alkaloids, platinum, taxanes, cytarabine, procarbazine, fludarabine, monoclonal antibodies
2. Other drugs: Statins, cyclosporine, metronidazole, dapsone, amiodarone

B. Nerve compression

1. Primary tumors: Sarcomas, neurofibromas
2. Compartment syndrome secondary to infection or trauma
3. Immobilization devices: Knee-high elastic stockings or wraps, pneumatic compression boots, casts
4. Prolonged bed rest without foot support
5. Heparinization, which predisposes a stretched nerve to intraneural bleeding
6. Chronic pressure from crossing legs

C. Brain: Trauma, tumor, infection, cerebral vascular accident (see Chapter 146)

D. Systemic disease
1. Paraneoplastic syndrome: Symmetric or asymmetric sensory neuropathy (see Appendix M)
2. Diabetes mellitus (see Chapter 151)
3. HIV/AIDS
4. Multiple sclerosis
5. Hypothyroidism (see Chapter 158)
6. Chronic renal failure: Uremia (see Chapter 86)
7. Collagen vascular disease
8. Amyotrophic lateral sclerosis
9. Postpolio syndrome
10. Hereditary conditions: Charcot-Marie-Tooth disease
11. HZV (see Chapter 22)
12. Vitamin deficiencies: B_1, B_9, B_{12} (see Chapters 115 and 116)
E. Toxic etiologies
1. Alcoholic neuropathy
2. Heavy metal exposure: Lead
3. Pesticides
4. Bacterial toxins: Botulinum, tetanus
F. Fracture or trauma (see Chapter 102)
1. Peroneal nerve trauma
2. Vertebral, tibial, or femoral fracture
3. Knee: Post–total knee replacement, tear of lateral collateral ligament
4. Femoral head dislocation
G. Lumbar etiology: Spinal stenosis, nerve root compression, radiculopathy
H. Idiopathic polyneuritis
1. Guillain-Barré syndrome
2. Paraproteinemia and macroglobulinemia
I. Myelopathy secondary to radiation to sacral plexus: Late effect seen one to two years after radiation

VI. Treatment: Directed by etiology of foot drop (Bethoux et al., 2014; Carolus et al., 2019; George & Boyce, 2014; Krishnamurthy & Ibrahim, 2019; Nath & Somasundaram, 2017; Poage et al., 2016)
A. Ankle–foot orthosis (AFO): A mechanical brace worn on the lower leg and foot
1. Two opposing views exist regarding the effect of AFO on overall muscle strength.
   a) Loss of strength in the ankle flexors may result because of disuse.
   b) AFO will stimulate the patient to walk, thereby activating paretic muscles.
2. Studies have shown that long-term use of neuroprosthesis or AFO significantly enhanced functional ability and reintegration.
3. Pneumatic power AFO device showed that fluid power control with a pneumatic built into the AFO allowed for ankle and foot motion during stance.
4. Currently, AFO is the gold standard for foot drop management.
B. Implanted and surface functional electrical stimulation (FES): Devices produce short bursts of electrical pulses to elicit muscle contractions primarily during the swing phase of gait.
1. FES was shown to have orthotic benefit for up to 11 months in progressive and non-progressive disorders that caused foot drop.
2. Long-term use of FES improves walking performance, even when the stimulator is off. FES strengthens the activation of the motor cortical areas and their residual descending pathways, which leads to an increase in walking speed.

3. FES has been shown to be an effective alternative to AFO.

C. Surgical interventions

1. It can repair trauma-induced injury to the dorsiflexors.
2. Posterior tibial tendon transfer has shown benefit.
3. Outcome of nerve grafting or nerve transfer is better if performed within four to seven months, with a graft length less than or equal to 12 cm.
4. Lumbar surgery can be performed for decompression of malignant and nonmalignant sources.

D. Physical and occupational rehabilitation therapy: To optimize function and prevent long-term morbidities such as contractures

E. Pain management, including adjuvant drugs (see Appendices E, F, and Q)

VII. Follow-up: Dependent on etiology and treatment plan

VIII. Referrals

A. Rehabilitative services: For physical and occupational therapy
B. Neurosurgeon, plastic surgeon, or orthopedist: For surgical intervention
C. Neurologist: To evaluate cause or treat foot drop not responding to conventional treatment

The author would like to acknowledge Laurie Rice, RN, MSN, ANP-BC, for her contribution to this chapter that remains unchanged from the previous edition of this book.

References

Bethoux, F., Rogers, H.L., Nolan, K.J., Abrams, G.M., Annaswamy, T.M., Brandstater, M., … Kufta, C. (2014). The effects of peroneal nerve functional electrical stimulation versus ankle-foot orthosis in patients with chronic stroke. *Neurorehabilitation and Neural Repair, 28*(7), 688–697. https://doi.org/10.1177/1545968314521007

Bowley, M.P., & Doughty, C.T. (2019). Entrapment neuropathies of the lower extremity. *Medical Clinics of North America, 103*(2), 371–382. https://doi.org/10.1016/j.mcna.2018.10.013

Carolus, A.E., Becker, M., Cuny, J., Smektala, R., Schmieder, K., & Brenke, C. (2019). The interdisciplinary management of foot drop. *Deutsches Ärzteblatt International, 116*(20), 347–354. https://doi.org/10.3238/arztebl.2019.0347

Daniels, S.P., Feinberg, J.H., Carrino, J.A., Behzadi, A.H., & Sneag, D.B. (2018). MRI of foot drop: How we do it. *Radiology, 289*(1), 9–24. https://doi.org/10.1148/radiol.2018172634

Dolev, A., Robinson, D., & Yassin, M. (2018). A central nervous system tumor mimicking a lumbar spine pathology causing acute foot drop: A case report. *Journal of Orthopaedic Case Reports, 8*(5), 78–81. https://doi.org/10.13107/jocr.2250-0685.1222

George, S.C., & Boyce, D.E. (2014). An evidence-based structured review to assess the results of common peroneal nerve repair. *Plastic and Reconstructive Surgery, 134*(2), 302e–311e. https://doi.org/10.1097/PRS.0000000000000318

Krishnamurthy, S., & Ibrahim, M. (2019). Tendon transfers in foot drop. *Indian Journal of Plastic Surgery, 52*(1), 100–108. https://doi.org/10.1055/s-0039-1688105

Lomaglio, M., & Canale, B. (2017). Differential diagnosis and recovery of acute bilateral foot drop in a patient with a history of low back pain: A case report. *Physiotherapy Theory and Practice, 33*(6), 508–514. https://doi.org/10.1080/09593985.2017.1323358

Macki, M., Lim, S., Elmenini, J., Fakih, M., & Chang, V. (2018). Clinching the cause: A review of foot drop secondary to lumbar degenerative diseases. *Journal of the Neurological Sciences, 395,* 126–130. https://doi.org/10.1016/j.jns.2018.09.036

Nath, R.K., & Somasundaram, C. (2017). Gait improvements after peroneal or tibial nerve transfer in patients with foot drop: A retrospective study. *Eplasty, 17,* e31.

Poage, C., Roth, C., & Scott, B. (2016). Peroneal nerve palsy. *Journal of the American Academy of Orthopaedic Surgeons, 24*(1), 1–10. https://doi.org/10.5435/jaaos-d-14-00420

Rallis, D., Skafida, A., Alexopoulos, G., Petsanas, A., Foteinos, A., Katsoulakou, S., & Koutra, E. (2015). Clinical reasoning: A 51-year-old woman with acute foot drop. *Neurology, 84*(7), e48–e52 https://doi.org/10.1212/wnl.0000000000001261

Stevens, F., Weerkamp, N.J., & Cals, J.W.L. (2015). Foot drop. *BMJ, 350,* h1736. https://doi.org/10.1136/bmj.h1736

CHAPTER 137

Headache

Christa Seligman, MSN, APRN, AGNP-C

I. Definition: Pain referred to the surface of the head from deep structures (May, 2018; Onderwater et al., 2018)
   A. Self-limiting: Headache resolves without therapy within several months.
   B. Refractory: Headache is resistant to aggressive treatment regimens.
   C. Primary: Headache is the disease.
   D. Secondary: Headache is a symptom.

II. Physiology/Pathophysiology (Al-Ansari & Robertson, 2019; Castien & De Hertogh, 2019; Goadsby & Holland, 2019; González-Quintanilla & Pascual, 2019; Onderwater et al., 2018)
   A. Normal: The head provides the bony housing and protective covering for the brain.
      1. Intracranial: The cranial vault, including cranial nerves V, IX, and X; upper cervical nerves; venous sinuses; the dura at the skull base; and the dura arteries and the large arteries at the brain base, which give rise to the circle of Willis
      2. Extracranial: The skin, fascia, muscles, scalp blood vessels, paranasal spaces, external and middle ear, teeth, scalp, and facial muscles
      3. Sensation of pain is transmitted by pain receptors, which are located at the base of the brain in arteries and veins and throughout the meninges; extracranial vessels; muscles of the scalp, neck, and face; sinuses; eyes; and teeth.
   B. Pathophysiology
      1. The brain itself is almost totally insensitive to pain; however, damage to the venous sinuses or to the membranes covering the brain can cause intense pain.
      2. Headache pain may originate from either intracranial or extracranial structures. In brain tumors or metastases, the meninges and basal vessels are displaced and stretched, causing pain.
      3. Tension headaches may be from hypersensitivity to incoming C fiber input from the trigeminal nerve or tonic contraction of jaw muscles.
      4. Migraine may be from inhibition of cortical neuronal activity, reduction of cerebral blood flow, vasodilation of dural arteries, or release of vasoactive substances such as substance P or prostaglandins. Activation of certain neurons containing the neurotransmitter chemicals 5-HT and norepinephrine appears to result in vasodilation of intracranial and extracranial blood vessels.
      5. Cluster headache is thought to result from an autonomic function abnormality with increased parasympathetic drive and decreased sympathetic function. Attacks often begin during sleep, implicating a disorder of circadian rhythm.

III. Clinical features: The clinical features of headache are related to the type. History should elicit previous patterns to determine whether headaches are directly related to a disease or treatment. Table 137-1 describes the clinical characteristics of a variety of headaches. Most primary headaches can be diagnosed from a thorough history and physical examination. Tension headaches are the most common primary headache, whereas migraine headaches are the most common disabling primary headache worldwide. Many people have a combination of the different types of headache. Headache presents in 60% of people with brain tumors or brain metastasis (Andrijauskis et al., 2019; Castien & De Hertogh, 2019; Chiu et al., 2015; D'Antona & Matharu, 2019; Evans, 2019; Ferini-Strambi et al., 2019; Finocchi & Sassos, 2017; Goadsby & Holland, 2019; González-Quintanilla & Pascual, 2019; Guryildirim et al., 2019; Kahriman & Zhu, 2018; Magge & DeAngelis, 2015; May, 2018; Sutherland & Griffiths, 2017; Vgontzas & Burch, 2018; Walling, 2018; Wei et al., 2019; Yamani & Olesen, 2019).

A. Etiology (see Table 137-1)
1. Cancer related
   a) Headache related to brain tumor may be the result of increased ICP from mass effect or associated edema, which distorts nerve endings in the pain-sensitive dura.
   b) Pituitary tumor can cause headaches as a result of dural stretch and endocrine factors.
   c) Headache related to brain edema has been reported as a side effect of high-dose cranial radiation therapy.
   d) Headache has been reported as a side effect of intrathecal therapy.
   e) Various chemotherapies, including hormonal therapies, may induce headache.
   f) Lung cancer rarely presents with facial pain or headache from invasion or compression of the vagus nerve and circulating humoral factors.
   g) Anemia-mediated cerebral hypoxia may cause headache.

TABLE 137-1	Classification of Headaches
Primary	**Secondary**
Associated with substance abuse or withdrawal	Acute or chronic substance use or exposure Acute or chronic withdrawal (alcohol, drugs)
Cluster	Chronic paroxysmal hemicrania Cluster
Cranial neuralgia	Glossopharyngeal neuralgia Nervus intermedius neuralgia Occipital neuralgia Persistent pain of cranial nerve origin Superior laryngeal neuralgia Trigeminal neuralgia
Disorder of facial or cranial structures	Cranial bone Eye, ears, nose, and sinuses Teeth, jaws, and related structures Temporomandibular disease
Head trauma	Acute post-traumatic Chronic post-traumatic
Metabolic disorder	Dialysis Hypercapnia Hypoxia Mixed hypoxia and hypercapnia Other

(Continued on next page)

TABLE 137-1	Classification of Headaches *(Continued)*
Primary	**Secondary**
Migraine	Migraine disorders not listed Migraine with aura Migraine without aura Ophthalmologic migraine
New daily persistent headache	Bilateral Mild to moderate intensity Pressing and tightening quality
Noncephalic infection	Bacterial Viral Other infection
Nonvascular intracranial disorder	High cerebrospinal fluid pressure Inflammatory disease Intracranial infection Intracranial neoplasm Low cerebrospinal fluid pressure Related to intrathecal injection Sarcoidosis
Tension	Chronic tension type Episodic tension type
Vascular disorders	Acute ischemic cerebrovascular disorder Arterial hypertension Arteritis Carotid or vertebral artery Intracranial hematoma Subarachnoid hemorrhage Unruptured vascular malformation Venous thrombosis
Miscellaneous (no association with structural lesion)	Benign cough Benign exertional Cold stimulus External compression Idiopathic stabbing

Note. Based on information from Al-Ansari & Robertson, 2019; Burch, 2019; Evans, 2019; Goadsby, 2019; González-Quintanilla & Pascual, 2019; Walling, 2018; Yamani & Olesen, 2019.

2. Migraine
   a) This headache type is seen in approximately 15% of women and 6% of men.
   b) Common instigators may be red wine, menses, estrogen, lack of sleep, and stress.
3. Tension
   a) This headache type is associated with emotional or physical strain.
   b) It can also be associated with obstructive sleep apnea.
4. Cluster: This rare form of headache (less than 0.1% of all headaches) occurs three times more frequently in men than women.
5. Hypertensive headache
   a) Headache may be a symptom attributed to arterial hypertension only if blood pressure values are very high or rise quickly.
   b) Increased risk for stroke event is seen with hypertensive headache.

6. New daily persistent headache: This daily headache is unremitting from the moment of onset or very rapidly builds up to continuous pain.

7. Postconcussion headache

B. History

1. History of cancer and cancer treatment

2. Current medications: Prescribed, over the counter (e.g., supplements)

3. History of presenting symptoms: Precipitating factors, location, intensity, temporal issues (e.g., close to menses), duration, associated symptoms (e.g., nausea, syncope, visual changes, photophobia, phonophobia), prodromal signs (a period of indistinct symptoms occurring before the headache starts) that include visual auras or feeling tired, irritable, clumsy, or thirsty

4. Changes in ADLs

5. Past medical history: Head or neck trauma, infection, headache syndromes

6. Family history: Strong genetic component to migraine

7. Social history: Alcohol use, sleeping patterns

C. Signs and symptoms: Symptoms described as the "worst headache in my life," waking up with a headache, vomiting preceding headache, or headache induced by activities such as coughing, lifting, or bending over may be serious in nature.

1. Migraine: Typically occurs with repeated attacks lasting 4–72 hours with a normal physical examination

   a) Two of the following symptoms classify a headache as migraine: Unilateral, throbbing pain or pain increased by movement of moderate to severe intensity, plus one of these two features: nausea and vomiting, or phonophobia or photophobia.

   b) Migraine can be with or without aura.

   (1) With aura: Nausea, vomiting, photophobia, phonophobia, temporary visual disturbances, weakness (hemiplegic migraine), paresthesia, dysarthria, fatigue

   (2) Without aura: Muscle tension, neck pain

2. Cluster: Ptosis, miosis, lacrimation, rhinorrhea, motoric restlessness (pacing or rocking), facial flushing, unbearable stabbing or gnawing pain that is usually unilateral (called "suicide headache" because of severity of pain) and radiates to upper teeth, jaw, and neck

3. Tension: Described as band-like tightness that builds slowly; may be episodic or chronic, defined as more than 15 days per month; includes sleep disturbances, vertigo, a dull and oppressive pain that is usually diffuse in the frontal and parietal areas; can be associated with neck, scalp, or shoulder tenderness or stiffness

4. Drug induced (e.g., 5-HT$_3$ receptor antagonist agents ondansetron and granisetron, nitroglycerin, hormone therapy, stimulants): Dull, oppressive, stabbing pain that is usually diffuse

5. Post-traumatic: May be acute within days or chronic within weeks to months; dull, oppressive pain that is usually diffuse

6. Postjunctional: Tinnitus; vertigo; reduction of hearing; nausea; dull, knocking pain that is usually diffuse or in the occipital location

7. Trigeminal neuralgia: Weight loss; inability to talk; very intense stabbing, burning pain felt unilaterally over one or more branches of the trigeminal nerve; pain over the middle (V2: maxillary nerve) or lower (V3: mandibular nerve) branch (common)

8. Brain tumors or metastasis: Nausea, vomiting, papilledema (late sign), seizures, and dull, moderate-to-severe pain located in occipital or bifrontal region; unilateral facial pain commonly localized to the ear, jaw, and temporal region

        9. Neck pain

      10. Sleep disturbances

   D. Physical examination

      1. Vital signs indicating late signs of increased ICP

         a) Widening pulse pressure: Increased systolic, decreased diastolic pressures

         b) Bradycardia

         c) Severe hypertension

      2. Neurologic: Mental status, awareness, cognitive abilities, affect

         a) Confusion

         b) Decreased attention span

         c) Memory loss

         d) Ataxia with severe nausea and vomiting indicative of midline cerebellar hemorrhage

         e) Visual impairments indicative of possible acute glaucoma

         f) Psychological evaluation: Strong relationship between pain and depression

      3. HEENT

         a) Evidence of head trauma

         b) Skull tenderness indicating subdural hematoma

         c) Poor dentition, teeth grinding, jaw grinding

         d) Bogginess or tenderness of sinuses with sinus headache

         e) Papilledema with brain tumors or brain metastasis

         f) Palpate TMJ: Limited motion and crepitus present with joint disorder

         g) Dull tympanic membrane or fluid in ear with OM

         h) Possible conjunctiva injection present in cluster headache

         i) Possible lacrimation and rhinorrhea in cluster headache

         j) Palpate temporal area for tenderness indicating temporal arteritis

      4. Neck

         a) Nuchal rigidity indicating meningitis

         b) Tenderness to palpation of shoulders, neck, and occiput with tension headaches

         c) Decreased range of motion with tension headaches

         d) Carotid bruits

      5. Integument: Vesiculopapular rash indicating HZV

      6. Musculoskeletal: Evidence of misalignment or trauma on palpation

IV. Diagnostic tests (Evans, 2019; Guryildirim et al., 2019; Walling, 2018)

   A. Laboratory

      1. ESR: May be elevated in cancer-related headaches or temporal arteritis

      2. CBC

         a) Anemia

         b) Increased WBCs indicative of possible infection

         c) Marked leukocytosis indicative of possible acute leukemia, which can present with headache

      3. Chemistries to evaluate for renal failure or metabolic imbalances

      4. Drug screen: Cocaine and amphetamines can cause intracranial hemorrhage; opioids can cause rebound headache.

   B. Radiology

      1. CT scan or MRI of brain to assess for lesions, mass, or bleed

      2. Chest x-ray: Hypertrophic osteopathy may be present as a paraneoplastic syndrome of lung cancer (see Appendix M).

C. Other
  1. Lumbar puncture to evaluate for infection or leptomeningeal disease, as indicated: Observe opening pressure if suspicion of increased ICP.
  2. Temporal artery biopsy if arteritis is suspected

V. Differential diagnosis (González-Quintanilla & Pascual, 2019; Guryildirim et al., 2019; May, 2018; Ravishankar et al., 2017)
  A. Migraine
  B. Subarachnoid hemorrhage
  C. Meningitis (see Chapter 141)
  D. Subdural hematoma
  E. Stroke (see Chapter 146)
  F. Arteriovenous malformation
  G. Dental abnormalities
  H. Sinusitis (see Chapter 11)
  I. Acute glaucoma
  J. Hypertension (see Chapter 47)
  K. SLE (see Chapter 110)
  L. Trigeminal neuralgia
  M. Malignancy-related conditions
    1. Primary brain tumor
    2. Brain metastasis
    3. Meningeal involvement
    4. Non-Hodgkin lymphoma
    5. Neurosarcoidosis
  N. TMJ dysfunction
  O. Substance abuse
  P. Tension
  Q. Cluster
  R. Giant cell arteritis
  S. Ruptured aneurysm
  T. Pseudotumor cerebri

VI. Treatment (Al-Ansari & Robertson, 2019; Assarzadegan & Sistanizad, 2017; Burch, 2019; Chan & Goadsby, 2019; D'Antona & Matharu, 2019; Evans, 2019; Ferini-Strambi et al., 2019; Goadsby, 2019; Herd et al., 2019; Kahriman & Zhu, 2018; Long et al., 2020; May, 2018; Parikh & Silberstein, 2019; Rau & Dodick, 2019; Scripter, 2018; Tepper, 2019; Wei et al., 2019)
  A. Migraines
    1. Nonpharmacologic
      a) Avoidance of triggers, such as chocolate, cheese, citrus fruit, alcohol/red wine, stress, and others: Headache diary can help to assess triggers.
      b) Noninvasive brain stimulation: Preventive and abortive
        (1) Transcutaneous magnetic stimulation
        (2) Transcutaneous direct current stimulation
    2. Prophylactic: Each option should be given at least a two-month trial unless not tolerated.
      a) Beta-blockers
        (1) Propranolol: 40 mg PO daily, up to 40–160 mg PO daily in two divided doses
        (2) Metoprolol: 100 mg PO daily, up to 100–200 mg PO daily in two divided doses

      (3) Timolol: 20 mg PO daily, up to 20–30 mg PO daily in two divided doses

      (4) Nadolol: 80 mg PO daily, up to 240 mg PO daily

      (5) Atenolol: 100 mg PO daily

  b) ACE inhibitors: Enalapril: 2.5 mg PO daily to 20 mg PO two times a day

  c) ARBs: Candesartan: 8 mg PO daily up to 16 mg PO daily

  d) N-methyl-d-aspartic acid receptor antagonists (off label)

      (1) Memantine: Initiate at 5 mg PO daily; may increase up to 20 mg PO daily.

      (2) Use in refractory cases.

  e) Tricyclic antidepressants: Initiate with a low dose and increase weekly. Perform a baseline ECG, as this drug class can prolong the QT interval.

      (1) Amitriptyline: 10–50 mg PO at bedtime

      (2) Nortriptyline: 10–100 mg PO at bedtime

  f) Anticonvulsants

      (1) Divalproex sodium extended release: 500 mg PO daily for one week, up to 1,000 mg PO daily

      (2) Topiramate: 25 mg PO daily, up to maximum of 100 mg PO two times a day; should not use if history of kidney stones

  g) Serotonergic drugs: Cyproheptadine: 4–16 mg PO daily

  h) Botulinum toxin type A injections have been found to decrease both frequency and severity of migraines.

  i) Monoclonal antibodies: Calcitonin gene–related peptide receptor agonists

      (1) Erenumab: 70 mg/ml or 140 mg/ml subcutaneous injection monthly

      (2) Fremanezumab: 100 mg/ml or 120 mg/ml subcutaneous injection monthly; indicated for both migraine and cluster headache prevention

      (3) Fremanezumab-vfrm: 675 mg/3.5 ml subcutaneous injection quarterly

      (4) Galcanezumab: Loading dose of 240 mg/2 ml subcutaneous injection, then 120 mg/ml monthly

3. Acute attacks

  a) NSAIDs (see Appendix E)

  b) Triptans: These are contraindicated in patients with certain cardiovascular risk factors, including diabetes, hypertension, hyperlipidemia, obesity, and smoking.

      (1) Sumatriptan: 6 mg subcutaneous; may be repeated in one hour if initial dose is not effective; maximum 12 mg in 24 hours; available in nasal spray; single dose of 5, 10, or 20 mg administered in one nostril; greater than 20 mg does not provide greater effect; oral route: 25–100 mg tablet initially, maximum of 200 mg daily

      (2) Zolmitriptan: 1.25–2.5 mg PO every two hours; maximum 10 mg PO in 24 hours; available in a nasal spray 5 mg (one spray); may be repeated after two hours; also available as 2.5 mg disintegrating tablet with maximum of 10 mg daily

      (3) Rizatriptan: 5–10 mg PO; may be repeated in two hours; maximum 30 mg in 24 hours; dissolves on tongue without liquids

  c) Prednisone: 50–80 mg PO daily; tapered over 10–14 days

  d) Prochlorperazine: 10 mg IV or IM as a single dose

  e) Calcitonin gene-related peptide receptor antagonists: Ubrogepant 100 mg PO at onset of migraine attack; may repeat once in two hours if no relief

4. Alternative therapies: Acupuncture, herbal remedies, massage, aromatherapy, meditation

B. Tension headaches
   1. Episodic: NSAIDs (see Appendix E)
      a) Encourage patients to avoid medication overuse for headaches.
      b) Recommend reduction if headaches and analgesic use are more than 15 days per month.
   2. Chronic: NSAIDs and lifestyle changes
      a) Relaxation techniques
      b) Coping strategies to deal with stress
      c) Physiotherapy for musculoskeletal symptoms
      d) Amitriptyline: 10 mg PO every night; may increase to 30–50 mg
      e) Transcutaneous electrical nerve stimulation unit: Nonpharmacologic method to treat tension headaches that may be beneficial; includes biofeedback, cognitive behavioral therapy, and massage
C. Cluster headaches
   1. Acute
      a) Sumatriptan: 6 mg subcutaneous or 20 mg nasal spray; may be repeated in 24 hours
      b) Oxygen: 7 L/min for 15 minutes by face mask
   2. Prophylactic treatments
      a) Verapamil: 80–480 mg PO daily, regular or sustained release
      b) Dihydroergotamine solution: 1 mg IV, IM, or subcutaneous; may be repeated in one hour; maximum 2 mg IV or 3 mg IM or subcutaneous; available in nasal spray
      c) Prednisone: 50–80 mg PO daily, tapered over 10–14 days
      d) Melatonin: 10 mg PO at bedtime
      e) Divalproex sodium: 600–2,000 mg PO daily
      f) Topiramate: 25 mg PO daily for seven days; increased by 25 mg daily every week; maximum dose 200 mg daily
      g) Fremanezumab: 100 mg/ml or 120 mg/ml subcutaneous injection monthly; indicated for both migraine and cluster headache prevention
      h) Ergotamine: 2–4 mg PO daily in divided doses; maximum of 6 mg daily and 10 mg weekly
      i) Lithium: 300 mg PO two to three times a day to achieve therapeutic serum level
      j) Radiofrequency trigeminal rhizotomy may be beneficial if patient is refractory to all pharmacologic interventions.
      k) Noninvasive brain stimulation
D. Headache related to brain tumor or brain metastasis
   1. Primary brain tumors usually are managed with multimodal treatment of chemotherapy, radiation, and surgery.
   2. Metastatic disease usually is treated with radiation or stereotactic treatment.
      a) Dexamethasone is used to decrease edema of the brain arising from the lesions themselves or from treatment. Doses vary based on many factors.
      b) Initiate at 4 mg PO daily and assess. Monitor steroid use closely with goal to taper.
E. Consider medications to manage sleep disturbances.

VII. Follow-up: Dependent on etiology of headache (Walling, 2018)
   A. Hospitalize patients with acute onset and severe headache who have history of cancer or symptoms of ICP or meningitis.
   B. Follow-up of patients with brain tumors will be frequent depending on treatment.
   C. Follow up 7–14 days after initiating treatment for headaches.

VIII. Referrals (Castien & De Hertogh, 2019; Goadsby, 2019)

    A. Massage therapist or physical therapist: For musculoskeletal etiology for tension headaches

    B. Neurologist: For evaluation and treatment plan of transient neurologic dysfunction, unilateral headache with increasing frequency and severity, headache refractory to two or more therapies, or neurologic deficits associated with headache

    C. Neurosurgeon: For surgery of brain tumor or neurostimulator device

    D. Radiation or medical oncologist: For treatment of cancer

    E. Ophthalmologist: For consideration of papilledema, glaucoma testing

    F. Dentist: For TMJ problems

    G. Psychiatrist or psychologist: For patients with chronic, intractable, tension-type headaches who have undergone complete evaluation for etiology; depression may play a part in headaches.

The author would like to acknowledge Laurie Rice, RN, MSN, ANP-BC, for her contribution to this chapter that remains unchanged from the previous edition of this book.

References

Al-Ansari, A., & Robertson, N.P. (2019). Cluster headache: An overview of established and emerging treatments. *Journal of Neurology, 266*(11), 2890–2892. https://doi.org/10.1007/s00415-019-09548-x

Andrijauskis, D., Ciauskaite, J., Vaitkus, A., & Pajediene, E. (2019). Primary headaches and sleep disturbances: A cause or a consequence? *Journal of Oral and Facial Pain and Headache, 34*(1), 61–66. https://doi.org/10.11607/ofph.2405

Assarzadegan, F., & Sistanizad, M. (2017). Tolerability and efficacy of memantine as add on therapy in patients with migraine. *Iranian Journal of Pharmaceutical Research, 16*(2), 791.

Burch, R. (2019). Migraine and tension-type headache: Diagnosis and treatment. *Medical Clinics of North America, 103*(2), 215–233. https://doi.org/10.1016/j.mcna.2018.10.003

Castien, R., & De Hertogh, W. (2019). A neuroscience perspective of physical treatment of headache and neck pain. *Frontiers in Neurology, 10,* 276. https://doi.org/10.3389/fneur.2019.00276

Chan, C., & Goadsby, P.J. (2019). Recent advances in pharmacotherapy for episodic migraine. *CNS Drugs, 33*(11), 1053–1071. https://doi.org/10.1007/s40263-019-00665-9

Chiu, Y.-C., Hu, H.-Y., Lee, F.-P., & Huang, H.-M. (2015). Tension-type headache associated with obstructive sleep apnea: a nationwide population-based study. *Journal of Headache and Pain, 16,* 34. https://doi.org/10.1186/s10194-015-0517-5

D'Antona, L., & Matharu, M. (2019). Identifying and managing refractory migraine: Barriers and opportunities? *Journal of Headache and Pain, 20,* 89. https://doi.org/10.1186/s10194-019-1040-x

Evans, R.W. (2019). Diagnostic testing for migraine and other primary headaches. *Neurologic Clinics, 37*(4), 707–725. https://doi.org/10.1016/j.ncl.2019.08.001

Ferini-Strambi, L., Galbiati, A., & Combi, R. (2019). Sleep disorder–related headaches. *Neurological Sciences, 40*(Suppl. 1), 107–113. https://doi.org/10.1007/s10072-019-03837-z

Finocchi, C., & Sassos, D. (2017). Headache and arterial hypertension. *Neurological Sciences, 38*(Suppl. 1), 67–72. https://doi.org/10.1007/s10072-017-2893-x

Goadsby, P.J. (2019). Primary headache disorders: Five new things. *Neurology: Clinical Practice, 9*(3), 233–240. https://doi.org/10.1212/CPJ.0000000000000654

Goadsby, P.J., & Holland, P.R. (2019). An update: Pathophysiology of migraine. *Neurologic Clinics, 37*(4), 651–671. https://doi.org/10.1016/j.ncl.2019.07.008

González-Quintanilla, V., & Pascual, J. (2019). Other primary headaches: An update. *Neurologic Clinics, 37*(4), 871–891. https://doi.org/10.1016/j.ncl.2019.07.010

Guryildirim, M., Kontzialis, M., Ozen, M., & Kocak, M. (2019). Acute headache in the emergency setting. *RadioGraphics, 39*(6), 1739–1759. https://doi.org/10.1148/rg.2019190017

Herd, C.P., Tomlinson, C.L., Rick, C., Scotton, W.J., Edwards, J., Ives, N.J., … Sinclair, A.J. (2019). Cochrane systematic review and meta-analysis of botulinum toxin for the prevention of migraine. *BMJ Open, 9*(7), e027953. https://doi.org/10.1136/bmjopen-2018-027953

Kahriman, A., & Zhu, S. (2018). Migraine and tension-type headaches. *Seminars in Neurology, 38*(6), 608–618. https://doi.org/10.1055/s-0038-1673683

Long, B., Koyfman, A., & Gottlieb, M. (2020). Prochlorperazine for treatment of acute migraines in adults. *Academic Emergency Medicine, 27*(3), 243–244. https://doi.org/10.1111/acem.13864

Magge, R.S., & DeAngelis, L.M. (2015). The double-edged sword: Neurotoxicity of chemotherapy. *Blood Reviews, 29*(2), 93–100. https://doi.org/10.1016/j.blre.2014.09.012

May, A. (2018). Hints on diagnosing and treating headache. *Deutsches Ärzteblatt International, 115*(17), 299–308. https://doi.org/10.3238/arztebl.2018.0299

Onderwater, G.L.J., Van Dongen, R.M., Zielman, R., Terwindt, G.M., & Ferrari, M.D. (2018). Primary headaches. In F. Deisenhammer, C.E. Teunissen, & H. Tumani (Eds.), *Handbook of clinical neurology: Vol. 146* (pp. 267–284). https://doi.org/10.1016/B978-0-12-804279-3.00016-2

Parikh, S.K., & Silberstein, S.D. (2019). Preventive treatment for episodic migraine. *Neurologic Clinics, 37*(4), 753–770. https://doi.org/10.1016/j.ncl.2019.07.004

Rau, J.C., & Dodick, D.W. (2019). Other preventive anti-migraine treatments: ACE inhibitors, ARBs, calcium channel blockers, serotonin antagonists, and NMDA receptor antagonists. *Current Treatment Options in Neurology, 21*(4), 17. https://doi.org/10.1007/s11940-019-0559-0

Ravishankar, K., Evans, R.W., & Wang, S.-J. (Eds.). (2017). *Modern day management of headache: Questions and answers.* Jaypee Brothers Medical Publishers.

Scripter, C. (2018). Headache: Tension-type headache. *FP Essentials, 473,* 17–20.

Sutherland, H.G., & Griffiths, L.R. (2017). Genetics of migraine: Insights into the molecular basis of migraine disorders. *Headache: The Journal of Head and Face Pain, 57*(4), 537–569. https://doi.org/10.1111/head.13053

Tepper, S.J. (2019). Acute treatment of migraine. *Neurologic Clinics, 37*(4), 727–742. https://doi.org/10.1016/j.ncl.2019.07.006

Vgontzas, A., & Burch, R. (2018). Episodic migraine with and without aura: Key differences and implications for pathophysiology, management, and assessing risks. *Current Pain and Headache Reports, 22*(12), 78. https://doi.org/10.1007/s11916-018-0735-z

Walling, A. (2018). Headache: Headache emergencies. *FP Essentials, 473,* 21–25.

Wei, D.Y., Khalil, M., & Goadsby, P.J. (2019). Managing cluster headaches. *Practical Neurology, 19*(6), 521–528. https://doi.org/10.1136/practneurol-2018-002124

Yamani, N., & Olesen, J. (2019). New daily persistent headache: A systematic review on an enigmatic disorder. *Journal of Headache and Pain, 20,* 80. https://doi.org/10.1186/s10194-019-1022-z

CHAPTER 138

Paresthesia

Julie G. Walker, PhD, APRN, FNP-C

I. Definition: Abnormal neurologic sensations, which include numbness, tingling, burning, and hyperesthesia, that progress to burning or shooting pain and motor weakness caused by insult to the somatosensory system (Boyette-Davis et al., 2018; Boyette-Davis et al., 2015; Mu et al., 2017)

II. Physiology/Pathophysiology (Boyette-Davis et al., 2018; Boyette-Davis et al., 2015; Butler & Bronner, 2015; Kim et al., 2015; Sudiwala & Knox, 2019)

   A. Normal
   1. The PNS develops from neural crest cells and ectodermal placodes at the cranial level, forming cranial sensory ganglia and sense organs of the nose, ears, and eyes. Caudal development of the PNS arises from neural crest cells along the neural tube.
      a) Those nearest the cranium migrate to form enteric ganglia, which is responsible for gut motility.
      b) Those arising from the level of the trunk aid the development of dorsal root and sympathetic ganglia.
      c) Bilateral sensory fibers appearing from the dorsal root ganglia are responsible for proprioception and sensation of temperature and injury.
   2. Afferent (sensory) fibers within the PNS transmit sensory information from the skin and mucous membranes, proprioception from musculoskeletal structures, and visceral sensations to the CNS. Afferent fibers within the cranium transmit sensory information related to visual, olfactory, auditory, sensory, gustatory, and balance functions. These cell bodies are located in the PNS, form ganglia, and are without synapses.
   3. Efferent (motor) fibers within the PNS are responsible for transmitting impulses responsible for motor activation to the sympathetic and parasympathetic portions of the autonomic nervous system. These fibers are responsible for motor activation and have cell bodies contained in the CNS.
   4. Cranial nerves in the PNS take impulses to and from the brain (CNS) and may have afferent and/or motor functions. Spinal nerves take impulses to and from the spinal cord.

   B. Pathophysiology
   1. Disorders of either the CNS or PNS may cause paresthesia.
      a) In the PNS, paresthesia may be caused by immune activation related to changes in nerve fiber density or insult to the dorsal root ganglia and peripheral nerves.
      b) In the CNS, paresthesia may be caused by an elevation of neuronal activity within the spinal dorsal horn and deep spinal lamina neurons. An increase in brain thalamic activities associated with neuropathic pain and neuronal apoptosis may also lead to paresthesia.

2. Hyperfunction of the sensory system is characterized by a lower threshold to stimulation (hyperesthesia) or by a spontaneous discharge that leads to distortion of sensory input (paresthesia).

3. Changes in ion channels, cellular structure (mitochondria and DNA), and neuronal and glial cells; increased levels of glutamate (neurotransmitter) and cytokine production; and genetic predispositions contribute to sensory changes in the PNS.

III. Clinical features: Paresthesia reflects an abnormality affecting the sensory pathways anywhere between the peripheral sensory nervous system and the sensory cortex. A concise history is the fundamental diagnostic tool (Beran, 2015; Boyette-Davis et al., 2018; Ferraro et al., 2016; Kumar et al., 2018; Terpos et al., 2015; Zhou, 2019).

A. Etiology

1. Metabolic disturbances
2. Spinal cord, brain, brain stem lesion
3. Drug induced
4. Neuromuscular diseases
5. Vitamin deficiency: B_1, B_6, B_{12}, E, niacin
6. Infection related: HIV, Epstein-Barr virus

B. History: Obtain a clear description of the paresthesia.

1. History of cancer and cancer treatment
2. Current medications: Prescribed, over the counter, herbal, other supplements
3. History of presenting symptoms: Precipitating factors, onset, location, duration, character (e.g., numb, burning, tingling, shooting), alleviating and exacerbating factors, functional impairments (e.g., impaired dexterity, balance)
4. Changes in ADLs
5. Past medical history: Diabetes, hypertension, other cardiovascular diseases
6. Social history: Alcohol use, smoking, risk for falls

C. Signs and symptoms: Location and characteristics of symptoms may provide information as to the origin.

1. Focal site involvement: Peripheral cutaneous nerve, nerve root lesion, entrapment
2. Single limb or hemibody involvement: Central brain, spinal cord, brain stem lesion
3. Involvement of all limbs: Peripheral neuropathy, cervical cord, brain stem lesion, metabolic disorder
4. Transient or chronic: Transient paresthesia resolve once nerve compression (e.g., sitting cross-legged) is resolved. Chronic paresthesia are related to an underlying neurologic disease or traumatic nerve damage.
5. Corresponding symptoms may include anxiety, muscle spasms, pain, weakness, rash, and sensitivity to touch.
6. Symptoms that may require emergent care include difficulty breathing, difficulty walking, dizziness, loss of bowel and bladder control, loss of vision or acute vision change, paralysis, and slurred speech.

D. Physical examination: Perform a complete neurologic examination to evaluate for coexisting disorders.

1. Cognitive function: Orientation, concentration, memory, language, speech
2. Cranial nerve: Visual fields (see Appendix A)
3. Motor: Observe gait and stance, foot drop, and muscular atrophy. Give special attention to strength of wrists, fingers, and toes, as chronic sensory–motor neuropathy may result in weakness.
4. Deep tendon reflexes: Increased in CNS pathology; decreased in PNS pathology
5. Sensory: Nature and distribution of sensory change

  a) Mononeuropathy (disease of a single nerve) versus polyneuropathy (disease of multiple nerves)

  b) Lhermitte sign: Shooting, electric shock–type pain precipitated by flexion of cervical spine; pain down the spine that may radiate to one or more extremities; considered a sign of inflammation or lesion in posterior column of cervical spinal cord

  c) Glove-and-stocking distribution: Polyneuropathy; systemic sensory loss greater distally than proximally; symmetrically present in bilateral hands and feet

  d) Carpal tunnel syndrome: Mononeuropathy; median nerve compression occurring beneath the transverse carpal ligament at the wrist

  e) Ulnar neuropathy: Mononeuropathy; ulnar nerve compression occurring in the area of the olecranon process due to repetitive flexion or resting on the elbows

6. Pain distribution evaluation using dermatome pattern (see Appendix B)

7. Autonomic disturbances

  a) Postural hypotension

  b) Extremity coldness

  c) Impaired thermoregulatory sweating: Intolerance of cold or heat extremes, decreased ability to sweat

  d) Distended bladder or bowel: Disturbances of bowel and bladder function

8. Total Neuropathy Score: Used to quantify sensory, motor, and autonomic functions and to monitor changes over time

IV. Diagnostic studies: Choice of diagnostic studies will depend on the suspected cause of the paresthesia (Gondim et al., 2018; Mu et al., 2017; Zhou, 2019).

  A. Laboratory

  1. Serum chemistries for baseline and to assess for metabolic disorder

  2. Vitamins B_{12}, B_6, D, folate to evaluate for deficiencies

  3. Hgb A1c to evaluate for hyperglycemia

  4. Thyroid studies (e.g., TSH, free T_4) to evaluate for hypothyroidism

  5. SPEP and immunofixation if myeloma is suspected

  6. If indicated, syphilis, Epstein-Barr virus, VZV, human herpesvirus 6, CMV

  7. CSF studies depending on suspected etiology: Oligoclonal bands, IgG index, paraneoplastic antibodies, infectious workup (e.g., syphilis, Epstein-Barr virus, VZV, human herpesvirus 6, CMV)

  B. Radiology

  1. MRI of the involved site to evaluate for nerve compression

  2. MRI of spinal cord and brain to evaluate for mass or nerve compression

  C. Other

  1. Electromyography and nerve conduction studies to evaluate for evidence of denervation in affected muscles

  2. Skin biopsy with intraepidermal nerve fiber density evaluation, as indicated

V. Differential diagnosis (Beran, 2015; Ferraro et al., 2016; Gondim et al., 2018; Terpos et al., 2015; Vinik et al., 2017; Zhou, 2019)

  A. Metabolic disorders

  1. Diabetes mellitus: Polyneuropathy (see Chapter 151)

  2. Hypothyroidism (see Chapter 158)

  3. Uremia

  4. Chronic liver disease

  5. Vitamin B deficiency: B_1, B_6, B_{12}, folate deficiency (see Chapters 115 and 116), overdose

      6. Sarcoidosis

      7. Collagen vascular disease

      8. Vasculitis

      9. SLE (see Chapter 110)

      10. Myxedema (see Chapter 158)

      11. Multiple sclerosis

      12. Guillain-Barré syndrome

      13. Chronic inflammatory demyelinating polyradiculoneuropathy

      14. Chronic and recurrent immunologically mediated neuropathy

      15. AIDS-related neuropathy

      16. HZV radiculopathy (see Chapter 22)

  B. Neoplastic disorders

      1. Metastasis

      2. Paraneoplastic syndromes (see Appendix M)

      3. CIPN (see Chapter 143): Cisplatin, oxaliplatin, vinca alkaloids, taxanes, thalidomide, pomalidomide, lenalidomide, bortezomib, ixazomib

      4. Paraproteinemia: Distal symmetric sensorimotor polyneuropathy associated with multiple myeloma and Waldenström macroglobulinemia

      5. Surgery-induced neuropathy caused by severing of nerves: Axillary node dissection, neck dissection, thoracotomy, mastectomy

      6. Radiation-induced injury to nerve plexus: Brachial plexus, lumbar plexus

  C. Drug-induced or toxic disorders

      1. Alcohol

      2. Heavy metals: Lead, arsenic, thallium

         a) Industrial solvents: Hexacarbons, organophosphate

         b) Insecticides/herbicides

      3. Isoniazid

      4. Hydralazine

      5. Phenytoin

      6. Gold

      7. Chloroquine

      8. Nitrofurantoin

      9. Recreational drugs: Glue, nitrous oxide, cocaine, heroin

      10. Lidocaine

      11. Beta-alanine

  D. Other

      1. Malnutrition

      2. Dehydration

      3. FMS (see Chapter 101)

      4. Hyperventilation

      5. Lyme disease (see Chapter 104)

VI. Treatment: Dependent on the accurate diagnosis and treatment of the underlying cause (Mu et al., 2017; Terpos et al., 2015; Zhou, 2019; Ziegler & Fonseca, 2015)

  A. In the case of antitumor therapies, consider reducing the dose, increasing cycle length, or eliminating the causative agent.

  B. Provide education and treatment to maintain optimal blood glucose and blood pressure.

  C. Educate the patient regarding lifestyle changes, such as tobacco and alcohol cessation.

  D. Administer medications based on etiology and/or to relieve symptoms (see Appendix Q).

      1. Supplements: Alpha-lipoic acid, acetyl-L-carnitine

    2. Calcium channel blockade: Gabapentin, pregabalin

    3. Sodium channel blockades: Oxcarbazepine

    4. Serotonin-norepinephrine reuptake inhibitor: Duloxetine

    5. Tricyclic antidepressants: Amitriptyline, nortriptyline

    6. Topical agents: Capsaicin, lidocaine

    7. Opioids in combination with other agents for refractory cases

E. Surgical procedures

    1. For mononeuropathies (e.g., ulnar neuropathy, median nerve neuropathy), treatment should include decompression of the nerve either by noninvasive means (wrist or elbow splint to hold the limb in a neutral position) or surgical intervention if noninvasive means are unsuccessful (e.g., ulnar nerve transposition, carpal tunnel release).

    2. Plexopathies are treated pharmacologically and with physical therapy. In the case of traumatic injury, evidence has shown that early surgical resection of associated neuromas may alleviate pain.

VII. Follow-up: Dependent on the underlying cause of the paresthesia and its treatment

VIII. Referrals

A. Neurologist: For appropriate diagnostic testing and treatment

B. Neurosurgeon: To evaluate for surgical decompression or resection of brain lesions

C. Physical or occupational therapist: To maximize motor function and balance

The author would like to acknowledge Giselle J. Moore-Higgs, ARNP, PhD, AOCN®, for her contribution to this chapter that remains unchanged from the previous edition of this book.

References

Beran, R. (2015). Paraesthesia and peripheral neuropathy. *Australian Family Physician, 44*(3), 92–95. https://www.racgp.org.au/afp/2015/march/paraesthesia-and-peripheral-neuropathy

Boyette-Davis, J.A., Hou, S., Abdi, S., & Dougherty, P.M. (2018). An updated understanding of the mechanisms involved in chemotherapy-induced neuropathy. *Pain Management, 8*(5), 363–375. https://doi.org/10.2217/pmt-2018-0020

Boyette-Davis, J.A., Walters, E.T., & Dougherty, P.M. (2015). Mechanisms involved in the development of chemotherapy-induced neuropathy. *Pain Management, 5*(4), 285–296. https://doi.org/10.2217/pmt.15.19

Butler, S.J., & Bronner, M.E. (2015). From classical to current: Analyzing peripheral nervous system and spinal cord lineage and fate. *Developmental Biology, 398*(2), 135–146. https://doi.org/10.1016/j.ydbio.2014.09.033

Ferraro, F., Jacopetti, M., Spallone, V., Padua, L., Traballesi, M., Brunelli, S., ... Tamburin, S. (2016). Diagnosis and treatment of pain in plexopathy, radiculopathy, peripheral neuropathy and phantom limb pain. Evidence and recommendations from the Italian Consensus Conference on Pain on Neurorehabilitation. *European Journal of Physical and Rehabilitation Medicine, 52*(6), 855–866. https://www.minervamedica.it/en/journals/europa-medicophysica/article.php?cod=R33Y2016N06A0855

Gondim, F.A.A., Barreira, A.A., Claudino, R., Cruz, M.W., da Cunha, F., de Freitas, M.R.G., ... Schestatsky, P. (2018). Definition and diagnosis of small fiber neuropathy: Consensus from the Peripheral Neuropathy Scientific Department of the Brazilian Academy of Neurology. *Arquivos de Neuro-Psiquiatria, 76*(3), 200–208. https://doi.org/10.1590/0004-282x20180015

Kim, J.H., Dougherty, P.M., & Abdi, S. (2015). Basic science and clinical management of painful and non-painful chemotherapy-related neuropathy. *Gynecologic Oncology, 136*(3), 453–459. https://doi.org/10.1016/j.ygyno.2015.01.524

Kumar, A., Kaur, H., & Singh, A. (2018). Neuropathic pain models caused by damage to central or peripheral nervous system. *Pharmacological Reports, 70*(2), 206–216. https://doi.org/10.1016/j.pharep.2017.09.009

Mu, A., Weinberg, E., Moulin, D.E., & Clarke, H. (2017). Pharmacologic management of chronic neuropathic pain: Review of the Canadian Pain Society consensus statement. *Canadian Family Physician, 63*(11), 844–852. https://www.cfp.ca/content/63/11/844.long

Sudiwala, S., & Knox, S.M. (2019). The emerging role of cranial nerves in shaping craniofacial development. *Genesis, 57*(1), e23282. https://doi.org/10.1002/dvg.23282

Terpos, E., Kleber, M., Engelhardt, M., Zweegman, S., Gay, F., Kastritis, E., ... Palumbo, A. (2015). European Myeloma Network guidelines for the management of multiple myeloma-related complications. *Haematologica, 100*(10), 1254–1266. https://doi.org/10.3324/haematol.2014.117176

Vinik, A.I., Camacho, P.M., Davidson, J.A., Handelsman, Y., Lando, H.M., Leddy, A.L., ... Ziegler, D. (2017). American Association of Clinical Endocrinologists and American College of Endocrinology position statement on testing for autonomic and somatic nerve dysfunction. *Endocrine Practice, 23*(12), 1472–1478. https://doi.org/10.4158/ep-2017-0053

Zhou, L. (2019). Small fiber neuropathy. *Seminars in Neurology, 39*(5), 570–577. https://doi.org/10.1055/s-0039-1688977

Ziegler, D., & Fonseca, V. (2015). From guideline to patient: A review of recent recommendations for pharmacotherapy of painful diabetic neuropathy. *Journal of Diabetes and its Complications, 29*(1), 146–156. https://doi.org/10.1016/j.jdiacomp.2014.08.008

CHAPTER 139

Syncope

Corazon Lauren Delumpa, MSN, RN, FNP-C

I. Definition: A transient loss of consciousness often unwitnessed and accompanied by loss of postural tone, with rapid onset and a full, quick recovery (Brignole et al., 2018; Shen et al., 2017)

II. Physiology/Pathophysiology (Cheshire, 2017; Giada & Nordio, 2016)
   A. Normal: Cerebral perfusion is maintained relatively constant by an intricate and complex feedback system involving cardiac output, systemic vascular resistance, arterial pressure, cerebrovascular resistance with intrinsic autoregulation, and metabolic regulation.
   B. Pathophysiology
      1. Loss of consciousness occurs in response to an acute reduction in the cerebral blood flow sufficient to deprive the cerebral reticular neurons of substrate.
      2. CNS hypoperfusion may be the result of vasomotor instability, reduced cardiac output, or neurologically reduced cerebral perfusion.

III. Clinical features: The degree and duration of impaired consciousness are dependent on the severity and duration of the reduction of cerebral blood flow. The clinical features of syncope can be correlated with the underlying process. Typically, the individual returns spontaneously to his or her baseline status with no therapeutic intervention and does not experience prolonged confusion. Syncope can be either low or high risk and can be evaluated in the outpatient versus acute setting. Patients may present due to nonaccidental falls. Syncope is a common problem in all age groups (Cheshire, 2017; Giada & Nordio, 2016; Goldberger et al., 2019; Janus et al., 2017; Joy et al., 2017; Martow & Sandhu, 2019; Shen et al., 2017).
   A. Etiology: The most common diagnoses associated with syncope include electrolyte imbalance (e.g., dehydration, hyponatremia, hypokalemia) and dysrhythmia (e.g., ventricular tachycardia, atrial fibrillation). In one-half of cases, etiology remains unknown.
      1. Neurally mediated: Reflex
      2. Vasovagal syncope: A sudden decrease in arterial blood pressure and heart rate combine to produce CNS hypoperfusion.
         a) Most common type of syncope
         b) May occur in all age groups
      3. Carotid sinus syncope
      4. Situational syncope
         a) Acute hemorrhage
         b) Cough and/or sneeze
         c) GI stimulation: Swallow, defecation, visceral pain
         d) Micturition: Postmicturition
         e) Pain

      f) Excessive heat

      g) Venipuncture

      h) Fear of bodily injury

  5. Glossopharyngeal neuralgia

  6. Orthostatic hypotension syncope: Decrease in systolic blood pressure greater than 20 mm Hg or diastolic greater than 10 mm Hg during position change; stands after prolonged recumbency, or stands motionless for a prolonged period of time; may be symptomatic or asymptomatic

      a) Primary autonomic failure syndromes: Pure autonomic failure, multiple system atrophy, parkinsonian dysautonomia

      b) Secondary autonomic failure disturbances: Alcohol, diabetes, amyloidosis, volume depletion

      c) Drugs: Antidepressants, phenothiazines, beta- and alpha-blockers, vasodilators, nitroglycerin

  7. Cardiac syncope: Reduced cardiac output as a result of pump failure, mechanical obstruction, or dysrhythmia; usually predicts worse short- and long-term prognoses

      a) Dysrhythmia

         (1) Sinus node dysfunction: Bradycardia–tachycardia syndrome

         (2) AV conduction system disease

         (3) Paroxysmal supraventricular and ventricular tachycardias

         (4) Inherited syndromes: Long QT syndrome, Brugada syndrome

         (5) Implanted device: Pacemaker, implanted cardioverter defibrillator) malfunction

         (6) Drug induced

      b) Structural cardiac or cardiopulmonary disease

         (1) Obstructive cardiac valvular disease

         (2) Acute MI/ischemia

         (3) Obstructive cardiomyopathy

         (4) Atrial myxoma

         (5) Acute aortic dissection

         (6) Pericardial disease/tamponade

         (7) PE/PH

  8. Other

      a) Cerebrovascular steal syndromes: Neurologically reduced cerebral perfusion resulting from cerebrovascular disease or vasospasm

      b) Hyperventilation

      c) Hydrocephalus

      d) Migraine headache

      e) Narcolepsy

      f) GVHD

      g) Baroreceptor failure after radiation therapy

      h) Presenting symptom of malignancy

B. History

  1. History of cancer and cancer treatment

  2. Current medications: Prescribed, over the counter

  3. History of presenting symptoms: Precipitating factors, onset, duration, associated symptoms (e.g., tics, tremors, dystonia, numbness, seizures, pain)

  4. Changes in ADLs

  5. Past medical history: Cardiac disease, diabetes, migraine, stroke

C. Signs and symptoms: Dizziness, light-headedness, fainting with no memory of events

1. Vasovagal syncope
   a) It is usually preceded by a prodromal episode that may last 10–90 seconds and include lassitude, light-headedness, nausea, pallor, diaphoresis, salivation, blurred vision, decreased visual fields, and tachycardia.
   b) This is followed by loss of consciousness during which the individual has bradycardia, pale skin, diaphoresis, and dilated pupils.
   c) Abnormal movement, usually tonic or opisthotonic severe hyperextension, and spasticity have been noted. Patient may suffer from possible urinary incontinence.
   d) Recovery is usually rapid, but residual nervousness, dizziness, headache, nausea, pallor, and diaphoresis may be present.
   e) Syncope may recur, especially if the individual attempts to stand within the following 30 minutes.
2. Orthostatic hypotension syncope
   a) Loss of consciousness occurs when blood pressure drops at least 20–30 mm Hg systolic or 10 mm Hg diastolic when the patient moves from lying (or sitting) to standing.
   b) There is usually an absence of a prodromal episode, but the individual may have pallor and sweating.
3. Cardiac syncope
   a) Usually, the loss of consciousness is quick.
   b) Seizure-like activity and urinary and fecal incontinence may be seen as the duration of cerebral hypoperfusion increases.
   c) Typically, it occurs in patients older than 60 years, of male sex, or with history of cardiac disease; brief prodrome (i.e., palpitation) occurs during exertion or in supine position.
   d) Episodes are infrequent.
4. Noncardiac syncope
   a) Individual may or may not have a prodromal episode but may have pallor and sweating. Prodrome symptoms include nausea, vomiting, and feeling warmth.
   b) Usually, the loss of consciousness is quick.
   c) Typically, it occurs in patients of younger age with no known cardiac disease, syncope in standing position or position change, or with triggers (e.g., cough, laugh, micturition, during or after meal).
   d) Recurrence is frequent.
D. Physical examination
   1. Vital signs: Orthostatic measurements of blood pressure in supine and standing positions in both arms every 10 minutes
   2. Skin: Pallor or ecchymoses from trauma
   3. Oral: Tongue lesions; lateral lesions usually associated with a tonic–clonic seizure; anterior lesions usually associated with a fall
   4. Cardiac
      a) Irregular heartbeat indicating dysrhythmias: Ventricular tachycardia, bradycardia
      b) Murmurs indicating cardiac valve abnormalities
      c) Carotid bruits indicating vascular obstruction in the neck
   5. Neurologic: Coexisting signs indicating structural brain or peripheral nerve abnormalities (e.g., peripheral neuropathy)
      a) Cognitive function: Orientation, concentration, memory, language, speech
      b) Cranial nerve examination with visual fields (see Appendix A)
      c) Upright tilt table test to evaluate for vasovagal syncope

    d) Increased or decreased deep tendon reflexes depending on etiology

    e) Sensory functions decreased depending on etiology

IV. Diagnostic studies: Choice of diagnostic studies will depend on the suspected cause of the syncope. Initial syncope evaluation involves a thorough history and physical examination, ECG, and orthostatic vitals (Brignole et al., 2018; Martow & Sandhu, 2019; Shen et al., 2017).

 A. Laboratory

  1. CBC with differential to evaluate for sepsis and anemia

  2. Complete metabolic panel to evaluate for hydration status and electrolyte imbalance

  3. Cardiac enzymes to evaluate for MI

  4. Urinalysis and culture to evaluate for sepsis

  5. Blood cultures to evaluate for sepsis

  6. Serum drug screen to screen for barbiturate or sedative use

  7. Paraneoplastic panel to evaluate occult malignancy if history warrants

 B. Radiology

  1. Chest x-ray to evaluate for cardiomegaly or pleural effusion

  2. If there is focal neurologic findings or head injury: CT scan of brain without contrast, MRI of brain

  3. Routine cardiac MRI or cardiac angiography: Not beneficial unless suspicion of cardiac abnormality is high

 C. Other: 2017 American College of Cardiology/American Heart Association Task Force on Clinical Practice Guidelines/Heart Rhythm Society (ACC/AHA/HRS) Guideline for the Evaluation and Management of Patients With Syncope

  1. CV abnormality suspected

   a) Cardiac monitor: Implantable versus ambulatory external monitor

   b) Exercise stress testing

   c) Transthoracic echocardiogram with bubble study to evaluate for shunting

   d) Electrophysiological study

   e) ECG to evaluate for dysrhythmia

  2. Vasovagal syncope suspected: Tilt table testing

  3. Neurologic or neurodegenerative disease suspected: Autonomic testing, electroencephalogram

V. Differential diagnosis (Joy et al., 2017; Martow & Sandhu, 2019)

 A. Decreased cerebral blood flow

 B. Vasodepressor (vasovagal response)

 C. Transient cardiac dysrhythmia (see Chapter 45)

 D. Orthostatic hypotension (see Chapter 48)

 E. Carotid sinus syndrome

 F. Obstruction to flow

  1. Aortic/pulmonic valve stenosis

  2. Hypertrophic cardiomyopathy (see Chapter 41)

  3. Prosthetic valve dysfunction

  4. Atrial myxoma

  5. PE (see Chapter 33)

  6. PH (see Chapter 52)

 G. Situational syncope

  1. Micturition

  2. Cough (see Chapter 23)

  3. Defecation (see Chapter 55)

H. Altered composition of blood

I. Hypoglycemia

J. Anemia (see Chapters 113–119)

K. Sepsis

L. Hypothyroidism: Cardiovascular disease, other (see Chapter 158)

M. Psychogenic

N. Migraine headaches (see Chapter 137)

O. Hyperventilation

P. Glossopharyngeal neuralgia

Q. Vertebrobasilar insufficiency

R. Carotid artery compression by tumor

S. Subclavian or innominate artery stenosis: Scarring from surgery, radiation therapy, embolic event

T. Takayasu disease or Ménière disease

VI. Treatment: Dependent on accurate diagnosis and treatment of the underlying cause (Aleksandra et al., 2018; Brignole et al., 2018; Dehghan et al., 2019; Goldberger et al., 2019; Hockin et al., 2019; Shen et al., 2017)

A. Eliminate causative agent.

B. Treat the underlying cause.

C. Nonpharmacologic treatment

1. Safety education: Reposition gradually, fall prevention

2. Revocation of driving privileges depending on the cause of the syncope; possible symptom-free wait period before patient can start driving

3. Avoidance of triggers: Dehydration, alcohol, hot temperatures, crowds, prolonged sitting or standing, holding one's breath

4. Diet with 10 g of sodium and 2–3 liters of water

5. Counterpressure maneuvers: Leg crossing, squatting, lying supine, squeezing an object in the hand

6. Vertical/tilt training with supervision

7. Intermittent compression (0–60 mm Hg every four seconds) versus static compression stockings beneficial in passive orthostasis

8. Sleeping with the head of the bed elevated (greater than 10°) postulated to prevent nocturnal polyuria

D. Pharmacologic and interventional treatment

1. Fludrocortisone: Mineralocorticoid that increases renal sodium reabsorption and expanding plasma volume

2. Midodrine: Alpha-agonists to possibly increase peripheral vasoconstriction

3. Pacemakers: Used primarily for bradycardic arrhythmias for severe, recurrent, unpredictable syncope; age older than 40 years

4. Catheter ablation: Used for ventricular tachycardia or supraventricular tachycardia

VII. Follow-up: Dependent on the suspected underlying cause of the syncope

VIII. Referrals: Dependent on the suspected underlying cause of the syncope

A. Cardiologist: For cardiac evaluation

B. Neurologist: For neurologic evaluation

The author would like to acknowledge Giselle J. Moore-Higgs, ARNP, PhD, AOCN®, for her contribution to this chapter that remains unchanged from the previous edition of this book.

References

Aleksandra, B., Dariusz, D., Szymon, G., Blanka, B., Oliwia, C., Daria, K., … Nataliia, B. (2018). Non-pharmacological methods of treatment and prevention of vasovagal syncope. *Journal of Education, Health and Sport, 8*(11), 796–803. https://doi.org/10.5281/zenodo.3014892

Brignole, M., Moya, A., de Lange, F.J., Deharo, J.-C., Elliott, P.M., Fanciulli, A., … van Dijk, J.G. (2018). 2018 ESC guidelines for the diagnosis and management of syncope. *European Heart Journal, 39*(21), 1883–1948. https://doi.org/10.1093/eurheartj/ehy037

Cheshire, W.P., Jr. (2017). Syncope. *Continuum, 23*(2), 335–358. https://doi.org/10.1212/con.0000000000000444

Dehghan, B., Sabri, M.R., & Mansourian, M. (2019). Nonpharmacologic treatments alone are enough to prevent the neurally mediated syncope: A 3 years follow-up study. *International Journal of Preventive Medicine, 10,* 69. https://doi.org/10.4103/ijpvm.IJPVM_386_17

Giada, F., & Nordio, A. (2016). Syncope: First evaluation and management in the emergency department. In M. Zecchin & G. Sinagra (Eds.), *The arrhythmic patient in the emergency department: A practical guide for cardiologists and emergency physicians* (pp. 19–28). Springer. https://doi.org/10.1007/978-3-319-24328-3_2

Goldberger, Z.D., Petek, B.J., Brignole, M., Shen, W.-K., Sheldon, R.S., Solbiati, M., … Hamdan, M.H. (2019). ACC/AHA/HRS versus ESC guidelines for the diagnosis and management of syncope: JACC guideline comparison. *Journal of the American College of Cardiology, 74*(19), 2410–2423. https://doi.org/10.1016/j.jacc.2019.09.012

Hockin, B.C.D., Ruiz, I.A., Brar, G.K., & Claydon, V.E. (2019). Intermittent calf compression reverses lower limb pooling and improves cardiovascular control during passive orthostasis. *Autonomic Neuroscience, 217,* 102–113. https://doi.org/10.1016/j.autneu.2018.12.004

Janus, S.E., Hirai, T., Mathew, V., & Rabbat, M. (2017). Syncope from radiation-induced baroreceptor failure. *BMJ Case Reports, 2017.* https://doi.org/10.1136/bcr-2017-221925

Joy, P.S., Kumar, G., & Olshansky, B. (2017). Syncope: Outcomes and conditions associated with hospitalization. *American Journal of Medicine, 130*(6), 699–706.e6. https://doi.org/10.1016/j.amjmed.2016.12.030

Martow, E., & Sandhu, R. (2019). When is syncope arrhythmic? *Medical Clinics of North America, 103*(5), 793–807. https://doi.org/10.1016/j.mcna.2019.05.002

Shen, W.-K., Sheldon, R.S., Benditt, D.G., Cohen, M.I., Forman, D.E., Goldberger, Z.D., … Yancy, C.W. (2017). 2017 ACC/AHA/HRS guideline for the evaluation and management of patients with syncope: Executive summary: A report of the American College of Cardiology/American Heart Association Task Force on Clinical Practice Guidelines and the Heart Rhythm Society. *Journal of the American College of Cardiology, 70*(5), 620–630. https://doi.org/10.1016/j.jacc.2017.03.002

CHAPTER 140

Tremor

Kimberly A. Noonan, DNP, ANP-BC, AOCN®

I. Definition: An involuntary, rhythmic, oscillatory movement of a body part classified along two axes (Albanese & Del Sorbo, 2016; Bhatia et al., 2018; Louis, 2019)
   A. Tremor is considered a movement disorder that can develop in certain physiologic conditions, such as exposure to a cold environment or a fearful situation.
   B. The definition of tremor can be further classified as Axis I or Axis II.

II. Physiology/Pathophysiology (Albanese & Del Sorbo, 2016; Bhatia et al., 2018; Shanker, 2019)
   A. Normal
      1. The basal ganglia comprise a large mass of gray matter influenced by several parts of the CNS.
      2. The basal ganglia are devoted to motor activities.
      3. It is thought that the motor circuitry of the basal ganglia is involved in transferring information from the neocortex to the motor areas, in particular the premotor and supplementary motor areas, and that the corpus striatum serves as a repository of instructions for fragments of learned movements.
   B. Pathophysiology
      1. Pathophysiology differs based on etiology. Tremor is generated and mediated from the CNS and PNS.
      2. Tremor is generated by rhythmical discharges in a neuronal network and can continue on a feedback and feed-forward loop.
      3. The cerebello–thalamo–cortical pathway is involved in all pathologic tremors.
      4. Tremor results from alternating contractions of opposing muscle groups or from simultaneous contractions of agonist and antagonist muscles, with one group more forceful than the other.
      5. Movement disorders, including tremors, impair the regulation of voluntary motor activity without directly affecting strength, sensation, or cerebellar function. This includes hypokinetic and hyperkinetic disorders, which result from dysfunction of deep subcortical gray matter structures (e.g., basal ganglia).

III. Clinical features: Tremor is categorized by resting and movement disorders. It is the most common of all movement disorders, with Parkinson disease the most common resting tremor. The fixed recurring interval between movements differentiates tremor from other repetitive movements, and tremor is classified depending on pathophysiology (Albanese & Del Sorbo, 2016; Bhatia et al., 2018; Louis, 2014, 2019; Morgan et al., 2017; Schneider & Deuschl, 2014; van der Stouwe et al., 2016).
   A. The new classification of tremor is identified by Axis I and Axis II.

1. Axis I: Describes clinical characteristics of the patient and is associated with a syndrome or phenotype that leads to the identification of one or more etiologies
   a) Clinical characteristics such as age at onset, family history of tremor, and temporal evolution are taken into consideration.
   b) Tremor characteristics are included, such as body distribution and activation condition.
   c) Some Axis I syndromes may have multiple etiologies.
2. Axis II: Identifies the common diagnostic process of syndrome identification to base the diagnosis on the underlying etiology, including acquired, genetic, or idiopathic
3. This identification allows for the classification of tremor with no known etiology.

B. Types of tremor
1. Rest: Tremor occurs in a body part that is fully supported, relaxed, and not voluntarily activated (e.g., when the patient's hands exhibit a tremor as they are resting in their lap).
2. Action: Tremor occurs with voluntary muscle contraction during movement of the affected body part from one part to another.
   a) Kinetic tremor occurs during any voluntary movement.
   b) Postural tremor is observed when the patient tries to maintain a specific position (e.g., holding the arms out in front of the body).
   c) Isometric tremor occurs during muscle contraction against a stationary object (e.g., squeezing an object).
3. Anatomical distribution
   a) Focal: One body region affected
   b) Segmental: Two or more body parts in upper or lower body affected
   c) Hemitremor: One side of body affected
   d) Generalized: Upper and lower body affected

C. Etiology is based on circumstances of occurrence. Tremor syndromes may have multiple etiologies and can change characteristics.
1. Postural tremor
   a) Physiologic tremor
   b) Alcohol or drug withdrawal
   c) Metabolic disturbances
   d) Drug-induced tremor
   e) Psychogenic tremor
2. Resting tremor
   a) Parkinson disease
   b) Dystonic tremor
   c) Isolated rest tremor
   d) Progressive supranuclear palsy
   e) Drug-induced tremor
   f) Rubral tremor
   g) Psychogenic tremor
3. Action tremor
   a) Cerebellar lesions
   b) Essential tremor
   c) Orthostatic tremor
   d) Rubral tremor
   e) Primary writing tremor
   f) Neuropathic tremor
   g) Psychogenic tremor

D. History
1. History of cancer and cancer treatment
2. Current medications: Prescribed, over the counter
3. History of presenting symptoms: Precipitating factors, onset, location, duration, associated symptoms (e.g., holding drinks, eating, holding utensils, writing)
4. Changes in ADLs
5. Past medical history: Birth trauma, psychiatric disorders
6. Family history: Tremors, neurologic disorders, Parkinson disease
7. Social history: Caffeine intake, alcohol use, exercise, fatigue, stress

E. Physical examination: Perform a complete neurologic examination to assess the nature of the abnormal movements, extent of neurologic involvement, and presence of a coexisting disease. Tremor frequencies are determined by the amount of oscillation per second or cycles per seconds, known as hertz.
1. Cognitive function: Orientation, concentration, memory, language, speech
2. Cranial nerve examination with visual fields (see Appendix A)
3. Motor examination including gait and stance to characterize tremors
   a) Rest tremor: Have patient place arms in lap when sitting or at side while lying down.
      (1) Tremor seen in a limb while at rest
      (2) Usually slow: 3–7 hertz
      (3) Diminished with purposeful movement of the extremity
      (4) Associated with increased muscle tone
   b) Postural tremor: Have patient stretch arms out in front of body or use hands to raise cup to mouth; evaluate handwriting and ability to copy spirals.
      (1) Occurs in a limb during sustained posture or during movement; increases toward the end of the movement
      (2) Usually rapid: 7–11 hertz
      (3) More severe in the distal part of the extremity than in the proximal part
      (4) May occur during subsequent movement but should not increase in severity
   c) Action tremor: Have patient perform finger-to-nose maneuver. Tremor remains constant or abruptly increases at fixation of the terminal movement.
   d) Deep tendon reflexes: Increased or decreased depending on etiology
   e) Sensory: Increased or decreased depending on etiology

IV. Diagnostic studies (Bhatia et al., 2018; Deuschl et al., 2015; Hedera, 2017; Schneider & Deuschl, 2014; Shanker, 2019; van der Stouwe et al., 2016)
A. Laboratory
1. Toxicology studies: May reveal excessive amounts of medications or alcohol
2. Thyroid function test to evaluate for hyperthyroidism
3. Heavy metal testing: Mercury, arsenic, lead
4. Genetic testing for family history of tremor disorders, if indicated
5. Chemistries to detect metabolic abnormalities
6. Glucose to evaluate for hypoglycemia
B. Radiology: Usually not indicated
1. CT scan and/or MRI of head to detect brain lesions
2. If uncertain if essential tremor or isolated Parkinson disease, striatal dopamine transporter imaging (DaTscan) to detect striatal dopamine deficiency and differential essential tumor from Parkinson disease
C. Other: Electrophysiological test
1. Electromyography to evaluate nerve conduction abnormalities
2. Electroencephalography to assess for seizure activity

V. Differential diagnosis (Deuschl et al., 2015; Hedera, 2017; Morgan et al., 2017; Schneider & Deuschl, 2014; van der Stouwe et al., 2016)

   A. Essential tremors: Postural tremor accentuated by voluntary movement

   B. Cerebellar tremor: Tremor that usually includes side-to-side movement of arms and legs that interrupts an involuntary action, especially at the extremes of reach, and is absent at rest

   C. Parkinson tremor: Resting tremor that begins unilaterally in an upper or lower extremity

   D. Drug-induced tremor

      1. Sympathomimetic agents

      2. Bronchodilator: Theophylline

      3. Levodopa

      4. Corticosteroids

      5. Levothyroxine

      6. Tricyclic antidepressants

      7. Hypoglycemic agents

      8. Benzodiazepines

      9. Lithium

      10. Cimetidine: May increase essential tremors

      11. Chemotherapy agents: Cytarabine

      12. Caffeine

      13. Cardiac medications: Beta-blockers, calcium channel blockers

      14. Epinephrine

      15. Amphetamines

      16. Carbon monoxide

      17. Heavy metals: Mercury, lead, arsenic

   E. Rubral (midbrain) tremor

      1. An uncommon tremor that consists of a combination of rest and postural tremors caused by a lesion in the vicinity of the red nucleus (e.g., tumor, abscess, demyelination)

      2. Usually associated with other midbrain neurologic deficits, including third cranial nerve palsy and hemiparesis

   F. Peripheral neuropathy tremor: Irregular, rhythmic, proximal, distal tremors (see Chapter 143)

   G. Psychogenic tremors

VI. Treatment: Accurate diagnosis of the underlying causative factor will optimize treatment. It is less effective if the underlying cause cannot be treated or tremor is not accurately diagnosed; however, treatment may be effective in reducing the tremors and improving QOL (Bhatia et al., 2018; Deuschl et al., 2015; Hedera, 2017; Kreisler et al., 2019; Marsot et al., 2017; Schneider & Deuschl, 2015; Shanker, 2019; Sharma & Pandey, 2019).

   A. Essential tremor

      1. Beta-blockers

         a) Propranolol: 120–240 mg PO daily in extended-release formulation; effective and more convenient at once-daily dosing

         b) Metoprolol: Initiated low at 25 mg PO daily; titrated to effect

      2. Primidone: 50 mg PO daily; may be increased in 50 mg increments to usual dose of 250 mg daily PO in divided doses; doses up to 750 mg PO daily may be beneficial.

         a) Anticonvulsants: Gabapentin 100–300 mg PO three times a day; increased to 1,200–3,000 mg PO daily

         b) Pregabalin: 50 mg PO two to three times a day; titrated to 100 mg PO two to three times a day

      3. Topiramate: 25–50 mg PO daily; titrated to approximately 200–400 mg PO daily

      4. Botulinum toxin injections

      5. Behavioral therapy: Psychotherapy, biofeedback, hypnosis

      6. Surgical intervention: Stereotactic thalamotomy

  B. Cerebellar tremor: Difficult to treat; surgical interventions should be considered (e.g., stereotactic thalamotomy).

  C. Parkinson tremor

      1. Levodopa: 0.5–1 g PO daily in divided doses

      2. Carbidopa/levodopa: 10/100–25/250 mg PO three times a day; controlled-release formulation for patients not receiving levodopa: 50/200 mg PO every 12 hours

      3. Bromocriptine: 2.5 mg PO daily, up to 5–10 mg PO four times a day

      4. Amantadine: 100 mg PO two times a day, up to 100 mg PO three times a day

      5. Selegiline: 5 mg PO daily

      6. Trihexyphenidyl: 1 mg PO two times a day; titrated to 2 mg two to three times a day

      7. Benztropine: 0.5 mg PO two times a day; titrated to 1–2 mg two to three times a day

      8. Pramipexole: 0.125 mg PO three times a day; titrated to 1.5 mg three times a day

  D. Drug-induced tremor: Eliminate the causative agent, and consider alternative drugs.

  E. Rubral tremor: Provide symptomatic treatment only.

  F. Peripheral neuropathic tremor: Treat the underlying cause of neuropathy.

  G. Psychogenic tremor: Treat underlying psychiatric disorder.

VII. Follow-up: Dependent on the cause of the tremor and its treatment and should be monitored on a consistent basis (Bhatia et al., 2018)

VIII. Referrals: Dependent on the suspected underlying cause of the tremor

  A. Neurologist: For treatment plan

  B. Pharmacotherapist: To assist with multidrug therapy

  C. Psychiatrist: For psychological evaluation

  D. Physical or occupational therapist: To assist with alternative methods of ambulation and ADLs

The author would like to acknowledge Giselle J. Moore-Higgs, ARNP, PhD, AOCN®, for her contribution to this chapter that remains unchanged from the previous edition of this book.

References

Albanese, A., & Del Sorbo, F. (2016). Dystonia and tremor: The clinical syndromes with isolated tremor. *Tremor and Other Hyperkinetic Movements, 6,* 319. https://doi.org/10.7916/D8X34XBM

Bhatia, K.P., Bain, P., Bajaj, N., Elble, R.J., Hallett, M., Louis, E.D., ... Deuschl, G. (2018). Consensus Statement on the classification of tremors. From the task force on tremor of the International Parkinson and Movement Disorder Society. *Movement Disorders, 33*(1), 75–87. https://doi.org/10.1002/mds.27121

Deuschl, G., Petersen, I., Lorenz, D., & Christensen, K. (2015). Tremor in the elderly: Essential and aging-related tremor. *Movement Disorders, 30*(10), 1327–1334. https://doi.org/10.1002/mds.26265

Hedera, P. (2017). Emerging strategies in the management of essential tremor. *Therapeutic Advances in Neurological Disorders, 10*(2), 137–148. https://doi.org/10.1177/1756285616679123

Kreisler, A., Bouchain, B., Defebvre, L., & Krystkowiak, P. (2019). Treatment with botulinum neurotoxin improves activities of daily living and quality of life in patients with upper limb tremor. *Tremor and Other Hyperkinetic Movements, 9.* https://doi.org/10.7916/tohm.v0.640

Louis, E.D. (2014). Twelve clinical pearls to help distinguish essential tremor from other tremors. *Expert Review of Neurotherapeutics, 14*(9), 1057–1065. https://doi.org/10.1586/14737175.2014.936389

Louis, E.D. (2019). Tremor. *Continuum, 25*(4), 959–975. https://doi.org/10.1212/CON.0000000000000748

Marsot, A., Guilhaumou, R., Azulay, J.P, & Blin, O. (2017). Levodopa in Parkinson's disease: A review of population pharmacokinetics/pharmacodynamics analysis. *Journal of Pharmacy and Pharmaceutical Sciences, 20*(2), 226–238. https://doi.org/10.18433/J30H04

Morgan, J.C., Kurek, J.A., Davis, J.L., & Sethi, K.D. (2017). Insights into pathophysiology from medication-induced tremor. *Tremor and Other Hyperkinetic Movements, 7,* 442. https://doi.org/10.7916/D8FJ2V9Q

Schneider, S.A., & Deuschl, G. (2014). The treatment of tremor. *Neurotherapeutics, 11*(1), 128–138. https://doi.org/10.1007/s13311-013-0230-5

Shanker, V. (2019). Essential tremor: Diagnosis and management. *BMJ, 366,* l4485. https://doi.org/10.1136/bmj.l4485

Sharma, S., & Pandey, S. (2019). Treatment of essential tremor: Current status. *Postgraduate Medical Journal, 96*(1132), 84–93. https://doi.org/10.1136/postgradmedj-2019-136647

van der Stouwe, A.M.M., Elting, J.W., van der Hoeven, J.H., van Laar, T., Leenders, K.L., Maurits, N.M., & Tijssen, M.A.J. (2016). How typical are 'typical' tremor characteristics? Sensitivity and specificity of five tremor phenomena. *Parkinsonism and Related Disorders, 30,* 23–28, https://doi.org/10.1016/j.parkreldis.2016.06.008

CHAPTER 141

Meningitis

Marcel Smith, RN, MS, FNP-BC

I. Definition: A clinical syndrome that involves inflammation of the meninges, the three layers of membrane that surround the brain and spinal cord (Agnihotri, 2019)

II. Physiology/Pathophysiology (Agnihotri, 2019; LaPenna & Roos, 2019; Mount & Boyle, 2017)
   A. Normal
      1. The brain and spinal cord are protected by the skull, vertebrae, meninges, and CSF.
      2. Three layers of meninges surround the brain and spinal cord and assist in production and drainage of CSF.
   B. Pathophysiology
      1. CSF flows through the pia and arachnoid layers of the meninges; meningitis is a diffuse infection of these layers.
      2. Bacterial cell wall fragments are thought to release cytokines (e.g., TNF, IL-1β).
         a) This causes an inflammatory reaction with an influx of leukocytes into the subarachnoid space, forming a purulent exudate.
         b) The exposure of cells to this thickened exudate leads to cerebral edema, increased ICP, and neuronal damage.

III. Clinical features: Mortality from bacterial meningitis is high. Acute sequelae can include cranial nerve palsies, seizures, hydrocephalus, coma, and cerebral herniation. Acute meningitis from infectious causes usually does not recur. If the person survives the meningitis, chronic complications often occur, including sensorineural deafness, epilepsy, ataxia, hydrocephalus, cortical blindness, and cognitive deficits (Agnihotri, 2019; Akaishi et al., 2019; Figueiredo et al., 2018; LaPenna & Roos, 2019; McGill et al., 2016; Mount & Boyle, 2017; Obaro, 2019).
   A. Classification
      1. Acute (onset over hours to days) or chronic (symptoms persistent for more than four weeks): Most common cause of acute meningitis is bacterial or viral infection. The time from symptom onset to presentation for medical care tends to be shorter in bacterial meningitis.
      2. Chronic: Meningitis lasts for four weeks or longer and is a complex entity with both infectious and noninfectious causes.
   B. Etiology: The cause can be infection (e.g., viral, bacterial, fungal) or chemical irritation (i.e., aseptic meningitis). Meningitis may be acquired either in the community, via various invasive procedures, or as a result of head trauma. Most cases are a result of invasion by an infectious agent that has colonized elsewhere in the host. The infectious organism typically invades the submucosa of these sites by evading host defenses. Common patho-

gens are associated with immunologic deficits. Incubation period is variable depending on the pathogen (e.g., 1–10 days).

1. Organisms such as bacteria, fungi, or viruses enter the CNS by various routes.
   a) Nasopharynx: Most common site of entry in community-acquired meningitis
   b) Ear canal
   c) Bloodstream
   d) CNS
      (1) Surgery: Craniofacial
      (2) Indwelling reservoirs and shunts
      (3) Lumbar puncture or spinal tap
   e) Mucosal surfaces of the GI and GU tracts
2. Type of organisms
   a) Acute bacterial meningitis: Most common causes are the following.
      (1) Age 18–50 years: *Neisseria meningitides* (meningocuccus), *Streptococcus pneumoniae, Haemophilus influenzae*
      (2) Age older than 50 years: *S. pneumoniae, N. meningitides, Listeria monocytogenes,* aerobic gram-negative bacilli
      (3) Immunocompromised state: *L. monocytogenes,* aerobic gram-negative bacilli, *S. pneumoniae*
      (4) Head trauma, neurosurgery, or CSF shunts: *S. pneumoniae, H. influenzae,* group A streptococci, coagulase-negative staphylococci, *Staphylococcus aureus, Cutibacterium acnes* (specifically in shunts)
   b) Acute viral meningitis: Most common causes include enteroviruses, herpesviruses, and HIV.
   c) Chronic meningitis: Causes are via infectious or noninfectious sources.
      (1) Infectious: Bacteria, viruses, fungi, parasites
      (2) Noninfectious: Vasculitis, connective tissue disease, chemical exposure, neoplasm

C. History
   1. History of cancer and cancer treatment
   2. Current medications: Prescribed, over the counter
   3. History of presenting symptoms: Precipitating factors, location, duration
   4. Changes in ADLs
   5. Past medical history: Recent infection, lumbar puncture, indwelling CNS catheter or shunt, oropharyngeal, neurosurgical procedures or surgeries, sickle cell disease, vaccine history
   6. Social history: Recent foreign travel, incarceration, exposure to TB or tick bite, work with soil

D. Signs and symptoms: Almost all patients present with at least two of the four symptoms—headache, fever, neck stiffness, and altered mental status.
   1. Headache: Often bifrontal and associated with photophobia, nausea, and vomiting; can be acute onset; excruciating pain may make raising the head difficult.
   2. Neck stiffness
   3. Fever or chills
   4. Changes in cognition from lethargy to obtundation/coma
   5. Seizures: Approximately 30% of cases
   6. Rash: Associated with *N. meningitides*
   7. Nausea and vomiting: Vomiting may be severe and projectile; movement may cause nausea.
   8. Myalgias

9. Lower extremity weakness
10. Cranial nerve abnormalities: Hearing loss, diplopia
11. Lethargy or drowsiness

E. Physical examination
   1. Vital signs: Fever (101°F–104°F [38.3°C–40°C]), chills; most common with bacterial meningitis
   2. Neurologic: Altered cognitive function (e.g., mental cloudiness, stupor, coma)
      a) Kernig sign: The clinician flexes one of the patient's legs at the hip and knee, then straightens the knee, noting resistance and pain; approximately 50% of patients with meningitis have positive test.
      b) Brudzinski sign: With the patient recumbent, the clinician places his or her hands behind the patient's head and flexes the neck forward, noting resistance or pain and watching for flexion of the patient's hips and knees in reaction to the maneuver; approximately 50% of patients with meningitis have positive test (see Appendix D).
      c) Nuchal rigidity (i.e., resistance to forward neck flexion) can occur.
      d) Changes in strength (e.g., hemiparesis, paraparesis) or balance (e.g., ataxia, apraxia) can occur.
   3. Eye
      a) Photophobia, diplopia
      b) Papilledema
   4. Integument
      a) Petechiae and purpura lesions (with meningococcal meningitis)
      b) Nonblanching rash indicating infection with meningococcal organism
      c) Dry, flushed skin indicating fever
      d) Vesicles (oral and/or genital) indicating HSV

IV. Diagnostic tests (Agnihotri, 2019; Figueiredo et al., 2018, LaPenna & Roos, 2019; McGill et al., 2016; Obaro, 2019; Salazar & Hasbun, 2017)
   A. Laboratory
      1. CBC
         a) WBC count: Usually elevated with left shift; severe infection leading to potential leukopenia
         b) Platelet count to assess for thrombocytopenia prior to lumbar puncture
            (1) Spinal subdural hematoma can occur if thrombocytopenia is present and potentially can lead to permanent neurologic deficits, including paraplegia.
            (2) Guidelines for performing lumbar puncture in the presence of thrombocytopenia include the following.
               (a) If the platelet count is less than or equal to 50,000/mm^3 or rapidly dropping, transfuse platelets prior to performing lumbar puncture.
               (b) If DIC or prolonged PT and PTT is present, implement corrective measures (i.e., two units of fresh frozen plasma during lumbar puncture).
               (c) Review medications if on anticoagulation; consider risk associated with performing lumbar puncture.
      2. PT, PTT, and INR to assess risk of hemorrhage prior to lumbar puncture
      3. Blood cultures to assess for source of infection: Perform immediately and obtain two sets.
         a) Positive in 40%–60% of patients with *H. influenzae,* meningococcal meningitis, or pneumococcal meningitis
         b) Positive for organism in bacterial meningitis 50%–75% of the time

    4. Urine cultures to assess for source of infection

    5. Skin/wound culture if presence of wound or vesicles

  B. Radiology

      1. CT scan of the head: Complete prior to lumbar puncture if patient exhibits focal neurologic signs. Test is nondiagnostic but essential to rule out mass or lesion, which may cause herniation during lumbar puncture. Prompt diagnosis and initiation of treatment can significantly improve patient outcome, so steps should be taken to avoid delays in obtaining imaging.

      2. MRI of the head: Imaging is indicated when cerebral edema, abscess, or demyelination encephalitis is suspected or in patients with known or suspected CNS disease.

  C. Other: Lumbar puncture is used to obtain CSF and complete evaluation for meningitis and determine causative organism (see Table 141-1).

      1. CBC with differential

      2. Glucose

      3. Protein

      4. Gram stain and bacterial culture; viral culture

      5. Fungal culture, India ink preparation, cryptococcal antigen

      6. Cytology

      7. Elevated CSF lactate greater than 36 mg/dl in postoperative neurosurgical patients indicative of bacterial infection

      8. Opening pressure elevated in bacterial meningitis

TABLE 141-1   **Assessment of Cerebrospinal Fluid Results From Lumbar Puncture**

Parameter	Normal	Abnormalities Seen With Meningitis	Possible Causes
Color	Clear, colorless	Xanthochromia, yellow, cloudy	High protein, presence of red blood cells, increased cell count
Glucose	50–75 mg/dl (60% of blood glucose level)	< 40 mg/dl	Bacterial meningitis, tuberculous meningitis, carcinomatous meningitis
Opening pressure	100–180 mm Hg	> 200 mm Hg	Block of cerebrospinal fluid flow, hydrocephalus, mass, lesion
Protein	15–45 mg/dl (1% of serum protein)	> 60 mg/dl	Spinal block (accumulation of infectious material blocking cerebrospinal fluid flow), carcinomatosis tumors located in proximity to the dura, meningitis
Red blood cells	None	Blood-tinged, grossly bloody	Traumatic tap, subarachnoid hemorrhage
White blood cells	0–6/mm³	> 10/mm³	Bacterial infections (may have predominantly neutrophils), viral infections (may have predominantly lymphocytes), tuberculous meningitis (may have predominantly lymphocytes), metastatic neoplastic process

Note. Based on information from LaPenna & Roos, 2019; McGill et al., 2016; Obaro, 2019.

V. Differential diagnosis (Agnihotri, 2019; LaPenna & Roos, 2019)
   A. Septicemia
   B. Carcinomatous meningitis
   C. Brain abscess with parameningeal inflammation
   D. SCC (see Chapter 145)
   E. Brain mass
   F. Migraine headaches (see Chapter 137)
   G. Encephalitis
   H. Subarachnoid hemorrhage

VI. Treatment (Figueiredo et al., 2018; Fitzgerald & Waterer, 2019; LaPenna & Roos, 2019; Mount & Boyle, 2017; Robinson & Busl, 2019; Tunkel et al., 2017)
   A. If meningitis is suspected, hospitalize patient to conduct diagnostic workup, initiate treatment, and monitor hemodynamic stability.
      1. If patient is hemodynamically unstable, transfer to ICU.
      2. Patients with meningitis can develop alterations in cardiac function, impaired respiratory drive, increased ICP, and seizure.
      3. If acute bacterial meningitis is suspected, prompt initiation of empiric antimicrobial treatment is essential to decrease morbidity and mortality.
   B. Antibiotic therapy (see Appendix C)
      1. Empiric antimicrobial therapy should be initiated immediately after CSF or blood culture is obtained; however, certain clinical features may require obtaining a CT scan of the head before performing diagnostic lumbar puncture, including immunocompromised state, history of CNS disease, new-onset seizure, papilledema, altered consciousness, or focal neurologic deficit, particularly cerebellar or brain stem dysfunction.
      2. Empiric treatment for immunocompromised patients: Ceftriaxone 2 g IV every 12 hours, or cefepime 2 g IV every eight hours plus vancomycin 15–20 mg/kg IV every 12 hours to achieve trough vancomycin concentration of 15–20 mcg/ml (combination therapy for *S. pneumoniae*), plus or minus ampicillin 2 g IV every four hours
      3. Empiric antimicrobial treatment should be tailored to pathogens and susceptibilities PRN.
         a) Vancomycin plus a third-generation cephalosporin (e.g., ceftriaxone, cefotaxime) is recommended to treat patients aged 2–50 years.
         b) Vancomycin and ampicillin plus a third-generation cephalosporin are recommended for patients older than 50 years.
      4. Vancomycin and ceftazidime or cefepime are recommended for patients who have recently undergone a neurosurgical procedure or have indwelling shunts or reservoirs, head trauma, or CSF leak.
      5. Patients with fungal meningitis should be treated with amphotericin B 0.7–1 mg/kg IV daily with flucytosine 100 mg/kg PO daily given as four divided doses for two weeks, then fluconazole 6–12 mg/kg PO or IV daily for 10 weeks, followed by maintenance therapy with fluconazole 3–6 mg/kg PO daily for 6–12 months.
      6. Patients suspected of having viral-induced meningitis should be treated with broad-spectrum antibiotics until a bacterial cause of meningitis has been excluded.
      7. Patients should be empirically treated with suspected herpetic meningitis with acyclovir 10 mg/kg IV every eight hours for 10 days.
      8. When the results of CSF culture are obtained, and local antibiotic-susceptibility testing is available, direct antibiotic coverage toward the known pathogen.

       a) Optimal duration of therapy for bacterial meningitis is not known.

       b) Recommended duration of therapy is 7 days for *H. influenzae,* 10–14 days for *S. pneumoniae,* and 14–21 days for *L. monocytogenes.*

  C. Steroid therapy

    1. The use of steroids in adult patients with meningitis is controversial.

       a) Steroids are thought to protect the meninges from the effects of bacterial cell products (e.g., cytokines) or meningeal inflammation.

       b) The main positive effect has been fewer neurologic or otologic sequelae in children and infants.

    2. Steroids should be given with or just before antimicrobial therapy. Patients exhibiting signs of increased ICP or cerebral edema should be given steroids to help manage these effects.

    3. Recommended treatment

       a) Dexamethasone is given at 0.15 mg/kg PO every six hours for two to four days. Rifampin 600 mg PO daily should be considered as an addition to the antimicrobial regimen because dexamethasone decreases the penetration of vancomycin in the CSF.

       b) Continued dosing and appropriate tapering are debatable and should be based on the patient's clinical recovery.

  D. Offending agent: Remove the offending agent in patients with indwelling reservoirs, evidence of surgical abscess, or bone flap infection to prevent recurrence of infection and neurologic symptoms.

  E. Seizure precautions are indicated, especially for patients with impaired mental state (see Chapter 144).

  F. Life support: Mechanical ventilation may be required in instances of worsening cognitive function, altered respiratory patterns, and increased ICP.

VII. Follow-up

  A. Assess for return of function, and appropriately refer to supportive services.

  B. Closely observe during hospitalization and rehabilitation; follow-up depends on the severity of symptoms and time to recovery.

VIII. Referrals

  A. Neurologist/neurosurgeon: For invasive testing, surgery, or management of seizures

  B. Infectious disease specialist: If uncommon organism is causative agent

  C. Physical, occupational, or speech therapist: Dependent on degree of involvement

The author would like to acknowledge Soo-Hyun Lee-Kim, RN, MS, FNP-C, and Terri S. Armstrong, PhD, ANP-BC, FAANP, FAAN, for their contribution to this chapter that remains unchanged from the previous edition of this book.

References

Agnihotri, S.P. (2019). Central nervous system opportunistic infections. *Seminars in Neurology, 39*(3), 383–390. https://doi.org/10.1055/s-0039-1687842

Akaishi, T., Kobayashi, J., Abe, M., Ishizawa, K., Nakashima, I., Aoki, M., & Ishii, T. (2019). Sensitivity and specificity of meningeal signs in patients with meningitis. *Journal of General and Family Medicine, 29*(5), 193–198. https://doi.org/10.1002/jgf2.268

Figueiredo, A.H.H., Brouwer, M.C., & van de Beek, D. (2018). Acute, community acquired bacterial meningitis. *Neurologic Clinics, 36*(4), 809–820. https://doi.org/10.1016/j.ncl.2018.06.007

Fitzgerald, D., & Waterer, G.W. (2019). Invasive pneumococcal and meningococcal disease. *Infectious Disease Clinics of North America, 33*(4), 1125–1141. https://doi.org/10.1016/j.idc.2019.08.007

LaPenna, P.A., & Roos, K.L. (2019). Bacterial infections of the central nervous system. *Seminars in Neurology, 39*(3), 334–342. https://doi.org/10.1055/s-0039-1693159

McGill, F., Heyderman, R.S., Panagiotou, S., Tunkel, A.R., & Solomon, T. (2016). Acute bacterial meningitis in adults. *Lancet, 388*(10063), 3036–3047. https://doi.org/10.1016/S0140-6736(16)30654-7

Mount, H.R., & Boyle, S.D. (2017). Aseptic and bacterial meningitis: Evaluation, treatment, and prevention. *American Family Physician, 96*(5), 314–322. https://www.aafp.org/afp/2017/0901/p314.html

Obaro, S. (2019). Updating the diagnosis of bacterial meningitis. *Lancet Infectious Diseases, 19*(11), 1160–1161. https://doi.org/10.1016/S1473-3099(19)30549-3

Robinson, C.P., & Busl, K.M. (2019). Meningitis and encephalitis management in the ICU. *Current Opinion in Critical Care, 25*(5), 423–429. https://doi.org/10.1097/MCC.0000000000000640

Salazar, L., & Hasbun, R. (2017). Cranial imaging before lumbar puncture in adults with community-acquired meningitis: Clinical utility and adherence to the Infectious Diseases Society of America guidelines. *Clinical Infectious Diseases, 64*(12), 1657–1662. https://doi.org/10.1093/cid/cix240

Tunkel, A.R., Hasbun, R., Bhimraj, A., Byers, K., Kaplan, S.L., Scheld, W.M., ... Zunt, J.R. (2017). 2017 Infectious Diseases Society of America's clinical practice guidelines for healthcare-associated ventriculitis and meningitis. *Clinical Infectious Diseases, 64*(6), 701–706. https://doi.org/10.1093/cid/cix152

CHAPTER 142

Neurotoxicity

Mary Elizabeth Davis, DNP, RN, CHPN, AOCNS®

I. Definition: Exposure to neurotoxins that causes either direct damage to glial cells or neurons or indirect injury by alteration of the cellular microenvironment within the CNS or PNS (Magge & DeAngelis, 2015; Stone & DeAngelis, 2016)

II. Physiology/Pathophysiology (Alberti et al., 2019; Cavaletti et al., 2019; Clark, 2018; Fodale et al., 2017; Horta et al., 2019; Kuks & Snoek, 2018; McLeary et al., 2019; Olsen et al., 2019; Pardo et al., 2018; Stone & DeAngelis, 2016; Verlinde et al., 2016)
   A. Normal
      1. The nervous system controls the motor, sensory, autonomic, cognitive, and behavioral functions.
      2. The CNS includes the brain and spinal cord and is the main network of coordination and control for the body.
      3. The PNS is composed of motor and sensory nerves and ganglia outside the CNS and serves as a relay between the CNS and the rest of the body.
      4. The blood–brain barrier and blood–nerve barrier protect the CNS and PNS against potentially neurotoxic effects.
      5. The autonomic nervous system regulates the internal body, which is involuntary. The three major subdivisions of the autonomic nervous system are sympathetic, parasympathetic, and enteric.
      6. Cranial nerves are peripheral nerves that arise from the brain, with each nerve having motor or sensory function.
   B. Pathophysiology
      1. Cancer itself can cause neurotoxicity.
         a) A primary tumor or metastases can invade the brain, spine, leptomeninges, and PNS.
         b) Headaches, seizures, stroke, cognitive dysfunction, increased ICP/hydrocephalus, fatigue, and paraneoplastic syndrome can all result from tumor presence.
      2. Various cancer-directed chemotherapy, immunotherapy, and targeted agents are associated with specific neurotoxicity disorders, including headache, seizures, encephalopathies, myelopathy, neuropathies, and cerebrovascular events such as stroke.
         a) The mechanism of action behind headache occurrence is unknown but is thought to be related to drug penetrating the blood–brain barrier. It can occur as a side effect of immune-modulated cytokine release. Additionally, meningeal irritation and increased ICP can cause headaches.
         b) Seizures may be related to the toxic effect of the drug itself (e.g., busulfan, intrathecal cytarabine) or to changes in the microenvironment (e.g., agents that cause SIADH).

    c) Encephalopathy can occur acutely post-treatment with the drug or metabolites causing damage to the neural tissue (e.g., chemical meningitis), or from immune-related cytokine and chemokine release (e.g., CAR T-cell therapy, other immunotherapies).

    d) Myelopathy can be caused by cord compression, demyelinating disorders, infection, metabolic disorders, or radiation.

    e) The mechanism of action leading to peripheral neuropathy varies depending on the offending agent administered; damage to the DNA, mitochondria, and axon transport can occur. Commonly, damage to the microtubules disrupts axonal transport and degeneration of the nerve occurs.

    f) Antiangiogenic agents (e.g., bevacizumab) can cause vascular changes, resulting in intracranial hemorrhage, thromboembolic events, and reversible posterior leukoencephalopathy syndrome.

    g) Immune checkpoint inhibitors have been associated with PNS and CNS neurotoxicity, including headaches, neuropathies, encephalopathies, myasthenic syndromes, and Guillain-Barré–like syndromes. Exact etiology is not known.

    h) CAR T-cell therapy can trigger a cytokine storm/cytokine release syndrome, resulting in prominent neurologic symptoms starting with aphasia and progressing to seizures and severe encephalopathy.

  3. Radiation therapy can cause direct effects to the PNS or CNS, causing vascular damage, fibrosis of neural structures, plexopathies, and cerebral radiation necrosis. It may also cause disruption of the blood–brain barrier, transient demyelination, and a rise in ICP.

    a) Effects can be acute (days to a week), early delayed (four weeks to six months), or late delayed (six months to years after treatment).

    b) Pathophysiology of radiation fibrosis is not fully understood but likely involves acute damage causing microvascular injury and chronic changes creating an inflammatory environment. Ischemic changes may predispose cells to develop fibrosis.

  4. Surgery can cause neurotoxicity by a variety of mechanisms.

    a) Postcraniotomy neurotoxicity can result from direct injury to the brain or from pressure/compression from edema postoperatively.

    b) Anesthesia

      (1) Local anesthetic systemic toxicity is an acute complication of regional anesthesia and can cause CNS toxicity (e.g., seizures) and cardiovascular toxicity (e.g., arrhythmia, cardiovascular collapse). Local anesthetics, nerve blocks, or epidural anesthesia may also cause temporary or permanent nerve damage, radiculopathy, or neuropathy due to chemical injury, needle injury, or hematoma.

      (2) Exposure to general anesthetics is potentially harmful to the human brain and may cause consequent long-term cognitive deficits.

    c) Nerve damage due to surgery may occur from the intraoperative use of tourniquets, traction, or patient positioning causing compression, contusion, or ischemia.

III. Clinical features: Neurotoxicity is the second most common dose-limiting factor (behind myelosuppression) requiring cancer drug modification or discontinuation. It includes conditions such as headache, seizures, neuropathy, cognitive impairment, encephalopathy, cerebellar toxicity, myelopathy, stroke, radiation necrosis, stroke-like migraine attacks after radiation therapy syndrome, and plexopathies (Alberti et al., 2019; Baer et al., 2019; Cavaletti et al., 2019; Hoeffner, 2016; Horta et al., 2019; Kuks & Snoek, 2018; Neelapu, 2019; Pardo et al., 2018; Rajabally & Attarian, 2018; Ranjan & Schiff, 2018; Stone & DeAngelis, 2016).

A. Risk factors that influence toxic effects on the nervous system include the following.

    1. A drug's ability to pass through the blood–brain, blood–ocular, or blood–nerve barriers

    2. The route of administration: IV, intrathecal, intraventricular

    3. Dose of treatment administered: High-dose chemotherapy, high fraction/total dose radiation

    4. Cranial irradiation: Dosing and area of involved brain

    5. Duration of treatment and cumulative dose

    6. Prior or concurrent treatment: Chemotherapy, immunotherapy, surgery, radiation therapy

    7. Comorbidities: Alcohol abuse, diabetes mellitus, history of stroke or transient ischemic attack, cerebrovascular disease, hereditary conditions (e.g., Charcot-Marie-Tooth disease)

    8. Concomitant medications: Glucocorticosteroids, cytarabine, ifosfamide, antiepileptics, opioids, isoniazid, ethambutol, streptomycin, other aminoglycoside antibiotics

    9. Impaired renal or hepatic function

   10. Age: Very young, older adults

   11. Concomitant neurotoxic agents

   12. High tumor burden and elevated baseline inflammatory state: Increased risk of CAR T-cell–induced neurotoxicity

   13. Exposure to heavy metals, certain foods and food additives, pesticides, industrial or cleaning solvents

   14. Presence of underlying structural nervous system disorder: Brain aneurysm, trauma to brain

   15. Specific genetic polymorphisms that may enhance or reduce tendency to develop neurotoxicity related to chemotherapy: Apolipoprotein e4

   16. Intracranial infection

   17. Metabolic disorders: Hyponatremia, hypercalcemia, severe hypoglycemia

B. Etiology

    1. Headache

       a) Headache is a common neurologic complaint; etiology can be related to tumor mass effect, meningeal irritation, elevation of ICP, inflammation, or vasodilation or can have a psychogenic origin.

       b) Stroke-like migraine attacks after radiation therapy (SMART) is a rare syndrome from brain irradiation. It causes headaches, seizures, and intermittent reversible neurologic dysfunction. It is thought to be caused by vasculopathy or neuronal impairment within the trigeminal nerve that innervates cerebral blood vessels.

    2. Seizures can be an indicator of primary or metastatic brain tumors, vascular complications, surgical manipulation, infection, or the result of antineoplastic treatment. Encephalopathy caused by organ dysfunction can be the etiology of seizures.

    3. Neuropathy

       a) Peripheral neuropathy

          (1) Metabolic: Diabetes mellitus, renal failure, amyloidosis, porphyria

          (2) Hereditary: Charcot-Marie-Tooth disease

          (3) Immune mediated: Guillain-Barré syndrome, chronic inflammatory demyelinating neuropathy

          (4) Toxic neuropathies: Chemotherapy, drugs, alcohol, heavy metals, tick bites

          (5) Infections: HIV, Lyme disease, CMV, syphilis, leprosy, diphtheria

      (6) Compression: Optic nerve, carpal tunnel syndrome, ulnar neuropathy

      (7) Vasculitis: Polyarteritis nodosa, Churg-Strauss syndrome, cryoglobulinemia

      (8) Paraneoplastic: Lung cancer and thymoma (most common cause)

      (9) Nutritional: Vitamin B_{12}, B_1, or B_6 deficiencies

    b) Autonomic neuropathy from paraneoplastic syndrome

      (1) Associated with small cell lung cancer, thymoma, neuroblastoma, teratomas, lymphoma, and myeloma

      (2) Thought to be related to a cell-mediated autoimmune process in which specific antibodies target proteins expressed by the tumor and nervous system

      (3) May also be caused by inappropriate secretion of tumor-mediated hormones or cytokines causing symptoms

   c) SCC

      (1) Compression of the spinal cord from tumor invasion causes neuronal injury, edema, and/or ischemia.

      (2) Most common cancers for spinal cord metastases include breast, lung, and prostate.

   d) Tumor or edema causing pressure on the nerve resulting in focal neuropathies

   e) Polyneuropathy: Chronic inflammatory demyelinating polyneuropathy

      (1) Associated with hematologic malignancies (lymphomas) and melanoma; rare in other cancers

      (2) Etiology unknown; may be related to lymphomatous infiltration into peripheral nerves.; toxic and metabolic mechanism also suggested

4. Encephalopathy

   a) Acute encephalopathy can develop hours to days after treatment.

   b) Chronic encephalopathy is most commonly associated with intrathecally and intraventricularly administered agents (e.g., cytarabine, methotrexate, thiotepa), particularly when followed or combined with radiation.

      (1) The effect generally occurs six months to two years after therapy.

      (2) Neurologic dysfunction can progress to severe impairment, coma, or death.

   c) Posterior reversible encephalopathy syndrome or reversible posterior leukoencephalopathy syndrome

      (1) Most commonly associated with the use of calcineurin inhibitors, such as tacrolimus and cyclosporine, and other agents, such as methotrexate, cytarabine, bevacizumab, and gemcitabine

      (2) Reversible condition that requires either a dose reduction or withholding of the causative agent

      (3) Etiology unknown but thought to be related to vasogenic edema and breakdown of blood–brain barrier from dysregulation of cerebral blood pressure or endothelial dysfunction

5. Cerebellar toxicity

   a) Radiation directly to the cerebellum

   b) Chemotherapy agents: Cytarabine, 5-fluorouracil

   c) Cytokines: IFN-α, IL, TNF

6. Myelopathy

   a) Rare complication occurring from radiation to spinal cord; may be early (usually transient) or delayed (often progressive)

   b) Following direct instillation of chemotherapy into the spinal fluid

7. Cranial nerve palsies: Thought to be a direct effect of specific chemotherapy agents (e.g., vincristine, vinblastine)

C. History
  1. History of cancer and cancer treatment
  2. Current medications: Prescribed, over the counter
  3. History of presenting symptoms: Precipitating factors, location, duration
  4. Changes in ADLs
  5. Past medical history: Stroke, brain aneurysm, head trauma, diabetes mellitus
  6. Family history: Hereditary neurologic disorders (e.g., Charcot-Marie-Tooth disease)
D. Signs and symptoms
  1. Headache
    a) Tight feeling in head
    b) Associated symptoms: Photophobia, occipital pain, diplopia, nausea, vomiting
  2. Seizures
    a) Decreased level of consciousness
    b) Motor symptoms: Jerking or rigidity, eye deviation
    c) Associated symptoms
      (1) Aura: Strange odor, nausea, or particular feeling prior to seizure
      (2) Nausea
      (3) Headache
      (4) Weakness
      (5) Postictal state: Aphasia, weakness, temporary hemiparesis
      (6) Biting tongue or inside cheek
      (7) Urinary incontinence
      (8) Excessive salivation: Foaming at mouth
      (9) Blinking or empty gaze
  3. Neuropathy
    a) Peripheral neuropathy
      (1) Dysesthesia sensation in hands and/or feet usually in a glove-and-stocking distribution, often referred to as "pins and needles"
      (2) Numbness in hands or feet: Anesthesia, paresthesia
      (3) Itching or burning of hands and feet
      (4) Pain in hands or feet: Allodynia
      (5) Difficulty distinguishing temperature
      (6) Difficulty walking: Ataxia, steppage gait
      (7) Weakness in ankles: Can lead to foot drop
    b) Autonomic neuropathy
      (1) Abdominal pain
      (2) Constipation or obstipation
      (3) Impotence
      (4) Urinary retention
      (5) Light-headedness/dizziness
      (6) Palpitations
    c) SCC
      (1) Back pain
      (2) Motor or sensory weakness or loss
    d) Polyneuropathy
      (1) Usually, symmetric presentation
      (2) Pain, burning, numbness along course of nerves
      (3) Weakness in extremities
      (4) Loss of motor function
      (5) Autonomic symptoms may occur

4. Encephalopathy
   a) Acute or posterior reversible encephalopathy syndrome
      (1) Delirium, confusion, disorientation
      (2) Impairment in memory, learning, executive function, concentration, and attention
      (3) Difficulty following direction or completing tasks
      (4) Loss of ability to read or write
      (5) Difficulty naming objects
      (6) Headache, visual changes
      (7) Seizures
   b) Chronic leukoencephalopathy
      (1) Acute symptoms plus progressive cognitive dysfunction and dementia
      (2) Gait abnormalities
      (3) Urinary incontinence
      (4) Somnolence
      (5) Inability to perform ADLs
      (6) Lack of initiative and apathy
5. Cerebellar toxicity
   a) Headache
   b) Slurred speech: Dysarthria
   c) Difficulty with tasks requiring fine motor control, such as buttoning shirts or writing: Dysarthria, apraxia
   d) Gait disturbances/ataxia
   e) Confusion
   f) Nystagmus
6. Myelopathy
   a) Lower extremity weakness
   b) Sensory changes/paresthesia or loss of sensation in lower extremities
   c) Alterations in bowel or bladder function: Incontinence
   d) Possible symptom of back pain
   e) Temporary electric shock sensation radiating down the spine of upper limbs that occurs with neck flexion: Lhermitte sign
7. Cranial nerve palsies: Dependent on which cranial nerve is affected (see Appendix A)

E. Physical examination: Focus on neurologic examination guided by signs and symptoms.
  1. Neuropathy
    a) Peripheral neuropathy
       (1) Loss of position/vibration sense (e.g., in great toe or finger) indicating large sensory fiber loss
       (2) Loss of hot/cold and pain sensations indicating small sensory fiber loss
       (3) Loss of fine motor movement, such as the ability to pick up a coin or button a shirt
       (4) Absence of deep tendon reflexes: Areflexia
       (5) Foot drop or weak dorsiflexion indicating loss of strength
       (6) "Slap gait": Steppage
    b) Autonomic neuropathy
       (1) Cardiac: Orthostatic hypotension without compensatory increase in heart rate indicative of tachycardia or bradycardia
       (2) Vision: Sluggish pupillary response to light and accommodation
       (3) Abdominal: Decreased bowel sounds, bladder extension due to retention
       (4) Skin: Palms and soles evaluation for excessive sweating

    c) Focal/cranial neuropathies: Dependent on which nerve is affected (see Appendix A)

    d) Polyneuropathy: Symmetric findings of weakness (e.g., in hip flexion testing adduction and abduction; see symmetric weakness of distal muscles)

2. Encephalopathy
   a) Mental status: Poor recall, short- or long-term memory loss, altered attention, agitation, somnolence
   b) Neurocognitive testing: Poor executive function, difficulty following commands, slowed word retrieval and processing speed
   c) Impaired fine motor dexterity movement: Ability to button buttons, pick up coin from table
   d) Decreased cortical sensory function
      (1) Stereognosis: Place a familiar object in the patient's hand to determine difficulty in identifying objects by touching.
      (2) Two-point discrimination: Simultaneously using the sides of two pens, touch the skin, alternating irregularly with a one-point touch; patients normally can discriminate about 2–3 mm.
      (3) Graphesthesia: Trace symbols, shapes, and numbers on the skin and have the patient identify them.
   e) Slowed rapid alternating movements
   f) Posterior reversible encephalopathy syndrome
      (1) Vision changes: Cortical blindness, blurred vision, homonymous hemianopia (i.e., blindness of nasal half of the visual field of one eye and temporal half of the other)
      (2) Vital signs: Elevated blood pressure

3. Cerebellar toxicity
   a) Truncal ataxia: Inability to sit upright
   b) Ataxia: Unsteady gait, difficulty standing with feet together irrespective of eyes open or closed
   c) Dysarthria: Slurred speech
   d) Nystagmus noted with extraocular movement examination
   e) Altered Mini-Mental State Examination: Mental clouding or confusion
   f) Uncoordinated writing or drawing
   g) Dysdiadochokinesis: Inability to perform rapid alternating movements
   h) Altered movement accuracy: Dysmetria on finger-to-nose or heel-to-shin testing
   i) Hypotonia: Poor muscle tone or strength

4. Myelopathy
   a) Sensory loss: Often a discrete level or following a particular dermatome (see Appendix B)
   b) Radiating pain in radicular pattern (made worse with palpation)
   c) Decreased strength or muscle weakness in extremities
   d) Abnormal reflexes (hyper- or hyporeflexia), positive Babinski reflex, positive Hoffman sign (flexion of the thumb and index finger after flicking the middle finger), clonus, positive inverted supinator sign
   e) Abdominal: Distended bowel or bladder, hypoactive or absent bowel sounds
   f) Rectal: Decreased anal sphincter tone
   g) Lhermitte sign: Triggered by neck flexion and characterized by a brief unpleasant sensation of numbness, tingling, or often electric shock–like feelings from the neck to the spine and extremities
   h) Impaired coordination, abnormal gait

IV. Diagnostic tests: Performed in conjunction with history and physical examination (Baer et al., 2019; Dietrich & Klein, 2014; Huang & Wen, 2018; Janani & Avila, 2018)
  A. Laboratory
    1. Chemistry profile: Electrolyte imbalance and liver function abnormalities to evaluate for other causes of symptoms
    2. Ammonia level if encephalopathy is suspected
    3. Thyroid function test to evaluate for hypothyroidism and hyperthyroidism
    4. Vitamin B_{12} level to assess for nutritional deficiency: Presents with peripheral neuropathy or encephalopathy
    5. Toxicology panel to assess for toxins, as indicated
    6. ABGs to assess for hypoxia
    7. CBC to evaluate for anemia and increase in WBCs indicating infection
    8. Increased ESR possibly indicating inflammation
    9. Glucose or Hgb A1c to evaluate for diabetes
    10. SPEP to evaluate for gammopathy or myeloma
    11. Collagen-vascular screen, if indicated
    12. Autoimmune disorder suspected: Antinuclear antibody, rheumatoid factor, myasthenia workup
    13. Paraneoplastic syndrome suspected: Evaluation of CSF and serum for paraneoplastic antibodies (e.g., anti-Hu, anti-Yo, anti-CRMP5)
    14. CSF analysis for immune-mediated profile, including elevated protein, pleocytosis, oligoclonal bands, elevated IgG index, and synthesis rate; CSF culture if infection suspected
    15. Coagulation profile, as indicated, for suspected thrombosis formation
    16. Urinalysis and urine culture to assess for infection, especially in older adults with altered mental status
  B. Radiology
    1. Diffusion-weighted MRI
      a) Brain metastases usually appear hypo- or isointense.
        (1) Irregular thickening around the wall of the enhancing rim can help to differentiate from a brain abscess.
        (2) Brain metastases may be solitary or multifocal.
      b) Stroke-like migraine attacks after radiation therapy syndrome appear with focal thickening of the gyri within the affected cortex with contrast enhancement.
      c) Leukoencephalopathy is best imaged by MRI. Nonenhancing hypodensities can be seen in white matter. Chronic encephalopathy may produce progressive deep brain atrophy.
      d) An open-ring sign (contrast enhancement in a crescent shape) is suggestive of demyelination and can help differentiate between a brain mass and multiple sclerosis.
      e) Enhancing without vasogenic edema may be suggestive of an arterial or vascular infarction or venous malformations, which can mimic a tumor.
      f) Spine MRI can help diagnose metastatic disease, SCC, and leptomeningeal disease.
      g) Additional MRI techniques, such as spectroscopy or perfusion and diffusion tensor imaging, may be ordered to enhance diagnosis.
    2. CT scan with and without contrast
      a) CT may be helpful in those with a sudden change in neurologic examination to assess for bleeding, hydrocephalus, or herniation.
      b) CT can evaluate tumor extension into bone.

       c) Brain metastases are usually isodense on CT.
          (1) Assess for presence of vasogenic edema.
          (2) Tumors may appear hypodense with cystic or necrotic areas.
          (3) Most lesions enhance with iodinated contrast.
       d) Acute hemorrhage and blood clots usually appear hyperdense; as blood ages, it will appear less hyperdense.
       e) Acute infarction and ischemia usually reveal edema and a loss of differentiation between gray and white matter.
       f) Certain tumors, such as oligodendrogliomas, germ cell tumors, and meningiomas, may produce calcifications that can be seen on CT.
       g) Contrast enhancement from radiation necrosis may be difficult to distinguish from tumor reoccurrence or progression. A biopsy may be required.
   3. A PET scan may be helpful to distinguish recurrent tumor from inflammation and necrosis.
  C. Other
    1. Electroencephalogram can evaluate clinical and subclinical seizures in patients with known seizure disorder, mental status changes, or unresponsiveness.
      a) Patients with focal brain lesions can have electroencephalogram changes in conjunction with metabolic abnormalities, such as hepatic or renal failure and electrolyte imbalance.
      b) Electroencephalogram changes may also be seen with certain chemotherapy agents (e.g., busulfan, vincristine, ifosfamide), brain irradiation, and autoimmune and paraneoplastic syndromes.
    2. Lumbar puncture
      a) Lumbar puncture is useful in the diagnosis of neurotoxic conditions such as meningitis (e.g., carcinomatosis, viral, infectious), hydrocephalus, vasculitis, subarachnoid hemorrhage, CNS tumors, encephalitis, Guillain-Barré syndrome, and other demyelinating diseases.
      b) Careful consideration of potential increased ICP is warranted, as lumbar puncture is contraindicated because of risk of herniation.
    3. Nerve conduction tests and electromyography
      a) Tests may be helpful in the diagnosis of PNS disorders and in patients with paresthesia, sensory loss, peripheral pain, muscle weakness, or atrophy.
      b) Tests may reveal axonal neuropathy associated with certain chemotherapy classes (e.g., taxanes, vinca alkaloids, platinums, proteasome inhibitors, some monoclonal antibodies).
      c) They can also help to differentiate axonal versus demyelinating neuropathies.

V. Differential diagnosis (Alberti et al., 2019; Cavaletti et al., 2019; Jin & Shin, 2019)
  A. Acute neurologic event: Stroke (see Chapter 146), intracranial hemorrhage
  B. CNS lesions: Metastases, recurrent tumor, infection, vascular lesions, demyelinating lesions
  C. Pseudoprogression or somnolence syndrome
  D. Electrolyte imbalance (see Chapters 152–156)
  E. Infection
  F. SIADH (see Chapter 95)
  G. Diabetes mellitus (see Chapter 151)
  H. Autoimmune disease
  I. Vitamin B_{12} deficiency (see Chapter 115)
  J. Hereditary neuropathy: Charcot-Marie-Tooth disease
  K. Paraneoplastic syndromes (see Appendix M)

VI. Treatment: Effective treatment is not available for most neurotoxicities associated with chemotherapy, immunotherapy, and radiation therapy. Methods of prevention and careful monitoring are paramount to minimize the effects (Alberti et al., 2019; Baer et al., 2019; Cavaletti et al., 2019; Clark, 2018; Spain et al., 2019).

   A. Prevention
   1. Careful neurologic screening of patients with preexisting neurologic deficits allows for baseline assessment of functional status (e.g., a patient with Charcot-Marie-Tooth disease or diabetic neuropathy who is more likely to experience peripheral neuropathy).
   2. Patients receiving intraventricular therapy should undergo a cisternogram if obstruction is suspected.
      a) This study assesses normal CSF flow by injecting tracer into the reservoir system and observing for flow of tracer out of the ventricles, around the spinal cord, and up over the convexities of the brain.
      b) Injection of chemotherapy into the ventricular system with abnormal flow can lead to retention of the injected drug and rapid development of leukoencephalopathy.
   3. Careful treatment planning is necessary when intrathecal chemotherapy is administered concomitantly with radiation therapy or if radiation therapy precedes the administration of chemotherapy to reduce the risk and severity of encephalopathy.
   4. Steroids (e.g., dexamethasone) may help prevent or limit the incidence of acute encephalopathy associated with cranial radiation therapy.
   5. Prophylactic antiseizure medication may prevent seizures after cranial resection, with busulfan chemotherapy administration, and with CAR T-cell therapy.

   B. Monitoring
   1. If an underlying neuropathy exists in patients receiving an agent known to cause peripheral neuropathy (e.g., vincristine, cisplatin, paclitaxel, docetaxel, bortezomib, thalidomide), careful monitoring for the development of decreased intestinal motility and implementation of a bowel regimen should occur (see Chapter 55).
   2. If evidence of neurotoxicity occurs during treatment, the treatment should be modified or discontinued based on the severity/grade of symptoms. Continued treatment with the offending agent often leads to worsening of effects and the potential for irreversibility.
   3. Seizure precautions should be instituted for those with seizure history or those at increased risk (e.g., primary brain tumor, intracerebral hemorrhage).

   C. Treatment aimed at symptomatic improvement, supportive care, and return of baseline functioning
   1. Headache (see Chapter 137): Treatment should be personalized to the etiology.
   2. Seizure (see Chapter 144): Anticonvulsants should be personalized based on patient factors, comorbidities, tolerance, and concomitant therapy, as potential drug–drug interactions need to be considered.
   3. Peripheral neuropathy (see Chapter 143)
      a) No current approved medications exist to treat or reverse CIPN. Treatment strategies include regimen modification by altering dosing, cycles, timing, and/or duration. Discontinuing the offending medication may be necessary if neuropathy progresses. Medications may be used to treat the neuropathic pain (Appendix Q).
      b) Pain and discomfort can be managed with a range of medications, including anticonvulsants, antidepressants, analgesics, and supplements. Other treatments have been used, such as electrostimulation and heat and cold stimulation.

      c) For paraneoplastic syndrome–related autonomic neuropathy, treatment of the underlying malignancy is key. Steroids, plasma exchange, or IVIg may be treatment options.

    4. Encephalopathy: An interprofessional team approach should be taken with the aim of optimizing function, minimizing severity of side effects, and preserving QOL. Provision of care includes assisting with ADLs, providing nutritional support, maintaining fluid and electrolyte status, and limiting patient environmental stimuli.

      a) With acute encephalopathy, dose reductions or elimination of offending agent may be required.

      b) Methylene blue may be used to treat ifosfamide encephalopathy.

      c) With progressive encephalopathy, patients may require assistance or custodial care with basic needs and ADLs, as well as protection and prevention of self-injury to limit permanent dysfunction.

      d) With posterior reversible encephalopathy syndrome, blood pressure should be gradually reduced if elevated (see Chapter 47). A rapid decrease in blood pressure can increase the size of involved ischemia, require prompt treatment of seizures (see Chapter 144), and include treatment of electrolyte imbalance (see Chapters 152–156).

    5. Cerebellar toxicity: Carefully monitor for occurrence; stop treatment when recognized.

      a) Use of physical, speech, and occupational therapists often can decrease the extent of dysfunction.

      b) Provision of emotional and physical support during recovery allows for enhanced coping mechanisms for deficits that may be permanent.

    6. Myelopathy

      a) Early diagnosis is imperative in radiation myelopathy because treatment options are limited, and the condition can lead to paralysis.

      b) Steroid therapy may provide stabilization or partial improvement.

      c) Other regimens that may be of benefit are warfarin and hyperbaric oxygen.

  D. Patient and family education

    1. Ensure a safe environment.

    2. Teach patients skills to avoid injury.

      a) Loss of pain/temperature sensation: Instruct patients to use oven mitts and gardening gloves; decrease water temperature setting to prevent burns. Maintain good foot care and wear properly fitting shoes.

      b) Loss of vibration/position sense: Instruct patients to remove throw rugs and use night-lights; instruct on the use of visual cues.

      c) Weakness: Provide patients with assistive devices, such as braces, lightweight splints, walkers, or canes, to support muscle weakness and gait difficulties.

      d) Autonomic dysfunction: Educate patients about the importance of safety issues, including avoidance of extreme heat, dehydration, and alcohol consumption. Other measures include increasing fiber in the diet to prevent constipation, wearing waist-high elastic support hose to increase venous return, and sleeping with the head of the bed elevated.

VII. Follow-up

  A. Follow-up is dependent on an individual assessment of the patient's neurologic status, functional ability, support systems, and treatment options.

  B. An interprofessional approach to the plan of care should be standard.

VIII. Referrals

    A. Neurologist: For neurologic evaluation, diagnosis, and treatment options

    B. Physical, occupational, or speech therapist: Dependent on deficits

    C. Neurocognitive testing specialist: For cognitive therapy plan

    D. Social worker or psychiatrist: For psychological and psychosocial needs assessment

    E. Homecare or case management specialist: For home safety evaluation

    F. Behavioral specialist: For cognitive behavioral therapy

The author would like to acknowledge Eva Lu T. Lee, MSN, RN, ANP-BC, and Laurel Westcarth, MS, MBA, RN, ANP-BC, for their contribution to this chapter that remains unchanged from the previous edition of this book.

References

Alberti, P., Cavaletti, G., & Cornblath, D.R. (2019). Toxic neuropathies: Chemotherapy induced peripheral neurotoxicity. *Current Opinion in Neurology, 32*(5), 676–683. https://doi.org/10.1097/WCO.0000000000000724

Baer, B., Dudley, C.V., & Simons, R.M. (2019). Management principles associated with cytokine release syndrome. *Seminars in Oncology Nursing, 35*(5), 150931. https://doi.org/10.1016/j.soncn.2019.08.010

Cavaletti, G., Alberti, P., Argyriou, A.A., Lustberg, M., Staff, N.P., & Tamburin, S. (2019). Chemotherapy-induced peripheral neurotoxicity: A multifaceted, still unsolved issue. *Journal of the Peripheral Nervous System, 24*(Suppl. 2), S6–S12. https://doi.org/10.1111/jns.12337

Clark, M. (2018). Minimizing risk of cancer therapeutics. *Physical Medicine and Rehabilitation Clinics of North America, 29*(4), 701–719. https://doi.org/10.1016/j.pmr.2018.06.006

Dietrich, J., & Klein, J.P. (2014) Imaging of cancer therapy–induced central nervous system toxicity. *Neurologic Clinics, 32*(1), 147–157. https://doi.org/10.1016/j.ncl.2013.07.004

Fodale, V., Tripodi, V.F., Penna, O., Famà, F., Squadrito, F., Mondello, E., & David, A. (2017). An update on anesthetics and impact on the brain. *Expert Opinion on Drug Safety, 16*(9), 997–1008. https://doi.org/10.1080/14740338.2017.1351539

Hoeffner, E.G. (2016). Central nervous system complications of oncologic therapy. *Hematology/Oncology Clinics of North America, 30*(4), 899–920. https://doi.org/10.1016/j.hoc.2016.03.010

Horta, E., Bongiorno, C., Ezzeddine, M., & Neil, E.C. (2019). Neurotoxicity of antibodies in cancer therapy: A review. *Clinical Neurology and Neurosurgery, 188,* 105566. https://doi.org/10.1016/j.clineuro.2019.105566

Huang, R., & Wen, P.Y. (2018) Imaging neurologic manifestations of oncologic disease. In D. Schiff, I. Arrillaga, & P.Y. Wen (Eds.), *Cancer neurology in clinical practice: Neurological complications of cancer and its treatment* (3rd ed., pp. 13–32). Springer. https://doi.org/10.1007/978-3-319-57901-6_2

Janani, C.S., & Avila, E.K. (2018) Other diagnostic tools for neurological disease in cancer: EEG, EMG, and lumbar puncture. In D. Schiff, I. Arrillaga, & P.Y. Wen (Eds.), *Cancer neurology in clinical practice: Neurological complications of cancer and its treatment* (3rd ed., pp. 33–54). Springer. https://doi.org/10.1007/978-3-319-57901-6_3

Jin, P.H., & Shin, S.C. (2019). Neuropathy of connective tissue disease and other systemic diseases. *Seminars in Neurology, 39*(5), 651–668. https://doi.org/10.1055/s-0039-1688989

Kuks, J.B.M., & Snoek, J.W. (2018). An overview over nervous system and muscles. Technical investigations in neurology. In J.B.M Kuks & J.W. Snoek (Eds.), *Textbook of clinical neurology* (pp. 13–27). Springer.

Magge, R.S., & DeAngelis, L.M. (2015). The double-edged sword: Neurotoxicity of chemotherapy. *Blood Reviews, 29*(2), 93–100. https://doi.org/10.1016/j.blre.2014.09.012

McLeary, F., Davis, A., Rudrawar, S., Perkins, A., & Anoopkumar-Dukie, S. (2019). Mechanisms underlying select chemotherapeutic-agent-induced neuroinflammation and subsequent neurodegeneration. *European Journal of Pharmacology, 842,* 49–56. https://doi.org/10.1016/j.ejphar.2018.09.034

Neelapu, S.S. (2019). Managing the toxicities of CAR T-cell therapy. *Hematological Oncology, 37*(Suppl. 1), 48–52. https://doi.org/10.1002/hon.2595

Olsen, M.M., LeFebvre, K.B., & Brassil, K.J. (Eds.). (2019). *Chemotherapy and immunotherapy guidelines and recommendations for practice.* Oncology Nursing Society.

Pardo, I.D., Rao, D.B., Butt, M.T., Jortner, B.S., Valentine, W.M., Arezzo, J., ... Bolon, B. (2018). Toxicologic pathology of the peripheral nervous system (PNS): Overview, challenges, and current practices. *Toxicologic Pathology, 46*(8), 1028–1036. https://doi.org/10.1177/0192623318800707

Rajabally, Y.A., & Attarian, S.(2018). Chronic inflammatory demyelinating polyneuropathy and malignancy: A systematic review. *Muscle and Nerve, 57*(6), 875–883. https://doi.org/10.1002/mus.26028

Ranjan, S., & Schiff, D. (2018). Headache as complication of cancer. In D. Schiff, I. Arrillaga, & P.Y. Wen (Eds.), *Cancer neurology in clinical practice: Neurological complications of cancer and its treatment* (3rd ed., pp. 143–151). Springer. https://doi.org/10.1007/978-3-319-57901-6_8

Spain, L., Tippu, Z., Larkin, J.M., Carr, A., & Turajlic, S. (2019). How we treat neurological toxicity from immune checkpoint inhibitors. *ESMO Open, 4*(Suppl. 4), e000540. https://doi.org/10.1136/esmoopen-2019-000540

Stone, J.B., & DeAngelis, L.M. (2016). Cancer-treatment-induced neurotoxicity—Focus on newer treatments. *Nature Reviews Clinical Oncology, 13*(2), 92–105. https://doi.org/10.1038/nrclinonc.2015.152

Verlinde, M., Hollmann, M.W., Stevens, M.F., Hermanns, H., Werdehausen, R., & Lirk, P. (2016). Local anesthetic-induced neurotoxicity. *International Journal of Molecular Science, 17*(3), 339. https://doi.org/10.3390/ijms17030339

CHAPTER 143

Peripheral Neuropathy

Corazon Lauren Delumpa, MSN, RN, FNP-C

I. Definition: A condition of altered function and structure of the motor, sensory, or autonomic components of a peripheral nerve (Doughty & Seyedsadjadi, 2018; Stubblefield et al., 2009; Watson & Dyck, 2015)

II. Physiology/Pathophysiology (Boyette-Davis et al., 2018; Chan et al., 2019; Lees et al., 2017; Pop-Busui et al., 2017; Stubblefield et al., 2009; Valentine, 2020; Watson & Dyck, 2015)
 A. Normal
  1. PNS: Consists of the cranial and spinal nerves and their associated ganglia
   a) The cranial nerves have 12 pairs, which leave the brain, pass through foramina in the skull, and coordinate motor and sensory function of the head and neck region.
   b) The spinal nerves have 31 pairs, which leave the spinal cord and pass through the intervertebral foramina. Their names are derived from the vertebral level from which they exit (8 cervical, 12 thoracic, 5 lumbar, 5 sacral, and 1 coccygeal).
    (1) Each spinal nerve is connected to the spinal cord by two roots, the anterior root and the posterior root, which give rise to three functional types of fibers (see 1*c*).
    (2) The anterior root contains bundles of nerve fibers (efferent fibers) that carry nerve impulses away from the CNS. Efferent fibers go to the skeletal muscles, causing them to contract, and therefore are called *motor fibers*.
    (3) The posterior root contains bundles of nerve fibers (afferent fibers) that carry nerve impulses to the CNS. These fibers convey information about sensations of touch, pain, temperature, and vibration (sensory fibers).
    (4) Sensory and motor fibers of each spinal nerve supply and receive information from a specific body distribution (i.e., dermatome [see Appendix B]).
    (5) Nerve cell bodies within each fiber are situated within or near the spinal cord (ganglion). Axons extend from the cell body and connect to receptors at the level of the muscle and skin.
   c) The PNS consists of three functional divisions—sensory, motor, and autonomic.
    (1) The sensory nerves sense touch, pain, temperature, position, and vibration.
    (2) The motor nerves are responsible for voluntary movement, muscle tone, and coordination.
    (3) The autonomic nerves control intestinal mobility, blood pressure, and other involuntary muscles.
  2. Functional elements of peripheral nerve fibers
   a) Small fiber nerves (spinothalamic tract) are composed of microtubules, which act as the transport mechanism for proteins. They are unmyelinated and include nerves that sense pain and temperature.

b) Large fiber nerves (posterior column tract) are composed of neurofilaments, which serve as the framework of the axon. They are myelinated and include nerves that sense position and vibration along with motor control.

c) These small and large sensory fibers terminate at the level of the skin and muscle. The fiber then extends caudally to the dorsal root ganglion, where the cell body is located. It then connects either with the dorsal column (large fiber) or spinothalamic tract (small fiber) in the spinal cord. These tracts then act as a relay station to the sensory area of the brain.

B. Pathophysiology: Exact mechanism is unknown. Peripheral neuropathy is associated with numerous pathologic processes that can affect the nerve cells and nerve fibers. It may result from direct damage from neurotoxic drugs with mechanism varying within class of drugs. It is classically grouped into four categories of degeneration— Wallerian, axonal, neuronal, and segmental.

    1. Alterations in the cellular and molecular level

       a) Changes in sodium, potassium, and calcium ion channels

       b) Changes in neurotransmitters: Glutamate, norepinephrine, serotonin, cannabinoid, opioid, orexins

       c) Changes in the mitochondria and DNA

       d) Changes in intracellular signaling pathways: Mitogen-activated protein kinase, caspases

       e) Neuronal and glial changes: Innervation and astrocyte activation

       f) Increase of cytokines/chemokines: TNF, IL

    2. Different locations where immune cell responses can occur in CIPN

       a) Peripheral sensory axon and epidermis at terminal

       b) Dorsal root ganglion

       c) Spinal cord dorsal horn

    3. Indirect damage from compression or entrapment of a nerve associated with metastasis, herniated disc, fibroma, or compression fracture

III. Clinical features: Dysfunction occurs from inflammation, injury, or degeneration of the PNS. Direct damage to nerves and microvasculature results in varying levels of discomfort and pain. Neuropathic pain from painful neuropathies significantly affects QOL and should be routinely assessed. CIPN is a serious dose-limiting side effect and a major source of pain and debilitation (Chan et al., 2019; Doughty & Seyedsadjadi, 2018; Girach et al., 2019; Haryani et al., 2017; Staff et al., 2018; Stubblefield et al., 2009; Watson & Dyck, 2015).

A. Risk factors

    1. Age older than 55 years

    2. Concurrent use of neurotoxic drugs

    3. Chemotherapy agents and combinations: Platinum compounds, taxanes, vinca alkaloids, thalidomide, bortezomib, ixabepilone (list not all inclusive)

    4. Prior radiation

    5. Preexisting neuropathy or radiculopathy

    6. Malnutrition, vitamin deficiency (especially B_{12}), alcohol abuse, gastric surgery

B. Etiology

    1. Associated with numerous etiologies and can be classified according to anatomic involvement or distribution

       a) Single peripheral nerve

       b) Multiple peripheral nerves

       c) Symmetric or asymmetric

       d) Proximal or distal involvement

2. Infections/infectious processes: Syphilis, HIV, leprosy, diphtheria, Epstein-Barr virus, rabies, sarcoidosis, Lyme disease, HZV (postherpetic neuralgia)
3. Vascular compromise
4. Entrapment disease: Diabetes
5. Alcohol abuse
6. Vitamin deficiency
7. Toxic substances: Chemotherapy, immunotherapy
8. Metabolic disorders: Diabetes, hypothyroidism, acromegaly, uremia, liver disease
9. Neoplasms: Compression and infiltration by tumor, multiple myeloma, nonhereditary amyloidosis
10. Inflammatory/autoimmune: Acute idiopathic polyneuropathy (Guillain-Barré syndrome), chronic inflammatory demyelination polyneuropathy, multiple sclerosis, paraneoplastic neuropathy, Sjögren syndrome
11. Connective tissue processes/vasculitis: Polyarteritis nodosa, RA, SLE, scleroderma, ischemic neuropathies, critical care polyneuropathy, systemic necrotizing vasculitis, giant cell arteritis, Wegener granulomatosis
12. Industrial/environmental toxin exposure: Organic and industrial compounds, heavy metals
13. Trauma/injury: Compression, severance, contusion, stretching, crushing, ischemia, electrical, thermal, radiation (breast, brachial plexus, and spinal/cranial fields), drug injections, compression from prolonged pressure, herniated discs, osteophytes, fracture
14. Hereditary disorders: Motor and sensory neuropathies, autonomic types (I–IV), Friedreich ataxia, porphyria, amyloidosis, Charcot-Marie-Tooth disease
15. Occupation/hobbies/behaviors: Repetitive motion leading to compression or nerve entrapment

C. History
  1. History of cancer and cancer treatment
  2. Current medications: Prescribed, over the counter
  3. History of presenting symptoms: Precipitating factors, location, onset (acute or chronic), duration
  4. Changes in ADLs: Difficulty handling keys, tying shoes, or buttoning shirt; tripping and falling
  5. Past medical history: Diabetes, neurofibromatosis, HZV, significant weight loss
  6. Family history: Inherited peripheral neuropathy (e.g., Charcot-Marie-Tooth disease), diabetes
  7. Past surgical history: Gastric surgery (e.g., Whipple, bypass) leading to vitamin B_{12} deficiency
  8. Social history: Repetitive activities (e.g., prolonged keyboard use), alcohol use

D. Signs and symptoms: Subacute, acute, chronic, or progressive
  1. Motor
    a) Muscles of the feet and legs are affected earlier and more severely than that of the hands and forearms.
    b) Truncal and cranial muscles can be affected in more severe cases.
    c) Tremor, fasciculations, cramps, spasms, weakness, and paralysis can occur.
    d) Difficulties with fine motor activities are common.
    e) Gait disturbances due to pain, decreased sensation, and muscle fatigue can occur.
  2. Sensory
    a) Symptoms most often are felt in hands and feet (i.e., glove-and-stocking distribution).

    b) Symptoms are described as numbness and tingling (i.e., pins-and-needles sensation).

    c) Small fiber neuropathy is often more painful, is less responsive to treatment, and may not be detected on testing (i.e., electromyography).

    d) Large fiber neuropathy may cause electric shock–like sensations (i.e., Lhermitte syndrome).

    e) Pain can be sequential in nature (i.e., myalgia precedes painful sensation).

    f) Common clinical features of CIPN

        (1) CIPN is predominantly sensory, although certain agents cause motor and autonomic dysfunction.

        (2) Symptoms are temporally related to chemotherapy and may occur at any time during the course, even after discontinuation (known as "coasting").

        (3) Symptoms are usually symmetric but may be worse on one side.

        (4) Distal extremities are affected in a glove-and-stocking distribution.

    g) Terms and definitions that describe sensory loss or pain sensation

        (1) Analgesia: Complete insensitivity to painful stimuli

        (2) Hyperalgesia: Increased pain sensation

        (3) Hypoalgesia: Decreased sensitivity to painful stimuli

        (4) Allodynia: Pain resulting from a stimulus that normally does not provoke pain (e.g., contact with bed linens)

        (5) Dysesthesias: Hypersensitivity

    h) Terms and definitions that describe touch sensation

        (1) Anesthesia: Complete inability to perceive pain, temperature, touch, or vibration

        (2) Hyperesthesia: Increased touch sensation

        (3) Hypoesthesia: Decreased touch sensation

        (4) Hypesthesia: Diminished ability to perceive pain, temperature, touch, or vibration; a variant of hypoesthesia

        (5) Paresthesia: Abnormal touch sensation, such as burning, prickling, or formication (a sensation as if small insects were crawling on the body), often in the absence of an external stimulus

3. Autonomic

    a) Light-headedness when standing

    b) Acute abdominal distress: Could represent an ileus

    c) Constipation

    d) Overflow incontinence

    e) Urinary retention

    f) Obstipation: Severe constipation caused by intestinal obstruction (e.g., vincristine-induced ileus)

    g) Sexual impotence

    h) Anhidrosis: Lack of sweat, tears, and saliva

4. Cranial nerves (see Appendix A)

    a) Blurred vision (II)

    b) Hearing loss (VIII)

    c) Tinnitus (VIII)

    d) Facial pain (V)

    e) Facial palsy (VII)

    f) Changes in taste sensation (IX)

    g) Hoarseness/dysphagia (IX, X)

    h) Dizziness (VIII)

    i) Altered eye movements (III, IV, VI)

5. Deformities of distal extremities and/or skin changes seen in chronic polyneuropathies
   a) The feet and hands can become deformed. This is more commonly seen when disease begins in childhood.
   b) Feet are pulled into a position of talipes equinus (plantar deviation).
   c) Intrinsic muscles of the hands or feet may be weak.
E. Physical examination
  1. Vital signs
    a) Variability of heart rate can be lost.
    b) Orthostatic hypotension can occur without compensatory rise in heart rate.
    c) Hemodynamics: Check lying, sitting, and standing heart rate and blood pressure.
  2. Neurologic
    a) Motor function: Check voluntary movement of each extremity.
     (1) Check strength of extremities (e.g., hand grasps, plantar flexion and dorsiflexion of feet).
     (2) Compare distal versus proximal strength in extremities.
     (3) Loss with peripheral nerve injury usually is bilateral, and weakness is detected distally in feet (i.e., weakness of dorsiflexion) prior to upper extremity weakness.
     (4) Fine motor skills will be uncoordinated or unable to be performed. Evaluation cannot be performed in the presence of weakness (see Appendix D).
      (a) Rapid alternating movements
      (b) Finger-to-nose test
      (c) Heel-to-shin test
     (5) Gait
      (a) Inability to perform heel-toe walking with broad base stance indicates sensory ataxia with profound neuropathy.
      (b) Steppage gait is common and can occur with foot drop. It occurs when the hip and knee are elevated excessively high to lift the foot; the foot is brought down to the floor with a slap.
     (6) Check for entrapment syndromes (e.g., carpal tunnel syndrome, median nerve and ulnar nerve entrapment).
      (a) Muscle weakness of fingers and/or hands: Weak handgrip, difficulty in touching opposing thumb to each finger
      (b) Wasting of the thenar and/or intrinsic hand muscles
    b) Deep tendon reflexes: Diminution or loss is an invariable sign of peripheral nerve disease.
     (1) Assess for diminished or loss of tendon reflexes.
     (2) Absence indicates neuropathy of the lower motor neuron or profound sensory loss.
     (3) Loss usually occurs distally first.
    c) Sensory: Screening includes assessment of the spinothalamic tract (small fibers) and posterior column tracts (large fibers).
     (1) Compare sensations on symmetric parts of the body. If an area of decrease exists, map the exact borders (mapping dermatome—see Appendix B).
     (2) Compare distal to proximal sensation in extremities.
      (a) Spinothalamic tract: Pain, temperature, and light touch
       i. Pain: Evaluate whether patient perceives sharp stimulus. Use a broken cotton tip applicator or sterile safety pin.

        ii. Temperature: Test only if pain sensation is abnormal (fiber tracts are much the same). Ask patient to detect hot/cold temperature using two test tubes filled with hot and cold water or use a tuning fork for cold stimulus.

        iii. Light touch: Use a wisp of cotton to test superficial touch. The use of a 10 g monofilament test is useful in diabetic foot neuropathy testing.

   (b) Posterior column tract: Vibration, position, and tactile discrimination

        i. Vibration: Assess the patient's ability to feel vibration of a tuning fork (128 hertz) placed over a distal interphalangeal joint of the finger, then great toe; the time in which it is felt should be similar to that of the examiner.

        ii. Move distally to proximally. Compare right and left.

   (c) Joint position sense: Proprioception

        i. The ability to perceive joint motion and acceleration (movement of finger or big toe)

        ii. Abnormalities: Loss of position sense/proprioception (the brain cannot feel what the digit/finger is doing)

   (d) Ask the patient to discriminate between sharp and dull stimuli to assess superficial pain.

d) Autonomic

   (1) Pupils: Pupillary size may be affected (i.e., small- or medium-sized and unreactive pupils).

   (2) Cardiac

     (a) Variability of heart rate is lost.

     (b) Orthostatic hypotension is present without compensatory rise in heart rate.

   (3) Abdomen: Bowel sounds may be hypoactive and abdomen distended indicating an ileus.

e) Cranial nerves: Most neuropathies are bilateral (see Appendix A).

   (1) Optic nerve: Check visual acuity using the Snellen chart for decrease in vision.

   (2) Optic fundi: Assess ophthalmoscopically to rule out papilledema or optic neuritis.

   (3) Cranial nerves III, IV, and VI: Assess together by evaluating pupillary reactions, EOMs, and ptosis.

     (a) Oculomotor (III): Shows ptosis, dilated pupil. Note size, shape, and symmetry of pupillary response.

     (b) Trochlear (IV): Head often tilts slightly to the side opposite the eye with diplopia.

     (c) Trigeminal (V): Involvement is evident when patient complains of acute jaw pain.

   (4) Facial (VII): Assess for facial weakness, fasciculation, facial asymmetry, and peripheral facial palsy. Ask patient to lift eyebrows, frown, and bare teeth. Assess bilateral nasolabial folds for flattening.

   (5) Acoustic (VIII): Assess for decreased hearing acuity.

   (6) Glossopharyngeal (IX) and vagus (X)

     (a) Nerves may be affected when hoarseness is present because of vocal cord paralysis (dysphagia).

     (b) Asymmetry of the palate and pharynx may occur.

        (c) Patients will be unable to enunciate a difficult phrase that requires precise articulation (i.e., "The rain in Spain stays mainly in the plain").
3. Extremities
    a) Check for deformities of the hands and feet (e.g., shortened foot, heightened arches, flexed distal phalanges).
    b) Observe the intrinsic muscles of the hands and feet for wasting.
    c) If autonomic fibers are interrupted, the limbs are warm and pink.
4. Integument: Check for skin and nail changes.
    a) Skin may be light and shiny or have thickened subcutaneous tissue.
    b) Nails may be curved and rigid.
    c) Hair growth is diminished in denervated areas.
5. CIPN rating scales: Several scales are available for neuropathy, which allow for subjective rating by patients and objective rating by clinicians. The Total Neuropathy Score and the Functional Assessment of Cancer Therapy/Gynecologic Oncology Group–Neurotoxicity have been shown to have high interrater reliability.

IV. Diagnostic tests (Doughty & Seyedsadjadi, 2018; Watson & Dyck, 2015)
  A. Laboratory
    1. Vitamin B_{12} to evaluate for deficiency
    2. Homocysteine and/or MMA levels: Confirms deficiency in asymptomatic high-risk patients with low normal levels of vitamin B_{12}
    3. TSH to evaluate for hypothyroidism
    4. Electrolytes to evaluate for imbalance
    5. Renal and liver function studies to evaluate for renal and liver insufficiency
    6. CBC to evaluate for anemia
    7. SPEP to evaluate for myeloma or gammopathies
    8. Antibody profile (HIV), as indicated
    9. Hgb A1c, if diabetic
    10. ESR to evaluate for inflammation
    11. Rapid plasma test: A screening blood test for syphilis
    12. Consideration of antinuclear antibodies and rheumatoid factor to evaluate for autoimmune disease
  B. Radiology
    1. Not indicated, except to evaluate for CNS lesion
    2. MRI of the spine to evaluate lesions resulting from cord edema from radiation necrosis, scarring, or tumor
  C. Other: Based on discretion of clinician
    1. Baseline audiometric testing is required for patients receiving high-dose ototoxic drugs (e.g., cisplatin), especially those with preexisting hearing loss; pure-tone hearing and high- and low-frequency hearing should be evaluated.
    2. Electromyography is used to detect axonal neuropathy after four to six weeks (denervation changes) and muscle atrophy.
    3. Neurophysiology to identify location, severity, and type of the neuropathy (i.e., nerve conduction studies and quantitative sensory testing) provides an objective measurement and is used serially.

V. Differential diagnosis (Doughty & Seyedsadjadi, 2018; Watson & Dyck, 2015)
  A. Diabetes mellitus (see Chapter 151)
  B. Alcoholism/malnutrition
  C. Malignancy

1. Primary brain cancer
2. Spinal cord tumor
3. Neoplastic meningitis (see Chapter 141)
4. Paraneoplastic syndrome (see Appendix M)
5. SCC (see Chapter 145)

D. Vitamin deficiency (see Chapters 115 and 116)
E. Idiopathic
F. Guillain-Barré syndrome
G. Amyloidosis
H. Medication-induced damage: Nonchemotherapy drugs or chemotherapy drugs (see Table 143-1)
I. Radiation therapy: Spinal myelopathy
J. Nerve entrapment: Carpal tunnel syndrome, neurofibromas
K. Uremia

VI. Treatment: Dependent on the etiology of the peripheral neuropathy (Albers et al., 2014; Fallon et al., 2018; Gewandter et al., 2019; Hanai et al., 2017; Kleckner et al., 2019; Kneis et al., 2019; Li et al., 2019; Marineo, 2019; Matsuoka et al., 2019; McCrary et al., 2019; Sommer & Cruccu, 2017; Stone & Deangelis, 2016; Stubblefield et al., 2009; Trouvin & Perrot, 2019)

A. Treatment of CIPN includes dose reduction or drug discontinuation if the cause is medication related and the neuropathy is significant. The timing of symptom resolution is variable, and the neuropathy may be irreversible.

B. Nonpharmacologic treatment

1. Hearing loss: Patient may require hearing aid. Speak to the patient in an environment that minimizes extraneous noise and look directly at the patient when speaking.
2. Vision impairment: Do not use color description in patient education (i.e., identifying pills by color). Discourage abrupt head movements (e.g., quick turning).
3. Bowel management: Prophylactic bowel program is indicated at the initiation of chemotherapy with vinca alkaloids to prevent constipation (see Chapter 55).
4. Incontinence: Encourage regularly scheduled fluid intake and bladder evacuation; discourage delaying of urination (see Chapter 84).
5. Tactile changes
   a) Avoid extreme temperatures.
   b) Protect hands and feet in cold weather.
   c) Wear gloves when washing dishes and gardening.
   d) Use potholders when cooking.
   e) Use a night-light and remove throw rugs.
   f) Examine extremities for injury or pressure sores.
   g) Use shower chair, shower wand, and liquid soap.
   h) Cryotherapy may be beneficial; however, it is contraindicated with oxaliplatin administration, patients with cold agglutinin disease, cryoglobulinemia or those with extreme sensitivity to cold.
6. Acupuncture may be a safe adjunct for treatment of CIPN.
7. Wireless transcutaneous electrical nerve stimulation unit has been shown to improve symptoms of pain and cramping.
8. Scrambler therapy is a mode of electroanalgesia that stimulates C fibers and has been found to be helpful in chronic cancer-related pain states.
9. Gait changes
   a) Safety precautions should be evaluated for each patient. It may require use of cane or other assistive devices.

TABLE 143-1 Chemotherapy Agents Associated With Peripheral Neuropathy

Antineoplastic Agent	Associated Neuropathy										
	AIDP/CIDP	Autonomic	Cranial	Focal Noninflammatory Neck Myopathy	Median Nerve, CTS	Motor	Myalgias	Myopathy	Neuromuscular Junction	Plexopathy	Sensory
Bortezomib											X
Brentuximab						X					X
Carboplatin		X	Rare								X
Carfilzomib											X
Carmustine (BCNU)		X	X								
Cisplatin			X			X			X		X
Cytarabine (Ara-C)			X			X				X	X
Docetaxel		Mild				X					X
Doxifluridine (5-dFUrd)						X					X
Eribulin						X					X
Etoposide (VP-16)						X					X
5-Fluorouracil						Rare					
Gemcitabine								X			
Hexamethylmelamine						X					X
Interleukin-2					X						
Ipilimumab	X	X							X		
Methotrexate			X			X					X

(Continued on next page)

TABLE 143-1 Chemotherapy Agents Associated With Peripheral Neuropathy *(Continued)*

Antineoplastic Agent	Associated Neuropathy										
	AIDP/CIDP	Autonomic	Cranial	Focal Noninflammatory Neck Myopathy	Median Nerve, CTS	Motor	Myalgias	Myopathy	Neuromuscular Junction	Plexopathy	Sensory
Paclitaxel	Mild					X					X
Procarbazine						X					X
Rituximab							X				X
Selumetinib				X							
Teniposide (VM-26)						X					X
Thalidomide, lenalidomide, pomalidomide		X									X
Vinblastine		X	X			X					X
Vincristine		X	X			X					X
Vindesine		X	X			X					X
Vinorelbine	Mild		X			X					X

AIDP—acute inflammatory demyelinating polyradiculoneuropathy; CIDP—chronic inflammatory demyelinating polyradiculoneuropathy; CTS—carpal tunnel syndrome

Note. Based on information from Staff et al., 2017; Stone & DeAngelis, 2016.

   b) Exercise-based rehabilitation has been shown to be beneficial for CIPN with noted improvement in proprioception, balance, and mobility.

C. Pharmacologic treatment
   1. CIPN neuroprotective agents: No established agent exists that can be recommended for the prevention of CIPN. Several agents have been used with varying results (e.g., vitamin E, IV calcium and magnesium, glutamine, glutathione, N-acetylcysteine, oxcarbazepine, xaliproden).
   2. CIPN treatment (see Appendix Q)
      a) Antiepileptic drugs: Gabapentin, pregabalin
      b) Local anesthetic: 5% lidocaine patch, high-concentration transdermal 8% capsaicin, neuropathy compound cream (e.g., ketamine, amitriptyline, lidocaine)
      c) Antidepressants: Tricyclic antidepressants (e.g., amitriptyline, nortriptyline), serotonin nonrepinephrine reuptake inhibitors (e.g., duloxetine, venlafaxine) (see Appendix L)
      d) Opioids generally used in combination with other agents for neuropathic pain (see Appendix F): Tramadol, morphine, oxycodone
      e) Cannabis may have a role in cancer supportive care; mechanism of effect is not clearly understood and has not been sufficiently studied in CIPN.

VII. Follow-up
   A. Short term
      1. Baseline neurologic testing should be performed prior to starting neurotoxic agent and every three to six months.
      2. An ongoing neurologic examination while receiving active treatment is recommended.
   B. Long term
      1. Neurotoxic potential of chemotherapy should be considered with monitoring for ongoing sensory, motor, cranial, and autonomic changes during and after completion of cancer therapy.
      2. Toxic synergy between neurotoxic agents and hereditary or metabolic causes require ongoing monitoring.

VIII. Referrals
   A. Physical medicine and rehabilitation: To assist with ADLs and assistive devices
   B. Physical, occupational, and aquatic therapy: For muscle strengthening, range of motion skills, and provision of assistive devices
   C. Neurologist: For neurologic evaluation or refractory CIPN PRN
   D. Pain specialist: For management of refractory pain
   E. Social services and psychiatry: For counseling regarding loss of function or disability
   F. Homecare specialist: For home safety evaluation

The author would like to acknowledge Kathleen A. Grisdale, RN, MSN, APRN, BC, FNP, and Terri S. Armstrong, PhD, ANP-BC, FAANP, FAAN, for their contribution to this chapter that remains unchanged from the previous edition of this book.

References

Albers, J.W., Chaudhry, V., Cavaletti, G., & Donehower, R.C. (2014). Interventions for preventing neuropathy caused by cisplatin and related compounds. *Cochrane Database of Systematic Reviews, 2014*(3). https://doi.org/10.1002/14651858 .cd005228.pub4

Boyette-Davis, J.A., Hou, S., Abdi, S., & Dougherty, P.M. (2018). An updated understanding of the mechanisms involved in chemotherapy-induced neuropathy. *Pain Management, 8*(5), 363–375. https://doi.org/10.2217/pmt-2018-0020

Chan, A., Hertz, D.L., Morales, M., Adams, E.J., Gordon, S., Tan, C.J., ... Lustberg, M.B. (2019). Biological predictors of chemotherapy-induced peripheral neuropathy (CIPN): MASCC neurological complications working group overview. *Supportive Care in Cancer, 27*(10), 3729–3737. https://doi.org/10.1007/s00520-019-04987-8

Doughty, C.T., & Seyedsadjadi, R. (2018). Approach to peripheral neuropathy for the primary care clinician. *American Journal of Medicine, 131*(9), 1010–1016. https://doi.org/10.1016/j.amjmed.2017.12.042

Fallon, M., Giusti, R., Aielli, F., Hoskin, P., Rolke, R., Sharma, M., & Ripamonti, C.I. (2018). Management of cancer pain in adult patients: ESMO clinical practice guidelines. *Annals of Oncology, 29*(Suppl. 4), iv166–iv191. https://doi.org/10.1093/annonc/mdy152

Gewandter, J.S., Chaudari, J., Ibegbu, C., Kitt, R., Serventi, J., Burke, J., ... Mohile, N.A. (2019). Wireless transcutaneous electrical nerve stimulation device for chemotherapy-induced peripheral neuropathy: An open-label feasibility study. *Supportive Care in Cancer, 27*(5), 1765–1774. https://doi.org/10.1007/s00520-018-4424-6

Girach, A., Julian, T.H., Varrassi, G., Paladini, A., Vadalouka, A., & Zis, P. (2019). Quality of life in painful peripheral neuropathies: A systematic review. *Pain Research and Management, 2019,* 2091960. https://doi.org/10.1155/2019/2091960

Hanai, A., Ishiguro, H., Sozu, T., Tsuda, M., Yano, I., Nakagawa, T., ... Tsuboyama, T. (2017). Effects of cryotherapy on objective and subjective symptoms of paclitaxel-induced neuropathy: Prospective self-controlled trial. *Journal of the National Cancer Institute, 110*(2), 141–148. https://doi.org/10.1093/jnci/djx178

Haryani, H., Fetzer, S., Wu, C.-L., & Hsu, Y.-Y. (2017). Chemotherapy-induced peripheral neuropathy assessment tools: A systematic review. *Oncology Nursing Forum, 44*(3), E111–E123. https://doi.org/10.1188/17.ONF.E111-E123

Kleckner, A.S., Kleckner, I.R., Kamen, C.S., Tejani, M.A., Janelsins, M.C., Morrow, G.R., & Peppone, L.J. (2019). Opportunities for cannabis in supportive care in cancer. *Therapeutic Advances in Medical Oncology, 11.* https://doi.org/10.1177/1758835919866362

Kneis, S., Wehrle, A., Müller, J., Maurer, C., Ihorst, G., Gollhofer, A., & Bertz, H. (2019). It's never too late—Balance and endurance training improves functional performance, quality of life, and alleviates neuropathic symptoms in cancer survivors suffering from chemotherapy-induced peripheral neuropathy: Results of a randomized controlled trial. *BMC Cancer, 19*(1), 414. https://doi.org/10.1186/s12885-019-5522-7

Lees, J.G., Makker, P.G.S., Tonkin, R.S., Abdulla, M., Park, S.B., Goldstein, D., & Moalem-Taylor, G. (2017). Immune-mediated processes implicated in chemotherapy-induced peripheral neuropathy. *European Journal of Cancer, 73,* 22–29. https://doi.org/10.1016/j.ejca.2016.12.006

Li, K., Giustini, D., & Seely, D. (2019). A systematic review of acupuncture for chemotherapy-induced peripheral neuropathy. *Current Oncology, 26*(2), e147–e155. https://doi.org/10.3747/co.26.4261

Marineo, G. (2019). Inside the scrambler therapy, a noninvasive treatment of chronic neuropathic and cancer pain: From the gate control theory to the active principle of information. *Integrative Cancer Therapies, 18.* https://doi.org/10.1177/1534735419845143

Matsuoka, H., Iwase, S., Miyaji, T., Kawaguchi, T., Ariyoshi, K., Oyamada, S., ... Yamaguchi, T. (2019). Additive duloxetine for cancer-related neuropathic pain nonresponsive or intolerant to opioid-pregabalin therapy: A randomized controlled trial (JORTC-PAL08). *Journal of Pain and Symptom Management, 58*(4), 645–653. https://doi.org/10.1016/j.jpainsymman.2019.06.020

McCrary, J.M., Goldstein, D., Sandler, C.X., Barry, B.K., Marthick, M., Timmins, H.C., ... Park, S.B. (2019). Exercise-based rehabilitation for cancer survivors with chemotherapy-induced peripheral neuropathy. *Supportive Care in Cancer, 27*(10), 3849–3857. https://doi.org/10.1007/s00520-019-04680-w

Pop-Busui, R., Boulton, A.J.M., Feldman, E.L., Bril, V., Freeman, R., Malik, R.A., ... Ziegler, D. (2017). Diabetic neuropathy: A position statement by the American Diabetes Association. *Diabetes Care, 40*(1), 136–154. https://doi.org/10.2337/dc16-2042

Sommer, C., & Cruccu, G. (2017). Topical treatment of peripheral neuropathic pain: Applying the evidence. *Journal of Pain and Symptom Management, 53*(3), 614–629. https://doi.org/10.1016/j.jpainsymman.2016.09.015

Staff, N.P., Grisold, A., Grisold, W., & Windebank, A.J. (2017). Chemotherapy-induced peripheral neuropathy: A current review. *Annals of Neurology, 81*(6), 772–781. https://doi.org/10.1002/ana.24951

Stone, J.B., & Deangelis, L.M. (2016). Cancer-treatment-induced neurotoxicity—Focus on newer treatments. *Nature Reviews Clinical Oncology, 13*(2), 92–105. https://doi.org/10.1038/nrclinonc.2015.152

Stubblefield, M.D., Burstein, H.J., Burton, A.W., Custodio, C.M., Deng, G.E., Ho, M., ... Von Roenn, J.H. (2009). NCCN task force report: management of neuropathy in cancer. *Journal of the National Comprehensive Cancer Network, 7*(Suppl. 5), S1–S26. https://doi.org/10.6004/jnccn.2009.0078

Trouvin, A.-P., & Perrot, S. (2019). Functional and histological improvements of small nerve neuropathy after high-concentration capsaicin patch application. *PAIN Reports, 4*(4), e761. https://doi.org/10.1097/pr9.0000000000000761

Valentine, W.M. (2020). Toxic peripheral neuropathies: Agents and mechanisms. *Toxicologic Pathology, 48*(1), 152–173. https://doi.org/10.1177/0192623319854326

Watson, J.C., & Dyck, P.J.B. (2015). Peripheral neuropathy: A practical approach to diagnosis and symptom management. *Mayo Clinic Proceedings, 90*(7), 940–951. https://doi.org/10.1016/j.mayocp.2015.05.004

CHAPTER 144

Seizures

Julie G. Walker, PhD, APRN, FNP-C

I. Definition: A seizure is "a paroxysmal alteration of neurologic function caused by the excessive, hypersynchronous discharge of neurons in the brain" (Stafstrom & Carmant, 2015, p. 1). Chronic seizures without an apparent transient cause, such as fever or hypoxia, fall into the category of epilepsy (Stafstrom & Carmant, 2015).
   A. Focal: Originate in networks limited to one cerebral hemisphere
   B. Generalized: Rapidly engage networking distributed across both hemispheres

II. Physiology/Pathophysiology (Stafstrom & Carmant, 2015)
   A. Normal
      1. The right and left cerebral hemispheres are connected by a thick band of nerve fibers, the corpus callosum. Each hemisphere is divided into the frontal, temporal, parietal, and occipital lobes and the limbic system (see Table 144-1).
      2. A neuron is a nerve cell in the brain that has specialized projections called *dendrites* and *axons*. An electrochemical process allows neurons to communicate with each other. *Synapse* is the area where a signal passes from the neuron to another cell.

TABLE 144-1   **Anatomy and Physiology of the Brain[a]**

Anatomy	Functions
Frontal lobe	Contains motor cortex associated with voluntary skeletal movement and speech Emotions, affect, memory, and self-awareness location
Limbic system	Mediates certain patterns of behavior that determine survival (mating, fear, affection) Memory function, particularly short term, dependent on the limbic system Includes the olfactory pathway
Occipital lobe	Contains the vision center Allows for vision interpretation
Parietal lobe	Processes sensory data (tactile, visual, olfactory, auditory sensations) discrimination
Temporal lobe	Perceives and interprets sounds and determines source Integrates taste, smell, balance, behavior, emotion, and personality Location of memory retrieval

[a]Although the functional areas of the brain are still held to be generally true, advances in brain mapping and neurologic testing during awake craniotomies are finding the brain to be much more plastic than previously believed.

Note. Based on information from Duffau, 2018.

3. Neurotransmitters, such as gamma-aminobutyric acid, acetylcholine, serotonin, glutamate, and catecholamines, assist in the transmission of signals across the synapse.

4. Normally, a balance exists between excitatory and inhibitory functions of the brain related to homeostasis of genetic characteristics, signaling of neuronal structures, presence and function of neurotransmitters, electrolytes, membrane lipid peroxidation, and antioxidants.

B. Pathophysiology: A seizure occurs when there is a sustained repetitive depolarization of abnormally hyperactive and hypersensitive neurons.

    1. It may result from genetic changes affecting neuronal connectivity and ionic channel function or from disruptions in the structural integrity of the brain due to injury, disease (e.g., malignancy, stroke), or to treatments such as radiation or intrathecal therapy.

    2. It is now recognized that seizures are not only related to local pathology within the brain but are a result of pathology within networks arising from the neocortical, thalamocortical, limbic, and brain stem structures.

III. Clinical features: In adults, various comorbidities are associated with seizures and epilepsy. Signs and symptoms of seizures are diverse and may involve motor, sensory, cognitive, or autonomic events (Allone et al., 2017; Fisher et al., 2017; Gómez-Porro et al., 2018; Klugah-Brown et al., 2019; Lin & Avila, 2017; Nitta et al., 2019; Nowacki & Jirsch, 2017; Stafstrom & Carmant, 2015; Stephani et al., 2019; Thompson et al., 2020).

A. Classification: International League Against Epilepsy released an updated classification system for seizures in 2017, accounting for variations in onset (focal or generalized), difficulty in describing level of consciousness by patients and witnesses, difficult terminology, and seizure types excluded in the 1981 classification system.

    1. Focal onset

        a) Aware/impaired awareness

        b) Motor onset

            (1) Automatisms

            (2) Atonic

            (3) Clonic

            (4) Epileptic spasms

            (5) Hyperkinetic

            (6) Myoclonic

            (7) Tonic

        c) Nonmotor onset

            (1) Autonomic

            (2) Behavior arrest

            (3) Cognitive

            (4) Emotional

            (5) Sensory

        d) Focal to bilateral tonic–clonic

    2. Generalized onset

        a) Motor

            (1) Tonic–clonic

            (2) Clonic

            (3) Tonic

            (4) Myoclonic

            (5) Myoclonic–tonic–clonic

            (6) Myoclonic–atonic

            (7) Epileptic spasms

3. Unknown onset
  a) Motor
    (1) Tonic–clonic
    (2) Epileptic spasms
  b) Nonmotor: Behavior arrest
4. Unclassified

B. Etiology
  1. Primary and metastatic brain tumors
  2. Treatment complications
  3. Metabolic derangements related to cancer
  4. Paraneoplastic limbic encephalitis
  5. Meningoencephalitis

C. History: Source for history may be the patient or an individual who witnessed the event.
  1. History of cancer and cancer treatment
  2. Current medications: Prescribed, over the counter
  3. History of presenting symptoms: Precipitating factors, onset, duration, associated symptoms (e.g., postictal)
  4. Changes in ADLs
  5. Past medical history: Recent illness, history of seizures, undiagnosed seizures such as "blacking out" or "lost time," urinary incontinence, tongue biting, head trauma or other neurologic injury, psychiatric illness, depression, obesity
  6. Social history: Alcohol use, illicit drug use
  7. Family history: Seizures

D. Signs and symptoms: Signs and symptoms are dependent on the area of the cortex involved. Witnesses and healthcare providers need to document the following information.
  1. Preceding symptoms: An *aura* is a subjective phenomenon, such as visual, olfactory, or gustatory perceptions; alterations in skin sensation; or feelings of anxiety or fear, déjà vu, or nausea.
  2. Onset: Focal, generalized, motor, nonmotor, unknown
  3. Timing of episode: Nocturnal or early morning
  4. Duration of episode
  5. Impaired awareness or confusion
  6. Type of motor movement, if applicable: Frequent types of muscular involvement, including clonic, tonic, tonic–clonic, or myoclonic
  7. Sensory symptoms, if applicable: A perceptual experience not caused by an external stimulus
  8. Autonomic symptoms: Sensations associated with the involvement of the autonomic nervous system, including cardiovascular, respiratory, GI, vasomotor, or thermoregulatory functions
  9. Other symptoms: Eye or head movements, aphasia, urinary incontinence, tongue biting, other injury
  10. Post-seizure episode (postictal phenomena) is the recovery period and presents with transient deficits that may resolve within minutes to several hours.
    a) Symptoms include slurred speech, disorientation, altered responsiveness, loss of consciousness, fatigue, headache, and muscle soreness.
    b) Todd paralysis can occur, which is characterized as arm or leg weakness or paralysis, aphasia, visual changes, or cortical blindness.
  11. Pattern of seizure episodes should be ascertained, including frequency and presentation (stereotypical or variable).

E. Physical examination: Findings are dependent on the type of seizure and area of the cortex involved.

    1. Vital signs: Blood pressure, pulse, and respirations to assess hemodynamic and respiratory stability and to determine need for supportive measures

    2. Neurologic: After seizure, to determine baseline dysfunction and to differentiate between transient postictal changes, new deficits, or worsening residual deficits

        a) Mental status

            (1) Level of consciousness and alertness, general behavior, mood, ability to follow simple and complex commands

            (2) Language fluency, evidence of paraphasic errors, evidence of expressive or receptive aphasia, difficulty with naming, spelling, or repetition

            (3) Orientation to person, place, and time

            (4) Memory of recent and remote events

            (5) Ability to process new information

        b) Cranial nerve: Assess for transient, new, or exacerbated cranial nerve deficits (see Appendix A).

        c) Motor: Assess for muscle weakness, paralysis, or spasticity, which may be transient or permanent. Deficits may be seen with intracranial pathology involving the motor cortex in the frontal lobe.

        d) Reflex: Assess for hyperreflexia in the affected extremities and extensor plantar response. A Babinski reflex may be appreciated in postictal period and with upper motor neuron intracranial pathology.

        e) Sensory: Assess for deficits to light and sharp touch, temperature, vibration, position sense of fingers and toes, graphesthesia, stereognosis, extinction to double simultaneous stimuli, and evidence of positive Romberg. Deficits may be seen with intracranial pathology involving the sensory cortex in the parietal lobe or from neuropathy.

        f) Coordination: Assess for change in posture, gait, or coordination of movements such as finger-nose-finger, heel-to-shin, and rapid alternating movements. Deficits may be seen with intracranial pathology involving the sensory cortex in the parietal lobe, motor cortex in the frontal lobe, or from neuropathy.

    3. Integument: Needle track marks from possible substance abuse and for lacerations, bruises, or skeletal trauma, which may occur during a generalized seizure

    4. Oral: Trauma to lips, tongue, or buccal mucosa, which may occur during a generalized seizure

IV. Diagnostic tests (Nowacki & Jirsch, 2017; Stafstrom & Carmant, 2015)

    A. Laboratory

        1. Chemical profile to assess for metabolic imbalances: Diabetes and thyroid abnormalities, inflammatory disorders (e.g., infections), obesity

        2. Pregnancy test for women of childbearing age: Necessary before beginning anticonvulsants, as there are potentially harmful effects to the fetus

        3. Drug screen: Use of or withdrawal from substances (e.g., cocaine, crack cocaine, heroin) that can cause seizure activity

        4. Drug level of current anticonvulsant medication in patients with previous seizure history

        5. CBC to evaluate for thrombocytopenia, which could cause intracerebral hemorrhage

        6. Blood alcohol level: Excess level resulting in seizures

    B. Radiology: Brain CT to evaluate for a source of seizure activity (e.g., malignancy, head trauma); should be obtained in patients with no history or changes in seizure character

C. Other
    1. Electroencephalogram: Most helpful when obtained within 24 hours of the event
        a) Should be obtained urgently if patient has persistent alterations in mental status
        b) Helps to definitively differentiate seizure activity from psychogenic symptoms or motor activity due to neuromuscular conditions
        c) Helpful in predicting risk of seizure recurrence
    2. Lumbar puncture: If patient is febrile, has existing malignancy or unresolved postictal state, or is immunocompromised
        a) Values can reveal CNS metastasis or CNS infections.
        b) If increased ICP is suspected, CT scan must be reviewed prior to lumbar puncture to evaluate for mass or lesion, which may cause brain herniation during or after lumbar puncture.

V. Differential diagnosis (Berntsson et al., 2018; Magge & DeAngelis, 2015; Nowacki & Jirsch, 2017)
  A. Cerebrovascular event: Aneurysm, arteriovenous malformation
  B. Tumor
  C. Trauma
  D. Infection: Meningitis (see Chapter 141), abscess
  E. Migraine headache (see Chapter 137)
  F. Alcohol withdrawal
  G. Drug toxicity
  H. Eclampsia
  I. Chemotherapy side effects
    1. Immunotherapies: Blinatumomab, CAR T cells
    2. Vinca alkaloids: Vincristine, vinblastine, vindesine, vinorelbine
    3. HSCT: May be related to the cryopreservative dimethyl sulfoxide
    4. Platinum compounds: Cisplatin
    5. Antimetabolites: Fludarabine, nelarabine
    6. Intrathecal administration of any agent
  J. Brain metastasis
  K. Primary brain tumor
    1. Low-grade gliomas have the highest incidence of seizure, though all primary brain tumor patients are at risk.
    2. Seizure may be presenting symptom or herald a recurrent tumor.
  L. Psychiatric disorders (e.g., pseudoseizures): History may include frequent episodes despite antiepileptic drug therapy, high frequency, unusual triggers, extensive list of symptoms, previous psychiatric diagnosis, and detailed memory of events.
  M. Metabolic imbalance (see Chapters 152–156)
  N. Syncope (see Chapter 139)

VI. Treatment: Goals of treatment are to identify reversible etiologies of seizures and prevent further seizures. A growing body of evidence exists that genetic factors influence the response to antiepileptic agents and risk of adverse effects. For example, variations in the *CYP2C9* and *CYP2C19* genes affect phenytoin metabolism, increasing the risk of neurologic and cutaneous toxicities; however, current practice remains to monitor for signs of antiepileptic toxicities and obtain serum concentrations of drug as required (Abou-Khalil, 2019; Balestrini & Sisodiya, 2018; Bonney et al., 2017; Elia et al., 2017; Hocker, 2015; Ułamek-Kozioł et al., 2019).

A. CNS cancers
    1. Surgery for tumor resection
    2. Radiation therapy to potentially reduce mass effect
    3. Chemotherapy
B. Pharmacologic management
    1. Antiepileptic agents (see Table 144-2)
    2. Management of status epilepticus: Should be given in the appropriate monitored environment
       a) First-line treatment
          (1) Lorazepam: 0.1 mg/kg IV up to 4 mg/dose 5–10 minutes apart or
          (2) Diazepam: 20 mg rectally or 5 mg IV or
          (3) Midazolam: 10 mg IM
       b) Second-line treatment
          (1) Fosphenytoin: 20 mg phenytoin equivalent/kg IV or
          (2) Valproate sodium: 40 mg/kg IV
       c) Convulsive or nonconvulsive: If consciousness is severely impaired
          (1) First agent
              (a) Propofol 1–2 mg/kg load; 2–12 mg/kg/hr infusion or
              (b) Midazolam 0.1–2 mg/kg IV load; 0.1–2 mg/kg/hr infusion
          (2) Second agent
              (a) Pentobarbital 5–15 mg/kg IV load; 0.5–5 mg/kg/hr infusion or
              (b) Ketamine 1.5–4.5 mg/kg IV load; 2–7.5 mg/kg/hr infusion
       d) Nonconvulsive status with preservation of consciousness: Trial of one or two drugs not previously used (e.g., fosphenytoin, valproic acid levetiracetam, phenobarbital, lacosamide, topiramate)
C. Psychogenic events: Psychiatric management should be provided, as appropriate.
D. Ketogenic diet: A high-fat, adequate-protein, low-carbohydrate diet is used primarily to treat difficult-to-control (refractory) epilepsy in children. The diet mimics aspects of starvation by forcing the body to burn fats rather than carbohydrates.
    1. This method shows some promise in seizure management in adults.
    2. Some diets are severely restrictive, requiring inpatient management.
E. Patient education
    1. Driving restrictions (see www.epilepsy.com/epilepsy/rights_driving)
       a) Some states have laws requiring that physicians report people with seizures to the department of motor vehicles.
       b) States without reporting laws often require a seizure-free period of varying lengths before the patient legally can drive again.
    2. Report symptoms of toxicity (e.g., blurred vision, ataxia, drowsiness) to the healthcare provider.
    3. Limit or avoid potential precipitating factors while taking anticonvulsants.
    4. Report use of new prescriptions from other healthcare providers and over-the-counter drugs, as some drugs alter the metabolism of the anticonvulsant.
    5. Seizure medications are teratogenic. Caution patients to use some form of birth control.

VII. Follow-up (Thompson et al., 2020)
    A. Serum anticonvulsant level should be monitored as determined by patient condition, seizure control, and medication changes. Clinical status and seizure frequency are the most important factors to consider when determining the proper doses. Evaluate anticonvulsant level based on time of patient dosing.

TABLE 144-2	Commonly Used Antiepileptic Agents			
Drug Name	**Mechanism of Action**	**Efficacy by Seizure Type**	**Side Effects**	**Potential for Drug Interactions**
Brivaracetam	Binds to SV2A similar to levetiracetam but with higher affinity and selectivity	Focal onset	Somnolence, dizziness, fatigue, irritability Concurrent use of enzyme-inducing antiepileptic drugs speeds rate of clearance, resulting in increased concentration of enzyme-inducing antiepileptic drugs Teratogenicity unknown	Moderate
Cannabidiol	Exact mechanism of action unknown Bioavailability increased with high-fat meal	Seizures related to Lennox-Gastaut or Dravet syndrome	Sedation, fatigue, anorexia, diarrhea Teratogenicity unknown	High
Carbamazepine	Sodium channel blocker	Focal onset Generalized onset (tonic-clonic)	May exacerbate absence, myoclonic, and atonic seizures Nausea, headache, dizziness, sedation, fatigue, cognitive impairment, hyponatremia, weight gain, osteopenia Toxicity symptoms: Blurred vision, diplopia, nystagmus, unsteadiness incoordination, tremor Intermediate teratogenicity	High
Clonazepam/ clobazam	Affects $GABA_A$ receptor to increase frequency of chloride channel conduction	Generalized onset	Sedation, nystagmus, incoordination, dysarthria Teratogenicity unknown	High
Eslicarbazepine acetate	Sodium channel blocker	Focal onset	Similar to oxcarbazepine but less frequent	CYP3A4 inducer, thus reduces efficacy of oral contraceptives at high concentrations (greater than 900 mg daily)

(Continued on next page)

TABLE 144-2	Commonly Used Antiepileptic Agents *(Continued)*			
Drug Name	**Mechanism of Action**	**Efficacy by Seizure Type**	**Side Effects**	**Potential for Drug Interactions**
Ethosuximide	T-type calcium channel blocker	Generalized onset (absence seizures)	Nausea, abdominal pain, anorexia, vomiting, diarrhea, sedation, insomnia, nervousness, dizziness, fatigue, ataxia, behavior changes, headaches, psychosis, depression, hallucinations, rash, Stevens-Johnson syndrome, systemic lupus erythematosus, aplastic anemia, thrombocytopenia, agranulocytosis, autoimmune thyroiditis Teratogenicity unknown	Moderate
Felbamate	NMDA acid receptor blocker GABA promoter Sodium channel blocker	Focal onset Generalized onset	Anorexia, nausea, vomiting, insomnia, irritability, headache, weight loss Toxicities: Lethal aplastic anemia, hepatic failure Teratogenicity unknown	High CYP3A4 inducer, thus reduces efficacy of oral contraceptives
Gabapentin	Calcium channel blocker	Focal onset	Sedation, dizziness, ataxia, fatigue, weight gain, myoclonus, cognitive slowing, peripheral edema Low teratogenicity	Low
Lacosamide	Sodium channel blocker	Focal onset	Does not exacerbate absence or myoclonic seizures Dizziness, headache, nausea, vomiting, diplopia, fatigue, sedation (more likely at higher doses and when used with other sodium channel blockers), prolongation of PR interval Teratogenicity unknown	Low
Lamotrigine	Sodium channel blocker Other mechanisms unknown	Focal onset Generalized onset (tonic-clonic)	May exacerbate myoclonic seizures in some patients Slowing titration to avoid rash Dizziness, blurred vision, diplopia, unsteadiness, nausea, vomiting, headache, tremor Low teratogenicity	Moderate

(Continued on next page)

TABLE 144-2   Commonly Used Antiepileptic Agents (Continued)

Drug Name	Mechanism of Action	Efficacy by Seizure Type	Side Effects	Potential for Drug Interactions
Levetiracetam	Binds to SV2A, resulting in lower nonspecific neurotransmitter conduction	Focal onset Generalized onset	Somnolence, dizziness, asthenia, irritability, hostility, depression Low teratogenicity	Low
Oxcarbazepine	Sodium channel blocker	Focal onset	May exacerbate absence and myoclonic seizures Sedation, headache, fatigue, hyponatremia Toxicity symptoms: Dizziness, blurred vision, diplopia, nausea, vomiting, ataxia	CYP3A4 inducer weak and interaction potential low; can reduce efficacy of oral contraceptives at high concentrations (greater than 900 mg daily)
Perampanel	Selective AMPA glutamate receptor antagonist	Focal onset Generalized onset (tonic-clonic)	Accelerates the metabolism of levonorgestrel in oral contraceptives, dizziness, somnolence, headache, fatigue, ataxia, blurred vision, hostility (up to 20% of patients) Teratogenicity unknown	Moderate
Phenobarbital	Binds GABA$_A$ receptor	Focal onset Generalized onset (not nonmotor)	Sedation, disturbed concentration, depression, osteopenia, dupuytren contractures, plantar fibromatoses, frozen shoulder Highly teratogenic	High
Phenytoin	Sodium channel blocker	Focal onset Generalized onset (tonic-clonic)	May exacerbate myoclonic and absence seizures Cognitive changes Toxic reaction with ataxia, dysarthria, nystagmus, diplopia Hypersensitivity reaction with Stevens-Johnson syndrome, toxic epidermal necrolysis, fever, rash, lymphadenopathy, eosinophilia, hepatic and renal impairment Paradoxical increase in seizures in serum level greater than 30 mg/L Intermediate teratogenicity	High

(Continued on next page)

TABLE 144-2	Commonly Used Antiepileptic Agents *(Continued)*			
Drug Name	Mechanism of Action	Efficacy by Seizure Type	Side Effects	Potential for Drug Interactions
Pregabalin	Similar to gabapentin	Focal onset	May exacerbate myoclonic and absence seizures Dizziness, somnolence, increased appetite, weight gain, peripheral edema Teratogenicity unknown	Low
Primidone	Hepatic conversion to phenobarbital and phenylethylmalonamide	Focal onset Generalized onset (motor)	Same as phenobarbital plus severe toxic reaction with sedation, dizziness, ataxia, nausea, vomiting	High
Tiagabine	GABA reuptake inhibitor	Focal onset	May exacerbate absence and myoclonic seizures Dizziness, asthenia, nervousness, tremor, depression, emotional lability, dose-related nonconvulsive status epilepticus and encephalopathy Teratogenicity unknown	High
Topiramate	AMPA; kainite receptor antagonist GABA promoter Sodium channel blocker	Focal onset Generalized onset	Cognitive slowing, impaired attention and memory, impaired executive function, impaired fluency, sedation, fatigue, dizziness, ataxia, depression, decreased appetite, weight loss, distal paresthesia Less frequent side effects: Oligohidrosis, hyperthermia, metabolic acidosis, acute myopia, angle closure glaucoma, hyperammonemia (if combined with valproic acid) Intermediate teratogenicity	Low CYP3A4 inducer, thus reduces efficacy of oral contraceptives
Rufinamide	Sodium channel blocker	Generalized onset (associated with Lennox-Gastaut syndrome)	Dizziness, fatigue, somnolence, headache, vomiting, shortening of QT interval Teratogenicity unknown	Moderate

(Continued on next page)

TABLE 144-2   Commonly Used Antiepileptic Agents (Continued)

Drug Name	Mechanism of Action	Efficacy by Seizure Type	Side Effects	Potential for Drug Interactions
Valproic acid/ divalproex sodium	GABA potentiation T-type calcium channel blocker Sodium channel blocker	All types	Nausea, vomiting, anorexia, diarrhea, fatigue, sedation, tremor, weight gain, hair loss, peripheral edema, cognitive changes, thrombocytopenia, polycystic ovary syndrome, hyperandrogenism, insulin resistance In older adults: increased risk of parkinsonism, altered gait, dementia, brain atrophy (chronic use) Encephalopathy, hyperammonemia, hepatotoxicity, pancreatitis with polypharmacy Very high teratogenicity	High
Vigabatrin	GABA transaminase inhibitor	Focal onset	May exacerbate myoclonic and absence seizures Sedation, fatigue, dizziness, ataxia, irritability, behavior changes, psychosis, depression, weight gain, bilateral concentric constriction of visual fields Teratogenicity unknown	Low
Zonisamide	T-type calcium channel blocker Sodium channel blocker Inhibition of carbonic anhydrase activity	Focal onset	Sedation, ataxia, dizziness, nausea, fatigue, irritability, anorexia, weight loss, cognitive slowing (< topiramate), depression, psychosis, kidney stones Rarely Stevens-Johnson syndrome, toxic epidermal necrolysis, oligohidrosis, hyperthermia, metabolic acidosis Low teratogenicity	Moderate

AMPA—alpha-amino-3-hydroxy-5-methyl-4-isoxazolepropionic acid; CYP—cytochrome P450; GABA—gamma-aminobutyric acid; NMDA—N-methyl-D-aspartate; SV2A—synaptic vesicle glycoprotein 2A

Note. Based on information from Abou-Khalil, 2019; Balestrini & Sisodiya, 2018; Bonney et al., 2017; Elia et al., 2017; Hocker, 2015; Ułamek-Kozioł et al., 2019.

   B. Conduct CBC and serum chemistries with liver enzymes every six months to mon-
      itor renal and hepatic function and assess for myelosuppression or as medically
      indicated.
   C. Withdrawal of seizure medications can be considered for patients who are seizure-free
      for two years. Electroencephalography may be performed prior to discontinuation. Edu-
      cation regarding the risks and benefits of stopping medication should be undertaken and
      documented prior to tapering medication. Anticonvulsant medication should be tapered
      slowly, at the discretion of the prescribing healthcare provider.

VIII. Referrals (Stafstrom & Carmant, 2015)
   A. Neurologist: Refer all patients experiencing a first seizure, particularly with the following.
      1. Diagnosis of seizure is not certain.
      2. Change in seizures exists.
      3. Controlling seizures with medication is difficult.
      4. Special testing is in question.
      5. The patient is considering pregnancy.
      6. Neurologic examination reveals abnormalities.
   B. Hospital: Recommend emergency department evaluation if the following occur.
      1. First seizure
      2. Seizure lasting longer than five minutes or recurrent episode
      3. Generalized seizure without recovery
      4. Injury during seizure
   C. Tertiary epilepsy center: Referral is appropriate for patients who have had no satisfac-
      tory response after using two or three anticonvulsant medications.
   D. Psychiatric evaluation: Depression is known to be a frequent comorbidity of epilepsy,
      and recent research has found the relationship between epilepsy and depression to be
      bidirectional. Impaired function of the hippocampal and limbic systems in the brains of
      depressed people is a potential contributor to epilepsy.

*The author would like to acknowledge Eileen M. Le, RN, MSN, GNP-BC, NP-C, AOCNP®, for her
contribution to this chapter that remains unchanged from the previous edition of this book.*

References

Abou-Khalil, B.W. (2019). Update on antiepileptic drugs 2019. *Continuum, 25*(2), 508–536. https://doi.org/10.1212/con
   .0000000000000715

Allone, C., Lo Buono, V., Corallo, F., Pisani, L.R., Pollicino, P., Bramanti, P., & Marino, S. (2017). Neuroimaging and cognitive functions in temporal lobe epilepsy: A review of the literature. *Journal of the Neurological Sciences, 381,* 7–15.
   https://doi.org/10.1016/j.jns.2017.08.007

Balestrini, S., & Sisodiya, S.M. (2018). Pharmacogenomics in epilepsy. *Neuroscience Letters, 667,* 27–39. https://doi.org/10
   .1016/j.neulet.2017.01.014

Berntsson, S.G., Merrell, R.T., Amirian, E.S., Armstrong, G.N., Lachance, D., Smits, A., ... Melin, B.S. (2018). Glioma-relat-
   ed seizures in relation to histopathological subtypes: A report from the glioma international case-control study. *Journal
   of Neurology, 265*(6), 1432–1442. https://doi.org/10.1007/s00415-018-8857-0

Bonney, P.A., Boettcher, L.B., Burks, J.D., Baker, C., Conner, A.K., Fujii, T., ... Sughrue, M.E. (2017). Rates of seizure free-
   dom after surgical resection of diffuse low-grade gliomas. *World Neurosurgery, 106,* 750–756. https://doi.org/10.1016
   /j.wneu.2017.06.144

Duffau, H. (2018). The error of Broca: From the traditional localizationist concept to a connectomal anatomy of human
   brain. *Journal of Chemical Neuroanatomy, 89,* 73–81. https://doi.org/10.1016/j jchemneu.2017.04.003

Elia, M., Klepper, J., Leiendecker, B., & Hartmann, H. (2017). Ketogenic diets in the treatment of epilepsy. *Current Pharmaceutical Design, 23*(37), 5691–5701. https://doi.org/10.2174/1381612823666170809101517

Fisher, R.S., Cross, J.H., French, J.A., Higurashi, N., Hirsch, E., Jansen, F.E., ... Zuberi, S.M. (2017). Operational classification of seizure types by the International League Against Epilepsy: Position paper of the ILAE Commission for Classification and Terminology. *Epilepsia, 58*(4), 522–530. https://doi.org/10.1111/epi.13670

Gómez-Porro, P., Serrano, A.A., Toledano, R., García-Morales, I., & Gil-Nagel, A. (2018). Genetic (idiopathic) generalized epilepsy with occipital semiology. *Epileptic Disorders, 20*(5), 434–439. https://doi.org/10.1684/epd.2018.0994

Hocker, S.E. (2015). Status epilepticus. *Continuum, 21*(5), 1362–1383. https://doi.org/10.1212/con.0000000000000225

Klugah-Brown, B., Luo, C., Peng, R., He, H., Li, J., Dong, L., & Yao, D. (2019). Altered structural and causal connectivity in frontal lobe epilepsy. *BMC Neurology, 19*(1), 70. https://doi.org/10.1186/s12883-019-1300-z

Lin, A.L., & Avila, E.K. (2017). Neurologic emergencies in the patients with cancer: Diagnosis and management. *Journal of Intensive Care Medicine, 32*(2), 99–115. https://doi.org/10.1177/0885066615619582

Magge, R.S., & DeAngelis, L.M. (2015). The double-edged sword: Neurotoxicity of chemotherapy. *Blood Reviews, 29*(2), 93–100. https://doi.org/10.1016/j.blre.2014.09.012

Nitta, N., Usui, N., Kondo, A., Tottori, T., Terada, K., Araki, Y., ... Inoue, Y. (2019). Semiology of hyperkinetic seizures of frontal versus temporal lobe origin. *Epileptic Disorders, 21*(2), 154–165. https://doi.org/10.1684/epd.2019.1047

Nowacki, T.A., & Jirsch, J.D. (2017). Evaluation of the first seizure patient: Key points in the history and physical examination. *Seizure, 49,* 54–63. https://doi.org/10.1016/j.seizure.2016.12.002

Stafstrom, C.E., & Carmant, L. (2015). Seizures and epilepsy: An overview for neuroscientists. *Cold Spring Harbor Perspectives in Medicine, 5*(6), a022426. https://doi.org/10.1101/cshperspect.a022426

Stephani, C., Paulus, W., & Focke, N.K. (2019). Focal visual status epilepticus. *Epileptic Disorders, 21*(1), 102–107. https://doi.org/10.1684/epd.2019.1034

Thompson, N.J., McGee, R.E., Garcia-Williams, A., Selwa, L.M., Stoll, S.C., Johnson, E.K., & Fraser, R.T. (2020). The impact of depression self-management intervention on seizure activity. *Epilepsy and Behavior, 103,* 106504. https://doi.org/10.1016/j.yebeh.2019.106504

Ułamek-Kozioł, M., Czuczwar, S.J., Januszewski, S., & Pluta, R. (2019). Ketogenic diet and epilepsy. *Nutrients, 11*(10), 2510. https://doi.org/10.3390/nu11102510

CHAPTER 145

Spinal Cord Compression

Kathryn R. Waitman, DNP, MSN, FNP-C, AOCNP®

I. Definition: SCC is a neurologic emergency that occurs when the spinal cord or cauda equina is compromised by direct pressure, vertebral collapse, or both by metastatic spread and direct extension of a malignancy. Compression results in compromised neurologic function if not treated promptly (Boussios et al., 2018; Rucker, 2018).

II. Physiology/Pathophysiology (Rucker, 2018)
   A. Normal: The spinal cord begins at the foramen magnum and is a continuation of the medulla oblongata, terminating at L1–L2 of the vertebral column.
      1. Approximately 31 pairs of spinal nerves arise from the spinal cord and exit at each intervertebral foramen.
      2. Within the spinal cord, each spinal nerve separates into ventral and dorsal roots.
      3. Motor fibers of the ventral root carry impulses from the spinal cord to the muscles and glands of the body.
      4. Sensory fibers of the dorsal root carry impulses from sensory receptors of the body to the spinal cord.
      5. Impulses travel to the brain for interpretation.
   B. Pathophysiology
      1. Metastatic disease in the epidural space or outside of the spinal cord causes about 95% of all SCCs. Primary tumors arising from the vertebral column and supporting structures cause the remaining 5%.
         a) Tumors usually invade the epidural space anterior to the cord.
         b) The vertebral body at the level of cord compression often is destroyed or extensively involved.
         c) Cord compression eventually leads to spinal cord infraction.
      2. Tumor invades the epidural space through the following methods.
         a) Direct extension of tumor into the space following bony erosion of vertebral body: Lung, breast, and prostate cancers
         b) Lymph node growth through intervertebral foramina: Lymphoma
         c) Hematogenous spread from emboli
         d) Metastasis to the epidural space without bone involvement
      3. Neurologic deficits result from these mechanisms by the following.
         a) Direct compression of spinal cord/cauda equina
         b) Interruption of vascular supply to the spinal cord
         c) Compression resulting from vertebral collapse secondary to pathologic bone involvement and dislocation of the vertebral bodies

III. Clinical features: Manifestations vary with location of compression and degree of block. SCC is a poor prognostic sign, and most patients die within a year of diagnosis. Spinal emergencies and urgent conditions must be recognized early so that the diagnosis can be confirmed quickly, and treatment can be initiated to possibly prevent loss of function (Boussios et al., 2018; Khan et al., 2017; Laur et al., 2019; Lawton et al., 2019; Lo et al., 2015; NCI CTEP, 2017; Rucker, 2018).

A. Etiology
  1. Metastatic disease: Lung cancer, breast cancer, head and neck cancer, prostate cancer, renal cell cancer, multiple myeloma, melanoma, sarcoma, lymphoma
  2. Trauma
  3. Osteoporosis
  4. Fractured vertebrae

B. History: A complete history will note classic signs and symptoms of SCC (e.g., back pain). Be aware that the time interval between initial cancer diagnosis and development of SCC can be months to as long as 20 years.
  1. History of cancer and cancer treatment
  2. Current medications: Prescribed, over the counter
  3. History of presenting symptoms: Precipitating factors, location, duration, associated symptoms (e.g., back pain; symmetric weakness, numbness, tingling, or coldness of the extremities or affected areas; urinary difficulties; difficulty passing stool; difficulty walking)
  4. Changes in ADLs

C. Signs and symptoms: Early recognition and diagnosis of SCC cannot be overemphasized. The single critical prognostic factor in SCC is neurologic status at the time of diagnosis. The likelihood of full ambulation, sensation, and bowel and bladder control after treatment correlates with the extent of injury to the cord.
  1. Pain: Present in more than 95% of patients
    a) Can be persistent, local, radicular, or referred
    b) May be acute in onset but more commonly develops insidiously over weeks to months and predates any other symptoms; most commonly bilateral if in legs
    c) Localized pain: Described as constant, dull, aching, worse in the morning, and progressive; occurs in one or two vertebrae of the actual compression
    d) Radicular pain: Usually follows a dermatome (see Appendix B) of involved nerve roots and will increase with spinal movement; worsens with movement, coughing, and sneezing; may awaken patient at night
    e) Referred pain: Poorly localized because of involvement of multiple dermatomes
  2. Motor weakness: Seen in 60%–85% of patients; usually follows course of a nerve
    a) Degree dependent on level of compression
    b) Varies from unsteadiness to foot drop to paralysis
    c) Described as heaviness, spasticity, or stiffness
    d) Can progress to sexual dysfunction and paralysis
  3. Sensory loss: Seen in 40%–80% of patients at diagnosis
    a) Symptoms dependent on the level and degree of compression
    b) Usually starts as numbness and paresthesia but can progress to loss of sensation of light touch, pain, and heat
    c) Lhermitte sign: Experience of electric shock–like pain down the spine with neck flexion
  4. Autonomic dysfunction: Usually final symptom to occur

      a) Bladder and bowel dysfunction is present in approximately 40%–60% of patients at diagnosis.

      b) Urinary symptoms include hesitancy, retention, overflow, and incontinence.

      c) Bowel problems begin as difficulty expelling stool and loss of feeling and progress to constipation or incontinence.

      d) Impotence can occur.

      e) Ataxia, especially with back pain, suggests SCC.

  D. Physical examination

    1. Back: Percussion eliciting tenderness at level of compression

    2. Musculoskeletal and neurologic

      a) Increased radicular pain with straight leg raises with lumbar or thoracic compression

      b) Pain of cervical compression with neck flexion

      c) Decreased strength in affected extremities

      d) Loss of sensation for light touch, pain, or temperature in affected extremities

      e) Loss or decrease of positional sense: Proprioceptive loss

      f) Decreased deep tendon reflexes at level of compression and hyperactive below level of compression

      g) Decreased muscle coordination

      h) Unsteady gait

      i) Palpation of the spine elicits pain over compression

    3. Absence of sweating below level of compression

    4. Abdominal: Autonomic dysfunction

      a) Distended colon

      b) Palpable bladder

      c) Large postvoid residual urine volume

    5. Grading categories for spinal cord injury

      a) American Spinal Injury Association Impairment Scale

      b) Grades A–E, where A is complete loss of motor or sensory function in S4–S5, B–D are varying degrees of incomplete loss, and E is normal motor and sensory function

      c) NCI CTEP Common Terminology Criteria for Adverse Events grading and documentation for peripheral sensory neuropathy and motor neuropathy

IV. Diagnostic tests (Khan et al., 2017; Laur et al., 2019; Lavi et al., 2018; Lawton et al., 2019; Lo et al., 2015; Rucker, 2018)

  A. Laboratory: Laboratory tests are not typically indicated; however, calcium and serum albumin tests should be examined in patients with bone metastases due to potential hypercalcemia. Calcium should be corrected for low albumin.

  B. Radiology

    1. Spine radiographs

      a) Shows vertebral body collapse, pedicle erosion, or vertebral lesions in greater than 85% of epidural metastases

      b) Detects approximately 72% of epidural cord compressions

      c) May not show early SCC because 50% of vertebral bone must be destroyed before evident on films

      d) Not unusual to find multiple sites

      e) Small percentage of false-negative rates from lack of sensitivity or specificity

    2. MRI

      a) Currently recommended for spinal axis within 48–72 hours of presentation of back pain without neurologic abnormalities

      b) Replaced myelogram for detecting epidural SCC; entire spine readily imaged; more specific and sensitive to extradural, intradural, intramedullary, and extravertebral lesion diagnoses and can detect paraspinal masses

  3. CT scan

      a) Superior to MRI for evaluating vertebral stability and bone destruction; performed before surgical management of epidural cord compression

      b) Accurate in location of cord compression

      c) Mandatory for the following

         (1) MRI is nondiagnostic or unavailable.

         (2) Patient is obese (i.e., greater than 300 pounds).

         (3) Patient is unable to lie still.

         (4) Patient has claustrophobia, severe pain, scoliosis, or a pacemaker.

  4. Bone scan: May identify vertebral bony metastases or fractures

      a) Useful for patient follow-up

      b) Not specific to epidural tumors or SCC

      c) Can have false results secondary to specific disease processes

  5. Myelogram: Accurately determines upper and lower extent of lesion

      a) Ascertains if more than one lesion is present

      b) Uncomfortable and invasive to patient

      c) Risk of further neurologic deterioration from lumbar puncture

      d) Reserved for patients who have poor CT or MRI results, cannot undergo CT or MRI, or have uncontrolled pain

      e) Used to obtain CSF samples to rule out meningeal carcinomatosis

  6. PET-CT scan: Both sensitive and specific but less available than MRI; should not be used alone for diagnosis or treatment guidance

V. Differential diagnosis (Laur et al., 2019; Lavi et al., 2018)

  A. Transverse myelitis

  B. Ischemic myelomalacia

  C. Syphilis

  D. Multiple sclerosis

  E. Subacute combined degeneration of the cord

  F. Motor neuron disease

  G. Epidural abscess

  H. Spinal epidural hemorrhage, hematomyelia, abscess

  I. Acute disc protrusion: Pain relieved by sitting

  J. Chronic compressive myelopathy: Cervical spondylosis, lumbar stenosis

  K. Ankylosing spondylitis

  L. RA (see Chapter 108)

  M. Paget disease

  N. Muscle spasm

  O. Radiation myelopathy

  P. Trauma

  Q. Osteoporosis (see Chapter 106)

  R. Vertebral fracture

VI. Treatment: Timely treatment is imperative to preserve maximal function. Therapy decisions are made depending on type of tumor, level of compression, rapidity of onset or duration of symptoms, and availability of clinical experience. Treatment outcomes are better for lesions on the lower spine than upper spine. Therapy will not reverse fixed paralysis of more than

48 hours of duration (Boussios et al., 2018; Laufer & Bilsky, 2019; Lawton et al., 2019; Lo et al., 2015; Rucker, 2018; Tsagozis & Bauer, 2019).

  A. Glucocorticoids to reduce vasogenic edema, pain, and oncolytic effects (see Appendix K)
     1. Emergent compression: Dexamethasone 10 mg IV, then 4 mg IV or PO every six hours, tapered through the course of radiation therapy
     2. Partial compression or metastasis: Dexamethasone 4 mg PO every six hours, tapered through the course of radiation therapy
     3. Steroid taper safely managed with 10% dose reduction every two days
  B. Local radiation with or without chemotherapy
     1. Radiosensitive tumors
     2. Total dose of radiation therapy: 3,000–4,000 cGy
     3. Stereotactic body radiation therapy
  C. Surgery
     1. Nonradiosensitive tumors or following maximum dose of radiation therapy
       a) Usually, surgery is the last resort for patients with limited life expectancy.
       b) Often, patients are not candidates for surgery.
     2. Removal of neurofibroma, meningioma, or other extramedullary tumors
     3. Mandatory tissue diagnosis
       a) Unknown cause of SCC but possibility of abscess or hematoma
       b) Rarely can remove entire tumor
     4. Laminectomy: Relieves compression and stabilizes spine when patient has anticipated survival of longer than two to three months
       a) Surgical decompression: Anterolateral resection is the principal surgical treatment for epidural metastases arising from the vertebral body.
       b) Removal of posterior lesions
       c) Treatment of pathologic fractures caused by symptomatic spinal metastases
     5. Kyphoplasty or vertebroplasty for painful vertebral body fractures by stabilizing the vertebral body using bone cement
  D. Chemotherapy: Adjuvant treatment to radiation therapy or surgery
     1. Chemosensitive tumor: Lymphoma, neuroblastoma, germ cell tumor
     2. Recurrent tumor at previously irradiated site
     3. Patients who are not candidates for surgery
  E. Pain management
     1. Scheduled oral or parenteral opioids (see Appendix F)
     2. Epidural blocks
     3. Intrathecal opioids
     4. Trial of an anticonvulsant (e.g., gabapentin); may take four to six weeks for maximal effect (see Appendix Q)
     5. Steroids: For patients with vasogenic edema; can decrease pain secondary to reduction of mechanical cord compression (see Appendix K)

VII. Follow-up: Most important prognostic factor in SCC is pretreatment neurologic status (Boussios et al., 2018; Lawton et al., 2019).
  A. Short term
     1. Determine response to treatment, pain management, sphincter control, and motor function.
     2. Damage to urinary tract can result from urinary retention with bladder distention and injury to detrusor muscle. Evaluate for infection.
     3. Mechanical respiratory failure is possible in high cervical cord lesions. Evaluate breathing.
     4. Severe hypertension can occur in response to stimuli (see Chapter 47).

B. Long term
1. Monitor for neurologic dysfunction.
a) UTIs (see Chapter 89)
b) Pressure ulcers (see Chapter 15)
2. Assess existing neurologic status.
3. Assist patients with adjustment to existing motor and autonomic dysfunction.

VIII. Referrals
A. Radiation oncologist, neurosurgeon, neurologist, or oncologist: Dependent on treatment regimen
B. Homecare services: Physical therapist, home health aide

References

Boussios, S., Cooke, D., Hayward, C., Kanellos, F.S., Tsiouris, A.K., Chatziantoniou, A.A., ... Karathanasi, A. (2018). Metastatic spinal cord compression: Unraveling the diagnostic and therapeutic challenges. *Anticancer Research, 38*(9), 4987–4997. https://doi.org/10.21873/anticanres.12817

Khan, U.A., Shanholtz, C.B., & McCurdy, M.T. (2017). Oncologic mechanical emergencies. *Hematology/Oncology Clinics of North America, 31*(6), 927–940. https://doi.org/10.1016/j.hoc.2017.08.001

Laufer, I., & Bilsky, M.H. (2019). Advances in the treatment of metastatic spine tumors: The future is not what it used to be. *Journal of Neurosurgery: Spine, 30*(3), 299–307. https://doi.org/10.3171/2018.11.SPINE18709

Laur, O., Nandu, H., Titelbaum, D.S., Nunez, D.B., & Khurana, B. (2019). Nontraumatic spinal cord compression: MRI primer for emergency department radiologists. *RadioGraphics, 39*(6), 1862–1880. https://doi.org/10.1148/rg.2019190024

Lavi, E.S., Pal, A., Bleicher, D., Kang, K., & Sidani, C. (2018). MR imaging of the spine: Urgent and emergent indications. *Seminars in Ultrasound, CT and MRI, 39*(6), 551–569. https://doi.org/10.1053/j.sult.2018.10.006

Lawton, A.J., Lee, K.A., Cheville, A.L. Ferrone, M.L., Rades, D., Balboni, T.A., & Abrahm, J.L. (2019). Assessment and management of patients with metastatic spinal cord compression: A multidisciplinary review. *Journal of Clinical Oncology, 37*(1), 61–71. https://doi.org/10.1200/JCO.2018.78.1211

Lo, S.S.-M., Ryu, S., Chang, E.L., Galanopoulos, N., Jones, J., Kim, E.Y., ... Vassil, A.D. (2015). ACR Appropriateness Criteria® metastatic epidural spinal cord compression and recurrent spinal metastasis. *Journal of Palliative Medicine, 18*(7), 573–584. https://doi.org/10.1089/jpm.2015.28999.sml

National Cancer Institute Cancer Therapy Evaluation Program. (2017). *Common terminology criteria for adverse events* [v. 5.0]. https://ctep.cancer.gov/protocoldevelopment/electronic_applications/docs/CTCAE_v5_Quick_Reference_8.5x11.pdf

Rucker, Y. (2018). Spinal cord compression. In C.H. Yarbro, D. Wujcik., & B.H. Gobel (Eds.), *Cancer nursing: Principles and practice* (8th ed., pp 1153–1167). Jones and Bartlett Learning.

Tsagozis, P., & Bauer, H.C.F. (2019). Outcome of surgical treatment for spinal cord compression in patients with hematological malignancy. *International Journal of Spine Surgery, 13*(2), 186–191. https://doi.org/10.14444/6025

CHAPTER 146

Stroke

Patricia A. Obulaney, DNP, APRN, ANP-C,

and Kristin Ownby, PhD, RN, AOCN®, ANP-BC, ACHPN

I. Definition: An acute clinical event with an abrupt onset of a neurologic deficit indicative of focal CNS involvement attributed to cerebral circulation disturbance (Lin & Avila, 2017; Navi & Iadecola, 2018)

   A. The cerebral incident includes sudden onset with symptoms persisting for a minimum of 24 hours.

   B. An ischemic deficit that resolves rapidly without radiologic evidence of infarction is defined as a *transient ischemic attack.*

II. Physiology/Pathophysiology (Dearborn et al., 2014; Shao et al., 2019; Splittgerber, 2019)

   A. Normal

     1. Approximately 18% of total blood volume circulates in the brain.

     2. The brain is responsible for 20% of total body oxygen consumption.

     3. Arterial supply of the brain includes the following.

       a) Extracerebral vessels of the right carotid artery arising from right subclavian artery

       b) Left carotid artery arising from aortic arch

       c) Intracranial cerebral vessels including the internal carotid artery, which divides into the anterior cerebral and the middle cerebral arteries

       d) Two vertebral arteries, which arise from subclavian arteries and join to form the basilar artery, which gives rise to the posterior cerebral artery supplying the occipital lobes and brain stem

     4. The circle of Willis is a confluence of vessels that gives rise to all major cerebral arteries.

       a) It is fed by the paired internal carotid arteries and the basilar artery.

       b) When the circle is complete, it contains a posterior communicating artery on each side and an anterior communicating artery.

     5. Each major artery supplies a certain area of the brain. Sudden occlusion affects this area immediately, which can result in irreversible damage.

     6. Regulation of cerebral blood flow: Cerebral perfusion pressure is the difference between mean arterial pressure and ICP. Cerebral perfusion pressure is (mean arterial pressure − ICP). Normal values are 80–100 mm Hg.

       a) Autoregulation is the process by which the cerebral blood flow remains almost constant with a mean arterial pressure of 60–160 mm Hg.

       b) Pressures greater than 150–160 mm Hg can disrupt the blood–brain barrier.

       c) Extrinsic mechanisms influence cerebral blood flow, including respiratory gas tensions, temperature, viscosity, and autonomic influences.

B. Pathophysiology

1. Ischemic stroke involves cerebral artery occlusion by an emboli or thrombi, leading to brain tissue damage from an insufficient blood supply to a portion of the brain.
2. Hemorrhagic stroke occurs when a cerebral artery leaks blood, damaging adjacent brain tissue or from ruptured aneurysm.

III. Clinical features: Several syndromes mimic stroke. The two most common are hypoglycemia and postictal seizure. The patient's overall medical well-being, age, and condition are important factors in mortality and morbidity with intracerebral hemorrhage. Brain swelling and herniation are the most frequent causes of early mortality in patients with hemispheric stroke. Symptoms of stroke may be transient or persist for longer periods of time. Neurologic symptoms do not accurately reflect the presence or absence of infarction or the cause of the infarction. Treatment is dependent on the cause of symptoms (Bright et al., 2017; Caprio & Sorond, 2019; Guzik & Bushnell, 2017; Knight-Greenfield et al., 2019; Lin & Avila, 2017; Matthews et al., 2018; Meng et al., 2016; Morawo & Adams, 2019; Navi & Iadecola, 2018; Wilbers et al., 2020; Yew & Cheng, 2015).

A. Classification of stroke
1. Hemorrhagic: Intracerebral and subarachnoid
2. Ischemic: Systemic hypoperfusion, thrombotic, embolic

B. Risk factors
1. Atherosclerosis
2. Atrial fibrillation
3. Smoking
4. Diabetes mellitus
5. Hypertension
6. Coronary vessel disease
7. Hypercholesterolemia

C. Etiology
1. Cancer-related causes of ischemic stroke
   a) Thrombotic stroke: Most common in patients with cancer
   b) Nonbacterial thrombotic endocarditis or marantic endocarditis
   c) Infections: Progressive multifocal leukoencephalopathy
   d) Trousseau syndrome: Spontaneous venous thrombosis of upper and lower limbs associated with visceral carcinoma
   e) Urogenital, breast, head and neck, or GI cancer
   f) Lung or liver metastasis
   g) Occlusive disease from emboli, compression, or meningeal extension of cancer
   h) Radiation-induced accelerated atherosclerosis
   i) Surgical procedures: May promote release of emboli
   j) Intravascular coagulation
   k) Chemotherapy agents: cisplatin-based drugs, tamoxifen, cyclophosphamide, 5-fluorouracil, paclitaxel, L-asparaginase, thalidomide, bevacizumab, sunitinib, sorafenib (list not all-inclusive)
   l) Intrathecal administration of chemotherapy
   m) Intra-arterial chemotherapy for primary brain tumors
   n) Hyperviscous obstructions of arterial vessels
   o) Hyperleukocytic syndrome in acute myeloid leukemia
   p) Septic emboli
   q) Hormonal therapies including tamoxifen; androgen deprivation therapy
2. Cancer-related causes of hemorrhagic stroke
   a) DIC, especially in patients with leukemia

       b) Promyelocytic leukemia, lymphoma, melanoma, lung cancer

       c) Chemotherapy-induced thrombocytopenia

       d) Chronic lymphocytic leukemia and lymphoma: Can induce an autoimmune thrombocytopenia

       e) Primary brain tumors: Astrocytoma

       f) Blast crisis with acute leukemia

       g) Neoplastic infiltration of arteries causing aneurysm formation

  3. Primary fibrinolysis

  4. Infections

  5. Vitamin K deficiency due to poor nutrition or antibiotic therapy

  6. Hypertension

  7. Hypercholesterolemia

  8. Hypercoagulable state

  9. CAD

  10. Diabetes mellitus

  11. Dysrhythmia

D. History

  1. History of cancer and cancer treatments

  2. Current medications: Prescribed, over the counter

  3. History of presenting symptoms: Precipitating factors, onset, location, duration

  4. Changes in ADLs

  5. Past medical history: Transient ischemia attacks, CAD, hypertension, atrial fibrillation, atherosclerosis, hypercholesterolemia, diabetes mellitus

  6. Social history: Smoking, illicit drug use (cocaine)

  7. Family history: Cardiac disease

E. Signs and symptoms of ischemic or hemorrhagic stroke (see Table 146-1)

F. Physical examination: Follow physical examination outlined in the National Institutes of Health Stroke Scale to determine whether a patient is a candidate for tissue plasminogen activator with an acute ischemic stroke. The stroke scale can be used to screen acute strokes in general.

  1. Vital signs: Blood pressure for hypertension; evaluation for fever (ischemic neuronal injury is hastened by fever)

  2. Neurologic: Level of functioning after stroke

       a) Level of consciousness and alertness assessments: Ask patient to open and close eyes and then to grip and release nonparetic hand.

       b) Extraocular movement assessment for a normal gaze, a partial gaze palsy, or a forced deviation in which total gaze paresis cannot be overcome with an oculocephalic maneuver

       c) Confrontation test to assess peripheral vision

       d) Facial palsy, via asking patient to show teeth, raise eyebrows, or close eyes

       e) Pronator drift, by asking patient to hold arms straight forward, palms up, and eyes closed

          (1) Instruct patient to keep arms still while tapping the arms briskly downward.

          (2) If patient is unable to maintain the extension and supination, this suggests an insult to upper motor neurons.

       f) Lower extremity for drift, by holding the leg at 30°: Drift occurs if the leg falls before five seconds.

       g) Limb ataxia (cerebellar function), by performing heel-to-shin or finger-nose-finger test (see Appendix D)

       h) Primary sensory functioning (see Appendix D)

TABLE 146-1	Signs and Symptoms of Ischemic or Hemorrhagic Stroke
Region	**Signs and Symptoms**
Cerebellum	Profound headaches
Left Hemisphere	
Anterior cerebral artery	Right hemiparesis with variable involvement of face and upper and lower extremities Right-sided sensory loss in a pattern similar to that of the motor deficit Decreased stereognosis and graphesthesia Dysarthria (difficulty of speech) Aphasia, fluent and nonfluent Alexia (loss of ability to read) Agraphia (inability to write) Acalculia (inability to solve math problems) Apraxia (inability to perform purposeful movement)
Middle cerebral artery	Right hemiparesis with variable involvement of face and upper and lower extremities Broca, Wernicke, or global aphasia Apraxia Agrammatism (inability to speak grammatically correct) Dysphasia
Posterior cerebral artery	Hemiplegia or hemiparesis Alexia Apraxia Prosopagnosia (inability to recognize faces) Memory impairment Visual changes including homonymous hemianopia, visual agnosia, disorders of color vision
Vertebrobasilar stroke	Impaired balance and coordination Vertigo Nausea and vomiting Headaches Nystagmus Slurred speech Brain stem strokes Hemiparesis or quadriplegia Sensory loss affecting either the hemibody or all four limbs Diplopia Slurred speech Dysphagia Decreased level of consciousness Abnormal respirations
Hemorrhagic stroke	Neck pain Light sensitivity Nausea and vomiting Impaired level of consciousness Other findings depend on artery involved

(Continued on next page)

TABLE 146-1	Signs and Symptoms of Ischemic or Hemorrhagic Stroke *(Continued)*
Region	**Signs and Symptoms**
Right Hemisphere	
Anterior cerebral artery	Left hemiparesis with variable involvement of face and upper and lower extremities Left-sided sensory loss that is similar pattern to that of the motor deficit Left homonymous hemianopia Dysarthria Neglect of the side of environment Anosognosia (pretend ignorance of disease) Asomatognosia (forgetting or misperceiving the body) Loss of prosody of speech Flat affect
Middle cerebral artery	Dysphagia Broca, Wernicke, or global aphasia Apraxia Extinction Neglect of the side of the environment Impersistence Topographic memory Confabulation General confusion and delirium Allesthesia (perception of stimulus in opposite limb from one stimulated) Aprosody (loss of normal speech pitch and rhythm)
Posterior cerebral artery	–
Vertebrobasilar stroke	Diplopia Slurred speech Dysphagia Decreased level of consciousness Abnormal respirations
Hemorrhagic stroke	–

Note. Based on information from Knight-Greenfield et al., 2019; National Institutes of Health, n.d.; Urdaneta & Bhalla, 2019; Yew & Cheng, 2015.

> *i)* Fluency, comprehension, and presence of aphasia, by asking the patient to read sentences and describe pictures located on the National Institutes of Health Stroke Scale
> *j)* Dysarthria, by asking the patient to say "mama, tip-top, fifty-fifty, thanks, huckleberry, baseball player"
> *k)* Extinction and inattention with double simultaneous stimulation
> 3. HEENT: Auscultation of carotid arteries for bruits suggesting stenosis
> 4. Cardiovascular: Heart sounds for irregularity suggesting dysrhythmias
> 5. Pulmonary: Abnormal breath sounds for fluid overload or post-stroke pneumonia

IV. Diagnostic tests (Fugate & Rabinstein, 2015; Knight-Greenfield et al., 2019; Potter et al., 2019; Urdaneta & Bhalla, 2019; Yew & Cheng, 2015)
   A. Laboratory
      1. Acute phase
         a) In case of suspected ischemic stroke, blood glucose must be drawn prior to the administration of a thrombolytic agent. With a patient with cancer who is sus-

pected of thrombocytopenia, a platelet count is checked prior to administration of a thrombolytic. Other laboratory results can be pending if a thrombolytic is administered to a patient who has had an ischemic stroke.

    b) Coagulation profile: PT, aPTT, and INR to evaluate for coagulopathy as underlying cause of stroke

    c) Glucose level to evaluate for hypoglycemia

    d) Basic metabolic panel to provide baseline data and reveal conditions that mimic a stroke, such as hyponatremia

    e) LFTs as indicated if liver dysfunction is suspected

    f) ESR if a vasculitis-related disease is suspected

    g) CBC to evaluate for thrombocytopenia, leukemia, and polycythemia

    h) Toxicology to evaluate for drug-related cause of stroke (e.g., cocaine); used in identifying intoxicated patients with behaviors mimicking stroke

    i) Urine pregnancy test on all women of childbearing age with stroke symptoms

    j) Creatinine and BUN to evaluate for CKD, which is associated with higher risk of stroke

    k) Cardiac enzymes to evaluate for an association between stroke and underlying CAD

    l) Troponin as baseline to determine if patient is presenting with acute MI

    m) DIC panel to evaluate coagulopathy

  2. Postacute stroke

    a) Hypercoagulable state (generally for stroke patients younger than age 45 years): Antiphospholipid antibodies, lupus anticoagulant, protein C, protein S, factor V Leiden mutation, anticardiolipin antibodies, antithrombin III deficiency, prothrombin gene polymorphism

    b) Lipid profile to evaluate for hyperlipidemia

    c) Thyroid panel to evaluate for thyroid abnormalities contributing to or mimicking stroke

B. Radiology

  1. Acute phase

    a) Noncontrast brain CT scan to emergently evaluate for cerebral hemorrhage, subdural hematoma, and other intracerebral pathology prior to the administration of thrombolytic therapy

    b) Cerebral angiography to evaluate brain vascular anatomy

    c) Chest radiography, as indicated, for suspicion of pulmonary or cardiac disease

  2. Postacute phase

    a) Transcranial Doppler ultrasonography: Rapid and noninvasive technique to identify site of major arterial occlusion in a cerebral artery and to identify emboli

    b) Carotid Doppler to evaluate for carotid artery stenosis as a cause of stroke

    c) MRI/magnetic resonance angiography diffusion and perfusion studies to quantify region of infarcted tissue and affected artery

  3. Poststroke rehabilitation: Barium swallow to assess the severity of dysphagia

C. Other

  1. Acute phase: ECG to evaluate for dysrhythmias predisposing a patient to embolic events such as atrial fibrillation

  2. Postacute phase: Echocardiogram including transesophageal echocardiography to evaluate for cardioembolic etiology

  3. Lumbar puncture: Inspection of CSF for bilirubin recommended if subarachnoid hemorrhage is suspected with normal CT results

4. Screening for depression

5. Swallowing assessment poststroke: Dysphagia (common)

6. Poststroke rehabilitation: Voiding analysis to evaluate urinary incontinence, as indicated

V. Differential diagnosis (see Figure 146-1)

A. Systemic infection

B. Seizure (see Chapter 144)

C. Brain tumor

D. Hypoglycemia

E. Hyponatremia (see Chapter 155)

F. Positional vertigo (see Chapter 134)

G. Conversion disorder

VI. Treatment: Treatment is determined according to the cerebrovascular pathology and the exact etiology of the cerebral incident, which aid in determining eligibility to receive acute treatment for ischemic stroke. Admission to a facility, preferably one with stroke care specialization, is the optimal approach (Arnett el al., 2019; Caprio & Sorond, 2019; Gross et al., 2019; Guzik & Bushnell, 2017; Morawo & Adams, 2019; Muller et al., 2019; Powers et al., 2018; Shao et al., 2019; Tsiygoulis et al., 2018; Urdaneta & Bhalla, 2019; U.S. Preventive Services Task Force, 2016; Yew & Cheng, 2015).

A. Overall goals of stroke treatment

FIGURE 146-1   **Differential Diagnosis of Stroke**

Anterior Cerebral Artery Stroke	**Middle Cerebral Artery Stroke**	**Posterior Cerebral Artery Stroke**	**Vertebrobasilar Stroke**
• Amnesia • Brain abscess • Cardioembolic stroke • Carotid disease • Cavernous sinus syndrome • Cerebral aneurysm • Drug toxicity • Glioblastoma multiforme • Head injury • Herpes simplex encephalitis • Hypoglycemia • Intracranial hemorrhage • Low-grade astrocytoma • Meningioma • Metastatic disease to brain • Migraine variants • Primary brain tumor • Primary central nervous system lymphoma • Seizure and epilepsy • Subarachnoid hemorrhage • Subdural hematoma • Transient global viral encephalitis	• Conversion disorder • Focal seizure • Hypoglycemia • Migraine headache • Subdural headache • Tumor	• Basilar artery thrombosis • Cardioembolic stroke • Dissection syndromes • Intracranial hemorrhage • Metabolic disease • Migraine headache • Migraine variants • Posterior reversible encephalopathy syndrome	• Basilar meningitis • Basilar migraine • Central pontine myelinolysis • Cerebellopontine angle tumors • Metastatic disease to brain • Supratentorial hemispheric mass lesions with mass effect, herniation, and brain stem compression

Note. Based on information from Caprio & Sorond, 2019; Knight-Greenfield et al., 2019; Muller et al., 2019; Shao et al., 2019; Urdaneta & Bhalla, 2019; Yew & Cheng, 2015

1. Immediate goal is to reestablish blood flow to the brain to preserve the blood flow in ischemic area.
2. Localize and treat the cerebral bleed with hemorrhagic stroke treatment to minimize permanent brain injury. Urgent neurosurgical consult is warranted. Establish onset of initial stroke symptoms (see Table 146-1). Time of onset is tantamount to safely determine the patient's eligibility for thrombolytic therapy.
3. Determine if pathophysiologic etiology is intracerebral ischemic stroke or subarachnoid hemorrhage within three hours of symptom onset for optimal reduction of subsequent, permanent damage.
4. Ensure medical stability, including airway patency and blood pressure maintenance.
5. Screen ischemic stroke patients for contraindications to thrombolysis therapy.
6. Rehabilitate to independent self-care and encourage development of lifestyle changes to diminish the probability of a subsequent stroke.

B. Ischemic stroke thrombolysis
   1. IV thrombolysis: The recombinant tissue plasminogen activator (rtPA) produced by recombinant DNA improves outcomes in ischemic stroke (see Table 146-2).
      a) It is initiated only after appropriate neuroimaging study and thorough neurologic examination.
      b) Perform thromboaspiration or rtPA therapy for ischemic stroke once absence of hemorrhage has been substantiated. Thrombectomy, in which the clot is removed via mechanical clot extraction, is used in large-vessel ischemic stroke in viable patients requiring treatment after the recommended three-hour rtPA window has closed. Procedure is performed to reestablish cerebral blood flow for symptom improvement.
      c) Successful clot dissolution is dependent on patient age, clot composition, clot size, and arterial vascular occlusion location and type.
      d) For ischemic stroke patients with more than 4.5 hours after symptom onset, administer ASA within 48 hours of stroke onset, which may be used in combination with subcutaneous heparin for DVT prophylaxis.
   2. Thrombolysis exclusion criteria: According to American Heart Association/American Stroke Association guidelines, the following patients are not candidates for thrombolytic therapy within the 3–4.5-hour window of ischemic stroke.
      a) Patients older than 80 years
      b) All patients taking oral anticoagulants, regardless of INR
      c) Patients with elevated aPTT
      d) Patients with baseline National Institutes of Health Stroke Scale score greater than 25
      e) Patients with a history of stroke and diabetes
   3. Prior to rtPA administration, discuss with the patient and family the benefits and risks of thrombolytic therapy.
      a) Main benefit is functional outcome improvement by salvaging threatened brain tissue.
      b) Discuss potential risk for intracerebral hemorrhage, further deterioration of neurologic function deficits, coma, and possible death.
   4. The rtPA recommended dose is 0.9 mg/kg (maximum of 90 mg) over 60 minutes with 10% of total dose given as initial IV bolus over one minute.
   5. Postinfusion management
      a) After administration of rtPA, transfer patient to ICU or stroke unit for close monitoring.

TABLE 146-2 **Contraindications for Treatment With Recombinant Tissue Plasminogen Activator in Patients With Ischemic Stroke**

Clinical Assessment	Contraindications
Cancer related	Gastrointestinal malignancy within 21 days Intra-axial intracranial neoplasm
Imaging studies	Computed tomography scan showing major acute or multilobar infarction or subarachnoid or intracranial hemorrhage
Laboratory tests	Patient on anticoagulant and international normalized ratio greater than 1.7 Patient received heparin within previous 48 hours and activated partial thromboplastin time outside normal range Platelet count < 100,000/mm³ Blood glucose < 50 mg/dl (increases risk of poor outcome but not a contraindication)
Patient examination	Elevated blood pressure (systolic greater than 185 mm Hg and diastolic greater than 110 mm Hg) or aggressive medication intervention required to attain recommended blood pressure level Evidence of active bleeding or acute trauma Seizure with postictal residual neurologic impairments Patient or family members do not understand the potential risks and benefits from treatment Age greater than 80 years
Patient history	Head trauma, prior stroke, spinal or intracranial surgery, or myocardial injury within previous 3 months Gastrointestinal or urinary tract hemorrhage within previous 21 days Arterial puncture at a noncompressible site within previous 7 days Major surgery within previous 14 days History of previous intracranial hemorrhage History of aneurysm, or untreated arteriovenous malformation, infective endocarditis
Signs and symptoms	No assessable neurologic deficit Neurologic signs that clear naturally Slight neurologic signs not associated with other entities Stroke symptoms potentially corresponding with subarachnoid hemorrhage Symptom onset greater than 3 hours before treatment

Note. Based on information from Powers et al., 2018.

      b) Perform head CT scan or MRI 24 hours after thrombolysis to evaluate for asymptomatic hemorrhage.

      c) Avoid anticoagulant and antiplatelet therapy for 24 hours after rtPA.

      d) Potential complications include intracerebral hemorrhage, venous puncture site oozing, angioedema, systemic hemorrhage, and allergic reactions.

    6. Mechanical thrombectomy with a stent retriever for ischemic stroke: Criteria includes prestroke modified Rankin score of 0–1; occlusion occurring in the internal carotid artery or middle cerebral artery; age 18 years or older; National Institutes of Health stroke score of 6 or more; and treatment can be initiated within six hours of symptom onset.

  C. Antiplatelet therapy

    1. The only antiplatelet agent recognized as effective for early acute ischemic stroke is ASA.

    a) American Heart Association/American Stroke Association recommends initial ASA dose of 325 mg PO, thereafter 150–325 mg PO daily within 48 hours of stroke onset for patients who are not receiving IV heparin, rtPA, or oral anticoagulants.

    b) ASA should not be used as an alternative to IV thrombolysis or other acute therapy.

2. Clopidogrel 75 mg PO daily (in combination with ASA 81 mg PO daily) or ticlopidine 250 mg PO two times a day are alternatives for patients who are intolerant to ASA. These are more valuable after ischemic stroke to prevent a recurrent ischemic event in patients with atrial fibrillation.

3. For the treatment of acute ischemic stroke, heparin and LMWH have been evaluated and seem to offer no benefit compared to antiplatelet agent use.

D. Hemorrhagic stroke treatment

1. Admit or transfer the patient to ICU for diligent observation with both medical and surgical treatments. Head of bed is to remain elevated 30° with head midline.

2. Indication for surgery to treat bleed is dependent on the cerebral hemorrhage location.

3. Reverse any recent anticoagulation due to oral anticoagulants by correcting the INR quickly with vitamin K and fresh frozen plasma infusions, treating fever, and maintaining glucose at 140–180 mg/dl.

4. Prevent DVT development with the use of elastic stockings and sequential compression devices. Once the intracerebral bleed has been controlled, unfractionated heparin or low-dose subcutaneous LMWH should be considered for DVT prevention in individuals who are immobile for one to four days after hemorrhagic stroke onset.

5. Manage elevated ICP via osmotic diuretics (mannitol) and/or ventricular catheter drainage. Administer analgesia, maintain sedation, and control blood pressure.

6. Control hypertension according to patient factors such as baseline blood pressure, elevated ICP, the supposed cause of hemorrhage, and age. If blood pressure is severely elevated, lower blood pressure slowly to avoid tissue ischemia (see Chapter 47).

7. Control seizure activity rapidly with a benzodiazepine agent (lorazepam or diazepam).

    a) Give lorazepam 0.1 mg/kg IV at a rate of 2 mg/min as a loading dose, with a maximum dose of 4 mg. Follow the loading dose with a second dose in 10–15 minutes if needed. A maximum of 8 mg in a 24-hour period is accompanied by either phenytoin (PO) or fosphenytoin (IV) loading.

    b) Prophylactic seizure therapy is not recommended due to insufficient data.

    c) However, prophylactic anticonvulsant therapy is recommended to reduce seizure risk in patients with lobar hemorrhage (see Chapter 144).

E. Maintenance of medical stability

1. Perform continuous cardiac monitoring to observe for ischemic changes and dysrhythmias (see Chapter 45).

2. Control blood pressure (see Chapter 47).

    a) Recommendations for acute ischemic stroke indicate blood pressure should be treated only if extreme (systolic blood pressure greater than 220 mm Hg or diastolic blood pressure greater than 120 mm Hg) or if treating patients with comorbidity of ischemic coronary disease, heart failure, aortic dissection, hypertensive encephalopathy, or AKI.

    b) Lower blood pressure guardedly. Reduce by 15% during the first 24 hours after stroke onset.

        (1) IV labetalol is the drug of choice. Sequential imaging of the brain is essential for moderating blood pressure treatment.

(2) Antihypertensives can be initiated 24 hours after stroke onset in neurologically stable patients with known hypertension (prior to the event).

(3) Before initiating thrombolytics, maintain systolic blood pressure less than or equal to 185 mm Hg and diastolic blood pressure less than or equal to 110 mm Hg. Blood pressure is optimally kept less than 180/105 mm Hg for at least 24 hours after IV rtPA treatment.

(4) Blood pressure control in intracranial hemorrhage requires cautious moderation. Both subarachnoid hemorrhage and intracerebral hemorrhage are affected by blood pressure extremes. Elevated blood pressure can increase propensity for bleed, and low blood pressure will predispose to hypoperfusion of the brain. American Heart Association/American Stroke Association guidelines recommend the following measures.

   (a) If systolic blood pressure is greater than 200 mm Hg, consider aggressive reduction of blood pressure with continuous IV infusion of medication accompanied by blood pressure monitoring every five minutes.

   (b) If systolic blood pressure is greater than 180 mm Hg, mean arterial pressure greater than 130 mm Hg, and suspicion of elevated ICP, consider monitoring ICP and reducing blood pressure using intermittent or continuous IV medication, and maintain cerebral perfusion pressure in the range of 61–80 mm Hg.

   (c) If systolic blood pressure is greater than 180 mm Hg or mean arterial pressure greater than 130 mm Hg and no evidence or suspicion of elevated ICP, consider a modest reduction of blood pressure (e.g., target mean arterial pressure of 110 mm Hg or target blood pressure of 160/90 mm Hg) using intermittent or continuous IV medication, and reexamine the patient every 15 minutes.

   (d) Hypotension and hypovolemia are critical to systemic perfusion and should be corrected.

3. Maintain patent airway and oxygenation.

   a) Do not administer supplemental oxygen unless patient is hypoxic as indicated by pulse oximetry. Order supplemental oxygen if oxygen saturation is less than 94%.

   b) Elective intubation may be necessary to facilitate oxygenation of acute stroke patients with brain swelling or acutely elevated ICP.

4. Maintain glucose level (see Chapter 151).

   a) Hyperglycemia is associated with poor clinical outcome for individuals with acute ischemic stroke.

   b) American Heart Association/American Stroke Association guidelines recommend treating patients whose serum glucose is greater than 185 mg/dl with insulin and fluids.

   c) Correct hypoglycemia (blood glucose less than 60 mg/dl) with glucose administration.

5. Prevent aspiration. Keep patient NPO until assessment of gag reflex and swallowing ability with dysphagia.

   a) Administer IV isotonic saline solution at 50 ml/hr for hydration unless otherwise indicated.

   b) Assess nutritional status and fluid balance through intake and output.

   c) If the patient is dysphagic, total parenteral nutrition or tube feedings are warranted until the patient can swallow properly. Dysphagia may be temporary or permanent.

6. Treat fever with acetaminophen and cooling blankets (temperature greater than 100.4°F [38°C]) during acute phase of stroke to reduce poor outcome.

7. Maintain skin integrity with change in bowel or bladder control.

   a) Use Foley catheter initially until bladder training can be initiated (see Chapter 84).

   b) Initiate bowel schedule (see Chapter 55).

F. Stroke prevention

1. Primary prevention

   a) Healthy diet recommendations: Encourage increased intake of fruits and vegetables, whole grain foods with low glycemic load, monounsaturated fats, and omega-3 fatty acid consumption through fish, plant sources, or supplements. Mediterranean diet supplemented with nuts (e.g., almonds, walnuts, hazelnuts) or olive oil is optimal. Limit intake of red meat, sugar-sweetened beverages, saturated fat, and trans fat.

   b) Smoking cessation: Counsel the patient on a regular basis to quit tobacco use and recommend medication assistance, behavioral therapy, and support groups.

   c) Physical activity: Adults should participate in at least 150 minutes per week of moderate-intensity or 75 minutes per week of vigorous-intensity aerobic activity.

   d) Weight loss: Encourage weight loss. Optimal BMI is less than 25 kg/m².

   e) Alcohol: Promote modest alcohol consumption of one to two drinks a day for men and one drink a day for women.

   f) ASA: Recommend according to stroke versus bleeding risk of the individual. Low dose of 81 mg PO daily should be considered for patients aged 40–70 years, with higher atherosclerotic cardiovascular disease risk. Low-dose ASA should not be routinely recommended for adults older than 70 years or for adults of any age particularly if at high risk for bleeding.

   g) Hypertension control: Goal blood pressure should be less than 140 mm Hg systolic and less than 90 mm Hg diastolic for most patients. Goal for patients with diabetes and renal disease is less than 130 systolic and less than 80 diastolic (see Chapter 47). DASH (Dietary Approaches to Stop Hypertension) diet in conjunction with low sodium (less than 1,500 mg) diet aids blood pressure control.

   h) Dyslipidemia control: Estimate total cardiovascular risk and determine LDL goal. The U.S. Preventive Services Task Force recommends initiating statin treatment for most patients with 10-year atherosclerotic cardiovascular disease risk greater than 10% with at least one cardiovascular disease risk factor.

      (1) Recommend a statin if LDL cholesterol greater than or equal to 190 mg/dl and patient is aged 20–75 years.

      (2) Recommend lifestyle changes or implement statin therapy. Initiate fibrates if triglyceride greater than 200 mg/dl and HDL less than 40 mg/dl (see Chapter 44).

   i) Diabetes management: Goal Hgb A1c is less than or equal to 6.5 % for most patients (see Chapter 151).

2. Secondary prevention

   a) Antihypertensive therapy: American Heart Association/American Stroke Association guidelines recommend hypertensive treatment for all patients following ischemic stroke and transient ischemic attack (see Chapter 47).

   b) Maintain glycemic control in diabetics: Goal Hgb A1c is less than or equal to 6.5% for most patients (see Chapter 151).

   c) Treat dyslipidemia: If no cardiovascular events, target LDL should be less than 70 mg/dl (see Chapter 44).

   d) Antiplatelet therapy: Most patients with atherosclerotic stroke or transient ischemic attack require ASA with extended-release dipyridamole (25 mg/200 mg

PO two times a day) or clopidogrel alone (75 mg PO daily) to reduce the risk of secondary stroke. Discontinuing antiplatelet therapy in high-risk patients may increase stroke risk. For patients preparing for carotid endarterectomy, ASA dose of 81–325 mg PO daily is recommended prior to the procedure and continued if no contraindications exist.

e) Antiplatelet therapy for transient ischemic attack of atherothrombotic, lacunar (small-vessel occlusive type), noncardioembolic stroke, or cryptogenic type should include either clopidogrel (75 mg PO daily) alone or the combination of ASA plus extended-release dipyridamole (25 mg/200 mg PO two times a day) rather than ASA alone.

f) Atrial fibrillation (see Chapter 45): Anticoagulant or antiplatelet therapy should be used to reduce the risk of systemic embolization in patients with nonvalvular atrial fibrillation. Currently, American Heart Association recommends initiation of novel oral anticoagulants for the prevention of ischemic stroke and transient ischemic attack.

VII. Follow-up: Determined by severity, cause of the stroke, and if complications are present (Caprio & Sorond, 2019; Morawo & Adams, 2019; Muller et al., 2019)
   A. Short term: Schedule follow-up within six weeks of discharge. Evaluate for depression at each follow-up visit.
   B. Collaborative, organized poststroke care is advisable for an optimal outcome with follow-up at regular intervals.

VIII. Referrals (Caprio & Sorond, 2019)
   A. Neurologist and stroke team: Referral to neurosurgeon at time of onset to manage stroke and control or treat bleeding through necessary surgical interventions
   B. Interventional radiologist: If clot retrieval is feasible
   C. Speech pathologist: For assessment of swallowing, language impairments, or dysarthria
   D. Cardiology: If warranted
   E. Sleep disorder specialist: Sleep apnea testing
   F. Nutritionist: For assistance with identifying nutritive food sources, particularly during dysphagia
   G. Psychologist: For assessment and treatment of psychiatric status; for family counseling to aid with lifestyle adjustments needed for transition to home care
   H. Physical therapist: For evaluation of deficits and need for assistive devices
   I. Occupational therapist: For treatment of decreased cognitive or upper extremity function and the need for adaptive equipment
   J. Social services: For discharge planning and coordination of services
   K. Spiritual services: To facilitate fulfillment of spiritual needs per patient preference
   L. Urologist: For bladder training or treatment of incontinence

References

Arnett, D.K., Blumenthal, R.S., Albert, M.A., Buroker, A.B., Goldberger, Z.D., Hahn, E.J., ... Ziaeian, B. (2019). 2019 ACC/AHA guideline on the primary prevention of cardiovascular disease: A report of the American College of Cardiology/American Heart Association task force on clinical practice guidelines. *Circulation, 140*(11), e596–e646. https://doi.org/10.1161/CIR.0000000000000678

Bright, C.J., Hawkins, M.M., Guha, J., Henson, K.E., Winter, D.L., Kelly, J.S., ... Reulen, R.C. (2017). Risk of cerebrovascular events in 178962 five-year survivors of cancer diagnosed at 15 to 39 years of age: The TYACSS (Teenage and Young Adult Cancer Survivor Study). *Circulation, 135*(13), 1194–1210. https://doi.org/10.1161/CIRCULATIONAHA.116.025778

Caprio, F.Z., & Sorond, F.A. (2019). Cerebrovascular disease: Primary and secondary stroke prevention. *Medical Clinics of North America, 103*(2), 295–308. https://doi.org/10.1016/j.mcna.2018.10.001

Dearborn, J.L., Urrutia, V.C., & Zeiler, S.R. (2014). Stroke and cancer—A complicated relationship. *Journal of Neurology and Translational Neuroscience, 2*(1), 1039.

Fugate, J.E., & Rabinstein, A.A. (2015). Absolute and relative contraindications to IV rt-PA for acute ischemic stroke. *Neurohospitalist, 5*(3), 110–121. https://doi.org/10.1177/1941874415578532

Gross, B.A., Jankowitz, B.T., & Friedlander, R.M. (2019). Cerebral intraparenchymal hemorrhage: A review. *JAMA, 321*(13), 1295–1303. https://doi.org/10.1001/jama.2019.2413

Guzik, A., & Bushnell, C. (2017). Stroke epidemiology and risk factor management. *Continuum, 23*(1), 15–39. https://doi.org/10.1212/CON.0000000000000416

Knight-Greenfield, A., Nario, J.J.Q., & Gupta, A. (2019). Causes of acute stroke: A patterned approach. *Radiologic Clinics of North America, 57*(6), 1093–1108. https://doi.org/10.1016/j.rcl.2019.07.007

Lin, A.L., & Avila, E.K. (2017). Neurologic emergencies in the cancer patient: Diagnosis and management. *Journal of Intensive Care Medicine, 32*(2), 99–115. https://doi.org/10.1177/0885066615619582

Matthews, A., Stanway, S., Farmer, R.E., Strongman, H., Thomas, S., Lyon, A.R., ... Bhaskaran, K. (2018). Long term adjuvant endocrine therapy and risk of cardiovascular disease in female breast cancer survivors: Systematic review. *BMJ, 363,* k3845. https://doi.org/10.1136/bmj.k3845

Meng, F., Zhu, S., Zhao, J., Vados, L., Wang, L., Zhao, Y., ... Niu, Y. (2016). Stroke related to androgen deprivation therapy for prostate cancer: A meta-analysis and systematic review. *BMC Cancer, 16,* 180. https://doi.org/10.1186/s12885-016-2221-5

Morawo, A.O., & Adams, C.A. (2019). Early management of acute ischaemic stroke: A clinical perspective. *West African Journal of Medicine, 36*(3), 286–289.

Muller, C., Roizman, M., & Wong, A. (2019). Secondary prevention of ischaemic stroke. *Internal Medicine Journal, 49*(10), 1221–1228. https://doi.org/10.1111/imj.14454

National Institutes of Health. (n.d.). NIH stroke scale. https://www.stroke.nih.gov/resources/scale.htm

Navi, B.B., & Iadecola, C. (2018). Ischemic stroke in cancer patients: A review of an underappreciated pathology. *Annals of Neurology, 83*(5), 873–883. https://doi.org/10.1002/ana.25227

Potter, C.A., Vagal, A.S., Goyal, M., Nunez, D.B., Leslie-Mazwi, T.M., & Lev, M.H. (2019). CT for treatment selection in acute ischemic stroke: A code stroke primer. *RadioGraphics, 39*(6), 1717–1738. https://doi.org/10.1148/rg.2019190142

Powers, W.J., Rabinstein, A.A., Ackerson, T., Adeoye, O.M., Banbakidis, N.C., Becker, K., ... Tirschwell, D.L. (2018). 2018 guidelines for the early management of patients with acute ischemic stroke: A guideline for healthcare professionals from the American Heart Association/American Stroke Association. *Stroke, 49*(3), e46–e99. https://doi.org/10.1161/STR.0000000000000158

Shao, Z., Tu, S., & Shao, A. (2019). Pathophysiological mechanisms and potential therapeutic targets in intracerebral hemorrhage. *Frontiers in Pharmacology, 10,* 1079. https://doi.org/10.3389/fphar.2019.01079

Splittgerber, R. (2019). *Snell's clinical neuroanatomy.* Wolters Kluwer.

Tsiygoulis, G., Safouris, A., Kim, D.E., & Alexandrov, A.V. (2018). Recent advances in primary and secondary prevention of atherosclerotic stroke. *Journal of Stroke, 20*(2), 145–166. https://doi.org/10.5853/jos.2018.00773

Urdaneta, A.E., & Bhalla, P. (2019). Cutting edge acute ischemic stroke management. *Emergency Medical Clinics of North America, 37*(3), 365–379. https://doi.org/10.1016/j.emc.2019.03.001

U.S. Preventive Services Task Force. (2016). Statin use for the primary prevention of cardiovascular disease in adults: US Preventive Services Task Force recommendation statement. *JAMA, 316*(19), 1997–2007. https://doi.org/10.1001/jama.2016.15450

Wilbers, J., Sondag, L., Mulder, S., Siegerink, B., & van Dijk, E.J. (2020). Cancer prevalence higher in stroke patients than in the general population: The Dutch String-of-Pearls Institute (PSI) stroke study. *European Journal of Neurology, 27*(1), 85–91. https://doi.org/10.1111/ene.14037

Yew, K.S., & Cheng, E. (2015). Diagnosis of acute stroke. *American Family Physician, 91*(8), 528–536. https://www.aafp.org/afp/2015/0415/p528.html

Metabolic

CHAPTER 147

Fever

Christina Ferraro, MSN, APRN–CNP, BMTCN®

I. Definition (Beresford & Gosbell, 2016; Fernandes e Santana et al., 2019; Fernandez & Beeching, 2018; Meier & Lee, 2017)
   A. A single episode of elevated temperature is greater than or equal to 100.4°F (38°C).
   B. Fever of unknown origin (FUO) is described as a temperature greater than 101°F (38°C) that persists for three or more weeks without identified etiology despite one week of extensive investigation.

II. Physiology/Pathophysiology (Beresford & Gosbell, 2016; Fernandez & Beeching, 2018; Pasikhova et al., 2017; van der Velden et al., 2014; Walter et al., 2016)
   A. Normal
      1. Body temperature normally is controlled by the thermoregulatory center in the hypothalamus.
      2. Host defense involves both antigen-specific and antigen-independent mechanisms to reduce fever.
         a) Acquired or adaptive immunity involves antigen recognition by T and B lymphocytes.
         b) Innate immunity recognizes molecular markers through cellular effectors such as macrophages, neutrophils, mast cells, and natural killer cells.
   B. Pathophysiology
      1. Fever may be related to a disease state, infectious pathogen, or inflammation.
         a) The hypothalamus may be stimulated by pyrogens, including both endogenous and exogenous pyrogens. Pyrogens are substances that can induce fever.
            (1) Exogenous pyrogens stimulate fever, such as bacteria, virus, or fungi.
            (2) Endogenous pyrogen cytokines stimulate fever, such as IL-1, IL-6, and TNF.
         b) During fevers, heat loss mechanisms (e.g., vasodilation, sweating) assist in returning the temperature to normal levels.
      2. Febrile response may be induced by IL-1β production in the hypothalamus and brain stem.
      3. Bacterial lipopolysaccharides may induce fever mediated by pyrogenic cytokines such as IL-1β.
      4. Other mechanisms in the febrile response include prostaglandin activation, heme oxygenase pathway, and T-cell stimuli of the immune system.
      5. Bacteremia or any stimulus that rapidly increases the hypothalamic set point can produce rigors (see Figure 147-1).
         a) Cutaneous vasoconstriction occurs when the hypothalamus responds to a stimuli; thus, the patient feels cold.

FIGURE 147-1 **Common Bacterial Causes of Febrile Episodes in Neutropenic Patients**

Gram-Positive Cocci and Bacilli	**Gram-Negative Cocci and Bacilli**	**Anaerobic Cocci and Bacilli**

• *Staphylococcus* species
  – Coagulase positive (*Staphylococcus aureus*)
  – Coagulase negative (*Staphylococcus epidermidis* and others)
• *Streptococcus* species
  – *Streptococcus pneumoniae*
  – *Streptococcus pyogenes*
  – Viridans group
	• *Acinetobacter* species
	• *Escherichia coli*
	• *Enterobacter* species
	• *Haemophilus influenzae*
	• *Klebsiella* species
	• *Pseudomonas aeruginosa*
	• *Pseudomonas* species (other than *P. aeruginosa*)
	• *Proteus* species
		• *Bacteroides* species
		• *Clostridium* species

Note. Based on information from National Comprehensive Cancer Network, 2021a, 2021b; Taplitz, Kennedy, Bow, et al., 2018.

    b) Fever defervescence with decrease in body temperature causes cutaneous vasodilation. Drenching sweat usually terminates an episode of fever.

    c) Most common organisms are gram-positive cocci and bacilli with *Staphylococcus* species predominant.

    d) Gram-negative bacilli, such as *Escherichia coli*, *Pseudomonas aeruginosa*, and *Klebsiella pneumoniae*, are less frequent but more lethal.

6. *Candida* species (yeasts) are not as common but are more lethal than gram-positive organisms. Typically, these organisms enter the bloodstream via translocation across the GI tract.

7. Each degree of temperature results in approximately 7% increase in metabolic rate and increased demands on the heart.

    a) Endothermic changes are observed at 104°F (40°C) in the nucleus of cellular regenerations.

    b) Extreme temperature (108°F [41°C]) causes direct cellular damage.

    c) Vascular endothelium seems particularly susceptible to cell damage; thus, DIC usually results.

8. Drug fever is suspected when no other cause of fever can be found (see Figure 147-2).

    a) Onset appears 7–10 days after drug administration and reverses with discontinuation of the drug.

    b) Fever can occur as a result of hypersensitivity reaction, altered thermoregulatory mechanism, reaction to the drug's mechanism of action, or idiosyncratic reaction.

III. Clinical features: Fever may be caused by different diseases and remains one of the most reliable hallmarks of disease. Most fevers are associated with self-limited infections (usually viral) and have easily identified causes. In patients with cancer, FUO may occur without proven evidence of infection. Fever generally is increased in the evening and decreased in the morning. Patients can have a history of fevers that recur over months or years in the absence of an associated viral or bacterial infection. After exclusion of infection and malignancy, consideration must be given to uncommon disorders causing fever. FUO is caused by infections (30%–40%), malignancy (20%–30%), collagen vascular diseases (10%–20%), and miscellaneous diseases (15%–20%) (Beresford & Gosbell, 2016; Fernandes e Santana et al., 2019; Fernandez & Beeching, 2018; Gödel et al., 2018; Hill et al., 2018; Lyman et al., 2014; Meier & Lee, 2017; Pasikhova et al., 2017; van der Velden et al., 2014; Walter et al., 2016).

  A. Etiology

    1. Malignancy

2. Periodic fever syndromes
3. Bacterial infections: Common in the neutropenic host (see Figure 147-1)
4. Gram infections: Approximately 60%–70% of documented infections are gram-positive; gram-negative infection occurrence is increasing.
5. Viral infections
   a) The most common viruses in neutropenic hosts are HSV and VZV.
   b) CMV infections may occur in recipients of HSCT or those who have otherwise been immunosuppressed for long periods of time.
6. Fungal infections: Caused by the *Candida* or *Aspergillus* species and have been reported in up to one-third of patients who experience febrile neutropenia
7. Immune mechanisms: Connective tissue diseases, drug reactions, hemolytic anemia
8. CAR T-cell immunotherapy: Cytokine release syndrome is a systemic inflammatory reaction with symptoms including, but not limited to, fever, rigors, hypotension, and tachypnea.
9. Vascular inflammation or thrombosis
10. Inflammatory bowel disease
11. Cancer treatment related: Occurs during chemotherapy in 40%–70% of cases and may be related to the agent used or tumor destruction

B. History
1. History of cancer and cancer treatment
2. Current medications: Prescribed, over the counter
3. History of presenting symptoms: Precipitating factors, onset, duration, associated symptoms (e.g., headache; abdominal, back, and neck pain; rash; malaise; mental status changes)
4. Changes in ADLs
5. History of recent travel, insect bites, animal contact, toxic substance exposure, venipuncture, recent infections, treatment

---

FIGURE 147-2   **Drugs Implicated in the Development of Fever**

Common
- Amphotericin B
- Asparaginase
- Atropine
- Barbiturates
- Beta-lactam antibiotics
- Bleomycin
- Cephalosporins
- Diphenylhydantoin
- H_1 and H_2 antihistamines
- Interferon
- Interleukin-2
- Methyldopa
- Penicillin
- Phenytoin
- Procainamide
- Quinidine
- Salicylates
- Sulfonamides (including sulfa-containing laxatives)
- Thyroid agents

Less Common
- Allopurinol
- Azathioprine
- Cimetidine
- Hydralazine
- Imipenem
- Iodides
- Isoniazid
- Metoclopramide
- Minocycline
- Nifedipine
- Nonsteroidal anti-inflammatory drugs
- Rifampin
- Streptokinase
- Vancomycin

Rare
- Aminoglycosides
- Chloramphenicol
- Clindamycin
- Corticosteroids
- Macrolides
- Salicylates (therapeutic doses)
- Tetracyclines
- Vitamin preparations

Note. Based on information from Fernandez & Beeching 2018; Meier & Lee, 2017.

C. Signs and symptoms: Refer to specific disease chapters for further information.
   1. Diaphoresis
   2. Chills or rigors: Uncontrolled violent shaking or trembling may precede or accompany fever.
   3. Productive or nonproductive cough
   4. Myalgia
   5. Arthralgia
   6. Neutropenic patients: Unable to exhibit signs of infection (e.g., purulent drainage) except for fever

D. Physical examination
   1. Vital signs: Temperature elevation, tachycardia, tachypnea, hypotension, signs of sepsis
   2. Integument: Rashes, altered integrity, petechiae, pustular or vesicular lesions; venous access site monitoring for erythema, edema, or drainage
   3. HEENT
      a) Oral: Mucosal integrity, erythema, lesions, bleeding
      b) Ophthalmoscopic: Infections in the eye
      c) Sinus: Tender or opacified sinuses, facial pain, nasal drainage indicating sinusitis
   4. Pulmonary: Abnormal lung sounds suggesting pneumonia
   5. Cardiac: Abnormal heart sounds (e.g., friction rubs, murmurs) suggesting endocarditis
   6. Abdominal: Masses or organomegaly, pain, rebound tenderness
   7. Posterior thorax: Costovertebral tenderness indicating kidney infection
   8. Musculoskeletal: Connective tissue disorder
      a) Muscle strength against gravity and resistance
      b) Joint: Range of motion, swelling, tenderness, erythema, warmth
   9. Lymph node: Enlargement and tenderness indicating infection (see Appendix D)
   10. Genital and perirectal: Rash, ulceration, lesions, induration, tenderness
   11. Neurologic: Meningeal irritation, changes in mentation

IV. Diagnostic tests (Fernandes e Santana et al., 2019; Fernandez & Beeching, 2018; Lehrnbecher et al., 2017; Meier & Lee, 2017; Taplitz, Kennedy, & Flowers, 2018)
   A. Laboratory
      1. CBC with differential
         a) Calculate ANC (see Table 147-1) to evaluate for neutropenic fever.
         b) Increased bands or left shift suggests bacterial infection.
      2. LFTs to evaluate hepatic function and liver disease
      3. Uric acid to evaluate kidney function and presence of gout

TABLE 147-1   Definition of Neutropenia

Absolute Neutrophil Count

$$\frac{\text{white blood cell count} \times (\text{neutrophils} + \text{bands})}{100}$$

	Susceptibility to Infection
< 1,000/mm³	Expected increased susceptibility to infection
< 500/mm³	Greater risk for infection
< 100/mm³	Extreme risk for life-threatening infection

Note. Based on information from National Comprehensive Cancer Network, 2021a; Taplitz, Kennedy, Bow, et al., 2018; Taplitz, Kennedy, & Flowers, 2018.

4. Blood cultures to evaluate for bacteria, fungi, and viruses (peripheral and central lines as appropriate)
5. Viral titers to evaluate for hepatitis, Epstein-Barr virus, CMV, and parvovirus
6. Urinalysis and urine culture to evaluate for UTI
7. Stool cultures to evaluate for *Clostridium difficile*, ova, parasites, viruses, and fungi
8. Sputum cultures to evaluate for fungi, viruses, and *Legionella*; acid-fast smear for TB
9. Wound culture to evaluate for wound infection
10. Rheumatoid factor to evaluate for RA
11. ESR to evaluate for inflammatory, autoimmune, or malignant disease
12. Antinuclear antibodies to evaluate for SLE, polyarthritis, and lupoid hepatitis
13. Quantitative Ig levels and subclasses to evaluate for immune deficiency or allergies
14. Lyme disease titers to evaluate for diagnosis of Lyme disease
15. SPEP to evaluate for protein deficiency and other conditions such as malignancy causing fever
16. HIV antibody assay and viral load for patients at high risk
17. Thyroid panel to evaluate for thyroid diseases

B. Radiology
1. Chest radiography to evaluate for pulmonary infiltrates, consolidation, or nodules
2. Radiographs of bones: Specific for diagnosis suspected
3. High-resolution chest CT scan to evaluate for *Aspergillus* pulmonary infection and presence of abscess or tumor
4. Echocardiogram or transesophageal echocardiogram to evaluate for valvular disease
5. Bone scan to detect infection or malignancy
6. Gallium scan to evaluate benign or malignant neoplasms or inflammatory lesions
7. MRI to evaluate for intracranial, spinal, or soft tissue abnormalities

C. Other
1. Bronchoscopy with lavage or biopsy to evaluate for infection or malignant disease
2. Skin tests
   a) Tuberculin or purified protein derivative in patients who have been exposed to or suspected of having TB
   b) Delayed hypersensitivity skin tests (e.g., intradermal skin tests) to evaluate the patient's cellular immune response
      (1) This may be done in patients with infections that are recurrent or caused by unusual organisms or who may have delayed hypersensitivity.
      (2) Several skin tests can be used including *Candida*, purified protein derivative, mumps, tetanus toxoid, and *Trichophyton*.
3. Bone marrow biopsy and aspirate to evaluate for malignant disease or infection in the bone marrow
4. Other biopsies, as indicated
   a) Open lung biopsy to diagnose pulmonary disease, as indicated
   b) Lymph node biopsy to evaluate for malignant disease or infection
   c) Liver biopsy to evaluate for hepatic disease, malignancy, or infection
   d) Skin biopsy to evaluate for malignancy or infection

V. Differential diagnosis (Beresford & Gosbell, 2016; Fernandes e Santana et al., 2019; Fernandez & Beeching, 2018; Meier & Lee, 2017; Mikkilineni & Gea-Banacloche, 2019; Walter et al., 2016)
   A. Tumor fever is common in the following diseases.
      1. Lymphoma
      2. Acute leukemia

        3. Chronic leukemia

        4. Multiple myeloma

        5. Solid tumors

        6. Hodgkin lymphoma

        7. Osteogenic sarcoma

        8. Liver metastasis

  B. Drug fevers (see Figure 147-2)

  C. Nosocomial fever

  D. Early sign of septic shock (see Chapter 160)

  E. Infectious organisms (see Figure 147-1)

  F. PFAPA (periodic fever, aphthous stomatitis, pharyngitis, adenitis) syndrome

  G. Cyclic neutropenia

  H. Genetic disorders: Familial Mediterranean fever, hyperimmunoglobulin D syndrome

  I. Abscess

  J. TB (see Chapter 36)

  K. Endocarditis (see Chapter 46)

  L. Hepatobiliary infections

  M. Osteomyelitis

  N. Autoimmune diseases

  O. Hyperthyroidism (see Chapter 157)

VI. Treatment: The vast majority of fevers are associated with self-limited infections, most commonly with a viral etiology (Aapro et al., 2017; Beyar-Katz et al., 2017; Fernandez & Beeching, 2018; Lehrnbecher et al., 2017; Meier & Lee, 2017; Mikkilineni & Gea-Banacloche, 2019; NCCN, 2021a, 2021b; Pasikhova et al., 2017; Smith et al., 2015; Taplitz, Kennedy, Bow, et al., 2018; Taplitz, Kennedy, & Flowers, 2018)

  A. Treatment is dependent on etiology.

  B. Infectious Diseases Society of America guidelines describe recommendations for management of fever and neutropenia (see Table 147-2).

  C. Empiric antibiotic therapy: High-risk patients with febrile neutropenia (see Figure 147-3 and Appendix C)

      1. Hospitalization for IV empiric antibiotic therapy within one hour of admission without waiting for culture results

      2. Monotherapy with an antipseudomonal beta-lactam agent

         a) Cefepime: 2 g IV every eight hours

         b) Meropenem: 1 g IV every eight hours

         c) Piperacillin/tazobactam: 4.5 g IV every six hours if confirmed or suspected extended spectrum beta-lactamase

         d) Imipenem/cilastatin: 500 mg IV every six hours if confirmed or suspected extended spectrum beta-lactamase

         e) Other antimicrobials may be added for management of complications (hypotension and pneumonia) or if antimicrobial resistance is suspected or proven.

         f) Oral combination ciprofloxacin plus amoxicillin/clavulanate for low-risk patients should not be used if quinolone prophylaxis was used.

         g) Additional agents for documented infection should be added with resistant gram-positive organisms or if certain risk factors (e.g., serious catheter infection, MRSA, penicillin/cephalosporin-resistant pneumococci infection, hypotension or septic shock, soft tissue infection) are present: vancomycin, linezolid, daptomycin, quinupristin/dalfopristin.

TABLE 147-2	Infectious Diseases Society of America Guidelines: Executive Summary
Guideline	**Recommendation**
Initial antibiotic therapy	Low risk: Levofloxacin 500–750 mg PO or IV daily or ciprofloxacin 500–750 mg PO every 12 hours High risk: Monotherapy with antipseudomonal beta-lactam agent: cefepime, meropenem, imipenem
Modification of therapy during first week of therapy	Patient is afebrile in 3–5 days. • If etiology is identified, adjust therapy as appropriate. • If etiology is not identified, patient is low risk, and oral antibiotic has been initiated, continue therapy. • If the patient is low risk and IV therapy was initially begun, change to oral ciprofloxacin plus amoxicillin/clavulanate. • If the patient is at high risk initially, continue IV antibiotics. Persistent fever throughout the first 3–5 days • Reassess fever throughout day 3; if no clinical worsening, continue same antibiotics. • Stop vancomycin if cultures do not identify a causative organism. • If there is progressive illness, change antibiotics. Broaden to include coverage for resistant gram-negative, gram-positive, and anaerobic bacteria and fungi. • If patient is febrile after 5 days, consider adding an antifungal drug with or without change in antibiotic therapy.
Duration of antibiotic therapy	In patients with clinically or microbiologically documented infections, the duration of therapy is dictated by the particular organism and site. Appropriate antibiotics should continue for at least the duration of neutropenia (until ANC ≥ 500/mm³) or longer if clinically necessary. In patients with unexplained fever, the initial regimen should be continued until clear signs of marrow recovery with an increasing ANC ≥ 500/mm³. If an appropriate antibiotic treatment course has been completed and all signs of a documented infection have resolved, patients who remain neutropenic may resume oral fluoroquinolone prophylaxis until marrow recovery.
Antiviral drugs	Not recommended for routine use unless evidence of viral infection is identified Inactivated influenza vaccine yearly
Granulocyte transfusions	Not recommended for routine use
Colony-stimulating factors	Not recommended for routine use but may be considered if clinical condition of patient is predictive of poor outcome
Antibiotic prophylaxis	Low risk: Not routinely recommended for afebrile neutropenic patients because of antibiotic resistance High risk: Fluoroquinolone prophylaxis should be considered for high-risk patients with expected duration of prolonged or profound neutropenia (ANC ≤ 100/mm³) more than 7 days. Trimethoprim/sulfamethoxazole (single- or double-strength daily or double-strength 3 times per week) may be used to prevent *Pneumocystis jirovecii* pneumonia.
Prophylaxis	Patients undergoing allogeneic hematopoietic stem cell transplantation or who are at risk for profound, protracted neutropenia, such as those with AML/MDS: • Antifungal prophylaxis with an oral triazole or parenteral echinocandin (i.e., fluconazole 100 mg PO daily) • Antiviral prophylaxis (acyclovir 400 mg PO two times a day) • Anti-cytomegalovirus prophylaxis (letermovir 480 mg PO daily) • Hepatitis B reactivation prevention if indicated (entecavir)

AML—acute myeloid leukemia; ANC—absolute neutrophil count; MDS—myelodysplastic syndrome

Note. Based on information from National Comprehensive Cancer Network, 2021a, 2021b; Taplitz, Kennedy, Bow, et al., 2018.

FIGURE 147-3 **High-Risk and Low-Risk Patients With Fever and Neutropenia**

High Risk
- Age > 60 years
- Alteration in physical barrier (e.g., skin, oral mucosa)
- Comorbidities
- Exposure to pathogens
- Hepatic insufficiency
- Hypotension
- Immunocompromised
- Inpatient at time of fever development
- Invasive procedure
- Neurologic changes
- New-onset abdominal pain
- Pneumonia
- Prolonged neutropenia
- Renal insufficiency
- Use of equipment (e.g., ventilators)

Low Risk
- Absence of chronic obstructive pulmonary disease, diabetes, blood loss, dehydration, and fungal infections
- Age < 60 years
- Anticipate short duration of neutropenia
- Asymptomatic
- Mild to moderate symptoms
- No hepatic or renal insufficiency
- Outpatient status at time of fever development
- Stable vital signs

Note. Based on information from National Comprehensive Cancer Network, 2021b; Taplitz, Kennedy, Bow, et al., 2018.

    h) Fevers in high-risk patients lasting greater than or equal to 96 hours should initiate an azole antifungal (e.g., fluconazole, voriconazole), echinocandin (e.g., caspofungin, micafungin), or amphotericin B for empiric antifungal therapy along with further testing.

D. Vancomycin or amikacin may be added for patients at high risk for gram-positive or gram-negative organisms, respectively, who have no response to monotherapy in 48–72 hours.
    1. Vancomycin: 25–30 mg/kg for initial dose, then 15–20 mg/kg IV every 12 hours
    2. Amikacin: Dosing individualized with monitoring of levels

E. Antifungal prophylaxis with use of fluconazole, voriconazole, and posaconazole may be used in HSCT recipients or patients with leukemia receiving chemotherapy.

F. Oral antibiotic therapy, including a quinolone and a drug effective against gram-positive organisms, may be used for patients with neutropenic fever who are hemodynamically stable and at low risk for infection.
    1. Ciprofloxacin: 500–750 mg PO every 12 hours
    2. Levofloxacin: 500–750 mg PO daily

G. The use of G-CSF may be considered for high-risk patients with neutropenic fever in the primary or secondary prophylactic setting, but clinical benefits have not been clearly documented in the therapeutic setting.
    1. 5 mcg/kg subcutaneous daily
    2. Long-acting 6 mcg subcutaneous for one dose

H. Antipyretics often are used to minimize the discomforts of fever (e.g., chills, seizures, delirium). Adverse effects may limit their use.
    1. Acetaminophen: Drug is preferred for patients with gastric ulcers and clotting disorders.
        a) Doses of 325–650 mg PO every four hours may be used.
        b) Do not exceed 4,000 mg in a 24-hour period.
    2. NSAIDs: Drug should be used with caution in febrile neutropenia because these agents can mask fevers and compromise gastric mucosa, putting patients at risk of gram-negative sepsis (see Appendix E).

3. Corticosteroids: Side effects limit their use for controlling fever, but they may be used for high fever unresponsive to other interventions (see Appendix K).

I. Cytokine release syndrome from CAR T-cell or BiTE (bispecific T-cell engager) therapy
 1. Treat with tocilizumab IV 4–8 mg/kg actual body weight up to every eight hours, not to exceed 800 mg daily, for up to four doses. A maximum of three doses is allowed in a 24-hour period.
 2. Dexamethasone and other supportive therapies are also useful.

J. Maintain hydration with PO and IV fluids to prevent dehydration.

K. Physical methods of controlling body temperature
 1. Tepid baths, sponging
 2. Ice packs, cooling blankets
 3. Air conditioning, fans

VII. Follow-up (Walter & Carraretto, 2016; Walter et al., 2016)
 A. Frequent and repeated physical examinations are imperative to evaluate FUO.
 B. Hospitalization may be required to evaluate FUO, especially in neutropenic patients whose ANC is less than 500/mm³.
 C. Long-term cognitive or neurologic changes after prolonged fevers can occur and should be monitored.

VIII. Referrals: Referrals may be necessary to assist in evaluating FUO. Specialties to consider include infectious disease, pharmacy, hematology, pulmonary, cardiology, gastroenterology, dermatology, neurology, and rheumatology (Pasikhova et al., 2017; Walter & Carraretto, 2016; Walter et al., 2016).

The author would like to acknowledge Dawn Camp-Sorrell, MSN, FNP, AOCN®, for her contribution to this chapter that remains unchanged from the previous edition of this book.

References

Aapro, M., Boccia, R., Leonard, R., Camps, C., Campone, M., Choquet, S., ... Valero, V. (2017). Refining the role of pegfilgrastim (a long-acting G-CSF) for prevention of chemotherapy-induced febrile neutropenia: consensus guidance recommendations. *Supportive Care in Cancer, 25*(11), 3295–3304. https://doi.org/10.1007/s00520-017-3842-1

Beresford, R.W., & Gosbell, I.B. (2016). Pyrexia of unknown origin: Causes, investigation and management. *Internal Medicine Journal, 46*(9), 1011–1016. https://doi.org/10.1111/imj.13180

Beyar-Katz, O., Dickstein, Y., Borok, S., Vidal, L., Leibovici, L., & Paul, M. (2017). Empirical antibiotics targeting gram-positive bacteria for the treatment of febrile neutropenic patients with cancer. *Cochrane Database of Systemic Reviews, 2017*(6). https://doi.org/10.1002/14651858.CD003914.pub4

Fernandes e Santana, L., de Sousa Rodrigues, M., de Araújo Silva, M.P., Cordeiro de Brito, R.J.V., Mendonça Nicacio, J., de Castro Duarte, R.M.S., & Vieira Gomes, O. (2019). Fever of unknown origin—A literature review. *Revista da Associação Médica Brasileira, 65*(8), 1109–1115. https://doi.org/10.1590/1806-9282.65.8.1109

Fernandez, C., & Beeching, N.J. (2018). Pyrexia of unknown origin. *Clinical Medicine, 18*(2), 170–174. https://doi.org/10.7861/clinmedicine.18-2-170

Gödel, P., Shimabukuro-Vornhagen, A., & von Bergwelt-Baildon, M. (2018). Understanding cytokine release syndrome. *Intensive Care Medicine, 44*(3), 371–373. https://doi.org/10.1007/s00134-017-4943-5

Hill, J.A., Li, D., Hay, K.A., Green, M.L., Cherian, S., Chen, X., ... Turtle, C.J. (2018). Infectious complications of CD19-targeted chimeric antigen receptor–modified T-cell immunotherapy. *Blood, 131*(1), 121–130. https://doi.org/10.1182/blood-2017-07-793760

Lehrnbecher, T., Robinson, P., Fisher, B., Alexander, S., Ammann, R.A., Beauchemin, M., ... Sung, L. (2017). Guideline for the management of fever and neutropenia in children with cancer and hematopoietic stem-cell transplantation recipients: 2017 update. *Journal of Clinical Oncology, 35*(18), 2082–2094. https://doi.org/10.1200/JCO.2016.71.7017

Lyman, G.H., Abella, E., & Pettengell, R. (2014). Risk factors for febrile neutropenia among patients with cancer receiving chemotherapy: A systematic review. *Critical Reviews in Oncology/Hematology, 90*(3), 190–199. https://doi.org/10.1016/j.critrevonc.2013.12.006

Meier, K., & Lee, K. (2017). Neurogenic fever: Review of pathophysiology, evaluation, and management. *Journal of Intensive Care Medicine, 32*(2), 124–129. https://doi.org/10.1177/0885066615625194

Mikkilineni, L., & Gea-Banacloche, J.C. (2019). Infectious complication in oncology. In J. Abraham & J.L. Gulley (Eds.), *The Bethesda handbook of clinical oncology* (5th ed., pp. 477–503). Wolters Kluwer.

National Comprehensive Cancer Network. (2021a). *NCCN Clinical Practice Guidelines in Oncology (NCCN Guidelines®): Hematopoietic growth factors* [v.4.2021]. https://www.nccn.org/professionals/physician_gls/pdf/growthfactors.pdf

National Comprehensive Cancer Network. (2021b). *NCCN Clinical Practice Guidelines in Oncology (NCCN Guidelines®): Prevention and treatment of cancer-related infections* [v.1.2021]. https://www.nccn.org/professionals/physician_gls/pdf/infections.pdf

Pasikhova, Y., Ludlow, S., & Baluch, A. (2017). Fever in patients with cancer. *Cancer Control, 24*(2), 193–197. https://doi.org/10.1177/107327481702400212

Smith, T.J., Bohlke, K., Lyman, G.H., Carson, K.R., Crawford, J., Cross, S.J., ... Armitage, J.O. (2015). Recommendations for the use of WBC growth factors: American Society of Clinical Oncology clinical practice guideline update. *Journal of Clinical Oncology, 33*(28), 3199–3212. https://doi.org/10.1200/JCO.2015.62.3488

Taplitz, R.A., Kennedy, E.B., Bow, E.J., Crews, J., Gleason, C., Hawley, D.K., ... Flowers, C.R. (2018). Antimicrobial prophylaxis for adult patients with cancer-related immunosuppression: ASCO and IDSA clinical practice guideline update. *Journal of Clinical Oncology, 36*(30), 3043–3054. https://doi.org/10.1200/JCO.18.00374

Taplitz, R.A., Kennedy, E.B., & Flowers, C.R. (2018). Outpatient management of fever and neutropenia in adults treated for malignancy: American Society of Clinical Oncology and Infectious Diseases Society of America clinical practice guideline update summary. *Journal of Oncology Practice, 14*(4), 250–255. https://doi.org/10.1200/JOP.18.00016

van der Velden, W.J.F.M., Herbers, A.H.E., Netea, M.G., & Blijlevens, N.M.A. (2014). Mucosal barrier injury, fever and infection in neutropenic patients with cancer: Introducing the paradigm febrile mucositis. *British Journal of Haematology, 167*(4), 441–452. https://doi.org/10.1111/bjh.13113

Walter, E.J., & Carraretto, M. (2016). The neurological and cognitive consequences of hyperthermia. *Critical Care, 20,* 199. https://doi.org/10.1186/s13054-016-1376-4

Walter, E.J., Hanna-Jumma, S., Carraretto, M., & Forni, L. (2016). The pathophysiological basis and consequences of fever. *Critical Care, 20,* 200. https://doi.org/10.1186/s13054-016-1375-5

CHAPTER 148

Flu–Like Symptoms

Wendy H. Vogel, MSN, FNP, AOCNP®

I. Definition: A cluster of constitutional symptoms that may include fever, chills, rigors, headache, lethargy, anorexia, myalgias, arthralgias, nausea, abdominal discomfort, nasal stuffiness/congestion, and cognitive impairment (Keskin et al., 2019; Muehlbauer et al., 2018)

II. Physiology/Pathophysiology
   A. Normal (Furman & Davis, 2015; Grimaldi et al., 2016; Liu & Zhao, 2018; Muehlbauer et al., 2018; Shimabukuro-Vornhagen et al., 2018)
      1. When a pathogen enters the body, the body recognizes that the pathogen is "foreign" and stimulates the body's immune response.
      2. Nonspecific immunity
         a) Macrophages phagocytize the pathogen and release proinflammatory cytokines, including IL-1, IL-6, and TNF-α.
         b) These cytokines stimulate other immune cells to mount an acute phase response.
      3. Body response
         a) Cytokines release prostaglandin, triggering the physical characteristics of sickness behavior (e.g., reduced intake of food and water, reduced physical activity, increased sleep, weakness, inability to concentrate, decreased interest in surroundings and social interactions, anhedonia).
         b) Prostaglandin crosses the blood–brain barrier and increases the thermoregulatory "set point" (a narrow range of temperature around 98.6°F [37°C]). The site for temperature control in the brain is termed the *preoptic anterior hypothalamus.* Increased thermogenesis occurs, raising the body temperature (fever).
         c) The body responds to increased heat production by vasoconstriction, shivering (chills), rigors, curled-up posture, and piloerection.
         d) Once the endogenous pyrogen blood levels fall or are blocked by an antipyretic (e.g., acetaminophen), the set point returns to normal, and body temperature is lowered by vasodilation and sweating. Fever subsides.
   B. Pathophysiology
      1. Flu-like syndrome is thought to be initiated by immunotherapy agents (e.g., therapeutic cytokines), pathogens, or cancer treatments, which stimulate proinflammatory cytokines and the brain's temperature control (see Figure 148-1).
      2. The control mechanism may be suppressed in patients on steroids or anti-inflammatory agents.
      3. Flu-like symptoms may be part of a larger syndrome called *cytokine release syndrome.* At times, in the literature, these terms may be used interchangeably.

| FIGURE 148-1 | Oncology Agents That May Potentially Cause Flu-Like Symptoms |

- Antibiotics (e.g., amphotericin B, vancomycin)
- Antithymocyte globulin
- Azacitidine
- Bacillus Calmette-Guérin
- Bisphosphonates
- Bleomycin
- CAR T-cell therapy
- Cladribine
- Cytarabine
- Dacarbazine
- Decitabine
- 5-Fluorouracil
- Hematopoietic growth factors
- Interferons (e.g., alpha, beta, gamma)
- Interleukin-2
- L-asparaginase
- Monoclonal antibodies, often as part of an infusion reaction (e.g., rituximab, ibritumomab)
- Procarbazine
- Retinoids
- Tumor necrosis factor

Note. Based on information from Chavez et al., 2020; Muehlbauer et al., 2018; Riegler et al., 2019; Shimabukuro-Vornhagen et al., 2018.

III. Clinical features: The onset, duration, and severity of symptoms are related to the etiology (Grimaldi et al., 2016; Kroschinsky et al., 2017; Liu & Zhao, 2018; Muehlbauer et al., 2018).
   A. Etiology
      1. Drug induced (see Figure 148-1)
      2. Infection
      3. Immunocompromise
      4. Tumor fever
      5. Cytokine release syndrome
   B. History
      1. History of cancer and cancer treatment
      2. Current medications: Prescribed, over-the-counter, alternative therapies, supplements
      3. History of presenting symptoms: Precipitating factors, onset, timing, duration, associated symptoms (e.g., nausea and vomiting, diarrhea, sore throat, nasal discharge, cough, sputum production, dyspnea, dysuria)
      4. Changes in ADLs
      5. Past medical history: Comorbidities, anemia
      6. Recent exposure to similar illnesses such as flu or mononucleosis, recent travel
   C. Signs and symptoms
      1. Rigors
      2. Fever
      3. Malaise
      4. Myalgia
      5. Arthralgia
      6. Anorexia
      7. Nausea and vomiting
      8. Diarrhea
      9. Headache
      10. Thirst
      11. Abdominal pain
      12. Nasal stuffiness or congestion
      13. Cognitive impairment
      14. Symptoms progressing to various organ dysfunction: Oliguria, bronchospasm, arrhythmia, and renal insufficiency

    D. Physical examination
       1. Vital signs
         a) Elevated temperature, pulse, and respirations indicating infection
         b) Hypertension or hypotension
       2. Neurologic: Mental status (e.g., somnolence, confusion, irritability, seizures, decreased performance status)
       3. Integument: Hot, dry, or diaphoretic
       4. Lymph node: Adenopathy, usually with infectious etiology (see Appendix D)
       5. Pulmonary: Crackles and rhonchi indicative of infection, pleural rub indicative of effusion
       6. Abdominal: Increased bowel sounds, tenderness indicative of infection, especially rebound tenderness

IV. Diagnostic tests (Kroschinsky et al., 2017; Liu & Zhao, 2018)
    A. Laboratory
       1. If flu-like syndrome is expected with current therapy, then no further workup is needed.
       2. If fever persists or does not respond to acetaminophen or nonsteroidal agent, a full culture workup is indicated to rule out infection (see Chapter 147).
         a) Nasal or throat swabs, sputum cultures
         b) Blood cultures
         c) Urine cultures, if indicated
         d) Stool cultures, if indicated
       3. CBC if neutropenia or infection is suspected
       4. Chemistry panel and kidney function to evaluate for electrolytes and renal/liver insufficiency
       5. Coagulation panel to assess for deficits
       6. CRP and/or procalcitonin to assess for inflammation or marker for sepsis
       7. Rapid flu test, if indicated
    B. Radiology: Not indicated unless specific etiology is suspected

V. Differential diagnosis (Shimabukuro-Vornhagen et al., 2018)
    A. Infection (bacterial or fungal)
    B. Sepsis
    C. Toxic shock syndrome
    D. Febrile neutropenia (see Chapter 127)
    E. Drug induced (see Figure 148-1)
    F. Influenza, respiratory syncytial virus, adenovirus
    G. Common cold
    H. FMS (see Chapter 101)
    I. Tumor
    J. HZV (see Chapter 22)

VI. Treatment (Frey & Porter, 2016; Kroschinsky et al., 2017; Liu & Zhao, 2018; Muehlbauer et al., 2018; Shimabukuro-Vornhagen et al., 2018)
    A. Arthralgias/myalgias: Treat with exercise, warmth, and massage (see Chapters 96 and 100).
    B. Painful rigors and chills
       1. Meperidine: 25–50 mg IV every 15 minutes, not to exceed 100 mg in one hour
       2. Morphine: 1–5 mg IV every 15 minutes
       3. Monitor for hypotension.
       4. Additional warmed blankets, clothing, heating pads, or hot water bottles

C. Fever: Pharmacologic; avoid using ASA.
1. Acetaminophen: 650–975 mg PO every four hours, not to exceed 4,000 mg in a day
2. NSAIDs (see Appendix E)
D. For CAR T-cell–associated cytokine release syndrome: Tocilizumab 8–12 mg/kg IV may be indicated; see prescribing information.
E. Fever: Pursue nonpharmacologic comfort measures.
1. Sponge baths, tepid showers
2. Removal of extra blankets and clothing
3. Cooling blanket
F. Ensure adequate hydration for duration of fever. To determine recommended daily oral intake in ounces, divide patient's weight in pounds by two. IV hydration of 500–1,000 ml daily may be needed.
G. Ensure periods of uninterrupted rest.
H. If GI symptoms are present, give antiemetic and antidiarrheal agents (see Chapter 56 and Appendix P).
I. Teach patients and their families which symptoms to anticipate and which symptoms they should report.
J. If drug-related etiology
1. Consider premedication for prophylaxis and then around-the-clock dosing for 24–48 hours.
   a) Acetaminophen: 650 mg PO prior to drug dose, then every four hours, not to exceed 4,000 mg daily
   b) Ibuprofen: 400–800 mg PO prior to drug dose, then every four to six hours, not to exceed 2,400–3,200 mg daily
   c) Naproxen: 250–500 mg PO prior to drug dose, then every 12 hours
   d) Diphenhydramine: 25–50 mg PO prior to drug dose, then every six hours
   e) Famotidine: 20 mg IV every 12 hours
   f) Other NSAIDs (see Appendix E)
2. Consider bedtime dosing of medications causing flu-like syndrome.
3. To mitigate risk of CAR T-cell–associated cytokine release syndrome
   a) Cytoreduction prior to treatment with CAR T cells
   b) Dose adjustment by disease burden
K. Fatigue: Perform baseline assessment of cancer-related fatigue prior to onset of cancer treatment (see Chapter 163).
L. Anorexia: Encourage eating small, frequent meals with high-protein content (see Chapter 66).
M. Anemia related: Treat accordingly to type of anemia (see Chapters 113–118).

VII. Follow-up: Flu-like symptoms are generally self-limiting and do not require follow-up unless symptoms persist beyond the expected time frame. More severe toxicity will require hospital admission and close follow-up.

VIII. Referral: Generally not indicated unless organ damage/failure is suspected

References

Chavez, J.C., Jain, M.D., & Kharfan-Dabaja, M.J. (2020). Cytokine release syndrome and neurologic toxicities associated with chimeric antigen receptor T-cell therapy: A comprehensive review of emerging grading models. *Hematology/Oncology and Stem Cell Therapy, 13*(1), 1–6. https://doi.org/10.1016/j.hemonc.2019.05.005

Frey, N.V., & Porter, D.L. (2016). Cytokine release syndrome with novel therapeutics for acute lymphoblastic leukemia. *Hematology: American Society of Hematology Education Program Book, 2016,* 567–572. https://doi.org/10.1182/asheducation-2016.1.567

Furman, D., & Davis, M.M. (2015). New approaches to understanding the immune response to vaccination and infection. *Vaccine, 33*(40), 5271–5281. https://doi.org/10.1016/j.vaccine.2015.06.117

Grimaldi, C., Finco, D., Fort, M.M., Gliddon, D., Harper, K., Helms, W.S., ... Walker, M. (2016). Cytokine release: A workshop proceedings on the state-of-the-science, current challenges and future directions. *Cytokine, 85,* 101–108. https://doi.org/10.1016/j.cyto.2016.06.006

Keskin, H., Cadirci, K., Demirkazik, A., Akbulut, H., & Yalcin, B. (2019). Following chemotherapy: Serum cytokine (tumor necrosis factor, interleukin-2, interleukin-11), immunoglobulin, complement, vascular endothelial growth factor levels, and the systemic symptoms like capillary leak syndrome. *Biomarkers in Cancer, 11.* https://doi.org/10.1177/1179299X19854447

Kroschinsky, F., Stölzel, F., von Bonin, S., Beutel, G., Kochanek, M., Kiehl, M., & Schellongowski, P. (2017). New drugs, new toxicities: Severe side effects of modern targeted and immunotherapy of cancer and their management. *Critical Care, 21,* 89. https://doi.org/10.1186/s13054-017-1678-1

Liu, D., & Zhao, J. (2018). Cytokine release syndrome: grading, modeling, and new therapy. *Journal of Hematology and Oncology, 11,* 121. https://doi.org/10.1186/s13045-018-0653-x

Muehlbauer, P.M., Callahan, A., Zlott, D., & Dahl, B.J. (2018). Biotherapy. In C.H. Yarbro, D. Wujcik, & B.H. Gobel (Eds.), *Cancer nursing: Principles and practice* (8th ed., pp. 611–651). Jones and Bartlett Learning.

Riegler, L.L., Jones, G.P., & Lee, D.W. (2019). Current approaches in the grading and management of cytokine release syndrome after chimeric antigen receptor T-cell therapy. *Therapeutics and Clinical Risk Management, 15,* 323–335. https://doi.org/10.2147/TCRM.S150524

Shimabukuro-Vornhagen, A., Gödel, P., Subklewe, M., Stemmler, H.J., Schlößer, H.A., Schlaak, M., ... von Bergwelt-Baildon, M.S. (2018). Cytokine release syndrome. *Journal for Immunotherapy of Cancer, 6*(1), 56–70. https://doi.org/10.1186/s40425-018-0343-9

CHAPTER 149

Thirst

Kristine Dukart-Harrington, DNP, RN, AGNP-C, ACHPN

I. Definition: The conscious desire for water; a sensation that promotes attainment of minimal hydration needs (Nigro et al., 2018; Zehm et al., 2016)

II. Physiology/Pathophysiology (Augustine et al., 2019; Gizowski & Bourque, 2018; Leib et al., 2016; Lowell, 2019; Nigro et al., 2018; Zimmerman et al., 2019)
   A. Normal
   1. The thirst center, located in the hypothalamus, consists of neuronal cells, which function as osmoreceptors.
   2. Approximately 60% of the body is made up of water; it is involved in a wide range of basic functions.
   3. In the blood, water transports oxygen, nutrients, and waste products; it moistens mucous membranes, cools the body by perspiration, and is required for digestion of food.
   4. The main determinants for the maintenance of water homeostasis are the hormone arginine vasopressin and thirst.
   B. Pathophysiology
   1. An increase in osmotic pressure in the CSF of the third ventricle or in the circulating extracellular fluid promotes thirst.
   2. Intracellular dehydration, present in hypernatremia and hypercalcemia, is a common cause of increased osmolar concentration of the extracellular fluid.
   3. Other stimuli causing thirst are an increased production of angiotensin II, decreased cardiac output, and dryness of the mouth.
   4. Dehydration triggers thirst.
      a) Intracellular dehydration refers to the loss of water from inside the cells typically caused by increase in blood osmolality.
      b) Extracellular dehydration refers to decrease in the total blood volume.
      c) Intracellular can be corrected by drinking water, whereas extracellular requires both water and salt to regenerate the blood and correct osmolality.

III. Clinical features: Water intake is one of the most basic physiologic responses and is essential to life. Thirst is a subjective symptom that may be accompanied by dry lips and mouth, polydipsia, and polyuria. No consistent relationship exists between thirst/dry mouth and fluid status. Approximately 80%–90% of dying patients report significant thirst. Without any intake of fluid, death can occur after three to five days (Armstrong et al., 2016; Gizowski & Bourque, 2018; Leib et al., 2016; Zadák et al., 2018; Zehm et al., 2016).
   A. Etiology
   1. Decreased fluid intake

  2. Increased fluid output

  3. Poor fluid transport

  4. Medication induced

  5. Mouth breathing

  6. Electrolyte imbalance

  7. Hypothalamic–pituitary pathologic conditions

  8. Head and neck irradiation

  9. Anxiety

  10. GI cancer

  11. Sweating

 B. History

  1. History of cancer and cancer treatment

  2. Current medications: Prescribed (e.g., opioids), over the counter

  3. History of presenting symptoms: Precipitating factors, location, duration, associated symptoms (e.g., dry mouth, anxiety, depression, fever, night sweats, shortness of breath, mouth breathing, edema)

  4. Changes in ADLs

  5. History of intake and output

  6. Past medical history: Diabetes mellitus, heart disease, endocrine disease, kidney disease

  7. Family history: Diabetes mellitus, thyroid disease

 C. Signs and symptoms

  1. Polydipsia

  2. Polyuria

  3. Polyphagia

  4. Weakness

  5. Light-headedness

  6. Dry mouth

 D. Physical examination

  1. Weight loss or gain

  2. Vital signs: Hypotension and orthostatic with dehydration

  3. Integument

   a) Dry skin

   b) Poor skin turgor indicating dehydration or renal disease

  4. Oral: Dry mucous membrane, thick saliva, dry or cracked lips

  5. Neurologic: Confusion and lethargy indicating dehydration or electrolyte imbalance

  6. Cardiac: Murmur and gallop indicating anemia

  7. Pulmonary: Rales indicating CHF, bronchitis, or pneumonia

  8. Extremities: Pitting edema indicating potential CHF, third-spacing, renal disease, or malnutrition

IV. Diagnostic tests (Armstrong et al., 2016)

 A. Laboratory

  1. CBC to evaluate for anemia or occult volume depletion

  2. Urinalysis and urine electrolytes: An increase in sodium excretion greater than 20 mEq/24 hrs indicative of SIADH

  3. Glucose: Increase indicative of diabetes mellitus or thyroid disease

  4. BUN and creatinine to determine prerenal, intrinsic, or postrenal diseases

  5. Electrolytes: Hyponatremia seen in SIADH, hypokalemia, hypernatremia, hypercalcemia

    6. TSH: Decreased in hyperthyroidism

    7. Serum PTH: Increased in hyperparathyroidism

    8. Serum osmolality: Decreased in excessive fluid intake; increased in dehydration

    9. Urine osmolality: Increased (greater than 300 mOsm/kg) in SIADH

   10. Atrial natriuretic peptide: Measures dehydration defined by level (less than or equal to 15 pg/ml) and hyperosmolality (greater than or equal to 300 mOsm/kg)

  B. Radiology: Not indicated

V. Differential diagnosis (Nigro et al., 2018; Zadák et al., 2018; Zehm et al., 2016)

  A. Decreased fluid intake

    1. Anorexia (see Chapter 66)

    2. Dehydration

    3. Nausea and vomiting (see Chapter 63)

    4. Inability to feed self or ask for assistance

    5. Small bowel obstruction (see Chapter 67)

  B. Increased fluid output

    1. Diuresis

    2. Vomiting (see Chapter 63)

    3. Diarrhea (see Chapter 56)

    4. Fever (see Chapter 147)

    5. Diaphoresis

  C. Poor fluid transport

    1. Hemorrhagic or vasomotor shock (see Chapter 160)

    2. Hypoalbuminemia

    3. CHF (see Chapter 42)

  D. Medications

    1. Alcohol

    2. Antidepressants (see Appendix L)

    3. Cyclophosphamide: High dose can induce SIADH.

    4. Diuretics

    5. Lithium

    6. Opioids (see Appendix F)

    7. Parasympatholytics: Hyoscyamine, dicyclomine

    8. Steroids (see Appendix K)

    9. Belladonna alkaloid with anticholinergic properties/scopolamine

  E. Mouth breathing: Nasal obstruction or positioning

  F. Electrolyte imbalance (see Chapters 152–156)

  G. Pathologic conditions

    1. Aldosteronism

    2. Chronic glomerulonephritis

    3. Diabetes mellitus (see Chapter 151)

    4. Diabetes insipidus

    5. Hyperparathyroidism

    6. Hyperthyroidism (see Chapter 157)

    7. Multiple sclerosis

    8. SIADH (see Chapter 95)

    9. Primary polydipsia

  H. Terminal condition

  I. Radiation induced

VI. Treatment (Assy & Brand, 2018; Bruera et al., 2005; Caccialanza et al., 2018; Garcia et al., 2019; Puntillo et al., 2014; van Belzen et al., 2017; Vidal et al., 2016; VonStein et al., 2019; Zadák et al., 2018; Zehm et al., 2016)

    A. Treatment should be directed at the underlying cause of thirst; however, thirst may occur as a side effect of medications or during the terminal phase of life.

    B. Measure intake and output to assess altered balance in dehydration; large volume output will be present in SIADH (see Chapter 95).

    C. Encourage patient to take frequent sips of fluid or ice chips.

    D. Frequent oral assessment and care is needed for patients unable to take care of their own oral hygiene (every hour PRN). Family members/loved ones may want to participate in oral care in order to demonstrate care.

    E. Artificial saliva/topical interventions
        1. Glandosane® aerosol spray: Spray one or two times in mouth every hour PRN.
        2. Moisture oral swab sticks: Swab to oral tissue every hour PRN.
        3. Moisture sprays: Spray one or two times in mouth every hour PRN.
        4. Frozen gauze pads or ice to soothe dry mucous membranes

    F. Cholinergic agonist increases secretion of exocrine glands: Pilocarpine hydrochloride, initial dose of 5 mg PO three times a day; titrated up to 10 mg three times a day if not responding and if tolerating lower doses

    G. Mouth rinses
        1. One liter of water mixed with one-half tablespoon of salt and one-half tablespoon of baking soda: Gargle with solution PRN for dry mouth.
        2. Moisturizing mouthwash: Gargle PRN.

    H. Products to stimulate salivary flow such as dental chewing gum or sugarless gum

    I. Lubrication of the lips: Petroleum-based or vitamin E–based ointment or lip moisturizer

    J. Oral hygiene products
        1. Dry mouth toothpaste used after meals and at bedtime
        2. Portable battery-powered hand-held device that delivers oral irrigation or suction PRN for comfort
        3. Soft-bristle toothbrush
        4. Oral irrigator used with water or antibacterial rinses
        5. Lemon-glycerin swabs are not recommended because they decrease pH, drying mucous membranes and ultimately exhausting salivary glands over time, which can lead to increased xerostomia.

    K. Consider heated humidifiers for patients receiving high-flow oxygen therapy to decrease mouth and throat dryness.

    L. Some studies have identified benefits of acupuncture in patients experiencing xerostomia secondary to radiation, but evidence is insufficient overall. Clinical trials are currently ongoing.

    M. Hydration at or near the end of life can be controversial and requires a careful assessment of individualized patient needs, clinical needs for hydration (e.g., presence of symptoms that could be alleviated), and patient and family wishes.
        1. IV fluids are expensive and difficult to administer in home hospice settings due to lack of IV access.
        2. Hypodermoclysis (subcutaneous fluid infusions) can provide hydration for patients if the goal is to maintain cognitive status or relieve symptoms such as myoclonus or delirium.
        3. Family caregivers can be educated to administer hypodermoclysis in the home setting.

    a) Administer a mixture of normal saline or normal saline with 5% dextrose and 20 mEq of potassium at a rate of 500–1,500 ml/24 hrs subcutaneous.

    b) If necessary, to increase absorption of fluid from the subcutaneous site, add hyaluronidase 500 units to each liter.

    c) Contraindications to hypodermoclysis are anasarca (generalized edema along with ascites) and severe thrombocytopenia.

    d) IV fluids are medically unnecessary and have numerous disadvantages in end-stage disease (e.g., cough, pulmonary congestion, choking, edema).

N. Education for palliative treatment

    1. Explain that decreased oral intake is natural in the terminal phase and that most patients do not feel hunger or thirst. IV fluid may increase discomfort.

    2. Reassure the patient and family that thirst can be relieved by careful mouth care, sips of water, or ice. Studies demonstrate that artificial nutrition or hydration is not necessary to provide comfort or to alleviate thirst or dry mouth.

VII. Follow-up: Dependent on cause of thirst

VIII. Referral: Only needed if underlying condition warrants referral

The author would like to acknowledge Patrick J. Coyne, MSN, ACHPN, ACNS-BC, FAAN, FPCN, for his contribution to this chapter that remains unchanged from the previous edition of this book.

References

Armstrong, L.E., Kavouras, S.A., Walsh, N.P., & Roberts, W.O. (2016). Diagnosing dehydration? Blend evidence with clinical observations. *Current Opinion in Clinical Nutrition and Metabolic Care, 19*(6), 434–438. https://doi.org/10.1097/MCO.0000000000000320

Assy, Z., & Brand, H.S. (2018). A systematic review of the effects of acupuncture on xerostomia and hyposalivation. *BMC Complementary and Alternative Medicine, 18*(1), 57. https://doi.org/10.1186/s12906-018-2124-x

Augustine, V., Ebisu, H., Zhao, Y., Lee, S., Ho, B., Mizuno, G.O., ... Oka, Y. (2019). Temporally and spatially distinct thirst satiation signals. *Neuron, 103*(2), 242–249. https://doi.org/10.1016/j.neuron.2019.04.039

Bruera, E., Sala, R., Rico, M.A., Moyano, J., Centeno, C., Willey, J., & Palmer, J.L. (2005). Effects of parenteral hydration in terminally ill cancer patients: A preliminary study. *Journal of Clinical Oncology, 23*(10), 2366–2371. https://doi.org/10.1200/JCO.2005.04.069

Caccialanza, R., Constans, T., Cotogni, P., Zaloga, G.P., & Pontes-Arruda, A. (2018). Subcutaneous infusion of fluids for hydration or nutrition: A review. *Journal of Parenteral and Enteral Nutrition, 42*(2), 296–307. https://doi.org/10.1177/0148607116676593

Garcia, A.K.A., Fonseca, L.F., Furuya, R.K., Rabelo, P.D., & Rossetto, E.G. (2019). Effect of chewing gum on thirst: An integrative review. *Revista Brasileira de Enfermagem, 72*(2), 484–493. https://doi.org/10.1590/0034-7167-2018-0132

Gizowski, C., & Bourque, C.W. (2018). The neural basis of homeostatic and anticipatory thirst. *Nature Reviews Nephrology, 14*(1), 11–25. https://doi.org/10.1038/nrneph.2017.149

Leib, D.E., Zimmerman, C.A., & Knight, Z.A. (2016). Thirst. *Current Biology, 26*(24), R1260–R1265. https://doi.org/10.1016/j.cub.2016.11.019

Lowell, B.B. (2019). New neuroscience of homeostasis and drives for food, water, and salt. *New England Journal of Medicine, 380*(5), 459–471. https://doi.org/10.1056/NEJMra1812053

Nigro, N., Grossmann, M., Chiang, C., & Inder, W.J. (2018). Polyuria-polydipsia syndrome: A diagnostic challenge. *Internal Medicine Journal, 48*(3), 244–253. https://doi.org/10.1111/imj.13627

Puntillo, K., Nelson, J.E., Weissman, D., Curtis, R., Weiss, S., Frontera, J., ... Campbell, M. (2014). Palliative care in the ICU: Relief of pain, dyspnea, and thirst—A report from the IPAL-ICU advisory board. *Intensive Care Medicine, 40*(2), 235–248. https://doi.org/10.1007/s00134-013-3153-z

van Belzen, L., Postma, E.M., & Boesveldt, S. (2017). How to quench your thirst. The effect of water-based products varying in temperature and texture, flavour, and sugar content on thirst. *Physiology and Behavior, 180*, 45–52. https://doi.org/10.1016/j.physbeh.2017.08.007

Vidal, M., Hui, D., Williams, J., & Bruera, E. (2016). A prospective study of hypodermoclysis performed by caregivers in the home setting. *Journal of Pain and Symptom Management, 52*(4), 570–574.e9. https://doi.org/10.1016/j.jpainsymman .2016.04.009

VonStein, M., Buchko, B.L., Millen, C., Lampo, D., Bell, T., & Woods, A.B. (2019). Effect of a scheduled nurse intervention on thirst and dry mouth in intensive care patients. *American Journal of Critical Care, 28*(1), 41–46. https://doi.org /10.4037/ajcc2019400

Zadák, Z., Tichá, A., & Hyšpler, R. (2018). Electrolyte and water disorders in old age. *Vnitřní Lékařství, 64*(11), 1059–1066.

Zehm, A., Mullin, J., & Zhang, H. (2016). Thirst in palliative care #313. *Journal of Palliative Medicine, 19*(9), 1009–1010. https://doi.org/10.1089/jpm.2016.0205

Zimmerman, C.A., Huey, E.L., Ahn, J.S., Beutler, L.R., Tan, C.L., Kosar, S., ... Knight, Z.A. (2019). A gut-to-brain signal of fluid osmolarity controls thirst satiation. *Nature, 568*(7750), 98–102. https://doi.org/10.1038/s41586-019-1066-x

CHAPTER 150

Anaphylaxis

Christina Ferraro, MSN, APRN–CNP, BMTCN®

I. Definition (Aun et al., 2017; Bilò et al., 2019; LoVerde et al., 2018; Reber et al., 2017; Yu & Lin, 2018)
   A. An acute systemic reaction with the potential to be fatal
   B. Serious allergic reaction that presents rapidly
   C. Essentially unavoidable in medical practice and most often results from immunologic reactions
      1. Foods: An adverse immunologic response to a dietary protein
      2. Medications: A spectrum of immunologically mediated hypersensitivity reactions with a myriad of mechanisms and clinical presentations
      3. Insect stings: Systemic reactions secondary to insect bites or stings
      4. Physical factors/exercise: Exercise-induced anaphylaxis and food-dependent, exercise-induced anaphylaxis
      5. Immunotherapy injections: Administration of allergens to perform allergen-specific immunotherapy; attempts to reduce symptoms triggered by allergens and prevent recurrence of the disease in the long term
      6. Idiopathic: Spontaneous anaphylaxis in which no cause can be identified

II. Physiology/Pathophysiology (Bilò et al., 2019; LoVerde et al., 2018; Maker et al., 2019; Olsen et al., 2019; Reber et al., 2017)
   A. Normal
      1. The immune system is a highly organized network of cells, tissues, and organs that defend the body against attack.
      2. The immune system can hit wrong targets and cause allergic responses and diseases. B lymphocytes mature in the bone marrow, whereas T lymphocytes mature in the thymus.
      3. A healthy immune system is able to distinguish between the body's own cells (self) and foreign cells (nonself) using both innate and adaptive immune defenses.
         a) The cellular elements of blood, including the lymphocytes of the adaptive immune system, are derived from the hematopoietic stem cells in the bone marrow.
         b) The myeloid progenitor is the precursor of the granulocytes, macrophages, dendritic cells, and mast cells of the immune system.
         c) Macrophages are freely distributed in the body tissues, where they perform an essential role in innate immunity.
         d) Dendritic cells are able to take up an antigen and display it for recognition by lymphocytes.

    e) Immature dendritic cells can perform both phagocytic and macropinocytic functions, ingesting extracellular fluid and confronting pathogens.

    f) Mast cells differentiate in tissues and, when activated, release substances that affect vascular permeability.

    g) Granulocytes (containing granules in their cytoplasm) are relatively short lived but increase in numbers during immune responses, migrating to sites of infection or inflammation; neutrophils, eosinophils, and basophils are known collectively as *granulocytes.*

    h) Neutrophils are an important part of response to bacterial infection.

    i) Eosinophils increase in number in response to infections, particularly parasitic infection.

    j) Adaptive immune responses are produced when recirculating T cells recognize a specific antigen on the surface of a dendritic cell.

B. Pathophysiology

  1. Anaphylaxis results from the activation of mast cells and basophils.

  2. The activation of the cells is thought to involve crosslinking of IgE. Anaphylaxis reactions are mediated by IgE; anaphylactoid reactions are not. Both produce similar physiologic effects.

  3. The severity and systemic nature of the reaction distinguish anaphylaxis from other allergic reactions.

    a) When activated, mast cells and/or basophils release preformed mediators from secretory granules, including histamine and other substances.

    b) Downstream activation of phospholipase, cyclooxygenases, and lipoxygenases produces arachidonic acid metabolites, including prostaglandins, leukotrienes, and platelet-activating factor.

    c) Inflammatory cytokines (e.g., TNF-α) are also released, along with other cytokines and chemokines.

    d) These mediators are considered the genesis for the pathophysiology of anaphylaxis.

    e) Histamine release stimulates the following events.

      (1) Vasodilation

      (2) Increased vascular permeability

      (3) Increased heart rate

      (4) Cardiac contraction

      (5) Glandular secretion

        (a) Prostaglandin D2 stimulates

          i. Bronchoconstriction

          ii. Pulmonary and coronary vasoconstriction

          iii. Peripheral vasodilation

        (b) Leukotrienes stimulate

          i. Bronchoconstriction

          ii. Increased vascular permeability

          iii. Promotion of airway remodeling

        (c) Platelet-activating factor release potentiates

          i. Potent bronchoconstrictor

          ii. Increased vascular permeability

        (d) TNF-α release

          i. Activates neutrophils

          ii. Recruits other effector cells

          iii. Enhances chemokine synthesis

III. Clinical features: Anaphylaxis is a systemic reaction that may involve multiple organ systems. It occurs most frequently after exposure to allergens and subsequent release of mediators from mast cells and basophils. The prevalence of anaphylaxis is approximately 2% and rising; the lifetime risk is presumed to be 1%–3% with a mortality rate of approximately 1%. The rapidity of anaphylactic response predicts the likelihood of severe or life-threatening reactions; anaphylaxis often produces symptoms within 5–30 minutes, but some patients may not experience reactions for several hours (Aun et al., 2017, 2018; Bonamichi-Santos & Castells, 2018; Lee et al., 2017; LoVerde et al., 2018; Maker et al., 2019; Olsen et al., 2019; Yu & Lin, 2018).

A. Etiology
  1. Drugs: Antibiotics, NSAIDs, immunomodulators or immunotherapy agents, chemotherapy (e.g., monoclonal antibodies, platinums, taxanes), contrast dye and agents, anesthetics
  2. Food reactions: Peanuts, tree nuts, milk, eggs, shellfish
  3. Unknown causes
  4. *Anisakis* species: Parasitic nematodes
  5. Hymenoptera venom: Bees, yellow jacket family, stinging ants
  6. Food-dependent, exercise-induced anaphylaxis
  7. Chemicals and latex
  8. Vaccines
  9. Honey

B. History: The history is the most important tool for the clinician in determining a diagnosis of anaphylaxis.
  1. History of cancer and cancer treatment
  2. Current medications: Prescribed, over the counter
  3. History of presenting symptoms: Precipitating factors, onset, location, duration, urticaria, angioedema, flushing, pruritus, airway obstruction, GI symptoms, syncope, hypotension, exposure to potential allergens (e.g., foods, medications, insect bite)
  4. Changes in ADLs
  5. Past medical history: Allergy history
  6. Social history: Patient activities prior to the anaphylactic event (e.g., exercise, sexual activity)

C. Signs and symptoms
  1. Anaphylaxis is a generalized reaction.
  2. Patients can present with a variety of symptoms.
    a) Skin: Urticaria with hives, angioedema (swelling), erythema (flushing), pruritus (itching), conjunctivitis
    b) Respiratory
      (1) Upper airway: Nasal congestion, rhinorrhea, sneezing, hoarseness, cough, laryngeal edema
      (2) Lower airway: Bronchospasm, dyspnea, wheezing, chest tightness, impaired swallowing, dysphonia, stridor, obstruction
    c) GI: Nausea, vomiting, abdominal pain or cramping, diarrhea
    d) Neurologic: Light-headedness, dizziness, confusion, feeling of impending doom, seizures
    e) Cardiovascular: Syncope, tachycardia, chest pain, orthostasis, cardiac arrest
    f) Oral: Itching, tingling, or swelling of lips, tongue, or palate; mucous membrane edema

D. Physical examination
  1. Vital signs: Hypotension, tachypnea

2. Integument: Skin hives, rash, flushing, urticaria
3. HEENT: Angioedema around the eyes, swollen tongue or lips
4. Respiratory: Breath sounds for wheezing or stridor
5. GI: Abdomen tenderness
6. Neurologic: Confusion, mental status changes

E. Diagnostic clinical criteria for anaphylaxis: Anaphylaxis is highly likely when any one of the following three criteria exists.

1. Acute onset of illness (minutes to several hours), along with involvement of skin, mucosal tissue, or both, and at least one of the following

   a) Respiratory compromise: Dyspnea, wheezing, stridor
   b) Reduction in blood pressure or associated symptoms of end-organ dysfunction: Syncope, incontinence

2. Two or more of the following occurring rapidly after exposure to a likely allergen for a specific patient

   a) Involvement of skin and mucosal tissues: Hives, itch, swollen lips or tongue
   b) Respiratory compromise
   c) Reduction in blood pressure or associated symptoms
   d) Persistent GI symptoms: Abdominal cramps, abdominal pain, vomiting

3. Reduction in blood pressure after exposure to known allergen for specific patients: In adults, systolic blood pressure less than 90 mm Hg or greater than 30% decrease from patient's baseline

IV. Diagnostic tests: Tests may not be indicated. Diagnosis is based primarily on clinical symptoms and a detailed description of the acute episode (Carter et al., 2020; Castells, 2017a).

A. Laboratory: Serum markers of mast cell activation and degranulation, such as tryptase plasma levels, may be ordered; however, tryptase levels may not be elevated in all forms of anaphylaxis, such as food-associated anaphylaxis.

B. Radiology: Not indicated

C. Other

1. Administration of skin tests and/or performing in vitro IgE tests can detect the presence of IgE antibodies to an offending agent.
2. For the majority of medications, standardized skin tests do not exist or are not available.
3. Skin testing is more sensitive than in vitro testing and is the optimal procedure to determine most IgE-mediated causes of anaphylaxis.
4. Trained personnel should perform skin testing under supervision of a clinician experienced in the procedure and in a setting with appropriate emergency equipment readily available.

V. Differential diagnosis: With a positive history of exposure to offending agent, diagnosis is usually obvious (Bilò et al., 2019; Carter et al., 2020).

A. Hypotension (see Chapter 48)

1. Septic shock (see Chapter 160)
2. Vasopressor (vasovagal reaction)
3. Myocardial dysfunction or cardiogenic shock
4. Hypovolemic shock

B. Respiratory distress

1. Airway foreign body
2. Asthma or COPD exacerbation (see Chapter 28)

      3. PE (see Chapter 33)

      4. Vocal cord dysfunction

      5. Hyperventilation

  C. Postprandial collapse

      1. Monosodium glutamate ingestion

      2. Sulfite ingestion

      3. Scombroid fish poisoning

  D. Flushing syndrome

      1. Carcinoid tumor

      2. Postmenopausal hot flashes (see Chapter 90)

      3. Red man syndrome (associated with vancomycin)

  E. Miscellaneous

      1. Acute anxiety or panic attacks (see Chapter 161)

      2. Acute poisoning

      3. Hypoglycemia

      4. Seizure disorders (see Chapter 144)

      5. Systemic mastocytosis

      6. Hereditary angioedema

      7. Leukemia associated with excess histamine production

VI. Treatment (Bilò et al., 2019; Bonamichi-Santos & Castells, 2018; Carter et al., 2020; Castells, 2017a; Maker et al., 2019; Olsen et al., 2019; Sicherer & Simons, 2017; Tanno et al., 2019)

  A. Nonpharmacologic measures: Treatment of anaphylaxis should start with a rapid evaluation of the patient; airway, breathing, and circulation assessment is critical.

  B. Pharmacologic measures: If the patient meets any of the three criteria of anaphylaxis, the patient should receive immediate pharmacologic treatment.

      1. Epinephrine (1 mg/ml): 0.01 mg/kg up to a maximum of 0.5 mg IM every 5–15 minutes PRN

      2. Treatment of choice

  C. Maintenance of adequate oxygenation is crucial; altered mental status may reflect hypoxia. Measurement of oxygen levels using pulse oximetry and peak expiratory flow rates may help to guide therapy.

  D. Patients should be monitored continuously to detect treatment complications.

      1. Following epinephrine administration

        a) Place patient in a recumbent position and maintain patent airway.

        b) Administer oxygen (usually 8–10 L/min; lower concentrations may be needed for those with COPD).

        c) Procure IV access. Administer normal saline IV for replacement of fluids.

        d) Diphenhydramine (25–50 mg IV for adults and 1 mg/kg [up to 50 mg]) with famotidine (20 mg IV) is more efficacious than diphenhydramine alone; histamine H_1 and H_2 antagonists are slower in action compared to epinephrine and are considered a second-line therapy for anaphylaxis.

        e) Minimal evidence supports the use of H_1 and H_2 antihistamines in anaphylaxis.

        f) Manage bronchospasm resistant to epinephrine with nebulized albuterol. Add 2.5 or 5 mg of albuterol to 3 ml of normal saline; give PRN.

        g) If refractory hypotension is present, consider dopamine with continuous hemodynamic monitoring.

        h) For patients with history of asthma or those with severe or prolonged anaphylaxis, consider methylprednisolone dose pack.

        i) Hydrocortisone 5 mg/kg IV (approximately 250 mg) or methylprednisolone 1–2 mg/kg IV (approximately 125 mg) should be considered to reduce the risk of recurring or protracted anaphylaxis; dose may be repeated every six hours as required (see Appendix K).

        j) Fluid resuscitation may be required for hypotension following epinephrine; potent vasopressors may be required.

   2. Consider transportation to emergency department or ICU.

E. For patients experiencing cardiopulmonary arrest during anaphylaxis, high-dose epinephrine and prolonged resuscitation efforts should be pursued, especially in younger patients with healthy cardiovascular systems.

F. Observation periods must be individualized.

   1. Anaphylaxis may recur anywhere from 1–72 hours after the initial signs and symptoms, with the reported incidence of biphasic anaphylaxis varying from 1%–23%.

   2. No evidence-based information has identified patient characteristics that predict a recurrent episode of late-phase reaction; however, published reports propose potential risk factors.

      a) Initial phase severity

      b) Delayed or suboptimal doses of epinephrine during initial therapy

      c) Laryngeal edema or hypotension during initial phase

      d) Delayed symptomatic onset after antigen exposure

      e) History of biphasic anaphylaxis

   3. Little evidence exists to definitively state that systemic corticosteroids in the initial phase can prevent or weaken late-phase reactions.

   4. Observation periods after the complete resolution of uniphasic anaphylaxis must be individualized in the absence of reliable predictors of biphasic anaphylaxis.

   5. A 10-hour observation period may be sufficient; however, some published reports suggest 24 hours.

   6. Before discharge from the medical facility, all patients should be educated on how to avoid the precipitating allergen if identified.

G. Considerations in treatment

   1. Comorbidities and concurrent medications potentially affect the severity of anaphylactic reactions and the reaction to therapeutic treatment.

   2. Patients on beta-blockers may have diminished responses to epinephrine, an integral part of anaphylaxis treatment. Patients on beta-blockers may need glucagon IV administration (1 mg IV bolus or 1–5 mg/hr continuous infusion).

   3. Patients on ACE inhibitors and angiotensin receptor blockers may have affected compensatory physiologic responses to anaphylaxis, thus experiencing more severe reactions.

   4. Most responses are uniphasic, occurring within a short time after exposure to the offending agent; for some patients, reactions may be biphasic with an initial reaction to the allergen that responds to therapy, followed by a resurgence of the original symptoms.

H. Prevention

   1. Avoid offending antigen.

   2. If possible, consider skin testing and desensitization.

   3. Wear informational bracelet and have immediate access to epinephrine kit.

VII. Follow-up (Bilò et al., 2019; Castells, 2017a, 2017b)

A. Patients should be given epinephrine autoinjector medication with instruction on use for possible subsequent episodes of anaphylaxis.

    B. Patients should have ready access to emergency medical services for treatment after injection of additional epinephrine.

    C. If possible, patients should avoid exposure to triggers or have an immunologist evaluate for possible desensitization.

VIII. Referrals (Castells, 2017a, 2017b)

    A. All patients require a post-anaphylaxis diagnostic evaluation with an allergist-immunologist and should notify their primary care physician.

    B. Desensitization may be possible with the help of an immunologist.

The author would like to acknowledge Pamela Hallquist Viale, RN, MS, AOCNP®, for her contribution to this chapter that remains unchanged from the previous edition of this book.

References

Aun, M.V., Kalil, J., & Giavina-Bianchi, P. (2017). Drug-induced anaphylaxis. *Immunology and Allergy Clinics of North America, 37*(4), 629–641. https://doi.org/10.1016/j.iac.2017.06.002

Aun, M.V., Kalil, J., & Giavina-Bianchi, P. (2018). Adults and children with anaphylaxis in the emergency room: Why it is not recognized? *Current Opinions in Allergy and Clinical Immunology, 18*(5), 377–381. https://doi.org/10.1097/ACI.0000000000000469

Bilò, M.B., Martini, M., Tontini, C., Mohamed, O.E., & Krishna, M.T. (2019). Idiopathic anaphylaxis. *Clinical and Experimental Allergy, 49*(7), 942–952. https://doi.org/10.1111/cea.13402

Bonamichi-Santos, R., & Castells, M. (2018). Diagnoses and management of drug hypersensitivity and anaphylaxis in cancer and chronic inflammatory diseases: Reactions to taxanes and monoclonal antibodies. *Clinical Review in Allergy and Immunology, 54*(3), 375–385. https://doi.org/10.1007/s12016-016-8556-5

Carter, M.C., Akin, C., Castells, M.C., Scott, E.P., & Lieberman, P. (2020). Idiopathic anaphylaxis yardstick: Practial recommendations for clinical practice. *Annals of Allergy, Asthma and Immunology, 124*(1), 16–27. https://doi.org/10.1016/j.anai.2019.08.024

Castells, M. (2017a). Diagnosis and management of anaphylaxis in precision medicine. *Journal of Allergy and Clinical Immunology, 140*(2), 321–333. https://doi.org/10.1016/j.jaci.2017.06.012

Castells, M. (2017b). Drug hypersensitivity and anaphylaxis in cancer and chronic inflammatory diseases: The role of desensitizations. *Frontiers in Immunology, 8,* 1472. https://doi.org/10.3389/fimmu.2017.01472

Lee, S., Hess, E.P., Lohse, C., Gilani, W., Chamberlain, A.M., & Campbell, R.L. (2017). Trends, characteristics, and incidence of anaphylaxis in 2001–2010: A population-based study. *Journal of Allergy and Clinical Immunology, 139*(1), 182–188.e2. https://doi.org/10.1016/j.jaci.2016.04.029

LoVerde, D., Iweala, O.I., Eginli, A., & Krishnaswamy, G. (2018). Anaphylaxis. *Chest, 153*(2), 528–543. https://doi.org/10.1016/j.chest.2017.07.033

Maker, J.H., Stroup, C.M., Huang, V., & James, S.F. (2019). Antibiotic hypersensitivity mechanisms. *Pharmacy, 7*(3), 122. https://doi.org/10.3390/pharmacy7030122

Olsen, M.M., LeFebvre, K.B., & Brassil, K.J. (Eds.). (2019). *Chemotherapy and immunotherapy guidelines and recommendations for practice.* Oncology Nursing Society.

Reber, L.L., Hernandez, J.D., & Galli, S.J. (2017). The pathophysiology of anaphylaxis. *Journal of Allergy and Clinical Immunology, 140*(2), 335–348. https://doi.org/10.1016/j.jaci.2017.06.003

Sicherer, S.H., & Simons, F.E.R. (2017). Epinephrine for first-aid management of anaphylaxis. *Pediatrics, 139*(3), e20164006. https://doi.org/10.1542/peds.2016-4006

Tanno, L.K., Alvarez-Perea, A., & Pouessel, G. (2019). Therapeutic approach of anaphylaxis. *Current Opinions in Allergy and Clinical Immunology, 19*(4), 393–401. https://doi.org/10.1097/ACI.0000000000000539

Yu, J.E., & Lin, R.Y. (2018). The epidemiology of anaphylaxis. *Clinical Reviews in Allergy and Immunology, 54*(3), 366–374. https://doi.org/10.1007/s12016-015-8503-x

CHAPTER 151

Diabetes Mellitus, Types 1 and 2

Sandra Kurtin, PhD, ANP-C, AOCN®

I. Definition: A group of metabolic diseases associated with defects in insulin secretion, insulin action, or a combination of both, resulting in hyperglycemia (American Diabetes Association, 2019a)

II. Physiology/Pathophysiology (American Diabetes Association, 2019a; Kharroubi & Darwish, 2015; Kreider et al., 2018)
   A. Normal
      1. Pancreatic function is critical to breaking down protein, carbohydrates, and fats using digestive juices of the pancreas combined with juices from intestines.
      2. The pancreas secretes hormones that affect the level of glucose (sugar) in the blood.
      3. It also produces chemicals that neutralize stomach acids that pass from the stomach into the small intestine by using substances in pancreatic juice.
      4. The pancreas contains islets of Langerhans, which are tiny groups of specialized cells that are scattered throughout the organ. These cells secrete the following.
         a) Glucagon: Raises the level of glucose in the blood
         b) Insulin: Stimulates cells to use glucose
         c) Somatostatin: Regulates the secretion of glucagon and insulin
   B. Pathophysiology
      1. Chronic hyperglycemia from defects in insulin secretion (insulin deficiency), insulin action on target cells (insulin resistance), increased hepatic glucose production, or a combination results in the following.
         a) Secondary organ damage, including to the eyes, kidneys, nerves, heart, and vasculature
         b) Abnormal metabolism of protein, carbohydrates, and fats
         c) Insulin deficiency
            (1) Autoimmune destruction of beta cells in the pancreas resulting in inadequate insulin production
            (2) Most common in type 1 diabetes mellitus (T1DM)
         d) Insulin resistance: Inability of insulin to affect the target tissue, resulting in increased blood glucose
            (1) Decreased ability of insulin to facilitate glucose transport from the circulation to the intracellular space in skeletal and adipose tissue
            (2) Decreased ability of insulin to inhibit hepatic glucose production
         e) Increased hepatic glucose production, raising blood glucose levels

    f) Deficiencies in other enzymes secreted by the pancreas or intestines

        (1) Decreased incretin effects: Two primary incretin hormones are released by the intestines in the postprandial state that control plasma glucose concentrations: glucagon-like peptide-1 and glucose-dependent insulinotropic polypeptide.

        (2) Decreased amylin effects: A hormone coexpressed by beta cells in the pancreas, it delays gastric emptying, inhibits postprandial glucagon secretion (increased blood glucose), and acts as a satiety agent.

2. T1DM most commonly results from cell-mediated immune destruction of beta cells of the pancreas.

    a) Rate of destruction is variable; it tends to be indolent in adults.

    b) Approximately 85%–90% of patients will have evidence of autoantibodies detected with the initial fasting hyperglycemia test.

    c) Surrogate measures of beta cell destruction include the following.

        (1) Autoantibodies to islet cells, glutamate decarboxylase (GAD65), tyrosine phosphatases 1A-2 and 1A-2β, and zinc transporter protein (ZnT8A)

        (2) Strong HLA association: DQA, DQB, and DRB alleles

3. Type 2 diabetes mellitus (T2DM) is characterized by insulin resistance and relative (not absolute) insulin deficiency. Genetic defects of the beta cells include the following.

    a) Chromosome 12, human hepatocyte nuclear factor (HNF)-1α (maturity onset diabetes of the young [MODY] 3)

    b) Chromosome 7, glucokinase (MODY 2)

    c) Chromosome 20, HNF-4α (MODY 1)

    d) Chromosome 13, insulin promoter factor-1 (MODY 4)

    e) Chromosome 17, HNF-1β (MODY 5)

    f) Chromosome 2, NeuroD1 (MODY 6)

III. Clinical features: Incidence of diabetes worldwide has more than doubled in the past 30 years and is projected to increase by approximately 54% (from 285 million in 2010 to 439 million) by 2030; approximately 90% of these cases are expected to be T2DM. The highest increase in the incidence of diabetes is expected to be in developing countries, including China (highest), India, Pakistan, and Indonesia. People with diabetes are more prone to have unhealthy LDL cholesterol and are at increased risk for atherosclerotic cardiovascular disease (Alrifai et al., 2019; American Diabetes Association, 2019a; Kharroubi & Darwish, 2015; Ohishi, 2018; Rice Bradley, 2018; Yu et al., 2019; Zhu et al., 2017).

  A. Classification: Categorized by most common underlying causes and clinical course

    1. T1DM: Previously categorized as insulin-dependent diabetes or juvenile-onset diabetes

      a) It comprises 5%–10% of diabetes cases.

      b) Patients require insulin administration for survival.

    2. Idiopathic diabetes type 1

      a) It exhibits no clear evidence of autoimmune destruction; strong familial tendencies are noted.

      b) It is rare but is seen most often in patients of Asian or African American descent.

    3. T2DM: Previously categorized as noninsulin-dependent diabetes or adult-onset diabetes

      a) It comprises 90%–95% of diabetes cases.

      b) Patients generally do not require insulin administration for survival but may require insulin during short periods.

      c) This type is most often associated with genetic predisposition and lifestyle.

      d) The most common risk factor is obesity.

4. Gestational diabetes mellitus
   a) More than 200,000 cases are reported annually in the United States, approximately 7% of all pregnancies.
   b) Pregnant women are at a more than sevenfold increased risk for developing T2DM compared to women without gestational diabetes mellitus.
   c) Intrauterine hyperglycemia exposure predisposes the fetus to obesity, metabolic syndrome, and T2DM in early adulthood.
B. Risk factors
   1. Modifiable risk factors
      a) Elevated BMI: Overweight is BMI 25–30 kg/m^2, and obese is BMI greater than 30 kg/m^2
      b) Overweight and obesity: Strongest predictor of diabetes
      c) Weight gain: Early adulthood (ages 25–40 years) carries higher risk than weight gain after age 40 years.
      d) Higher visceral adiposity or waist circumference at any BMI (metabolic obesity): Associated with insulin resistance
      e) Sedentary lifestyle and physical inactivity
      f) Dietary factors: High consumption of red meats, high-fat foods, and refined/processed foods; excess alcohol use
      g) Hyperlipidemia
      h) Hypertension
      i) Smoking
      j) Inflammation
      k) Intrauterine environment
      l) Sleeping disorders
      m) Depression and certain antidepressant medications
      n) Environmental toxins: Endocrine disruptors (bisphenol A—common in air pollution)
   2. Nonmodifiable risk factors
      a) Age
      b) Gender: Female higher risk
      c) Ethnicity: Native American, Asian, Australian indigenous populations, Hispanic
      d) Familial history of diabetes: Lifestyle and genetic predisposition
      e) History of gestational diabetes: Sevenfold risk of developing T2DM
      f) Polycystic ovary syndrome
      g) Low-birth weight: Fetal malnutrition
      h) Viral factors: Congenital rubella, enterovirus, rotavirus, herpes viruses, CMV, endogenous retrovirus
C. Etiology: Genetic defects in insulin action
   1. Type A insulin resistance
   2. Leprechaunism
   3. Rabson-Mendenhall syndrome
   4. Lipoatrophic diabetes
   5. Diseases of the exocrine pancreas
      a) Pancreatitis
      b) Pancreatectomy
      c) Pancreatic neoplasms
      d) Cystic fibrosis
      e) Hemochromatosis

6. Endocrinopathies
    a) Acromegaly
    b) Cushing syndrome
    c) Pheochromocytoma
    d) Hyperthyroidism
    e) Aldosteronism
    f) Somatostatin-producing tumors
7. Drug- or chemical-induced diabetes or hyperglycemia
    a) Pentamidine
    b) Nicotinic acid
    c) Glucocorticoids
    d) Thyroid hormone
    e) Beta-adrenergic agonists
    f) Thiazides
    g) Phenytoin
    h) IFN-γ
    i) Immune checkpoint inhibitors
    j) TKIs: Nilotinib, dasatinib, imatinib
8. Viral infections: Upregulate the immune system
D. History
    1. History of cancer and cancer treatment, particularly regimens containing gluco-corticoids
    2. Current medications: Prescribed, over the counter
    3. History of presenting symptoms: Precipitating factors, onset, duration
    4. Changes in ADLs: Chronic vascular changes associated with diabetes may predispose the patient to cardiovascular disease, CKD, neuropathy, visual deficits, and muscle fatigue, all of which may interfere with ADLs.
    5. Past medical history: Infections, hypertension, increased triglyceride or cholesterol levels, weight change, hypomagnesemia
    6. Family history: Diabetes mellitus, cardiovascular disease, hyperlipidemia, fetal exposure to hyperglycemia
    7. Social history: Diet, exercise routines/habits, smoking, alcohol use
    8. Women: History of gestational diabetes
    9. History of existing T1DM or T2DM
        a) Date of diagnosis
        b) Current and previous treatment regimens for diabetes mellitus
        c) Serial Hgb A1c levels
        d) Episodes of diabetic ketoacidosis or hospitalization for diabetes-related complications
        e) Hypoglycemic episodes, including frequency and severity
        f) History of diabetes-associated complications
            (1) Microvascular disease
                (a) Retinopathy: Severity and managing ophthalmologist
                (b) Nephropathy: Severity and managing nephrologist
                (c) Neuropathy: Severity and managing neurologist
                    i. Sensory: History of falls, pain, and foot ulcers
                    ii. Autonomic: History of sexual dysfunction and gastroparesis
            (2) Macrovascular disease
                (a) Coronary heart disease: Dyslipidemia, hypertension, atherosclerosis
                (b) Peripheral arterial disease

        (c) Cerebrovascular disease: transient ischemic attacks, strokes, thrombosis

        (d) Managing cardiologist or neurologist

E. Signs and symptoms

1. Clinical manifestations are dependent on the rapidity of onset, level of severity, result of hyperglycemia, and secondary metabolic and vascular changes.

    a) Manifestations may be indolent in T2DM with more severe symptoms associated with the chronicity and/or level of hyperglycemia.

    b) T1DM is generally associated with a rapid onset and more severe symptoms until insulin dosing is initiated and sustained.

    c) Patients undergoing pancreatectomy or Whipple procedure will develop insulin dependence immediately following surgery and will require lifelong insulin support.

2. Symptoms will be more pronounced in patients with preexisting cardiovascular, kidney, neurologic, or cerebrovascular disease.

3. Common presenting symptoms

    a) Hyperglycemia

    b) Polyuria

    c) Polydipsia

    d) Tremors

    e) Visual changes

    f) Extreme hunger

    g) Unusual weight loss

    h) Extreme fatigue and irritability

    i) Frequent infections

    j) Cuts and bruises that are slow to heal

    k) Tingling or numbness in the hands or feet

    l) Recurring skin, gum, or bladder infections

4. Late signs and symptoms due to microvascular or macrovascular disease

    a) Visual changes

    b) Peripheral neuropathy

F. Physical examination

1. Vital signs: Weight; BMI; blood pressure, including orthostatic measures if indicated; hypertension with early nephropathy

2. HEENT

    a) Funduscopic examination to evaluate for microaneurysms, venous loops, hard exudates, or soft exudates indicating retinopathy

    b) New vessels in the eye or vitreous hemorrhage possibly indicating proliferative retinopathy

    c) Palpation of thyroid gland to evaluate for nodules or enlargement

3. Lymph: Generally normal unless recurrent infections (see Appendix D)

4. Cardiac

    a) Presence of murmurs, gallops, or rubs indicating possible underlying microvascular or macrovascular disease

    b) Possible peripheral edema with cardiac disease or nephropathy

    c) Decreased dorsalis pedis and posterior tibial pulses on palpation typically indicative of peripheral vascular disease

5. Abdominal: Truncal adiposity, injection-site ecchymoses for patients on insulin, borderline hepatomegaly

6. Musculoskeletal: Focal muscle or joint pain indicative of possible underlying focal or generalized neuropathy

7. Foot: Open areas, calluses, or fungal infection on skin and nails
8. Neurologic: May reveal focal mononeuritis
   a) Presence or absence of patellar or Achilles reflexes, assessment of ankles for depression or loss of ankle jerks indicating distal polyneuropathy
   b) Evaluation of proprioception, which is decreased with peripheral nerve damage
   c) Vibration: Use of 128 hertz tuning fork; typically decreased with peripheral nerve damage
   d) Monofilament sensation: Use of 10 g monofilament pressure sensation at the distal plantar aspect of both great toes and metatarsal joints; decreased with peripheral nerve damage
9. Integument: Acanthosis nigricans (tan or brown raised areas on the sides of the neck, armpits, and groin; may also occur on the hands, elbows, and knees); more common in obese patients
10. Psychiatric: Agitation or somnolence with more severe hyperglycemia or hypoglycemia

IV. Diagnostic tests (Akhtar et al., 2020; Chen et al., 2019)
   A. Laboratory testing is the primary diagnostic technique used for T1DM and T2DM.
      1. Fasting plasma glucose: Blood glucose level drawn after fasting (no caloric intake for eight hours)
      2. Hgb A1c: Measures nonreversible glycosylation of the Hgb molecule, which is directly related to blood glucose concentrations over two to three months
         a) Findings indicating an increased risk for diabetes are an indication to institute preventive measures.
            (1) Fasting plasma glucose of 100–125 mg/dl (3.6–6.9 mmol/L)
            (2) Two-hour 75 g oral glucose tolerance test plasma glucose of 140–190 mg/dl indicative of impaired glucose tolerance
            (3) Hgb A1c 5.7%–6.4%
         b) Diagnostic criteria for diabetes: Any of the following criteria is diagnostic.
            (1) Hgb A1c greater than or equal to 6.5% (48 mmol/mol): The test should be performed in a laboratory using a method that is National Glycohemoglobin Standardization Program certified and standardized to the Diabetes Control and Complications Trial assay.
            (2) Fasting plasma glucose greater than 126 mg/dl (7 mmol/L): Fasting is defined as no caloric intake for at least eight hours.
            (3) Two-hour 75 g oral glucose tolerance test plasma glucose greater than or equal to 200 mg/dl (11.1 mmol/L)
            (4) Random plasma glucose greater than or equal to 200 mg/dl (11.1 mmol/L) in patients with symptoms of hyperglycemia or hyperglycemic crisis
      3. Complete metabolic panel
         a) Serum creatinine and estimated GFR are used to estimate the level of kidney damage.
         b) Assess at diagnosis and then as clinically indicated for the presence and severity of CKD defined as one or more of the following.
            (1) GFR less than 60 ml/min/1.73 m^2
            (2) Albuminuria: Urine albumin greater than 30 mg in 24 hours or urine albumin-to-creatinine ratio greater than 30 mg/g
            (3) Abnormalities in urine sediment, histology, or imaging suggestive of kidney damage
            (4) Renal tubular disorders: Nondiabetic glomerular or interstitial disease

(5) History of kidney transplantation
(6) Severity of CKD
    (a) Stage 1: GFR greater than or equal to 90 ml/min
    (b) Stage 2: GFR 60–89 ml/min
    (c) Stage 3 (moderate): GFR 30–59 ml/min
    (d) Stage 4 (severe): GFR 15–29 ml/min
    (e) Renal failure: GFR less than 15 ml/min or dialysis
    (f) The preferred estimating equation in the United States is the CKD-EPI 2009 creatinine equation, which is more accurate than the earlier Modification of Diet in Renal Disease equation, particularly for eGFR values greater than 60 ml/min/1.73 m^2 (see www.kidney.org/content/ckd-epi-creatinine-equation-2009).

4. Urine for microalbuminuria: Albumin-to-creatinine ratio with spot urine collection based on two to three specimens collected over three to six months
   a) Normal urine albumin: less than 30 mcg/mg creatinine
   b) Microalbuminuria: 30–299 mcg/mg creatinine; earliest indication of diabetic nephropathy
   c) Macroalbuminuria: greater than or equal to 300 mcg/mg creatinine; associated with progression to CKD or end-stage renal disease
   d) Factors that may alter albuminuria measures: Exercise within a 24-hour period, infection, fever, CHF, hyperglycemia
5. CBC to evaluate for presence of infection
6. Vitamin D level to evaluate for deficiency
7. Testosterone levels in men to evaluate for erectile dysfunction
8. TSH in patients with T1DM: Hypothyroidism can induce hyperglycemia.
9. Vitamin B_{12} level: If on metformin, which can induce deficiency
10. Liver function at baseline and to monitor for abnormalities

B. Radiology
   1. Renal ultrasound in presence of severe kidney disease
   2. Bone density scan to evaluate for possible osteoporosis

C. Other
   1. ECG for patients who present with symptoms suggestive of dysrhythmias, electrolyte imbalances, or severe hyperglycemia
   2. Echocardiogram or stress test at baseline

V. Differential diagnosis (American Diabetes Association, 2019a)
  A. Drugs, chemicals, and toxins causing secondary diabetes mellitus
    1. Diuretics: Thiazides, furosemide
    2. Antihypertensive agents: Beta-blockers, clonidine, diazoxide
    3. Hormones: Oral contraceptives, glucocorticoids, adrenocorticotropic hormone, aldosterone, alpha-adrenergic agonists, growth hormone, glucagon, progesterone
    4. Psychoactive agents: Lithium, atypical antipsychotics
    5. Antiepileptic drugs: Phenytoin
    6. Antineoplastic agents: Streptozocin, L-asparaginase, mithramycin
    7. Antiprotozoal drugs: Pentamidine
    8. Nicotinic acid: Niacin
    9. Cyclosporine
    10. Theophylline
  B. Renal tubular disease
  C. Diabetes insipidus

    D. Cushing disease

    E. Pheochromocytoma

    F. Acromegaly

    G. Severe stress secondary to trauma, burns, or infections

    H. Pancreatitis (see Chapter 77)

    I. Cirrhosis (see Chapter 69)

    J. Paraneoplastic syndrome (see Appendix M)

VI. Treatment: Refer to a comprehensive review of overall management of diabetes at https://professional.diabetes.org/content-page/practice-guidelines-resources (American Diabetes Association, 2019a, 2019b; Arnold et al., 2016; Kirwan et al., 2017; Kreider et al., 2018; Sesti et al., 2018; Skugor, 2017; Sterrett et al., 2016; Storey et al., 2017; Strain et al., 2018; Tillman & Kim, 2018).

    A. Prevention/delay of T2DM in at-risk patients: Intensive lifestyle modification programs

        1. Weight loss of approximately 7% of body weight

        2. Increased physical activity: Moderate activity for greater than or equal to 150 min/week

        3. Metformin therapy for patients at high risk: Initial dose of 500 mg PO daily, titrated upward based on laboratory values and assessment of GI distress

           a) Aforementioned laboratory measures, or

           b) BMI greater than 35 kg/m^2, age older than 60 years, or history of gestational diabetes mellitus

           c) Monitoring of renal function

    B. Lifestyle management and disease self-management education

        1. Referral to a diabetes self-management education and support program

        2. Individualized medical nutrition therapy

           a) Weight loss diet should be implemented in any patient who exceeds suggested BMI, which varies by ethnicity.

              (1) BMI is 25–30 kg/m^2 in majority of population; obese is BMI greater than 30 kg/m^2.

              (2) BMI greater than 23 kg/m^2 in Asian Americans

              (3) BMI greater than 26 kg/m^2 in African Americans

           b) Goals include the following.

              (1) Achieve and maintain body weight goals.

              (2) Attain individualized glycemic, blood pressure, and lipid goals.

              (3) Delay or prevent the complications of diabetes.

           c) Carbohydrates are the primary source of postprandial glucose. Glucose content in carbohydrates varies.

              (1) The plate method of estimating carbohydrate content in foods is a useful tool.

              (2) Instruct patients to fill one-half of their plate with vegetables, excluding potatoes and corn.

              (3) Fill one-quarter or less of the plate with fish, poultry, lean red meat, meat substitutes, nuts, or seeds.

              (4) Fill one-quarter of the plate with whole grains, legumes, fruit, or low-fat dairy.

           d) Protein goals in patients with cancer are estimated to be 1–1.5 g/kg. These levels may need to be lower in patients with CKD or renal impairment.

           e) Limiting dietary fat is recommended to reduce the risk of microvascular and macrovascular disease.

              (1) Saturated fats should be less than 7% of total calories.

              (2) Decreased intake of trans fat leads to lower LDL and higher HDL.

  f) Alcohol intake should be limited to one drink or less a day for women, two drinks or less a day for men.

  g) Salt intake should be limited to less than 2,300 mg daily for the general population but may need further modification in the presence of diabetes-associated comorbidities.

  h) Patients with cancer may require additional calories and protein based on their nutritional status, ability to swallow, and concurrent symptoms such as diarrhea, nausea, vomiting, anorexia, weight loss, or constipation.

3. Diabetic nutritional supplements

  a) Boost Glucose Control® (8 oz): 190 calories, 16 g protein, 16 g carbohydrates, 4 g sugar

  b) Glucerna® (8 oz): 200 calories, 10 g protein, 27 g carbohydrates, 6 g sugar

  c) Carnation® Breakfast Essentials™, No Sugar Added (1 packet with 8 oz whole milk): 220 calories, 12 g protein, 24 g carbohydrates, 20 g sugar

  d) Enterex® Diabetic (8 oz): 237 calories, 12 g protein, 27 g carbohydrates, less than 1 g sugar

  e) Scandishake® Sweetened with Aspartame (with 8 oz whole milk): 600 calories, 16 g protein, 53 g carbohydrates, 9 g sugar

  f) Isosource® Original (20 oz bottle): 260 calories, 40 g protein, 25 g carbohydrates, 0 g sugar

  g) Slim-Fast® Low Carb (11 oz): 190 calories, 20 g protein, 6 g carbohydrates, 1 g sugar

4. Exercise

  a) Patients should be evaluated for underlying cardiovascular, pulmonary, musculoskeletal, or retinal risk prior to initiating an exercise program.

  b) Goal is 150 min/week of moderate-intensity exercise (brisk walking) spread over at least three days per week. Shorter durations (minimum 75 min/week) of vigorous intensity or interval training may be sufficient for younger and more physically fit individuals.

  c) Patients should engage in resistance training unless contraindicated. It may be contraindicated in patients with severe retinopathy because of the risk of triggering vitreous hemorrhage.

  d) Patients should be instructed on the signs and symptoms of hyperglycemia or hypoglycemia, which may result from moderate exercise.

   (1) Patients with T1DM and poor glycemic control may develop progressive hyperglycemia with moderate activity.

   (2) Patients with T1DM on insulin may develop hypoglycemia. Additional carbohydrate intake prior to exercise is recommended.

  e) Patients with neuropathy may need modified exercise programs (e.g., chair exercises) to avoid injury.

  f) All patients should be instructed to wear proper footwear for exercise to prevent foot injuries.

5. Patients should be encouraged to stop smoking to limit the risk of microvascular and macrovascular complications.

6. Immunizations should be current.

  a) Annual influenza vaccine

  b) Pneumococcal polysaccharide vaccine: Vaccination should be repeated if the first dose was given prior to age 65 years or in the instance of immunocompromised state (e.g., CKD, nephrotic syndrome, transplantation).

  c) Hepatitis B vaccine series

C. Glycemic control

    1. Target range for Hgb A1c is less than or equal to 7% (plasma glucose is 150 mg/dl) for most patients with diabetes mellitus.

        a) It is less than 6.5% (plasma glucose is 130 mg/dl) for patients with no risk of coronary heart disease, long life expectancy, and expected short duration of diabetes mellitus (e.g., drug induced).

        b) Less stringent guidelines of less than 8% (plasma glucose is 183 mg/dl) may be appropriate for patients with tendency for hypoglycemia, those with limited life expectancy, or those with advanced microvascular or macrovascular complications.

    2. Oral therapies (see Table 151-1): Refer to American Diabetes Association guidelines for detailed management strategies, including special populations.

        a) Metformin (unless contraindicated): Long-term use of metformin may be associated with biochemical vitamin B_{12} deficiency.

        b) Newly diagnosed patients with T2DM and Hgb A1c greater than or equal to 1.5% above glycemic target or severe hyperglycemia and/or symptoms at diagnosis: Add basal insulin.

        c) If noninsulin therapy at maximum tolerated dose does not meet target blood glucose after three months of therapy, add second oral agent, glucagon-like peptide-1 receptor agonist, or insulin.

        d) Treatment should be individualized based on comorbidities and the risk of adverse events including hypoglycemia.

    3. Insulin therapy: Refer to American Diabetes Association guidelines for detailed management strategies, including special populations.

        a) All patients with T1DM require insulin therapy, and the majority of patients with T2DM will require insulin subcutaneously over the course of their disease.

        b) Types of insulin

            (1) Rapid acting: Humalog®, NovoLog®, Apidra®

                (a) Onset: 5–15 minutes

                (b) Peak: 30–90 minutes

                (c) Duration: Less than 5 hours

            (2) Short acting: Regular

                (a) Onset: 30–60 minutes

                (b) Peak: 2–3 hours

                (c) Duration: 5–8 hours

            (3) Intermediate, basal: Neutral protamine Hagedorn (NPH)

                (a) Onset: 2–4 hours

                (b) Peak: 4–10 hours

                (c) Duration: 10–16 hours

            (4) Long acting, basal

                (a) Insulin glargine: Lantus®

                    i. Onset: 2–4 hours

                    ii. Peak: None

                    iii. Duration: 20–24 hours

                (b) Insulin detemir: Levemir®

                    i. Onset: 3–8 hours

                    ii. Peak: None

                    iii. Duration: 5–24 hours

                (c) Premixed insulin: 70% NPH/30% regular

                    i. Onset: 30–60 minutes

ii. Peak: Dual

iii. Duration: 10–16 hours

c) Insulin management guidelines are described in detail in the American Diabetes Association guidelines. A typical starting insulin dose for metabolically stable patients with T1DM is 0.5 units/kg daily divided into two doses: 50% as pran-

TABLE 151-1	Oral Diabetic Therapy			
Drug Class	**Route and Agents**[a]	**Mechanism of Action**	**Advantages**	**Disadvantages**
Alpha-glucosidase inhibitors	Oral • Acarbose • Miglitol	Decreases rate of carbohydrate (polysaccharide) digestion in the small intestine Decreases post-prandial glycemic excursion	No hypoglycemia Weight neutral	Common and frequently severe gastrointestinal side effects Three-times-daily dosing
Amylin mimetic	Subcutaneous • Pramlintide	Decreases excess postprandial glucagon secretion Increases satiety Slows gastric emptying	No weight gain	Expensive Injectable Gastrointestinal upset
Biguanides	Oral • Metformin	Decreases hepatic glucose output Decreases intestinal glucose absorption Increases insulin action	No hypoglycemia High efficacy No weight gain, possible weight loss Decreased cardiovascular disease events	Gastrointestinal side effects Contraindicated in chronic kidney disease Lactic acidosis (very rare) Vitamin B_{12} deficiency
Dipeptidyl peptidase-4 (DPP-4) inhibitors	Oral • Alogliptin • Sitagliptin • Saxagliptin • Linagliptin	Incretin enhancer Decreases endogenous glucagon-like peptide-1 (GLP-1) degradation Increases active GLP-1 concentration Increases insulin secretion Decreases glucagon secretion	Oral, once-daily dosing Few side effects Intermediate efficacy Weight neutral No hypoglycemia	Dose adjustment necessary in chronic kidney disease Rare: Angioedema, pancreatitis Alogliptin, saxagliptin: Risk of congestive heart failure Joint pain
Glinides	Oral • Nateglinide • Repaglinide	Increases insulin secretion	Short duration allowing for action only during postprandial period	Dosing prior to every meal (three times daily) Hypoglycemia Weight gain

(Continued on next page)

TABLE 151-1	Oral Diabetic Therapy *(Continued)*			
Drug Class	**Route and Agents**[a]	**Mechanism of Action**	**Advantages**	**Disadvantages**
GLP-1 mimetics	Subcutaneous • Exenatide • Dulaglutide • Liraglutide • Semaglutide	Increases post-prandial insulin secretion Decreases excess postprandial glucagon secretion Increases satiety Slows gastric emptying	No hypoglycemia Possible weight loss Liraglutide: Once-daily dosing, atherosclerotic cardiovascular disease benefit Semaglutide and extended-release exenatide: Atherosclerotic cardiovascular disease benefit	Gastrointestinal side effects Requires renal dose adjustment Injectable Exenatide: twice-daily dosing (once-weekly dosing in phase 3 clinical trials) U.S. Food and Drug Administration Black Box warning for class: Potential for thyroid malignancy
Sodium glucose cotransporter-2 (SGLT2) inhibitors	Oral • Canagliflozin • Dapagliflozin • Empagliflozin • Ertugliflozin	Inhibits glucose reabsorption in proximal tubule of the kidney leading to glycosuria, which lowers the blood glucose concentration, lowers blood pressure, and leads to some weight loss	Intermediate efficacy Low risk of hypoglycemia Canagliflozin, empagliflozin: Atherosclerotic cardiovascular disease benefit and congestive heart failure benefit	Requires renal dose adjustment Genitourinary symptoms Risk for diabetic ketoacidosis Increased low density lipoprotein Canagliflozin: U.S. Food and Drug Administration Black Box warning for risk of amputation
Sulfonylureas (second generation)	Oral • Glimepiride • Glyburide • Glipizide • Glimepiride	Increases insulin secretion from beta cells	High efficacy Well tolerated	Hypoglycemia (usually mild) Weight gain Dose adjustment necessary in chronic kidney disease; glyburide not recommended
Thiazolidinediones	Oral • Pioglitazone • Rosiglitazone	Decreases insulin resistance in skeletal muscle and adipose tissue	No hypoglycemia Improved lipid profile pioglitazone only (increased high density lipoprotein cholesterol, decreased triglycerides) Benefit in nonalcoholic steatosis	Fluid retention, weight gain, edema Bone fractures Increased low density lipoprotein cholesterol Contraindicated in heart failure Some evidence that rosiglitazone may increase risk of myocardial infarction

[a]For agent-specific dosing recommendations, please refer to manufacturer prescribing information.

Note. Based on information from American Diabetes Association, 2019a; Skugor, 2017.

dial insulin given to control blood glucose after meals, and 50% as basal insulin to control glycemia in the periods between meal absorption.
   d) Check fasting glucose daily.
      (1) Increase dose by two units every three days until fasting levels are consistently in target range (70–130 mg/dl).
      (2) Increase dose up to four units every three days for sustained blood glucose greater than 180 mg/dl.
      (3) If hypoglycemia occurs, reduce bedtime dose by four units or 10%, whichever is greater.
      (4) Blood glucose should be checked before meals, at bedtime, before exercise, if hypoglycemia is suspected, and under special circumstances.
   e) Recheck Hgb A1c after two to three months.
      (1) Hgb A1c less than 7%: Continue current regimen, and repeat every three months.
      (2) Hgb A1c greater than 7% and blood glucose within target: Check blood glucose before lunch, dinner, and bedtime.
         (a) Prelunch greater than target range: Add rapid-acting insulin at breakfast.
         (b) Predinner blood glucose greater than target range: Add NPH insulin at breakfast and rapid-acting insulin at lunch.
         (c) Prebedtime blood glucose greater than target range: Add rapid-acting insulin at dinner.
         (d) Initial dose can begin at four units and adjust by two units every three days until blood glucose is in target range.
      (3) Select medications that may lower Hgb A1c levels to treat comorbidities, illness, or symptoms.
         (a) Antibiotics: Clarithromycin B, levofloxacin, ciprofloxacin
         (b) Antipsychotics: Aripiprazole, lithium
         (c) Hypertension: Atenolol, bisoprolol, diltiazem, nifedipine
         (d) Antidepressants: Doxepin
         (e) Pain: Morphine, fentanyl, oxycodone, pregabalin
         (f) Anticonvulsants: Fosphenytoin, phenytoin
         (g) Bronchodilator: Theophylline
         (h) Gout: Probenecid
         (i) Parkinson agent: Selegiline
         (j) Immunosuppressant: Tacrolimus
         (k) Smoking cessation: Varenicline
         (l) TB: Rifampin
         (m) PPIs
4. Hypoglycemia: Plasma glucose less than 70 mg/dl
   a) It is most often associated with insulin administration.
   b) Moderate hypoglycemia can be treated with one of the following.
      (1) 15–20 g glucose
      (2) 4 oz (½ cup) regular soda
      (3) 2 tbsp raisins
      (4) 4–5 saltine crackers
      (5) 4 tsp sugar
      (6) 1 tbsp honey or corn syrup
      (7) Emergency glucagon kit
   c) Severe hypoglycemia: Requires the assistance of another person to administer emergency glucagon

D. Prevention and treatment of disease-related secondary effects and complications

1. Coronary heart disease

   a) Antiplatelet agents: Prevention of microvascular or macrovascular changes

      (1) Low-dose ASA: 81 mg PO daily for patients at increased risk for cardiovascular disease

      (2) Age and gender: Men older than 50 years or women older than 60 years with one or more risk factors (see Risk Factors)

      (3) ASA: Not recommended for prevention in patients without risk factors because of risk of bleeding

      (4) Clopidogrel: 75 mg PO daily for patients with an ASA allergy

      (5) Combination of ASA and clopidogrel: May be recommended for patients with a history of acute coronary syndrome

   b) Smoking cessation: Advise all patients not to smoke.

   c) Hypertension (see Chapter 47) and/or dyslipidemia (see Chapter 44)

      (1) Systolic blood pressure 140–160 mm Hg or diastolic blood pressure 90–100 mm Hg: Lifestyle management, including reducing sodium and increasing potassium intake, moderation of alcohol intake, and increased physical activity, should be practiced for three months. If no improvement, institute pharmacologic management.

      (2) Systolic pressure greater than 160 mm Hg or diastolic pressure greater than 100 mm Hg: Institute pharmacologic therapy

      (3) Home blood pressure monitoring is recommended as part of the diabetes self-management program.

      (4) Dyslipidemia target range is LDL less than 100 mg/dl for any patient with diabetes mellitus.

2. Nephropathy

   a) It occurs in 20%–40% of patients with diabetes mellitus.

   b) Primary mechanisms of reducing risk are glycemic control and control of hypertension.

   c) Persistent albuminuria is associated with diabetic nephropathy and cardiovascular risk.

   d) Adjustment of medications, including chemotherapy dosing, may be necessary based on GFR and creatinine clearance.

3. Retinopathy

   a) It is a vascular complication of T1DM or T2DM. Onset is most common five years after onset of diabetes.

   b) Retinopathy is strongly associated with duration of diabetes, chronic hyperglycemia, nephropathy, and hypertension.

   c) It is the most frequent cause of onset of new blindness in adults aged 24–70 years.

   d) Prevention is based on effective glycemic control and control of hypertension.

      (1) Dilated and comprehensive ophthalmic examination is recommended at the time of diagnosis of diabetes.

      (2) It should include fundus examination and retinal photography.

      (3) Repeat examinations as indicated based on any changes.

   e) Treatment

      (1) No treatments are currently available for reversal of visual loss due to microvascular damage.

      (2) Effective diabetes management may reduce progressive microvascular changes.

    (3) Laser photocoagulation surgery has been shown to reduce the progression of retinopathy. It should be considered for patients who have a high risk for retinopathy, existing proliferative or nonproliferative retinopathy, or evidence of macular edema.

    (4) Recombinant vascular endothelial growth factor injections may be used in patients with macular edema.

4. Peripheral neuropathy (see Chapter 143)

a) Peripheral neuropathy may be caused by diabetes, comorbid conditions (e.g., various malignancies), medications (e.g., chemotherapy agents), metabolic deficiencies (e.g., vitamin B_{12}), CKD, vasculitis, or chronic inflammatory demyelinating neuropathy.

b) Symptoms may be subtle or asymptomatic yet may predispose the patient to falls and foot or other injuries.

c) No effective treatments exist to reverse underlying nerve damage.

5. Foot care

a) General foot care instructions should be provided to all patients with diabetes, including strategies to prevent injuries.

    (1) Daily foot examinations

    (2) Reporting of loss of protective sensation

    (3) Daily skin (foot) and nail care

    (4) Well-fitting shoes

    (5) Preventive management of foot deformities (e.g., hammertoes, bunions) and calluses by a healthcare professional trained in diabetes management

b) Effective diabetes management may reduce the risk of foot ulcers and amputations.

c) High-risk factors for ulcers or amputations due to injury or vascular disease

    (1) Previous amputation or history of foot ulcers

    (2) Presence of peripheral neuropathy

    (3) Presence of peripheral vascular disease

    (4) Poorly controlled hypertension

    (5) Foot deformity

    (6) Nail changes: Fungal infections, ingrown toenails

    (7) Visual impairment

    (8) History of falls

    (9) Poor glycemic control

    (10) Continued tobacco use

d) Screening for peripheral arterial disease should occur, particularly in patients with evidence of macrovascular disease and those who smoke.

VII. Follow-up (American Diabetes Association, 2019a)

  A. Diabetes (T1DM and T2DM) requires a comprehensive interprofessional approach for effective management.

  B. Self-care strategies are critical for effective monitoring and control.

  C. The frequency of follow-up and the members of the healthcare team involved will vary widely based on the severity of symptoms, patient and caregiver self-management skills, and presence of comorbid conditions, including cancer and cancer treatment.

  D. Typical follow-up is every three months to evaluate Hgb A1c if glucose is controlled.

VIII. Referrals: Individualized based on patient risk factors, disease status, and needs (American Diabetes Association, 2019a)

A. Primary care provider: To manage glucose levels

B. Endocrinologist: If Hgb A1c remains greater than or equal to 7% after three months of intensified regimen

C. Nephrologist: For patients with stage 3 or greater CKD

D. Ophthalmologist
    1. Annual eye examination to evaluate for retinal disease
    2. Patients with evidence of proliferative or nonproliferative diabetic retinopathy

E. Clinical dietitian: To assist with diet

F. Diabetes educator: For further refinement of regimen for persistent elevated Hgb A1c and for evaluation of diet, exercise, glycemic control measures, and how to use glucose monitor for serial plasma glucose levels

G. Cardiologist: For cardiac-induced complications such as CHF, peripheral vascular disease, or uncontrolled hypertension

H. Podiatrist: For neurologic impairment, foot ulcers, or chronic nail problems

I. Urologist: For erectile dysfunction and low testosterone levels

J. Vascular surgeon: For severe peripheral vascular disease needing surgeon

K. Psychologist/psychiatrist: For lifestyle changes, depression, anxiety, or eating disorders PRN

L. Smoking cessation program

M. Periodontist: For comprehensive periodontal examination

N. Occupational or physical therapist: For patients with visual impairment, severe peripheral vascular disease, or amputations

References

Akhtar, M., Taha, N.M., Nauman, A., Mujeeb, I.B., & Al-Nabet, A.D.M.H. (2020). Diabetic kidney disease: Past and present. *Advances in Anatomic Pathology, 27*(2), 87–97. https://doi.org/10.1097/PAP.0000000000000257

Alrifai, T., Ali, F.S., Saleem, S., Ruiz, D.C.M., Rifai, D., Younas, S., & Qureshi, F. (2019). Immune checkpoint inhibitor induced diabetes mellitus treated with insulin and metformin: Evolution of diabetes management in the era of immunotherapy. *Case Reports in Oncological Medicine, 2019*, 8781347. https://doi.org/10.1155/2019/8781347

American Diabetes Association. (2019a). Comprehensive medical evaluation and assessment of comorbidities: Standards of medical care in diabetes—2019. *Diabetes Care, 42*(Suppl. 1), S34–S45. https://doi.org/10.2337/dc19-S004

American Diabetes Association. (2019b). Diabetes advocacy: Standards of medical care in diabetes—2019. *Diabetes Care, 42*(Suppl. 1), S182–S183. https://doi.org/10.2337/dc19-S016

Arnold, P., Scheurer, D., Dake, A.W., Hedgpeth, A., Hutto, A., Colquitt, C., & Hermayer, K.L. (2016). Hospital guidelines for diabetes management and the Joint Commission-American Diabetes Association inpatient diabetes certification. *American Journal of the Medical Sciences, 351*(4), 333–341. https://doi.org/10.1016/j.amjms.2015.11.024

Chen, T.K., Knicely, D.H., & Grams, M.E. (2019). Chronic kidney disease diagnosis and management: A review. *JAMA, 322*(13), 1294–1304. https://doi.org/10.1001/jama.2019.14745

Kharroubi, A.T., & Darwish, H.M. (2015). Diabetes mellitus: The epidemic of the century. *World Journal of Diabetes, 6*(6), 850–867. https://doi.org/10.4239/wjd.v6.i6.850

Kirwan, J.P., Sacks, J., & Nieuwoudt, S. (2017). The essential role of exercise in the management of type 2 diabetes. *Cleveland Clinic Journal of Medicine, 84*(7 Suppl. 1), S15–S21. https://doi.org/10.3949/ccjm.84.s1.03

Kreider, K.E., Gabrielski, A.A., & Hammonds, F.B. (2018). Hyperglycemia syndromes. *Nursing Clinics of North America, 53*(3), 303–317. https://doi.org/10.1016/j.cnur.2018.04.001

Ohishi, M. (2018). Hypertension with diabetes mellitus: Physiology and pathology. *Hypertension Research, 41*(6), 389–393. https://doi.org/10.1038/s41440-018-0034-4

Rice Bradley, B.H. (2018). Dietary fat and risk for type 2 diabetes: A review of recent research. *Current Nutrition Reports, 7*(4), 214–226. https://doi.org/10.1007/s13668-018-0244-z

Sesti, G., Antonelli Incalzi, R., Bonora, E., Consoli, A., Giaccari, A., Maggi, S., … Ferrara, N. (2018). Management of diabetes in older adults. *Nutrition, Metabolism and Cardiovascular Diseases, 28*(3), 206–218. https://doi.org/10.1016/j.numecd.2017.11.007

Skugor, M. (2017). Medical treatment of diabetes mellitus. *Cleveland Clinic Journal of Medicine, 84*(7 Suppl. 1), S57 S61. https://doi.org/10.3949/ccjm.84.s1.07

Sterrett, J.J., Bragg, S., & Weart, C.W. (2016). Type 2 diabetes medication review. *American Journal of the Medical Sciences, 351*(4), 342–355. https://doi.org/10.1016/j.amjms.2016.01.019

Storey, S., Von Ah, D., & Hammer, M.J. (2017). Measurement of hyperglycemia and impact on health outcomes in people with cancer: Challenges and opportunities. *Oncology Nursing Forum, 44*(4), E141–E151. https://doi.org/10.1188/17.Onf.E141-e151

Strain, W.D., Hope, S.V., Green, A., Kar, P., Valabhji, J., & Sinclair, A.J. (2018). Type 2 diabetes mellitus in older people: A brief statement of key principles of modern day management including the assessment of frailty. A national collaborative stakeholder initiative. *Diabetic Medicine, 35*(7), 838–845. https://doi.org/10.1111/dme.13644

Tillman, F., & Kim, J. (2018). Select medications that unexpectedly lower HbA1c levels. *Journal of Clinical Pharmacology and Therapeutics, 43*(4), 587–590. https://doi.org/10.1111/jcpt.12689

Yu, L., Liu, J., Huang, X., & Jiang, Q. (2019). Adverse effects of dasatinib on glucose-lipid metabolism in patients with chronic myeloid leukaemia in the chronic phase. *Scientific Reports, 9,* 17601. https://doi.org/10.1038/s41598-019-54033-0

Zhu, B., Hershberger, P.E., Kapella, M.C., & Fritschi, C. (2017). The relationship between sleep disturbance and glycaemic control in adults with type 2 diabetes: An integrative review. *Journal of Clinical Nursing, 26*(23-24), 4053–4064. https://doi.org/10.1111/jocn.13899

CHAPTER 152

Hypocalcemia/Hypercalcemia

Sandra Kurtin, PhD, ANP-C, AOCN®

I. Definitions (NCI CTEP, 2017)
   A. Hypocalcemia: A disorder characterized by laboratory test results indicating a low concentration of calcium (Ca^{2+}) (corrected for albumin) in the blood
   1. Grade 1
      a) Corrected serum Ca^{2+} of less than LLN–8 mg/dl
      b) Less than LLN–4 mEq/L
      c) Ionized Ca^{2+} less than LLN–2 mEq/L
   2. Grade 2
      a) Corrected serum Ca^{2+} less than 8–7 mg/dl
      b) Less than 3.5–4 mEq/L
      c) Ionized Ca^{2+} less than 1.8–2 mEq/L; symptomatic
   3. Grade 3: Hospitalization indicated
      a) Corrected serum Ca^{2+} less than 7–6 mg/dl
      b) Less than 3–3.5 mEq/L
      c) Ionized Ca^{2+} less than 1.6–1.8 mEq/L
   4. Grade 4: Life-threatening consequences
      a) Corrected serum Ca^{2+} less than 6 mg/dl
      b) Less than 3 mEq/L
      c) Ionized Ca^{2+} less than 1.6 mEq/L
   B. Hypercalcemia: A disorder characterized by laboratory test results indicating an elevation in the concentration of calcium (corrected for albumin) in the blood
   1. Grade 1
      a) Corrected serum Ca^{2+} greater than ULN–11.5 mg/dl
      b) Greater than ULN–5.8 mEq/L
      c) Ionized Ca^{2+} greater than ULN–3 mEq/L
   2. Grade 2
      a) Corrected serum Ca^{2+} greater than 11.5–12.5 mg/dl
      b) Greater than 5.8–6.2 mEq/L
      c) Ionized Ca^{2+} greater than 3–3.2 mEq/L; symptomatic
   3. Grade 3: Hospitalization indicated
      a) Corrected serum Ca^{2+} greater than 12.5–13.5 mg/dl
      b) Greater than 6.2–6.8 mEq/L
      c) Ionized Ca^{2+} greater than 3.2–3.6 mEq/L
   4. Grade 4: Life-threatening consequences
      a) Corrected serum Ca^{2+} greater than 13.5 mg/dl
      b) Greater than 6.8 mEq/L
      c) Ionized Ca^{2+} greater than 3.6 mEq/L

II. Physiology/Pathophysiology (Berndt et al., 2016; Body et al., 2017; Reagan et al., 2014; Smogorzewski et al., 2016; Song, 2017)

A. Normal: Ranges from 4.5–5.5 mEq/L or 9–11 mg/dl

1. Corrected Ca^{2+} is serum Ca^{2+} + [0.8 × (4 − serum albumin)].

2. Approximately 99% of the body's calcium is concentrated in the skeletal system (bone and teeth) as hydroxyapatite crystal.

3. The remainder is present in the soft tissues (0.6%), the extracellular fluid (0.1%), and the plasma (0.03%) (serum Ca^{2+}).

4. Of extacellular Ca^{2+}, 40% is protein bound, 48% is free (ionized Ca^{2+}), and the remaining 12% is compounded with anions (phosphate, lactate, citrate, bicarbonate).

5. Ionized Ca^{2+} is the physiologically active component of extracellular (blood and plasma) Ca^{2+}.

6. Extracellular Ca^{2+} is regulated by complex interactions between three primary organs (skeleton, kidney, and intestines) and PTH, vitamin D, and calcitonin.

   a) Skeleton: Provides a reserve pool of calcium

      (1) Ca^{2+} deposition or release from the bone

      (2) 500 mg of Ca^{2+} released daily from the bone with similar amount deposited as new bone formation

   b) Intestines

      (1) Ca^{2+} absorption or release from the GI tract, primarily the duodenum

      (2) Average daily intake of 1,000 mg of Ca^{2+} with 200 mg absorbed in the duodenum and upper intestines and 800 mg excreted in the urine (200 mg daily), bile (200 mg daily), and pancreatic and intestinal (feces) secretions

   c) Kidneys: Filter approximately 10 g of Ca^{2+} daily, with 200 mg excreted in the urine

   d) PTH and parathyroid receptor protein (PTHrP) and calcium-sensing receptor (CaSR): Increased serum Ca^{2+}

      (1) Stimulates bone resorption of Ca^{2+} via stimulation of osteoclasts and kidney reabsorption of Ca^{2+} in the ascending loop of Henle and distal nephron

      (2) Augments intestinal absorption of calcium

      (3) Activates renal hydroxylation of 25-hydroxyvitamin D (25[OH]D) to 1,25-dihydroxyvitamin D (1,25[OH]$_2$D, calcitriol)

      (4) CaSR: Senses the plasma Ca^{2+} concentration and modifies PTH secretion accordingly

      (5) PTHrP: Rare in normal calcium balance; is upregulated in humoral hypercalcemia of malignancy

   e) Vitamin D: 1,25(OH)$_2$D (calcitriol) exerts an endocrine effect on vitamin D receptors in the kidney, small intestine, and bone.

      (1) Enhances renal tubular reabsorption of Ca^{2+}

      (2) Enhances absorption of Ca^{2+} in the small intestine

      (3) Increases osteoclastogenesis via stimulation of receptor activator of nuclear factor kappa-B ligand after binding to vitamin D receptor sites on osteoclasts

   f) Calcitonin: Decreases serum Ca^{2+}

      (1) Produced by the thyroid

      (2) Promotes Ca^{2+} transfer from the plasma to the bones

   g) Serum protein: Primarily in the form of albumin; binds calcium

   h) Acid-base balance

      (1) Acidosis: Ca^{2+} released from serum protein; increased serum Ca^{2+}

      (2) Alkalosis: Ca^{2+} bound to serum protein; decreased serum Ca^{2+}

   i) Anion phosphorus: Inhibits calcium absorption

7. Calcium function

    a) Neuromuscular activity: Transmission of nerve impulses and contraction of skeletal muscles

    b) Cardiac (myocardial) contractility

    c) Cellular permeability

        (1) Increased calcium decreases cellular permeability.

        (2) Decreased calcium increases cellular permeability.

    d) Thrombosis: Promotes blood clotting by converting prothrombin into thrombin

    e) Formation and strengthening of teeth and bone

B. Pathophysiology

    1. Calcium imbalances generally are a result of calcium shifting to or from the primary compartments.

        a) Intestines: Increased or decreased absorption

        b) Kidneys: Increased excretion or reabsorption

        c) Skeleton: Shifting of calcium out of or into the bones

        d) Serum albumin: Increased or decreased binding of calcium with secondary effect on free calcium

        e) Abnormal shifting of calcium: Result of processes that affect the intake, absorption, or excretion of calcium

        f) Levels: Regulated by the complex interaction among these compartments and a variety of biochemical substances or processes, including PTH, vitamin D, calcitonin, albumin, and acid-base levels

    2. Decreased serum Ca^{2+}: Hypocalcemia

        a) Decreased PTH level: Inhibits calcium release from bones and decreases renal calcium absorption

        b) Excitability of the skeletal, smooth, and cardiac muscles

    3. Increased serum Ca^{2+}: Hypercalcemia

        a) Decreased GI peristalsis and GI motility

        b) Enhanced hydrochloric acid, gastrin, and pancreatic enzyme release

        c) Decreased cellular permeability

        d) Osteolytic hypercalcemia: Occurs as local osteoclast-activating cytokines (e.g., IL-1, IL-6, PTHrP) lead to increased receptor activator of nuclear factor kappa-B ligand expression on osteoblasts and receptor activator of nuclear factor kappa-B–mediated bone resorption, causing release of transforming growth factor-beta and increased PTHrP expression on tumor cells and leading to increased Ca^{2+}, decreased PTH, decreased $1,25(OH)_2D$, increased phosphate, and hypercalciuria

        e) In granulomatous disease: Elevated circulating levels of $1,25(OH)_2D$ by activated macrophages leading to hyperabsorption of Ca^{2+} in the intestines and resulting in increased Ca^{2+}

III. Clinical features: Onset of calcium imbalances may be acute (less than 48 hours), such as in tumor lysis syndrome or AKI, or chronic (greater than 48 hours), such as in vitamin D deficiency, exposure to bisphosphonates, or in the case of genetic disorders. Primary hyperparathyroidism and malignancy account for the majority of hypercalcemia cases. Hypocalcemia is less common but is usually symptomatic and requires treatment (Berndt et al., 2016; Body et al., 2017; Feldenzer & Sarno, 2018; Marcucci et al., 2018; Schattner et al., 2016; Smogorzewski et al., 2016; Zagzag et al., 2018).

A. Etiology: Hypocalcemia

    1. Common in patients in the ICU

        a) Trauma setting (70%–80%) and hospitalized patients (10%–18%)

    b) Crystalloids, citrated blood products, contrast dye, hyperventilation, immobilization

  2. Hypoparathyroidism

    a) Genetic syndromes: *PTH* gene mutation, DiGeorge syndrome, *CASR* gene mutation

    b) Acquired hypoparathyroidism: Damage or destruction of the parathyroid gland such as parathyroidectomy, autoimmune disorders (rare), hypomagnesemia, radiation, iron or copper overload

  3. Vitamin D deficiency

    a) Low vitamin D production: Lack of ultraviolet light exposure

    b) End-stage liver disease: Diminished hydroxylation of vitamin D

    c) CKD: Ineffective hydroxylation of 25-hydroxycholecalciferol leading to reduced intestinal absorption and renal reabsorption

    d) Vitamin D malabsorption: Decreased biliary salts, increased GI transit time, mucosal disease in the GI tract

    e) Vitamin D resistance: Rickets

  4. Malabsorption

    a) Ca^{2+} deficit resulting from lack of Ca^{2+} intake is rare.

    b) Vitamin D must be present for calcium absorption from GI tract.

    c) Inadequate protein intake inhibits the body's utilization of calcium.

    d) Chronic diarrhea interferes with adequate calcium absorption.

    e) Celiac disease and bypass procedures occur.

  5. Rapid transfusion of citrated blood: Binds with free Ca^{2+}; leads to decreased ionized Ca^{2+}

  6. Hyperphosphatemia: Binds free Ca^{2+}, such as in pancreatitis, tumor lysis syndrome, and sepsis

  7. Hypomagnesemia: Inhibits PTH secretion, which is common in malnourishment with ethanol abuse

  8. Hypoalbuminemia/hypoproteinemia: Most common cause of low serum Ca^{2+}

    a) Nephrotic syndrome

    b) Hepatic cirrhosis

    c) GI malabsorption or protein leak

  9. Alkalosis: Increases calcium protein binding

 10. Renal dysfunction: Renal failure causing phosphorus and calcium retention

 11. Acute pancreatitis

    a) Hypoalbuminemia

    b) Precipitation of calcium with fatty acids from mesenteric fat necrosis and lipolysis

 12. Gadolinium contrast: Used for MRI; may temporarily interfere with serum Ca^{2+}

 13. Plasmapheresis

 14. Medications

    a) Phosphate laxatives, oral phosphate compounds

    b) Drugs that deplete magnesium: Diuretics, cisplatin, aminoglycosides

    c) Drugs that inhibit bone resorption of Ca^{2+}: Bisphosphonates, mithramycin, calcitonin

    d) PPIs

    e) H_2 antagonists

    f) Foscarnet: Trisodium phosphonoformate

    g) Pentamidine

    h) Ketoconazole

    i) Chemotherapy agents: Cisplatin, asparaginase, doxorubicin

B. Etiology: Hypercalcemia
1. Hyperparathyroidism
    a) Increased osteoclast-mediated bone resorption moves Ca^{2+} into the extracellular fluid.
    b) Primary hyperparathyroidism: Approximately 50% of cases of hypercalcemia in the general population
        (1) Benign adenoma of the parathyroid gland: Most common cause of primary hyperparathyroidism (80%–85% of cases)
        (2) Multiple endocrine neoplasia type 1 and 2
        (3) Parathyroid carcinoma: Rare
2. Increased intestinal Ca^{2+} absorption occurs with vitamin D overdose or milk-alkali syndrome (prolonged intake of calcium carbonate together with milk products usually greater than 4 g of Ca^{2+} daily).
3. Hypercalcemia of malignancy: Present in 10%–25% of patients; particularly common in late-stage disease and at the end of life (last four to six weeks)
    a) Humoral hypercalcemia of malignancy: Approximately 80% of cases
        (1) Common tumor types: Squamous cell, renal, breast, and ovarian carcinomas; non-Hodgkin lymphoma
        (2) Mechanism: Upregulation of PTHrP increased bone resorption and decreased osteoclast bone formation leading to shift of Ca^{2+} to the extracellular fluid
    b) Local osteolytic hypercalcemia: Approximately 20% of cases
        (1) Common tumor types: Breast and prostate carcinoma, multiple myeloma, lymphoma, leukemia
        (2) Subtypes
            (a) Osteolytic: Most common in multiple myeloma; approximately 15%–20% of patients develop hypercalcemia.
            (b) Osteoblastic: Variety of tumors
            (c) Mixed: Common in breast cancer with humoral component
        (3) $1,25(OH)_2D$-induced hypercalcemia in lymphoma: Malignant cells produce 1-alpha-hydroxylase, which converts $25(OH)D$ to $1,25(OH)_2D$, leading to increased Ca^{2+}.
        (4) Ectopic secretion of PTH: Rare
4. Multiple endocrine neoplasia
5. Prolonged immobilization or bone fractures: Cause bone loss of calcium
6. Acidosis: Ca^{2+} unbound from protein
7. Milk-alkali syndrome: Chronic intake of calcium supplements, especially taken with vitamin D, that may activate the kidney CaSR, causing a reactive diuresis and subsequent decrease in GFR and increase in tubular reabsorption of calcium
8. Granulomatous disease: TB, sarcoidosis, histoplasmosis, coccidiomycosis, *Pneumocystis*, leprosy, eosinophilic granulomatosis, inflammatory bowel disease
9. Medications
    a) Lithium
    b) Excessive use of calcium supplements, calcium salts, and antacids causing potential increase in serum Ca^{2+} level
    c) Thiazide diuretics decreasing the excretion of calcium
    d) Steroids mobilizing calcium absorption from the bone
    e) Accidental overdose of vitamin D
    f) Excessive doses of vitamin A: greater than 500 IU daily over prolonged periods
C. History

1. History of cancer and cancer treatment
2. Current medications: Prescribed, over the counter, in particular calcium-containing compounds, vitamin D, magnesium, and phosphate
3. History of presenting symptoms: Precipitating factors, location, duration
4. Changes in ADLs
5. Past medical history
   a) Hypocalcemia: Parathyroidectomy, rare familial parathyroid disorders, celiac disease, gastric bypass procedures
   b) Hypercalcemia: Immobility, fractures, rare familial parathyroid disorders, endocrine abnormalities, receiving treatment for osteoporosis
D. Signs and symptoms (see Table 152-1): Clinical manifestations are dependent on the rapidity of onset (acute [less than 48 hours] or chronic [greater than 48 hours]) and the level of severity.
E. Physical examination (see Table 152-1)
   1. Vital signs

TABLE 152-1	Most Common Clinical Manifestations of Hypocalcemia/Hypercalcemia	
Organ/System	**Hypocalcemia**	**Hypercalcemia**
Cardiovascular	Prolonged QT interval Hypotension Congestive heart failure	Bradycardia First-degree heart block Short QT interval Bundle branch block Hypertension Cardiac arrest (rare)
Gastrointestinal	Gastric ulcers	Anorexia Dry mouth, thirst Nausea, vomiting, constipation
General	Malaise, weakness, dry skin, brittle nails, cataracts	Malaise, weakness
Neuromuscular	Tetany Paresthesias: circumoral, fingers, toes Cramping: extremities or abdominal muscles Chvostek sign Convulsions Laryngeal or bronchial spasm Hyperreflexia Seizures Papilledema	Muscle weakness Hyporeflexia, hypotonia Myalgia Arthralgia Bone pain Chondrocalcinosis
Neuropsychiatric	Emotional disturbances, irritability Depression	Memory loss, lack of concentration Headache Drowsiness Irritability Paranoia, hallucinations Ataxia Speech defects
Renal	Hypercalciuria	Nephrolithiasis Polyuria

Note. Based on information from Body et al., 2017; Smogorzewski et al., 2016; Zagzag et al., 2018.

    a) Heart rate: Bradycardia with hypercalcemia

    b) Blood pressure: Hypotension with hypocalcemia; hypertension with hypercalcemia

    c) Temperature: Normal to slightly elevated

    d) Weight: Variable changes based on fluid status and appetite

    e) Pain: Muscle cramping, tetany in hypocalcemia; bone pain is common with hypercalcemia of malignancy.

    f) General: Fatigued, withdrawn, or irritable patient

2. HEENT

    a) Dry mouth noted with hypercalcemia

    b) Papilledema noted with hypocalcemia

3. Cardiac: Displaced apical pulse and peripheral edema suggestive of CHF with hypocalcemia

4. Pulmonary

    a) Bronchial or laryngeal spasm with hypocalcemia

    b) Rales indicating CHF with hypocalcemia

    c) Stridor or laryngeal spasm with hypocalcemia

5. Abdominal: Increased muscular tone/spasticity of the abdominal muscles possible with hypocalcemia; abdominal fullness/distention due to constipation possible with hypercalcemia

6. Neurologic: Observation of gait and analysis of reflexes (critical)

    a) Hypocalcemia: Chvostek sign (muscle twitching noted after tapping the facial nerve) and Trousseau sign (spasm of the fingers and hands following constriction of circulation of the upper arm, such as with a blood pressure cuff) (see Appendix D)

    b) Deep tendon reflexes: Hyporeflexia, muscle weakness, and hypotonia possible with hypercalcemia; hyperreflexia with hypocalcemia

    c) Speech deficits with hypercalcemia

    d) Ataxia typically present with hypercalcemia

7. Musculoskeletal: Pain noted on palpation of joints, muscles, or bony prominences

8. Psychiatric/mood: Speech, demeanor, understanding and reaction to questions, articulation of thoughts

9. Integument: Dry skin or brittle nails in hypocalcemia

IV. Diagnostic tests (Jacobi, 2019; Song, 2017)

  A. Laboratory

    1. Hypocalcemia

      a) Corrected serum Ca^{2+} less than 8.4 mg/dl with albumin less than 4 g/dl

        (1) Ionized Ca^{2+} 1.09–1.29 mEq/L: Reduction in protein-bound calcium only

        (2) Ionized Ca^{2+} less than 1.09 mEq/L

          (a) Ionized hypocalcemia: Most common in trauma/ICU settings

          (b) True hypocalcemia

      b) PTH

        (1) PTH less than 29 pmol/L: Hypoparathyroidism

        (2) PTH greater than 29 pmol/L: Evaluate vitamin D level.

          (a) 1,25(OH)$_2$D less than 20 pg/ml: Suggestive of nutritional deficiency, malabsorption, drug-induced increased metabolism, or increased loss (e.g., nephrotic syndrome, biliary cirrhosis)

          (b) Decreased production: Hepatic or kidney disease, rickets, pseudohypoparathyroidism

          (c) 1,25(OH)$_2$D 20–76 pg/ml: Suggestive of hyperphosphatemia, hypomagnesemia, acute pancreatitis, or drug effects

2. Hypercalcemia
   a) Corrected serum Ca^{2+} greater than 10 mg/dl with albumin 5.2 g/dl: Pseudohypercalcemia
   b) Corrected serum Ca^{2+} greater than 10 mg/dl with albumin 4–5.2 g/dl: Evaluate PTH level.
      (1) PTH elevated or high: Greater than 65 pmol/L
         (a) Primary hyperparathyroidism
         (b) Secondary hyperparathyroidism, malabsorption, renal failure
         (c) Lithium induced
      (2) PTH 65 pmol/L: Evaluate vitamin D level.
         (a) 1,25(OH)$_2$D greater than 55 pg/ml
            i. Vitamin D intoxication
            ii. Tumor production of vitamin D
            iii. Sarcoidosis
         (b) Normal 1,25(OH)$_2$D is 10–55 pg/ml
            i. Endocrine dysfunction
            ii. Increased bone release
            iii. Thiazide diuretics
            iv. Milk-alkali syndrome
B. Radiology
   1. Plain films for evaluation of lytic lesions or fractures
   2. MRI of the brain and/or spine to evaluate neurologic symptoms
   3. Baseline chest x-ray to evaluate for CHF
   4. Ultrasound of thyroid to evaluate for enlargement, nodules, or masses
C. Other
   1. ECG: Indicated for grade 3–4 hypocalcemia or hypercalcemia
      a) Hypocalcemia: Prolonged QT interval
      b) Hypercalcemia: Bradycardia, first-degree heart block, short QT interval, bundle branch block
   2. EGD to evaluate for ulcers

V. Differential diagnosis of calcium imbalance (Body et al., 2017; Body et al., 2018; Kontogeorgos et al., 2020; Musri et al., 2019; Nasser et al., 2019; Schattner et al., 2016; Smogorzewski et al., 2016; Zagzag et al., 2018)
   A. Hypocalcemia
      1. Malabsorption: Chronic diarrhea (see Chapter 56), small bowel resection, pelvic irradiation
      2. Renal failure/insufficiency: Most common cause (see Chapter 86)
      3. Hypoparathyroidism
      4. Alkalosis
      5. Hypoalbuminemia
      6. Vitamin D deficiency
      7. Hyperphosphatemia (see Chapter 156)
      8. Medullary carcinoma of the thyroid
      9. Malnutrition
      10. Pancreatitis (see Chapter 77)
      11. Tumor lysis syndrome
      12. Bisphosphonate medications and other bone remodeling agents
   B. Hypercalcemia
      1. Hyperparathyroidism: Primary or secondary

    2. Adrenal insufficiency: Addison disease

    3. Thyrotoxicosis

    4. Malignancy: Paraneoplastic syndrome (see Appendix M) or bone metastasis; most common in breast and lung cancer, myeloma, and lymphomas

    5. Hypophosphatemia (see Chapter 156)

    6. Granulomatous disease: TB (see Chapter 36), sarcoidosis

    7. Immobility

    8. Familial hypocalciuric hypercalcemia

    9. Endocrine disorders: Multiple endocrine neoplasia

    10. Medication

VI. Treatment (Feldenzer & Sarno, 2018; Jacobi, 2019; Marcucci et al., 2018; Reagan et al., 2014; Reid et al., 2015; Schattner et al., 2016; Smogorzewski et al., 2016; Zagzag et al., 2018)

  A. Primary goals of treatment of calcium imbalance include the following.

    1. Prevent life-threatening conditions (e.g., cardiac arrest, flaccid paralysis, AKI, rhabdomyolysis [see Chapter 159]).

    2. Normalize the serum Ca^{2+} level.

    3. Identify and treat the underlying causes.

  B. The approach to treatment will require consideration of underlying characteristics of the patient that confer higher risk.

    1. Risk of increased or decreased Ca^{2+} is greater in older patients.

    2. Other risk factors are impaired renal or hepatic function, organic heart disease, and underlying neuromuscular disease.

  C. Hypocalcemia

    1. Mainstay of treatment is Ca^{2+} replacement and correction of hypomagnesemia, the most common cause of hypocalcemia.

    2. Initial treatment will depend on severity and the presence of symptoms.

      a) Mild, asymptomatic hypocalcemia: Oral replacement with elemental calcium 1–3 g daily in divided doses is sufficient.

        (1) Calcium carbonate, 40% elemental Ca^{2+}: Most common calcium supplement; requires stomach acid for absorption and should be taken with a meal

        (2) Calcium gluconate, 21% elemental Ca^{2+}: Best absorbed supplemental calcium; does not require the presence of extra stomach acid to dissolve

      b) Severe hypocalcemia (serum Ca^{2+} less than 7–7.5 mg/dl, ionized Ca^{2+} less than 1.6 mEq/L) or symptomatic hypocalcemia with neuromuscular findings: Treat urgently with IV calcium.

        (1) Calcium gluconate (preferred) 1–2 g in 50 ml dextrose 5% in water over 20–30 minutes, not to exceed 200 mg/min

        (2) Calcium chloride 500 mg to 1 g (5–10 ml of a 10% solution) IV every one to three days depending on patient response; maximum rate of 1 ml/min

        (3) Calcium chloride should be given via a central line because of a higher incidence of thrombophlebitis.

      c) Replacement of vitamin D in patients with deficiency: Required for absorption of Ca^{2+}

        (1) Foods: Vitamin D–fortified milk, fish, and egg yolks

        (2) 10–15 minutes of sunlight exposure to the skin daily

        (3) Oral replacement

          (a) Os-Cal 500® 500 mg calcium carbonate plus vitamin D 400 IU/tablet; other formulations available

        (b) Ages 50–70 years: Recommended 400 IU daily

        (c) Age older than 70 years: Recommended 600 IU daily

        (d) Dosing for hypoparathyroidism, nephrotic syndrome, and CKD: Varies widely; generally 50,000 IU twice weekly until vitamin D level 20–30 ng/ml

    (4) Calcitriol

        (a) Hypoparathyroidism, postsurgical or idiopathic

            i. Initial dose is 0.25 mcg PO daily in the morning.

            ii. Dose may be increased at two- to four-week intervals.

            iii. Usual dose range is 0.5–2 mcg PO once daily.

        (b) Pseudohypoparathyroidism

            i. Initial dose is 0.25 mcg PO daily in morning.

            ii. Dose may be increased at two- to four-week intervals.

            iii. Usual dose range is 0.5–2 mcg PO once daily.

D. Hypercalcemia

  1. Assessment of the severity of symptoms and serum Ca^{2+} will determine treatment.

  2. Hypercalcemia due to abnormal parathyroid function: Treat the underlying cause.

    a) High intact parathyroid level: Most likely primary hyperparathyroidism; may require surgical treatment

    b) Low intact parathyroid level: Most likely due to malignancy

  3. Hypercalcemia of malignancy: Primary strategies include dilution (hydration), increased excretion of Ca^{2+} (loop diuretics), inhibition of bone resorption, and decreased intestinal absorption of Ca^{2+}.

    a) Mild (corrected serum Ca^{2+} less than 12 mg/dl), either asymptomatic or mild symptoms

      (1) Eliminate any supplements containing Ca^{2+}.

      (2) Increase oral hydration.

      (3) Limit oral intake of calcium-rich foods.

      (4) Maintain weight-bearing activities as tolerated.

    b) Moderate (corrected serum Ca^{2+} is 12.5–13.5 mg/dl, ionized Ca^{2+} greater than 3.2–3.6 mEq/L), symptomatic, or severe (corrected serum Ca^{2+} greater than 13.5 mg/dl, ionized Ca^{2+} greater than 3.6 mEq/L): Requires aggressive management

      (1) Moderate: May be treated in outpatient setting

      (2) Severe: Generally, requires hospitalization for aggressive hydration and cardiac monitoring

  4. Hydration, diuresis, and binding agents

    a) Aggressive hydration: Goal is to dilute Ca^{2+} concentration in extracellular fluid and increase urine output.

      (1) 0.9% saline 200–500 ml/hr initially (rate as tolerated based on age and underlying disease), continued at lower rate until serum Ca^{2+} is corrected

      (2) Patients who are older adults, frail, or have cardiomyopathy or pulmonary disease: Generally require hospitalization for close monitoring of fluid and electrolyte status

    b) Diuresis (after initial hydration): Increased Ca^{2+} excretion

      (1) Loop diuretics (furosemide) 40–80 mg IV every six hours based on urine output and serial serum Ca^{2+} measures

      (2) Serial electrolyte measures: Ca^{2+}, potassium, sodium, magnesium, and phosphate to detect depletion due to diuresis; replaced as indicated

    c) Bisphosphonates: Inhibition of bone resorption, IV bisphosphonates first-line therapy, then denosumab for bisphosphonate-refractory hypercalcemia of malignancy

(1) Dose and infusion rate adjustments for creatinine clearance

(2) Pamidronate 60–90 mg IV over 2–24 hours with adequate hydration; repeated after seven days for sustained hypercalcemia

(3) Zoledronic acid 4 mg IV over a minimum of 15 minutes with adequate hydration; repeated after seven days for sustained hypercalcemia

(4) Common adverse events: Flu-like symptoms, fever, osteonecrosis of the jaw (with prolonged use), AKI

d) Calcitonin: Inhibition of bone resorption

(1) Initial: 4 IU/kg subcutaneous or IM every 6–12 hours

(2) Continued treatment: May increase after one to two days to 8 IU/kg every 12 hours; diminished effects after 48 hours because of tachyphylaxis

(3) Common adverse events: Flushing, injection-site reaction, nausea, rhinitis, sinusitis

e) Steroids (see Appendix K)

(1) Inhibition of bone resorption and increased tubular reabsorption

(2) Most effective in hematologic malignancies and hypercalcemia as a result of abnormal vitamin D metabolism

f) Dialysis: May be necessary for more severe cases

VII. Follow-up

A. Hypocalcemia

1. Mild/asymptomatic

a) Patients may be followed on an outpatient basis with serial serum Ca^{2+} levels at intervals determined by severity and identified causes.

b) Patients should be instructed on the signs and symptoms of hypocalcemia, management with oral supplements, and when to notify a healthcare provider.

2. Severe

a) Serial monitoring of serum Ca^{2+} should occur every four to six hours until corrected.

b) Subsequent monitoring will be determined based on status of the underlying causes.

c) Patients converted to oral replacement should be monitored within one to two weeks of conversion, then as clinically indicated.

B. Hypercalcemia

1. Mild/asymptomatic

a) Patients may be followed on an outpatient basis with serial serum Ca^{2+} levels at intervals determined by severity and identified causes.

b) Patients should be instructed on the signs and symptoms of hypercalcemia, management with oral supplements, and when to notify a healthcare provider.

2. Severe

a) Serial monitoring of serum Ca^{2+} should occur every four to six hours until corrected.

b) Subsequent monitoring will be determined based on status of the underlying causes and expected relapse.

3. Continued treatment of hypercalcemia of malignancy and commonly associated underlying bone disease will require continued monitoring of serum Ca^{2+} prior to each dose of bisphosphonate.

4. Monthly infusions of bisphosphonates for up to two years and then reevaluation should occur for patients with osteoblastic/osteolytic bone disease due to malignancy.

5. Routine dental examinations should be performed to monitor for osteonecrosis of the jaw.

VIII. Referrals
  A. Primary care physician: For management of oral supplements and further evaluation and treatment of the underlying causes for hypocalcemia and hypercalcemia
  B. Specialists: Referral based on underlying cause (i.e., suspected thyroid malignancy may require referral to surgeon for biopsy and/or neck surgery)
  C. Endocrinologist: If unable to determine underlying cause or if patient inadequately responds to treatment

References

Berndt, T.J., Thompson, J.R., & Kumar, R. (2016). The regulation of calcium, magnesium, and phosphate excretion by the kidney. In K. Skorecki, G.M. Chertow, P.A. Marsden, A.S.L. Yu, & M.W. Taal (Eds.), *Brenner and Rector's the kidney* (10th ed., pp. 185–203). Elsevier.

Body, J.-J., Niepel, D., & Tonini, G. (2017). Hypercalcaemia and hypocalcaemia: Finding the balance. *Supportive Care in Cancer, 25*(5), 1639–1649. https://doi.org/10.1007/s00520-016-3543-1

Body, J.-J., von Moos, R., Niepel, D., & Tombal, B. (2018). Hypocalcaemia in patients with prostate cancer treated with a bisphosphonate or denosumab: Prevention supports treatment completion. *BMC Urology, 18,* 81. https://doi.org/10.1186/s12894-018-0393-9

Feldenzer, K.L., & Sarno, J. (2018). Hypercalcemia of malignancy. *Journal of the Advanced Practitioner in Oncology, 9*(5), 496–504. https://doi.org/10.6004/jadpro.2018.9.5.4

Jacobi, J. (2019). Management of endocrine emergencies in the ICU. *Journal of Pharmacy Practice, 32*(3), 314–326. https://doi.org/10.1177/0897190019834771

Kontogeorgos, G., Welin, L., Fu, M., Hansson, P.-O., Landin-Wilhelmsen, K., & Laine, C.M. (2020). Hyperparathyroidism in men—Morbidity and mortality during 21 years' follow-up. *Scandinavian Journal of Clinical and Laboratory Investigation, 80*(1), 6–13. https://doi.org/10.1080/00365513.2019.1683763

Marcucci, G., Cianferotti, L., & Brandi, M.L. (2018). Clinical presentation and management of hypoparathyroidism. *Best Practice and Research Clinical Endocrinology and Metabolism, 32*(6), 927–939. https://doi.org/10.1016/j.beem.2018.09.007

Musri, F.Y., Mutlu, H., Eryilmaz, M.K., Salim, D.K., Tazegul, G., & Coşkun, H.Ş. (2019). Hypercalcemia associated with squamous cell carcinoma of renal pelvis: A case and review of the literature. *Journal of Cancer Research and Therapeutics, 15*(8 Suppl.), S170–S172. https://doi.org/10.4103/0973-1482.187236

Nasser, S.M., Sahal, A., Hamad, A., & Elazzazy, S. (2019). Effect of denosumab versus zoledronic acid on calcium levels in cancer patients with bone metastasis: A retrospective cohort study. *Journal of Oncology Pharmacy Practice, 25*(8), 1846–1852. https://doi.org/10.1177/1078155218820927

National Cancer Institute Cancer Therapy Evaluation Program. (2017). *Common terminology criteria for adverse events* [v.5.0]. https://ctep.cancer.gov/protocoldevelopment/electronic_applications/docs/CTCAE_v5_Quick_Reference_5x7.pdf

Reagan, P., Pani, A., & Rosner, M.H. (2014). Approach to diagnosis and treatment of hypercalcemia in a patient with malignancy. *American Journal of Kidney Diseases, 63*(1), 141–147. https://doi.org/10.1053/j.ajkd.2013.06.025

Reid, I.R., Bristow, S.M., & Bolland, M.J. (2015). Calcium supplements: Benefits and risks. *Journal of Internal Medicine, 278*(4), 354–368. https://doi.org/10.1111/joim.12394

Schattner, A., Dubin, I., Huber, R., & Gelber, M. (2016). Hypocalcaemia of malignancy. *Netherlands Journal of Medicine, 74*(6), 231–239. http://www.njmonline.nl/getpdf.php?id=1732

Smogorzewski, M.J., Stubbs, J.R, & Yu, A.S.L. (2016). Disorders of calcium, magnesium, and phosphate balance. In K. Skorecki, G.M. Chertow, P.A. Marsden, A.S.L. Yu, & M.W. Taal (Eds.), *Brenner and Rector's the kidney* (10th ed., pp. 601–636). Elsevier.

Song, L. (2017). Calcium and bone metabolism indices. In G.S. Makowski (Ed.), *Advances in clinical chemistry: Vol. 82* (pp. 1–46). Elsevier. https://doi.org/10.1016/bs.acc.2017.06.005

Zagzag, J., Hu, M.I., Fisher, S.B., & Perrier, N.D. (2018). Hypercalcemia and cancer: Differential diagnosis and treatment. *CA: A Cancer Journal for Clinicians, 68*(5), 377–386. https://doi.org/10.3322/caac.21489

CHAPTER 153

Hypokalemia/Hyperkalemia

Sandra Kurtin, PhD, ANP-C, AOCN®

I. Definitions (NCI CTEP, 2017; Palaka et al., 2019)
   A. Hypokalemia: A disorder characterized by laboratory results indicating a low concentration of potassium in the blood
      1. Grade 1: Less than LLN–3 mEq/L
      2. Grade 2: Less than LLN–3 mEq/L; symptomatic; intervention indicated
      3. Grade 3: Less than 2.5–3 mEq/L; hospitalization indicated
      4. Grade 4: Less than 2.5 mEq/L; life-threatening consequences
   B. Hyperkalemia: A disorder characterized by laboratory results indicating an elevation in the potassium concentration in the blood; associated with renal failure or sometimes with medications such as diuretics
      1. Grade 1: Greater than ULN–5.5 mEq/L
      2. Grade 2: Greater than 5.5–6 mEq/L
      3. Grade 3: Greater than 6–7 mEq/L; hospitalization indicated
      4. Grade 4: Greater than 7 mEq/L; life-threatening consequences

II. Physiology/Pathophysiology (Capasso et al., 2019; Ellison & Farrar, 2018; Gumz et al., 2015; Hunter & Bailey, 2019; Mount, 2016a, 2016b; Palmer, 2015; Palmer & Clegg, 2019)
   A. Normal: Normal serum potassium (K^+) ranges from 3.5–5 mEq/L.
      1. K^+ is the most abundant intracellular cation.
      2. Approximately 97% of potassium is located within the cells (intracellular fluid), and 2%–3% is located within the extracellular fluid.
      3. Skeletal muscle contains as much as 75% of the body's potassium, which may be released to the extracellular fluid after moderate exercise or muscle damage, causing transient hyperkalemia.
      4. Potassium is constantly moving into and out of the cells based on the body's needs via the sodium–potassium–chloride ion pump.
      5. More than 98% of total body potassium is intracellular, chiefly in muscle.
      6. Healthy individuals excrete all of the potassium they eat and absorb from the GI tract. Normal daily potassium intake is 40–60 mEq.
      7. The majority of potassium is excreted in the urine (80%–90%; 20–120 mEq daily), the remainder (10%) is excreted in the stool.
      8. Long-term regulation of potassium is modulated by the following.
         a) Regulation of renal excretion occurs through feedback mechanisms within the cells of the distal nephron, lumen-negative voltage (regulated by sodium, potassium, and chloride ions), and open K^+ channels within the target cells.
         b) In the sodium–potassium–ATPase enzyme complex, ATPase density within various tissues mediates intracellular K^+ uptake against the electrochemical gradient.

9. Potassium function

   a) Has a critical role in cellular function, neuromuscular activity, and cardiac conduction

   b) Regulates hormone secretion and action, vascular tone, systemic blood-pressure control, and GI motility

   c) Promotes the transmission and conduction of nerve impulses and the contraction of skeletal, cardiac, and smooth muscles

   d) Maintains intracellular osmolality and balance (i.e., electrical neutrality) between hydrogen and sodium within the cell

   e) Maintains a stable resting membrane potential for transmitting and conducting nerve impulses

   f) Plays a role in depositing glycogen in skeletal and liver cells in response to insulin secretion

   g) Promotes enzyme action for cellular metabolism

   h) Assists in maintenance of acid-base balance: Potassium deficit is associated with alkalosis, whereas potassium excess is associated with acidosis.

B. Pathophysiology

   1. Decreased or increased extracellular K^+ levels may occur without actual loss of total body K^+ through processes that result in potassium shifting from the extracellular fluid into or out of the cell into the extracellular fluid. These include both acute and chronic etiologies.

      a) Acute

         (1) Factors that enhance movement of K^+ into the cell, such as insulin, beta-catecholamines, and alkalosis

         (2) Factors that inhibit cell uptake of K^+

            (a) Acidosis: K^+ moves out of the cell in exchange for hydrogen; continued renal excretion results in hypokalemia.

            (b) Alpha-catecholamines

            (c) Cell damage: Anabolic cellular activity increases the demand for intracellular K^+, which can cause K^+ depletion, such as in cellular repair following trauma or injury.

         (3) Factors that enhance movement of K^+ out of the cell

            (a) Hyperosmolality: Increased sodium intake

            (b) Hypovolemia: Stimulates the renin–angiotensin system, which leads to secretion of aldosterone and K^+ excretion via the kidneys

      b) Chronic: Primarily due to the effect on ATP pump density

         (1) Increased K^+ movement: Thyroid hormones, adrenal steroids, exercise, growth

         (2) Impaired or decreased K^+ regulation in diabetic ketoacidosis with existing hypokalemia: The administration of insulin will shift K^+ into the cell and lead to more severe hypokalemia.

         (3) Chronic renal failure: Impaired renal regulation of K^+

   2. Pseudohypokalemia may occur with leukocytosis because of an increased uptake of K^+ by WBCs after the blood specimen has been drawn or in patients with leukocytosis. Increased ambient temperatures and delayed processing of the laboratory specimens contribute to this process.

III. Clinical features: Most cases of hypokalemia result from replenished GI or urinary losses (e.g., vomiting, diarrhea, diuretic therapy). Hyperkalemia is most often a result of impaired urinary potassium excretion from renal insufficiency or drugs that inhibit the renin–

angiotensin–aldosterone system. A serum K^+ level less than 2.5 mEq/L or greater than 7 mEq/L can cause cardiac arrest. Thus, serum K^+ values must be closely monitored (Capasso et al., 2019; Ellison & Farrar, 2018; Hunter & Bailey, 2019; Mount, 2016a; NCI CTEP, 2017; Palaka et al., 2019; Palmer, 2020; Palmer & Clegg, 2019).

A. Etiology: Hypokalemia
1. Decreased potassium intake
   a) Malnutrition
   b) Discontinued supplementation in the presence of chronic hypokalemia
2. Nonrenal potassium loss
   a) GI loss: Vomiting, diarrhea
   b) Surgical drains
   c) Suction
   d) Excessive sweating
3. Renal potassium loss
   a) Diuretics: Loop and thiazide
   b) Renal tubular damage or dysfunction: Autoimmune causes are most common, such as Sjögren syndrome or lupus.
   c) Primary hyperreninism: Raised renin and aldosterone concentrations
      (1) Malignant hypertension
      (2) Renal artery stenosis
      (3) Renin-secreting tumor
   d) Hyperaldosteronism
      (1) Primary: Conn syndrome, congenital adrenal hyperplasia, glucocorticoid-suppressible hyperaldosteronism
      (2) Secondary: Hypovolemia, cardiac failure, hepatic failure
   e) Non-Fanconi inherited syndromes: Associated with alkalosis, hypomagnesemia, hypovolemia, and secondary aldosteronism
      (1) Bartter syndrome
      (2) Gitelman syndrome
   f) Renal Fanconi syndrome
      (1) Chemotherapy: Cisplatin
      (2) Antiretroviral therapies
      (3) Tubular damage caused by light chain in myeloma
      (4) Acute tubular necrosis
   g) Hypomagnesemia: Prevents compensatory renal reabsorption of potassium
   h) Hypercalcemia
   i) Antibiotics: Penicillin analogs, amphotericin
   j) Villous adenomas
   k) Ureterosigmoidostomy
4. Redistributive: Total body potassium is normal but intracellular concentration is increased (e.g., insulin, beta-2 agonists).
5. Tumor related
   a) Lysozymuria with acute leukemia
   b) Mineralocorticoid excess syndrome
   c) Primary hyperaldosteronism: Adrenal carcinoma
   d) Renin-producing tumors: Extremely rare
   e) Ectopic adrenocorticotropin syndrome
   f) Intracellular shifts (pseudohypokalemia) in the setting of high WBC count
6. Antimicrobial and antifungal agents: Aminoglycosides, amphotericin B
B. Etiology: Hyperkalemia

1. True hyperkalemia
   a) Excessive potassium intake in susceptible patients
   b) Cell damage: Tumor lysis, rhabdomyolysis, hemolysis
   c) Diabetic ketoacidosis, hyperosmolar hyperglycemic states
   d) Lactic acidosis
   e) Toxins and drugs: Digoxin
   f) Intense exercise: Possible transient hyperkalemia
2. Pseudohyperkalemia
   a) Leukocytosis
   b) Thrombocytosis
   c) Laboratory techniques
      (1) Repeated fist clenching prior to venipuncture
      (2) Hemolysis from a small-gauge needle
      (3) Delayed processing of sample or samples kept on ice or at high ambient temperatures during transport to the laboratory
      (4) Hyperventilation
   d) Familial: Chromosome 16 abnormality
3. Redistribution
   a) Inorganic acids cause K^+ efflux (hydogen influx on buffering).
   b) Diabetic ketoacidosis: K^+ leaves the cells as a result of insulin deficiency.
   c) Lactic acidosis with cellular ischemia (cellular ATP decreased) leads to K^+ efflux.
4. Medication related
   a) Medications that target the renin–angiotensin–aldosterone axis
      (1) Renin: NSAIDs, cyclo-oxygenase inhibitors, aliskiren, beta-blockers
      (2) Angiotensin: ACE inhibitors, ARBs
      (3) Aldosterone: Spironolactone, canrenone, eplerenone, drospirenone
      (4) Renal tubule: Amiloride, triamterene, trimethoprim, pentamidine, nafamostat
   b) Calcineurin inhibitors: Cyclosporine, tacrolimus
   c) Inhibition of sodium epithelial channels
      (1) Trimethoprim: Particularly with concomitant use of ACE inhibitor or angiotensin receptor blockers or in the presence of renal insufficiency or hyporeninemic hypoaldosteronism
      (2) Pentamidine
      (3) Amiloride
      (4) Triamterene
      (5) Nafamostat
      (6) Spironolactone
      (7) Eplerenone
5. Renal retention of potassium
   a) Primary decrease in mineralocorticoids
      (1) Low renin aldosteronism: Diabetes mellitus
      (2) Drug-related inhibition of the renin–angiotensin–aldosterone system
   b) Heparin treatment
   c) Addison disease
   d) Decrease in delivery of sodium to the distal nephron
      (1) Oliguric AKI
      (2) Acute glomerulonephritis
      (3) Gordon syndrome
6. Blood transfusions

C. History
1. History of cancer and cancer treatment
2. Current medications: Prescribed, over the counter, with particular attention to use of diuretics, laxatives, digoxin, cyclosporine, tacrolimus, cyclooxygenase-2 inhibitors, NSAIDs, ACE inhibitors, angiotensin receptor blockers, trimethoprim/sulfamethoxazole, penicillin, K^+ supplements, salt substitutes, licorice intake, and other medications or supplements known to affect K^+ balance
3. History of presenting symptoms: Precipitating factors, location, duration
4. Changes in ADLs
5. Past medical history
    a) Hypokalemia: Diabetes mellitus, kidney disease, hypertension, anorexia, bulimia
    b) Hyperkalemia: Diabetes mellitus, kidney disease, hyperaldosteronism, Cushing syndrome
6. Family history: Familial hypokalemic alkalosis (Bartter and Gitelman syndromes) or familial hyperkalemic periodic paralysis
D. Signs and symptoms (see Table 153-1)
1. Clinical manifestations are dependent on the rapidity of onset (acute [less than 48 hours] or chronic) and the level of severity.
2. Acute-onset (less than 48 hours) or grade 3–4 imbalances are most often associated with severe cardiovascular consequences.
E. Physical examination

TABLE 153-1   Common Clinical Manifestations of Hypokalemia and Hyperkalemia

Organ/System	Hypokalemia	Hyperkalemia
Cardiovascular	Postural hypotension Increased sensitivity to digitalis Premature atrial and ventricular contractions Electrocardiogram changes: ST-segment depression Broad, flat T waves QT prolongation (more common with potassium ion [K^+] < 2.7 mEq/L) Long QT syndrome/torsades de pointes—more common with low K^+ and low magnesium	Early electrocardiogram changes: ST-T segment depression K^+ = 5.5–6.5 mEq/L: Tall, peaked T waves with narrow base, best seen in precordial leads K^+ = 6.5–8 mEq/L: Peaked T waves, prolonged PR interval, decreased P waves, widening of QRS complex K^+ greater than 8 mEq/L: Absent P waves, intraventricular blocks, bundle branch block, progressive widening of QRS, ventricular fibrillation, asystole
Gastrointestinal	Anorexia, nausea, vomiting Decreased bowel motility, ileus	Nausea Intermittent intestinal colic or diarrhea
Neuromuscular	Muscle weakness, particularly in proximal muscles (quadriceps) Paresthesias or severely tender muscles	Vague muscular weakness—common early sign Flaccid muscle paralysis—first noticed in the legs, later in the trunk or arms Paresthesias of the face, tongue, feet, and hands—common; are the result of stimulation of pain receptors
Renal	Sodium chloride retention Polyuria due to polydipsia Phosphaturia	Increased urinary ammonium excretion

Note. Based on information from Ellison & Farrar, 2018; Mount, 2016a; Palmer & Clegg, 2019.

1. Vital signs
   a) Heart rate: Irregular rhythm, bradycardia in hyperkalemia
   b) Blood pressure: Postural hypotension with decreased K⁺; hypertension may be present initially with increased K⁺ with rapidly ensuing hypotension.
   c) Temperature: Normal to slightly elevated
   d) Weight: Gain (hyperkalemia) or loss (hypokalemia)
   e) Pain: Painful musculature (hypokalemia) and paresthesia (both)
2. HEENT: Dry oral mucosa; altered speech in severe hyperkalemia
3. Cardiac: Rate and rhythm
   a) Weak pulse suggestive of hypokalemia
   b) Irregular heart rate suggestive of dysrhythmia; can be associated with either hypokalemia or hyperkalemia
4. Pulmonary
   a) Hypokalemia: Pulmonary muscle paralysis with diminished respiratory effort.
   b) Hyperkalemia: Pulmonary muscles spared in early hyperkalemia; hyperventilation in metabolic acidosis
5. Abdominal: Abdominal distention, decreased bowel sounds, and pain in hypokalemia
6. Neurologic: Careful evaluation of cranial nerves (although CNS is often spared), reflexes, gait, grip strength, flexion, dorsiflexion; mental changes common with both electrolyte imbalances (see Appendix A)
7. Musculoskeletal: Muscle pain
   a) Hypokalemia: Diminished strength in the quadriceps is common.
   b) Hyperkalemia: Vague muscle weakness is most common in early hyperkalemia with rapid progression to flaccid muscle paralysis spreading from the legs to the trunk and arms.

IV. Diagnostic tests: A basic or complete metabolic panel and CBC with differential and platelet count are commonly ordered in follow-up visits or urgent visits as the initial screening and will provide the basis for additional testing (Dromigny & Robert, 2017; Hunter & Bailey, 2019; Mount, 2016a; Palmer & Clegg, 2019; Wang et al., 2020).
   A. Laboratory: Hypokalemia with serum K⁺ less than 3.5 mEq/L
      1. Plasma electrolytes including magnesium; magnesium decreases with potassium decrease.
      2. Urine electrolytes including urine K⁺
         a) Urine K⁺ less than 15 mEq/L: Likely extrarenal loss of serum K⁺
         b) Urine K⁺ greater than 15 mEq/L: Likely renal loss of serum K⁺
         c) Urine K⁺ level may vary in intracellular shift of K⁺.
      3. Serum BUN and creatinine to evaluate renal function
      4. Serum and urine osmolality to calculate the transtubular K⁺ gradient (TTKG)
         a) Calculation of the TTKG will help to distinguish true potassium imbalance as well as the presence of an anion gap.
         b) TTKG is (urine K⁺ × serum osmolality) / (serum K⁺ × urine osmolality).
            (1) TTKG 3–4 is hypokalemia.
            (2) TTKG 6–7 is hyperkalemia.
      5. Serum bicarbonate to distinguish acidosis versus alkalosis and renal tubular necrosis
         a) Sodium bicarbonate less than 25 mEq/L is acidosis.
            (1) Chronic hypokalemia: Check urine ammonium level.
            (2) Urine ammonium less than 40 mcg/dl: Suggests distal renal tubular necrosis
            (3) Urine ammonium greater than 100: Suggests GI loss, glue sniffing, or acetazolamide

       b) Serum bicarbonate greater than 25 mEq/L is alkalosis.

          (1) Urine chloride greater than 20 mEq/L

          (2) Urine calcium/creatinine ratio

             (a) Greater than 0.20: Suggests loop diuretic, Bartter syndrome

             (b) Less than 0.15: Suggests thiazide diuretic, Gitelman syndrome

          (3) Urine chloride less than 10 mEq/L: GI loss

    6. Serum aldosterone and renin levels for patients with high extracellular blood volume and hypertension

       a) Low/low: Check serum cortisol.

          (1) High: Suggests Cushing syndrome

          (2) Normal: Suggests Liddle syndrome, licorice ingestion, or apparent mineralocorticoid excess

       b) Low/high: Suggests adrenal problem such as adenoma hyperplasia, primary aldosteronism, or glucocorticoid-remediable hyperaldosteronism

       c) High/high: Suggests renal artery stenosis, malignant hypertension, or renin-producing tumor

    7. Glucose level elevated with uncontrolled diabetes

B. Laboratory: Hyperkalemia with serum K+ greater than 5.5 mEq/L

    1. CBC: WBC greater than 100,000/mm^3 or platelets greater than 1,000,000/mm^3; likely pseudohyperkalemia

    2. Normal CBC: Check urine K+.

       a) Urine K+ less than 40 mEq/L: Decreased K+ excretion

          (1) Serum creatinine greater than 2 mg/dl: Renal failure

          (2) Serum creatinine less than 2 mg/dl: Check serum aldosterone.

             (a) Aldosterone less than 2 ng/dl supine: Suggests hypoaldosteronism

             (b) Aldosterone greater than 2 ng/dl supine

                i. Drug effect: Heparin, ACE inhibitor/angiotensin receptor blocker, ketoconazole

                ii. Inadequate distal tubular delivery of sodium primary renal secretory defect: SLE, sickle cell disease, renal transplantation, obstructive nephropathy, amyloid deposition

       b) Urine K+ greater than 20 mEq/L

          (1) Increased K+ intake or endogenous K+ release suggests hemolysis, GI bleeding, or catabolic state.

          (2) Normal K+ intake: Check pH.

             (a) pH less than 7.35: Acidosis

             (b) pH greater than 7.35

                i. Glucose greater than 200 mg/dl: Suggests insulin deficiency

                ii. Glucose less than 200 mg/dl: Evaluate creatine phosphokinase, uric acid, and serum phosphorus.

                 • Normal: Drug related

                 • Elevated: Tissue release

    3. Electrolytes: Magnesium increases with potassium increase.

C. Radiology: Chest x-ray may be indicated for evaluation of respiratory symptoms.

D. Other: Evaluate ECG for dysrhythmia or altered wave conduction.

    1. Hypokalemia: ST-segment depression, T-wave flattening, and an increase in amplitude of the U wave are associated with hypokalemia.

    2. Hyperkalemia: Peaking of the T wave, ST-segment depression, widening of the PR interval, and widening of the QRS interval are sequential changes of progressively

severe hyperkalemia; right bundle branch block and right precordial ST-segment elevations may also be seen.

V. Differential diagnosis of potassium imbalance (Ellison & Farrar, 2018; Hunter & Bailey, 2019; Mount, 2016a; Palmer & Clegg, 2019)
  A. Hypokalemia
    1. Malnutrition
    2. Hypomagnesemia (Chapter 154)
    3. Renal failure or renal tubular acidosis (see Chapter 86)
    4. Primary or secondary hyperaldosteronism
    5. Metabolic alkalosis
    6. Paraneoplastic syndrome (see Appendix M)
    7. GI loss: Diarrhea, vomiting, fistula, NG suctioning (see Chapters 56 and 63)
    8. Anabolic state: Rapidly proliferating tumor, secondary to G-CSF administration
    9. Pseudohyperkalemia
    10. Iatrogenic/medication induced
    11. Thyrotoxicosis
  B. Hyperkalemia
    1. Iatrogenic/medication induced
    2. Renal failure (see Chapter 86)
    3. Dehydration
    4. Metabolic acidosis
    5. Diabetes mellitus/insulin deficiency (see Chapter 151)
    6. Primary (e.g., Addison disease) or secondary (e.g., adrenal metastases, ACE inhibitors) hypoaldosteronism
    7. Laboratory/sampling error
    8. Hypocalcemia (see Chapter 152)
    9. Thermal or electrical burns
    10. Rhabdomyolysis (see Chapter 159)
    11. Tumor lysis syndrome

VI. Treatment (Cupisti et al., 2018; Mount, 2016a; NCI CTEP, 2017; Palmer, 2020; Palmer & Clegg, 2019)
  A. Primary goals of treatment of potassium imbalance
    1. Prevent life-threatening conditions (e.g., cardiac arrest, flaccid paralysis, rhabdomyolysis).
    2. Normalize K^+ levels.
    3. Identify and treat the underlying causes.
  B. Considerations for the approach to treatment
    1. Rapidity of onset (acute vs. chronic) and severity (e.g., changes on ECG, tumor lysis syndrome, rhabdomyolysis) of the underlying cause will dictate the approach to treatment.
    2. Underlying characteristics of the patient that confer higher risk include the following.
      a) Age: Risk of increased or decreased K^+ greater in older patients
      b) Comorbidities: Organic heart disease, impaired renal function, diabetes
      c) Current medications: Antiarrhythmics, antihypertensives, insulin
    3. Tailor correction of K^+ imbalance to pathophysiology of the underlying cause to avoid overcorrection or under correction (e.g., redistribution).
    4. Carefully evaluate the excess or deficit and monitor the replacement.

C. Hypokalemia
1. Mainstay of treatment is K⁺ replacement.
2. Goal is to rapidly raise the serum K⁺ to a safe range, then replace at a slower rate over days to weeks.
    a) Serum K⁺ 3–3.5 mEq/L: Asymptomatic
        (1) Oral replacement may be used in asymptomatic patients (see Table 153-2 for oral agents). An oral dose of 75 mEq of K⁺ will increase serum K⁺ by 1–1.4 mEq/L in 60–90 minutes.
        (2) Patients with heart failure, cardiac arrhythmias, MI, or ischemic heart disease; patients taking digoxin; and patients with hepatic disease may not tolerate serum K⁺ less than 4 mEq/L.
    b) Serum K⁺ less than 3 mEq/L or symptomatic patients with serum K⁺ less than 3.5 mEq/L not able to tolerate oral replacement

---

TABLE 153-2   **Common Oral Formulations for Potassium Chloride Replacement**

Formulation	Available Agents	Clinical Considerations
Controlled Release		
Microencapsulated tablets or capsules	Klor-Con® M10: 10 mEq (750 mg) Klor-Con M15: 15 mEq (scored; 1,125 mg) Klor-Con M20: 20 mEq (scored; 1,500 mg) Generic • Oral tablet, extended release: 8 mEq, 10 mEq, 15 mEq, 20 mEq • Oral capsule, extended release: 8 mEq, 10 mEq	Tablets: Swallow tablets whole; do not chew. Capsules: Contents may be opened and sprinkled on a spoonful of applesauce or pudding. Capsule should be swallowed immediately without chewing.
Wax-matrix extended-release tablets	K-Tab® 10 mEq (750 mg) Klor-Con 8: 8 mEq (600 mg) Klor-Con 10: 10 mEq (750 mg)	Swallow whole; do not chew.
Immediate Release		
Potassium chloride (K⁺Cl⁻) powder	Epiklor™: 20 mEq/packet (30s, 100s) (sugar free; orange flavor) Epiklor/25: 25 mEq/packet (30s, 100s) (sugar free; orange flavor) Klor-Con: 20 mEq/packet (30s, 100s) (sugar free; fruit flavor) Klor-Con/25: 25 mEq/packet (30s, 100s) (sugar free; fruit flavor)	Dissolved (one packet) in 4–5 oz of water or another beverage prior to administration More expensive than elixir Convenient
Potassium chloride (K⁺Cl⁻) tablets	K-Tab 10 mEq Klor-Con 10 mEq, 20 mEq	K-Tab: Swallow tablets whole; do not crush, chew, or suck on tablet. Klor-Con: Swallow tablets whole; do not crush, chew, or suck on tablet. Tablet may be broken in half and each half swallowed separately; the whole tablet may be dissolved in about 4 oz of water (allow approximately 2 minutes to dissolve, stir well, and drink immediately).

Note. Based on information from IBM Micromedex, n.d.

        (1) IV K⁺ replacement is recommended, although this limits the rapidity with which the serum K⁺ can be corrected because of limits in the amount of K⁺ infused per hour.

        (2) The usual IV dose of potassium chloride replacement is 10 mEq/hr.

        (3) Higher rates of infusion require cardiac monitoring and are generally reserved for the ICU or emergency department settings in medical emergencies.

        (4) Concentrations of K⁺ greater than 40 mEq/L should be administered via a central line to prevent phlebitis.

        (5) All IV infusions of potassium-containing solutions should be administered using a controlled infusion device to eliminate the potential for inadvertent rapid infusion, which may be fatal.

        (6) The IV solution should be dextrose-free to avoid transient reduction in serum K⁺ due to endogenous insulin secretion.

3. Strategies to limit potassium loss

    a) Minimize use of potassium-sparing diuretics.

    b) Limit sodium intake.

    c) PPIs may help to reduce the effects of metabolic alkalosis secondary to upper GI losses.

4. Replacement of magnesium is necessary in the presence of hypomagnesemia (see Chapter 154).

5. Dietary intake of potassium-rich foods or fluids is recommended for patients with chronic hypokalemia.

    a) Greater than 1,000 mg (25 mEq/100 g): Dried figs, molasses, seaweed, dry soybeans, dry beans

    b) 500–1,000 mg (12.5–24 mEq/100 g): Dried fruits (e.g., dates, prunes, raisins), nuts, avocados, bran cereals, wheat germ, lima beans, potatoes

    c) Greater than 250 mg less than 500 mg (6.2–12 mEq/100 g)

        (1) Vegetables: Spinach, tomatoes, broccoli, winter squash, beets, carrots, cauliflower, sweet potatoes

        (2) Fruits: Bananas, cantaloupe, kiwis, mangoes, peach, watermelon, pomegranate, pineapple

        (3) Meats: Beef, pork, veal, lamb, trout, salami, ham, chicken, turkey

D. Hyperkalemia

1. Patients with nonemergent hyperkalemia: Grade 1–2

    a) Provide dietary counseling.

    b) Discontinue drugs that interfere with renal excretion of K⁺ including over-the-counter drugs (e.g., NSAIDs).

    c) Ensure effective diuretic therapy (loop diuretics for GFR less than 30 ml/min).

    d) Give oral sodium bicarbonate to treat metabolic acidosis.

    e) Consider potassium-binding drugs.

2. Patients with grade 3–4 or those at risk due to comorbid conditions generally require hospitalization for cardiac monitoring.

    a) Hyperkalemia in patients with ECG changes is a medical emergency.

    b) Serum K⁺ greater than or equal to 6.5 mEq/L should be treated aggressively and includes 12-lead ECG, admission to the hospital, continuous cardiac monitoring, and immediate treatment.

3. Three primary goals of treatment of hyperkalemia

    a) Antagonism of cardiac effects to stabilize myocardial cell membrane

      (1) Give IV calcium gluconate 10 ml of 10% infused over two to three minutes under continuous ECG monitoring.

      (2) Use with caution in patients taking digoxin.

      (3) Do not administer in solutions containing bicarbonate to avoid precipitation.

      (4) This does not significantly affect K⁺ levels.

    b) Redistribution of K⁺ into the cells to decrease extracellular K⁺

      (1) Insulin and glucose: 10 units IV of regular insulin followed immediately by 50 ml of 50% dextrose (25 g of glucose)

        (a) Effect on K⁺ occurs within 20–30 minutes, with peak at 30–60 minutes and duration of four to six hours.

        (b) Expected change in serum K⁺ is 0.5–1.2 mEq/L.

        (c) Hypoglycemia may occur; infusion of 10% dextrose solution may be necessary. These patients require intensive monitoring.

      (2) Use of beta-adrenergic agonist agents

        (a) Activate the sodium–potassium–ATPase channels.

        (b) Albuterol: Inhaled albuterol (nebulized) at doses of 10–20 mg in 4 ml of normal saline inhaled over 10 minutes can reduce serum K⁺ by 0.5–1 mEq/L with onset at 30 minutes, peak at 90 minutes, and duration of two to six hours.

      (3) The use of sodium bicarbonate for hyperkalemia is no longer recommended.

    c) Increased rate of K⁺ excretion

      (1) Diuretics

        (a) Oral diuretics with the highest bioavailability and lowest potential for renal impairment (e.g., torsemide)

        (b) IV agents with the lowest potential for hepatic toxicity (e.g., furosemide)

        (c) Combinations of loop and thiazide diuretics

      (2) Dialysis: Hemodialysis is the preferred mode when rapid correction of hyperkalemia is necessary.

VII. Follow-up

  A. Ongoing monitoring of K⁺ levels is necessary to detect rebound effects (hyperkalemia) or ineffective replacement (hypokalemia).

  B. Continue monitoring of underlying abnormality to prevent recurrent imbalance.

  C. Assess for resolution of clinical signs and symptoms.

  D. Patients taking medications known to affect K⁺ or magnesium levels (e.g., cisplatin, EGFR inhibitors, diuretics) will require frequent monitoring.

VIII. Referrals

  A. Hospital/critical care unit physician: In cases of severe K⁺ imbalance (K⁺ less than 2.5 mEq/L or greater than 6.5–7 mEq/L), emergent situations require admission to a hospital/critical care unit for cardiac monitoring and more aggressive interventions (e.g., dialysis).

  B. Consider complexity of cause of imbalance: Some causes (e.g., diet, dehydration, medication) may be relatively simple to correct. However, in individuals with complex medical problems (e.g., unstable diabetes mellitus, bronchogenic carcinoma with adrenal metastasis, acid-base imbalance, HIV/AIDS), consultation and close collaboration with a physician are needed.

  C. Nephrologist: Refer for possible dialysis with hyperkalemia and renal failure.

  D. Oncologist/hematologist: Refer if tumor lysis syndrome is causing hyperkalemia.

E. Endocrinologist: Refer for suspected mineralocorticoid disorders.

F. Nutritionist: In patients who have hyperkalemia secondary to renal failure, a diet in which sodium and K⁺ intake is carefully monitored must be initiated.

G. Psychiatrist: Specialist is appropriate for patients in whom alcoholism or eating disorders have been identified.

References

Capasso, A., Benigni, A., Capitanio, U., Danesh, F.R., Di Marzo, V., Gesualdo, L., ... Capasso, G. (2019). Summary of the International Conference on Onco-Nephrology: An emerging field in medicine. *Kidney International, 96*(3), 555–567. https://doi.org/10.1016/j.kint.2019.04.043

Cupisti, A., Kovesdy, C.P., D'Alessandro, C., & Kalantar-Zadeh, K. (2018). Dietary approach to recurrent or chronic hyperkalaemia in patients with decreased kidney function. *Nutrients, 10*(3), 261. https://doi.org/10.3390/nu10030261

Dromigny, J.-A., & Robert, E. (2017). Stability of blood potassium: Effects of duration, temperature and transport during 10 hours storage of human whole blood in serum and plasma. *Annales de Biologie Clinique, 75*(4), 369–374. https://doi.org/10.1684/abc.2017.1255

Ellison, D., & Farrar, F.C. (2018). Kidney influence on fluid and electrolyte balance. *Nursing Clinics of North America, 53*(4), 469–480. https://doi.org/10.1016/j.cnur.2018.05.004

Gumz, M.L., Rabinowitz, L., & Wingo, C.S. (2015). An integrated view of potassium homeostasis. *New England Journal of Medicine, 373*(1), 60–72. https://doi.org/10.1056/NEJMra1313341

Hunter, R.W., & Bailey, M.A. (2019). Hyperkalemia: Pathophysiology, risk factors and consequences. *Nephrology Dialysis Transplantation, 34*(Suppl. 3), iii2–iii11. https://doi.org/10.1093/ndt/gfz206

IBM Micromedex. (n.d.). Micromedex drug reference. https://www.micromedexsolutions.com

Mount, D.B. (2016a). Disorders of potassium balance. In K. Skorecki, G.M. Chertow, P.A. Marsden, A.S.L. Yu, & M.W. Taal (Eds.), *Brenner and Rector's the kidney* (10th ed., pp. 559–599). Elsevier.

Mount, D.B. (2016b). Transport of sodium, chloride, and potassium. In K. Skorecki, G.M. Chertow, P.A. Marsden, A.S.L. Yu, & M.W. Taal (Eds.), *Brenner and Rector's the kidney* (10th ed., pp. 144–184). Elsevier.

National Cancer Institute Cancer Therapy Evaluation Program. (2017). *Common terminology criteria for adverse events* [v.5.0]. https://ctep.cancer.gov/protocoldevelopment/electronic_applications/docs/CTCAE_v5_Quick_Reference_5x7.pdf

Palaka, E., Grandy, S., Darlington, O., McEwan, P., & van Doornewaard, A. (2019). Associations between serum potassium and adverse clinical outcomes: A systematic literature review. *International Journal of Clinical Practice, 74*(1), e13421. https://doi.org/10.1111/icjp.13421

Palmer, B.F. (2015). Regulation of potassium homeostasis. *Clinical Journal of the American Society of Nephrology, 10*(6), 1050–1060. https://doi.org/10.2215/cjn.08580813

Palmer, B.F. (2020). Potassium binders for hyperkalemia in chronic kidney disease—Diet, renin-angiotensin-aldosterone system inhibitor therapy, and hemodialysis. *Mayo Clinic Proceedings, 95*(2), 339–354. https://doi.org/10.1016/j.mayocp.2019.05.019

Palmer, B.F., & Clegg, D.J. (2019). Physiology and pathophysiology of potassium homeostasis: Core curriculum 2019. *American Journal of Kidney Diseases, 74*(5), 682–695. https://doi.org/10.1053/j.ajkd.2019.03.427

Wang, X., Han, D., & Li, G. (2020). Electrocardiographic manifestations in severe hypokalemia. *Journal of International Medical Research, 48*(1). https://doi.org/10.1177/0300060518811058

CHAPTER 154

Hypomagnesemia/
Hypermagnesemia

Sandra Kurtin, PhD, ANP-C, AOCN®

I. Definitions (NCI CTEP, 2017)
   A. Hypomagnesemia: A disorder characterized by laboratory results indicating a low concentration of magnesium (Mg^{2+}) in the blood and referred to as magnesium deficiency
      1. Grade 1: Mg^{2+} less than LLN–1.2 mg/dl; less than LLN–1 mEq/L
      2. Grade 2: Mg^{2+} less than 1.2–0.9 mg/dl; less than 0.8–1 mEq/L
      3. Grade 3: Mg^{2+} less than 0.9–0.7 mg/dl; less than 0.6–1 mEq/L
      4. Grade 4: Mg^{2+} less than 0.7 mg/dl; less than 0.6 mEq/L; life-threatening consequences
   B. Hypermagnesemia: A disorder characterized by laboratory results indicating an elevation in the concentration of magnesium in the blood
      1. Grade 1: Mg^{2+} greater than ULN–3 mg/dl; greater than ULN–2.46 mEq/L
      2. Grade 2: Not specified
      3. Grade 3: Mg^{2+} greater than 3–8 mg/dl; greater than 2.46–6.6 mEq/L
      4. Grade 4: Mg^{2+} greater than 8 mg/dl; greater than 6.6 mEq/L; life-threatening consequences

II. Physiology/Pathophysiology (Ahmed & Mohammed, 2019; Berndt et al., 2016; Costello et al., 2016; Gröber, 2019; Izzedine & Perazella, 2017; Lo Piano et al., 2019; Smogorzewski et al., 2016; Van Laecke, 2019)
   A. Normal: Normal serum Mg^{2+} ranges 1.8–3 mg/dl.
      1. Normal daily intake of Mg^{2+} is 300 mg or 228–323 mg daily (female/male); recommended daily allowance is 320 mg for females and 420 mg for males.
      2. The skeleton stores 50%–60% of Mg^{2+}.
         a) Part of the hydroxyapatite crystalline structure: 60% within the hydration shell and 30% on the crystal surface
         b) Serves as a reservoir for maintaining Mg^{2+} homeostasis
      3. It is the second most plentiful intracellular cation and has similar functions, causes of imbalances, and clinical manifestations as potassium.
         a) Majority of intracellular Mg^{2+} is bound to ATP; thus, Mg^{2+} is an obligate cofactor in all reactions that require ATP.
         b) It acts directly on the myoneural junction.
         c) It is closely associated with imbalances of potassium, calcium, phosphate, and sodium.
      4. Only 1% is in extracellular fluid.

       a) Approximately 30% is protein bound and approximately 60% is ionized (free).

       b) Ionized magnesium is primarily involved in neuromuscular activity and other physiologic processes.

   5. Mg^{2+} is absorbed in the colon, predominantly in the small intestine.

       a) It is primarily a passive paracellular process regulated by active absorption of sodium and water, followed by Mg^{2+} and other ions.

       b) Transcellular absorption of Mg^{2+} in the colon is regulated by TRPM6, which regulates epithelial uptake of Mg^{2+}.

   6. Approximately 60% is excreted in feces and 40% via the kidneys.

       a) Renal reabsorption of Mg^{2+} in the ascending loop of Henle and the distal collecting duct plays a key role in correcting Mg^{2+} loss/deficiency.

       b) The glomeruli filter 80% of total plasma Mg^{2+}. Approximately 90% of the filtered Mg^{2+} is reabsorbed.

          (1) Passive paracellular mechanism: 15% in the proximal tubule and 70% in the thick ascending loop of Henle

          (2) Transcellular transport: 10% in the distal collecting duct

             (a) The remaining 3%–5% is excreted in the urine in the presence of hypomagnesemia; this can be reduced to 0.5%–1% to conserve Mg^{2+}.

             (b) Diuretics or agents that block EGFR inhibitor agents may contribute to Mg^{2+} deficiency.

   7. Mg^{2+} homeostasis is controlled by a complex balance among intestinal uptake of Mg^{2+}, exchange within the bone, and renal excretion of Mg^{2+}.

       a) Transcellular movement of Mg^{2+} is, in part, regulated by TRPM6.

          (1) It is expressed in the colon and the distal convoluted tubule.

          (2) This plays a key role in the absorption of Mg^{2+} in the colon and active renal reabsorption of Mg^{2+}.

          (3) Mutations in TRPM6 are thought to explain rare genetic hypomagnesemia syndromes.

       b) Extracellular calcium-sensing receptor may affect Mg^{2+} hemostasis through its effect on calcium and PTH.

   8. Functions of magnesium

       a) Cofactor in many enzymatic processes, including protein and DNA synthesis, energy metabolism, and regulation of ion channels

       b) Influences neuromuscular activity, including myocardial contractility

       c) Influences the use of protein and other electrolytes, including potassium and calcium

B. Pathophysiology

   1. Mg^{2+} imbalances are generally a result of changes in Mg^{2+} balance in three primary organ systems.

       a) Intestines: Increased or decreased absorption

       b) Kidneys: Increased excretion or reabsorption

       c) Skeleton: Shifting of magnesium out of or into the bones

   2. It is broadly categorized into renal or extrarenal causes and acute or chronic onset.

   3. Physiologic decrease of renal tubule reabsorption of Mg^{2+} occurs within the proximal tubule (volume expansion), thick ascending limb, and distal convoluted tubule.

   4. Renal causes of Mg^{2+} imbalance

       a) Disorders of potassium and calcium and processes involve ATP (sodium–potassium–ATPase) or renal processing of Mg^{2+}.

       b) TRPM6 dysregulation of Mg^{2+} can occur as a result of various proteins, acid-base balance, or medications, which affect renal excretion of Mg^{2+}.

(1) Increased TRPM6 expression or activity leads to decreased urinary excretion of Mg^{2+}: EGFR for activated C-kinase 1, alkalosis, 17-beta-estradiol.

(2) Decreased TRPM6 expression or activity leads to increased urinary excretion of Mg^{2+}: Acidosis, tacrolimus/cyclosporine, thiazide diuretics.

5. Extrarenal causes of Mg^{2+} imbalance

 a) Decreased intestinal absorption of magnesium

 (1) Increased luminal force in the intestines may result in Mg^{2+} wasting through increased excretion in the stool.

 (2) Mutations in the TRPM6 are rare.

 b) Nutritional deficiency

III. Clinical features: Hypomagnesemia usually indicates significant whole-body magnesium depletion. Hypermagnesemia is rare but can be manifested in renal failure when patients are taking magnesium-containing medications or in acute rhabdomyolysis. Magnesium levels are typically not measured as a part of routine blood testing. Identification of imbalance requires recognizing risk factors or clinical manifestations (Ahmed & Mohammed, 2019; Berndt et al., 2016; Boyle et al., 2017; Gröber, 2019; Izzedine & Perazella, 2017; Kostov, 2019; Lo Piano et al., 2019; Smogorzewski et al., 2016; Van Laecke, 2019; J. Wang et al., 2018; R. Wang et al., 2017).

 A. Etiology: Hypomagnesemia

 1. Decreased intake/absorption

 a) Nutritional deficiency: Inadequate Mg^{2+} intake

 (1) Alcoholism: Approximately 20%–30% of alcoholics are Mg^{2+} deficient because of poor nutritional intake and impaired Mg^{2+} renal absorption.

 (2) Parenteral nutrition: Aggressive parenteral feeding in malnourished patients may result in hyperinsulinemia and rapid uptake of glucose, water, phosphate, potassium, and Mg^{2+}.

 b) Intestinal malabsorption

 (1) Malabsorption disease associated with Mg^{2+} wasting: Celiac disease, Whipple disease, inflammatory bowel disease

 (2) Surgical resection of the distal small intestine, jejunoileal bypass

 (3) Diabetes mellitus: Mg^{2+} deficiency is present in 13%–47% of patients with type 2, likely due to multiple factors such as decreased intake, poor intestinal absorption because of gastroparesis, and increased renal loss.

 c) GI loss: Diarrhea, GI fistula

 d) Cutaneous loss

 (1) Prolonged intense exertion: Marathon runners

 (2) Severe burns: Early cutaneous loss may exceed 1 g daily.

 2. Renal losses

 a) Polyuria

 (1) Hyperglycemia

 (2) Functional insulin deficiency

 b) Extracellular fluid volume expansion leading to decreased sodium and water reabsorption and eventually to secondary increased Mg^{2+} excretion

 c) Prolonged administration of magnesium-free IV fluids

 d) Medications

 (1) Diuretics

 (a) Loop diuretics: sodium-potassion-chloride cotransporter inhibition in the ascending loop inhibits Mg^{2+} reabsorption.

 (b) Thiazide diuretics: Decreased TRPM6 expression in the distal tubule leads to increased Mg^{2+} excretion.

        (2) Tubular nephrotoxins

            (*a*) Cisplatin 50 mg/m^2: Hypomagnesemia may persist for four to five months after drug is discontinued, for many years in some cases. It also may inhibit intestinal Mg^{2+} absorption.

            (*b*) Aminoglycosides: Most often after more than two weeks of therapy, it is associated with loss of Mg^{2+}, potassium, calcium, and development of tetany.

            (*c*) IV pentamidine: It causes Mg^{2+} and calcium wasting. Onset is after nine days of treatment and persists for up to two months after the drug is discontinued.

        (3) EGFR inhibitors

            (*a*) Hypomagnesemia occurs in up to 50% of patients receiving EGFR inhibitors (e.g., cetuximab, panitumumab).

            (*b*) Median time to onset is 99 days and persists up to three months after drug is discontinued.

            (*c*) EGFRs located in the distal loop and distal convoluted tubule normally increase TRPM6 expression or activity, leading to decreased urinary excretion of Mg^{2+}; EGFR inhibitors block this mechanism, causing Mg^{2+} wasting.

      e) Hypercalcemia of malignancy leads to renal wasting of Mg^{2+}.

    3. Redistribution: Hungry bone disease associated with hypocalcemia secondary to severe hypoparathyroidism, leading to decreased bone resorption and increased sequestration of calcium and Mg^{2+} for bone formation

B. Etiology: Hypermagnesemia

    1. Hypermagnesemia is relatively rare in the absence of acute or chronic renal injury.

    2. Decreased renal excretion of Mg^{2+}

      a) Renal excretion of Mg^{2+} can be increased to adjust for excess levels of Mg^{2+}.

      b) Decreased renal excretion of Mg^{2+} is generally a result of decreased GFR.

        (1) GFR less than 20 ml/min leads to impaired renal excretion of Mg^{2+}.

        (2) Older adult patients with borderline GFR and increased Mg^{2+} intake may develop hypermagnesemia.

    3. Increased intake

      a) Magnesium-containing antacids, cathartics, enemas; high doses of IV magnesium salts

      b) Increased risk in the presence of inflammatory bowel disease, bowel obstruction, or perforation

    4. Lithium

    5. Rhabdomyolysis

C. History

    1. History of cancer and cancer treatment

    2. Current medications: Prescribed; over the counter, especially the use of magnesium-containing antacids, laxatives, cathartics, and loop diuretics; PPIs; digoxin

    3. History of presenting symptoms: Precipitating factors, onset, duration

    4. Changes in ADLs

    5. Past medical history

      a) Hypomagnesemia: Diabetes, intestinal surgeries, chronic pyelonephritis, metastatic bone disease with hypercalcemia, cardiac disease (e.g., MI, CHF, arrhythmias)

      b) Hypermagnesemia: Chronic renal failure

    6. Family history: Bartter syndrome, familial hypercalciuric hypomagnesemia with nephrocalcinosis, autosomal dominant hypoparathyroidism, Gitelman syndrome,

familial hypomagnesemia with secondary hypocalcemia, isolated familial hypomagnesemia

D. Signs and symptoms: Clinical manifestations are dependent on the rapidity of onset (acute
[less than 48 hours] or chronic) and the level of severity (see Table 154-1).

E. Physical examination
　1. Vital signs
　　　a) Heart rate
　　　　　(1) Increased with hypomagnesemia
　　　　　(2) Decreased with hypermagnesemia
　　　b) Blood pressure: Hypotension is the most common early sign of hypermagnesemia.
　　　c) Temperature: It is based on underlying disease and severity of Mg^{2+} imbalance.
　　　d) Weight: It is variable based on underlying disease and severity of Mg^{2+} imbalance.
　　　e) Pain: It may be present because of neuromuscular effects of Mg^{2+} imbalance.
　　　f) General: Patients may appear fatigued and thin in the presence of malabsorp-
　　　　tion syndromes.
　　　g) The patient may report anxiety or depression.
　2. HEENT
　　　a) Poor dentition or gum retraction present in nutritional deficiencies
　　　b) Vertical nystagmus with hypomagnesemia
　　　c) Pupillary dilation with hypermagnesemia
　3. Pulmonary: Diminished effort in the presence of smooth muscle paralysis in grades
　　3–4 hypomagnesemia
　4. Abdominal: May be normal; diminished bowel sounds indicative of possible ileus
　　in hypermagnesemia
　5. Neurologic
　　　a) Observation of gait

TABLE 154-1　Most Common Clinical Manifestations of Hypomagnesemia and Hypermagnesemia

Organ/System	Hypomagnesemia	Hypermagnesemia
Cardiovascular	Hypertension Ventricular tachyarrhythmias Nonspecific T-wave changes Prolonged QT interval	Hypotension Sinus bradycardia Prolonged PR interval Widened QRS complex Complete heart block Cardiac arrest due to asystole
Neuromuscular	Tetany-like symptoms Tremors Twitching of face Spasticity Increased tendon reflexes Seizures Trousseau and Chvostek signs Vertical nystagmus	Lethargy Confusion Coma Smooth muscle paralysis (urinary reten- tion, intestinal ileus, pupillary dilation)
Renal/electrolyte	Hypokalemia Hypocalcemia	Elevated creatinine Decreased creatinine clearance
Skeletal	Decreased bone mass	–

Note. Based on information from Berndt et al., 2016; Costello et al., 2016; Smogorzewski et al., 2016.

      b) Hyperreflexia with hypomagnesemia

      c) Hypomagnesemia: Chvostek sign (muscle twitching noted after tapping the facial nerve) and Trousseau sign (spasm of the fingers and hands following constriction of circulation of the upper arm, such as with a blood pressure cuff) (see Appendix D)

  6. Musculoskeletal: Pain with palpation of muscles in the presence of tetany

IV. Diagnostic tests (Costello et al., 2016; Smogorzewski et al., 2016)

  A. Laboratory

    1. Given the minimal Mg^{2+} in the extracellular fluid, standard laboratory measures of Mg^{2+} (serum Mg^{2+}) are thought to poorly reflect true total body Mg^{2+} stores.

    2. Ionized Mg^{2+} is generally less than protien-bound Mg^{2+} because of protein binding.

    3. Urinary fractional excretion of Mg^{2+} (FEMg) is calculated using a random urine specimen.

      a) FEMg (urine Mg^{2+} × plasma creatinine concentration) / (0.7 × serum Mg^{2+} × urine creatinine concentration) × 100

      b) FEMg greater than 2% with normal GFR is inappropriate Mg^{2+} loss.

        (1) Evaluate common causes of renal loss.

        (2) If no renal loss, extrarenal causes can be identified.

    4. Full chemistry panel to evaluate calcium, potassium, phosphate, albumin, creatinine, and serum protein: Hypokalemia and hypocalcemia with low magnesium; hypercalcemia and decreased creatinine clearance with increased magnesium

  B. Radiology: Testing based on presenting symptoms

    1. Renal ultrasound may be ordered in the presence of AKI to evaluate kidneys.

    2. Avoid contrast dye in the presence of impaired renal function with hypermagnesemia.

  C. Other: ECG indicated for grades 3–4

    1. Hypomagnesemia: Ventricular tachycardia, nonspecific T waves, prolonged QT interval

    2. Hypermagnesemia: Sinus bradycardia, prolonged PR, widened QRS, complete heart block, asystole

V. Differential diagnosis of magnesium imbalance (Gröber, 2019; Lo Piano et al., 2019; Van Laecke, 2019)

  A. Hypomagnesemia

    1. Malabsorption

    2. Malnutrition

    3. Hyperparathyroidism

    4. Iatrogenic/medications

    5. Parenteral alimentation

    6. Hypocalcemia (see Chapter 152)

    7. Hypokalemia (see Chapter 153)

    8. Hyperthyroidism (see Chapter 157)

    9. Hyperaldosteronism

   10. SIADH (see Chapter 95)

  B. Hypermagnesemia

    1. Renal insufficiency or failure (see Chapter 86)

    2. Excess intake: magnesium-containing antacids/laxatives

    3. Diabetic ketoacidosis (severe dehydration) (see Chapter 151)

    4. Adrenal insufficiency

    5. Rhabdomyolysis (see Chapter 159)

VI. Treatment (Ahmed & Mohammed, 2019; Berndt et al., 2016; Costello et al., 2016; Lo Piano et al., 2019; Olza et al., 2017; Smogorzewski et al., 2016)

A. Primary goal is treatment of magnesium imbalance.

    1. Prevent life-threatening conditions (e.g., cardiac arrest, flaccid paralysis, rhabdomyolysis).

    2. Normalize Mg^{2+} level.

    3. Identify and treat the underlying causes.

B. Considerations in the approach to treatment

    1. Rapidity of onset: Acute versus chronic

    2. Severity

    3. Underlying characteristics of the patient that confer higher risk

        a) Age: Risk of increased or decreased Mg^{2+} is greater in older patients.

        b) Organic heart disease, impaired renal function, diabetes, seizure disorders, concurrent hypokalemia or hypocalcemia

        c) Medications: Antiarrhythmics, calcium-containing medications, diuretics, lithium

    4. Tailor correction of Mg^{2+} imbalance to pathophysiology of the underlying cause to avoid overcorrection or undercorrection.

C. Hypomagnesemia

    1. Mainstay of treatment is Mg^{2+} replacement.

    2. Correction of calcium (see Chapter 152), potassium (see Chapter 153), and sodium (see Chapter 155) imbalances is necessary.

    3. Mild hypomagnesemia (grade 1–2), asymptomatic, and not at high risk

        a) Increase oral intake of magnesium-rich foods, such as green vegetables, nuts, legumes, bananas, grapefruit, oranges, peanut butter, chocolate, tap water, mineral water, and dairy foods.

            (1) Diabetic diet should include magnesium 200–400 mg for adults.

            (2) Dose in Mg^{2+} deficiency is 100–600 mg daily.

        b) Oral Mg^{2+} salts: Common dosing is 54–483 mg elemental Mg^{2+} daily in divided doses.

            (1) Magnesium oxide 140 mg (85.5 mg elemental Mg^{2+})

            (2) Magnesium oxide 400 mg (241.3 mg elemental Mg^{2+})

            (3) Magnesium gluconate 500 mg (27 mg elemental Mg^{2+})

            (4) Magnesium amino acids chelate 500 mg (100 mg elemental Mg^{2+})

            (5) Magnesium chloride hexahydrate 535 mg (64 mg elemental Mg^{2+})

        c) Doses may need to be increased in patients with intestinal Mg^{2+} malabsorption.

        d) Common adverse events include diarrhea at higher doses (greater than 300 mg daily elemental Mg^{2+}).

    4. Potassium-sparing diuretics for renal Mg^{2+} wasting

    5. Moderate to severe or with sustained underlying etiology: Intestinal malabsorption, EGFR inhibitor therapy, parenteral nutrition

        a) IV administration is most common in the oncology setting.

        b) Rates of IV infusion should not exceed 1.2 mEq/min (1.5 ml of a 10% solution).

        c) Asymptomatic: Give 4 g magnesium sulfate in 250 ml or 500 ml over four to six hours. Recheck serum magnesium levels after six to eight hours.

        d) Symptomatic but stable: Give 2 g magnesium sulfate in 100 ml over 20 minutes, then 4 g in 250 ml over two to four hours.

        e) Symptomatic and unstable: Give 2 g magnesium sulfate in 20 ml of normal or half-normal saline over two minutes, then 2 g in 100 ml over 20 minutes, then 2–4 g in 250 ml over two to four hours.

        f) Titration of replacement dosing is based on effective replacement and treatment of the underlying etiology.

g) IV replacement should continue one to two days beyond correction of the serum Mg^{2+} for effective replenishment of intracellular stores.

h) Common adverse events: Facial flushing, hypotension, loss of deep tendon reflexes, tetany if concurrent hypocalcemia

6. Total parenteral nutrition maintenance

a) The maintenance dose used in adults is 1–3 g daily (8–24 mEq, 4–12 mmol).

b) Up to 6 g daily may be required in select patients, such as those with short bowel syndrome.

7. Careful monitoring of patients with compromised renal function is required to avoid hypermagnesemia.

D. Hypermagnesemia

1. Any magnesium-containing medications should be discontinued.

2. Saline diuresis with furosemide (20–80 mg PO or IV in divided doses) may enhance renal excretion.

3. Hemodialysis may be required in presence of acute or chronic renal failure.

4. Severe with cardiac findings: IV calcium

a) 1 g calcium chloride infused via a central line over two to five minutes

b) 1 g calcium gluconate via a peripheral line over two to five minutes

c) May repeat after five minutes if necessary

VII. Follow-up

A. Frequency of laboratory and clinical monitoring will be determined by the etiology of the magnesium sulfate imbalance and effectiveness of interventions to correct it.

B. Concurrent follow-up for calcium, potassium, and sodium imbalances is necessary.

C. Patients with mild hypomagnesemia on oral replacement

1. Confirm that the cause of the imbalance has been corrected.

2. Check that serum potassium level is within normal range.

3. Check serum Mg^{2+} one to two weeks after oral replacement based on risk.

4. Evaluate tolerance of oral replacement.

D. Patients with severe hypomagnesemia or at high risk for adverse events

1. Patients with symptomatic hypomagnesemia (e.g., ventricular tachyarrhythmias, seizures) will require hospitalization for emergent treatment.

2. Follow-up is determined by frequent monitoring following discharge depending on continued IV replacement or transition to oral replacement.

E. Patients with sustained underlying disease (e.g., malabsorption, renal wasting) or exposure to medications for treatment (e.g., cisplatin, EGFR inhibitor, pentamidine) and secondary hypomagnesemia

1. A combination of oral and IV Mg^{2+} replacement may be required.

2. Frequency of renal and electrolyte monitoring is determined by severity, symptoms, and treatment schedule.

3. Increased diarrhea with oral replacement for patients on EGFR inhibitor therapy may make this an ineffective route and add to intolerance (e.g., EGFR-induced diarrhea).

4. Regular monitoring of serum Mg^{2+} levels should continue.

F. Patients with renal failure and secondary hypermagnesemia: Frequency of monitoring is determined by dialysis schedule or renal follow-up.

VIII. Referrals

A. Specialists: Referral based on underlying cause (e.g., acute renal failure, intestinal malabsorption, alcoholism, medication abuse)

B. Nephrologist: For patients with acute or chronic renal failure with hypermagnesemia

C. Endocrinologist: For patients with diabetes
D. Clinical dietitian: For instruction on diets for patients with malabsorption syndromes, malnutrition, or diabetes
E. Alcohol treatment program/behavioral health specialist: For patients with alcoholism
F. Behavioral health specialist: For patients abusing laxatives or enemas
G. Gastroenterologist: To evaluate for possible underlying gastroesophageal disease if abuse of antacids containing magnesium sulfate
H. Cardiologist: For follow-up for arrhythmias

References

Ahmed, F., & Mohammed, A. (2019). Magnesium: The forgotten electrolyte—A review on hypomagnesemia. *Medical Sciences, 7*(4), 56. https://doi.org/10.3390/medsci7040056

Berndt, T.J., Thompson, J.R., & Kumar, R. (2016). The regulation of calcium, magnesium, and phosphate excretion by the kidney. In K. Skorecki, G.M. Chertow, P.A. Marsden, A.S.L. Yu., & M.W. Taal (Eds.), *Brenner and Rector's the kidney* (10th ed., pp. 185–203). Elsevier.

Boyle, N.B., Lawton, C., & Dye, L. (2017). The effects of magnesium supplementation on subjective anxiety and stress—A systematic review. *Nutrients, 9*(5), 429. https://doi.org/10.3390/nu9050429

Costello, R., Wallace, T.C., & Rosanoff, A. (2016). Magnesium. *Advances in Nutrition, 7*(1), 199–201. https://doi.org/10.3945/an.115.008524

Gröber, U. (2019). Magnesium and drugs. *International Journal of Molecular Sciences, 20*(9), 2094. https://doi.org/10.3390/ijms20092094

Izzedine, H., & Perazella, M.A. (2017). Adverse kidney effects of epidermal growth factor receptor inhibitors. *Nephrology Dialysis Transplantation, 32*(7), 1089–1097. https://doi.org/10.1093/ndt/gfw467

Kostov, K. (2019). Effects of magnesium deficiency on mechanisms of insulin resistance in type 2 diabetes: Focusing on the processes of insulin secretion and signaling. *International Journal of Molecular Sciences, 20*(6), 1351. https://doi.org/10.3390/ijms20061351

Lo Piano, F., Corsonello, A., & Corica, F. (2019). Magnesium and elderly patient: The explored paths and the ones to be explored: A review. *Magnesium Research, 32*(1), 1–15. https://www.jle.com/10.1684/mrh.2019.0453

National Cancer Institute Cancer Therapy Evaluation Program. (2017). *Common terminology criteria for adverse events* [v.5.0]. https://ctep.cancer.gov/protocoldevelopment/electronic_applications/docs/CTCAE_v5_Quick_Reference_5x7.pdf

Olza, J., Aranceta-Bartrina, J., González-Gross, M., Ortega, R.M., Serra-Majem, L., Varela-Moreiras, G., & Gil, Á. (2017). Reported dietary intake, disparity between the reported consumption and the level needed for adequacy and food sources of calcium, phosphorus, magnesium and vitamin D in the Spanish population: Findings from the ANIBES study. *Nutrients, 9*(2), 168. https://doi.org/10.3390/nu9020168

Smogorzewski, M.J., Stubbs, J.R., & Yu, A.S.L. (2016). Disorders of calcium, magnesium, and phosphate balance. In K. Skorecki, G.M. Chertow, P.A. Marsden, A.S.L. Yu., & M.W. Taal (Eds.), *Brenner and Rector's the kidney* (10th ed., pp. 601–636). Elsevier.

Van Laecke, S. (2019). Hypomagnesemia and hypermagnesemia. *Acta Clinica Belgica, 74*(1), 41–47. https://doi.org/10.1080/17843286.2018.1516173

Wang, J., Um, P., Dickerman, B.A., & Liu, J. (2018). Zinc, magnesium, selenium and depression: A review of the evidence, potential mechanisms and implications. *Nutrients, 10*(5), 584. https://doi.org/10.3390/nu10050584

Wang, R., Chen, C., Liu, W., Zhou, T., Xun, P., He, K., & Chen, P. (2017). The effect of magnesium supplementation on muscle fitness: A meta-analysis and systematic review. *Magnesium Research, 30*(4), 120–132. https://doi.org/10.1684/mrh.2018.0430

CHAPTER 155

Hyponatremia/ Hypernatremia

Sandra Kurtin, PhD, ANP-C, AOCN®

I. Definitions (NCI CTEP, 2017)
  A. Hyponatremia: A disorder characterized by laboratory test results indicating a low concentration of sodium (Na^+) in the blood
    1. Grade 1: Less than LLN–130 mEq/L
    2. Grade 2: 125–129 mEq/L and asymptomatic
    3. Grade 3: Less than 125–129 mEq/L symptomatic; 120–124 mEq/L regardless of symptoms
    4. Grade 4: Less than 120 mEq/L; life-threatening consequences
  B. Hypernatremia: A disorder characterized by laboratory test results indicating an elevation in the concentration of sodium in the blood
    1. Grade 1: Greater than ULN–150 mEq/L
    2. Grade 2: Greater than 150–mEq/L
    3. Grade 3: Greater than 155–160 mEq/L; hospitalization indicated
    4. Grade 4: Greater than 160 mEq/L; life-threatening consequences

II. Physiology/Pathophysiology (Capasso et al., 2019; Ellison & Farrar, 2018; Itzchak & Skorecki, 2016; Mount, 2016; Seay et al., 2020; Selmer et al., 2016; Whelton, 2016)
  A. Normal: Normal range is 135–145 mEq/L.
    1. Na^+ is the most abundant extracellular cation.
    2. Extracellular fluid volume is dependent on sodium concentration.
    3. Plasma sodium concentration is an index of total body fluid osmolality.
    4. Sodium concentration is regulated by multiple factors.
      a) Sodium intake
      b) Urinary excretion of sodium
      c) Hormones
        (1) ADH (vasopressin): Promotes water retention
          (a) Release of ADH in response to a decrease in blood volume or an increase in serum osmolality results in an increase in the permeability of cells lining the renal tubules.
          (b) This leads to increased reabsorption of water, restoration of blood volume, increased concentration of urine, and normalization of osmolality.
          (c) When blood volume is low, the juxtaglomerular cells of the kidney release renin.

          (d) Renin spurs the synthesis of angiotensin I, which then is converted to angiotensin II. This, in turn, stimulates the secretion of aldosterone, which promotes reabsorption of Na$^+$ and water.

     (2) Aldosterone: Promotes Na$^+$ retention primarily through reabsorption in the distal nephron

   d) Extrarenal control mechanisms

     (1) Atrial natriuretic peptide: Inhibits Na$^+$ reabsorption; released by the cardiac atria in response to stretch; increases Na$^+$ excretion by suppressing the renin–angiotensin–aldosterone mechanism

     (2) Angiotensin II and sympathetic nerve stimulation

     (3) Tonicity-responsive enhancer: Binding protein/vascular endothelial growth factor type C (TonEBP/VEGF-C)–dependent mechanism, enhancing electrolyte clearance via VEGF-C/VEGFR-3–mediated modulation of the lymph capillary network in the skin

  5. Functions of sodium

   a) Neuromuscular activity: Transmission and conduction of nerve impulses

   b) Body fluids

     (1) Sodium is largely responsible for the osmolality of vascular fluids.

     (2) Doubling the sodium level gives the approximate serum osmolality.

     (3) Regulation of body fluid: Increased sodium levels cause water retention.

   c) Cellular function

     (1) Sodium–potassium pump: Continuous shift of sodium into cells (depolarization occurs) and potassium shift out of cells (repolarization occurs) maintains water balance and neuromuscular activity.

     (2) Enzyme activity

   d) Acid-base balance: Sodium combines readily with chloride or bicarbonate to regulate the acid-base balance.

 B. Pathophysiology

  1. Hyponatremia: Occurs in a three-step process

   a) Osmotic pressure is higher inside the cells.

   b) Water moves into the cellular cytoplasm.

   c) This results in a decrease in overall plasma volume, and the patient may exhibit signs and symptoms of hypovolemia.

  2. Hypernatremia

   a) Most prominent cause of hypernatremia is free water deficit, which leads to hypovolemia and increased plasma osmolality (i.e., water loss is greater than Na$^+$ loss).

   b) A hyperosmolar state draws fluid from the intracellular to the extracellular compartment.

III. Clinical features: Disturbances of sodium concentration result in most cases from abnormalities of water homeostasis. Hyponatremia represents a relative excess of water compared to sodium. The more acute (less than 48 hours) the greater the risk of complications and the need for aggressive treatment. Hypernatremia is most often caused by unreplaced water lost from the GI tract, skin, or urine. Hypernatremia caused by water loss is dehydration. This differs from hypovolemia, which is loss of water and salt (Capasso et al., 2019; Cavusoglu et al., 2019; Ellison & Farrar, 2018; Filippatos et al., 2016; Itzchak & Skorecki, 2016; Kieneker et al., 2018; Mente et al., 2018; NCI CTEP, 2017; Seay et al., 2020; Selmer et al., 2016; Zhu et al., 2018).

 A. Etiologies: Hyponatremia

  1. The etiologies of hyponatremia may be categorized based on the excess loss of sodium or gain of water.

    2. Hypovolemic: Associated with extracellular fluid volume deficit; deficits of total body water and sodium, with the deficit of sodium relatively greater

       a) Renal loss: Diuretics, particularly thiazide diuretics; salt-losing nephritis; adrenal insufficiency; osmotic diuresis

       b) Nonrenal loss

          (1) Loss of GI fluids: Diarrhea, emesis, increased ostomy output

          (2) Sweating

          (3) Third-spacing of fluids: Burns, pancreatitis, peritonitis, rhabdomyolysis

          (4) Addison disease: Hypoaldosteronism or adrenal insufficiency

          (5) Osmotic diuresis

          (6) Cystic fibrosis

          (7) Metabolic acidosis

    3. Euvolemic: Associated with normal extracellular fluid volume; low serum sodium level with no evidence of hypovolemia or edema

       a) SIADH

       b) Psychogenic polydipsia: Compulsive water drinking

       c) Hypothyroidism: Vasopressin dependent

       d) Drugs: Direct stimulation of vasopressin release or factors that enhance its action, such as tricyclic antidepressants, cyclophosphamide, cisplatin, vincristine, vinblastine, nicotine, sulfonylurea, IL-2, SSRIs, and opioids

       e) CNS disorders: Subarachnoid hemorrhage, tumors, meningitis, stroke, trauma, multiple sclerosis

       f) Tumors: Pancreatic tumors, small cell carcinoma, bronchogenic carcinoma, duodenal tumors, neuroendocrine carcinomas, adenoid cystic carcinomas, undifferentiated carcinomas

       g) Redistributive: Mannitol infusion, hyperglycemia, surgical irrigation fluids

       h) Emotional stress

       i) Pulmonary processes: Aspergillosis, pneumonia, TB, pulmonary tumors, abscess

    4. Hypervolemic: Associated with extracellular fluid volume excess; both total body sodium and total body water increased to a great extent

       a) Heart failure: Reduced cardiac output

       b) Liver failure: Systemic vasodilation

       c) Nephrotic syndrome

       d) Renal failure: Acute and chronic

    5. Pseudohyponatremia: Rare; measurement artifact from reduced plasma water

       a) Excess lipids: Triglycerides

       b) Abnormal proteins: IgM

B. Etiologies: Hypernatremia

    1. Almost always reflects excessive water loss and/or the inability to adequately replace water

    2. Lesions in the CNS affecting thirst, CNS tumors, CNS infections, traumatic brain injury

    3. Inability to obtain or drink fluids: Disability, communication problems (common in older adults)

    4. Excessive water loss without adequate replacement

       a) Burns, hyperthermia

       b) Respiratory disease, hyperventilation

       c) Diabetes insipidus

       d) Diabetes mellitus

    5. Impaired vasopressin mechanisms: Decreased secretion or lack of effect on the kidneys

      6. Medications: Lithium, lactulose, hypertonic saline, sodium bicarbonate

C. History

    1. History of cancer and cancer treatment

    2. Current medications: Prescribed, over the counter, especially diuretics

    3. History of presenting symptoms: Precipitating factors, location, onset, severity, duration

    4. Changes in ADLs: History of urine output and fluid intake

    5. Past medical history: Headaches, use of tap water enemas, recent surgery, trauma, pregnancy

    6. Past medical history for hyponatremia: COPD, older age, hypertension, diabetes, cardiovascular disease, psychiatric disorders

D. Signs and symptoms (see Table 155-1)

    1. It is dependent on the rapidity of onset (acute vs. chronic) and level of severity.

    2. Acute onset (less than 48 hours) or grades 3–4 imbalances are most often associated with severe CNS symptoms.

E. Physical examination (see Table 155-1)

    1. Vital signs

       a) Tachycardia: Hypovolemic or fluid overload states

       b) Blood pressure

          (1) Hypotension: Volume depletion

          (2) Hypertension: May be associated with CNS changes

       c) Temperature: Low-grade fever with hypernatremia

       d) Weight: Loss or gain indicative of possible change in fluid status

       e) Pain: May be present with muscle twitching or tremors

TABLE 155-1   **Common Clinical Manifestations of Hyponatremia and Hypernatremia**

Organ/System	Hyponatremia	Hypernatremia
Cardiovascular	Tachycardia Hypotension Atrial fibrillation	Tachycardia Hypertension
Central nervous system	Headaches Agitation, lethargy, confusion, depression Seizures Severe or acute onset: Delirium, signs of increased intracranial pressure (focal weakness, hemiparesis, ataxia, papilledema, coma)	Restlessness Generalized weakness Low-grade temperature Severe or acute onset: Disorientation, hallucinations, lethargy, irritability and hyperreactive when stimulated, seizures, coma
Gastrointestinal	Anorexia Taste alterations	Thirst; rough, dry tongue Anorexia Nausea, vomiting
Integumentary	Xerosis, pallor, diminished turgor (hypovolemic, euvolemic) Dry mucous membranes	Xerosis Dry, sticky mucous membranes Flushing
Neuromuscular	Muscle cramps, muscle twitching	Muscle twitching, tremor Hyperreflexia
Pulmonary	Dyspnea on exertion	–

Note. Based on information from Cavusoglu et al., 2019; Ellison & Farrar, 2018; Itzchak & Skorecki, 2016.

2. HEENT
   a) Hyponatremia: Dry mouth, inability to produce tears
   b) Hypernatremia: Dry, sticky mucous membranes; rough, dry tongue
3. Integument: Xerosis, skin turgor (will vary based on extracellular fluid state), flushing
4. Cardiac
   a) Capillary refill decreased, neck JVD, depending on etiology of sodium imbalance
   b) In hyponatremia: Irregular pulse indicating dysrhythmia
5. Neurologic: Behavior changes, mental status
   a) Muscle strength, twitching, tremors, and weakness
   b) Mental status, confusion, speech changes
   c) Deep tendon reflexes: Diminished (hyponatremia); hyperreflexia (hypernatremia)
   d) Ataxia (hypernatremia), history of falls (chronic hyponatremia)

IV. Diagnostic tests (Ellison & Farrar, 2018; Itzchak & Skorecki, 2016; Rhee et al., 2019)
   A. Laboratory: Hyponatremia
      1. Serum Na^+ less than 135 mEq/L is hyponatremia.
         a) Corrected Na^+ is $([Na^+] + 0.016) \times (glucose - 100)$.
         b) Sodium deficit (mEq) is $([Na^+]$ goal $- [Na^+]$ plasma$) \times$ total body water (weight $\times$ 60%).
      2. Serum osmolality
         a) Serum osmolality (calculated): $(2 \times [Na^+]) + BUN/2.8 + glucose/18$
         b) Serum osmolality less than 275 mOsm/kg water: True hyponatremia
            (1) Evaluate clinical hydration and urine Na^+.
            (2) Hypervolemic with urine Na^+ less than 10 mEq/L: Most common with organ failure (e.g., heart, liver, renal)
            (3) Hypervolemic with urine Na^+ greater than 20 mEq/L: Most common with renal failure
            (4) Hypovolemic with urine Na^+ less than 10 mEq/L: Most common with extrarenal loss
            (5) Hypovolemic with urine Na^+ greater than 20 mEq/L: Most common with renal loss
            (6) Euvolemic: Normal total body sodium
         c) Serum osmolality greater than 295 mOsm/kg water: Pseudohyponatremia
            (1) Hyperosmolar: Suggests hyperglycemia, mannitol
            (2) Iso-osmolar: Suggests hyperlipidemia, proteinemia
      3. Serum glucose: Hyperglycemia may affect Na^+ shift.
      4. BUN and creatinine to evaluate renal function, volume status
      5. Serum albumin: Decrease suggests nephrotic syndrome.
      6. TSH to detect hypothyroidism
      7. Serum electrolytes: Magnesium and potassium levels may shift with hyponatremia.
   B. Laboratory: Hypernatremia
      1. Hypernatremia always represents a state of hyperosmolality.
      2. Serum sodium greater than 145 mEq/L indicates hypernatremia.
         a) Corrected is $([Na^+] + 0.016) \times (glucose - 100)$.
         b) Free water deficit is $([Na^+]/140) - 1) \times$ total body water.
         c) Fractional excretion of Na^+ (FENa) is (Na^+) urine $+$ creatinine plasma $/(Na^+)$ plasma $+$ creatinine urine.
            (1) Less than 1% is prerenal (hypovolemia).
            (2) Greater than 2% is intrinsic renal disorder.

3. Measure serum osmolality, urine osmolality, and urine Na$^+$.
   a) Urine/plasma osmolality ratio greater than 0.7 with urine Na$^+$ less than 10 mEq/L: Suggests extrarenal loss
   b) Urine/plasma osmolality ratio greater than 0.7 with urine Na$^+$ greater than 20 mEq/L: Suggests renal loss or iatrogenic
   c) Urine/plasma osmolality ratio less than 0.7 with urine Na$^+$ greater than 20 mEq/L: Suggests excessive water intake or iatrogenic
   d) Urine/plasma osmolality ratio less than 0.7 with variable urine Na$^+$: Suggests CNS disease, congenital or acquired vasopressin disorders

C. Radiology
   1. Chest x-ray for baseline assessment for underlying cause and fluid status
   2. CT scan of the head for patients exhibiting CNS symptoms

D. Other: ECG to evaluate for atrial fibrillation
   1. Hyponatremia has been independently associated with the occurrence of atrial fibrillation.
   2. Patients with preexisting heart failure are at an increased risk.

V. Differential diagnosis (Cavusoglu et al., 2019; Filippatos et al., 2016; Gankam Kengne & Decaux, 2018; Itzchak & Skorecki, 2016; Wang et al., 2018; Whelton, 2016; Zhu et al., 2018)
   A. Pseudohyponatremia: Hyperproteinemia, dyslipidemia (see Chapter 44), multiple myeloma
   B. SIADH (see Chapter 95): Medication-induced SIADH (e.g., cyclophosphamide, vinblastine, vincristine)
   C. GI loss: Nausea, vomiting, diarrhea, suctioning (see Chapters 56 and 63)
   D. Dilutional hyponatremia/increased extracellular volume: CHF, renal failure (see Chapters 42 and 86)
   E. Hypoaldosteronism: Primary or secondary
   F. Adrenal insufficiency, Cushing syndrome
   G. Severe burns
   H. Hypothyroidism (see Chapter 158)
   I. Nephrotic syndrome (see Chapter 91)
   J. Pancreatitis (see Chapter 77), peritonitis, rhabdomyolysis (see Chapter 159)
   K. Mineralocorticoid deficiency
   L. Drug induced: Thiazides, SSRIs, norepinephrine reuptake inhibitors, carbamazepine, oxcarbazepine, ecstasy, lamotrigine, duloxetine
   M. Bicarbonaturia
   N. Stress
   O. Cirrhosis (see Chapter 69)
   P. Hyperglycemia (see Chapter 151): Hyperglycemia pulls water out of the cells into the extracellular fluid. Serum Na$^+$ concentrations fall in proportion to the dilution caused by the hyperglycemia.
   Q. Sweating, strenuous exercise
   R. Ketonuria
   S. Dehydration secondary to renal and nonrenal losses or inadequate fluid intake
   T. Nephrogenic diabetes insipidus
   U. CNS malignancy/metastases
   V. Hyperaldosteronism: Primary or secondary
   W. Hyperosmotic coma
   X. Oral ingestion of excess salts

VI. Treatment: Therapy is directed toward restoring Na^+ and extracellular fluid volume balance (Bankir et al., 2017; Capasso et al., 2019; Ellison & Farrar, 2018; Gralla et al., 2017; Itzchak & Skorecki, 2016; Seay et al., 2020).

   A. The underlying cause should be determined and treated while restoring sodium and fluid balance: SIADH (see Chapter 95), hyperglycemia (see Chapter 151), hypothyroidism (see Chapter 158), hypoaldosteronism/adrenal insufficiency.

   B. Restoration of sodium and fluid balance will be determined by the specific imbalance, onset, and severity of symptoms.

      1. Correction of hypovolemia

        a) Sodium chloride 0.9% or colloids are recommended.

        b) Rate of correction should not exceed 12 mEq/L in 24 hours.

        c) Caution should be used when administering solutions with dextrose 5% in water (D_5W).

        d) In patients with mild hypovolemia and hypernatremia, oral hydration to replace free water is preferred. Otherwise, use 0.45% saline followed by D_5W IV.

        e) Encourage euvolemic patients with hypernatremia to drink water or give D_5W IV to enhance excretion of excess Na^+.

        f) Hypernatremia associated with hypervolemia may require loop diuretics, such as furosemide 20 mg PO or IV daily, to promote excretion of excess Na^+. In patients with renal failure, dialysis may be indicated.

        g) Calculate water deficit in liters to determine initial therapy: $(0.6 \times weight) \times ([Na^+] - 140)$.

      2. Hyponatremia: Replace sodium.

        a) Determine if the hyponatremia onset is acute (less than 48 hours) or chronic (onset greater than 48 hours).

        b) Acute and symptomatic hyponatremia

          (1) Severe: Sodium replacement must be administered carefully to avoid osmotic demyelination syndrome—not to exceed 0.5–1 mEq/L/hr or 12 mEq/L/24 hrs.

          (2) Frequent serial monitoring of serum Na^+, urinary free water, and Na^+ excretion should be maintained until serum Na^+ greater than 120 mEq/L.

          (3) Hypertonic saline solution (3% sodium) should be administered cautiously—not to exceed 1 ml/kg/hr.

          (4) Tolvaptan: Initiate therapy inpatient to closely monitor serum Na^+. Initial dose is 15 mg PO daily. Titrate to desired serum Na^+. Increase every 24 hours or more slowly to 30 mg PO daily. Maxium dose is 60 mg daily.

          (5) Conivaptan: Initiate loading dose of 20 mg IV over 30 minutes, then continuous infusion 20 mg over 24 hours for one to four days. Titrate to desired serum Na^+. Maxium dose is 40 mg daily as a continuous infusion. Serum Na^+ should be closely monitored.

        c) Chronic hyponatremia

          (1) Patients with hypotonic hyponatremia are generally asymptomatic.

          (2) Symptomatic: Hypovolemic; exercise caution with Na^+ replacement.

          (3) Symptomatic: Hypervolemic or euvolemic

            (a) Restrict water intake, generally 800 ml daily.

            (b) Add furosemide to increase solute delivery to the distal tubule to improve free water excretion.

            (c) In CHF (hypervolemic hyponatremia), cardiac output is less effective, leading to decreased GFR and warranting water and Na^+ restriction (see Chapter 42).

            (d) The combination of decreased GFR and low Na^+ stimulates secretion of ADH and aldosterone, causing further retention of water and salt.

            (e) Effective management of hypervolemia of any cause must include Na^+ restriction.

    3. Hypernatremia

        a) Correct underlying cause of water loss.

        b) Replace fluids and then electrolytes.

        c) Restore severely hypovolemic patients to euvolemia with isotonic saline (0.9%) followed by 0.45% saline or D_5W.

        d) Rate of replacement is dependent on severity of volume depletion, as well as cardiac and renal status.

        e) Clinical parameters for adequate volume replacement are stabilization of blood pressure and heart rate and restoration of adequate urine output (less than 25 ml/hr indicates inadequate renal perfusion).

        f) Implement sodium restriction.

            (1) Average daily requirement of Na^+ is 2–4 g; however, the average amount consumed is 8–15 g.

            (2) A cautious restriction would be 1–3 g of Na^+ and 0.5–1.5 L of water daily; degree of restriction is dependent on severity of hyponatremia and extent of extracellular fluid excess.

        g) Serum Na^+ will increase gradually over several days.

    4. Comfort measures for dry mouth include ice chips, sips of water, mouth care, and lip moisturizer.

VII. Follow-up

    A. Follow-up varies depending on severity of imbalance and the patient's overall medical condition.

    B. Initial monitoring for severe and symptomatic patients will be hourly or more frequently.

    C. As the patient reaches a euvolemic state and becomes asymptomatic, monitoring will extend gradually until the patient is stable with effective treatment of the underlying etiology.

VIII. Referrals

    A. Referrals for appropriate follow-up are based on the underlying cause of the sodium and/or fluid imbalance.

    B. Dietitian: For reinforcement of dietary sodium and water intake

    C. Endocrinologist: For sodium imbalances that result from hypoaldosteronism or hyperaldosteronism, hypoadrenalism or hyperadrenalism, hypothyroidism, or poorly controlled diabetes

    D. Nephrologist: Recommended for patients with renal failure or nephrotic syndrome or for patients in need of dialysis

References

Bankir, L., Perucca, J., Norsk, P., Bouby, N., & Damgaard, M. (2017). Relationship between sodium intake and water intake: The false and the true. *Annals of Nutrition and Metabolism, 70*(Suppl. 1), 51–61. https://doi.org/10.1159/000463831

Capasso, A., Benigni, A., Capitanio, U., Danesh, F.R., Di Marzo, V., Gesualdo, L., ... Capasso, G. (2019). Summary of the International Conference on Onco-Nephrology: An emerging field in medicine. *Kidney International, 96*(3), 555–567. https://doi.org/10.1016/j.kint.2019.04.043

Cavusoglu, Y., Kaya, H., Eraslan, S., & Yilmaz, M.B. (2019). Hyponatremia is associated with occurrence of atrial fibrillation in outpatients with heart failure and reduced ejection fraction. *Hellenic Journal of Cardiology, 60*(2), 117–121. https://doi.org/10.1016/j.hjc.2018.03.006

Ellison, D., & Farrar, F.C. (2018). Kidney influence on fluid and electrolyte balance. *Nursing Clinics of North America, 53*(4), 469–480. https://doi.org/10.1016/j.cnur.2018.05.004

Filippatos, T.D., Liamis, G., Christopoulou, F., & Elisaf, M.S. (2016). Ten common pitfalls in the evaluation of patients with hyponatremia. *European Journal of Internal Medicine, 29,* 22–25. https://doi.org/10.1016/j.ejim.2015.11.022

Gankam Kengne, F., & Decaux, G. (2018). Hyponatremia and the brain. *Kidney International Reports, 3*(1), 24–35. https://doi.org/10.1016/j.ekir.2017.08.015

Gralla, R.J., Ahmad, F., Blais, J.D., Chiodo, J., III, Zhou, W., Glaser, L.A., & Czerwiec, F.S. (2017). Tolvaptan use in cancer patients with hyponatremia due to the syndrome of inappropriate antidiuretic hormone: A post hoc analysis of the SALT-1 and SALT-2 trials. *Cancer Medicine, 6*(4), 723–729. https://doi.org/10.1002/cam4.805

Itzchak, N.S., & Skorecki, K.L. (2016). Disorders of sodium balance. In K. Skorecki, G.M. Chertow, P.A. Marsden, A.S.L. Yu., & M.W. Taal (Eds.), *Brenner and Rector's the kidney* (10th ed., pp. 390–458). Elsevier.

Kieneker, L.M., Eisenga, M.F., Gansevoort, R.T., de Boer, R.A., Navis, G., Dullaart, R.P.F., ... Bakker, S.J.L. (2018). Association of low urinary sodium excretion with increased risk of stroke. *Mayo Clinic Proceedings, 93*(12), 1803–1809. https://doi.org/10.1016/j.mayocp.2018.05.028

Mente, A., O'Donnell, M., Rangarajan, S., McQueen, M., Dagenais, G., Wielgosz, A., ... Yusuf, S. (2018). Urinary sodium excretion, blood pressure, cardiovascular disease, and mortality: A community-level prospective epidemiological cohort study. *Lancet, 392*(10146), 496–506. https://doi.org/10.1016/s0140-6736(18)31376-x

Mount, D.B. (2016). Transport of sodium, chloride, and potassium. In K. Skorecki, G.M. Chertow, P.A. Marsden, A.S.L. Yu., & M.W. Taal (Eds.), *Brenner and Rector's the kidney* (10th ed., pp. 144–184). Elsevier.

National Cancer Institute Cancer Therapy Evaluation Program. (2017). *Common terminology criteria for adverse events* [v.5.0]. https://ctep.cancer.gov/protocoldevelopment/electronic_applications/docs/CTCAE_v5_Quick_Reference_5x7.pdf

Rhee, C.M., Ayus, J.C., & Kalantar-Zadeh, K. (2019). Hyponatremia in the dialysis population. *Kidney International Reports, 4*(6), 769–780. https://doi.org/10.1016/j.ekir.2019.02.012

Seay, N.W., Lehrich, R.W., & Greenberg, A. (2020). Diagnosis and management of disorders of body tonicity—Hyponatremia and hypernatremia: Core curriculum 2020. *American Journal of Kidney Diseases, 75*(2), 272–286. https://doi.org/10.1053/j.ajkd.2019.07.014

Selmer, C., Madsen, J.C., Torp-Pedersen, C., Gislason, G.H., & Faber, J. (2016). Hyponatremia, all-cause mortality, and risk of cancer diagnoses in the primary care setting: A large population study. *European Journal of Internal Medicine, 36,* 36–43. https://doi.org/10.1016/j.ejim.2016.07.028

Wang, D., Lai, J., Lu, S., Huang, M., Hu, S., & Xu, Y. (2018). Rapid-onset hyponatremia and delirium following duloxetine treatment for postherpetic neuralgia: Case report and literature review. *Medicine, 97*(46), e13178. https://doi.org/10.1097/md.0000000000013178

Whelton, P.K. (2016). Hyponatremia in the general population. What does it mean? *Nutrition, Metabolism and Cardiovascular Diseases, 26*(1), 9–11. https://doi.org/10.1016/j.numecd.2015.10.008

Zhu, Y., Zhang, J., Li, Z., Liu, Y., Fan, X., Zhang, Y., & Zhang, Y. (2018). Association of sodium intake and major cardiovascular outcomes: A dose-response meta-analysis of prospective cohort studies. *BMC Cardiovascular Disorders, 18,* 192. https://doi.org/10.1186/s12872-018-0927-9

CHAPTER 156

Hypophosphatemia/ Hyperphosphatemia

Sandra Kurtin, PhD, ANP-C, AOCN®

I. Definitions (Megapanou et al., 2020; NCI CTEP, 2017)
   A. Hypophosphatemia: A disorder characterized by laboratory test results indicating a low concentration of phosphate in the blood; currently graded in the Common Terminology Criteria for Adverse Events with general parameters and not discrete values
      1. Grade 1: Laboratory finding only; interventions not indicated
      2. Grade 2: Oral replacement therapy indicated
      3. Grade 3: Severe or medically significant but not immediately life threatening; hospitalization or prolongation of existing hospitalization indicated
      4. Grade 4: Life-threatening consequences
   B. Hyperphosphatemia: A disorder characterized by laboratory test results indicating an elevation in the concentration of phosphate in the blood; currently graded in the Common Terminology Criteria for Adverse Events with general parameters and not discrete values
      1. Grade 1: Laboratory finding only; interventions not indicated
      2. Grade 2: Noninvasive intervention indicated
      3. Grade 3: Severe or medically significant but not immediately life threatening; hospitalization or prolongation of existing hospitalization indicated
      4. Grade 4: Life-threatening consequences; urgent intervention indicated (e.g., dialysis)

II. Physiology/Pathophysiology (Berndt et al., 2016; Eaton & Pooler, 2018; Kraft, 2015; Leung & Crook, 2019; McClure et al., 2017; Michigami et al., 2018; Michigami & Ozono, 2019; Moore et al., 2015; Nadkarni & Uribarri, 2014; Smogorzewski et al., 2016; Stremke & Hill Gallant, 2018; Suki & Moore, 2016)
   A. Normal: Serum phosphorus (phosphate; PO_4) ranges from 2.5–4.5 mg/dl in adults; PO_4 is a major anion that has its highest concentration in the intracellular fluid.
      1. PO_4 homeostasis is dependent on movement among four primary body compartments: intestines, skeleton, intracellular space, and kidneys.
         a) Total body PO_4 is 500–800 mg.
         b) Approximately 85% is in the skeleton, 14% is in the soft tissues, and 1% is in the extracellular fluid and other tissues.
         c) Extracellular fluid PO_4 is approximately 600 mg: 60% as organic (phospholipids) and 30% as inorganic PO_4.
            (1) Approximately 85%–90% of plasma PO_4 is filtered by the kidneys: 50% is ionized or free, 40% is complexed with other cations (calcium is most common), and 10% is bound to protein.

(2) Approximately 70% of the filtered PO_4 is reabsorbed in the proximal tubules by NPt2a and NPt2c transporters.

d) Excretion of PO_4 is 800 mg daily by the kidneys and 150 mg daily in the colon.

2. The shifting of phosphate within and between these compartments is regulated by dietary phosphate intake, phosphate transporters, and urinary phosphate excretion.

a) Phosphorus intake

(1) Dietary intake of phosphorus varies by food group: grain products (29.3%); meats/poultry/fish (25.2%); milk and milk products (21%); sugars, sweeteners, beverages (7.1%); vegetables (6.7%); legumes/nuts/seeds (4.8%); eggs (3.4%); fruits (2%); fats/oils (0.3%).

(2) Intestines can only absorb inorganic PO_4; organic PO_4 in food must be hydrolyzed in the gut prior to absorption.

(3) The average daily PO_4 intake in a Western diet is 1,500 mg; approximately 70% of PO_4 is absorbed by healthy people eating a mixed diet.

(4) Approximately 60% of this is absorbed by the intestine (primarily the jejunum) through active transport and paracellular diffusion.

(5) Approximately 150–200 mg of phosphorus is secreted daily by the colon.

(6) Intestinal absorption is mediated by sodium–phosphate cotransporters and is enhanced by $1,25(OH)_2D$ (calcitriol).

b) Phosphate transporters and hormones

(1) PO_4 is transported across cell membranes by sodium–phosphate cotransporters expressed in the kidney and intestinal epithelium.

(2) Kidneys express type II sodium-dependent phosphate transporters, NaPiIIa, and NaPiIIc and actively reabsorb PO_4 in the proximal tubules.

(3) Intestines express both type II (NaPiIIb) and III (PiT-1 and PiT-2) sodium-dependent phosphate transporters. NaPiIIb is encoded by the gene *SLC34A2*.

(4) Transcellular transport accounts for approximately 50% of total PO_4 transport in the intestines, the majority of which (greater than 90%) is regulated by NaPiIIb.

(5) $1,25(OH)_2D$, PTH, and dietary phosphorus intake regulate transcellular sodium-dependent PO_4 transport in the intestine.

c) Phosphatonins: A class of proteins that decrease extracellular fluid PO_4 concentrations by inhibiting renal tubule reabsorption of PO_4. Fibroblast growth factor 23 (FGF23), a protein secreted by osteoblasts and osteocytes, is most common.

(1) Implicated in several hereditary PO_4 disorders

(2) Increased FGF23: Hypophosphatemia

(3) Decreased FGF23: Hyperphosphatemia

(4) FGF23 increased in CKD

d) Urinary phosphate excretion

(1) Virtually all serum PO_4 is filtered at the glomerulus.

(a) Approximately 20% of the filtered PO_4 load is excreted.

(b) Approximately 80% of filtered PO_4 load is reabsorbed by the renal tubules.

(2) Reabsorption is facilitated by PO_4 cotransporters and hormones.

(3) Interactions between the NaPiIIa and the sodium–hydrogen exchanger regulatory factor 1 (NHERF-1) modulate the amount of NaPiIIa and NaPiIIc present on the surface of the proximal tubular cell.

(a) Upregulation: Increased PO_4 uptake

(b) Downregulation: Decreased PO_4 uptake

3. Phosphorus and calcium have similar and opposite effects.
   a) Both electrolytes need vitamin D for intestinal absorption and are present in bones and teeth.
   b) PTH acts on phosphorus and calcium differently. PTH decreases serum phosphorous levels by stimulating the renal tubules to excrete phosphorus, and it increases serum calcium levels by pulling calcium from the bone.
4. Functions of phosphorus
   a) Neuromuscular activity: Normal nerve and muscle activity
   b) Skeletal: Bone and teeth formation, strength, and durability
   c) Cellular activities
      (1) Maintenance of cell membrane integrity as phospholipids
      (2) Synthesis of DNA and RNA
      (3) Transfer as phosphorylated intermediates
      (4) Regulation of proteins by phosphorylation/dephosphorylation.
      (5) Storage of metabolic energy, formation of ATP
   d) Components of nucleic acids
   e) Formation of 2,3-diphosphoglycerate, an RBC enzyme responsible for delivering oxygen to tissues
   f) Facilitates utilization of B vitamins
   g) Maintenance of acid-base balance in body fluids
B. Pathophysiology: Decreased (hypophosphatemia) or increased (hyperphosphatemia)
   1. Acute: Onset less than 48 hours; most often due to renal impairment (e.g., AKI) secondary to electrolyte or acid-base imbalances or hormone abnormalities (e.g., respiratory acidosis, metabolic acidosis, tumor lysis syndrome, hemolytic anemia, hypoparathyroidism)
   2. Chronic: Greater than 48 hours; primarily due to CKD; prolonged hyperphosphatemia may lead to acute tissue calcification and hypocalcemia; chronic hypophosphatemia may result in osteomalacia as a result of vitamin D deficiency.

III. Clinical features: PO_4 imbalances are generally a result of changes in the PO_4 concentration in the primary compartments (e.g., intestinal, bone, intracellular, renal) (Kraft, 2015; Leung & Crook, 2019; Megapanou et al., 2020; Merhi et al., 2017; Smogorzewski et al., 2016).
A. Etiology: Hypophosphatemia
   1. Incidence is highest in patients hospitalized in the ICU (28%–34%). It can be as high as 80% in the presence of sepsis and 28%–30% in chronic alcoholism.
   2. Decreased intestinal absorption
      a) Malnutrition, alcoholism, malabsorption
      b) GI loss: Diarrhea, vomiting
      c) Aluminum-containing antacids
      d) Vitamin D–mediated disorders: Decreased $1,25(OH)_2D$ leads to decreased PO_4 and calcium absorption.
      e) CKD
      f) Chronic liver disease
   3. Intracellular shifts: Redistribution
      a) Respiratory alkalosis: Intracellular shift of PO_4
      b) Refeeding syndrome: Consists of metabolic disturbances that occur as a result of reinstitution of nutrition to patients who are starved or severely malnourished
      c) Burns: Increased PO_4 utilization for tissue building
      d) Diabetic ketoacidosis
         (1) Glycosuria and polyuria increase PO_4 excretion.

(2) Dextrose infusion with insulin causes a PO_4 shift into the cells, decreasing the serum PO_4 level.

   e) Hungry bone syndrome: Postparathyroidectomy

4. Increased urinary phosphate excretion

   a) Primary and secondary hyperparathyroidism leads to increased PTH and increased PO_4 excretion and calcium reabsorption.

   b) Increased production or activity of phosphatonins

      (1) Increased production of FGF23 leads to decreased intestinal absorption of PO_4 and calcium.

      (2) Rare syndromes of PO_4 renal wasting: X-linked hypophosphatemia, autosomal dominant hypophosphatemic rickets (e.g., *FGF23* mutations), autosomal recessive hypophosphatemic rickets (e.g., *DMP1* and *ENPP1* mutations)

      (3) Tumor-induced osteomalacia: Acquired paraneoplastic syndrome is most common in mesenchymal tumors that express and secrete FGF23 (see Appendix M).

   c) Kidney transplantation: Hypophosphatemia is present in up to 90% of recipients after kidney transplantation and may persist for up to one year due to hyperparathyroidism, increased FGF23 expression, decreased $1,25(OH)_2D$, and immunosuppressive medications.

   d) Hereditary syndromes associated with phosphate wasting: *SLC34A3* mutations; *SLC34A1* mutations; *NHERF1* mutations; *KLOTHO* mutations

   e) Medications

      (1) Diuretics: Acetazolamide, loop diuretics, thiazide diuretics

      (2) Corticosteroids: Decreased intestinal absorption and increased urinary excretion of PO_4

   f) Fanconi syndrome: Impaired proximal tubule reabsorption of PO_4, glucose, calcium, uric acid, bicarbonate, other organic compounds

      (1) Acquired: Monoclonal gammopathies, amyloidosis, toxins (e.g., antineoplastic agents, antiviral agents, aminoglycosides, anticonvulsants)

      (2) Genetic: Wilson disease, cystinosis

   g) Miscellaneous

      (1) Tumor consumption of PO_4, leukemic blast crisis, aggressive lymphomas

      (2) Sepsis

      (3) Heat stroke

      (4) Diabetic ketoacidosis

      (5) Surgeries: Hepatectomy, colorectal surgery

B. Etiology: Hyperphosphatemia

1. Increased phosphorus intake: Bowel preparations containing sodium phosphorus are the most common cause. Greatest risk factors are older age, female gender, renal impairment, dehydration, bowel obstruction, hypertension, and concurrent ACE inhibitor and NSAID use.

2. Intracellular shifts: Redistribution

   a) Respiratory acidosis: Increased PO_4 due to renal resistance to PTH and hypocalcemia

   b) Metabolic alkalosis: Increased PO_4 due to reduced glycolysis and PO_4 utilization

   c) Tumor lysis syndrome: Increased PO_4 due to rapid release of intracellular PO_4 during cellular breakdown

   d) Rhabdomyolysis

   e) Hemolytic anemia

        f) Bisphosphonate administration: Increased PO_4 due to PO_4 distribution and decreased PO_4 renal excretion

        g) Catabolic state

    3. Decreased renal excretion

        a) CKD (most common); increased PO_4 due to increased PTH and FGF23

        b) Hypoparathyroidism, pseudohypoparathyroidism

        c) Acromegaly

        d) Tumoral calcinosis: *FGF23* inactivating gene mutation; *GALNT3* mutation with aberrant FGF23 glycosylation; *KLOTHO* inactivating mutation with FGF23 resistance; bisphosphonates

C. History

    1. History of cancer and cancer treatment

    2. Current medications: Prescribed, over the counter, especially agents containing phosphate or calcium, diuretics, insulin

    3. History of presenting symptoms: Precipitating factors, onset, duration

    4. Changes in ADLs

    5. Past medical history

        a) Hypophosphatemia: Malnutrition, alcoholism, vitamin D deficiency, hyperparathyroidism, diabetes

        b) Hyperphosphatemia: CKD, hypoparathyroidism

    6. Family history: Hereditary forms of hypophosphatemia

D. Signs and symptoms

    1. Hypophosphatemia

        a) Anorexia

        b) Dysphagia

        c) Muscle weakness

        d) Tremors

        e) Paresthesia

        f) Bone pain

        g) Seizure

    2. Hyperphosphatemia

        a) Nausea

        b) Diarrhea

        c) Abdominal cramps

        d) Muscle weakness

E. Physical examination

    1. Vital signs

        a) Heart rate: May be increased with hyperphosphatemia; possible thready pulse with hypophosphatemia

        b) Blood pressure: Variable

        c) Temperature: Variable

        d) Weight: Variable based on fluid retention or excretion and presence of renal insufficiency or other underlying disorders

        e) Pain: May be present with severe hypophosphatemia in the presence of tumor lysis syndrome or rhabdomyolysis

        f) General: Normal patient appearance with mild PO_4 imbalances; possible lethargy and fatigue in more severe cases

    2. HEENT: Possible dry mouth present with underlying CKD, diabetic ketoacidosis, or dehydration; possible poor dentition and gum retraction in chronic alcoholism or malnutrition

3. Cardiac: Systolic ejection murmurs as possible symptoms of cardiomyopathy (left ventricular hypertrophy); valve disease with hyperphosphatemia in the presence of CKD

4. Pulmonary: Hyperventilation indicative of possible severe hypophosphatemia

5. Neurologic: Observation of gait and analysis of reflexes (e.g., hyporeflexia with hypophosphatemia, hyperreflexia with hyperphosphatemia)

6. Musculoskeletal: Presence of bone pain with palpation of bony prominences with hypophosphatemia

IV. Diagnostic tests (Smogorzewski et al., 2016)
  A. Laboratory
    1. Hypophosphatemia: Serum PO_4 less than 2.5 mg/dl
      a) Serum PO_4 levels may not adequately reflect true PO_4 stores.
      b) Urine PO_4 greater than 100 mg/24 hours: Excess renal loss indicative of hyperparathyroidism, tubular defects, hypokalemia, or ketoacidosis
      c) Urine PO_4 less than 100 mg/24 hours
        (1) Phosphate deficiency: Phosphate binders, malabsorption, vitamin D deficiency, hyperosmolar states
        (2) Intracellular shift
          (*a*) pH greater than 7.45: Alkalosis
          (*b*) pH 7.35–7.45: Non–pH-related shifts
            i. Glucose administration, total parenteral nutrition, refeeding syndrome
            ii. Hormone mediated: Insulin, corticosteroids
    2. Hyperphosphatemia: Serum PO_4 greater than 5.2 mg/dl
      a) Urine PO_4 greater than 1,500 mg/24 hours
        (1) Increased PO_4 load: Check LDH, uric acid, and creatine phosphokinase.
          (*a*) If elevated: Likely cellular destruction—rhabdomyolysis, hemolysis, tumor lysis, neoplastic cell turnover (e.g., leukemia, lymphoma)
          (*b*) If normal: Parenteral or enteral administration, vitamin D intoxication
        (2) Redistribution of PO_4: Check bicarbonate. If less than 22 mEq/L, it suggests respiratory acidosis, diabetic ketoacidosis, lactic acidosis, or tissue ischemia.
      b) Urine PO_4 less than 1,500 mg/24 hours
        (1) Creatinine clearance less than 25 ml/min: Acute or chronic renal failure
        (2) Creatinine clearance greater than 25 ml/min: Decreased tubular clearance
          (*a*) Calcium ions less than 8.5 mg/dl: Check PTH. PTH less than 29 pmol/L indicates hypoparathyroidism.
          (*b*) Calcium ions 8.5–10.4 mg/dl: This may suggest hyperthyroidism, hypomagnesemia, dehydration, or hyperthermia.
    3. Vitamin D levels: $1,25(OH)_2D$ deficiency is associated with hypophosphatemia.
  B. Radiology: Baseline and follow-up DEXA scan to evaluate for bone loss
  C. Other: ECG indicated with severe PO_4 imbalance, which may be associated with concurrent calcium and potassium imbalance; hypophosphatemia potentially indicative of ventricular tachyarrhythmias

V. Differential diagnosis (Florenzano et al., 2020)
  A. Hypophosphatemia
    1. Malnutrition/malabsorption
    2. Hyperparathyroidism
    3. Hypercalcemia (see Chapter 152)

4. Hypomagnesemia (see Chapter 154)
5. Alkalosis
6. Vitamin D deficiency
7. Inadequate PO_4 replacement in total parenteral nutrition
8. Poorly controlled diabetes mellitus (see Chapter 151)
9. Iatrogenic: Diuretics, phosphate-binding antacids

B. Hyperphosphatemia
1. Renal insufficiency/failure: Most common cause (see Chapter 86)
2. Iatrogenic: Oral phosphate supplements, phosphate laxatives
3. Hypoparathyroidism
4. Tumor lysis syndrome
5. Rhabdomyolysis (see Chapter 159)

VI. Treatment (Kraft, 2015; Leung & Crook, 2019; Marcuccilli et al., 2017; McClure et al., 2017; NCI CTEP, 2017; Sekar et al., 2018; Smogorzewski et al., 2016)

A. Primary goals of treatment of PO_4 imbalance
1. Prevent life-threatening conditions (e.g., AKI, tumor lysis syndrome, cardiac arrest, flaccid paralysis, and rhabdomyolysis).
2. Normalize PO_4 level.
3. Identify and treat the underlying causes.

B. Considerations for approach to treatment
1. Rapidity of onset: Acute versus chronic
2. Severity: Underlying characteristics of the patient that confer higher risk include older age, underlying kidney disease, underlying cardiomyopathy, and diabetes.

C. Hypophosphatemia
1. First priority is to establish the cause and treat any underlying disorder.
2. Mainstay of treatment is PO_4 replacement.
3. Mild asymptomatic or chronic hypophosphatemia
   a) Oral replacement salts
      (1) Moderate to severe: 1,000–2,000 mg daily
      (2) Neutra-Phos® capsules or powder: 250 mg PO_4, 164 mg sodium, 278 mg potassium
      (3) Neutra-Phos K capsules: 250 mg PO_4, 164 mg sodium, 556 mg potassium
      (4) K-Phos® Neutral tablets: 250 mg PO_4, 298 mg sodium, 45 mg potassium
      (5) Uro-KP-Neutral® tablets: 250 mg PO_4, 250.5 mg sodium, 50 mg potassium
   b) Duration of therapy will be determined by the underlying cause and efficacy of replacement therapy.
   c) Adverse events: Diarrhea, hyperkalemia (potassium salts), volume overload (sodium) salts
   d) Foods rich in PO_4
      (1) Milk is high in PO_4 content (0.9 mg/ml or inorganic PO_4).
      (2) Other foods: Cheese, meat, poultry, fish, eggs, grains, nuts, dry beans, peas, lentils, green leafy vegetables
4. PO_4 may be added to total parenteral nutrition and dialysis solutions.
5. IV PO_4 solutions must be administered with caution because of potential hypocalcemia and must be selected based on the combined salts.
   a) Potassium phosphate: Avoid in patients with hyperkalemia.
   b) Sodium phosphate: Avoid in patients with hypernatremia.
   c) It is generally reserved for severe deficiency and administered in the intensive care setting.

6. Patients at high risk for infection should be monitored.

D. Hyperphosphatemia

1. Patients should avoid carbonated beverages and other foods high in PO_4 content.

2. Patients with severe hyperphosphatemia (PO_4 greater than 7 mg/dl): Aluminum-based phosphate binders may be used for up to four weeks with concurrent dialysis.

3. Calcium–phosphate binders: Elemental calcium from calcium-based phosphate binders should not exceed 1,500 mg daily, and the total intake of elemental calcium, including dietary calcium, should not exceed 2,000 mg daily.

   a) PO_4 5–7 mg/dl: Calcium carbonate 1–2 g with each meal

      (1) Increase dose gradually to reduce serum PO_4 levels to normal; stop dose escalation when calcium ions greater than or equal to 11 mg.

      (2) If calcium carbonate is given in high doses, use vitamin D replacement with caution to avoid hypercalcemia and hyperphosphatemia.

4. Non-calcium binding agents

   a) Sevelamer hydrochloride: Preferred in dialysis patients with severe vascular and other soft-tissue calcifications

   b) Lanthanum carbonate: Non-calcium, naturally occurring, metal-based binder; hepatic elimination not dependent on renal function; may improve bone remodeling and lower FGF23 levels; expensive

   c) Iron-based phosphate binders: Sucroferric oxyhydroxide and ferric citrate approved for use in patients with end-stage renal disease

   d) Sodium–hydrogen exchanger 3 inhibitors in clinical trials

5. Vitamin D_2 or D_3 in small amounts (400–800 IU/day) may be used with caution to prevent nutritional vitamin D deficiency.

6. Hyperphosphatemia associated with tumor lysis syndrome or hemolytic anemia (see Chapter 117) will require treatment of the underlying cause.

VII. Follow-up

A. Frequency of laboratory and clinical monitoring will be determined by the etiology of the PO_4 imbalance and effectiveness of interventions to correct it.

B. Concurrent follow-up for calcium, potassium, and sodium imbalances is necessary.

C. Patients with mild hypophosphatemia on oral replacement

1. Confirm that the cause of the imbalance has been corrected.

2. Check serum calcium and vitamin D levels while correcting PO_4.

3. Check PO_4 one to two weeks after initiating oral replacement based on risk.

4. Evaluate tolerance of oral replacement.

D. Patients with severe hypophosphatemia at high risk for adverse events

1. Patients with symptomatic hypophosphatemia (e.g., ventricular tachyarrhythmias, seizures) will require hospitalization for emergent treatment.

2. Follow-up will require frequent monitoring following discharge depending on continued IV replacement or transition to oral replacement.

E. Patients with sustained underlying disease (e.g., CKD on dialysis) malabsorption

1. Frequent monitoring is indicated based on the status of the underlying disease.

2. Severity, symptoms, and treatment schedule will determine frequency of monitoring of renal and electrolyte parameters.

VIII. Referrals

A. Primary care physician: For management of oral supplements and further evaluation and treatment of the underlying causes for hypophosphatemia and hyperphosphatemia

B. Specialists: Referral based on underlying cause (e.g., AKI, intestinal malabsorption, alcoholism, medication abuse)

C. Nephrologist: For patients with hyperphosphatemia due to acute or chronic renal failure

D. Endocrinologist: For patients with diabetes

E. Clinical dietitian: For patients with malabsorption syndromes, malnutrition, or diabetes

F. Alcohol treatment program/behavioral health specialist: For patients with alcoholism

G. Cardiologist: For follow-up for patients with chronic hypophosphatemia and underlying cardiac disease

References

Berndt, T.J., Thompson, J.R., & Kumar, R. (2016). The regulation of calcium, magnesium, and phosphate excretion by the kidney. In K. Skorecki, G.M. Chertow, P.A. Marsden, A.S.L. Yu., & M.W. Taal (Eds.), *Brenner and Rector's the kidney* (10th ed., pp. 185–203). Elsevier.

Eaton, D.C., & Pooler, J.P. (2018). *Vander's renal physiology* (9th ed.). McGraw-Hill Education.

Florenzano, P., Cipriani, C., Roszko, K.L., Fukumoto, S., Collins, M.T., Minisola, S., & Pepe, J. (2020). Approach to patients with hypophosphatamia. *Lancet: Diabetes and Endocrinology, 8*(2), 163–174. https://doi.org/10.1016/S2213-8587(19)30426-7

Kraft, M.D. (2015). Phosphorus and calcium: A review for the adult nutrition support clinician. *Nutrition in Clinical Practice, 30*(1), 21–33. https://doi.org/10.1177/0884533614565251

Leung, J., & Crook, M. (2019). Disorders of phosphate metabolism. *Journal of Clinical Pathology, 72*(11), 741–747. https://doi.org/10.1136/jclinpath-2018-205130

Marcuccilli, M., Chonchol, M., & Jovanovich, A. (2017). Phosphate binders and targets over decades: Do we have it right now? *Seminars in Dialysis, 30*(2), 134–141. https://doi.org/10.1111/sdi.12568

McClure, S.T., Chang, A.R., Selvin, E., Rebholz, C.M., & Appel, L.J. (2017). Dietary sources of phosphorus among adults in the United States: Results from NHANES 2001–2014. *Nutrients, 9*(2). 95. https://doi.org/10.3390/nu9020095

Megapanou, E., Florentin, M., Milionis, H., Elisaf, M., & Liamis, G. (2020). Drug-induced hypophosphatemia: Current insights. *Drug Safety, 43*(3), 197–210. https://doi.org/10.1007/s40264-019-00888-1

Merhi, B., Shireman, T., Carpenter, M.A., Kusek, J.W., Jacques, P., Pfeffer, M., ... Bostom, A. (2017). Serum phosphorus and risk of cardiovascular disease, all-cause mortality, or graft failure in kidney transplant recipients: An ancillary study of the FAVORIT trial cohort. *American Journal of Kidney Diseases, 70*(3), 377–385. https://doi.org/10.1053/j.ajkd.2017.04.014

Michigami, T., Kawai, M., Yamazaki, M., & Ozono, K. (2018). Phosphate as a signaling molecule and its sensing mechanism. *Physiological Reviews, 98*(4), 2317–2348. https://doi.org/10.1152/physrev.00022.2017

Michigami, T., & Ozono, K. (2019). Roles of phosphate in skeleton. *Frontiers in Endocrinology, 10,* 180. https://doi.org/10.3389/fendo.2019.00180

Moore, L.W., Nolte, J.V., Gaber, A.O., & Suki, W.N. (2015). Association of dietary phosphate and serum phosphorus concentration by levels of kidney function. *American Journal of Clinical Nutrition, 102*(2), 444–453. https://doi.org/10.3945/ajcn.114.102715

Nadkarni, G.N., & Uribarri, J. (2014). Phosphorus and the kidney: What is known and what is needed. *Advances in Nutrition, 5*(1), 98–103. https://doi.org/10.3945/an.113.004655

National Cancer Institute Cancer Therapy Evaluation Program. (2017). *Common terminology criteria for adverse events* [v.5.0]. https://ctep.cancer.gov/protocoldevelopment/electronic_applications/docs/CTCAE_v5_Quick_Reference_5x7.pdf

Sekar, A., Kaur, T., Nally, J.V., Rincon-Choles, H., Jolly, S., & Nakhoul, G.N. (2018). Phosphorus binders: The new and the old, and how to choose. *Cleveland Clinic Journal of Medicine, 85*(8), 629–638. https://doi.org/10.3949/ccjm.85a.17054

Smogorzewski, M.J., Stubbs, J.R, & Yu, A.S.L. (2016). Disorders of calcium, magnesium, and phosphate balance. In K. Skorecki, G.M. Chertow, P.A. Marsden, A.S.L. Yu., & M.W. Taal (Eds.), *Brenner and Rector's the kidney* (10th ed., pp. 601–636). Elsevier.

Stremke, E.R., & Hill Gallant, K.M. (2018). Intestinal phosphorus absorption in chronic kidney disease. *Nutrients, 10*(10), 1364. https://doi.org/10.3390/nu10101364

Suki, W.N., & Moore, L.W. (2016). Phosphorus regulation in chronic kidney disease. *Methodist DeBakey Cardiovascular Journal, 12*(Suppl. 4), 6–9. https://doi.org/10.14797/mdcj-12-4s1-6

CHAPTER 157

Hyperthyroidism

Sandra Kurtin, PhD, ANP-C, AOCN®

I. Definitions (Bel Lassen et al., 2019; Sharma & Stan, 2019)
  A. Hyperthyroidism: A disorder characterized by excessive levels of thyroid hormone (i.e., T_4 and T_3) in the body
  B. Thyrotoxicosis: The clinical manifestations of hyperthyroidism
  C. Thyroid storm: Abrupt onset of thyrotoxicosis (rare)
  D. Graves disease: An autoimmune disease frequently causing hypertrophy of the extraocular muscles with ophthalmopathy

II. Physiology/Pathophysiology (Ross et al., 2016; Sharma & Stan, 2019; Sheehan, 2016)
  A. Normal
    1. The thyroid gland is a butterfly-shaped organ located in the neck with two distinct lobes joined by isthmus tissue.
    2. It is regulated by a combination of hormones in a feedback loop—the hypothalamic–pituitary–thyroid axis.
      a) Thyrotropin-releasing hormone is secreted by the hypothalamus and is carried by the portal vein to the anterior pituitary and stimulates release of TSH.
      b) TSH acts directly on the thyroid to stimulate thyroid hormone biosynthesis and secretion.
      c) T_4 (thyroxine): 85%; carries four iodine atoms
        (1) Prohormone: Requires activation to T_3 for biologic activity
        (2) Conversion to T_3 is catalyzed by a group of selenoproteins— deiodinases (D1, D2).
        (3) Thyroid hormone is inactivated primarily by deiodinase 3 (D3), which removes one iodine group, forming compounds that will not bind to thyroid hormone receptors in the cells.
      d) T_3 (triiodothyronine): 15%; carries three iodine atoms
        (1) Majority of T_4 and T_3 transported in serum is bound to carrier proteins and serves as a reservoir for thyroid hormone. Bound thyroid hormone does not exert the same effect on target cells.
        (2) Thyroid hormone–binding globulin is the main carrier, accounting for 75% of bound T_4 and all of bound T_3.
        (3) Thyroxine-binding prealbumin and albumin are responsible for the remaining 25% of bound T_4.
        (4) Free thyroid hormone: 0.03%–0.04% of T_4 is free hormone; 0.3%–0.4% of T_3 is free hormone and the metabolically active form of thyroid hormones.
          (a) Free T_4 and T_3 enter target cells primarily via passive diffusion.

        (b) T_4 and T_3 exert a negative feedback on thyrotropin-releasing hormone secretion from the hypothalamus and on TSH secretion from the pituitary.

      e) Transporter proteins: Monocarboxylate transporter 8 (MCT8), MCT10, organic anion transporting polypeptide (OATP1C1)

      f) Genomic activation of thyroid hormone: T_4 and T_3 exert effects primarily via binding to and activating nuclear receptor proteins that cause expression of thyroid hormone–responsive genes.

   3. Iodine

      a) Thyrocytes concentrate iodine against a gradient to synthesize thyroid hormone requiring the activity of sodium–iodide symporter protein.

      b) Abnormalities of sodium–iodide symporter protein are implicated in many pathologic states involving the thyroid.

      c) Iodine concentrated in the thyrocytes is converted to tyrosine residues via thyroid peroxidase enzyme, a selenoprotein.

         (1) Excess iodine exposure can block thyroid peroxidase enzyme activity, leading to decreased TSH and hypothyroidism.

         (2) Iodine deficiency with subsequent iodine exposure can lead to increased TSH and hyperthyroidism.

   4. Primary functions of thyroid hormones

      a) Increase the basal metabolic rate

      b) Stimulate metabolism of carbohydrates, fat, and protein

      c) Stimulate thermogenesis

B. Pathophysiology

   1. Hyperthyroidism occurs as a result of excess production or uncontrolled release of preformed thyroid hormones (T_4 and T_3), causing overstimulation of target cells and secondary metabolic changes.

   2. Causes of imbalances of thyroid hormone secretion or production

      a) Infiltrative processes of the thyroid gland

      b) Infiltrative processes of the pituitary or hypothalamus (rare)

      c) Exogenous manipulation of thyroid receptors or binding proteins

      d) Genetic defects in transporter proteins

III. Clinical features: Most common hyperthyroid conditions are Graves disease and toxic multinodular goiter. Thyroid storm is rare, presenting as a life-threatening exacerbation of hyperthyroidism (Bai et al., 2020; Bel Lassen et al., 2019; Del Rivero et al., 2020; Gherbon et al., 2019; Guerri et al., 2019; Hussain et al., 2017; Ishii, 2017; Jabrocka-Hybel et al., 2015; Ross et al., 2016; Sharma & Stan, 2019).

  A. Etiology

   1. Infiltrative processes of the thyroid gland

      a) Toxic multinodular goiter: Increased thyroid hormone production

      b) Plummer disease in patients with iodine deficiency

      c) Toxic adenoma: Increased thyroid hormone production

      d) Metastatic thyroid carcinoma: Increased thyroid hormone production

   2. Infiltrative processes of the pituitary or hypothalamus: Primary pituitary tumors (rare)

   3. Exogenous manipulation of thyroid receptors or binding proteins

      a) Graves disease: Increased thyroid hormone production; autoimmune antibodies bind and stimulate TSH receptor, activating thyroid hormone synthesis.

      b) TSH-mediated thyrotoxicosis/secondary hyperthyroidism: Increased thyroid hormone production

     c) Subacute thyroiditis (uncontrolled release of thyroid hormone): De Quervain thyroiditis

   4. Drug-induced hyperthyroidism

     a) Amiodarone

     b) IFN and IL-2

     c) Alemtuzumab

     d) Ipilimumab

     e) Immune checkpoint and TKIs

     f) Ifosfamide

     g) Other medications: Phenobarbital, rifampin, phenytoin, carbamazepine

   5. Iodine excess: Increased thyroid hormone production; excess ingestion of kelp seaweed

   6. Genetic defects in transporter proteins: Rare condition; nonautoimmune hyperthyroidism with autosomal dominant inheritance caused by mutations in *TSHR* (OMIM gene: 603373; OMIM disease: 609152, 603373)

B. History

   1. History of cancer and cancer treatment: Particular attention to immune checkpoint inhibitors

   2. Current medications: Prescribed, over the counter, especially drugs known to contribute to hyperthyroidism (e.g., anticoagulants, bisphosphonates, antiarrhythmic agents, phenobarbital, rifampin); compliance with antithyroid medications in patients with history of hypothyroidism

   3. History of presenting symptoms: Precipitating factors, onset, duration

   4. Changes in ADLs

   5. Past medical history: Graves disease, multinodular goiter, previous history of thyroid disorders with pregnancy/delivery or other surgeries, underlying cardiovascular disease, atrial fibrillation, osteoporosis, coagulopathy, hip fractures, vertebral fractures

   6. Social History: Tobacco use

C. Signs and symptoms

   1. Clinical manifestations are dependent on the rapidity of onset and severity.

     a) Majority of signs and symptoms are a result of hypermetabolic state.

     b) Many patients with chronic hyperthyroidism may have subclinical manifestations. Symptoms will be more pronounced in patients with preexisting cardiovascular or bone disease and in patients with insulin resistance.

     c) Apathetic hyperthyroidism (e.g., weight loss, anorexia, depression) is often confused with other etiologies in older patients.

   2. Most common clinical manifestations of hyperthyroidism

     a) General: Nervousness, fatigue, heat intolerance, excessive sweating, insomnia, weight loss, hair loss, fever

     b) Cardiovascular: Palpitations

     c) Dermatologic: Hair loss, warm and moist skin, palmar erythema, acropathy (swelling of the fingers)

     d) GI: Diarrhea, vomiting

     e) GU: Oligomenorrhea, infertility

     f) HEENT: Photophobia, eye irritation, diplopia

     g) Neuromuscular: Weakness, poor concentration, and seizures possibly present in thyroid storm

     h) Respiratory: Exertional dyspnea, tachypnea

D. Physical examination

   1. Vital signs

a) Heart rate: Tachycardia

b) Blood pressure: Systolic hypertension (hypotension in late stages due to multi-organ failure) with widened pulse pressure

c) Temperature: Increased

d) Weight: Weight loss common due to hypermetabolic state in acute cases; possible weight gain in chronic setting

e) Pain: May be present

f) General: Potentially agitated, thin, or fatigued patient

2. HEENT

a) Exophthalmos, which may be present with Graves disease

b) Eye irritation possible in thyroiditis.

c) Assessment for staring gaze, lid lag, and lid retention

d) Thyroid: Smoothness, nodules, and masses, tender or nontender

   (1) Thyroid is usually enlarged two to three times normal size in Graves disease.

   (2) Multiple nodules typically are present in toxic adenoma and multinodular goiter.

3. Cardiac: Findings consistent with CHF in sustained or severe hyperthyroidism such as JVD, displaced apical impulse, or peripheral edema; bruit or thrill possible with carotids with Graves disease

4. Pulmonary: Exertional dyspnea or hyperventilation indicative of possible severe hyperthyroidism

5. Abdominal: Increased bowel sounds, or abdominal tenderness; diminished bowel sounds, abdominal distention, and pain with impending ileus in thyroid storm

6. Neurologic: Hyperreflexia, fine tremors; gait observation for unsteadiness

7. Musculoskeletal: Presence of pretibial myxedema or pain with palpation of bony prominences; possible presence of proximal muscle weaknesss

IV. Diagnostic tests (Ross et al., 2016; Sheehan, 2016)

A. Laboratory: The most useful test to begin screening is TSH.

1. TSH normal range is 0.5–5 mIU/L. If less than 0.5 mIU/L, perform the following.

a) Measure free T_3/T_4.

   (1) It is elevated in hyperthyroidism, Graves disease, and multinodular goiter.

   (2) Small changes in free T_3 and/or free T_4 will result in very large changes in TSH.

   (3) It is normal in subclinical thyroiditis.

   (4) T_3/T_4 ratio is greater than 20 in Graves disease.

   (5) T_4 elevation greater than T_3 is more common in nonthyroidal illnesses (decreased conversion of T_4 to T_3).

b) Apply clinical findings if no clear etiology.

2. Other tests, as indicated: Thyroid peroxidase enzyme antibodies, TSH receptor antibodies, and thyroglobulin testing may help to differentiate diagnosis.

3. Baseline CBC with differential and a liver profile including bilirubin and transaminases to monitor for secondary effects of thyrotoxicosis

4. Serum calcium, PTH: Patients undergoing thyroidectomy will need to have oral calcium and calcitriol supplementation.

5. Lipid panel: Hyperthyroidism typically results in low total and IIDL cholesterol concentrations.

6. Serum glucose elevated with hyperthyroidism

B. Radiology
    1. Thyroid ultrasound to evaluate thyroid nodules
    2. Radioactive iodine (RAI) uptake to differentiate if no clear etiology
        a) Exposure to iodine contrast within one to two months of testing or iodine-rich diets (seaweed/kelp) will interfere with the accuracy of the test.
        b) RAI is contraindicated in women who are pregnant or breastfeeding.
        c) Diffuse uptake: Graves disease
        d) "Hot spots" with otherwise normal uptake and suppression of extranodal tissue: Multinodular goiter
        e) Low uptake: Subacute thyroiditis
    3. Chest x-ray at baseline to evaluate early cardiopulmonary disease
C. Other: Echocardiogram, ECG, Holter monitor, or myocardial perfusion studies to obtain baseline for any patient, particularly older adults, noted to have hyperthyroidism; atrial fibrillation and supraventricular tachyarrhythmia possible

V. Differential diagnosis (Ishii, 2017; Ross et al., 2016)
  A. Graves disease
  B. Multinodular goiter
  C. Solitary toxic nodule
  D. Thyroiditis
  E. TSH-secreting pituitary adenoma
  F. Choriocarcinoma
  G. Dermoid malignancy of ovary
  H. Other conditions that can mimic hyperthyroidism
    1. Anxiety (see Chapter 161)
    2. Depression (see Chapter 162)
    3. Panic disorder
    4. Pheochromocytoma
    5. Uncontrolled diabetes mellitus (see Chapter 151)
    6. Myasthenia gravis
    7. Orbital tumors
    8. Pregnancy
    9. Menopause (see Chapter 90)

VI. Treatment (Asban et al., 2020; Bartalena et al., 2016; Biondi & Cooper, 2019; Burch & Cooper, 2015; Castinetti et al., 2018; Chiha et al., 2015; Corvilain et al., 2018; Hussain et al., 2017; Ross et al., 2016; Sharma & Stan, 2019)
  A. Primary goals are to suppress the release of additional T_3 and T_4, reduce the effects of circulating free T_3 and free T_4, and control or treat life-threatening symptoms.
  B. Interventions are based on the severity of symptoms and patient characteristics.
  C. Individual patient characteristics should be considered in the selection of treatment (see individual therapies for considerations).
  D. Thyroid-directed therapy: Suppress release of additional T_3 and T_4 and control symptoms associated with circulating thyroid hormone.
    1. RAI (iodine-131) therapy
        a) Treatment of choice for patients without contraindications: Pregnancy or of childbearing age without confirmed contraception (females), breastfeeding, poor performance status, unable to comply with radiation safety guidelines
            (1) Administered orally as a single dose based on thyroid size
            (2) Peak effect in three to six months: RAI-induced euthyroid state

b) Requires pregnancy testing 48 hours prior to administration and confirmation of contraception

c) Requires lifelong thyroid replacement therapy

d) Short-term increase in circulating T_3 and T_4 levels potential to exacerbate thyrotoxicosis

    (1) Administration of thioamides with RAI inhibits thyroid hormone synthesis.

    (2) It may be indicated in patients presenting with severe symptoms, complex comorbidities that may cause life-threatening consequences, or free T_4 levels two to three times normal (see antithyroid medication).

2. Antithyroid medication

  a) It is useful in patients in whom RAI or surgery is contraindicated or not easily accessible to the patient and in female patients with mild disease; doses are higher in thyroid storm or severe symptoms and are titrated for maintenance.

  b) Thioamide

    (1) Methimazole: 15–60 mg PO daily, divided into three doses and given at eight-hour intervals

    (2) Drug of choice due to superior toxicity profile (less neutropenia and agranulocytosis), cost, and frequency of dosing

    (3) Propylthiouracil: 300–600 mg PO three times a day; higher doses for thyroid storm

    (4) Should include follow-up in four to six weeks to verify euthyroid state

      (a) Include assessment of free T_4 and total T_3.

      (b) If still thyrotoxic, titrate dose and continue monitoring at four- to six-week intervals.

    (5) Maintenance dosing: Required for patients who have not received RAI or thyroidectomy with titration of the dose to maintain the euthyroid state

      (a) Relapse is most common in the first three to six months but may occur as late as 40 years.

      (b) Most common side effects include skin reactions, arthralgias, GI effects, sialadenitis, and agranulocytosis (more common with propylthiouracil).

    (6) Beta-blockers: Decrease heart rate and systolic blood pressure, muscle weakness, and tremor

      (a) Propranolol: 60–80 mg PO every four hours

        i. Consider invasive monitoring in patients with CHF.

        ii. Drug blocks conversion of T_4 to T_3 in high doses.

      (b) Atenolol: 25–50 mg PO daily; alternative beta-blocker with once-daily dosing (beta-1 selective)

  c) Iodine: Saturated solution of potassium iodide

    (1) Give five drops (0.25 ml or 250 mg) PO every six hours, not to exceed 12 times daily.

    (2) Do not start until one hour after antithyroid drugs.

  d) Hydrocortisone: 300 mg IV load, then 100 mg every eight hours for prophylaxis against relative adrenal insufficiency for short duration; not indicated for long-term therapy

3. Thyroidectomy

  a) Useful for symptomatic debulking in large tumors and patients who are not candidates for RAI or have coexisting hyperparathyroidism

  b) Contraindications: Substantial comorbidity such as cardiopulmonary disease, end-stage cancer, or other debilitating disorders, or lack of access to a high-volume thyroid surgeon; pregnancy a relative contraindication

    c) Provides prompt and definitive control of hyperthyroidism
    d) Requires experienced surgeon, usually one with a high volume of thyroid surgeries
    e) Requires lifelong thyroid replacement therapy

E. Life-threatening symptoms: Thyroid storm is a rare, most often iatrogenic, multisystem disorder characterized by tachycardia, arrhythmias, CHF, hypotension, hyperpyrexia, agitation, delirium, psychosis, stupor, and coma, as well as nausea, vomiting, diarrhea, and hepatic failure.

  1. Factors increasing the risk for thyroid storm include abrupt cessation of antithyroid drugs, thyroid or nonthyroidal surgery in a patient with unrecognized or inadequately treated thyrotoxicosis, acute illnesses unrelated to thyroid disease, and, rarely, following RAI.

  2. Treatment is aimed at controlling each symptom and underlying comorbidity while simultaneously implementing antithyroid treatments.

F. Graves ophthalmopathy

  1. An inflammatory eye disease associated with autoimmune thyroid disorders; most often Graves disease

  2. Common features: Lid retraction, soft tissue inflammation, proptosis, diplopia, corneal exposure, optic nerve irritation

  3. Risk factors: RAI, smoking, high pretreatment T_3 values (greater than 325 ng/dl), high serum pretreatment TSH receptor antibody levels, hypothyroidism following RAI treatment

  4. Prevention and treatment

    a) Rapid induction and maintenance of euthyroid state for patients with hyperthyroidism presenting with Graves ophthalmopathy or at high risk for Graves ophthalmopathy

    b) Smoking cessation counseling

VII. Follow-up

A. Goal is to maintain euthyroid state.

B. Frequency of monitoring of thyroid hormone levels will be determined by the severity of symptoms and clinical findings at the onset of hyperthyroid state, the approach to treatment, underlying comorbid conditions, and patient characteristics.

  1. Acute phase: Frequent monitoring of T_3 and free T_4 levels in select patients to evaluate effective control of hyperthyroid state

  2. Following primary antithyroid treatment

    a) RAI

      (1) Follow up within four weeks. If persistent thyrotoxicosis continues, monitor free T_4 monthly until euthyroid state is achieved, then every three to six months for the first year, then TSH and free T_4 yearly.

      (2) For hepatic profile, including bilirubin and transaminases for monitoring of secondary effects of thyrotoxicosis and treatment, obtain monthly for the first three months.

    b) Surgery

      (1) Follow up within four weeks. If persistent thyrotoxicosis continues, monitor monthly until euthyroid state is achieved, then every three to six months.

      (2) Obtain hepatic profile including bilirubin and transaminases to monitor for secondary effects of thyrotoxicosis and treatment.

      (3) Patients undergoing thyroidectomy will need to have oral calcium and calcitriol supplementation.

    c) Antithyroid drugs

        (1) Administer thyroid hormones every two to four weeks until euthyroid state is achieved, then as clinically indicated.

        (2) Obtain CBC with differential and platelet count in patients taking propylthiouracil.

        (3) For hepatic profile, including bilirubin and transaminases to monitor for secondary effects of thyrotoxicosis and treatment, obtain monthly for the first three months, with any dose change, or as clinically indicated based on comorbidities and symptoms.

        (4) Monitor for osteoporosis and cardiovascular disease.

    3. Patients on beta-blockers: Follow-up ECG may be indicated for persistent arrhythmias.

    4. Surgical follow-up, as indicated

VIII. Referrals

    A. Primary care physician: For management of oral supplements and further evaluation and treatment of the underlying causes for hyperthyroidism

    B. Endocrinologist: For diagnosis and initiation of treatment and continued monitoring

    C. Ophthalmologist: For patients with more than mild ophthalmic signs and symptoms

    D. Tobacco cessation program/behavioral health specialist: For patients who are smokers

    E. Cardiologist: For follow-up in patients with underlying cardiac disease and for those on continued beta-blockers

    F. Other specialists: Referral based on underlying cause and treatment (i.e., thyroid carcinoma, thyroidectomy)

    G. Hospital admission: If thyroid storm occurs, for surgery, or for patients with severe presenting symptoms

References

Asban, A., Anue, A., Xie, R., & Chen, H. (2020). Increasing use of thyroidectomy as definitive treatment for hyperthyroidism. *Journal of Surgical Research, 246,* 435–441. https://doi.org/10.1016/j.jss.2019.09.020

Bai, X., Chen, X., Wu, X., Huang, Y., Zhuang, Y., & Lin, X. (2020). Immune checkpoint inhibitor-associated thyroid dysfunction: A disproportionality analysis using the WHO adverse drug reaction database, VigiBase. *European Journal of Endocrinology, 182*(1), 1–9. https://doi.org/10.1530/eje-19-0535

Bartalena, L., Chiovato, L., & Vitti, P. (2016). Management of hyperthyroidism due to Graves' disease: Frequently asked questions and answers (if any). *Journal of Endocrinology Investigation, 39*(10), 1105–1114. https://doi.org/10.1007/s40618-016-0505-x

Bel Lassen, P., Kyrilli, A., Lytrivi, M., & Corvilain, B. (2019). Graves' disease, multinodular goiter and subclinical hyperthyroidism. *Annales d'Endocrinologie, 80*(4), 240–249. https://doi.org/10.1016/j.ando.2018.09.004

Biondi, B., & Cooper, D.S. (2019). Thyroid hormone suppression therapy. *Endocrinology and Metabolism Clinics of North America, 48*(1), 227–237. https://doi.org/10.1016/j.ecl.2018.10.008

Burch, H.B., & Cooper, D.S. (2015). Management of Graves disease: A review. *JAMA, 314*(23), 2544–2554. https://doi.org/10.1001/jama.2015.16535

Castinetti, F., Albarel, F., Archambeaud, F., Bertherat, J., Bouillet, B., Buffier, P., ... Borson-Chazot, F. (2018). Endocrine side-effects of new anticancer therapies: Overall monitoring and conclusions. *Annales d'Endocrinologie, 79*(5), 591–595. https://doi.org/10.1016/j.ando.2018.07.005

Chiha, M., Samarasinghe, S., & Kabaker, A.S. (2015). Thyroid storm: An updated review. *Journal of Intensive Care Medicine, 30*(3), 131–140. https://doi.org/10.1177/0885066613498053

Corvilain, B., Hamy, A., Brunaud, L., Borson-Chazot, F., Orgiazzi, J., Hachmi, L.B., ... Lussey-Lepoutre, C. (2018). Treatment of adult Graves' disease. *Annales d'Endocrinologie, 79*(6), 618–635. https://doi.org/10.1016/j.ando.2018.08.003

Del Rivero, J., Cordes, L.M., Klubo-Gwiezdzinska, J., Madan, R.A., Nieman, L.K., & Gulley, J.L. (2020). Endocrine-related adverse events related to immune checkpoint inhibitors: Proposed algorithms for management. *Oncologist, 25*(4), 290–300. https://doi.org/10.1634/theoncologist.2018-0470

Gherbon, A., Frandes, M., Lungeanu, D., Nicula, M., & Timar, R. (2019). Transient hyperthyroidism following the ingestion of complementary medications containing kelp seaweed: A case-report. *Medicine, 98*(37), e17058. https://doi.org/10.1097/md.0000000000017058

Guerri, G., Bressan, S., Sartori, M., Costantini, A., Benedetti, S., Agostini, F., ... Bertelli, M. (2019). Hypothyroidism and hyperthyroidism. *Acta Biomedica, 90*(Suppl. 10), 83–86. https://doi.org/10.23750/abm.v90i10-S.8765

Hussain, Y.S., Hookham, J.C., Allahabadia, A., & Balasubramanian, S.P. (2017). Epidemiology, management and outcomes of Graves' disease—Real life data. *Endocrine, 56*(3), 568–578. https://doi.org/10.1007/s12020-017-1306-5

Ishii, M. (2017). Endocrine emergencies with neurologic manifestations. *Continuum, 23*(3), 778–801. https://doi.org/10.1212/con.0000000000000467

Jabrocka-Hybel, A., Bednarczuk, T., Bartalena, L., Pach, D., Ruchała, M., Kamiński, G., ... Hubalewska-Dydejczyk, A. (2015). Amiodarone and the thyroid. *Endokrynologia Polska, 66*(2), 176–186. https://doi.org/10.5603/ep.2015.0025

Ross, D.S., Burch, H.B., Cooper, D.S., Greenlee, M.C., Laurberg, P., Maia, A.L., ... Walter, M.A. (2016). 2016 American Thyroid Association guidelines for diagnosis and management of hyperthyroidism and other causes of thyrotoxicosis. *Thyroid, 26*(10), 1343–1421. https://doi.org/10.1089/thy.2016.0229

Sharma, A., & Stan, M.N. (2019). Thyrotoxicosis: Diagnosis and management. *Mayo Clinic Proceedings, 94*(6), 1048–1064. https://doi.org/10.1016/j.mayocp.2018.10.011

Sheehan, M.T. (2016). Biochemical testing of the thyroid: TSH is the best and, oftentimes, only test needed—A review for primary care. *Clinical Medicine and Research, 14*(2), 83–92. https://doi.org/10.3121/cmr.2016.1309

CHAPTER 158

Hypothyroidism

Rebecca A. Hawkins, MSN, ARNP

I. Definition (Chaker et al., 2017; Hartman, 2015)
   A. A decrease in the function of the thyroid or the thyroid gland that causes a reduced production of thyroid hormone and results in low serum thyroid hormone levels that alters the body's natural function
   B. Subclinical hypothyroidism: Abnormal biochemical measurement of thyroid hormones (elevated TSH and normal T_4 and T_3 serum levels) without specific clinical symptoms of thyroid diseases

II. Physiology/Pathophysiology (Chaker et al., 2017; Chiovato et al., 2019; Hartman, 2015; Hennessey, 2017)
   A. Normal
      1. The thyroid gland secretes predominantly T_4; T_3 results from the conversion of T_4 to T_3 by nonthyroidal tissues.
      2. Thyroid hormones (T_4 and T_3) are released under the control of the pituitary, which releases TSH.
      3. The pituitary is under a classic negative feedback regulation by thyroid hormone circulation.
      4. The hypothalamus regulates pituitary release of TSH by secreting thyrotropin-releasing hormone.
      5. Thyroid hormones play an important role in regulating energy balance and metabolism of glucose and lipids.
      6. Thyroid hormones influence protein synthesis and cell growth.
      7. Thyroid hormones affect renal clearance of water load by their effects on the GFR.
   B. Pathophysiology
      1. Primary hypothyroidism
         a) It is caused by impaired thyroid function.
         b) The hypothalamus responds with increased output of thyrotropin-releasing hormone, which triggers primary thyrotropin (TSH) secretion, stimulating thyroid gland enlargement, goiter formation, and synthesis of T_3 instead of T_4.
      2. Secondary hypothyroidism
         a) It is caused by hypothalamic–pituitary dysfunction.
         b) TSH response is inadequate.
         c) Gland remains normal or reduced in size.
         d) T_3 and T_4 synthesis are equally reduced.
      3. Thyroid disorders have been associated with insulin resistance resulting from altered insulin secretion and altered lipid levels leading to diabetes mellitus and dyslipidemia.

4. Hypothyroidism can result in decreased cardiac contractility, decreased cardiac output, increased peripheral resistance, and decreased renal flow.

III. Clinical features: Hypothyroidism prevalence in the U.S. general population varies between 0%–7% (depending on the definition). It occurs more frequently in women, older adults (older than 65 years), and Caucasians (although ethnic data are scarce). Iodine deficiency is the most common cause of hypothyroidism worldwide. Thyroid disease can increase the risk of cardiovascular disease, diabetes, infertility, and osteoporosis. Subclinical hypothyroidism occurs in approximately 3%–12% of the population. The most common physical finding is a goiter (Chaker et al., 2017; Chiovato et al., 2019; Duntas & Yen, 2019; Hartman, 2015; Jonklaas, 2016; Kim & Park, 2014; Mammen, 2019; Okosieme et al., 2016; Peeters, 2017; Taylor et al., 2019).

A. Etiology: From cancer, cancer treatments, or other conditions such as autoimmune

1. Primary hypothyroidism is caused by thyroid hormone deficiency and is the most common form.

   a) Idiopathic

   b) Radioactive iodine treatment for hyperthyroidism

   c) Thyroiditis: Autoimmune or subacute; Hashimoto disease

   d) Iodine deficiency: Rare in the United States

   e) Drug induced: Lithium, amiodarone, sunitinib, rifampin, thalidomide, IFN-α, IL-2, TKIs, antiepileptic drugs, second-line treatment of multidrug resistant TB

   f) Cancer of the thyroid with thyroidectomy

   g) Infiltrative disorders of the thyroid: Amyloidosis

   h) Thyroidectomy for goiters

   i) Thyroid dysgenesis

   j) Radiation treatment for head and neck cancers

2. Secondary or tertiary (central) hypothyroidism is caused by TSH deficiency.

   a) Hypothalamic dysfunction

   b) Pituitary dysfunction

   c) Pituitary tumors

   d) Head trauma

   e) Resistance to TSH or thyrotropin-releasing hormone

   f) Drug induced: Dopamine, somatostatins, glucocorticosteroids, retinoid X receptor selective ligands

3. Thyroiditis is associated with several autoimmune diseases; all patients should be screened for hypothyroidism who have the following.

   a) Vitiligo: Lack of pigmentation of the skin

   b) RA

   c) Addison disease

   d) Diabetes mellitus

   e) Pernicious anemia

4. Hypothalamus etiology

   a) Hypothalamic tumors

   b) History of surgery or radiation to the hypothalamus

B. History

1. History of cancer and cancer treatment

2. Current medications: Prescribed, over the counter

3. History of presenting symptoms: Precipitating factors, onset, duration

4. Changes in ADLs

5. Past medical history: Cardiovascular disease, diabetes, renal insufficiency, RA, anemia

C. Signs and symptoms: Clinical hypothyroidism symptoms are more severe, whereas sub-clinical hypothyroid symptoms are less serious and may be absent. Symptoms are highly variable depending on age of onset, duration, and severity of thyroid hormone deficiency.

1. Fatigue, lethargy
2. Cold intolerance
3. Constipation
4. Depressed appetite
5. Slight weight gain (late symptom)
6. Muscle cramps or weakness
7. Mental sluggishness
8. Heavy menstrual periods or abnormal bleeding
9. Hoarseness
10. Dyspnea on exertion
11. Angina
12. Depression
13. Decrease in hearing
14. Paresthesia
15. Hair loss
16. Nerve entrapment syndrome
17. Ataxia
18. Infertility
19. Diastolic hypertension

D. Physical examination

1. Vital signs: Blood pressure to assess for diastolic hypertension; potential slow pulse rate
2. Integument
   a) Dry, brittle hair
   b) Dry, rough skin
   c) Hair loss
3. HEENT
   a) Periorbital edema
   b) Thyroid not palpable unless goiter present
   c) Hoarseness
   d) Assessment for hearing loss (see Appendix D)
4. Cardiac
   a) Abnormal sounds: S_3, S_4, to muffled sounds of CHF
   b) Decreased capillary refill indicating poor perfusion
5. Pulmonary: Rales or rhonchi indicating heart failure
6. Neurologic: Hyporeflexia

IV. Diagnostic tests: Thyroid dysfunction is common in adults and can be diagnosed accurately by laboratory testing (Chaker et al., 2017; Duntas & Yen, 2019; Hartman, 2015; Jonklaas, 2016; Jonklaas et al., 2014; Mammen, 2019; Okosieme et al., 2016).

A. Laboratory (see Table 158-1)

1. TSH
   a) Normal range is 0.35–4 mIU/ml; controversy exists regarding ULN.
   b) It is recommended as first-line screening.
   c) TSH can detect low levels of the normal range and is highly sensitive.
   d) A rise in the TSH will precede other abnormalities in thyroid function tests when diagnosing primary hypothyroidism.

TABLE 158-1	Diagnosis of Hypothyroidism Disorders	
Thyroid-Stimulating Hormone	**Thyroxine (T$_4$)**	**Diagnosis**
High: > 5.5 mIU/ml	Low	Primary hypothyroidism
Borderline: 5.1–10 mIU/ml	Low or borderline	Questionable subclinical hypothyroidism versus normal variant hypothyroidism
Normal: 0.35–5.5 mIU/ml	Low	Euthyroid sick syndrome[a]

[a]Alterations in thyroid function tests in patients who have nonthyroidal disease

Note. Based on information from Chaker et al., 2017; Hartman, 2015; Jonklaas, 2016; Jonklaas et al., 2014; Okosieme et al., 2016.

     e) TSH should be monitored during thyroid hormone replacement.

     f) Subclinical hypothyroidism has normal levels of T$_3$ and T$_4$ with moderately elevated TSH of 5–10 mIU/L.

     g) Overt hypothyroidism is a level greater than 10 mIU/L.

  2. Total T$_4$ (serum T$_4$)

     a) Total T$_4$ measures all T$_4$ bound to protein.

     b) It can be affected by alterations in plasma proteins (i.e., from liver disease, malnutrition, chronic illness).

     c) Total T$_4$ is a more expensive test for monitoring or screening hypothyroidism.

     d) It can be used to confirm hypothyroidism, although it is not as sensitive as TSH. It is useful if TSH level is abnormally high or low to confirm diagnosis.

     e) Total T$_4$ is less helpful in monitoring patients on replacement therapy.

  3. Free T$_4$

     a) It measures the metabolically active form of T$_4$, which is a better indicator of thyroid status than total T$_4$.

     b) Traditionally, this is a first-line screening test, but it is now used to confirm TSH assay.

     c) Free T$_4$ should be used when diagnosing secondary hypothyroidism (TSH is low or normal; free T$_4$ is low), which is caused by TSH deficiency from hypothalamus. Thus, TSH assay is not a sensitive diagnostic test.

  4. Serum T$_3$: This is not useful test for diagnosis or monitoring.

  5. Thyroid peroxidase enzyme autoantibody immunoassays

     a) Immunoassays are antithyroid antibody markers.

     b) It is the most sensitive test for detecting autoimmune thyroid dysfunction.

     c) Immunoassays will elevate before the TSH.

  6. If secondary hypothyroidism is suspected, check other pituitary axis levels (e.g., gonadotropin/sex steroid, adrenocorticotropic hormone/cortisol).

  7. Hgb and hematocrit testing should be performed to rule out anemia, which is common with hypothyroidism. ACD is the most common type. Ferritin, folate, vitamin B$_{12}$, transferrin, iron, and iron saturation are typically normal.

  8. Lipid panel: Increased values are associated with hypothyroidism.

  9. Glucose: It may be elevated with hypothyroidism. Hgb A1c may be indicated.

B. Radiology to rule out pituitary-hypothalamic pathology

  1. CT scan or MRI of sella/pituitary to evaluate for pituitary or hypothalamic etiology

  2. Chest x-ray to evaluate for CHF and cardiomegaly, which is associated with hypothyroidism

      3. Thyroid scan (nuclear medicine) to evaluate for nodules

      4. Ultrasound of thyroid to evaluate for nodules

V. Differential diagnosis (Chiovato et al., 2019; Duntas & Yen, 2019; Hartman, 2015)
   A. Treatment related
      1. Radioactive iodine (iodine-131)
      2. Surgery: Total or subtotal thyroidectomy
      3. Propylthiouracil
      4. External beam radiation: Mantle field or thyroid field
      5. Antineoplastic agents: Bexarotene, IFN, IL-2, ipilimumab, nivolumab, pembrolizumab, cemiplimab, avelumab, durvalumab, atezolizumab, sorafenib, lenalidomide, thalidomide
   B. Autoimmune
      1. Primary disease: Atrophic thyroiditis; no goiter
      2. Hashimoto thyroiditis: Goiter present
   C. Idiopathic thyroid failure
   D. Congenital thyroid failure
   E. Iodine insufficiency: Rare
   F. Secondary hypothyroidism from pituitary or hypothalamic dysfunction
   G. Drug induced: Lithium, iodine compounds, antithyroid medications
   H. Fluid overload
   I. Glomerulonephritis
   J. Nephrotic syndrome (see Chapter 91)

VI. Treatment: Patients may exhibit symptoms of hyperthyroidism if overtreated and symptoms of hypothyroidism if undertreated. Patients with adequate treatment are euthyroid. Therapy is long term and usually lifelong with thyroid replacement medications (Chaker et al., 2017; Chiovato et al., 2019; Duntas & Yen, 2019; Hartman, 2015; Jonklaas, 2016; Jonklaas et al., 2014; Magri et al., 2019; Okosieme et al., 2016; Taylor et al., 2019).
   A. Continuous replacement therapy: Adjust dose according to clinical response and laboratory findings.
   B. Thyroid replacement medications
      1. Levothyroxine (T_4 replacement) should be taken on an empty stomach.
         a) Initial dose is 1.6 mcg/kg PO daily (usual range: 50–200 mcg PO daily) in young, healthy patients.
         b) Older adults and individuals with CAD should start at 25 mcg PO daily.
         c) Younger patients can begin at full dose.
         d) Dose adjustments are made by evaluating TSH. If level remains elevated, increase by 12–25 mcg PO daily in older patients every two to four weeks. In younger patients, adjust the dose by 25 mcg PO every two to four weeks.
         e) Substances that may interfere with absorption of levothyroxine and should be used with caution.
            (1) Cholestyramine
            (2) Ferrous sulfate
            (3) Calcium carbonate
            (4) Antacids containing aluminum hydroxide
            (5) Magnesium
            (6) Zinc
            (7) Fiber
            (8) Caffeine

        (9) Sucralfate

        (10) Sertraline hydrochloride

        (11) Raloxifene

        (12) Omeprazole

    f) Drugs that affect thyroid binding and should be used with caution: Anticonvulsants

    g) Drugs that may accelerate levothyroxine metabolism and should be used with caution

        (1) Rifampin

        (2) Sertraline hydrochloride

        (3) Phenytoin

        (4) Carbamazepine

        (5) Estrogen hormone replacement therapy

    h) Drugs affected by levothyroxine

        (1) Drug effect enhanced: Warfarin and amitriptyline

        (2) Drug effect decreased: Propranolol

  2. Sodium liothyronine (T_3 replacement): Rarely used because of short half-life

    a) Maintenance dose is 25–75 mcg PO daily. The usual range is 15–37.5 mcg PO daily. It is also available in injectable form.

    b) Initiate at 25 mcg PO and increase by 12.5–25 mcg every one to two weeks.

  3. Liotrix: Mixture of T_4 and T_3

    a) It is a 4:1 mixture of T_4 and T_3 (75 mcg/18.75 mcg).

    b) Treatment is used to mimic normal physiology and primarily used for those patients who do not respond to T_4 replacement alone.

  4. Desiccated thyroid: It is rarely recommended because contents are variable. It is more difficult to be precise with dosing.

    a) Maintenance dose is 60–120 mg PO daily.

    b) Initiate at 30 mg PO daily and increase by 15 mg every two to three weeks.

    c) It was previously ordered in grains; 1 grain is 60 mg.

C. If hypoadrenalism is diagnosed, give cortisone acetate prior to initiating replacement therapy.

D. Routine use of levothyroxine in subclinical hypothyroidism remains controversial. If the patient is symptomatic, has dyslipidemia, or TSH greater than 10 mIU/L, a three- to six-month trial can be considered. Otherwise, monitor TSH levels.

E. Treat other associated diseases such as dyslipidemia (see Chapter 44) and diabetes (see Chapter 151).

F. Patient education

  1. Emphasize to patients the importance of taking medications as prescribed, probably for life.

  2. Teach patients regarding foods and beverages that hamper the absorption of replacement medication, such as fatty meals and coffee.

  3. Thyroid hormone should be taken prior to breakfast with water. Bedtime dosing can be tried as an alternative with problems of morning dosing.

  4. Thyroid preparations are not identical in bioavailability; therefore, instruct patients not to switch preparations.

VII. Follow-up (Chiovato et al., 2019; Duntas & Yen, 2019)

  A. The half-life of T_4 is 7–10 days. It takes approximately five half-lives (35–50 days or five to seven weeks) to reach steady state. Check TSH blood level every six to eight weeks of thyroid replacement therapy until level normalizes, as well as with each dose adjustment.

  B. Once level is normalized and the patient is stable, check level every six months to annually.

C. Symptoms should improve within two weeks and resolve within three to six months.

D. For primary hypothyroidism, aim for a TSH level less than 2.5 mIU/L.

VIII. Referral: An endocrinologist visit should be scheduled for the following.

A. Patients younger than age 18 years

B. Patients who are unresponsive to therapy or need T_3/T_4 replacement therapy

C. Older adult patients with comorbidities and polypharmacy

D. Cardiac patients for close monitoring

E. Patients with goiters, nodules, structural thyroid changes, or other endocrine disorders

References

Chaker, L., Bianco, A.C., Jonklaas, J., & Peeters, R.P. (2017). Hypothyroidism. *Lancet, 390*(10101), 1550–1562. https://doi.org/10.1016/S0140-6736(17)30703-1

Chiovato, L., Magri, F., & Carle, A. (2019). Hypothyroidism in context: where we've been and where we're going. *Advances in Therapy, 36*(Suppl. 2), 47–58. https://doi.org/10.1007/s12325-019-01080-8

Duntas, L.H., & Yen, P.M. (2019). Diagnosis and treatment of hypothyroidism in the elderly. *Endocrine, 66*(1), 63–69. https://doi.org/10.1007/s12020-019-02067-9

Hartman, K. (2015). Thyroid disorders in the oncology patient. *Journal of the Advanced Practitioner in Oncology, 6*(2), 99–106. https://doi.org/10.6004/jadpro.2015.6.2.2

Hennessey, J.V. (2017). The emergence of levothyroxine as a treatment for hypothyroidism. *Endocrine, 55*(1), 6–18. https://doi.org/10.1007/s12020-016-1199-8

Jonklaas, J. (2016). Update on the treatment of hypothyroidism. *Current Opinion in Oncology, 28*(1), 18–25. https://doi.org/10.1097/CCO.0000000000000242

Jonklaas, J., Bianco, A.C., Bauer, A.J., Burman, K.D., Cappola, A.R., Celi, F.S., ... Sawka, A.M. (2014). Guidelines for the treatment of hypothyroidism: Prepared by the American Thyroid Association task force on thyroid hormone replacement. *Thyroid, 24*(12), 1670–1751. https://doi.org/10.1089/thy.2014.0028

Kim, Y.A., & Park, Y.J. (2014). Prevalence and risk factors of subclinical thyroid disease. *Endocrinology and Metabolism, 29*(1), 20–29. https://doi.org/10.3803/EnM.2014.29.1.20

Magri, F., Chiovato, L., Croce, L., & Rotondi, M. (2019). Thyroid hormone therapy for subclinical hypothyroidism. *Endocrine, 66*(1), 27–34. https://doi.org/10.1007/s12020-019-02039-z

Mammen, J.S. (2019). Interpreting elevated TSH in older adults. *Current Opinion in Endocrine and Metabolic Research, 5*, 68–73. https://doi.org/10.1016/j.coemr.2019.04.001

Okosieme, O., Gilbert, J., Abraham, P., Boelaert, K., Dayan, C., Gurnell, M., ... Vanderpump, M. (2016). Management of primary hypothyroidism: Statement of the British Thyroid Association executive committee. *Clinical Endocrinology, 84*(6), 799–808. https://doi.org/10.1111/cen.12824

Peeters, R.P. (2017) Subclinical hypothyroidism. *New England Journal of Medicine, 376*(26), 2556–2565. https://doi.org/10.1056/NEJMcp1611144

Taylor, P.N., Eligar, V., Muller, I., Scholz, A., Dayan, C., & Okosieme, O. (2019). Combination thyroid hormone replacement; Knowns and unknowns. *Frontiers in Endocrinology, 10*, 706. https://doi.org/10.3389/fendo.2019.00706

CHAPTER 159

Rhabdomyolysis

Rachael Fornwalt, MSN, AG–ACNP

I. Definition: A potentially life-threatening syndrome resulting from the dissolution or destruction of skeletal muscle with a subsequent release of intracellular components (e.g., electrolytes, myoglobin, other sarcoplasmic proteins) into the circulation (Cervellin et al., 2017; Fernandes & Davenport, 2019; McKenna et al., 2019; Petejova & Martinek, 2014; Stahl et al., 2020)

II. Physiology/Pathophysiology (Cervellin et al., 2017; Heard & Barker, 2016; Kim et al., 2016; Makic, 2019; Petejova & Martinek, 2014; Zutt et al., 2014)
   A. Normal
      1. Excitation of skeletal muscle results in energy-consuming muscular contraction. Intracellular myosin, actin, calcium, sodium, potassium, and acetylcholine work in concert to fuel the muscle by producing ATP.
      2. During normal muscle relaxation and contraction, numerous pumps found within the sarcolemma (myocyte) regulate the electrochemical charge of skeletal muscle cell membranes and regulate the membranes' cellular electrochemical gradients.
         a) The intercellular sodium is maintained at 10 mEq/L by a sodium–potassium ATP pump (sodium–potassium–ATPase), and the potassium concentration is preserved at 150 mEq/L.
         b) This gradient pulls sodium to the interior of the cell in exchange for calcium by a separate ion exchange channel. The gradient, along with an active calcium exchanger, regulates calcium entry into the sarcoplasmic reticulum and mitochondria.
         c) During rest, low levels of calcium are maintained, allowing for the increase needed during muscle contraction.
   B. Pathophysiology
      1. Extreme muscular demand or dysfunction depletes normal energy stores.
         a) As a result, phosphocreatine is transferred to adenosine diphosphate, leading to the production of excess energy by the secondary production of ATP.
         b) This enzymatic process is driven by creatine kinase and ultimately results in an overabundance of phosphocreatine and creatine kinase, leading to muscular damage and breakdown.
      2. With muscle injury and ATP depletion comes dysregulation of normal ion pump regulation, resulting in an unregulated increase in intracellular calcium.
         a) The excess intracellular calcium leads to persistent muscle contraction and energy depletion.
         b) Eventually, destruction of the myofibrillar network occurs, resulting in disintegration of the myocyte.

3. With myocyte destruction and muscle necrosis, large quantities of intracellular electrolytes (e.g., potassium, calcium, phosphate), enzymes (e.g., creatinine kinase, LDH, AST, aldolase), proteins (e.g., myoglobin) and purine metabolites (e.g., uric acid) are released into the systemic circulation. In large quantities, these intracellular components act as toxins, leading to electrolyte imbalances, hypovolemia, metabolic acidosis, coagulation defects, and AKI.

4. Multiple factors contribute to AKI induced by rhabdomyolysis.

   a) Unbound myoglobin in the urine interacts with the Tamm-Horsfall protein in the thick ascending limb of the loop of Henle, leading to precipitate formation, a process favored by acidic urine.

   b) Myoglobin itself can be toxic to the proximal renal tubules secondary to the myoglobin-induced release of hydroxyl free oxygen radicals reducing renal perfusion.

   c) Fluid sequestration within damaged muscle leads to volume depletion and renal vasoconstriction by activation of the renin–angiotensin system, vasopressin, and the sympathetic nervous system.

   d) Vascular mediators such as endothelin-1, thromboxane A$_2$, TNF-α, and F$_2$-isoprostanes further reduce renal blood flow.

III. Clinical features: Rhabdomyolysis is a relatively rare and complex syndrome that can have significant morbidity and mortality risks. Exertional rhabdomyolysis is the combination of muscle symptoms and substantial rise in serum creatine kinase in the setting of exercise. Most cases of exertional rhabdomyolysis are caused by heat-related injuries (e.g., heat stroke, heat injury). The severity of illness ranges from asymptomatic elevations in serum muscle enzymes to life-threatening disease–associated enzyme elevations, electrolyte imbalances, and AKI (Arnautovic & Tereziu, 2019; Cervellin et al., 2017; Fernandes & Davenport, 2019; Heytens et al., 2019; Kim et al., 2016; Kruger & Han, 2017; Makic, 2019; McKenna et al., 2019; Rawson et al., 2017; Stahl et al., 2020; Tarnopolsky, 2018; Wen et al., 2019; Zutt et al., 2014).

A. Risk factors

1. Extreme muscular activity
2. Infections or viral illness
3. Alcoholism or excessive alcohol consumption
4. Exposure to temperature extremes
5. Carbon monoxide exposure: Leads to insufficient muscle energy production
6. High-dose statin therapy alone or in combination
7. High-dose IFN or chemotherapy
8. Uncontrolled diabetes
9. Sickle cell disease or trait
10. Seizure disorder
11. Illicit drug use

B. Etiology

1. Trauma: A direct result of burns, physical assault, automobile accidents, struggling against restraints, torture, high-voltage electrical injury, crush injuries from natural disasters, or Taser gun injury
2. Prolonged immobilization: Reperfusion of damaged tissue after a period of ischemia and the release of necrotic material into the circulation once pressure is relieved
3. Physical overexertion/excessive muscular activity: Marathon runners, weight lifters, people with severe agitation or delirium tremors
4. Drugs and toxins (see Figure 159-1)
5. Infection: Tissue hypoxia, bacterial invasion of muscle, low oxidative and glycolytic enzyme activity, activation of lysosomal enzymes, endotoxins

| **FIGURE 159-1** | **Drugs and Toxins Associated With Rhabdomyolysis** |

Prescription	**Nonprescription**	**Toxins**
• Amiodarone	• Alcohol	• Bee venom
• Amphetamines	• Caffeine	• Benzene
• Antipsychotics	• Cocaine	• Carbon monoxide
• Barbiturates	• Designer "bath salts"	• Hemlock
• Benzodiazepine	• Ecstasy	• Mushrooms
• Chemotherapy drugs	• Heroin	• Snake venom
• Ciprofloxacin	• LSD	• Spider venom
• Colchicines	• Marijuana	
• Corticosteroids	• Phencylidine (PCP)	
• Cyclosporine	• Toluene (glue sniffing)	
• Erythromycin		
• Fibrates		
• Imatinib mesylate		
• Iron dextran		
• Isoniazid		
• Leuprolide acetate		
• Lithium		
• Phenytoin		
• Propofol		
• Protease inhibitors		
• Quinine		
• Salicylates		
• Serotonin antagonists		
• Statins		
• Sulfamethoxazole		
• Theophylline		

Note. Based on information from Cervellin et al., 2017; Fernandes & Davenport, 2019; Makic, 2019; Wen et al., 2019; Zutt et al., 2014.

    a) Associated viral infections include HSV, HIV, CMV, VZV, influenza A and B, Coxsackievirus, Epstein-Barr virus, parainfluenza, adenovirus, echovirus, and West Nile virus.

    b) Bacterial infections include *Legionella, Salmonella, Streptococcus, Staphylococcus aureus, Leptospira, Coxiella burnetii, Mycoplasma,* and *Escherichia coli.*

  6. Autoimmune inflammatory myopathies/connective tissue disorders

  7. Genetic disorders (see Figure 159-2)

  8. Severe electrolyte imbalances: Hyponatremia, hypernatremia, hypokalemia, hypophosphatemia

  9. Endocrine abnormalities: Hypothyroidism, hyperthyroidism, diabetic ketoacidosis, nonketotic hyperosmolar diabetic coma, pheochromocytoma

  10. Snake and spider bites

  11. Alcohol abuse

C. History

  1. History of cancer and cancer treatment

  2. Current medications: Prescribed, over the counter, herbal supplements

  3. History of presenting symptoms: Precipitating factors, onset, location, duration

  4. Changes in ADLs

  5. Past medical history: Renal insufficiency, viral infections, bacterial infections, diabetes, hypothyroidism/hyperthyroidism, pheochromocytoma, inflammatory myopathies, asthma, seizures, previous episode of rhabdomyolysis, recent trauma, sickle cell disease

| FIGURE 159-2 | Genetic Disorders Associated With Rhabdomyolysis |

Abnormal Lipid Metabolism
- Carnitine deficiency
- Carnitine palmitoyltransferase deficiency I and II

Disorders of Carbohydrate Metabolism
- Lactate dehydrogenase
- Myophosphorylase (McArdle disease)
- Phosphofructokinase (Tarui disease)
- Phosphoglycerate kinase
- Phosphoglycerate mutase
- Phosphorylase kinase

Other Genetic Disorders
- Duchenne muscular dystrophy
- Malignant hyperthermia
- Mitochondrial disorders
- Myoadenylate deaminase deficiency
- Succinate dehydrogenase

Note. Based on information from Fernandes & Davenport, 2019; Heytens et al., 2019; Rawson et al., 2017; Tarnopolsky, 2018.

6. Dietary history: Ingestion of wild mushrooms and dietary supplements; high concern with weight loss and performance-enhancing drugs

7. Social history: Alcohol use, illicit drug use, smoking, exercise patterns and tolerance, domestic abuse

8. Family history: Parent or sibling with history of exercise intolerance or rhabdomyolysis; genetic disorders of carbohydrate and lipid metabolism

D. Signs and symptoms: Clinical presentation may be vague and nonspecific depending on muscle damage.

   1. Muscle pain, weakness, and swelling: Reported in approximately 50% of patients

     a) Muscle swelling may not become apparent until after rehydration with IV fluids.

     b) Postural muscles of the thighs, calves, and lower back are most common sites.

     c) Other muscular symptoms include stiffness and cramping.

     d) It is prominent in proximal muscle groups, such as thighs and shoulders and the lower back and calves.

   2. Tea-colored urine (from myoglobinuria): Hallmark sign of rhabdomyolysis

   3. Decreased or absent urinary output

   4. Nausea and/or vomiting

   5. Fever

   6. Mental status changes

   7. Malaise/fatigue

   8. Right upper quadrant abdominal pain

E. Physical examination

   1. Vital signs: Fever, tachycardia, tachypnea, hypotension/hypertension

   2. Cardiovascular: Bradycardia, tachycardia, or an irregular rhythm, which may be present secondary to electrolyte imbalances

   3. Pulmonary: Increased respiratory rate or shortness of breath needed to increase waste product excretion

   4. Abdominal: Right upper quadrant tenderness indicative of possible hepatic inflammation or failure

   5. Posterior thorax: Dorsal costovertebral region tenderness and pain on palpation

   6. Musculoskeletal

     a) Perform full body visual inspection, including side, back, and frontal views. Assess for swelling and evidence of compartment syndrome or injury.

     b) Palpate all major muscle groups for mass effect, tenderness, and temperature.

     c) Measure any discrepancies and document muscle weakness.

7. Neurologic: Electrolyte imbalance and/or urea-induced encephalopathy resulting in confusion, agitation, lethargy, hyporeflexia/hyperreflexia, or balance instability

8. Integument: Indurated skin, edematous extremity, or discoloration or blistering of skin due to ischemia in patients who are comatose

IV. Diagnostic tests (Cervellin et al., 2017; Fernandes & Davenport, 2019; Heard & Barker, 2016; Kim et al., 2016; Kruger & Han, 2017; Makic, 2019; Rawson et al., 2017; Stahl et al., 2020; Zutt et al., 2014)

  A. Laboratory

    1. Serum creatine kinase (particularly CK-MM): It is usually five times ULN. Creatine kinase begins to rise within 2–12 hours of muscle injury and peaks within 24–72 hours. Risk of AKI increases with creatine kinase greater than 15,000 U/L.

    2. CBC: Evaluate for decreased platelet count with DIC occurring as a late complication, increased WBCs with infection, or decreased RBCs with sickle cell disease or anemia.

    3. PT, PTT: If abnormal, obtain DIC panel with D-dimer.

    4. Chemistries: Hyperkalemia, hyperphosphatemia, hypermagnesemia, and hypocalcemia are most common. Low BUN-to-creatinine ratio may be seen because the plasma creatinine tends to rise more rapidly in rhabdomyolysis than other types of renal failure.

    5. Uric acid: Purine release from damaged muscle results in hyperuricemia.

    6. Urinalysis

      a) Myoglobin may not be detected until serum levels exceed 1,500–3,000 ng/ml.

      b) If the urine dipstick is positive for Hgb but RBCs are absent on microscopic examination, myoglobinuria should be assumed.

      c) Urine sediment may have pigmented brown granular casts, brown debris, or renal tubular epithelial cells.

    7. Serum myoglobin: Measurement has a low sensitivity and usually is not helpful.

    8. Evaluation of urine electrolytes can be utilized to determine renal tubule functional integrity.

    9. Blood alcohol level or urine drug screen may be indicated to confirm exposure to specific drugs.

    10. Genetic panel, if warranted

  B. Radiology: It is not indicated unless the area of muscle undergoing rhabdomyolysis needs to be identified. If imaging is needed, MRI has high sensitivity for detecting muscle damage compared to CT and ultrasound.

  C. Other

    1. ECG to evaluate for conduction abnormalities and evidence of hyperkalemia: PR interval prolongation, peaked T waves, widened QRS complex

    2. ABGs: Metabolic acidosis and hypoxia frequently are seen.

V. Differential diagnosis (Arnautovic & Tereziu, 2019; Fernandes & Davenport, 2019; Heard & Barker, 2016; Heytens et al., 2019; McKenna et al., 2019; Rawson et al., 2017; Stahl et al., 2020; Tarnopolsky, 2018; Zutt et al., 2014)

  A. Connective tissue disorders

  B. Viral infections

  C. Bacterial infections

  D. Spider or snake bite

  E. Inflammatory myopathy

  F. Hematuria/hemoglobinuria (see Chapter 82)

G. MI (see Chapter 49)

H. Renal colic

I. Drug induced (see Figure 159-1)

J. Genetic disorders (see Figure 159-2)

K. Trauma

L. Severe electrolyte imbalances (see Chapters 152–156)

VI. Treatment: Primary aim of treatment is early rehydration. Damaged muscle tissue may sequester up to 12 L of fluid, resulting in hypovolemia. Early intervention decreases the incidence of AKI (Cervellin et al., 2017; Fernandes & Davenport, 2019; Heard & Barker, 2016; Kim et al., 2016; Kruger & Han, 2017; Makic, 2019; Petejova & Martinek, 2014; Zutt et al., 2014).

A. Aggressive rehydration is considered the standard of care in preventing AKI. Initiate fluid replacement with normal saline at rate of 1–2 L/hr and maintain urine output at 200–300 ml/hr.

1. No evidence is available to identify the optimal type of fluid for resuscitation, but solutions containing potassium and lactate should be avoided because of the increased risk of hyperkalemia and lactic acidosis.

2. If injury is from trauma or crush injury, begin fluid resuscitation before extrication. Continue fluids until creatine kinase level decreases to less than or equal to 1,000 U/L.

3. A urinary catheter should be inserted to monitor output.

4. Patients with significant electrolyte imbalances and ECG changes or significant comorbidities should be monitored in the ICU.

B. Diuretics: The use of diuretics remains controversial and is restricted to patients who are fluid depleted.

1. Proposed benefits of mannitol include an increase in renal blood flow and GFR to draw fluid from the interstitial compartment to the intravascular compartment. Mannitol is a free radical scavenger. A 20% infusion of mannitol at 0.5 g/kg over a 15-minute period followed by an infusion of 0.1 g/kg/hr is reasonable. Urine and serum pH levels must be monitored. Plasma osmolality and the osmolar gap should be monitored. Discontinue mannitol if adequate diuresis is not achieved or if the osmolar gap is greater than 55 mOsm/kg.

2. Loop diuretics may increase urinary flow and decrease the risk of myoglobin precipitation, but no study has demonstrated a clear benefit in patients with rhabdomyolysis. Loop diuretics may worsen hypocalcemia because they can induce calciuria and increase the risk of cast formation.

3. Diuretics are contraindicated in patients with oliguria or anuria.

C. Hyperuricemia: Treat with urinary alkalization to maintain urinary pH greater than or equal to 6.5 by the addition of one or two ampoules of sodium bicarbonate per liter.

1. Urinary alkalization increases uric acid and myoglobin solubility, inhibition of lipid peroxidation, and correction of hyperkalemia; however, some consider it controversial because of its potential to worsen hypocalcemia.

2. If urine pH does not rise after four to six hours of treatment, discontinue alkalization.

D. Hyperkalemia: IV sodium bicarbonate, glucose and insulin therapy, and inhaled beta-2 agonist act to drive extracellular potassium into the intracellular compartment. The use of ion-exchange resins (e.g., kayexalate) is effective but can take hours (see Chapter 153). Calcium administration acts to stabilize cardiac membranes with severe hyperkalemia with ECG changes; however, if calcium is administered with coexisting hyperphosphatemia, it may bind with extracellular phosphate, leading to metastatic calcification.

E. Hyperphosphatemia: Oral binders can be used when serum levels exceed 7 mg/dl, but this usually does not require treatment and is rarely of clinical significance (see Chapter 156).

F. Hypocalcemia: To avoid the late occurrence of hypercalcemia, calcium supplementation should be avoided unless significant signs and symptoms develop (see Chapter 152).

G. Metabolic acidosis: Treat with aggressive hydration. Bicarbonate administration may be detrimental and could worsen hypocalcemia.

H. DIC: Treatment of the underlying cause usually results in resolution. It may require fresh frozen plasma, vitamin K, or platelets (see Chapter 120).

I. Discontinue any drugs leading to exacerbation.

J. Dialysis may be lifesaving for patients with hyperkalemia, acidosis, or oliguric renal failure with fluid overload.

K. Returning to training and exercise through a basic rehabilitation protocol after suffering exercise-induced rhabdomyolysis should be encouraged.

VII. Follow-up (Fernandes & Davenport, 2019; Heard & Barker, 2016)

A. Follow up with primary care and any specialist consulted during inpatient treatment within one week.

B. Follow-up laboratory tests include CBC, electrolytes, renal function, liver function, uric acid level, urinalysis, and, most importantly, serum creatine kinase level.

C. After discharge for exertional rhabdomyolysis, serum creatine kinase and renal function should be monitored closely (e.g., every 72 hours until serum creatine kinase returns to a safe level). Failure of the serum creatinine kinase to normalize could indicate an underlying myopathy, and additional workup may be needed.

VIII. Referrals

A. Surgeon: For consideration of fasciotomy if compartment syndrome is a threat or if muscle biopsy is needed to confirm the diagnosis of rhabdomyolysis

B. Nephrologist: To help manage renal failure and if dialysis is needed

C. Geneticist: When genetic or metabolic abnormalities are thought to be the cause

D. Social worker: In cases of domestic or child abuse

E. Cardiologist: To assist in the management of arrhythmias

The author would like to acknowledge Kelley Duncan Mayden, MSN, FNP, AOCNP®, for her contribution to this chapter that remains unchanged from the previous edition of this book.

References

Arnautovic, J.Z., & Tereziu, S. (2019). Evaluation of clinical outcomes in hospitalized patients with exertional rhabdomyolysis. *Journal of the American Osteopathic Association, 119*(7), 428–434. https://doi.org/10.7556/jaoa.2019.079

Cervellin, G., Comelli, I., Benatti, M., Sanchis-Gomar, F., Bassi, A., & Lippi, G., (2017). Non-traumatic rhabdomyolysis: Background, laboratory features, and acute clinical management. *Clinical Biochemistry, 50*(12), 656–662. https://doi.org/10.1016/j.clinbiochem.2017.02.016

Fernandes, P.M., & Davenport, R.J. (2019). How to do it: Investigate exertional rhabdomyolysis (or not). *Practical Neurology, 19*(1), 43–48. https://doi.org/10.1136/practneurol-2018-002008

Heard, H., & Barker, J. (2016). Recognizing, diagnosing, and treating rhabdomyolysis. *Journal of the American Academy of Physician Assistants, 29*(5), 29–32. https://doi.org/10.1097/01.JAA.0000482294.31283.fe

Heytens, K., De Ridder, W., De Bleecker, J., Heytens, L., & Baets, J. (2019). Exertional rhabdomyolysis: Relevance of clinical and laboratory findings, and clues for investigation. *Anaesthesia and Intensive Care, 47*(2), 128–133. https://doi.org/10.1177/0310057X19835830

Kim, J., Lee, J., Kim, S., Ryu, H.Y., Cha, K.S., & Sung, D.J. (2016). Exercise induced rhabdomyolysis mechanisms and prevention: A literature review. *Journal of Sport and Health Science, 5*(3), 324–333. https://doi.org/10.1016/j.jshs.2015.01.012

Kruger, D., & Han, J. (2017). Assessing acquired rhabdomyolysis in adults. *Journal of the American Academy of Physician Assistants, 30*(1), 20–26. https://doi.org/10.1097/01.JAA.0000510986.14286.fd

Makic, M.B.F. (2019). Rhabdomyolysis: Recognizing risks. *Journal of PeriAnesthesia Nursing, 34*(6), 1282–1283. https://doi.org/10.1016/j.jopan.2019.08.001

McKenna, M.C., Kelly, M., Boran, G., & Lavin, P. (2019). Spectrum of rhabdomyolysis in an acute hospital. *Irish Journal of Medical Science, 188*(4), 1423–1426. https://doi.org/10.1007/s11845-019-01968-y

Petejova, N., & Martinek, A. (2014). Acute kidney injury due to rhabdomyolysis and renal replacement therapy: A critical review. *Critical Care, 18,* 224. https://doi.org/10.1186/cc13897

Rawson, E.S., Clarkson, P.M., & Tarnopolsky, M.A. (2017). Perspectives on exertional rhabdomyolysis. *Sports Medicine, 47*(Suppl. 1), S33–S49. https://doi.org/10.1007/s40279-017-0689-z

Stahl, K., Rastelli, E., & Schoser, B. (2020). A systematic review on the definition of rhabdomyolysis. *Journal of Neurology, 267*(4), 877–882. https://doi.org/10.1007/s00415-019-09185-4

Tarnopolsky, M.A. (2018). Myopathies related to glycogen metabolism disorders. *Neurotherapeutics, 15*(4), 915–927. https://doi.org/10.1007/s13311-018-00684-2

Wen, Z., Liang, Y., Hao, Y., Delavan, B., Huang, R., Mikailov, M., ... Liu, Z. (2019). Drug-induced rhabdomyolysis atlas (DIRA) for idiosyncratic adverse drug reaction management. *Drug Discovery Today, 24*(1), 9–15. https://doi.org/10.1016/j.drudis.2018.06.006

Zutt, R., van der Kooi, A.J., Linthorst, G.E., Wanders, R.J.A., & de Visser, M. (2014). Rhabdomyolysis: Review of the literature. *Neuromuscular Disorders, 24*(8), 651–659. https://doi.org/10.1016/j.nmd.2014.05.005

CHAPTER 160

Shock

Rachael Fornwalt, MSN, AG–ACNP

I. Definition: Shock is characterized by a pathologically low blood pressure that results in end-organ hypoperfusion. It occurs when the body's normal homeostatic compensatory mechanisms fail, leading to systemic tissue hypoxia and organ dysfunction (Landsberg, 2018; Marini & Dries, 2019; Singer et al., 2016; Standl et al., 2018).

II. Physiology/Pathophysiology (Bellumkonda et al., 2018; Geisen et al., 2019; Hendy & Bubenek-Turconi, 2016; Landsberg, 2018; Marini & Dries, 2019; Procter, 2020; Standl et al., 2018; Watts & Marie Ditto, 2019)

A. Normal: Cardiac output (blood flow) is the volume of blood ejected by the left ventricle per minute.

1. Cardiac output is the product of heart rate and stroke volume.

   a) Stroke volume is determined by three components—preload, contractility, and afterload.

   b) Stroke volume and systemic vascular resistance work together to deliver oxygen and nutrients to peripheral tissue and return metabolic waste products for removal.

   c) Cardiac output must match metabolic requirements to maintain homeostasis.

2. Circulatory flow originates in the heart. The volume of blood leaving the left side of the heart during contractions must equal that returning on the right.

   a) Preload is the tension developed by the stretching of myocardial fibers. It is affected by circulating blood volume, venous capacitance, body posture, intracavity pressures (e.g., thoracic cavity, abdominal cavity), ventricular compliance, heart rate, and atrial contraction.

   b) Contractility, also known as inotropy, is the strength of ventricular contraction.

   c) Afterload is the ventricular wall tension required to eject the stroke volume during systole. It is dependent on wall thickness and ventricular radius.

      (1) An increase in ventricular radius, such as dilation of the ventricle, will increase afterload.

      (2) Alternatively, an increase in wall thickness, such as ventricular hypertrophy, will reduce afterload.

3. Force of ventricle contraction is related to the following.

   a) Volume of blood in the ventricles

   b) Ability of the ventricle wall to distend or stretch in response to ventricle filling

   c) Vascular resistance or the mechanical property of the vascular system opposing flow of blood into the vascular bed: Systemic vascular resistance is affected by vessel diameter, compliance of the systemic circulation, blood viscosity, and hematocrit.

    4. Humoral factors play a role at the cellular level through direct cardiovascular and renal effects, and indirectly on central and peripheral adrenergic transmission.

        a) Renin–angiotensin system: Produces angiotensin I and angiotensin II; ACE promotes vasoconstriction to maintain arterial pressure and releases aldosterone for sodium and water retention.

        b) Vasopressin: Hormone released by the pituitary gland in response to changes in blood volume and/or osmotic pressure; vasopressin has an antidiuretic effect and vasoconstriction action with a general effect of retaining water in the circulation.

        c) Beta-adrenergic amines (e.g., epinephrine, norepinephrine): Increases myocardial contractibility and heart rate and triggers release of corticosteroids from the adrenal gland, glucose from the liver, and renin from the kidneys

  B. Pathophysiology

    1. Hypoperfusion triggers inflammatory and clotting cascades.

    2. WBCs are activated by hypoxic vascular endothelial cells, which bind to the endothelium and release damaging substances (e.g., reactive oxygen species, proteolytic enzymes) and inflammatory mediators (e.g., cytokines, leukotrienes, TNF). These mediators bind to cell surface receptors and activate nuclear factor kappa B, leading to production of additional cytokines and nitric oxide, a potent vasodilator leading to further vasoplegia.

    3. The body uses compensatory mechanisms, such as vasoconstriction and increased heart rate, to restore arterial pressure and blood flow to vital organs.

III. Clinical features: Shock is a life-threatening condition of circulatory failure. Initially, shock is reversible but can rapidly become irreversible, resulting in multiorgan failure. The main characteristic of shock is reduced perfusion of vital tissues. As perfusion declines and oxygen delivery to cells is insufficient for aerobic metabolism, cells shift to anaerobic metabolism, which subsequently increases production of carbon dioxide and elevates blood lactate levels. Cellular function declines, and without prompt reversal of shock, irreversible cell damage and death occur (Bellumkonda et al., 2018; Campbell et al., 2014; Geisen et al., 2019; Hendy & Bubenek-Turconi, 2016; Landsberg, 2018; Marini & Dries, 2019; Singer et al., 2016; Standl et al., 2018).

  A. Types of shock

    1. Hypovolemic shock is caused by loss of preload as a result of acute blood loss (hemorrhage) or third-spacing illnesses. Loss of preload leads to decreased central venous pressure, and right ventricular and left ventricular end-diastolic pressure, causing reduced stroke volume and cardiac output. This decrease in cardiac output triggers increased sympathetic activity, which leads to tachycardia and increased systemic vascular resistance.

    2. Cardiogenic shock begins with an acute cardiac injury that results in decreased cardiac output and stroke volume, leading to hypotension, decreased peripheral perfusion, and coronary ischemia. The body's attempt to compensate results in peripheral vasoconstriction increasing afterload to the left ventricle, which further exacerbates myocardial dysfunction.

        a) Acute cardiac injury then triggers a systemic inflammatory response, causing vasodilation by increasing circulating levels of nitric oxide, peroxynitrite, and proinflammatory cytokines. These humoral mediators further decrease cardiac output and stroke volume by impairing contractility.

        b) Myocardial dysfunction also increases left ventricle end-diastolic pressure causing pulmonary edema and hypoxia, which can worsen myocardial ischemia.

3. Distributive shock can be caused by sepsis, anaphylaxis, adrenal crisis, severe pancreatitis, or neurogenic shock. It results in inappropriate arteriolar vasodilation and increased capillary permeability, which leads to decreased systemic vascular resistance and effective circulating volume and results in hypotension. Increased sympathetic activity is triggered by hypotension causing tachycardia and increased cardiac output.

4. Mixed physiology shock

   a) Distributive shock can commonly occur concurrently with heart failure, as infection and sepsis can decompensate preexisting heart failure and cause cytokine-mediated myocardial depression. These patients will typically present with warm edematous extremities and pulmonary edema of varying severity.

   b) Hypovolemic shock can occur when patients with preexisting heart failure, typically individuals with chronic decompensated heart failure, develop hemorrhagic shock or third-spacing physiology (less common).

B. Etiology

   1. Hypovolemic

      a) Hemorrhagic: Greater than 30% loss of blood volume

      b) Nonhemorrhagic: Common causes

         (1) External: Vomiting, diarrhea, burns, polyuria

         (2) Internal: Third-spacing states such as ascites, severe pancreatitis, and after large abdominal surgery

   2. Cardiogenic

      a) Myocardial disease

         (1) Acute MI: greater than 80% of patients with cardiogenic shock

            (a) Greater than 40% loss of left ventricular mass

            (b) Less than 40% loss of left ventricular mass with recurrent, refractory arrhythmia

            (c) Right ventricular infarction

            (d) Mechanical complications: Papillary muscle free-wall rupture, ventral septal defect

         (2) Acute decompensated heart failure

            (a) Chronic heart failure with acute decompensation

            (b) Initial presentation of acute heart failure: Myocarditis, peripartum cardiomyopathy, Takotsubo cardiomyopathy

         (3) Postcardiotomy shock

         (4) Other causes: Dynamic left ventricular outflow tract obstruction, myocardial depression in sepsis (e.g., mixed shock picture), myocardial contusion (e.g., blunt force trauma)

      b) Valve disease: Stenosis, regurgitation, prosthetic valve failure

      c) Electrical disease: Bradyarrhythmia, atrial/ventricular tachyarrhythmia

      d) Extracardiac disease: Obstructive shock

         (1) Pulmonary vascular

            (a) PE

            (b) PH

         (2) Mechanical

            (a) Constrictive pericarditis

            (b) Cardiac tamponade

            (c) Tension pneumothorax

            (d) Restrictive cardiomyopathy

3. Distributive
   a) Septic shock
      (1) Sepsis is defined as life-threatening organ dysfunction caused by a dysregulated host response to infection.
      (2) Septic shock is a subset of sepsis in which the body's underlying circulatory and cellular/metabolic abnormalities are profound enough to substantially increase mortality.
   b) Anaphylactic: A serious, generalized or systemic, allergic, or hypersensitivity reaction that can be life threatening or fatal
   c) Adrenal failure: Lack of cortisol and mineralocorticoids; may be the result of an abrupt stress in patients with adrenal insufficiency or more commonly due to abrupt withdrawal of steroids
   d) Neurogenic shock: Lack of sympathetic tone caused by any spinal cord injury or stroke; blood vessels no longer receive sympathetic inputs and respond by dilating.

C. Signs and symptoms
   1. Cardinal signs and symptoms
      a) Hypotension: Systolic blood pressure less than 90 mm Hg measured or a relative drop in systolic pressure from baseline by greater than 40 mm Hg
      b) Oliguria: May accompany orthostatic hypotension, poor skin turgor, absence of axillary perspiration, and dry mucous membranes
      c) Changes in mentation: Progression through agitation, irritability, confusion, delirium, and obtundation
      d) Altered skin temperature: Cool and clammy but may be flushed and hyperemic in early or terminal shock
   2. Subtle signs and symptoms are not conclusive and may be described in addition to the cardinal signs.
      a) Hematemesis and/or hematochezia
      b) Melena, vomiting, diarrhea, and/or abdominal pain
      c) Light-headedness, dizziness
      d) Productive cough, chills, myalgias
      e) Dyspnea, chest pain or palpitations, tachypnea
      f) Headache, photophobia, abnormal mentation

D. History
   1. History of cancer and cancer treatments
   2. Current medications: Prescribed, over the counter, supplements
   3. History of presenting symptoms: Precipitating factors, onset, duration, associated factors (e.g., recent infection, bleeding, trauma, allergen exposure)
   4. Changes in ADLs
   5. Past medical history: Cardiac disease, syncope
   6. Social history: Illicit drug use or intoxication

E. Physical examination
   1. Vital signs
      a) Temperature: Fever or hypothermia (greater than 38.5°C [101.3°F] or less than 35°C [95°F])
      b) Hypotension: Systolic blood pressure less than 90 mm Hg measured or a relative drop in systolic pressure from baseline by greater than 40 mm Hg; patients with history of uncontrolled hypertension may show signs of end-organ hypoperfusion despite mean arterial pressure greater than 65 mm Hg or systolic blood pressure greater than 90 mm Hg.

2. Cardiac
    a) Tachycardia
    b) Bradycardia indicative of possible conduction system disease or AV nodal blockade
    c) Murmur indicative of aortic stenosis, acute mitral or aortic regurgitation, or ventricular septal defect
    d) S_3 suggestive of CHF or S_4 suggestive of decreased ventricular compliance as seen in MI or acute ischemia
    e) Elevated jugular venous pressure, which could indicate right-sided heart failure, constrictive pericarditis, cardiac tamponade, fluid overload without heart failure, or SVC obstruction or flat neck veins suggestive of distributive shock
3. Mental status: Delirium and/or global decreased mentation likely in the setting of poor cerebral perfusion
4. Pulmonary
    a) Tachypnea, presence of rales, and rhonchi, which may indicate infection or heart failure
    b) Unilateral diminished breath sounds indicative of possible large pleural effusion, pneumothorax, or hemothorax
5. Abdomen
    a) Presence of ascites, tenderness, distention, firmness, hepatomegaly, splenomegaly, penetrating injury, and the presence or absence of bowel sounds
    b) Increasing abdominal distention or pain indicative of possible internal organ injury and bleeding or disease progression in some malignancies
6. Integument
    a) Presence of purpuric lesions (internal bleeding or blunt trauma) and infected wounds (source of sepsis)
    b) Poor skin turgor and pallor with decreased perfusion
    c) Patients with distributive shock present with warm extremities; patients with cardiogenic shock present with cool extremities.
7. Extremities: Presence of peripheral edema related to cardiac failure

IV. Diagnostic tests (Hendy & Bubenek-Turconi, 2016; Landsberg, 2018; Marini & Dries, 2019; Rhodes et al., 2017)
    A. Laboratory
        1. CBC with differential: WBC count greater than 12,000/mm³ or less than 4,000/mm³ can point toward infection as the cause of shock, as can a left shift or bandemia. Evaluation of Hgb and platelet count help to determine if bleeding is a source of shock.
        2. Comprehensive chemistry panel with liver panel, renal function, and electrolyte levels: Elevated liver enzymes and creatinine may reflect organ damage and abnormal glucose; alterations to serum sodium, potassium, and calcium may reflect adrenal dysfunction.
        3. Coagulation values: PT, PTT, INR, fibrinogen and D-dimer are necessary to detect the development of sepsis-induced DIC or for adequate resuscitation in hemorrhagic shock.
        4. Cardiac enzymes to evaluate for MI: N-terminal prohormone BNP elevated in heart failure
        5. ABGs and lactate levels to evaluate for presence and severity of acidosis: Central venous oxygen saturations may be helpful to trend during resuscitation or to differentiate mixed shock states.
        6. Type and crossmatch to prepare blood products if bleeding

7. Amylase and lipase if necrotizing pancreatitis is suspected cause of shock
8. Urinalysis
    a) Leukocytosis indicative of infection
    b) Protein or casts suggestive of renal failure or disease
9. Two sets of blood cultures should be sent (aerobic and anaerobic). No correlation has been found between fevers and yield of positive cultures. Cultures should be sent from central line or peripherally if concern for vascular access as source of sepsis.
10. Urine culture and sputum culture should be sent if urinary or pulmonary source of sepsis is suspected.
11. Gram stain: Specimens should be collected at all possible sites of infection—pleural fluid, peritoneal fluid, stool, and any open wounds.
12. Cortisol to evaluate for adrenal insufficiency or relative adrenal insufficiency
B. Radiology
1. Chest x-ray to evaluate for presence of pneumonia, acute respiratory distress syndrome, pleural effusion, or pulmonary edema
2. Other imaging studies, as determined by clinical suspicion from examination and history
3. CT angiogram to evaluate for areas of bleeding, if necessary
C. Other
1. 12-lead ECG to evaluate for ischemic changes
2. Echocardiogram to assess global right and left ventricular function, acute valve failure or tamponade: Hypovolemic and distributive shock states cause under filling of the right and left ventricles, which will appear hyperdynamic with an increased ejection fraction.

V. Differential diagnosis: Dependent on the suspected type of shock (Campbell et al., 2014; Gutierrez et al., 2018; Landsberg, 2018; Singer et al., 2016)
A. Hemorrhagic
1. Trauma: Blunt or crush injury
2. GI bleed: Upper or lower
3. Ruptured aneurysm: Abdomen, left ventricle
4. Fracture: Large bone of the pelvis (see Chapter 102)
5. Hemorrhagic pancreatitis
6. Ruptured liver or spleen hematoma
7. Aortic dissection
B. Hypovolemic
1. Heat stroke
2. Burns: Stevens-Johnson syndrome, toxic epidermal necrolysis
3. Third spacing of fluid: Illness, malignancy, postoperative, capillary leak syndrome
4. Pancreatitis (see Chapter 77)
5. GI disturbances: Vomiting (see Chapter 63), diarrhea (see Chapter 56)
C. Cardiogenic
1. MI involving greater than 40% of the left ventricle (see Chapter 49)
2. Atrial fibrillation and atrial flutter (see Chapter 45)
3. Myocarditis
4. Prolonged ischemia following bypass surgery
5. Valvular defects
6. Septal defects
7. PE (see Chapter 33)
8. Tension pneumothorax (see Chapter 31)

9. Pericarditis (see Chapter 50)

10. PH (see Chapter 52)

11. Cardiac tamponade (see Chapter 50)

12. Hypertrophic cardiomyopathy (see Chapter 41)

D. Distributive shock

   1. Sepsis

   2. Anaphylaxis (see Chapter 150)

   3. Adrenal crisis

   4. Myxedema coma

   5. Capillary leak syndrome (see Chapter 35)

   6. Cancer: Carcinoid or paraneoplastic syndrome; post-HSCT immune reconstitution, CAR T-cell–related cytokine release syndrome

   7. Neurogenic shock: Spinal cord injury

VI. Treatment (Annane et al., 2018; Bellumkonda et al., 2018; Bissell & Mefford, 2020; Campbell et al., 2014; Chakravarthy et al., 2018; Landsberg, 2018; Rhodes et al., 2017; Russell, 2019; Semler et al., 2018; Singer et al., 2016; Standl et al., 2018; Venkatesh & Cohen, 2019; Watts & Marie Ditto, 2019)

A. Hypovolemic shock

   1. Establish IV access. Large-bore peripheral IV (minimum two) or central line should be used if necessary. In cases of hemorrhagic shock, large bore catheters may be required for rapid transfusion of blood products.

   2. Rapid administration of balanced crystalloid fluid (lactated Ringer's solution) via 500–1,000 ml boluses should be given until heart rate, blood pressure, and urine output return to normal.

     a) Patients may require up to 6–12 liters of fluid, especially in third-spacing states (e.g., severe pancreatitis).

     b) Monitor for fluid overload.

   3. Hemorrhagic shock is managed with rapid transfusion of blood products. Persistent tachycardia and/or ongoing bleeding should be considered under resuscitation.

   4. When patients require massive transfusion, or greater than four units of packed RBCs in one hour or six units in a 12-hour period, platelets and fresh frozen plasma should be transfused 1:1 with packed RBCs (or one dose of pooled platelets depending on institution). Calcium should also be repleted during massive transfusion protocol, as citrate in the blood products results in citrate chelation of serum calcium and can lead to severe hypocalcemia.

   5. Hemorrhagic shock not responsive to resuscitation may require additional vasopressors support; however, rapid infusion of blood products is the mainstay of treatment.

B. Cardiogenic shock

   1. Rapid transfer to a tertiary or quaternary medical center with critical care management, mechanical circulatory support, and interprofessional team care is necessary to achieve good clinical outcomes.

   2. Coronary revascularization for patients with acute coronary syndrome and cardiogenic shock is the cornerstone of treatment. Guidelines recommend early percutaneous coronary intervention or coronary artery bypass grafting for all patients with cardiogenic shock as a result of acute coronary syndrome.

   3. After percutaneous coronary intervention, dual antiplatelet therapy should be administered to all patients without bleeding complications.

   4. Inotropic agents should be used to normalize the cardiac index, such as dopamine, dobutamine, milrinone, or epinephrine. If hypotension is present despite inotro-

pic therapy, vasoactive agents such as vasopressin, phenylephrine, or norepinephrine should be added.

5. Mechanical circulatory support should be considered for patients who are not
responding to aggressive medical management. These temporary mechanical support devices include pulsatile pumps (e.g., intra-aortic balloon pumps), left atrium
to femoral artery pumps, left ventricle to aorta axial pumps, and right atrium or
central vein to a systemic artery pump with oxygenation (also known as venoarte-
rial extracorporeal membrane oxygenation).

6. Patients with biventricular failure or severe isolated RV failure and cardiogenic shock
may require right ventricular mechanical support.

C. Distributive shock

1. Rapid identification, intervention, and early detection of organ dysfunction are
essential for improved outcomes in sepsis.

   a) Utilization of the qSOFA score, an abbreviated version of the Sequential Organ
   Failure Assessment (SOFA) score, can aid in detection of imminent sepsis.

   b) The qSOFA is composed of the following.

      (1) Alteration of mental status

      (2) Respiratory rate greater than 22 breaths per minute

      (3) Systolic blood pressure less than 100 mm Hg

   c) Scores range from 0–3 points. Patients with two or more points at the onset of
   infection have increased risk of death or prolonged hospital stay.

2. Airways should be stabilized and maintained. High-flow nasal cannula can be utilized for hypoxic respiratory failure. Mechanical ventilation may be indicated for
acute respiratory distress syndrome or inadequate compensation for metabolic acidosis.

3. Establish IV access. Large-bore peripheral IV or central line may be used if necessary.

4. Initiate fluid resuscitation with rapid infusion of normal saline or balanced crystalloid solution. Lactated ringers or Plasma-Lyte are preferred in all shock states.

   a) Fluid resuscitation with at least 30 ml/kg of IV crystalloid fluid is given within
   the first three hours. Lactated Ringer's or Plasma-Lyte is the fluid of choice for
   resuscitation. Balanced crystalloids have demonstrated lower rates of death from
   any cause, need for initiation of renal replacement therapy, or persistent renal
   dysfunction when compared to the use of saline.

   b) Fluid challenge technique (500–1,000 ml bolus over one hour) should be used
   when fluid administration demonstrates a continued hemodynamic benefit.

   c) Monitor for fluid overload.

5. Albumin can be utilized in addition to crystalloids for initial resuscitation and subsequent intravascular volume repletion in patients who require substantial amounts
of crystalloids; however, use of albumin has demonstrated no mortality benefit compared to crystalloids.

6. Maintain mean arterial pressure greater than 65 mmHg.

   a) Norepinephrine is the vasopressor of choice.

   b) Vasopressin (maximum dose 0.04 U/min) or epinephrine are recommended
   second-line pressor to norepinephrine when single-agent pressor is inadequate
   to maintain mean arterial pressure greater than 65 mm Hg or to decrease norepinephrine dosage.

   c) Dopamine is not recommended as first- or second-line vasopressor and should
   only be considered in select patients with low risk of tachyarrhythmias or absolute bradycardia. No evidence exists to support low-dose dopamine for renal
   protection.

    d) Dobutamine is recommended in patients with evidence of persistent hypoperfusion despite adequate fluid resuscitation and the use of vasopressor agents. It should be discontinued in the setting of worsening hypotension or arrhythmias.

    e) Arterial line placement is used to monitor pressure closely for rapid titration of vasopressors.

  7. Treat with broad empiric antibiotic coverage (see Appendix C).

    a) Administration of IV antimicrobials should be initiated within one hour of recognition of symptoms for both sepsis and septic shock.

      (1) Initial selection of antimicrobial therapy must be broad enough to cover all likely pathogens.

      (2) A thorough review of the patient's history, clinical status, and local epidemiologic factors must be completed prior to choosing antibiotics.

      (3) Important factors to consider include site of infection, concomitant underlying diseases, chronic organ failures, indwelling devices, the presence of immunosuppression or other forms of immunocompromise, recent known infection or prior colonization with specific drug-resistant pathogens, and the receipt of antimicrobials within the previous three months.

    b) Infectious disease specialists should be consulted when dealing with multidrug resistant organisms.

    c) A broad-spectrum carbapenem (e.g., imipenem/cilastatin, meropenem, doripenem) or extended-range penicillin/beta-lactamase inhibitor combination (e.g., piperacillin/tazobactam, ticarcillin/clavulanate) are typical first-line antibiotic choices.

    d) Vancomycin or other anti-MRSA antibiotics can be used when significant risk factors for MRSA exist, or in patients with significant mucositis or indwelling lines.

    e) Addition of a macrolide or fluoroquinolone should be considered for patients with risk of infection with *Legionella* species.

    f) Antifungal therapy should be considered for patients with risk factors for invasive fungal infections, such as immunocompromised status, prolonged invasive vascular devices, total parenteral nutrition, necrotizing pancreatitis, recent major abdominal surgery, prolonged administration of broad-spectrum antibiotics, prolonged hospital/ICU admission, recent fungal infection, and multisite colonization. Empiric use of an echinocandin (e.g., micafungin, caspofungin) is preferred in patients with septic shock, those who have recently been treated with other antifungal agents, or those with a history of *Candida glabrata* or *Candida krusei* infection.

    g) Aminoglycosides can be used for multidrug resistant organisms or in patients with refractory shock despite broad spectrum antibiotics coverage.

D. Monitor renal function. Hemodialysis may be necessary if AKI occurs.

E. Consider stress dose steroids; however, this has shown no mortality benefit in patients who are not adrenally insufficient (see Appendix K).

  1. Patients at risk for adrenal insufficiency or on chronic steroids should receive a trial of corticosteroids.

  2. In patients with refractory shock or requiring rapidly rising pressor support, corticosteroids should be considered, as there has been no demonstrated increase in mortality.

  3. Recent evidence suggests that hydrocortisone in combination with fludrocortisone may reduce mortality in septic shock, but confirmatory study is necessary.

F. Treat suspected anaphylaxis.

1. Epinephrine is first-line treatment for anaphylaxis. Epinephrine 0.3–0.5 mg of 1:1,000 epinephrine should be administered via IM route. Do not exceed 0.5 mg per injection. Repeated doses can be given every 5–10 minutes PRN.

   a) During respiratory and/or circulatory arrest, epinephrine should be administered intravenously.

   b) If severe anaphylactic reactions occur, continuous infusion epinephrine may need to be administered at a rate of 5–15 mcg/min.

2. Provide supplemental oxygen. If needed, perform cardiopulmonary resuscitation and secure airway.

3. Secure IV access. Administer IV resuscitation with 0.9% saline or lactated Ringer's. Aggressive fluid resuscitation combats the significant plasma leak associated with anaphylaxis. Monitor for fluid overload.

4. Infusions of glucagon have been used to treat anaphylaxis refractory to epinephrine in patients on beta-blockers. The recommended dose of glucagon is 1–5 mg IV administered over five minutes and followed by an infusion of 5–15 mg/min titrated to clinical response.

5. Antihistamine may be used as adjuncts but should not be used as first-line treatment for anaphylaxis. Diphenhydramine 25–50 mg IV or IM may be given every six hours PRN. Maximum daily dose is 400 mg.

6. Inhaled bronchodilators can be administered for bronchospasm, such as albuterol 2.5 ml of 0.5% nebulized solution.

7. Corticosteroids have a delayed onset and should not be used as first-line treatment for anaphylaxis. Dosing of corticosteroids should be 1–2 mg/kg IV per dose of methylprednisolone.

VII. Follow-up

A. Inpatient hospitalization in an ICU is necessary to manage the signs, symptoms, and complications of shock.

B. Monitor for multiorgan organ system failure/recovery using laboratory tests (e.g., serum creatinine, bilirubin), fraction of inspired oxygen rate, and Glasgow coma score.

VIII. Referrals

A. Cardiologist: To evaluate cardiac function and recommend supportive measures

B. Nephrologist: To evaluate for AKI and recommend management

C. Pulmonologist: To evaluate current lung function, perform bronchoscopy if clinically indicated, and recommend management of pulmonary disease or symptoms

D. Infectious disease specialist: To recommend antibiotics and antifungal medication

E. Gastroenterologist: To manage acute GI hemorrhage

F. Interventional radiologist or surgeons: For control of bleeding or source control for infection

The author would like to acknowledge Dana L. Viviano, RN, BSN, for her contribution to this chapter that remains unchanged from the previous edition of this book.

References

Annane, D., Renault, A., Brun-Buisson, C., Megarbane, B., Quenot, J.-P., Siami, S., ... Bellissant, E. (2018). Hydrocortisone plus fludrocortisone for adults with septic shock. *New England Journal of Medicine, 378*(9), 809–818. https://doi.org/10.1056/NEJMoa1705716

Bellumkonda, L., Gul, B., & Masri, S.C. (2018). Evolving concepts in diagnosis and management of cardiogenic shock. *American Journal of Cardiology, 122*(6), 1104–1110. https://doi.org/10.1016/j.amjcard.2018.05.040

Bissell, B.D., & Mefford, B. (2020). Pathophysiology of volume administration in septic shock and the role of the clinical pharmacist. *Annals of Pharmacotherapy, 54*(4), 388–396. https://doi.org/10.1177/1060028019887160

Campbell, R.L., Li, J.T.C., Nicklas, R.A., & Sadosty, A.T. (2014). Emergency department diagnosis and treatment of anaphylaxis: A practice parameter. *Annals of Allergy, Asthma and Immunology, 113*(6), 599–608. https://doi.org/10.1016/j.anai.2014.10.007

Chakravarthy, M., Tsukashita, M., & Murali, S. (2018). A targeted management approach to cardiogenic shock. *Critical Care Clinics, 34*(3), 423–437. https://doi.org/10.1016/j.ccc.2018.03.009

Geisen, M., Cecconi, M., & Rhodes, A. (2019). Assessment of cardiac filling and blood flow. In J.E. Parrillo & R.P. Dellinger (Eds.), *Critical care medicine: Principles of diagnosis and management in the adult* (5th ed., pp. 29–39). Elsevier.

Gutierrez, C., McEvoy, C., Mead, E., Stephens, R.S., Munshi, L., Detsky, M., … Nates, J.L. (2018). Management of the critically ill adult chimeric antigen receptor-T cell therapy patient: A critical care perspective. *Critical Care Medicine, 46*(9), 1402–1410. https://doi.org/10.1097/CCM.0000000000003258

Hendy, A., & Bubenek-Turconi, S.I. (2016). The diagnosis and hemodynamic monitoring of circulatory shock: Current and future trends. *Journal of Critical Care Medicine, 2*(3), 115–123. https://doi.org/10.1515/jccm-2016-0018

Landsberg, J.W. (2018). *Manual for pulmonary and critical care medicine.* Elsevier.

Marini, J.J., & Dries, D.J. (2019). *Critical care medicine: The essentials and more* (5th ed.). Wolters Kluwer.

Procter, L.D. (2020). Shock. In R.S. Porter (Ed.), *Merck manual: Professional version.* https://www.merckmanuals.com/professional/critical-care-medicine/shock-and-fluid-resuscitation/shock

Rhodes, A., Evans, L.E., Alhazzani, W., Levy, M.M., Antonelli, M., Ferrer, R., … Dellinger, R.P. (2017). Surviving sepsis campaign: International guidelines for management of sepsis and septic shock: 2016. *Critical Care Medicine, 45*(3), 486–552. https://doi.org/10.1097/CCM.0000000000002255

Russell, J.A. (2019). Vasopressor therapy in critically ill patients with shock. *Intensive Care Medicine, 45*(11), 1503–1517. https://doi.org/10.1007/s00134-019-05801-z

Semler, M.W., Self, W.H., Wanderer, J.P., Ehrenfeld, J.M., Wang, L., Byrne, D.W., … Rice, T.W. (2018). Balanced crystalloids versus saline in critically ill adults. *New England Journal of Medicine, 378*(9), 829–839. https://doi.org/10.1056/NEJMoa1711584

Singer, M., Deutschman, C.S., Seymour, C.W., Shankar-Hari, M., Annane, D., Bauer, M., … Angus, D.C. (2016). The third international consensus definitions for sepsis and septic shock (Sepsis-3). *JAMA, 315*(8), 801–810. https://doi.org/10.1001/jama.2016.0287

Standl, T., Annecke, T., Cascorbi, I., Heller, A.R., Sabashnikov, A., & Teske, W. (2018). The nomenclature, definition and distinction of types of shock. *Deutsches Ärzteblatt International, 115*(45), 757–768. https://doi.org/10.3238/arztebl.2018.0757

Venkatesh, B., & Cohen, J. (2019). Hydrocortisone in vasodilatory shock. *Critical Care Clinics, 35*(2), 263–275. https://doi.org/10.1016/j.ccc.2018.11.005

Watts, M.M., & Marie Ditto, A. (2019). Anaphylaxis. *Allergy and Asthma Proceedings, 40*(6), 453–456. https://doi.org/10.2500/aap.2019.40.4270

Miscellaneous

CHAPTER 161

Anxiety

Elena C. Prendergast, DNP, APRN, FNP-C, ACHPN,
and Constance Dahlin, MSN, ANP-BC, ACHPN, FPCN, FAAN

I. Definition (American Psychiatric Association, 2013; DeMartini et al., 2019; Glass et al., 2018)
   A. Anxiety is feelings of distress and tension with or without a known stimulus.
   B. Anxiety is an expected state in life and can be divided into two categories.
      1. An acute, severe wave of intense anxiety with impressive cognitive, physiologic, and behavioral components
      2. A low-grade persistent distress consisting of restlessness or being on edge, difficulty in concentrating, irritability, muscle tension, and altered sleep that interferes with psychosocial functioning
   C. The American Psychiatric Association recognized an aspect of anxiety that can relate to patients with cancer called *anxiety disorder due to another medical condition*. This diagnosis explains that the disorder is related to the circumstances of the direct pathophysiologic consequences of a medical condition, is not explained by a mental disorder, and affects the social and occupational situations of the patient as well as his or her general functioning.
   D. Generalized anxiety disorder is characterized by excessive and persistent worrying that is hard to control, causes significant distress, and occurs on more days than not for at least six months.

II. Physiology/Pathophysiology (Glass et al., 2018)
   A. Normal: The CNS contains several neurotransmitters. These include dopamine, norepinephrine, and serotonin. Stable mood is noted in individuals who have the correct metabolism and balance of the neurotransmitters.
   B. Pathophysiology: Anxiety is not well understood but is thought to result from dysregulated physiologic systems, likely inappropriate activation of the sympathetic nervous system involving the following.
      1. Altered levels of neurotransmitters, which cause neurobiologic reactions
         a) Norepinephrine: Increased levels
         b) Serotonin (5-HT): Decreased levels
         c) Gamma-aminobutyric acid: Decreased levels
      2. Hormonal systems such as the hypothalamus, pituitary, and adrenal glands that disrupt normal processes, yielding symptoms of panic, sweating, and sense of dread
      3. Brain structures such as the amygdala, hippocampus, and frontal lobe that cause disruption, yielding feelings of unreality, lack of focus, or lack of contact with other people
      4. Cardiovascular abnormalities secondary to dysregulation of the autonomic nervous system that cause disruption in cardiac tissue, yielding symptoms of distress

III. Clinical features: Anxiety is thought to result from biochemical imbalances and can range from mild to panic. Panic attacks usually reach a peak within 10 minutes then slowly resolve spontaneously. Generalized anxiety is characterized by chronic uncontrollable worry that interferes with functioning and is often accompanied by restlessness and disturbed sleep. Generalized anxiety disorder is the most common mental disorder in primary care settings and considered to be a potentially chronic illness (Chen et al., 2019; DeMartini et al., 2019; Gatto et al., 2016; Glass et al., 2018; Lichtenstein et al., 2019; Loving & Dahlin, 2019; NCCN, 2021; Pary et al., 2019; Pitman et al., 2018; Salman et al., 2019).

A. Types of anxiety disorders
1. Generalized anxiety disorder: Chronic uncontrollable nervousness, fearfulness, or sense of worry that lasts six months or longer
2. Post-traumatic stress disorder: Onset after a traumatic event, resembling panic when there is a trigger related to the initial event
3. Phobic disorders
4. Four different types of anxiety commonly thought to be present in patients with cancer
   a) Situational
   b) Psychiatric
   c) Organic
   d) Existential

B. Etiology: Multiple medical conditions
1. Cancer with hormone-producing tumors (e.g., pheochromocytoma), adrenal tumors
2. Cardiovascular conditions: CHF, angina, mitral valve prolapse, new onset of severe hypertension or dysrhythmias
3. Endocrine disorders: Hyperthyroidism, hypothyroidism, hyperglycemia, hypoglycemia, carcinoid syndrome, Cushing syndrome, diabetes
4. Immune and autoimmune conditions: HIV/AIDS, infections, SLE
5. Hematologic conditions: Anemia
6. Metabolic disorders: Hyponatremia, hyperkalemia
7. Respiratory disorders: Hypoxia, pneumonia, PE, asthma
8. Neurologic disorders: Brain lesions, encephalopathy, seizure disorders, cerebrovascular accident, multiple sclerosis, dementia
9. Withdrawal from sedatives, benzodiazepines, or alcohol; use of steroids, stimulants, or neuroleptics
10. Psychological distress from a potential cancer diagnosis or disease progression, the necessary tests and procedures for workup, and/or cancer treatment
11. Treatment issues: Uncontrolled pain or other symptoms
12. Hereditary link: Family history

C. History
1. History of cancer and cancer treatment
2. Current medications: Prescribed, over the counter
3. History of presenting symptoms: Precipitating factors, onset, duration, alleviating factors, associated symptoms (e.g., worry, fear, foreboding thoughts, associated somatic complaints)
4. Changes in ADLs
5. Past medical history: Coping with stress, panic attacks, sexual abuse, psychiatric disorders
6. History of psychosocial situations or anticipated changes: Adaptation to cancer, living conditions, emotional stress

D. Signs and symptoms

    1. Affective symptoms
       a) Nervous behaviors: Pacing, picking, frequent movement, inability to sit still
       b) Edginess
       c) Panic
       d) Terror
    2. Behavioral responses
       a) Avoidance
       b) Compulsions
    3. Cognitive or psychological responses
       a) Recurrent thoughts or worries about diagnosis and treatment
       b) Apprehension about changes in role and function
       c) Obsessions with aspects of care
       d) Fears and worry about the future and death
       e) Thoughts of physical or emotional damage to self
    4. Physical symptoms: Autonomic responses
       a) Tachycardia
       b) Tachypnea or dyspnea
       c) Diaphoresis
       d) Light-headedness/dizziness
       e) Headache
       f) Palpitations, chest pain, tightness
       g) GI distress or "butterflies" in stomach
       h) Restlessness
       i) Difficulty concentrating
       j) Sleep disturbances
  E. Physical examination
    1. General observations: Behaviors and movements such as rapid speech, tremors, and restlessness
    2. Vital signs: Elevated heart rate, blood pressure, respiratory rate, and temperature for possible infection
    3. Integument: Endocrine disorders
       a) Dry, patchy skin with thyroid abnormalities
       b) Facial puffiness with Addison disease
       c) Increased skin pigmentation with Addison disease
       d) Decreased skin turgor with hypernatremia
    4. Oral: Nutritional deficiencies
       a) Dry mouth
       b) Poor dentition
       c) Smooth, glossy, red tongue suggesting vitamin B_{12} and folate deficiencies
    5. Cardiac: Dysrhythmias, cardiac disease
       a) Irregular heartbeat
       b) Abnormal heart sounds
    6. Pulmonary: Decreased air exchange suggestive of pneumonia, pleural effusions, and embolus
    7. Neurologic: Cranial nerve palsies and neuropathies with cranial nerve testing (see Appendix A)

IV. Diagnostic studies (American Psychiatric Association, 2013; NCCN, 2021; Zvolensky et al., 2018)
  A. Laboratory

    1. CBC to assess Hgb and potential infections

    2. Chemistry profile to assess for electrolyte imbalances

    3. TSH to detect thyroid abnormalities

    4. Glucose level to detect hypoglycemia/hyperglycemia

    5. Folate, ferritin, and vitamin B_{12} to detect nutrition deficiencies

    6. Drug screening, such as cocaine

    7. Oxygen saturation to detect hypoxia

  B. Radiology: Depending on examination, may need chest x-ray to rule out pneumonia, pleural effusion, or PE

  C. Other

    1. May need ECG to evaluate for dysrhythmia

    2. Assessment tools for anxiety and depression

      a) Anxiety Sensitivity Index: 16-item self-reported psychological questionnaire used to identify whether a patient is experiencing a general sense of worry or has specific concerns related to symptoms of stress

      b) Depression screening: Anxiety and depression often seen together

V. Differential diagnosis (Gatto et al., 2016; Glass et al., 2018; Latas et al., 2019; Salman et al., 2019)

  A. Endocrine disorders

    1. Hyperglycemia or hypoglycemia (see Chapter 151)

    2. Hyperthyroidism or hypothyroidism (see Chapters 157 and 158)

    3. Carcinoid syndrome

  B. Metabolic disorders

    1. Anemia (see Chapters 113–119)

    2. Hyperkalemia (see Chapter 153)

    3. Hyponatremia (see Chapter 155)

  C. Cardiac disorders

    1. CHF (see Chapter 42)

    2. MI (see Chapter 49)

    3. Atrial fibrillation (see Chapter 45)

    4. Premature ventricular contractions (see Chapter 45)

  D. Pulmonary conditions

    1. Pleural effusion (see Chapter 29)

    2. Pneumonia (see Chapter 30)

    3. PE (see Chapter 33)

    4. Pulmonary edema (see Chapter 32)

    5. Asthma (see Chapter 28)

  E. Immune disorders: Infections, SLE (see Chapter 110)

  F. Rare tumors: Pheochromocytoma, islet cell tumors

  G. Neurologic conditions

    1. Encephalopathy

    2. Brain lesions

    3. Seizure disorders (see Chapter 144)

  H. Withdrawal from alcohol, sedatives, or opioids

  I. Medication induced: Caffeine, steroids, decongestants, bronchodilators, stimulants, thyroid hormone

  J. Uncontrolled symptoms: Pain and dyspnea common

  K. Sleep disorders

  L. Psychological conditions

    1. Stress from workup: Claustrophobia from MRI

2. Fear, particularly in regard to cancer, treatment, and the future
3. Panic disorder
4. Depression/suicidal ideation (see Chapter 162)

VI. Treatment (Chen et al., 2019; DeMartini et al., 2019; Gatto et al., 2016; Glass et al., 2018; Lichtenstein et al., 2019; Loving & Dahlin, 2019; NCCN, 2021; Pary et al., 2019; Pitman et al., 2018; Salman et al., 2019; Salt et al., 2017; Vallerand & Sanoski, 2020)
   A. Treatment must be viewed from the perspective that anxiety in patients with cancer is dynamic and will ebb and flow during treatment, follow-ups, and disease progression. Nonpharmacologic approaches should be used before pharmacologic approaches, particularly with attention to polypharmacy.
   B. Treat per patient request to cope with ongoing diagnosis, particularly as disease advances and patients are faced with end-of-life issues. Some patients will only be able to cope with the issues at hand and not future issues. Thus, the provider must take care not to provide too much information or prescribe more interventions for a patient who is already too anxious and overwhelmed, unless the patient requests otherwise.
   C. Proactively treat patients for anxiety prior to cancer diagnostic testing, such as CT scan or MRI.
   D. Treat uncontrolled symptoms, such as pain or dyspnea.
   E. Discontinue or reduce the dose of potential contributing medications, such as steroids and/or psychostimulants.
   F. Encourage cessation of nicotine. Treat nicotine withdrawal with patch, gum, or sprays. Taper dose according to use and do not exceed maximum dosage and duration.
   G. Encourage abstinence from caffeine.
   H. Treat opioid or benzodiazepine withdrawal with a tapered approach. Cut by one-fourth dose every three to four days.
   I. Pharmacologic therapy
      1. Age dependent: Because of altered metabolism and polypharmacy, use low doses in older adults.
      2. Consider treating anxiety and depression together because they often are a dyad of symptoms.
      3. Common medications used (see Table 161-1)
         a) Short term: Benzodiazepines increase the level of the gamma-aminobutyric acid system to decrease anxiety.
         b) First-line treatment: SSRIs increase the activity of the 5-HT system to reduce anxiety.
         c) Second-line treatment: Tricyclic antidepressants downregulate norepinephrine to reduce anxiety symptoms.
         d) Antipsychotics or azapirones should be considered for refractory symptoms.
   J. Nonpharmacologic therapy
      1. Engage in proactive supportive discussion with patients about their information needs, how they want information provided, and the need for support people to accompany them to visits to alleviate fear.
      2. Provide ongoing education, support, and counseling to patients and families about concrete information to prevent fear of the unknown and acknowledge feelings and fears.
      3. Provide structure and opportunity for control of treatment decisions.
      4. Patient and family education are needed to understand the following.
         a) Anxiety and related manifestations
         b) Medications and side effects
         c) Interference of anxiety on ability to learn, communicate, and problem-solve

TABLE 161-1	Commonly Used Anxiolytic Agents		
Agent	**Conventional Dosages**	**Maximal Dosage**	**Route**
Antihistamines			
Hydroxyzine	25–50 mg every 4–6 hours	150–300 mg daily	PO, IM
Atypical Antipsychotic			
Risperidone	1–3 mg every 12–24 hours	6 mg daily	PO
Azapirones			
Buspirone	5–20 mg three times a day	60 mg daily	PO
Benzodiazepines: Short-Term Therapy			
Alprazolam	0.25–0.5 mg three times a day; titrated to maximum	4 mg daily	PO
Clonazepam (not FDA-approved for anxiety)	0.25–1 mg twice a day	30 mg daily	PO
Diazepam	2.5–10 mg every 4–12 hours	60 mg daily	PO, IV
Lorazepam	0.5–2 mg three times or four times a day	8 mg daily	PO, IV
Oxazepam	10–15 mg three times or four times a day	60 mg daily	PO
Temazepam	15–30 mg at bedtime (labeled for insomnia)	30 mg daily	PO
Selective Serotonin Reuptake Inhibitors: First-Line Therapy			
Citalopram	10–40 mg daily	40 mg daily	PO
Escitalopram	5 mg daily	20 mg daily	PO
Fluoxetine[a]	10–80 mg daily	80 mg daily	PO
Paroxetine[a]	10–60 mg daily	60 mg daily	PO
Sertraline	25–200 mg daily	200 mg daily	PO
Tricyclic Antidepressants			
Imipramine	10–25 mg daily	200 mg daily	PO
Mirtazapine	5–15 mg at night	45 mg daily	PO

[a] Lowers tamoxifen levels

FDA—U.S. Food and Drug Administration; IM—intramuscular; IV—intravenous; PO—by mouth

Note. Based on information from Gatto et al., 2016; Glass et al., 2018; Loving & Dahlin, 2018.

5. Psychotherapy includes counseling, spiritual care, cognitive behavioral therapy, and hypnotherapy.
6. Stress management includes exercise, relaxation, massage, distraction, music and art therapy, yoga, and visualization. Cancer centers, as well as the YMCA/YWCA, offer many support programs, including Livestrong Foundation coping sessions.
7. Environmental manipulation includes safety evaluation of home. Control of daily schedule often is lost to therapy regimens.

8. Adjust and decrease intake of products containing caffeine, such as soda, coffee, and chocolate. Minimize alcohol use.

9. Offer appropriate disease-specific support groups for patients and families who may want to discuss anxieties and fears with other individuals.

VII. Follow-up

A. Assess for side effects and regimen adherence one week following initiation of medications.

B. Depending on medication prescribed, evaluate at three weeks and PRN.

VIII. Referrals

A. Pain specialist: If pain is the major focus of stress, for interventional approaches or general consult to promote proactive management, as well as reassurance of attending to pain reduction

B. Psychologist: To provide counseling, support, and education on behavioral techniques to manage anxiety

C. Psychiatrist: To help with ongoing medication management of stress and anxiety, as well as treatment for panic episodes and suicidal thoughts

D. Social worker: To assess living conditions and family dynamics adding to stress and anxiety and to offer resources to alleviate stress

E. Pharmacist: To review medications for polypharmacy and side effects

F. Physical or occupational therapist: To offer safe exercise strategies and interventions for ongoing management

G. Spiritual provider, chaplain, or parish nurse: To offer spiritual support and counseling and a place to voice concerns

References

American Psychiatric Association. (2013). *Diagnostic and statistical manual of mental disorders* (5th ed.).

Chen, T.-R., Huang, H.-C., Hsu, J.-H., Ouyang, W.-C., & Lin, K.-C. (2019). Pharmacological and psychological interventions for generalized anxiety disorder in adults: A network of meta-analysis. *Journal of Psychiatric Research, 118*, 73–83. https://doi.org/10.1016/j.jpsychires.2019.08.014

DeMartini, J., Patel, G., & Fancher, T.L. (2019). Generalized anxiety disorder. *Annals of Internal Medicine, 170*(7), ITC49–ITC64. https://doi.org/10.7326/AITC201904020

Gatto, M., Thomas, P., & Berger, A. (2016). Anxiety. In C. Dahlin, P.J. Coyne, & B.R. Ferrell (Eds.), *Advanced practice palliative nursing* (pp. 301–310). Oxford University Press.

Glass, S.P., Pollack, M.H., Otto, M.W., Wittmann, C.W., & Rosenbaum, J.F. (2018). Anxious patients. In T.A. Stern, O. Feudenreich, F.A. Smith, G.L. Fricchione, & J.F. Rosenbaum (Eds.), *Massachusetts General Hospital handbook of general hospital psychiatry* (7th ed., pp. 123–139). Elsevier.

Latas, M., Vučinić Latas, D., & Spasić Stojaković, M. (2019). Anxiety disorders and medical illness comorbidity and treatment implications. *Current Opinion in Psychiatry, 32*(5), 429–434. https://doi.org/10.1097/YCO.0000000000000527

Lichtenstein, A.H., Jolliffe, A.B., & Ameli, R. (2019). Psychiatric symptom management in adult and pediatric cancer patients: Anxiety, delirium, and depression. In A.M. Berger, P.S. Hinds, & C.M. Puchalski (Eds.), *Handbook of supportive oncology and palliative care: Whole-person adult and pediatric care* (pp. 131–150). Springer.

Loving, N.G., & Dahlin, C.M. (2019). Anxiety, depression, and delirium. In M. Matzo & D.W. Sherman (Eds.), *Palliative care nursing: Quality care to the end of life* (5th ed., pp. 545–578). Springer.

National Comprehensive Cancer Network. (2021). *NCCN Clinical Practice Guidelines in Oncology (NCCN Guidelines®): Distress management* [v.2.2021]. https://www.nccn.org/professionals/physician_gls/pdf/distress.pdf

Pary, R., Sarai, S.K., Micchelli, A., & Lippmann, S. (2019). Anxiety disorders in older patients. *Primary Care Companion for CNS Disorders, 21*(1), 18nr02335. https://doi.org/10.4088/PCC.18nr02335

Pitman, A., Suleman, S., Hyde, N., & Hodgkiss, A. (2018). Depression and anxiety in patients with cancer. *BMJ, 361,* k1415. https://doi.org/10.1136/bmj.k1415

Salman, J., Wolfe, E., & Patel, S.K. (2019). Anxiety and depression. In B.R. Ferrell & J.A. Paice (Eds.), *Oxford textbook of palliative nursing* (5th ed., pp. 309–318). Oxford University Press.

Salt, S., Mulvaney, C.A., & Preston, N.J. (2017). Drug therapy for symptoms associated with anxiety in adult palliative care patient. *Cochrane Database of Systematic Reviews, 2017*(5). https://doi.org/10.1002/14651858.CD004596.pub3

Vallerand, A.H., & Sanoski, C.A. (2020). *Davis's drug guide for nurses* (17th ed.). F.A. Davis Company.

Zvolensky, M.J., Garey, L., Fergus, T.A., Gallagher, M.W., Viana, A.G., Shepherd, J.M., ... Schmidt, N.B. (2018). Refinement of anxiety sensitivity measurement: The Short Scale Anxiety Sensitivity Index (SSASI). *Psychiatry Research, 269,* 549–557. https://doi.org/10.1016/j.psychres.2018.08.115

CHAPTER 162

Depression

Elena C. Prendergast, DNP, APRN, FNP-C, ACHPN,
and Constance Dahlin, MSN, ANP-BC, ACHPN, FPCN, FAAN

I. Definition (American Psychiatric Association, 2013; Shapero et al., 2018)
   A. Depression is a mood disorder with both psychological (e.g., mood is low, inability to think or make decisions) and somatic symptoms (e.g., altered sleep, fatigue, slowed movements, decreased energy) that alter mood, affect, and personality.
   B. Depression is defined as an episode of two weeks or longer in which there is a loss of interest or pleasure in almost all activities.
   C. Situational depression may occur as a result of various circumstances, including a diagnosis of cancer.
   D. The American Psychiatric Association recognizes depression as a depressive disorder due to another medical condition, which relates to the patient with cancer. This explains that the disorder is related to the circumstances of the direct pathophysiologic consequences of a medical condition, is not explained by a mental disorder, and affects the social interaction of the patient.

II. Physiology/Pathophysiology (Bialek et al., 2019; Li et al., 2016)
   A. Normal: The CNS contains several neurotransmitters, including dopamine, norepinephrine, and serotonin. Stable mood is noted in individuals who have the correct metabolism and balance of the neurotransmitters.
   B. Pathophysiology
      1. Depression results from disruption of neurotransmitters in the CNS.
      2. Many theories suggest that it is caused by insufficient levels of dopamine, norepinephrine, and serotonin, which results in imbalances of neurochemicals, imbalances of neuroendocrine levels, and perhaps alterations in neuroanatomy.

III. Clinical features: Depression is a leading cause of global burden. Multifactorial causes and various etiologies lead to depression. The challenge is that a majority of patients with cancer meet the criteria of depression from their disease condition and treatment without factoring in their mood. Depression may be mild or severe depending on signs and symptoms exhibited, as well as length of time symptoms have been present. Virtually every class of medication can potentially induce or worsen depression (Fernandez-Robles et al., 2018; Folstein et al., 1975; Li et al., 2016; Lichtenstein et al., 2019; Loving & Dahlin, 2019; Michaelides & Zis, 2019; Nasreddine et al., 2005; Ragguett et al., 2019; Pitman et al., 2018; Schuch & Stubbs, 2019; Shapero et al., 2018).
   A. Etiology
      1. Physical causes
         a) Medical conditions

        (1) Endocrine disorders: Hypothyroidism, hyperparathyroidism, diabetes, Cushing disease, Addison disease

        (2) Cardiovascular conditions: CHF, dysrhythmias, infarction

        (3) Neurologic conditions: Dementia, cerebrovascular accident

        (4) Immune disorders: HIV/AIDS, Epstein-Barr virus

        (5) Cancer diagnosis: Lung cancer, due to poor prognosis; pancreatic cancer, due to symptom burden; brain cancer, due to changes in cognitive functioning

        (6) Other: SLE, pain, anemia, alcoholism

    b) Medication induced

        (1) Various chemotherapy agents: Vinca alkaloids, platins, taxanes

        (2) Other cancer treatments: Hormones, immunotherapies, opioids, steroids, inhibitors of kinase-signaling enzymes

        (3) Medications for comorbid conditions: Opioids, benzodiazepines, antihypertensives, cimetidine

    c) Sensory deprivation

    d) Sleep deprivation

  2. Psychological causes

    a) Unresolved conflict or grief

    b) Loss of independence

    c) Change in living situations

    d) Financial situation

    e) Changes in body image

  3. Social causes

    a) Isolation because of disease

    b) Loss of family and friends

    c) Loss of employment

    d) Preexisting conflicted relationships

  4. Biologic causes

    a) Family history

    b) Previous episodes of depression

    c) Neurotransmission deficiencies

    d) CNS effects of cytokines

B. History

  1. History of cancer and cancer treatment

  2. Current medications: Prescribed, over the counter

  3. History of presenting symptoms: Precipitating factors, onset, duration, alleviating factors, associated symptoms (e.g., changes in appetite, sleep, energy, weight, and cognitive functioning; previous episodes of depression or feeling "blue" or "down")

  4. Changes in ADLs

  5. Family history: Other psychiatric symptoms or disorders, depression

  6. Social history: Alcohol use, tobacco use, illicit drug use

C. Signs and symptoms: Triad of symptoms—change in mood, disturbances in self-perception of the environment and future, and regulative physical and behavioral symptoms

  1. Change in mood: Depressed mood

  2. Flat affect

  3. Slow or agitated movements

  4. Injuries: Intentional or unintentional

  5. Breath and sweat that smell of alcohol

  6. Perceptual disturbance of oneself, the environment, and the future

  7. Pain

8. Social avoidance
9. Changes in sleep patterns
10. Changes in sexual drive
11. Lack of interest or pleasure in activities
12. Excessive guilt
13. Lack of energy
14. Lack of concentration
15. Changes in appetite: Increased or decreased
16. Changes in self-worth or self-esteem
17. Increased use or abuse of substances
18. Vegetative and behavioral signs: Lack of focus, crying, staring, irritability
19. At least four accompanying symptoms constitutes diagnosis of depression: Appetite changes; sleep changes; weight changes; psychomotor changes; decreased energy; feelings of worthlessness or guilt; difficulty thinking, concentrating, or decision-making; recurrent thoughts of death; and suicidal ideation or attempts.

D. Physical examination
    1. Cardiac: Cardiac irregularities indicating dysrhythmias
    2. Pulmonary: Changes in breath sounds (e.g., rales, wheezes, rub)
        a) Infection
        b) Obstructive disease
    3. Integument: Dryness or poor skin turgor suggestive of dehydration
    4. Neurologic
        a) Confusion or altered mental status suggesting dementia
        b) Tremors suggestive of neurologic disease, such as Parkinson disease
    5. Cognitive assessment
        a) Mental status examination to screen for cognitive impairment as opposed to depression
            (1) Visuospatial/executive function: Have the patient draw a clock and connect dots.
            (2) Orientation: Ask the patient to identify the day, month, year, season, and setting.
            (3) Memory/recall: Name three items for the patient. Have the patient repeat to remember for later.
            (4) Attention/calculation: Instruct the patient to count backward from 100 by serial 7s, and name patterns of numbers or pictures.
            (5) Abstraction: Ask the patient to identify commonality between two words, such as banana and apple, sandal and boot, or plane and train.
            (6) Language: Instruct the patient to perform the following tasks.
                (a) Identify objects.
                (b) Follow a command.
                (c) Write a sentence.
                (d) Copy a sentence.
        b) Evaluate psychological areas.
            (1) Self-worth
            (2) View of life
            (3) Ability to engage in life
            (4) Ability to find joy in life versus inability to find any joy in life
            (5) Feelings of hopelessness versus optimism
            (6) Interest in world around the patient versus lack of interest
            (7) Suicidality or expression of ideation

IV. Diagnostic studies (Chovan, 2016; Lichtenstein et al., 2019; Loving & Dahlin, 2019; NCCN, 2021; Salman et al., 2019; Wang & Gorenstein, 2013)
   A. Laboratory
      1. CBC to evaluate for dehydration and anemia
      2. Glucose level to evaluate for hyperglycemia suggestive of diabetes
      3. Thyroid profile to evaluate for hypothyroidism
      4. Vitamin B_{12} and folate levels to evaluate for vitamin deficiencies
      5. LFTs for baseline liver function and to evaluate liver failure
      6. BUN and creatinine to evaluate renal function
      7. Venereal Disease Research Laboratory test in older adults to evaluate for syphilis
      8. Enzyme-linked immunosorbent assay (ELISA) or Western blot for HIV testing
      9. Epstein-Barr nuclear antigen for Epstein-Barr virus
   B. Radiology
      1. If short of breath: Chest x-ray to evaluate for infection and lung mass
      2. CT scan of head to evaluate for cerebrovascular accident, tumor, or other brain disorders
   C. Other tests
      1. ECG to evaluate for dysrhythmia
      2. Oxygen saturation to evaluate for hypoxia suggestive of respiratory disorders, such as COPD
   D. Possible depression assessment tools
      1. Screening has not been proven to improve depression outcomes in patients with cancer.
      2. Beck Depression Inventory: Patients complete a 21-item multiple choice questionnaire on how they had been feeling in the past week. A value of 0–3 is assigned for each answer, and the total score is compared to a key to determine the depression's severity.
      3. Simple screening questions
         a) Are you depressed?
         b) In the last month, have you been bothered by feeling down, depressed, hopeless, or in poor spirits?
         c) In the last month, have you been bothered by lack of interest or pleasure in doing things?
         d) Do you feel that life is not worth living?
         e) Have you thought about harming yourself?
         f) Are you thinking about suicide or taking your life?
         g) Do you have a plan?
         h) Have you attempted suicide?

V. Differential diagnosis (Bialek et al., 2019; NCCN, 2021; Salman et al., 2019)
   A. Psychosocial distress: Grief, loss, spiritual distress
   B. Dehydration
   C. Anemia (see Chapters 113–119)
   D. Hypothyroidism (see Chapter 158)
   E. Vitamin deficiencies: Vitamin B_{12} and folate (see Chapters 115 and 116)
   F. Liver failure
   G. Renal failure (see Chapter 83)
   H. Cardiac disease: CHF (see Chapter 42), dysrhythmia (see Chapter 45), MI (see Chapter 49)
   I. Neurologic disorders: Dementia, cerebrovascular accident (see Chapter 146), Parkinson disease, multiple sclerosis, brain lesions, epilepsy

    J. Endocrine disorders: Diabetes mellitus (see Chapter 151), Cushing disease, Addison disease

    K. Respiratory disease: COPD (see Chapter 28)

    L. Infection: HIV, Epstein-Barr virus

    M. Untreated pain or other symptoms: Nausea (see Chapter 63), insomnia

    N. Alcoholism

    O. Anxiety and stress (see Chapter 161)

    P. Cancer

    Q. Medication induced

        1. Antihypertensive drugs: Clonidine, methyldopa, reserpine, beta-blockers, diltiazem

        2. Steroids

        3. Digitalis

        4. H_2 antagonists

        5. Isoniazid

        6. Neuroleptic drugs

        7. Multiphasic oral contraceptives

        8. Sedative–hypnotic drugs

    R. Medication withdrawal

    S. Bipolar disorder

VI. Treatment (Fernandez-Robles et al., 2018; Lichtenstein et al., 2019; Loving & Dahlin, 2019; NCCN, 2021; Ragguett et al., 2019; Riordan et al., 2019; Salman et al., 2019; Schuch & Stubbs, 2019; Schwasinger-Schmidt & Macaluso, 2019)

    A. Treat underlying symptoms, such as pain, dyspnea, and nausea and vomiting, with appropriate opioids and antiemetics. This may help to lift depression and feelings of hopelessness as the patient feels better (see Chapters 24 and 63).

    B. Correct underlying conditions, such as infection, nutritional issues, anemia (see Chapters 113–118), dehydration, and thyroid conditions (see Chapters 157 and 158).

    C. Discontinue potential medications that can cause depression.

    D. Treat symptoms accompanying appropriate medication withdrawal.

    E. Treat other psychiatric conditions, such as anxiety and mood disorders (see Chapter 161).

    F. Pharmacologic therapy: Most antidepressant therapy takes three to four weeks for onset of action to elicit visible changes (see Appendix L).

        1. Consider comorbid conditions in addition to cancer when choosing treatment.

           a) Avoid tricyclic antidepressants in cardiac disease, SSRIs in GI disease, and atypical antidepressants in renal disease.

           b) Dosing considerations exist in hepatic disease.

        2. Psychostimulants may provide quicker relief (within a few days). Patients who exhibit a positive response probably will respond to SSRIs.

           a) Start SSRIs and wean off psychostimulant within two to three weeks when it starts to take effect.

           b) If no response to psychostimulant, try another class of medication.

        3. A medication effective for both anxiety and depression may be needed because both symptoms are seen together.

        4. Mirtazapine may help with depression, anorexia, and insomnia.

        5. Consider side effect profile for older adult patients with cancer.

        6. Medication should not be changed until a trial of six to eight weeks has been given to measure the progress unless the patient is experiencing intolerable side effects. Verify patient is taking medication correctly.

7. Antidepressant therapy should be continued for six months to one year (or longer if necessary) because of risk of recurrence of depression. Patients with two or more episodes of depression should be considered for indefinite maintenance treatment.

8. Taper antidepressant medication when discontinuing instead of abruptly withdrawing.

G. Nonpharmacologic therapy

1. Psychotherapy: Cognitive or behavioral approaches; found to be most effective with pharmacologic management

2. Music therapy

3. Movement therapy: Exercise

4. Pet therapy for self-worth

5. Group activities

6. Acupressure, acupuncture: Working in collaboration with oncology team

7. Massage therapy

8. Patient and family education

    a) Depression and its causes

    b) Risk factors for patients with cancer or chronic disease because of the diagnosis and effect of its treatment

    c) Medication, onset of effect, and side effects

    d) Ongoing safety plan for emergency assistance if the patient is suicidal

9. Exercise programs

H. Interventional therapy: Electroconvulsive therapy is generally reserved for treatment-resistant depression unresponsive to medication or for patients in whom the use of antidepressants is medically contraindicated.

VII. Follow-up

A. Assess patient one week following medication initiation to monitor adherence and side effects. Readminister depression survey and reevaluate suicidality. If the patient is suicidal, immediately arrange for psychiatric evaluation and admission.

B. Assess and evaluate response to medication in three weeks. Readminister depression survey and reevaluate suicidality. If the patient is suicidal, immediately arrange for psychiatric evaluation and admission.

C. Perform monthly reassessment and evaluation of medication along with support.

D. Patients should be monitored closely after termination of treatment since relapse is common.

VIII. Referrals

A. Psychiatrist: For moderate to severe depression and poor response to pharmacologic therapy and/or electroconvulsive therapy

B. Psychologist, psychiatrist, or social worker: Studies show that antidepressant medications concomitant with psychotherapy are efficacious for treatment of depression.

C. Psychiatric emergency service: For urgent evaluation of patients with suicidal intent

References

American Psychiatric Association. (2013). *Diagnostic and statistical manual of mental disorders* (5th ed.).

Bialek, K., Czarny, P., Strycharz, J., & Sliwinski, T. (2019). Major depressive disorders accompanying autoimmune disease—Response to treatment. *Progress in Neuro-Psychopharmacology and Biologic Psychiatry, 95,* 109678. https://doi.org/10.1016/j.pnpbp.2019.109678

Chovan, J.D. (2016). Depression and suicide. In C. Dahlin, P.J. Coyne, & B.R. Ferrell (Eds.), *Advanced practice palliative nursing* (pp. 321–330). Oxford University Press.

Fernandez-Robles, C.G., Irwin, K.E., Pirl, W.F., & Greenberg, D.B. (2018). Patients with cancer. In T.A. Stern, O. Freudenreich, F.A. Smith, G.L. Fricchione, & J.F. Rosenbaum (Eds.), *Massachusetts General Hospital handbook of general hospital psychiatry* (7th ed., pp. 349–358). Elsevier.

Folstein, M.F., Folstein, S.E., & McHugh, P.R. (1975). "Mini-mental state": A practical method for grading the cognitive state of patients for the clinician. *Journal of Psychiatric Research, 12*(3), 189–198. https://doi.org/10.1016/0022-3956(75)90026-6

Li, M., Kennedy, E.B., Byrne, N., Gérin-Lajoie, C., Katz, M.R., Keshavarz, H., ... Green, E. (2016). Management of depression in patients with cancer: A clinical practice guideline. *Journal of Oncology Practice, 12*(8), 747–756. https://doi.org/10.1200/JOP.2016.011072

Lichtenstein, A.H., Jolliffe, A.B., & Ameli, R. (2019). Psychiatric symptom management in adult and pediatric cancer patients: Anxiety, delirium, and depression. In A.M. Berger, P.S. Hinds, & C.M. Puchalski (Eds.), *Handbook of supportive oncology and palliative care: Whole-person adult and pediatric care* (pp. 131–150). Springer.

Loving, N.G., & Dahlin, C.M. (2019). Anxiety, depression, and delirium. In M. Matzo & D.W. Sherman (Eds.), *Palliative care nursing: Quality care to the end of life* (5th ed., pp. 545–578). Springer.

Michaelides, A., & Zis, P. (2019). Depression, anxiety and acute pain: Links and management challenges. *Postgraduate Medicine, 131*(7), 438–444. https://doi.org/10.1080/00325481.2019.1663705

Nasreddine, Z.S., Phillips, N.A., Bédirian, V., Charbonneau, S., Whitehead, V., Collin, I., ... Chertkow, H. (2005). The Montreal Cognitive Assessment, MoCA: A brief screening tool for mild cognitive impairment. *Journal of the American Geriatrics Society, 53*(4), 695–699. https://doi.org/10.1111/j.1532-5415.2005.53221.x

National Cancer Comprehensive Network. (2021). *NCCN Clinical Practice Guidelines in Oncology (NCCN Guidelines®): Distress management* [v.2.2021]. https://www.nccn.org/professionals/physician_gls/pdf/distress.pdf

Pitman, A., Suleman, S., Hyde, N., & Hodgkiss, A. (2018). Depression and anxiety in patients with cancer. *BMJ, 361*, k1415. https://doi.org/10.1136/bmj.k1415

Ragguett, R.-M., Tamura, J.K., & McIntyre, R.S. (2019). Keeping up with the clinical advances: Depression. *CNS Spectrums, 24*(Suppl. 1), 25–37. https://doi.org/10.1017/S1092852919001159

Riordan, P.A., Briscoe, J., Uritsky, T.J., Jones, C.A., & Webb, J.A. (2019). Top ten tips palliative care clinicians should know about psychopharmacology. *Journal of Palliative Medicine, 22*(5), 572–579. https://doi.org/10.1089/jpm.2019.0106

Salman, J., Wolfe, E., & Patel, S.K. (2019). Anxiety and depression. In B.R. Ferrell & J.A. Paice (Eds.), *Oxford textbook of palliative nursing* (5th ed., pp. 309–318). Oxford University Press.

Schuch, F.B., & Stubbs, B. (2019). The role of exercise in preventing and treating depression. *Current Sports Medicine Reports, 18*(8), 299–304. https://doi.org/10.1249/JSR.0000000000000620

Schwasinger-Schmidt, T.E., & Macaluso, M. (2019). Other antidepressants. In M. Macaluso & S.H. Preskorn (Eds.), *Handbook of experimental pharmacology: Vol. 250. Antidepressants: From biogenic amines to new mechanisms of action* (pp. 325–355). Springer. https://doi.org/10.1007/164_2018_167

Shapero, B.G., Cassano, P., Papakostas, G.I., Fava, M., & Stern, T.A. (2018). Depressed patients. In T.A. Stern, O. Freudenreich, F.A. Smith, G.L. Fricchione, & J.F. Rosenbaum (Eds.), *Massachusetts General Hospital handbook of general hospital psychiatry* (7th ed., pp. 69–81). Elsevier.

Wang, Y.-P., & Gorenstein, C. (2013). Psychometric properties of the Beck Depression Inventory-II: A comprehensive review. *Brazilian Journal of Psychiatry, 35*(4), 416–431. https://doi.org/10.1590/1516-4446-2012-1048

CHAPTER 163

Fatigue

Jennifer A. Tschanz, MSN, FNP, AOCNP®, ACHPN

I. Definition: Self-perceived sensation of tiredness or exhaustion (Mustian et al., 2016; Narayanan & Escalante, 2017; NCCN, 2020)
   A. Recent fatigue: Symptoms lasting less than a month
   B. Prolonged fatigue: Symptoms lasting more than a month
   C. Chronic fatigue: Fatigue alone lasting more than six months
   D. Chronic fatigue syndrome: Clinically evaluated, unexplained persistent or relapsing fatigue plus four or more associated symptoms
   E. Cancer-related fatigue: Distressing, persistent, subjective sense of physical, emotional, and/or cognitive tiredness or exhaustion related to cancer or cancer treatment that is not proportional to recent activity and interferes with usual functioning

II. Physiology/Pathophysiology: Exact pathophysiology is not known (Bower, 2014, 2019; O'Higgins et al., 2018; Saligan et al., 2015; Wang & Woodruff, 2015; Yang et al., 2019; Zielinski et al., 2019).
   A. Normal: The body perceives normal energy without a feeling of tiredness. An individual is able to perform ADLs without difficulty and feels refreshed after rest.
   B. Pathophysiology: Cancer-related fatigue is the result of multiple, interactive, altered processes that can be classified as central or peripheral mechanisms based on the system affected.
      1. *Central fatigue* refers to impairments in the ability of the CNS to generate signals that control voluntary movement. Symptoms originate from failure to transmit CNS neuronal impulses and are characterized by inability to complete physical and mental tasks requiring self-motivation and internal cues without notable cognitive failure or motor weakness.
      2. *Peripheral fatigue* refers to muscle exhaustion or inability to perform a task during exertion. It arises from impairments in the peripheral nerves and contracting muscles, such as neuromuscular junction defects, altered muscle metabolites, and peripheral changes in the muscle.
      3. Proposed altered pathways contributing to cancer-related fatigue development and severity include cytokine dysregulation, hypothalamic–pituitary–adrenal axis disruption, circadian rhythm disruption, serotonin dysregulation, vagal afferent nerve activation, muscle metabolism dysregulation, ATP dysregulation, and contractile changes of the muscle.
      4. Inflammation is thought to play a strong role in cancer-related fatigue development. Cancer tumor or cancer therapy can release proinflammatory cytokines that act centrally on the brain causing fatigue and behavioral changes, known as "sickness behavior." These proinflammatory cytokines can also act peripherally by destroying muscle cells, leading to fatigue.

III. Clinical features: Patterns of fatigue must be correlated with symptoms, laboratory data, physical examination findings, and life demands/activities to diagnose cause. Fatigue is a major symptom associated with multiple factors and diseases, including acute and chronic diseases. Cancer-related fatigue differs from fatigue reported by individuals without cancer. It is more severe, more incapacitating, and more persistent than noncancer-related fatigue. Cancer-related fatigue also is not relieved by rest. Fatigue is one of the most distressing symptoms related to cancer and its treatment, affecting 15%–90% of patients with cancer overall and more than 75% of those with advanced cancer or bone metastasis. Fatigue can persist after active treatment is completed as moderate to severe fatigue in survivors. Cancer-related fatigue can be a dose-limiting toxicity (Blitshteyn & Chopra, 2018; Bower, 2014; Bower et al., 2014; Brahmer et al., 2018; Ebede et al., 2017; Koornstra et al., 2014; Mohandas et al., 2017; Narayanan & Escalante 2017; Wang & Woodroff, 2015; Zielinski et al., 2019).

A. Etiology

1. As a symptom or result of cancer

   a) Not present in all patients with advanced disease; not seen at presentation in most early-stage malignancies

   b) Multiple mechanisms suggested and multiple etiologies likely in patients with advanced disease

   (1) Cachexia and anorexia

   (2) Endocrine effects when tumor secretes hormones or interferes with normal endocrine function

   (3) Hypoxia as a result of circulatory or respiratory impairment

   (4) Anemia

   (a) Vessel erosion: Colon cancer, gastric cancer, cervical cancer

   (b) Bone marrow involvement

   (c) Liver involvement

   (d) Inadequate intake or absorption of protein, iron, or folate

   (e) Induction of chemotherapy or radiation therapy

   (5) Renal involvement: May interfere with EPO production

   (6) CNS involvement

   (7) Fluid or electrolyte imbalance

   (8) Infection

   (9) Liver metastasis

   (10) Pain

   (11) Heightened immune system activity in response to tumor

   (12) Uncontrolled symptoms

   (13) PE/pulmonary thrombosis

   (14) Possible sign of disease progression

2. As a side effect of cancer treatment

   a) Bolus chemotherapy–induced fatigue: Peaks within a few days after treatment and gradually declines to lowest point occurring at the next treatment

   b) Molecularly targeted therapy: Monoclonal antibodies, TKIs

   c) Cytokines: IFN, IL-2

   d) Chemotherapy-induced anemia

   e) Steroid-induced muscle mass loss: Prednisone, dexamethasone

   f) Muscle mass loss/deconditioning as a result of decreased physical activity

   g) Decreased endocrine function related to surgery, radiation therapy, chemotherapy, androgen deprivation therapy, antiestrogen therapy, or immune checkpoint inhibitor therapy (e.g., anti–CTLA-4, PD-1 inhibitor, PD-L1 inhibitor)

   h) Sleep disruption

        i) Changes in neurotransmitters
        j) Fluid or electrolyte imbalance
        k) Inadequate nutrition
        l) Infection
        m) Neuropathy
        n) Radiation therapy–induced fatigue: Occurs during the second or third week of treatment, peaks near the end of treatment, and gradually declines (most dramatically in the first four weeks after treatment)
        o) Surgery: Postoperative fatigue
        p) HSCT
   3. Comorbid factors
        a) Cardiac disease: CAD, valve disorder
        b) Respiratory disease: COPD
        c) Neuromuscular disease: Multiple sclerosis, post-polio syndrome
        d) Disorders of the immune system: RA, SLE, Sjögren syndrome
        e) Clinical depression or anxiety
        f) Chronic fatigue syndrome
        g) Anemia
        h) Bleeding unrelated to cancer or cancer treatment
        i) Hormone deficiencies unrelated to cancer or cancer treatment
        j) Hormone excesses unrelated to cancer or cancer treatment
        k) Side effects of medications: Opioids, sedatives, hypnotics, histamine blockers
        l) Acute or chronic renal failure
        m) Liver problems: Cirrhosis, hepatitis
        n) Infection unrelated to cancer or cancer treatment
        o) Obstructive sleep apnea
B. History
   1. History of cancer and cancer treatment: Assess patient's self-report, adjusting timing to type and pattern of treatment; use as cornerstone.
   2. Current medications: Prescribed, over the counter, vitamins, herbal treatments, supplements
   3. History of presenting symptoms: Precipitating factors, onset, duration, associated symptoms (e.g., sleep disturbances, continual sadness, loss of appetite)
        a) Direct questions to relevant time frames, and assess usual and highest levels of fatigue experienced by the patient.
        b) Recommend screening for fatigue at cancer diagnosis, throughout treatment, following completion of cancer treatment, and annually throughout survivorship.
   4. Changes in ADLs: Focus on impact of fatigue rather than the decrease in performing activities.
   5. Past medical history: Depression, childhood adversity, comorbid diseases, trait anxiety, tendency to catastrophize
   6. Family history: Depression or recent losses
   7. Social history: Isolation, loneliness, alcohol use, illicit drug use
C. Signs and symptoms
   1. Cognitive ability
        a) Difficulty concentrating and processing information
        b) Short-term memory loss
        c) Speech difficulty: Problems with finding or combining words
   2. Activity
        a) Change in activity resulting from cancer treatment

        b) Decrease in discretionary activities (e.g., recreation, pastimes); likely takes place before decrease ADLs

    3. Role function

        a) Change in work, play, or study habits

        b) Decline in family interaction

        c) Change in community volunteer activities

        d) Shift in social interaction, such as using the telephone rather than visiting

    4. Affect

        a) Normal transient sadness reflecting patient feeling "out of sorts"

        b) Normal grieving process triggered by patient feeling loss of function as a result of fatigue

        c) Use of synonymous terms, such as weary, sluggish, dragged-out, heavy limbs, slow, tired

D. Physical examination: No specific examination exists to assess fatigue. Focus on identifying abnormalities that point to specific contributing factors that can be managed.

    1. Neurologic: Mental status, cranial nerves (see Appendix A), balance, coordination, sensation, and reflexes to evaluate for brain metastases, brain tumor, SCC, and neuropathy

    2. HEENT: Mouth or throat lesions, enlarged thyroid, unusual discharge from throat or sinuses, and fluid or discharge in ears to evaluate for hypothyroidism, sinusitis, and infection

    3. Musculoskeletal: Focal or generalized weakness, muscle mass loss, joint pain, warm or edematous joints, muscle pain, muscle twitching, new limitations in range of motion, or bone pain indicating arthritis, bone metastases, or FMS

    4. Pulmonary: Adventitious sounds that may indicate pulmonary edema, COPD, or pneumonia

    5. Cardiac: Abnormal heart sounds and JVD that may indicate CHF, anemia, pericarditis, or cardiac tamponade

    6. Abdominal: Hepatomegaly, ascites, pain, tenderness, and abnormal bowel sounds that may indicate obstruction, venous congestion, hepatitis, and cirrhosis

    7. GU: Lesions, pain, unusual discharge, or pelvic mass that may indicate STI or pelvic inflammatory disease

    8. Integument: Jaundice, poor turgor, changes in hair, rash, scratch marks, and lesions that suggest cellulitis, liver disease, dehydration, and hypothyroidism

    9. Lymph: Presence of lymphadenopathy suggesting tumor or infection (see Appendix D)

IV. Diagnostic tests: To determine treatable causes of fatigue (Bower et al., 2014; Brahmer et al., 2018; Ebede et al., 2017; Mustian et al., 2016; Nakano et al., 2018; Wang & Woodruff, 2015; Zielinski et al., 2019)

A. Laboratory

    1. CBC to evaluate for anemia, thrombocytopenia, and neutropenia

    2. Thyroid function panel to evaluate for hypothyroidism or hyperthyroidism

    3. Comprehensive metabolic panel to evaluate for electrolyte imbalances and renal function

    4. Liver function panel to evaluate for abnormalities indicating cirrhosis, hepatitis, or hepatic failure

    5. Urinalysis to evaluate for infection

    6. ESR to evaluate for inflammatory state

    7. Creatine kinase to evaluate muscle pain or weakness

    8. In males, evaluation of testosterone level if hypogonadism is suspected

9. Other appropriate laboratories to confirm or evaluate for primary diagnosis and treatable comorbidities: Epstein-Barr virus, glucose, hepatitis panel

B. Radiology: As appropriate

V. Differential diagnosis: Malignancy and side effects of cancer treatment exclude patients from receiving a diagnosis of chronic fatigue syndrome (Blitshteyn & Chopra, 2018; Richman et al., 2019; Zielinski et al., 2019).

A. Sepsis

B. Dehydration

C. Electrolyte imbalances (see Chapters 152–156)

D. Menopause (see Chapter 90)

E. Sleep disturbances
   1. Sleep apnea (see Chapter 34)
   2. GERD (see Chapter 71)

F. Endocrine disorders
   1. Hypothyroidism (see Chapter 158)
   2. Diabetes mellitus (see Chapter 151)
   3. Pituitary insufficiency
   4. CKD (see Chapter 86)
   5. Hepatic failure

G. Infectious diseases
   1. Endocarditis (see Chapter 46)
   2. Epstein-Barr virus
   3. Hepatitis (see Chapter 74)

H. Cardiopulmonary diseases
   1. CHF (see Chapter 42)
   2. COPD (see Chapter 28)
   3. Pulmonary fibrosis
   4. Peripheral vascular disease (see Chapter 51)

I. Medication use
   1. Sedatives
   2. Analgesics
   3. Hypnotics
   4. Antidepressants (see Appendix L)
   5. Substance abuse
   6. Supplements

J. Psychological disorders
   1. Depression (see Chapter 162)
   2. Anxiety (see Chapter 161)

K. Neurologic impairment: Central and peripheral

VI. Treatment (Bennett et al., 2016; Bower, 2014; Bower et al., 2014; Ebede et al., 2017; Hilfiker et al., 2018; Kelley & Kelley, 2017; Larun et al., 2019; Meneses-Echávez et al., 2015; Mohandas et al., 2017; Mustian et al., 2017; Nakano et al., 2018; NCCN, 2020; Richman et al., 2019; Vilchynska & Beard, 2016; Wang & Woodruff, 2015; Wu et al., 2019)

A. Detection and correction of underlying problems
   1. Determine if fatigue is related to disease recurrence or progression.
   2. Treat infection.
   3. Treat chemotherapy-induced anemia (see Chapters 113–118).
   4. Correct fluid and electrolyte imbalances (see Chapters 152–156).

    5. Correct hormone imbalances.

    6. Correct metabolic and nutritional problems (e.g., diabetes; see Chapter 151), hypothyroidism (see Chapter 158).

    7. Treat clinical depression (see Chapter 162).

    8. Optimize management and minimize self-care burden.

B. Preparatory information

    1. Provide information to patients who are beginning treatment to help them to understand fatigue, interpret it appropriately (i.e., as a treatment side effect rather than a symptom of metastatic cancer), and plan for it. This will decrease disruption in their usual activities.

    2. Include specific information about patterns of fatigue.

    3. Encourage maintaining a diary to determine patterns of energy and fatigue and plan activities accordingly.

    4. Provide reassurance that treatment-related fatigue does not necessarily indicate progression of disease.

    5. During and after cancer treatment, exercise and psychological interventions should be considered as first-line treatments for cancer-related fatigue. Beneficial effects have been observed as compared to pharmaceutical options.

    6. Prepare patients who are completing treatment for persistence of fatigue.

        a) Continue assessment in post-treatment visits.

        b) Assess high levels of post-treatment fatigue against emerging data on late effects of treatment (e.g., cardiomyopathy, declines in endocrine function, persistent symptoms disrupting sleep).

        c) Evaluate post-treatment fatigue in relation to patterns emerging by type of treatment.

    7. At end of life

        a) Fatigue is an expected symptom that can vary in intensity.

        b) Consider eliminating nonessential activities to conserve energy for valued activities.

C. Physical activity

    1. Benefits

        a) Observation studies show that individuals who participate in at least three to five hours of moderate activity per week experience better outcomes and have fewer side effects, including fatigue.

        b) Exercise may reduce cancer-related fatigue by increasing cardiorespiratory fitness, muscle function, psychological well-being, and physical fitness, as well as decreasing inflammation and improving autonomic nervous system function by increasing heart rate variability.

    2. Base exercise prescription on individual assessment of functional capacity and limitations (e.g., physical therapy, exercise physiology, cardiac or pulmonary rehabilitation program).

    3. Prescribe a moderate level of activity.

        a) Encourage moderate aerobic exercise (e.g., fast walking, cycling, swimming) combined with strength and resistance training (e.g., weightlifting).

        b) Begin at a slow pace and progress to moderate intensity.

        c) Consider safety (e.g., risk of falls, limitations due to metastasis or comorbid conditions, anemia, thrombocytopenia, fever or active infection, comorbid illnesses) and refer to physical therapist if needed.

D. Mind–body interventions may reduce fatigue based on stress reduction.

    1. Yoga

    2. Acupuncture

    3. Other: Touch therapy (e.g., biofield therapies), massage, music therapy, Reiki, qigong

4. Relaxation sessions have been noted to be more effective during cancer-related therapy than after completion of treatment.

E. Psychological interventions: Cognitive behavioral therapy, psychoeducational therapy, supportive expressive therapy

1. These interventions may decrease fatigue by increasing and improving coping techniques for managing challenging situations and activities and promoting self-care management.

2. Examples include support groups, counseling, and journal writing.

F. Energy conservation

1. Base level of conservation on individual patient knowledge of patterns of fatigue and activity.

2. Set priorities for maintaining, transferring/delegating, changing, postponing, and abandoning activities.

3. Involve a physical or occupational therapist to help identify alternative ways (e.g., use of assistive devices) of performing desired activities.

4. Learn how to effectively manage other side effects and symptoms (e.g., pain, nausea).

5. Attend one activity at a time.

G. Promoting sleep

1. Limit sleep disruptions (e.g., hospital noise, family interruptions, pain, medication administration).

2. Avoid stimulants (e.g., caffeine-containing medications or foods) prior to sleep.

3. Implement adequate hygiene (e.g., clean bed) and usual bedtime routine, dim lighting, and encourage patients to spend time out of bed prior to sleeping.

4. Use hypnotics appropriately (e.g., short-term basis, lowest effective dose, avoidance of drug interactions, evaluation of side effects).

5. Use appropriate behavioral techniques (e.g., relaxation, imagery).

6. Limit naps to less than an hour to minimize interference with nighttime sleep quality

7. Use bright white light therapy.

8. Treat obstructive sleep apnea (see Chapter 34).

H. Pharmacologic treatment

1. Weak but positive indications for use of psychostimulants exists in patients with advanced disease. Limited evidence of effectiveness has been found in patients without disease after completing therapy.

   a) Methylphenidate: Give 10 mg PO two times a day. Optimal dosing and schedule have not been established for use in patients with cancer.

   b) Modafinil: Give 100 mg PO daily for seven days, and then increase to 200 mg daily.

2. Trial of antidepressants for six to eight weeks may be beneficial if depression is noted with cancer-related fatigue (see Appendix L).

3. If anemia is related to deficiency of vitamin B_{12}, folate, or iron, consider supplementation (see Chapters 115, 116, and 118).

4. A progestational steroid, such as megestrol acetate, may help stimulate appetite for cancer-related fatigue due to anorexia/cachexia (see Chapter 66).

VII. Follow-up

A. Assess outcome of interventions.

1. Compare current level of fatigue to previous levels.

2. Assess target of intervention (e.g., sleep, exercise level, Hgb/hematocrit level).

3. Remember that complex problems (e.g., fatigue) will generate complex intervention plans.

B. Fatigue should be continually assessed through post-treatment visits.

VIII. Referrals: Select resources based on etiology of problem or desired result of intervention.
- A. Physical therapist, exercise physiologist, or rehabilitation program: To encourage exercise
- B. Physical or occupational therapist, homecare organization: To provide home evaluation or consultation for workplace ergonomics to promote energy conservation
- C. Mental health providers: To provide emotional support and cognitive behavioral therapy
- D. Sleep laboratory team: To evaluate for sleep disorders or apnea
- E. Pain/palliative care management teams: To manage side effects
- F. Endocrinologist: To manage adrenal gland or thyroid gland problems
- G. Infectious disease team: To manage sepsis or cellulitis

The author would like to acknowledge Diane G. Cope, PhD, ARNP-BC, AOCNP®, for her contribution to this chapter that remains unchanged from the previous edition of this book.

References

Bennett, S., Pigott, A., Beller, E.M., Haines, T., Meredith, P., & Delaney, C. (2016). Educational interventions for the management of cancer-related fatigue in adults. *Cochrane Database of Systematic Reviews, 2016*(11). https://doi.org/10.1002/14651858.CD008144.pub2

Blitshteyn, S., & Chopra, P. (2018). Chronic fatigue syndrome: From chronic fatigue to more specific syndromes. *European Neurology, 80*(1–2), 73–77. https://doi.org/10.1159/000493531

Bower, J.E. (2014). Cancer-related fatigue—Mechanisms, risk factors, and treatments. *Nature Reviews Clinical Oncology, 11*(10), 597–609. https://doi.org/10.1038/nrclinonc.2014.127

Bower, J.E., Bak, K., Berger, A., Breitbart, W., Escalante, C.P., Ganz, P.A., ... Jacobsen, P.B. (2014). Screening, assessment, and management of fatigue in adult survivors of cancer: An American Society of Clinical Oncology clinical practice guideline adaptation. *Journal of Clinical Oncology, 32*(17), 1840–1850. https://doi.org/10.1200/JCO.2013.53.4495

Bower, J.E. (2019). The role of neuro-immune interactions in cancer-related fatigue: Biobehavioral risk factors and mechanisms. *Cancer, 125*(3), 353–364. https://doi.org/10.1002/cncr.31790

Brahmer, J.R., Lacchetti, C., Schneider, B.J., Atkins, M.B., Brassil, K.J., Caterino, J.M., ... Thompson, J.A. (2018). Management of immune-related adverse events in patients treated with immune checkpoint inhibitor therapy: American Society of Clinical Oncology clinical practice guideline. *Journal of Clinical Oncology, 36*(17), 1714–1768. https://doi.org/10.1200/JCO.2017.77.6385

Ebede, C.C., Jang, Y., & Escalante, C.P. (2017). Cancer-related fatigue in cancer survivorship. *Medical Clinics of North America, 101*(6), 1085–1097. https://doi.org/10.1016/j.mcna.2017.06.007

Hilfiker, R., Meichtry, A., Eicher, M., Balfe, L.N., Knols, R.H., Verra, M.L., & Taeymans, J. (2018). Exercise and other non-pharmaceutical interventions for cancer-related fatigue in patients during or after cancer treatment: A systematic review incorporating an indirect-comparisons meta-analysis. *British Journal of Sports Medicine, 52*(10), 651–658. https://doi.org/10.1136/bjsports-2016-096422

Kelley, G.A., & Kelley, K.S. (2017). Exercise and cancer-related fatigue in adults: A systematic review of previous systematic reviews with meta-analysis. *BMC Cancer, 17*, 693. https://doi.org/10.1186/s12885-017-3687-5

Koornstra, R.H.T., Peters, M., Donofrio, S., van den Borne, B., & de Jong, F.A. (2014). Management of fatigue in patients with cancer—A practical overview. *Cancer Treatment Reviews, 40*(6), 791–799. https://doi.org/10.1016/j.ctrv.2014.01.004

Larun, L., Brurberg, K.G., Odgaard-Jensen, J., & Price, J.R. (2019). Exercise therapy for chronic fatigue syndrome. *Cochrane Database Systematic Reviews, 2019*(10). https://doi.org/10.1002/14651858.CD003200.pub8

Meneses-Echávez, J.F., González-Jiménez, E., & Ramírez-Vélez, R. (2015). Effects of supervised multimodal exercise interventions on cancer-related fatigue: Systematic review and meta-analysis of randomized controlled trials. *Biomed Research International, 2015*, 328636. https://doi.org/10.1155/2015/328636

Mohandas, H., Jaganthan, S.K., Mani, M.P., Ayyar, M., & Rohini Thevi, G.V. (2017). Cancer-related fatigue treatment: An overview. *Journal of Cancer Research and Therapeutics, 13*(6), 916–929. https://doi.org/10.4103/jcrt.JCRT_50_17

Mustian, K.M., Alfano, C.M., Heckler, C., Kleckner, A.S., Kleckner, I.R., Leach, C.R., ... Miller, S.M. (2017). Comparison of pharmaceutical, psychological, and exercise treatments for cancer-related fatigue: A meta-analysis. *JAMA Oncology, 3*(7), 961–968. https://doi.org/10.1001/jamaoncol.2016.6914

Mustian, K.M., Cole, C.L., Lin, P.J., Asare, M., Fung, C., Janelsins, M.C., ... Magnuson, A. (2016). Exercise recommendations for the management of symptom clusters resulting from cancer and cancer treatments. *Seminars in Oncology Nursing, 32*(4), 383–393. https://doi.org/10.1016/j.soncn.2016.09.002

National Comprehensive Cancer Network. (2020). *NCCN Clinical Practice Guidelines in Oncology (NCCN Guidelines®): Cancer-related fatigue* [v.1.2021]. https://www.nccn.org/professionals/physician_gls/pdf/fatigue.pdf

Nakano, J., Hashizume, K., Fukushima, T., Ueno, K., Matsuura, E., Ikio, Y., … Kusuba, Y. (2018). Effects of aerobic and resistance exercises on physical symptoms in cancer patients: A meta-analysis. *Integrative Cancer Therapies, 17*(4), 1048–1058. https://doi.org/10.1177/1534735418807555

Narayanan, S., & Escalante, C.P. (2017). Clinical assessment and management of cancer-related fatigue. *Journal of Clinical Outcomes Management, 24*(5), 217–228. https://www.mdedge.com/jcomjournal/article/145928/clinical-assessment-and-management-cancer-related-fatigue

O'Higgins, C.M., Brady., B., O'Connor, B., Walsh, D., & Reilly, R.B. (2018). The pathophysiology of cancer-related fatigue: Current controversies. *Supportive Care in Cancer, 26*(10), 3353–3364. https://doi.org/10.1007/s00520-018-4318-7

Richman, S., Morris, M.C., Broderick, G., Craddock, T.J.A., Klimas, N.G., & Fletcher, M.A. (2019). Pharmaceutical interventions in chronic fatigue syndrome: A literature-based commentary. *Clinical Therapeutics, 41*(5), 798–805. https://doi.org/10.1016/j.clinthera.2019.02.011

Saligan, L.N., Olson, K., Filler, K., Larkin, D., Cramp, F., Sriram, Y., … Mustian, K. (2015). The biology of cancer-related fatigue: A review of the literature. *Supportive Care in Cancer, 23*(8), 2461–2478. https://doi.org/10.1007/s00520-015-2763-0

Vilchynska, T., & Beard, B. (2016). Cancer-related fatigue in palliative care: A global perspective. *International Journal of Palliative Nursing, 22*(5), 244–252. https://doi.org/10.12968/ijpn.2016.22.5.244

Wang, X.S., & Woodruff, J.F. (2015). Cancer-related and treatment-related fatigue. *Gynecologic Oncology, 136*(3), 446–452. https://doi.org/10.1016/j.ygyno.2014.10.013

Wu, C., Zheng, Y., Duan, Y., Lai, X., Cui, S., Xu, N., … Lu, L. (2019). Nonpharmacological interventions for cancer-related fatigue: A systematic review and Bayesian network meta-analysis. *Worldviews on Evidence-Based Nursing, 16*(2), 102–110. https://doi.org/10.1111/wvn.12352

Yang, S., Chu, S., Gao, Y., Ai, Q., Liu, Y., Li, X., & Chen, N. (2019). A narrative review of cancer-related fatigue (CRF) and its possible pathogenesis. *Cells, 8*(7), 738. https://doi.org/10.3390/cells8070738

Zielinski, M.R., Systrom, D.M., & Rose, N.R. (2019). Fatigue, sleep, and autoimmune and related disorders. *Frontiers in Immunology, 10*, 1827. https://doi.org/10.3389/fimmu.2019.01827

CHAPTER 164

Phlebitis

Laurl A. Matey, MSN, RN–BC, CHPN

I. Definition: Inflammation of a vein (Amano & Shimizu, 2018; Di Nisio et al., 2018; Kim et al., 2019; Nyika et al., 2018)
   A. Superficial thrombophlebitis
      1. Thrombophlebitis: One or more clots in a superficial vein with inflammation of the vein wall
      2. Mondor disease: An uncommon disorder of superficial thrombophlebitis in the anterolateral thoracoabdominal wall, usually benign and self-limiting
   B. Pylephlebitis: Septic thrombophlebitis of the portal vein system
   C. Suppurative (septic) thrombophlebitis: Venous thrombosis associated with vein cannulation and in the setting of bacteremia
   D. Phlebitis
      1. Mechanical irritation of the vein wall from the presence of a catheter
      2. Chemical irritation from high acidic or alkaline solution

II. Physiology/Pathophysiology (Di Nisio et al., 2018; Ho et al., 2018; Nyika et al., 2018)
   A. Normal
      1. Veins have three layers, as well as valves, to prevent backward circulation.
      2. The portal vein is formed by the union of the superior mesenteric and splenic veins. The portal system moves blood from the GI tract to the liver.
   B. Pathophysiology
      1. Superficial phlebitis
         a) Superficial phlebitis occurs spontaneously or secondarily to some form of irritant or trauma. Dehydration may contribute because of increased blood viscosity.
         b) Superficial thrombophlebitis includes the presence of a thrombus of the superficial tributary veins; superficial vein thrombosis includes the axial veins, with increased risk for extension to the deeper vein system.
         c) Inflammatory process is initiated by the release of serotonin, bradykinin, and histamine, causing vasodilation, vascular permeability, and protein and plasma shift toward the interstitial space and leading to edema.
         d) Platelet aggregation is stimulated by histamine resulting in inflammation along the vein wall, causing erythema and a palpable vascular cord.
      2. Pylephlebitis: Usually a result of an infection, ischemic bowel, or ascites, which results in venous stasis of the portal venous system
      3. Suppurative thrombophlebitis: Inflammation and pus formation within the vein wall

III. Clinical features: Superficial thrombophlebitis of the lower limbs is common, estimated at 0.64 per 1,000 diagnosed annually. It affects women more than men, increases in incidence with age for both genders, and is closely associated with concurrent DVT or PE at diagnosis or within the first three months after diagnosis. Suppurative thrombophlebitis is uncommon in the absence of venipuncture or catheterization and is suspected when persistent bacteremia is present after 72 hours of antimicrobial therapy. Phlebitis and thrombosis of the lower extremity superficial veins is generally a benign self-limiting disorder (Cannegieter et al., 2015; Di Nisio et al., 2018; Frappé et al., 2014; Ho et al., 2018; Nyika et al., 2018).

A. Etiology
   1. Current or recent IV catheter use
   2. Irritant medications or solutions
   3. Infection or dehydration
   4. DVT
   5. Hypercoagulable state or malignancy
   6. Varicose veins, vein excision/ablation, prior thrombosis
   7. Venous stasis
   8. Immobilization

B. History
   1. History of cancer and cancer treatment
   2. Current medications: Prescribed, over the counter
   3. History of presenting symptoms: Precipitating events, location, duration, associated symptoms (e.g., fever, pain)
   4. Changes in ADLs
   5. Recent history of IV therapy

C. Signs and symptoms
   1. Warmth, erythema, tenderness, and swelling along vein wall
   2. Hard cord-like area along the vein
   3. Purulent drainage
   4. Fever
   5. Pain at the location of involved vein

D. Physical examination
   1. Vital signs: Temperature to evaluate for fever
   2. Extremities: Inflammation of the vein on palpation; area of induration measurement; presence of a cord when extremity is raised suggestive of thrombus
   3. Abdominal: Abdomen tenderness or organomegaly on palpation

IV. Diagnostic tests (Bonar et al., 2017; Di Nisio et al., 2018; Frappé et al., 2014)
   A. Laboratory
      1. Cultures of any purulent drainage
      2. CBC, platelets, ANC: Leukocytosis may occur.
      3. Anticoagulation studies, as indicated
         a) Protein C and protein S levels to assess for deficiency
         b) Antithrombin III
         c) Prothrombin mutation
         d) Homocysteine levels
         e) Factor V Leiden mutation
         f) IgG, IgM, IgA anticardiolipin antibodies
      4. Blood cultures to isolate organism, in the presence of fever with abdominal pain or as indicated
   B. Radiology
      1. CT scan of abdomen to evaluate for abscess, obstruction, ascites, or portal vein thrombosis

2. Duplex ultrasound to evaluate for the presence, location, and the extent of vein thrombosis (either superficial or deep venous thrombosis)

V. Differential diagnosis (Bonar et al., 2017; Cannegieter et al., 2015; Di Nisio et al., 2018)
   A. DVT (see Chapter 43)
   B. Extravasation from vesicant agents
   C. Inflammatory bowel disease, infarction, or obstruction (see Chapter 67)
   D. Cutaneous TB
   E. Erythema nodosum
   F. Nodular granulomatous phlebitis
   G. Diverticulitis (see Chapter 70)
   H. Insect bite
   I. Lymphangitis
   J. Blood clotting disorders

VI. Treatment (Beyer-Westendorf et al., 2017; Di Nisio et al., 2018; Kim et al., 2019)
   A. Uncomplicated superficial thrombophlebitis: Goal is reduction of symptoms and prevention of extension into venous system.
      1. Elevation, warm or cool soaks: If phlebitis from a peripherally inserted catheter (PICC) is not resolved within 48–72 hours, consider discontinuing line.
      2. Prophylactic dose fondaparinux should be considered for patients with leg involvement and low risk anatomical for DVT; efficacy may vary depending on underlying risk factors.
      3. Vein ligation should be considered for patients with recurrent thrombophlebitis.
   B. Pain: Administer NSAIDs (see Appendix E).
   C. Pylephlebitis
      1. Consider anticoagulation if patient is in a hypercoagulable state (see Chapter 122).
      2. Order antibiotics per blood culture results (see Appendix C). Pylephlebitis is often polymicrobial.
   D. Suppurative phlebitis: Remove source, order antibiotics, and consider anticoagulation therapy.

VII. Follow-up: Assess the peripheral phlebitis in 48–72 hours to ensure healing.

VIII. Referral: Refer to a dermatologist or internist for consultation if poor healing.

The author would like to acknowledge Dawn Camp-Sorrell, MSN, FNP, AOCN®, for her contribution to this chapter that remains unchanged from the previous edition of this book.

References

Amano, M., & Shimizu, T. (2018). Mondor's disease: A review of the literature. *Internal Medicine, 57*(18), 2607–2612. https://doi.org/10.2169/internalmedicine.0495-17

Beyer-Westendorf, J., Schellong, S.M., Gerlach, H., Rabe, E., Weitz, J.I., Jersemann, K., ... Bauersachs, R. (2017). Prevention of thromboembolic complications in patients with superficial vein thrombosis given rivaroxaban or fondaparinux: The open-label, randomised, non-inferiority SURPRISE phase 3b trial. *Lancet Haematology, 4*(3), e105–e113. https://doi.org/10.1016/S2352-3026(17)30014-5

Bonar, R.A., Lippi, G., & Favaloro, E.J. (2017). Overview of hemostasis and thrombosis and contribution of laboratory testing to diagnosis and management of hemostasis and thrombosis disorders. In E.J. Favaloro & G. Lippi (Eds.), *Methods in molecular biology: Vol. 1646. Hemostasis and thrombosis: Methods and protocols* (pp. 3–27). Springer. https://doi.org/10.1007/978-1-4939-7196-1_1

Cannegieter, S.C., Horváth-Puhó, E., Schmidt, M., Dekkers, O.M., Pedersen, L., Vandenbroucke, J.P., & Sørensen, H.T. (2015). Risk of venous and arterial thrombotic events in patients diagnosed with superficial vein thrombosis: A nationwide cohort study. *Blood, 125*(2), 229–235. https://doi.org/10.1182/blood-2014-06-577783

Di Nisio, M., Wichers, I.M., & Middeldorp, S. (2018). Treatment for superficial thrombophlebitis of the leg. *Cochrane Database of Systematic Reviews, 2018*(2). https://doi.org/10.1002/14651858.CD004982.pub6

Frappé, P., Buchmuller-Cordier, A., Bertoletti, L., Bonithon-Kopp, C., Couzan, S., Lafond, P., ... Décousus, H. (2014). Annual diagnosis rate of superficial vein thrombosis of the lower limbs: The STEPH community-based study. *Journal of Thrombosis and Haemostasis, 12*(6), 831–838. https://doi.org/10.1111/jth.12575

Ho, V.T., Rothenberg, K.A., McFarland, G., Tran, K., & Aalami, O.O. (2018). Septic pulmonary emboli from peripheral suppurative thrombophlebitis: A case report and literature review. *Vascular and Endovascular Surgery, 52*(8), 633–635. https://doi.org/10.1177/1538574418779469

Kim, J.H., Kwon, H.Y., & Durey, A. (2019). Thrombophlebitis of superior mesenteric vein with bacteremia of *Gemella sanguinis* and *Streptococcus gordonii*. *Journal of Microbiology, Immunology and Infection, 52*(4), 672–673. https://doi.org/10.1016/j.jmii.2018.06.001

Nyika, M.L., Mukona, D., & Zvinavashe, M. (2018). Factors contributing to phlebitis among adult patients admitted in the medical-surgical units of a central hospital in Harare, Zimbabwe. *Journal of Infusion Nursing, 41*(2), 96–102. https://doi.org/10.1097/NAN.0000000000000265

Appendices

Appendix A. Cranial Nerves

Cranial Nerve	Function	Examination Technique	Deficit Examples
I. Olfactory	Sensory: Smell	Test ability to identify aromatic odors one nostril at a time. Patient must have eyes closed. Use substances such as tobacco, alcohol, peppermint, or lemon. Commercially prepared smell kits are available.	Inflammation of the mucous membranes, allergic rhinitis, and excessive smoking that may interfere with ability to smell Abnormalities: Trauma or olfactory tract lesion; viral infections
II. Optic	Sensory: Visual acuity and visual fields	Test acuity with Snellen chart and Rosenbaum near-vision chart. Perform ophthalmoscopic examination of fundi. Test peripheral fields by confrontation. Cover one eye at a time and have patient look at your eye. Have patient point to the finger that is moving. Compare patient's response to the time you first noted the movement. Check pupillary reaction to light.	Decreased visual acuity from drugs or compression from tumor of nerve, eye, or optic radiation within the brain Retinal ischemia, cataracts, glaucoma, nystagmus
III. Oculomotor	Motor: Raising eyelids, extraocular movement	Assess pupillary reaction to accommodation; note ability to follow moving objects.	Inability to adduct, elevate, and depress the eye Ptosis and nonreactive pupil
IV. Trochlear	Motor: Eye movement	Observe extraocular movements in the six cardinal points of gaze: (1) to the right, (2) upward to the right of midline, (3) downward to the right of midline, (4) to the left, (5) upward to the left of the midline, and (6) downward to the left of the midline.	Unable to perform extraocular movements Unilateral third-nerve palsy Horner syndrome as a result of bronchogenic carcinoma with superior cervical ganglion involvement
V. Trigeminal	Motor: Jaw Sensory: Ophthalmic branch, maxillary branch, mandibular branch	Inspect face for muscle atrophy and tremors. Palpate jaw for strength with jaw clenched. Test for superficial pain and touch sensation with patient's eyes closed. Test corneal reflex if previous test results are abnormal.	Loss of corneal reflex with or without impaired sensation suggestive of cerebellopontine angle tumors Numbness of face indicating possible neuropathy or brain stem tumor Trismus indicating possible oral cavity or oropharyngeal tumor Trismus or muscle spasm of mandible indicating possible drug reaction, such as with phenothiazine Deviation of mandible related to possible paralysis after a stroke

(Continued on next page)

Appendix A. Cranial Nerves *(Continued)*

Cranial Nerve	Function	Examination Technique	Deficit Examples
VI. Abducens	Motor: Lateral eye movement	Observe for lateral eye movement.	Nerve VI is the first function to be lost in the presence of increased intracranial pressure.
VII. Facial	Motor: Muscles of face Sensory: Anterior tongue, ear canal, postauricular area	Inspect symmetry of facial features. Ask patient to smile, wrinkle forehead, show teeth, and close eyes. Test ability to identify salty and sweet tastes.	Weakness of face Fasciculation Facial asymmetry indicative of possible stroke, tumor, nerve compression, or inflammatory paralysis Inability to raise eyebrows, squeeze eyes shut, or purse lips indicative of possible peripheral facial palsy (lower motor neuron) and central facial palsy (upper motor neuron)
VIII. Acoustic 1. Vestibular 2. Cochlear or auditory	Sensory: Hearing acuity, equilibrium	Test hearing acuity with whisper test. Compare bone and air conduction (Rinne test). Test sound lateralization (Weber test).	Ototoxic drugs that alter hearing acuity Hearing loss or impairment from tumors in the external auditory canal, middle ear, inner ear, or central auditory pathways or secondary to chemotherapy, cerumen impaction, chronic infection, or radiation damage Vertigo from lesions of the vestibular, visual, or somatosensory system or vestibular dysfunction Weber test: Sound lateralizes to the poor ear in conduction loss. Sound lateralizes to the good ear in sensorineural loss. Bone conduction greater than air conduction indicates organ damage.
IX. Glossopharyngeal	Motor: Swallowing Sensory: Gag, taste	Test ability to identify sour and bitter tastes. Test gag reflex.	Difficulty swallowing indicative of possible tumor obstruction or stroke Neurologic impairments affecting swallowing
X. Vagus	Motor: Phonation and swallowing Sensory: Sensation behind ear and external ear canal	Inspect palate and uvula for symmetry with speech sounds. Observe gag reflex. Evaluate speech quality.	Difficulty swallowing indicative of possible neurologic impairment, obstruction, or stroke Asymmetry of the uvula indicative of possible stroke or severe mucositis Hoarseness indicative of possible injury to the recurrent laryngeal nerve

(Continued on next page)

Appendix A. Cranial Nerves *(Continued)*

Cranial Nerve	Function	Examination Technique	Deficit Examples
XI. Spinal accessory	Motor: Turning head and shrugging shoulders	Test trapezius muscle strength. Test sternocleidomastoid muscle strength.	Decreased strength from tumor invasion, injury, or surgery Inability to shrug shoulders
XII. Hypoglossal	Motor: Movement of tongue	Inspect tongue for symmetry, tremors, and atrophy. Inspect tongue movement. Test tongue strength.	Tongue deviating to side of weakness indicative of possible stroke or tumor Difficulty controlling tongue or difficulty chewing and swallowing indicative of stroke, severe mucositis, or tumor invasion Fasciculation of tongue indicative of a lower motor neuron lesion

Note. Based on information from Ball, J.W., Dains, J.E., Flynn, J.A., Solomon, B.S., & Stewart, R.W. (2019). *Seidel's guide to physical examination: An interprofessional approach* (9th ed.). Elsevier Mosby; Bickley, L.S. (2020). *Bates' guide to physical examination and history taking* (13th ed.). Lippincott Williams and Wilkins.

Appendix B. Dermatomes of the Body

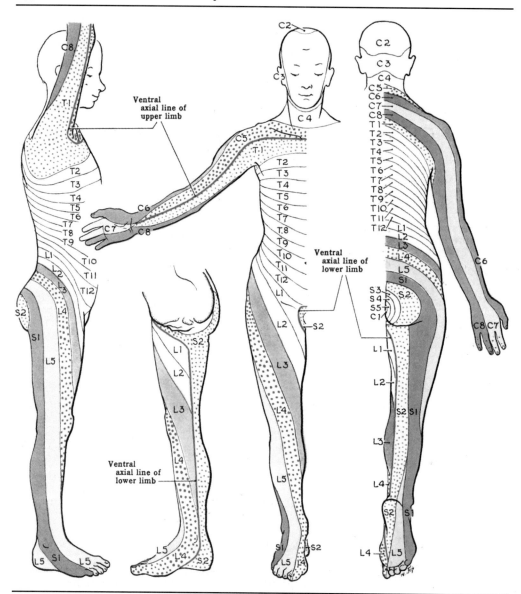

Note. From "An Atlas of Anatomy/by Regions," by J.C.B. Grant, 1962 (https://commons.wikimedia.org/wiki/File:Grant_1962_663.png), licensed under CC BY-SA 3.0 (https://creativecommons.org/licenses/by-sa/3.0/deed.en).

Appendix C. Antibiotics and Treatment of Selected Organisms[a]

Site of Infection	Most Common Etiology	Primary Antibiotics	Alternative Antibiotics
Brain			
Meningitis, aseptic	Enterovirus	None; IV fluids and analgesics	–
Meningitis, bacterial	*Streptococcus pneumoniae, Pseudomonas aeruginosa*, meningococci, *Listeria*, gram-negative bacilli	Empiric therapy: Ceftriaxone 2 g IV every 12 hours or cefepime 2 g IV every 8 hours and vancomycin 15–20 mg/kg actual body weight every 12 hours to achieve trough vancomycin concentration of 15–20 mcg/ml (combination therapy for *S. pneumoniae*) +/- ampicillin 2 g IV every 4 hours Tailor therapy to pathogens and susceptibilities, as necessary.	Extended-spectrum beta-lactamases resistance suspected: Switch ceftriaxone to meropenem 2 g IV every 8 hours.
Breast			
Mastitis	*Staphylococcus aureus*	Dicloxacillin 500 mg PO every 6 hours or cephalexin 500 mg every 6 hours	MRSA suspected: TMP/SMX double strength (160 mg/800 mg) 1–2 tablets PO two times a day Vancomycin • Dosing: 15–20 mg/kg IV every 12 hours • Goal trough: 15–20 mcg/ml
Ear			
Otitis externa	*S. aureus, Pseudomonas*	Acetic acid 2% otic solution, 3–5 drops instilled into affected ear(s) every 4–6 hours Ciprofloxacin 0.2%/hydrocortisone 1% otic solution, 3 drops instilled into affected ear(s) two times a day Ciprofloxacin 0.3%/dexamethasone 0.1% otic solution, 4 drops into affected ear(s) two times a day Ofloxacin 0.3% otic solution, 10 drops instilled into affected ear(s) daily Polymyxin B, neomycin, and hydrocortisone otic suspension, 3–4 drops instilled into affected ear(s) three to four times a day Duration of therapy generally 7–14 days	Systemic therapy should only be reserved for cellulitis, immunocompromised populations, and systemic symptoms. Dicloxacillin 500 mg PO four times a day Ciprofloxacin 500 mg PO two times a day Consider IV antipseudomonal beta-lactam agents for necrotizing otitis externa.
Otitis media	*S. pneumoniae, Haemophilus influenzae*	Amoxicillin 80–90 mg/kg/day PO every 12 hours Cefdinir 14 mg/kg/day; can split into two divided doses	Ceftriaxone 50 mg/kg IM or IV daily for 1–3 days; maximum 1 g daily

(Continued on next page)

Appendix C. Antibiotics and Treatment of Selected Organisms[a] *(Continued)*

Site of Infection	Most Common Etiology	Primary Antibiotics	Alternative Antibiotics
Ear *(cont.)*			
Mastoiditis	*S. aureus, Enterobacteriaceae*	Imipenem 500 mg IV every 6 hours and vancomycin 20 mg/kg IV every 12 hours to achieve trough vancomycin concentration of 15–20 mcg/ml	–
Eye			
Conjunctivitis	*Staphylococcus, Streptococcus, H. influenzae, Moraxella*	Polymyxin B and TMP ophthalmic solution 1–2 drops into affected eye(s) four times a day for 7 days Ofloxacin ophthalmic solution, 1–2 drops into affected eye(s) four times a day for 7 days	Gentamicin ophthalmic ointment applied four times a day to affected eye for 7 days or solution, 1–2 drops four times a day for 7 days Erythromycin ophthalmic ointment applied four times a day to affected eye(s) for 7 days Ointments may blur vision for 10–20 minutes after application.
Gastrointestinal			
Cholecystitis, biliary sepsis, common duct obstruction	*Enterobacteriaceae enterococcus*	Community acquired, mild to moderate: Ceftriaxone 1 g IV daily +/- metronidazole 500 mg IV every 12 hours Severe community-acquired and any severity healthcare acquired: Piperacillin/tazobactam 3.375 g IV every 6 hours or meropenem 1 g IV every 8 hours or cefepime 1 g IV every 8 hours plus metronidazole 500 mg IV every 12 hours	Empirically add vancomycin to other agents for healthcare acquired. • Dosing: 15 mg/kg IV every 12 hours • Goal trough: 15–20 mcg/ml
Diverticulitis	*Enterobacteriaceae*	Mild to moderate: Ceftriaxone 1 g IV daily plus metronidazole 500 mg IV every 12 hours or ertapenem 1 g IV daily	Ciprofloxacin 400 mg IV every 12 hours plus metronidazole 500 mg IV every 12 hours
Gastroenteritis	*Clostridium difficile*	Initial infection, nonsevere and severe: Vancomycin 125 mg PO four times a day for 10 days or fidaxomicin 200 mg PO two times a day for 10 days If agent unavailable or resistant, metronidazole 500 mg PO three times a day for 10–14 days First recurrence • Vancomycin 125 mg PO four times a day for 10 days if metronidazole was used for the initial episode	Initial infection, complicated by hypotension, sepsis, or ileus: Vancomycin 500 mg PO four times a day with metronidazole 500 mg IV every 8 hours

(Continued on next page)

Appendix C. Antibiotics and Treatment of Selected Organisms[a] *(Continued)*

Site of Infection	Most Common Etiology	Primary Antibiotics	Alternative Antibiotics
Gastrointestinal *(cont.)*			
Gastroenteritis *(cont.)*		• Or a prolonged tapered and pulsed vancomycin regimen if a standard regimen was used for the initial episode (e.g., 125 mg PO four times a day for 10–14 days, two times a day for 7 days, once daily for a week, and then every 2–3 days for 2–8 weeks) • Or fidaxomicin 200 mg PO two times a day for 10 days if vancomycin was used for the initial episode	
Peritonitis (spontaneous bacterial peritonitis)	*E. enterococcus*	Cefotaxime or ceftazidime 2 g IV every 8 hours or ceftriaxone 2 g IV daily	Piperacillin/tazobactam 3.375 g IV every 6 hours for severe infection
Secondary (e.g., bowel perforation)	*E. enterococcus*	Mild to moderate: Ceftriaxone 1 g IV daily plus metronidazole 500 mg IV every 12 hours or ertapenem 1 g IV daily Severe: Piperacillin/tazobactam 3.375 g IV every 6 hours or cefepime 1 g IV every 8 hours plus metronidazole 500 mg IV every 12 hours	Ciprofloxacin 400 mg IV every 12 hours plus metronidazole 500 mg IV every 12 hours
Genitourinary			
Prostatitis, acute	*Enterobacteriaceae*	Ciprofloxacin 500 mg PO two times a day for 4–6 weeks or levofloxacin 500 mg PO daily for 4–6 weeks	TMP/SMX double strength (160 mg/800 mg) 1 tablet PO two times a day
Prostatitis, chronic	*Enterobacteriaceae*	Ciprofloxacin 500 mg PO twice a day for 4–6 weeks or levofloxacin 500 mg PO every 24 hours for 4–6 weeks	TMP/SMX double strength (160 mg/800 mg) 1 tablet PO two times a day
Urinary tract infection (cystitis and pyelonephritis)	*Escherichia coli*	Uncomplicated cystitis: TMP/SMX double strength (160 mg/800 mg), 1 tablet PO two times a day for 3 days or nitrofurantoin monohydrate 100 mg PO two times a day for 5–7 days Pyelonephritis: Ciprofloxacin 500 mg PO two times a day or TMP/SMX double strength (160 mg/800 mg) PO two times a day Minimum duration of therapy is generally 7–14 days for pyelonephritis and complicated cystitis; agent should be narrowed based on antimicrobial susceptibilities.	Levofloxacin 750 mg PO daily Ceftriaxone 1 g IV every 24 hours, then transition to an oral agent based on antimicrobial susceptibilities

(Continued on next page)

Appendix C. Antibiotics and Treatment of Selected Organisms[a] *(Continued)*

Site of Infection	Most Common Etiology	Primary Antibiotics	Alternative Antibiotics
Heart			
Bacterial endo-carditis	*Streptococcus, S. aureus*	*Streptococcus* species: Penicillin G 2–3 million units IV every 4–6 hours or ceftriaxone 2 g IV every 24 hours +/- gentamicin 3 mg/kg IV every 24 hours MSSA: Nafcillin or oxacillin 2 g IV every 4 hours or cefazolin 2 g IV every 8 hours Various other pharmacotherapeu-tic options exist based on caus-ative bacteria. Duration of therapy is generally 2–6 weeks.	Vancomycin indicated in patients unable to tolerate penicillin or ceftriaxone or with MRSA • Dosing: 15 mg/kg IV every 12 hours • Goal trough: 15–20 mcg/ml for *Staphylococcus* and 10–15 mcg/ml for *Streptococcus*
Hemoglobinopathy			
Acute chest syndrome (e.g., sickle cell)	*S. pneumoniae, H. influenzae,* atypical organ-isms (e.g., *Myco-plasma, Chla-mydia pneumo-niae*)	Severe community-acquired pneu-monia: Amoxicillin/clavulanate 500 mg/125 mg PO two times a day and azithromycin 500 mg PO on day 1, then 250 mg PO daily on days 2–5	Ceftriaxone 1–2 g IV every 24 hours plus clarithro-mycin 500 mg PO two times a day; or azithromy-cin 500 mg PO on day 1, then 250 mg PO daily on days 2–5
Lung			
Community-acquired pneu-monia	*S. pneumoniae, H. influenzae, Mycoplasma*	Amoxicillin 1 g PO three times a day or azithromycin 500 mg PO on day 1, then 250 mg PO daily on days 2–5; or ceftriaxone 1–2 g IV every 24 hours and azithromycin 500 mg PO on day 1, then 250 mg PO daily on days 2–5 Minimum duration of therapy is 5 days. Severe: Minimum duration of ther-apy is 7 days.	Severe: Amoxicillin/clavula-nate 875 mg/125 mg PO two times a day and azi-thromycin 500 mg PO on day 1, then 250 mg PO daily on days 2–5, or levo-floxacin 750 mg PO daily
Pharynx			
Pharyngitis	Group A *Strepto-coccus*	Penicillin V 500 mg PO two times a day or 250 mg PO four times a day for 10 days	Clindamycin 300 mg PO three times a day for 10 days or azithromy-cin 500 mg PO on day 1, then 250 mg PO daily on days 2–5
Sinuses			
Sinusitis	*S. pneumoniae, H. influenzae*	Amoxicillin/clavulanate 875 mg/125 mg PO every 12 hours for 5–7 days	Moxifloxacin 400 mg PO daily for 5–7 days

(Continued on next page)

Appendix C. Antibiotics and Treatment of Selected Organisms[a] *(Continued)*

Site of Infection	Most Common Etiology	Primary Antibiotics	Alternative Antibiotics
Skin			
Cellulitis (non-purulent)	Group A *Streptococcus, S. aureus*	PO therapy: Dicloxacillin 500 mg every 6 hours or cephalexin 500 mg every 6 hours IV therapy: Oxacillin 2 g every 4 hours or cefazolin 1 g every 8 hours	MRSA suspected: TMP/SMX double strength (160 mg/800 mg) 1–2 tablets PO two times a day Vancomycin • Dosing: 15–20 mg/kg IV every 12 hours • Goal trough: 15–20 mcg/ml
Systemic			
Sepsis, not neutropenic	Aerobic gram-negative bacilli, gram-positive cocci	Antimicrobials with antipseudomonal activity indicated: Piperacillin/tazobactam 3.375 g IV every 6 hours Confirmed or suspected extended-spectrum beta-lactamases: Imipenem 500 g IV every 6 hours or meropenem 1–2 g IV every 8 hours Vancomycin • Dosing: 25–30 mg/kg for one dose, then 15–20 mg/kg IV every 12 hours • Goal trough: 15–20 mcg/ml	If vancomycin-resistant *Enterococcus* species is suspected, consider linezolid or daptomycin instead of vancomycin.
Sepsis, neutropenic	Aerobic gram-negative bacilli, gram-positive cocci	Antimicrobials with antipseudomonal activity indicated: Cefepime 2 g IV every 8 hours or piperacillin/tazobactam 4.5 g IV every 6 hours Confirmed or suspected extended-spectrum beta-lactamases: Imipenem 500 g IV every 6 hours or meropenem 1–2 g IV every 8 hours Vancomycin • Dosing: 25–30 mg/kg for one dose, then 15–20 mg/kg IV every 12 hours • Goal trough: 15–20 mcg/ml	If vancomycin-resistant *Enterococcus* species is suspected, consider linezolid or daptomycin instead of vancomycin.
Venous access devices	*S. aureus*	MSSA: Cefazolin 2 g IV every 8 hours or oxacillin 2 g IV every 4 hours MRSA • Vancomycin 15–20 mg/kg IV every 12 hours • Goal trough: 15–20 mcg/ml	Remove access device with persistent fever or positive blood culture. Consider transthoracic echocardiogram or transesophageal echocardiogram to evaluate infective endocarditis.

[a] This table is not a comprehensive antibiotic listing and should only be used as a guide. Several agents listed require dose reductions in renal impairment. Vancomycin and aminoglycosides require therapeutic drug monitoring. Consider obtaining allergy history prior to selecting antimicrobial therapy. Duration of therapy for these agents is highly variable and depends on the type, severity, and etiology of infection.

IM—intramuscular; IV—intravenous; MRSA—methicillin-resistant *Staphylococcus aureus*; MSSA—methicillin-susceptible *Staphylococcus aureus*; PO—by mouth; TMP/SMX—trimethoprim/sulfamethoxazole

Appendix C. Antibiotics and Treatment of Selected Organisms[a] *(Continued)*

Note. Based on information from Alfonso, S.A., Fawley, J.D., & Lu, X.A. (2015). Conjunctivitis. *Primary Care: Clinics in Office Practice, 42*(3), 325–345. https://doi.org/10.1016/j.pop.2015.05.001; Baddour, L.M., Wilson, W.R., Bayer, A.S., Fowler, V.G., Jr., Tleyjeh, I.M., Rybak, M.J., ... Taubert, K.A. (2015). Infective endocarditis in adults: Diagnosis, antimicrobial therapy, and management of complications: A scientific statement for healthcare professionals from the American Heart Association. *Circulation, 132*(15), 1435–1486. https://doi.org/10.1161/CIR.0000000000000296; Chow, A.W., Benninger, M.S., Brook, I., Brozek, J.L., Goldstein, E.J.C., Hicks, L.A., ...File, T.M., Jr. (2012). Executive summary: IDSA clinical practice guideline for acute bacterial rhinosinusitis in children and adults. *Clinical Infectious Diseases, 54*(8), 1041–1045. https://doi.org/10.1093/cid/cir1043; Facciorusso, A., Antonino, M., Orsitto, E., & Sacco, R. (2019). Primary and secondary prophylaxis of spontaneous bacterial peritonitis: Current state of the art. *Expert Review of Gastroenterology and Hepatology, 13*(8), 751–759. https://doi.org/10.1080/17474124.2019.1644167; Freifeld, A.G., Bow, E.J., Sepkowitz, K.A., Boeckh, M.J., Ito, J.L., Mullen, C.A., ... Wingard, J.R. (2011). Clinical practice guideline for the use of antimicrobial agents in neutropenic patients with Cancer: 2010 update by the Infections Diseases Society of America. *Clinical Infectious Diseases, 52*(4), e56–e93. https://doi.org/10.1093/cid/cir073; Gaddey, H.L., Wright, M.T., & Nelson, T.N. (2019). Otitis media: Rapid evidence review. *American Family Physician, 100*(6), 350–356; Griffiths, M.J., McGill, F., & Solomon, T. (2018). Management of acute meningitis. *Clinical Medicine, 18*(2), 164–169. https://doi.org/10.7861/clinmedicine.18-2-164; Gupta, K., Hooton, T.M., Naber, K.G., Wullt, B., Colgan, R., Miller, L.G., ... Soper, D.E. (2011). International clinical practice guidelines for the treatment of acute uncomplicated cystitis and pyelonephritis in women: A 2010 update by the Infectious Diseases Society of America and the European Society for Microbiology and Infectious Diseases. *Clinical Infectious Diseases, 52*(5), e103–e120. https://doi.org/10.1093/cid/ciq257; Howard, J., Hart, N., Roberts-Harewood, M., Cummins, M., Awogbade, M., & Davis, B. (2015). Guideline on the management of acute chest syndrome in sickle cell disease. *British Journal of Haematology, 169*(4), 492–505. https://doi.org/10.1111/bjh.13348; Liu, C., Bayer, A., Cosgrove, S.E., Daum, R.S., Fridkin, S.K., Gorwitz, R.J., ... Chambers, H.F. (2011). Clinical practice guidelines by the Infectious Diseases Society of America for the treatment of methicillin-resistant *Staphylococcus aureus* infections in adults and children: Executive summary. *Clinical Infectious Diseases, 52*(3), 285–292. https://doi.org/10.1093/cid/cir034; Metlay, J.P., & Waterer, G.W. (2020). Update in adult community-acquired pneumonia: Key points from the new American Thoracic Society/Infectious Diseases Society of America 2019 guideline. *Current Opinion in Pulmonary Medicine, 26*(3), 203–207. https://doi.org/10.1097/MCP.0000000000000671; Moran, G.J., Krishnadasan, A., Mower, W.R., Abrahamian, F.M., LoVecchio, F., Steele, M.T., ... Talan, D.A. (2017). Effect of cephalexin plus trimethoprim-sulfamethoxazole vs cephalexin alone on clinical cure of uncomplicated cellulitis: A randomized clinical trial. *JAMA, 317*(20), 2088–2096. https://doi.org/10.1001/jama.2017.5653; National Comprehensive Cancer Network. (2021). *NCCN Clinical Practice Guidelines in Oncology (NCCN Guidelines®): Prevention and treatment of cancer-related infections* [v.1.2021]. https://www.nccn.org/professionals/physician_gls/pdf/infections.pdf; Prat, L.I., Wilson, P., Freeman, S.C., Sutton, A.J., Cooper, N.J., Roccarina, D., ... Gurusamy, K.S. (2019). Antibiotic treatment for spontaneous bacterial peritonitis in people with decompensated liver cirrhosis: A network meta-analysis. *Cochrane Database Systematic Reviews, 2019*(2). https://doi.org/10.1002/14651858.CD013120.pub2; Rees, J., Abrahams, M., Doble, A., & Cooper, A. (2015). Diagnosis and treatment of chronic bacterial prostatitis and chronic prostatitis/chronic pelvic pain syndrome: A consensus guideline. *BJU International, 116*(4), 509–525. https://doi.org/10.1111/bju.13101; Rhodes, A., Evans, L.E., Alhazzani, W., Levy, M.M., Antonelli, M., Ferrer, R., ... Dellinger, R.P. (2017). Surviving sepsis campaign: International guidelines for management of sepsis and septic shock: 2016. *Intensive Care Medicine, 43*(3), 304–377. https://doi.org/10.1007/s00134-017-4683-6; Rybak, M.J., Lomaestro, B.M., Rotscahfer, J.C., Moellering, R.C., Jr., Craig, W.A., Billeter, M., ... Levine, D.P. (2009). Vancomycin therapeutic guidelines: A summary of consensus recommendations from the Infectious Diseases Society of America, the American Society of Health-System Pharmacists, and the Society of Infectious Diseases Pharmacists. *Clinical Infectious Diseases, 49*(3), 325–327. https://doi.org/10.1086/600877; Shulman, S.T., Bisno, A.L., Clegg, H.W., Gerber, M.A., Kaplan, E.L., Lee, G., ... Van Beneden, C. (2012). Clinical practice guideline for the diagnosis and management of group A streptococcal pharyngitis: 2012 update by the Infectious Diseases Society of America. *Clinical Infectious Diseases, 55*(10), 1279–1282. https://doi.org/10.1093/cid/cis847; Stevens, D.L., Bisno, A.L., Chambers, H.F., Dellinger, E.P., Goldstein, E.J., Gorbach, S.L., ... Wade, J.C. (2014). Practice guidelines for the diagnosis and management of skin and soft tissue infections: 2014 update by the Infectious Diseases Society of America. *Clinical Infectious Diseases, 59*(2), 147–159. https://doi.org/10.1093/cid/ciu444; Szmuilowicz, J., & Young, R. (2019). Infections of the ear. *Emergency Medicine Clinics of North America, 37*(1), 1–9. https://doi.org/10.1016/j.emc.2018.09.001; Tunkel, A.R., Hasbun, R., Bhimraj, A., Byers, K., Kaplan, S.L., Scheld, W.M., ... Zunt, J.R. (2017). 2017 Infectious Diseases Society of America's clinical practice guidelines for healthcare-associated ventriculitis and meningitis. *Clinical Infectious Diseases, 64*(6), e34–e65. https://doi.org/10.1093/cid/ciw861.

Appendix D. Physical Examination Techniques

Boas point: Evaluative test to determine the presence of gastric ulcer
• Technique: Palpate the spinal column.
• Tenderness left of the 12th vertebra is indicative of gastric ulcer.

Brudzinski sign: Evaluative test for meningitis
• Technique: With the patient supine, place one hand behind the patient's head and place other hand on the patient's chest. Then, raise the patient's head (with the hand behind the head) while the hand on the chest restrains the patient and prevents the patient from rising.
• Positive sign: Flexion of the patient's lower extremities (hips and knees) occurs.

Carnett sign: Evaluative test for acute abdominal wall pain
• Technique: With the patient supine, ask the patient to lift the head and shoulders from the examination table to tense abdominal muscles. Or ask the patient to raise both legs with straight knees.
• Negative sign: The abdominal pain decreases when the patient is asked to lift the head or raise legs, indicating an intra-abdominal cause of pain.
• Positive sign: The abdominal wall and not the abdominal cavity is the source of pain.

Chvostek sign: Evaluative test for hypocalcemia
• Technique: Tap the facial nerve.
• Positive sign: Twitching of muscles around the mouth, nose, or eyes can occur.

Courvoisier sign: Evaluative test for gallbladder disorder
• Technique: Palpate the right upper quadrant.
• Palpable mass at the center reflects a palpable enlarged gallbladder.

Cullen sign: Evaluative test for intraperitoneal hemorrhage suggestive of acute pancreatitis
• Assess for ecchymosis and edema in the subcutaneous tissue around the umbilicus.

Fluid wave: Evaluative test for ascites
• Technique: Procedure requires three hands; consequently, assistance from the patient or another examiner is needed. Ask the patient to lie supine. Ask the patient or another examiner to press the edge of the hand and forearm firmly along the vertical midline of the abdomen. This position helps to stop the transmission of a wave through the adipose tissue. Place your hands on each side of the abdomen and strike one side sharply with your fingers. Feel for the wave impulse with the fingers of the other hand.
• Positive sign: Feeling a fluid wave may indicate ascites; however, this test is not conclusive because a fluid wave can be detected in patients without ascites or not detected in patients with ascites.

Grey Turner sign: Evaluative test for retroperitoneal bleeding suggestive of acute pancreatitis
• Technique: Assess for ecchymosis of the flank.

Hepatojugular reflux: Used to examine the function of jugular veins
• Technique: Adjust the position of the patient for the highest level of pulsation identified in the lower neck. Exert firm and sustained pressure with your hand over the patient's right upper quadrant for up to 60 seconds. Watch for an increase in the jugular venous pressure during this maneuver. If the right upper quadrant is tender, use another abdominal area.
• A rise of more than 1 cm is abnormal.

Homan sign: Evaluative test for deep venous thrombosis
• Technique: Flex the patient's knee slightly with one hand and dorsiflex the foot with the other hand.
• Positive sign: Complaint of calf pain indicates thrombosis.

Iliopsoas muscle test: Evaluative test for appendicitis
• Technique: Ask the patient to lie supine and place your hand over the lower thigh. Ask the patient to raise the leg, flexing at the hip, while you push downward against the leg.
• Positive sign: Lower quadrant pain is experienced.

Jugular vein measurement: Indicates volume and pressure in the right side of the heart
• Technique: Ask the patient to slowly lean back into a supine position. Using a ruler, measure the vertical distance between the angle of Louis (manubriosternal joint) and the highest level of jugular vein pulsation on both sides. Record the measurement. Note symmetry of right and left jugular veins.
• Positive sign: Measurement greater than 2 cm distention on one side suggests localized abnormality. Bilateral distention indicates cardiac etiology.

(Continued on next page)

Appendix D. Physical Examination Techniques (Continued)

Murphy sign: Evaluative test for gallbladder disease
- Technique: Ask the patient to breathe out and gently place the hand below the costal margin on the right side at the midclavicular line, the approximate location of the gallbladder. Ask the patient to breathe in.
- Positive sign: Pain on inspiration during palpation causes the patient to stop breathing or winces with a catch in breath. To confirm positive results, repeat procedure on left side. Pain will not be elicited.

Neurologic-specific tests: Evaluation for accuracy of movements and coordination; evaluation of fine motor skills
- Techniques
  - Finger-to-finger test: Ask the patient to use the index finger and alternately touch his or her nose and your index finger. Position your index finger approximately 18 inches from the patient and change the location of your finger several times.
  - Finger-to-nose test: Ask the patient to close his or her eyes and touch his or her nose with the index finger of each hand.
  - Graphesthesia: Write a single number or simple letter on the skin, usually the palm. Patient should be able to recognize writing on the skin by sensation of touch.
  - Heel-to-shin test: Technique can be performed with patient standing, sitting, or supine. Ask the patient to run his or her heel of one foot up and down the shin of the opposite leg. Repeat with the other leg.
  - Rapid rhythmic alternating movements: To evaluate fine motor skills and coordination, ask the seated patient to pat their knees with both hands, alternately turning up the palm and the back of the hands, or have the patient touch the thumb to each finger on the same hand, sequentially from the index finger to the little finger and back.
  - Stereognosis: Ask the patient to identify an object placed in their hand (e.g., key, comb).
  - Two-point discrimination: Using the two ends of an opened paper clip or other object, alternate randomly between touching the patient with one or two points on the area being tested (e.g., finger, arm, leg, toe). Patient should be able to distinguish between one or two points felt.
- Positive sign: Abnormal movement or incoordination of movement occurs.

Obturator muscle test: Evaluative test for a ruptured appendix or a pelvic abscess
- Technique: Ask the patient to lie supine and flex the right leg at the hip and knee to 90°. Hold the leg just above the knee, grasp the ankle, and rotate the leg laterally and medially.
- Positive sign: Pain in the hypogastric region indicates irritation of the obturator muscle.

Pulsus paradoxus: Evaluative test for cardiac tamponade, constrictive pericarditis, or chronic obstructive pulmonary disease
- Technique: Ask the patient to breathe easily and as normally as possible. Apply sphygmomanometer and inflate until no sounds are audible. Deflate cuff gradually until sounds are audible only during expiration and note the pressure. Deflate cuff further until sounds are audible during inspiration and note the pressure.
- Positive sign: A difference greater than 10 mm Hg; paradoxical pulse is exaggerated.
- Associated findings include low blood pressure and a weak, rapid pulse.

Rinne test: Evaluative hearing test for air and bone conduction
- Technique: To measure bone conduction, place the base of the vibrating tuning fork against patient's mastoid bone. Time the interval and ask the patient to tell you when the sound is no longer heard, noting the time in seconds. To measure air conduction, position the vibrating tuning fork 1–2 cm from the auditory canal, and ask the patient to tell you when the sound is no longer heard. Continue to time the interval to determine the length of time the sound is heard by air conduction. Compare the number of seconds the sound is heard by bone conduction versus air conduction.
- Negative sign: Bone conduction is heard longer than air conduction in affected ear, indicating conductive hearing loss.
- Positive sign: The air conduction is heard longer or louder than bone conduction in affected ear, indicating sensorineural hearing loss.

Scratch test: Evaluative test for hepatomegaly
- Technique: With stethoscope over the liver, lightly scratch the abdominal surface moving toward the liver. The sound will be magnified over the liver.
- Positive sign: Liver size is greater than 4–8 cm in the midsternal line and liver span is greater than 8 cm.

(Continued on next page)

Appendix D. Physical Examination Techniques *(Continued)*

Stemmer sign: Evaluative test for lymphedema
- Technique: Pinch the skin on the upper surface of the toes or fingers. In a healthy person, a fold of skin can be pinched and lifted up at the base of the second toe or middle finger.
- Positive sign: The skin fold cannot be raised.

Straight leg raise (Lasegue sign): Evaluative test to determine if herniated disk is possible cause of back pain; often located at fifth lumbar spinal nerve
- Technique: With the patient lying down on their back on examination table, lift the patient's leg while the knee is straight. Test can be more specific by dorsiflexing the ankle and asking patient to lift head to flex cervical spine.
- Positive sign: Sciatic pain and pain radiating down the leg (radiculopathy) occurs when the straight leg is at an angle between 30°–70°.

Tilt test: Evaluative test to determine the cause of fainting spells or syncope
- Technique: Place patient in head-up position; tilt for up to 45 minutes.
- Positive sign: Test can precipitate vasovagal syncope with associated bradycardia and hypotension.

Trousseau sign: Evaluative test for hypocalcemia
- Technique: Apply sphygmomanometer and inflate midway between systolic and diastolic pressures.
- Positive sign: Spasm of the hand occurs during three to four minutes of exercise while the cuff is inflated.

Weber test: Evaluative test for lateralization of sound
- Technique: Place the base of vibrating tuning fork on the midline vertex of the patient's head. Ask the patient if the sound is heard equally in both ears or is better in one ear.
- Positive sign: Lateralization to affected ear indicates hearing loss. Lateralization to better ear, unless conductive loss, indicates sensorineural hearing loss.

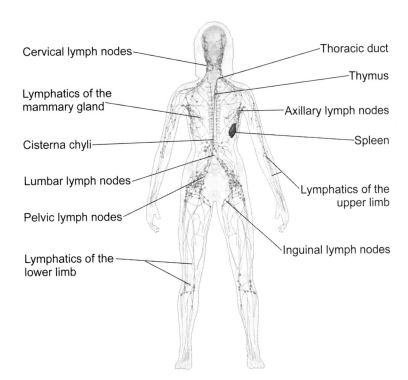

Cervical lymph nodes — Thoracic duct — Thymus — Lymphatics of the mammary gland — Axillary lymph nodes — Cisterna chyli — Spleen — Lumbar lymph nodes — Lymphatics of the upper limb — Pelvic lymph nodes — Inguinal lymph nodes — Lymphatics of the lower limb

Note. Based on information from Ball, J.W., Dains, J.E., Flynn, J.A., Solomon, B.S., & Stewart, R.W. (2019). *Seidel's guide to physical examination: An interprofessional approach* (9th ed.). Elsevier Mosby; Bickley, L.S. (2020). *Bates' guide to physical examination and history taking* (13th ed.). Lippincott Williams and Wilkins; Blausen.com. (2014). Medical gallery of Blausen Medical 2014. *WikiJournal of Medicine, 1*(2). https://doi.org/10.15347/wjm/2014.010.

Appendix E. Anti-Inflammatory Oral Agents

Drug	Usual Dose	Maximum Daily Dose
Aspirin	650 mg every 4 hours	4,000 mg
Celecoxib	200–400 mg every 12–24 hours	400 mg the first day, followed by an additional 200 mg dose if needed on the first day; on subsequent days, 200 mg two times daily, as needed
Diclofenac	50 mg three times a day	150 mg
Etodolac	200 mg every 4–6 hours	1,200 mg
Ibuprofen	400 mg every 6 hours	3,200 mg
Indomethacin	25–50 mg three or four times a day	200 mg
Meloxicam	7.5–15 mg	15 mg
Naproxen	250 mg every 6–8 hours	1,250 mg (acute); 1,000 mg (chronic)
Naproxen sodium	275 mg every 8 hours	1,375 mg (acute); 1,100 mg (chronic)

[a] Products listed are examples; the list is not all-inclusive.

Note. Based on information from Fallon, M., Giusti, R., Aielli, F., Rolke, R., Sharma, M., & Ripamonti, C.I. (2018). Management of cancer pain in adult patients: ESMO clinical practice guidelines. *Annals of Oncology, 29*(Suppl. 4), IV166–IV191. https://doi.org/10.1093/annonc/mdy152; Katzung, B.G. (Ed.). (2018). *Basic and clinical pharmacology* (14th ed.). McGraw-Hill; Lexicomp. (n.d.). Lexi-drugs [Login required]. http://online.lexi.com; Wolters Kluwer Health. (n.d.). Facts and Comparisons®. https://www.wolterskluwercdi.com/facts-comparisons-online/databases.

Appendix F. Dose Equivalents for Opioid Analgesics and Methadone Dosing[a,b]

Drug	Route/Dose	Selected Formulations[c,d]
Morphine	Oral: 30 mg Parenteral: 10 mg	CR/ER tablet: 15 mg, 30 mg, 60 mg, 100 mg, 200 mg IR tablet: 15 mg, 30 mg Oral solution (IR): 10 mg/5 ml; 100 mg/5 ml
Oxycodone	Oral: 20 mg	CR/ER tablet: 10 mg, 15 mg, 20 mg, 30 mg, 40 mg, 60 mg, 80 mg IR tablet: 5 mg, 10 mg, 15 mg, 20 mg, 30 mg Oral solution (IR): 5 mg/5 ml, 100 mg/5 ml
Hydromorphone	Oral: 7.5 mg Parenteral: 1.5 mg	CR/ER tablet: 8 mg, 12 mg, 16 mg, 32 mg IR tablet: 2 mg, 4 mg, 8 mg Oral solution (IR): 1 mg/ml
Fentanyl	Parenteral: 0.1 mg Transdermal, transmucosal: see Selected Formulations[e]	Transdermal patch: 12 mcg/hr, 25 mcg/hr, 50 mcg/hr, 75 mcg/hr, 100 mcg/hr Transmucosal lozenge: 200 mcg, 400 mcg, 600 mcg, 800 mcg, 1,200 mcg, 1,600 mcg
Codeine	200 mg[f]	IR tablet: 15 mg, 30 mg, 60 mg
Tramadol	300 mg[g]	CR/ER tablet: 100 mg, 200 mg, 300 mg IR tablet: 50 mg, 100 mg

Methadone Dose Conversions

CAUTION: Equianalgesic dosing is highly variable depending on a multitude of factors. Always consult with pain or palliative care specialist if unfamiliar with methadone prescribing.

Oral Morphine Dose	Dose Conversion or Ratio
< 60 mg	2–7.5 mg methadone daily
60–199 mg	10:1 morphine: methadone (and patient age < 65 years)
≥ 200 mg	20:1 morphine: methadone (and/or patient age > 65 years)

[a] Recommended doses may not apply to patients who weigh less than 50 kg, with renal insufficiency, with hepatic insufficiency, or with other conditions affecting drug metabolism and kinetics.

[b] This is not an all-inclusive list.

[c] CR and ER formulations are generally dosed every 8–12 hours.

[d] IR formulation is generally dosed every 3–6 hours, as needed, depending on pain severity, renal function, prior tolerance of opioids, age, and other factors.

[e] Fentanyl: transdermal patch conversion 50–60 oral morphine daily = 25 mcg/hr transdermal patch. Patch should be placed every 72 hours (can consider placing every 48 hours in certain clinical scenarios [e.g., end of dose failure with every 72-hour dosing]). Doses > 25 mcg/hr should not be used in opioid-naïve patients. Do NOT convert mcg for mcg among fentanyl products (i.e., patch, lozenge, injectable, buccal tablet). See the package insert for additional dosing calculations and clinical guidance.

[f] Codeine doses greater than 65 mg often are not appropriate because of diminishing incremental analgesia with increasing doses but continually increasing nausea, constipation, and other side effects.

[g] Tramadol is associated with serotonin syndrome. Use with caution in combination with linezolid, selective serotonin reuptake inhibitors, selective norephinephrine reuptake inhibitors, tricyclic antidepressants, monoamine oxidase inhibitors, triptans, 5-HT$_3$ antagonists, dextromethorphan, and amphetamines (not an all-inclusive list).

Note. Published tables vary in the suggested doses that are equianalgesic to morphine. Clinical response is the criterion that must be applied for each patient; titration to clinical responses is necessary. Because there is not complete cross-tolerance among these drugs, it is usually necessary to use a lower-than-equianalgesic dose when changing drugs and to reiterate to response.

CR—controlled release; ER—extended release; 5-HT$_3$—5-hydroxytryptamine-3 (serotonin receptor); IR—immediate release

Based on information from Chou, R., Fanciullo, G.J., Fine, P.G., Adler, J.A., Ballantyne, J.C., Davies, P., … Miaskowski, C. (2009). Clinical guidelines for the use of chronic opioid therapy in chronic noncancer pain. Journal of Pain, 10(2), 113–130. e22. https://doi.org/10.1016/j.jpain.2008.10.008; Fallon, M., Giusti, R., Aielli, F., Rolke, R., Sharma, M., & Ripamonti, C.I. (2018). Management of cancer pain in adult patients: ESMO clinical practice guidelines. *Annals of Oncology, 29*(Suppl. 4), IV166–IV191. https://doi.org/10.1093/annonc/mdy152; Katzung, B.G. (Ed.). (2018). *Basic and clinical pharmacology* (14th ed.). McGraw-Hill; Lexicomp. (n.d.). Lexi-drugs [Login required]. http://online.lexi.com; National Comprehensive Cancer Network. (2021). *NCCN Clinical Practice Guidelines in Oncology (NCCN Guidelines®): Adult cancer pain* [v.2.2021]. http://www.nccn.org/professionals/physician_gls/pdf/pain.pdf; Wolters Kluwer Health. (n.d.). Facts and Comparisons®. https://www.wolterskluwercdi.com/facts-comparisons-online/databases.

Appendix G. Topical Nasal Steroids

Action: Aerosol preparations deliver corticosteroids to the airways with minimal systemic absorption.

Indications: For relief of nasal congestion from environmental allergens causing allergic rhinitis

Contraindications: Hypersensitivity to the product

Special considerations: The development of localized infections of the nose and pharynx with *Candida albicans* has been reported. The incidence may increase when the patient is immunocompromised.

Examples[a]

Drug	Adult Dosage
Beclomethasone	1 spray per nostril two, three, or four times a day (2–4 sprays daily)
Budesonide	2 sprays per nostril two times a day or 4 sprays daily
Ciclesonide	2 sprays per nostril daily
Flunisolide	2 sprays per nostril two, three, or four time a day (4–8 sprays daily)
Fluticasone propionate	2 sprays per nostril daily
Mometasone furoate monohydrate	2 sprays per nostril daily
Triamcinolone	2 sprays per nostril daily

[a]Products listed are examples; the list is not all-inclusive.

Note. Based on information from Fallon, M., Giusti, R., Aielli, F., Rolke, R., Sharma, M., & Ripamonti, C.I. (2018). Management of cancer pain in adult patients: ESMO clinical practice guidelines. *Annals of Oncology, 29*(Suppl. 4), IV166–IV191. https://doi.org/10.1093/annonc/mdy152; Lexicomp. (n.d.). Lexi-drugs [Login required]. http://online.lexi.com; Wolters Kluwer Health. (n.d.). Facts and Comparisons®. https://www.wolterskluwercdi.com/facts-comparisons-online/databases.

Appendix H. Antihistamines

Action: Antihistamines are reversible, competitive H_1 antagonists that reduce or prevent most of the physiologic effects of histamine. They do not prevent histamine release or bind with histamine that already has been released.

Indications: Antihistamines are used to relieve the manifestations of immediate-type hypersensitivity reactions. They also may be used as a sedative, antiemetic, antitussive, or antiparkinsonian agent, adjuncts to pre- or postoperative analgesic therapy, and to combat motion sickness and allergic rhinitis (running nose, sneezing, itching nose, and watery eyes).

Examples[a]

Generation	Agent	Usual Daily Dose	Maximum Daily Dose
First (more anticholinergic, more sedating, and more frequent dosing than second generation)	Chlorpheniramine	4 mg PO every 4–6 hours	24 mg
	Cyproheptadine	4 mg PO three times daily	0.5 mg/kg or 32 mg
	Dexchlorpheniramine	2 mg PO every 4–6 hours	12 mg
	Diphenhydramine	PO: 25 mg every 4–6 hours or 50 mg every 6–8 hours, as needed IV: 10–50 mg IV every 6 hours as needed	PO or IV: 200 mg Although doses as high as 300 mg and 400 mg have been approved in some labels respectively, these doses are associated with higher likelihood of adverse effects.
	Hydroxyzine	25 mg PO three to four times a day	100 mg
Second	Cetirizine	10 mg PO	10 mg
	Desloratadine	5 mg PO	5 mg
	Fexofenadine	180 mg PO	180 mg
	Levocetirizine	5 mg PO	5 mg
	Loratadine	10 mg PO	10 mg

[a] Products listed are examples; the list is not all-inclusive.

H_1—histamine 1; IV—intravenous; PO—by mouth

Note. Based on information from Katzung, B.G. (Ed.). (2018). *Basic and clinical pharmacology* (14th ed.). McGraw-Hill; Lexicomp. (n.d.). Lexi-drugs [Login required]. http://online.lexi.com; Wolters Kluwer Health. (n.d.). Facts and Comparisons®. https://www.wolterskluwercdi.com/facts-comparisons-online/databases.

Appendix I. Decongestants

Action: Decongestants stimulate alpha-adrenergic receptors of vascular smooth muscle, and some have a beta-adrenergic property. The alpha-adrenergic effects cause intense vasoconstriction when applied directly to the mucosal membrane. Systemically, the products have similar muted effects and result in mucosal membrane shrinkage, which promotes drainage, improves ventilation, and reduces a stuffy feeling.

Indications: For the temporary relief of nasal congestion. Topical nasal decongestants should be limited to three days of therapy to prevent rebound congestion.

Contraindications
- Monoamine oxidase inhibitor therapy
- Hypersensitivity or idiosyncrasy to sympathomimetic amines (insomnia, dizziness, weakness, tremor, or dysrhythmias)
- Severe hypertension and coronary artery disease (especially with oral preparation)

Special considerations: Administer with caution in older adults and patients with the following.
- Hyperthyroidism
- Diabetes mellitus
- Cardiovascular disease: Coronary artery disease, ischemic heart disease, hypertension
- Increased intraocular pressure
- Prostatic hypertrophy

Examples[a]

Drug	Adult Dose
Topical Preparations	
Naphazoline	1–2 sprays or drops in each nostril as needed; no more than 4 doses in 24 hours
Oxymetazoline	2–3 sprays or drops (0.05%) in each nostril two times a day or every 10–12 hours (2 doses in 24 hours)
Phenylephrine regular strength and extra strength (0.125%, 0.5%, and 1%)	2–3 sprays or drops in each nostril; repeated every 3–4 hours (0.5%); 1% solution should be repeated no more than every 4 hours.
Tetrahydrozoline	2–4 drops (0.1%) in each nostril every 3–4 hours as needed or 3–4 sprays every 4–6 hours as needed (8 doses in 24 hours)
Xylometazoline	2–3 sprays or drops (0.1%) in each nostril every 8–10 hours (3 doses in 24 hours)
Oral Preparations	
Phenylephrine	10 mg tablet PO every 4 hours (maximum 60 mg daily)
Pseudoephedrine	• Immediate release: 30–60 mg PO every 4–6 hours, as needed • 12-hour extended release: 120 mg PO every 12 hours, as needed • 24-hour extended release: 240 mg PO every 24 hours, as needed • Long-acting tablet: 120 mg PO every 12 hours • Maximum dose: 240 mg daily

[a] Products listed are examples; the list is not all-inclusive.

Note. Based on information from Katzung, B.G. (Ed.). (2018). *Basic and clinical pharmacology* (14th ed.). McGraw-Hill; Lexicomp. (n.d.). Lexi-drugs [Login required]. http://online.lexi.com; Wolters Kluwer Health. (n.d.). Facts and Comparisons®. https://www.wolterskluwercdi.com/facts-comparisons-online/databases.

Appendix J. Antiviral Agents[a]

Agent	Usual Daily Dose[b]
Acyclovir	Prophylaxis: 400–800 mg PO twice a day or 250 mg/m^2 IV every 12 hours Treatment: 400–800 mg PO five times a day or 5–10 mg IV every 8 hours
Famciclovir	Prophylaxis: 250–500 mg PO two times a day Treatment: 500 mg PO two to three times a day
Valacyclovir	Prophylaxis: 500–1,000 mg PO one or two times a day Treatment: 1,000 mg PO three times a day

[a] Products listed are examples; the list is not all-inclusive.

[b] Dose varies based on etiology.

PO—by mouth

Note. Based on information from Lexicomp. (n.d.). Lexi-drugs [Login required]. http://online.lexi.com.

Appendix K. Corticosteroid Preparations[a]

Oral/Injectable Preparations

- Dexamethasone: tablet, oral solution, injectable
- Hydrocortisone: tablet, oral solution, injectable
- Methylprednisolone: tablet, injectable
- Prednisone: tablet, oral solution

Corticosteroid	Equivalent Dose (mg)
Dexamethasone	0.75
Hydrocortisone	20
Methylprednisolone	4
Prednisone	5

Oral to IV conversions are 1:1.

Topical Preparations

Group 1. Highest Potency
- Betamethasone dipropionate in optimized vehicle 0.05% ointment
- Clobetasol propionate 0.05% cream, ointment
- Halobetasol propionate 0.05% cream, ointment
- Diflorasone diacetate 0.05% ointment

Group 2. High Potency
- Amcinonide 0.1% cream, ointment, lotion
- Betamethasone dipropionate 0.05% cream, ointment
- Desoximetasone 0.25% cream, ointment, gel (0.05%)
- Fluocinonide 0.05% cream, ointment, gel, solution
- Halcinonide 0.1% cream, ointment
- Triamcinolone acetate cream, ointment 0.5%

Group 3. Medium-High Potency
- Amcinonide 0.1% cream
- Betamethasone dipropionate 0.05% cream
- Diflorasone diacetate 0.05% cream

Group 4. Medium Potency
- Desoximetasone 0.05% cream
- Flurandrenolide 0.05% ointment
- Hydrocortisone butyrate 0.1% ointment
- Hydrocortisone valerate 0.2% ointment
- Mometasone furoate 0.1% cream, ointment
- Triamcinolone acetonide 0.1% ointment

Group 5. Low Potency
- Alclometasone dipropionate 0.05% cream
- Betamethasone valerate 0.1% cream
- Flurandrenolide 0.05% cream
- Fluocinolone acetonide 0.025% cream
- Hydrocortisone butyrate 0.1% cream
- Hydrocortisone valerate 0.2% cream
- Triamcinolone acetonide 0.1% cream, lotion

Group 6. Mild Potency
- Desonide 0.05% cream
- Fluocinolone acetonide 0.01% solution

Group 7. Lowest Potency
- Dexamethasone 0.1% ointment, gel
- Hydrocortisone 0.5%, 1%, and 2.5% cream, ointment, lotion

[a] It is recommended to be familiar with and use one agent from each category, making the selection on the basis of cost, cosmetic acceptability, and efficacy. Products listed are examples; the list is not all-inclusive.

Note. Based on information from Goodheart, H.P., & Gonzalez, M.E. (Eds.). (2016). *Goodheart's photoguide to common pediatric and adult skin disorders: Diagnosis and management* (4th ed.). Wolters Kluwer Health; Katzung, B.G. (Ed.). (2018). *Basic and clinical pharmacology* (14th ed.). McGraw-Hill; Lexicomp. (n.d.). Lexi-drugs [Login required]. http://online.lexi.com.

Appendix L. Psychotropic Oral Agents[a]

Classification/ Drug	Doses[b]	Side Effects	Comments
Serotonin-Norepinephrine Reuptake Inhibitors, Tricyclic (primary serotonin, mixed norepinephrine and serotonin uptake)			
Amitriptyline	Starting: 10–50 mg daily as a single dose or in divided doses Maximum: 300 mg daily in divided doses	Somnolence, xerostomia, blurred vision, constipation, urinary hesitancy, confusion, orthostasis, weight gain, sexual disturbances	Can be used for neuropathic pain
Clomipramine	Starting: 12.5–50 mg daily as a single dose Maximum: 150–250 mg daily in divided doses		Can be used for neuropathic pain
Doxepin	Starting: 25–50 mg daily as a single dose or in divided doses Maximum: 300 mg daily in divided doses		Available in capsule, oral liquid, and topical formulations Can be used for neuropathic pain
Imipramine	Starting: 10–75 mg daily as a single dose or in divided doses Maximum: 300 mg daily in divided doses		Can be used for neuropathic pain
Serotonin-Norepinephrine Reuptake Inhibitors, Tricyclic (secondary)			
Desipramine	Starting: 12.5–50 mg daily as a single dose or in divided doses Maximum: 300 mg daily in divided doses	Somnolence, dysgeusia, xerostomia, blurred vision, constipation, urinary hesitancy, confusion, orthostasis, weight gain, sexual disturbances	Can be used for neuropathic pain
Nortriptyline	Starting: 10–25 mg daily as a single dose Maximum: 150 mg once daily or in divided doses		Available in capsule and oral liquid formulations Can be used for neuropathic pain
Serotonin-Norepinephrine Reuptake Inhibitors, Nontricyclic (third-generation heterocyclic; serotonin and norepinephrine)			
Desvenlafaxine	Starting: 50 mg once daily Maximum: Manufacturer states that no benefit exists > 50 mg once daily, although doses up to 400 mg once daily have been studied and have been shown to be effective.	Nausea, insomnia, hyperhidrosis	Extended-release formulation Can be used for neuropathic pain
Duloxetine	Starting: 30–60 mg once daily or divided into two doses Maximum: 120 mg daily divided into two doses	Constipation, decreased appetite, xerostomia, hyperhidrosis, nausea, somnolence	Delayed-release formulation Can be used for neuropathic pain
Levomilnacipran	Starting: 20 mg once daily Maximum: 120 mg once daily	Nausea, orthostasis	Dose reduce for creatinine clearance < 60 ml/min
Milnacipran[c]	Starting: 50 mg two times daily Maximum: 100 mg two times daily	Nausea, headache, insomnia, hot flashes	Indicated for fibromyalgia

(Continued on next page)

Appendix L. Psychotropic Oral Agents[a] *(Continued)*

Classification/ Drug	Doses[b]	Side Effects	Comments
Serotonin-Norepinephrine Reuptake Inhibitors, Nontricyclic (third-generation heterocyclic; serotonin and norepinephrine) *(cont.)*			
Venlafaxine	Starting: 37.5–75 mg once daily (immediate-release or extended-release formulations) Maximum: 225–300 mg once daily (extended release) or in 3–4 divided doses (immediate release)	Nausea, somnolence, sweating, dizziness, anxiety, sexual disturbances, hypertension	Available in immediate- and extended-release formulations Immediate-release doses > 37.5 mg should be divided in at least two daily doses. Can be used for neuropathic pain
Monoamine Oxidase Inhibitors (serotonin, norepinephrine, dopamine)			
Phenelzine	Starting: 15 mg three times daily Maximum: 90 mg daily in divided doses, although may slowly reduce dose over several weeks once maximum benefit is attained	Headache, drowsiness, xerostomia, weight gain, postural hypotension, sexual disturbances, neuropathy	Give vitamin B_6 50 mg PO every day to avoid neuropathy. Interacts with tyramine found in fermented foods and beverages, and serotonergic agents resulting in serotonin syndrome
Tranylcypromine	Starting: 10–30 mg daily in divided doses Maximum: 60 mg daily in divided doses		
Selective Serotonin Reuptake Inhibitors			
Citalopram	Starting: 10–20 mg daily Maximum: 40 mg daily	Insomnia or somnolence depending on agent, tremor, diarrhea, nausea, decreased libido/ sexual dysfunction	Available in oral solution
Escitalopram	Starting: 5–10 mg daily Maximum: 60 mg daily		Available in oral solution
Fluoxetine	Starting: 10–20 mg daily Maximum: 80 mg daily		Long half-life; taper over at least 4 weeks. Available in oral solution and weekly delayed-release formulation Do not prescribe with tamoxifen.
Fluvoxamine	Starting: 50 mg daily Maximum: 300 mg daily in divided doses		Sustained- or extended-release formulations available
Sertraline	Starting: 25–50 mg daily Maximum: 300 mg daily		–
Paroxetine	Starting: 10 mg daily Maximum: 75 mg daily in divided doses (one daily dose if controlled-release formulation is utilized)		Available in tablet, oral suspension, and controlled-release formulations Do not prescribe with tamoxifen. Sustained or extended-release formulations available

(Continued on next page)

Appendix L. Psychotropic Oral Agents[a] *(Continued)*

Classification/ Drug	Doses[b]	Side Effects	Comments
Norepinephrine-Dopamine Reuptake Inhibitors (norepinephrine, some dopamine)			
Bupropion[d]	Starting: 100 mg daily as a single dose Maximum: 450 mg daily as a single dose or in divided doses	Tachycardia, headache, insomnia, weight loss, nausea, tremor, seizures (high doses)	Contraindicated in patients with history of seizure disorder, anorexia/bulimia Useful in patients with sexual dysfunction Useful in patients with desire to stop smoking Immediate-release formulation is dosed two to three times a day. Sustained-release formulation is dosed every 12 hours. Extended-release formulation is dosed every 24 hours.
Serotonin Antagonist and Reuptake Inhibitors (serotonin, 5-HT$_2$ antagonists)			
Mirtazapine	Starting: 15 mg once daily at bedtime Maximum: 45 mg once daily (prescribing information); 60 mg (clinical trials)	Somnolence, xerostomia, increased appetite	Available in orally disintegrating tablets
Trazodone	Starting: 50 mg daily as a single dose Maximum: 600 mg daily in divided doses (400 mg daily in patients with cardiovascular disease)	Somnolence, xerostomia	Not FDA approved for use in pediatric patients
Serotonin Dopamine Receptor Antagonists			
Olanzapine	Starting: 5 mg daily Maximum: 20 mg daily	Xerostomia, somnolence, increased appetite, weight gain, extrapyramidal reactions, metabolic abnormalities (e.g., hyperprolactinemia)	Available in orally disintegrating tablets and IM injection
Risperidone	Starting: 0.25–0.5 mg once daily Maximum: 3 mg once daily or divided into two daily doses (higher for other psychiatric indications) 1 mg PO two times daily up to 16 mg daily		Available in orally disintegrating tablets, oral solution, and IM injection

[a] Products listed here are examples; the list is not all-inclusive. Onset of action of all agents is generally 2–4 weeks. Many agents are associated with increased risk of suicidal thoughts and behavior in children, adolescents, and young adults, so should be monitored closely within 4–8 weeks after initiation of therapy and in the setting of dosage adjustments.

[b] Psychotropic agents listed are used for a variety of different diagnoses, so starting and maximum doses may differ depending on indication. Doses are often started low and slowly titrated over several weeks to desired effect. Use caution in combination with other serotonergic and dopaminergic agents due to risk of serotonin syndrome and neuroleptic malignant syndrome, respectively.

[c] Not indicated for depressive or other mental disorders

[d] Doses expressed as the hydrochloride salt. Bupropion hydrochloride 150 mg is equivalent to approximately bupropion hydrobromide 174 mg.

CNS—central nervous system; FDA—U.S. Food and Drug Administration; 5-HT$_2$—5-hydroxytryptamine-2; IM—intramuscular; GI—gastrointestinal; PO—by mouth

Note. Based on information from Katzung, B.G. (Ed.). (2018). *Basic and clinical pharmacology* (14th ed.). McGraw-Hill; Lexicomp. (n.d.). Lexi-drugs [Login required]. http://online.lexi.com; Wolters Kluwer Health. (n.d.). Facts and Comparisons®. https://www.wolterskluwercdi.com/facts-comparisons-online/databases..

Appendix M. Paraneoplastic Syndromes[a]

Disorder	Finding	Associated Malignancy
Cutaneous		
Acanthosis nigricans	Hyperpigmentation and velvety hyperkeratosis on flexural surfaces	Gastrointestinal (GI) adenocarcinoma
Acquired ichthyosis	Generalized dry scaling of the skin with accentuation over the shins	Hodgkin lymphoma
Amyloidosis	Pink or yellow elevated nodules, translucent papules, waxy appearance	Multiple myeloma, macroglobulinemia
Dermatomyositis	Scaly violaceous papules overlying bony prominences of the hands, periorbital skin, scalp, lateral thighs, periungual telangiectasia, and ragged cuticles; myopathy usually present with a progressive, symmetric, proximal weakness	Ovarian, lung, breast, gastric, uterine, colorectal, or pancreatic cancer
Erythroderma	Diffuse and generalized erythema of the skin involving more than 92% of body surface area	Lymphoid T-cell lymphoma (most common)
Gardner syndrome	Multiple epidermoid cysts, desmoid tumors, fibroma, and lipoma; hallmark is intestinal polyposis of the colon and rectum.	Colon adenocarcinoma
Neurofibromatosis	Neurofibroma, axillary freckling	Neurofibrosarcoma, pheochromocytoma, leukemia
Palmar hyperkeratosis	Keratoderma of palms and soles; yellow, symmetric smooth bilateral thickening; tylosis	Squamous cell esophageal cancer, Hodgkin lymphoma, leukemia, breast cancer
Paraneoplastic acrokeratosis (Bazex syndrome)	Hyperkeratotic lesions on nose, ears, palms, and soles	Upper aerodigestive tract
Paraneoplastic pemphigus	Generalized mucocutaneous blistering	Lymphoma, thymoma, chronic lymphocytic leukemia, sarcoma, bronchogenic squamous cell carcinoma
Pyoderma gangrenosum	Irregular ulcer with an overhanging border and necrotic base	Acute myeloid leukemia
Sweet syndrome (acute febrile neutrophilic dermatosis)	Tender erythematous plaques	Acute myeloid leukemia, lymphoma, genitourinary cancers, breast cancer, stomach cancer
Tripe palm	Velvety thickening of palms with ridged appearance	Gastric cancer, bronchogenic lung cancer

(Continued on next page)

Appendix M. Paraneoplastic Syndromes[a] *(Continued)*

Disorder	Finding	Associated Malignancy
Endocrine		
Acromegaly	Overproduction of growth hormone	Carcinoid tumor, pheochromocytoma, pancreatic cancer
POEMS syndrome	Polyneuropathy, organomegaly, endocrinopathy, monoclonal protein, skin abnormalities	Multiple myeloma
Sign of Leser-Trélat	Multiple pruritic seborrheic keratosis with inflammatory base	GI adenocarcinoma, breast cancer, lung cancer
Carcinoid syndrome	Flushing, diarrhea, bronchospasm	GI, laryngeal, lung, breast, ovarian, or testicular cancer
Cushing syndrome	Excessive production of ectopic adrenocorticotropic hormone; increased pigmentation; hypokalemia	Small cell lung cancer, thymoma, pancreatic cancer, carcinoid tumor, pheochromocytoma, thyroid cancer
Gynecomastia	Increase in breast tissue	Lung cancer, adrenal cancer, testicular cancer, hepatoma, breast cancer in men
Hypercalcemia	Increased serum calcium level	Breast, lung, kidney, ovarian, or oral cancer
Hyperpyrexia and fever	Increase in temperature, release of pyrogens from the tumor, inability to detoxify endogenous endotoxin	Hepatic metastasis, Hodgkin lymphoma, lymphoma, sarcoma
Hyperthyroidism	Decreased thyroid-stimulating hormone, increased triiodothyronine and thyroxine	Lung cancer
Hypocalcemia	Decreased serum calcium, decreased parathyroid hormone–related protein	Bone metastasis from cancer of the lung, prostate, breast, ovary, head and neck, bladder, or kidney
Hypoglycemia	Decreased serum glucose level	Fibrosarcoma; mesothelioma; hepatoma; GI adenocarcinoma; breast, lung, kidney, or ovarian cancers
Hypophosphatemia	Decreased serum phosphorus	Mesenchymal tumors (arising from connective or fibrous tissue)
Nephrotic syndrome	Massive edema with proteinuria hypoalbuminemia	Hodgkin lymphoma
Syndrome of inappropriate antidiuretic hormone	Hyponatremia from excessive urine output	Small cell lung cancer, carcinoid tumor, esophageal cancer, duodenal cancer, colon cancer, pancreatic cancer, prostate cancer, thymoma, lymphoma, oral cancer

(Continued on next page)

Appendix M. Paraneoplastic Syndromes[a] *(Continued)*

Disorder	Finding	Associated Malignancy
Eyes		
Cancer-associated retinopathy	Abnormal visual acuity, color vision abnormalities, central or ring-like scotomata	Small cell lung cancer, gynecologic cancers, breast cancer, osteosarcoma, Warthin tumor of parotid gland, prostate cancer, pancreatic neuroendocrine tumor, small bowel cancer, bladder cancer, laryngeal cancer, lymphomas (systemic follicular cell lymphoma), colon adenomas
Melanoma-associated retinopathy	Shimmering, flickering, or pulsating photopsia; night blindness; loss of peripheral vision	Melanoma
Hematologic		
Antiphospholipid syndrome	Thrombus, treatment resistant to anticoagulation	Mesothelioma
Disseminated intravascular coagulation	Thromboplastin-like agent fibrinolytic system activation, increased fibrin degradation products	Acute promyelocytic leukemia, prostate cancer
Eosinophilia	Increased number of eosinophils	Pancreatic cancer
Immunoglobulin M	Elevation of immunoglobulin M	Waldenström lymphoma
Hypercoagulability	Disruption of clotting factors, such as protein C, protein S, tissue plasminogen factor, and antithrombin III	Adenocarcinoma, multiple myeloma
Lymphoproliferative disorders	Increased white blood cell or platelet count	Non-Hodgkin and Hodgkin lymphomas, liposarcoma, hepatocellular carcinoma
Polycythemia	Increased red blood cell count	Pancreatic cancer, carcinoid tumor
Trousseau syndrome	Deep venous thrombosis	Lung, colon, pancreatic, breast, ovarian, or prostate cancer
Thrombocytosis	Elevation of platelets	Ovarian cancer
Vasculitis	Thrombosis arterioles, purpuric ulcer, necrotic lesion of extremities	Multiple myeloma
Musculoskeletal		
Hypertrophic osteoarthropathy, pulmonary hypertrophic osteoarthropathy	Digital clubbing and tenderness along the distal long bones	Non-small cell lung cancer, lung metastasis
Joint pain	Enlarged joints	Pancreatic cancer

(Continued on next page)

Appendix M. Paraneoplastic Syndromes[a] *(Continued)*

Disorder	Finding	Associated Malignancy
Neurologic		
Lambert-Eaton myasthenic syndrome	Mediator of voltage-gated calcium channel antibodies, proximal muscle weakness of limbs	Bladder, kidney, breast, stomach, colon, prostate, gallbladder, or small cell lung cancer; lymphoma; sarcoma; thymoma
Limbic encephalitis	Short-term memory loss, seizures	Lung, ovarian, or testicular cancer; thymoma
Motor neuronopathy	Disorder of anterior horn cells	Lymphoma
Paraneoplastic cortical cerebellar degeneration	Injury to the Purkinje cells of the cerebellum, ataxia, dysarthria, dysphagia, dementia	Small cell lung, breast, ovarian, genitourinary, colon, or prostate cancer; sarcoma; neuroblastoma; Hodgkin lymphoma; lymphoma
Sensory neuropathy	Affects the cell bodies of sensory neurons in dorsal root ganglion	Carcinomas

[a] Syndromes listed are examples; the list is not all-inclusive. Paraneoplastic syndromes can affect a variety of body systems, including endocrine, hematologic, epithelial, nervous, renal, gastrointestinal, immunologic, and musculoskeletal. They are most commonly associated with cancer of the lung, breast, or stomach. Diagnosis is difficult because signs and symptoms represent other clinical abnormalities. Treatment is based on removing the underlying cancer with cancer treatment or suppressing the mediator causing the syndrome.

Note. Based on information from Bellan, M., Sainaghi, P.P., & Pirisi, M. (2018). The real evidence for polymyalgia rheumatic as a paraneoplastic syndrome. *Reumatismo, 70*(2), 117. https://doi.org/10.4081/reumatismo.2018.1148; Boddu, P., Villlines, D., & Aklilu, M. (2016). Paraneoplastic leukocytosis and thrombocytosis as prognostic biomarkers in non-small cell lung cancer. *Chinese Journal of Lung Cancer, 19*(11), 725–730. https://doi.org/10.3779/j.issn.1009-3419.2016.11.02; Bussat, A., Langner-Lemercier, S., Salmon, A., & Mouriaux, F. (2018). Paraneoplastic syndromes in ophthalmology. *Journal Français d'Ophtalmologie, 41*(5), e181–e185. https://doi.org/10.1016/j.jfo.2018.03.002; Dimitriadis, G.K., Angelousi, A., Weickert, M.O., Randeva, H.S., Kaltsas, G., & Grossman, A. (2017). Paraneoplastic endocrine syndromes. *Endocrine-Related Cancer, 24*(6), R173–R190. https://doi.org/10.1530/ERC-17-0036; Dispenzieri, A., Kourelis, T., & Buadi, F. (2018). POEMS syndrome: Diagnosis and investigative work-up. *Hematology/Oncology Clinics of North America, 32*(1), 119–139. https://doi.org/10.1016/j.hoc.2017.09.010; Dumansky, Y.V., Syniachenko, O.V., Stepko, P.A., Yehudina, Y.D., & Stoliarova, O.Y. (2018). Paraneoplastic syndrome in lung cancer. *Experimental Oncology, 40*(3), 239–242; Kordyś, M., Przeździecka-Dołyk, J., Turno-Kręcicka, A., & Misiuk-Hojło, M. (2018). Immunopathogenesis of ophthalmological paraneoplastic syndromes: Recent findings. *Advances in Clinical and Experimental Medicine, 27*(10), 1431–1439. https://doi.org/10.17219/acem/73860; Rosenfeld, M.R., & Dalmau, J. (2018). Paraneoplastic neurologic syndromes. *Neurologic Clinics, 36*(3), 675–685. https://doi.org/10.1016/j.ncl.2018.04.015; Viau, M., Renaud, M.-C., Gregoire, J., Sebastianelli, A., & Plante, M. (2017). Paraneoplastic syndromes associated with gynecological cancers: A systematic review. *Gynecologic Oncology, 146*(3), 661–671. https://doi.org/10.1016/j.ygyno.2017.06.025; Wick, M.R., & Patterson, J.W. (2019). Cutaneous paraneoplastic syndromes. *Seminars in Diagnostic Pathology, 36*(4), 211–228. https://doi.org/10.1053/j.semdp.2019.01.001.

Appendix N. Antihistamine/Decongestant Oral Combinations[a]

Antihistamine	Decongestant	Adult Dose
Cetirizine 5 mg	Pseudoephedrine 120 mg	1 tablet every 12 hours
Cetirizine 10 mg	Pseudoephedrine 240 mg	1 tablet every 24 hours
Chlorpheniramine 4 mg	Phenylephrine 10 mg	1 tablet every 4–6 hours (maximum 6 tablets daily)
Desloratadine 2.5 mg	Pseudoephedrine 120 mg	1 tablet every 12 hours
Desloratadine 5 mg	Pseudoephedrine 240 mg	1 tablet every 24 hours
Fexofenadine 60 mg	Pseudoephedrine 120 mg	1 tablet every 12 hours
Fexofenadine 180 mg	Pseudoephedrine 240 mg	1 tablet every 24 hours
Loratadine 5 mg	Pseudoephedrine 120 mg	1 tablet every 12 hours
Loratadine 10 mg	Pseudoephedrine 240 mg	1 tablet every 24 hours

[a] Products listed are examples; the list is not all-inclusive.

Note. Based on information from Katzung, B.G. (Ed.). (2018). *Basic and clinical pharmacology* (14th ed.). McGraw-Hill; Lexicomp. (n.d.). Lexi-drugs [Login required]. http://online.lexi.com; Wolters Kluwer Health. (n.d.). Facts and Comparisons®. https://www.wolterskluwercdi.com/facts-comparisons-online/databases.

Appendix O. Tumor Markers[a]

Tumor Marker	Application in Cancer	Comments
Antigens		
Alpha-fetoprotein	Testicular cancer, choriocarcinoma, cancers of the pancreas, colon, lung, stomach, biliary system, and liver	Also elevated in cirrhosis, hepatitis, and liver injury
Carcinoembryonic antigen	Cancers of the breast, lung, prostate, pancreas, stomach, colon, and rectum	Elevated in smokers, chronic obstructive pulmonary disease, pancreatitis, hepatitis, and inflammatory bowel disease
Cancer antigen (CA) 19-9	Cancers of the pancreas, colon, and stomach	–
CA-125	Cancers of the ovary, pancreas, breast, and colon	–
CA 27-29	Breast cancer	–
Cluster of differentiation 20 (CD20)	Non-Hodgkin lymphoma	Determines if targeted therapy is appropriate
Prostate-specific antigen	Prostate cancer	Often used as a screening tool for prostate cancer
Enzymes		
Creatine kinase	Breast, colon, ovarian, prostate, and small cell lung cancers	–
Lactic dehydrogenase	Lymphoma, seminoma, acute leukemia, and metastatic cancer	Also elevated in hepatitis and myocardial infarction
Prostatic acid phosphatase	Metastatic cancers of the prostate, myeloma, lung cancer, and osteogenic sarcoma	–
Gene/Chromosome		
ALK gene rearrangement	Non-small cell lung cancer, anaplastic large cell lymphoma	–
BCR-ABL fusion gene	Chronic myeloid leukemia	–
BRAF mutation	Cutaneous melanoma, colorectal cancer	–
Cytokeratin fragments 21-1	Lung cancer	–
Human epididymis protein 4 (HE4)	Ovarian cancer	–
KIT	Gastrointestinal stromal tumor, mucosal melanoma	–
KRAS mutation	Colorectal cancer, non-small cell lung cancer	–
S-100	Melanoma	–

(Continued on next page)

Appendix O. Tumor Markers[a] *(Continued)*

Tumor Marker	Application in Cancer	Comments
Growth Factors		
Epidermal growth factor receptor	Non-small cell lung cancer	Used for treatment base; experimental in several solid tumors
Human epidermal growth factor receptor 2 (HER2)	Breast cancer	Amplified in 20%–40% of breast cancers. Positive indicates more aggressive tumor and is used in treatment planning; experimental for ovarian and endometrial cancers
Hormones		
Adrenocorticotropic hormone	Cancers of the lung, prostate, gastrointestinal tract, and neuroendocrine system	Also elevated in Cushing disease
Antidiuretic hormone	Small cell lung cancer, adenocarcinomas	Also elevated in syndrome of inappropriate secretion of antidiuretic hormone and in pneumonia and porphyria
Calcitonin	Medullary thyroid cancer, small cell lung cancer, breast cancer, carcinoid tumor	–
Estrogen receptors	Breast cancer	Used to evaluate prognosis and base treatment
Human chorionic gonadotropin (beta-HCG)	Choriocarcinoma, germ cell testicular cancers, ectopic production in cancers of the stomach, pancreas, lung, colon, and liver	Also elevated in pregnancy
Parathyroid hormone	Ectopic hyperparathyroidism from cancers of the kidney, lung (squamous cell), pancreas, and ovary and myeloma	Also elevated in primary hyperparathyroidism
Progesterone receptors	Breast cancer	Used to evaluate prognosis and base treatment
Thyroglobulin	Thyroid cancer	–
Metabolic Products		
5-Hydroxyindoleacetic acid	Carcinoid tumors	Catabolized product of serotonin; levels can be affected by certain foods (e.g., bananas, walnuts) and medications (e.g., acetaminophen, guaifenesin, heparin, tricyclic antidepressants).
Vanillylmandelic acid	Neuroblastoma, adrenal tumors	–

(Continued on next page)

Appendix O. Tumor Markers[a] *(Continued)*

Tumor Marker	Application in Cancer	Comments
Proteins		
Beta-2 microglobulin	Multiple myeloma, lymphoma	–
Chromogranin A	Carcinoid tumors, neuroendocrine tumors	Protein produced by tumor cells
Serum immunoglobulin (Ig)	Multiple myeloma, lymphoma	Also elevated in connective tissue disease, benign monoclonal gammapathy, and chronic renal failure
IgA	IgA multiple myeloma	Also elevated in connective tissue disease, benign monoclonal gammapathy, and chronic renal failure
IgE	IgE multiple myeloma	Also elevated in connective tissue disease, benign monoclonal gammapathy, and chronic renal failure
IgG	IgG multiple myeloma	Also elevated in connective tissue disease, benign monoclonal gammapathy, and chronic renal failure
IgM	Waldenström macroglobulinemia	Also elevated in connective tissue disease, benign monoclonal gammapathy, and chronic renal failure

[a]Tumor markers listed are examples; the list is not all-inclusive.

Note. Based on information from Holdenrieder, S. (2016). Biomarkers along the continuum of care in lung cancer. *Scandinavian Journal of Clinical and Laboratory Investigation, 245*(Suppl.), S40–S45. https://doi.org/10.1080/00365513.2016.1208446; Jeong, S., Park, M.-J., Song, W., & Kim, H.-S. (2020). Current immunoassay methods and their applications to clinically used biomarkers of breast cancer. *Clinical Biochemistry, 78,* 43–57. https://doi.org/10.1016/j.clinbiochem.2020.01.009; Morrison, T., Booth, R.A., Hauff, K., Berardi, P., & Visram, A. (2019). Chapter one: Laboratory assessment of multiple myeloma. In G.S. Makowski (Ed.), *Advances in Clinical Chemistry: Vol. 89* (pp. 1–58). *Springer.*. https://doi.org/10.1016/bs.acc.2018.12.001; Nagpal, M., Singh, S., Singh, P., Chauhan, P., & Zaidi, M.A. (2016). Tumor markers: A diagnostic tool. *National Journal of Maxillofacial Surgery, 7*(1), 17–20. https://doi.org/10.4103/0975-5950.196135; Yan, Y.-B. (2016). Creatine kinase in cell cycle regulation and cancer. *Amino Acids, 48*(8), 1775–1784. https://doi.org/10.1007/s00726-016-2217-0.

Appendix P. Antiemetics Therapy[a]

Classification	Drug	Dosing	Comments
Anticholinergics Common side effects: Dry mouth, sedation, blurred vision, restlessness	Scopolamine	Patch: 0.5 mg daily placed every three days	Drug may irritate skin. Drug may be difficult to obtain.
Antipsychotics Mechanism of action: Dopamine antagonist in the CTZ, esophagus, and stomach Common side effects: Drowsiness, dry mouth	Haloperidol	0.5–2 mg PO or IV every 4–6 hours	EPS is more common in young patients. Drug may have additive effects. Drug may prolong QTc interval; use with caution in patients with cardiac disorders and on other QTc-prolonging medications. Drug is effective for breakthrough/refractory CINV.
	Olanzapine	2.5–5 mg tablet PO at bedtime	Drug protects from both acute and delayed CINV.
Benzodiazepines Mechanism of action: CNS depressant; interferes with afferent nerves from cerebral cortex; sedative Common side effects: Sedation, amnesia, confusion	Lorazepam	0.5–2 mg PO, sublingually, or IV every 4–6 hours	Drug is useful for anticipatory nausea and vomiting. Use with caution in patients with hepatic and renal dysfunction.
Cannabinoids Mechanism of action: Suppresses pathways to vomiting center (speculated) Common side effects: Sedation, dizziness, dysphoria, dry mouth, disorientation, impaired concentration, orthostatic hypotension, tachycardia	Dronabinol	5–10 mg PO two times a day; can be dosed up to four times a day	Drug may be difficult to obtain in outpatient setting. Older adults are susceptible to CNS effects. Generally, it is used as third-line antiemetic therapy.
Phenothiazines Mechanism of action: Blocks dopamine receptor in the CTZ; inhibits vomiting center by blocking autonomic afferent impulses via vagus nerve Common side effects: Sedation, orthostatic hypotension, dizziness, drowsiness	Prochlorperazine	5–10 mg PO or IV every 4–6 hours 25 mg rectal suppository every 12 hours	Administer IV dose over 15–30 minutes. Do not exceed 5 mg/min with IV dose. CNS effects can be more pronounced in older adult patients.
	Promethazine	12.5–25 mg PO or IV every 4–6 hours 25 mg rectal suppository every 6 hours	IV concentration should not exceed 25 mg/ml and should not be infused at a rate > 25 mg/min. Drug should be diluted to 50 ml or into IV tubing of large volume IV. IV administration can cause significant tissue damage if extravsates.

(Continued on next page)

Appendix P. Antiemetics Therapy[a] (Continued)

Classification	Drug	Dosing	Comments
Phenothiazines (cont.)	Trimethoben-zamide	300 mg PO three or four times a day 200 mg IM three or four times daily	–
Neurokinin-1 Receptor Antagonist Common side effects: Head-ache, flushing	Aprepitant	125 mg PO on day 1, 80 mg on days 2 and 3 of che-motherapy	Drug is used for CINV in combi-nation with a 5-HT$_3$ antagonist and corticosteroid.
	Aprepitant	100 mg or 130 mg IV once	Give IV over 15–30 minutes. Drug is used for CINV in combi-nation with a 5-HT$_3$ antagonist and corticosteroid.
	Fosaprepitant	150 mg IV once	Give IV over 20–30 minutes. Drug is used for CINV in combi-nation with a 5-HT$_3$ antagonist and corticosteroid.
Serotonin Inhibitors Mechanism of action: Sero-tonin receptor (5-HT$_3$) antagonist Common side effects: head-ache, constipation	Dolasetron	100 mg PO	IV form is no longer recom-mended because of potential for cardiac side effects. Drug is useful for postoperative nausea and vomiting.
	Granisetron	1–2 mg PO daily or 1 mg PO two times a day Maximum 1 mg IV daily 3.1 mg transder-mal patch applied every 7 days	Drug may prolong QTc interval. Drug is useful for postoperative nausea and vomiting.
	Ondansetron	CINV: 8–16 mg IV or PO daily (dura-tion dependent on chemotherapy regimen sched-ule) Other indications: 4–16 mg PO daily as a single dose or divided into 2–3 doses Maximum daily dose of 24 mg	Avoid in patients with history of congenital long QT syndrome. Maximum IV dose is 16 mg due to risk of torsades de pointes. Drug is useful for postoperative nausea and vomiting. Drug is useful in pregnancy-associated nausea and vom-iting.
	Palonosetron	0.25 mg IV	No redosing 7 days after treat-ment. Receptor binding affinity is 30 times higher than that of other 5-HT$_3$ antagonists.

(Continued on next page)

Appendix P. Antiemetics Therapy[a] *(Continued)*

Classification	Drug	Dosing	Comments
Somatostatin Analog Mechanism of action: Unknown Common side effects: Local skin reactions, headache, hypothyroidism, cardiac toxicity	Octreotide	100 mcg subcutaneously two times a day, up to a maximum of 300 mcg three times a day	Drug is used as a palliative agent in the treatment of malignant bowel obstruction. It has no U.S. Food and Drug Administration indication for use in nausea and vomiting.
Steroids Mechanism of action: Antiprostaglandin synthesis activity Common side effects: Insomnia, euphoria, anxiety, hypertension, edema, facial flushing	Dexamethasone	4–12 mg IV or PO daily as a single dose or in divided doses	Limit course and/or taper as necessary to prevent adverse effects (e.g., hyperglycemia, hypothalmus-pituitary-adrenal axis suppression).
Substituted Benzamide Mechanism of action: Dopamine antagonist; accelerates gastric emptying and small-bowel transit; blocks dopamine receptors in the CTZ Common side effects: EPS, somnolence	Metoclopramide	10–20 mg PO or IV every 4–6 hours	EPS is more common in young patients. Drug may be given with diphenhydramine. Use with caution in patients with renal dysfunction.

[a] Not an all-inclusive list

CINV—chemotherapy-induced nausea and vomiting; CNS—central nervous system; CTZ—chemoreceptor trigger zone; EPS—extrapyramidal symptoms; IM—intramuscular; IV—intravenous

Note. Based on information from Lexicomp. (n.d.). Lexi-drugs [Login required]. http://online.lexi.com; National Comprehensive Cancer Network. (2020). *NCCN Clinical Practice Guidelines in Oncology (NCCN Guidelines®): Antiemesis* [v.1.2021]. https://www.nccn.org/professionals/physician_gls/pdf/antiemesis.pdf; Wolters Kluwer Health. (n.d.). Facts and Comparisons®. https://www.wolterskluwercdi.com/facts-comparisons-online/databases.

Appendix Q. Adjuvant Drugs for Neuropathic Cancer Pain[a]

Category	Drug/Dose	Indications
Anesthetics, local	Cutaneous 2.5% lidocaine and 2.5% prilocaine cream Lidocaine 5%–10% cream Capsaicin 0.025% and 0.075% cream	Refractory neuropathic pain, allodynia, hyperesthesia, postherpetic neuralgia, diabetic neuropathy, postsurgical neuropathy
Anticonvulsants	Gabapentin 300–900 mg PO three to four times a day (maximum dose 3,600 mg daily) Pregabalin 50 mg tablet PO two times a day (maximum dose 300 mg daily)	Lancinating dysesthesia, paroxysmal lancinating pain, plexopathies, postherpetic neuralgia; peripheral neuropathy, diabetic neuropathy, chemotherapy-induced neuropathy
Antidepressants	Tricyclics (amitriptyline, desipramine, nortriptyline), serotonin-norepinephrine reuptake inhibitors (venlafaxine, duloxetine), and other agents can be utilized. See Appendix I for drug-specific dosing references.	Lancinating dysesthesia, diabetic neuropathy, postherpetic neuralgia, postmastectomy pain, chemotherapy-induced neuropathy
Corticosteroids	Dexamethasone 4–16 mg tablet PO daily in divided doses Prednisone 60–80 mg tablet PO daily in divided doses	Spinal cord compression, brain metastasis, bone and nerve pain, brachial and lumbosacral plexopathies
N-methyl-D aspartate antagonists	Ketamine	Adjuvant to other agents for neuropathic pain as a last resort; consult with pain management specialist.
Skeletal muscle relaxant	Baclofen 5 mg tablet PO every 8 hours initially, titrate to 150 mg daily in divided doses	Spinal spasticity

[a] Products listed are examples; the list is not all-inclusive.

PO—by mouth

Note. Based on information from Fallon, M., Giusti, R., Aielli, F., Rolke, R., Sharma, M., & Ripamonti, C.I. (2018). Management of cancer pain in adult patients: ESMO clinical practice guidelines. *Annals of Oncology, 29*(Suppl. 4), IV166–IV191. https://doi.org/10.1093/annonc/mdy152; Katzung, B.G. (Ed.). (2018). *Basic and clinical pharmacology* (14th ed.). McGraw-Hill; Lexicomp. (n.d.). Lexi-drugs [Login required]. http://online.lexi.com; National Comprehensive Cancer Network. (2021). *NCCN Clinical Practice Guidelines in Oncology (NCCN Guidelines®): Adult cancer pain* [v.2.2021]. http://www.nccn.org/professionals/physician_gls/pdf/pain.pdf; Wolters Kluwer Health. (n.d.). Facts and Comparisons®. https://www.wolterskluwercdi.com/facts-comparisons-online/databases.

Index

The letter *f* after a page number indicates that relevant content appears in a figure; the letter *t*, in a table.